MW01154154

Medical Radiology

Diagnostic Imaging

Series Editors

Hans-Ulrich Kauczor
Paul M. Parizel
Wilfred C. G. Peh

The book series *Medical Radiology – Diagnostic Imaging* provides accurate and up-to-date overviews about the latest advances in the rapidly evolving field of diagnostic imaging and interventional radiology. Each volume is conceived as a practical and clinically useful reference book and is developed under the direction of an experienced editor, who is a world-renowned specialist in the field. Book chapters are written by expert authors in the field and are richly illustrated with high quality figures, tables and graphs. Editors and authors are committed to provide detailed and coherent information in a readily accessible and easy-to-understand format, directly applicable to daily practice.

Medical Radiology – Diagnostic Imaging covers all organ systems and addresses all modern imaging techniques and image-guided treatment modalities, as well as hot topics in management, workflow, and quality and safety issues in radiology and imaging. The judicious choice of relevant topics, the careful selection of expert editors and authors, and the emphasis on providing practically useful information, contribute to the wide appeal and ongoing success of the series. The series is indexed in Scopus.

Mark Davies • Steven James
Rajesh Botchu
Editors

Imaging of the Foot and Ankle

Techniques and Applications

Second Edition

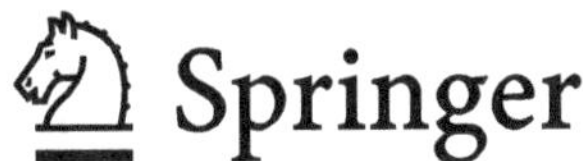

Editors
Mark Davies
Department of Musculoskeletal Radiology
Royal Orthopaedic Hospital
Birmingham, UK

Steven James
Department of Musculoskeletal Radiology
Royal Orthopaedic Hospital
Birmingham, UK

Rajesh Botchu
Department of Musculoskeletal Radiology
Royal Orthopaedic Hospital
Birmingham, UK

ISSN 0942-5373 ISSN 2197-4187 (electronic)
Medical Radiology
ISSN 2731-4677 ISSN 2731-4685 (electronic)
Diagnostic Imaging

ISBN 978-3-031-38608-4 ISBN 978-3-031-38609-1 (eBook)
https://doi.org/10.1007/978-3-031-38609-1

This Springer imprint is published by the registered company Springer Nature Switzerland AG
The registered company address is: Gewerbestrasse 11, 6330 Cham, Switzerland

Paper in this product is recyclable.

Preface

Musculoskeletal imaging continues to evolve since the first edition of this book published 20 years ago. The foot and ankle is one of the anatomical sites imaged by orthopedic surgeons, rheumatologists, and other musculoskeletal clinicians. It is necessary to continually update the knowledge of all working in this field. As before, the book takes a dual approach with the first part dealing with the full range of techniques available for imaging foot and ankle pathologies, including contribution on radiographs, ultrasound, computed tomography, and MR imaging. The second part comprising 18 chapters discusses the optimal application of these techniques to specific pathologies, highlighting practical solutions to everyday clinical problem.

The editors are grateful to the international panel of authors for their contribution to this second edition that aims to provide a comprehensive overview of current imaging of the foot and ankle.

Birmingham, UK Mark Davies
Birmingham, UK Steven James
Birmingham, UK Rajesh Botchu

Contents

Part I

Imaging Techniques and Procedures

Radiography

Basil Zia Khan, Radoslaw Rippel,
and Ramy Mansour

Contents

B. Z. Khan · R. Rippel · R. Mansour (✉)
Oxford University Hospitals NHS Foundation Trust, Oxford, UK
e-mail: Ramymansour@hotmail.co.uk

Abstract

The aim of this chapter is to explore the use of radiography in imaging the ankle and foot. It provides a basic overview of the anatomy of the ankle and foot. This is followed by a discussion on the various radiographic projections that are encountered in current clinical practice. The benefits as well as limitations of each projection are also discussed throughout the chapter. By the end of the chapter, the reader should have an understanding of the processes involved in taking ankle and foot radiographs and how to interpret them.

1 Anatomy of the Ankle

The ankle provides a connection between the distal end of the leg and foot. It is a common site of pathology, both acute and chronic. The ankle is made of three joints, the talocrural, subtalar, and distal tibiofibular joint. The talocrural joint, otherwise known as the mortise joint, is an example of a hinge joint. It involves the distal end of the tibia and fibula and the dome of the talus. It is responsible for plantarflexion and dorsiflexion of the foot. The subtalar joint, otherwise known as the talocalcaneal joint, comprises three areas where the talus and calcaneus articulate. These

Med Radiol Diagn Imaging (2023)
https://doi.org/10.1007/174_2023_396,

Published Online: 11 April 2023

are the anterior, middle, and posterior articulations/facets. The posterior facet is the largest out of the three. The subtalar joint is a form of a gliding synovial joint or plane joint where the articulating surfaces slide over each other. The floor of the middle facet gives rise to a horizontal eminence known as the sustentaculum tali (talar shelf). This is where the tibiocalcaneal ligament, plantar calcaneonavicular ligament, medial talocalcaneal ligament, part of the deltoid ligament, and flexor hallucis longus tendon attach. The subtalar joint allows for inversion and eversion of the foot.

2 Ankle Radiographs

Radiography of the ankle is commonly used as a diagnostic test to assess traumatic or nontraumatic ankle pain (Stiell et al. 1995). An ankle radiograph series typically consists of the mortise and lateral views (discussed below) (Croft et al. 2015). Other less commonly requested ankle radiograph projections include the horizontal beam lateral, anterior posterior, and stress views. Radiographs of the ankle may also be used to follow up patients (e.g., healing of fractures) (Resnick 2002).

2.1 The Mortise Projection

This radiograph provides detailed assessment of the distal tibia, distal fibula, talus, proximal fifth metatarsal, and talocrural joint. The foot is dorsiflexed; this can be done with the aid from a 90° pad placed on the plantar aspect of the foot. This is followed by rotating the ankle medially by a factor of 15–20°. The internal rotation should be done at the level of the hip rather than the ankle. In instances where internal rotation is not possible, the beam is adjusted and angled 15–20° medially. The beam is centered at the midway point between both the malleoli (Whitley et al. 2005). The projection should demonstrate the lower third of the tibia and fibula and the talocrural joint space. This projection is ideal for assessing malleolar fractures, distal tibial or fibular shaft fractures, base of fifth metacarpal fractures, and dislocations of the talocrural joint. Figure 1 shows how the mortise view is obtained in weight-bearing and non-weight-bearing projections (Fig. 2).

2.2 The Lateral Projection

This radiograph makes up the second image commonly obtained when undertaking an ankle radiograph series. The foot is placed with the medial surface facing toward the ceiling. A pad is placed under the lateral border of the foot creating a 15° elevation. The X-ray beam is centered over the medial malleolus (Whitley et al. 2005). This view in particular allows for assessment of the calcaneus, base of fifth metatarsal, talus, navicular, and distal tibia and fibula. It is important to note that minimally displaced fibular fractures may only be apparent on this view, and extra caution should be exercised. In addition, this dedicated view is very useful in assessing the Bohler's angle for calcaneal crush fractures (Lau et al. 2021). It also allows evaluation for fractures of the anterior process of the calcaneus and avulsion fractures of the talar head (Figs. 3 and 4).

2.3 Horizontal Beam Lateral Projection

This projection is useful when patient mobility is limited and when they are unable to weight bear. The patient can sit or lie supine with the foot held in dorsiflexion. Unlike the mortise view, there is

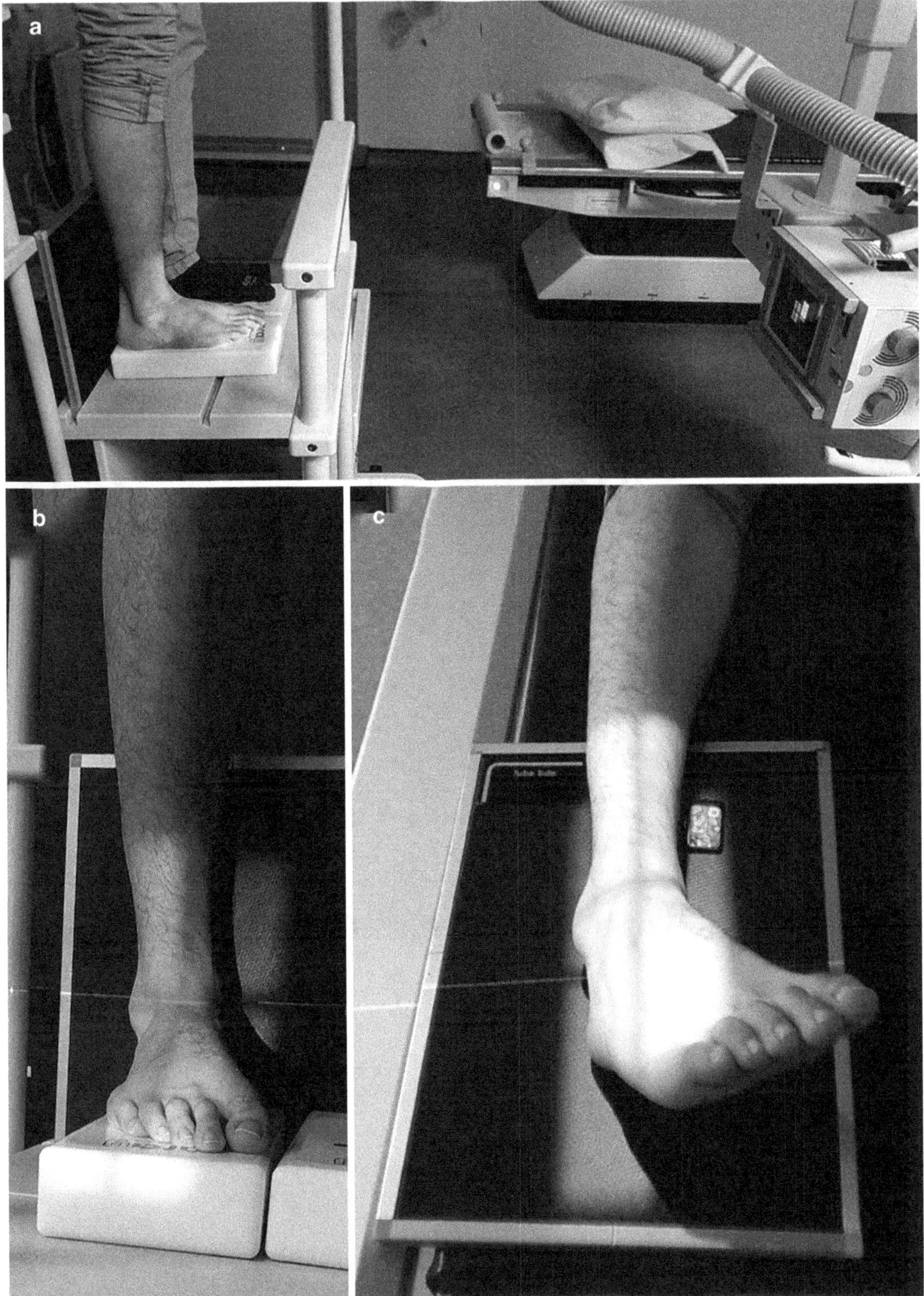

Fig. 1 (**a**, **b**) Demonstrate how a weight-bearing mortise projection of the ankle is taken. (**c**) Demonstrates a mortise view of the ankle in a non-weight-bearing position

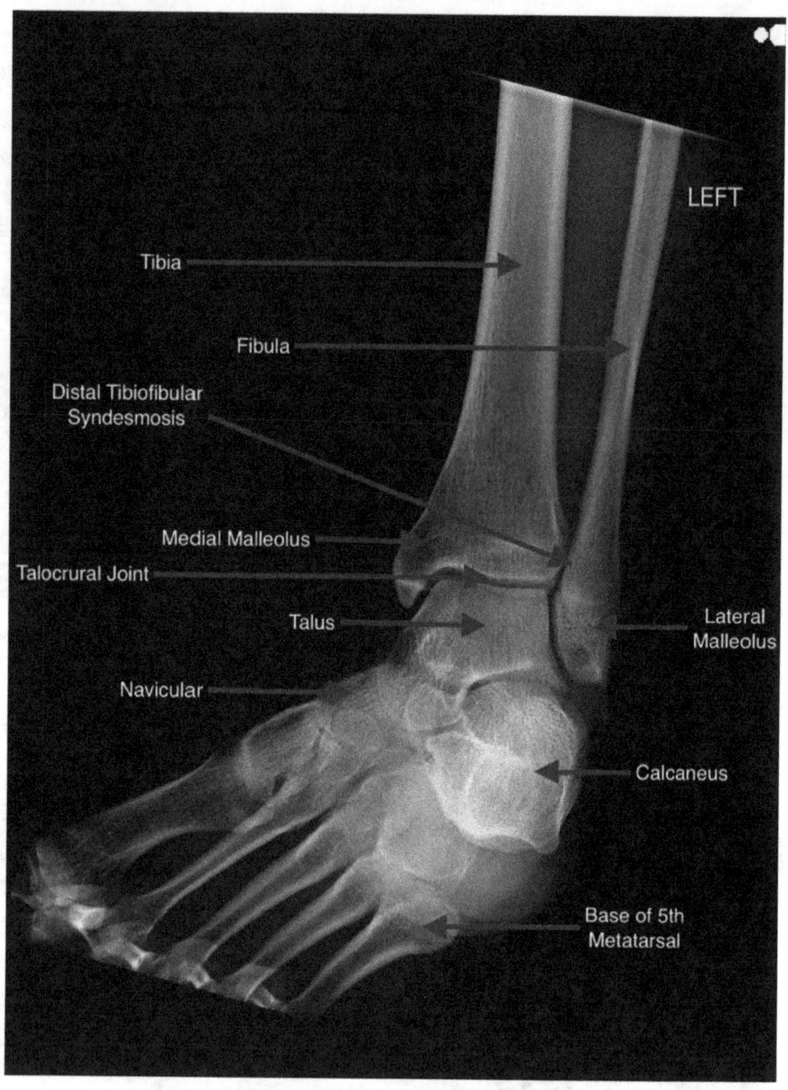

Fig. 2 Mortise view in ankle series

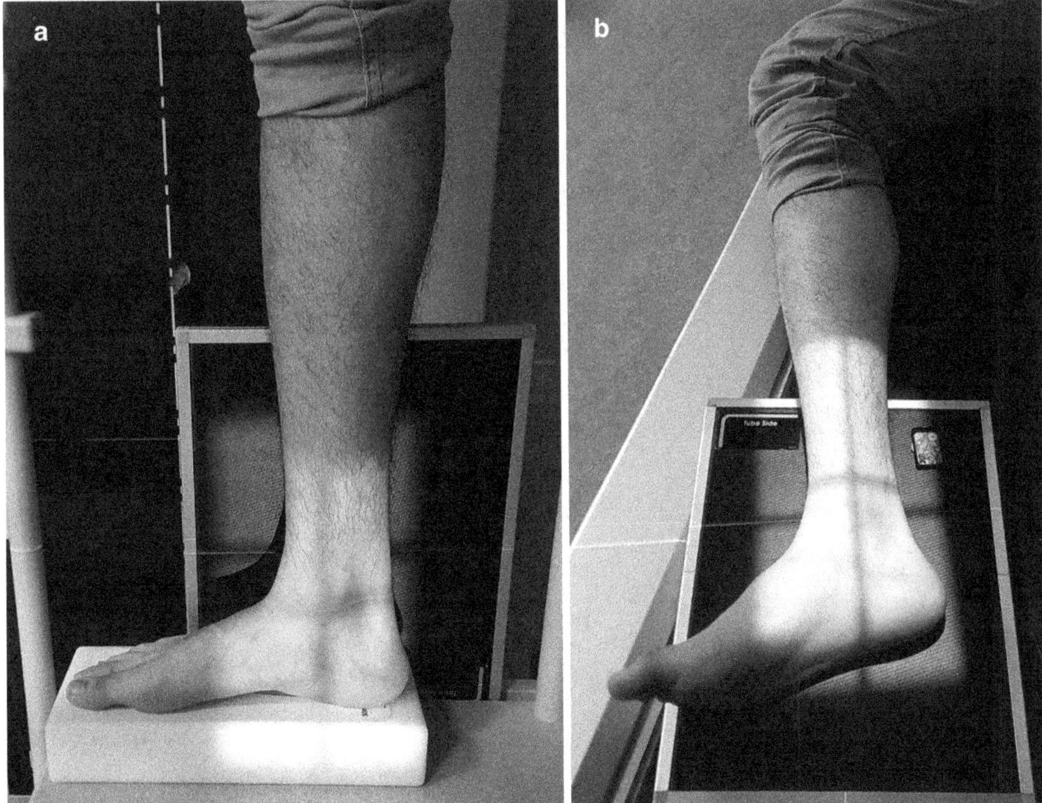

Fig. 3 (**a**) Demonstrates a weight-bearing lateral view. (**b**) Demonstrates a non-weight-bearing lateral view

no internal rotation of the foot. The imaging plate can be placed on the medial or lateral aspect of the foot. The X-rays are centered around the lateral or medial malleoli. Figure 5 shows how this projection is obtained (Fig. 6).

2.4 Anteroposterior Stress Projection

This projection is less commonly encountered in clinical practice. The aim is to apply stress to the ankle joint in order to assess for subluxation. The patient sits or lies supine. The foot is held in a similar position to the basic AP projection; however, stress is applied by the clinician, inverting the foot. The imaging plate is placed underneath the foot. The X-rays are centered around the midway point between both malleoli (Whitley et al. 2005). Figure 7 demonstrates how an AP stress projection of the ankle is taken.

2.5 Lateral Stress Projection

Similar to the AP stress projection, this view allows assessment of subluxation of the ankle joint, particularly in the anterior direction. The

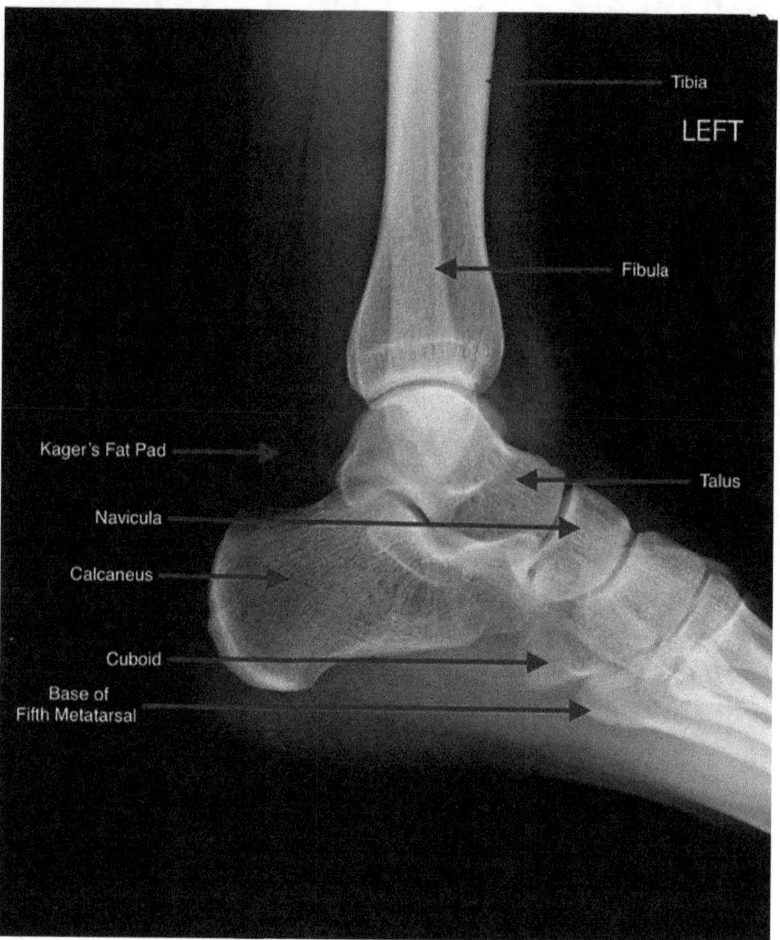

Fig. 4 Lateral ankle radiograph

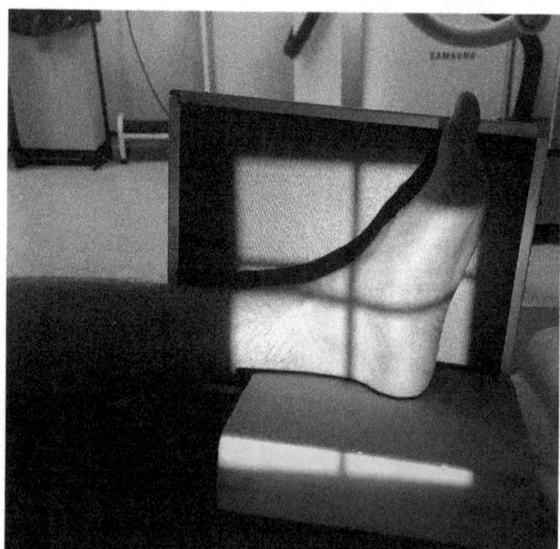

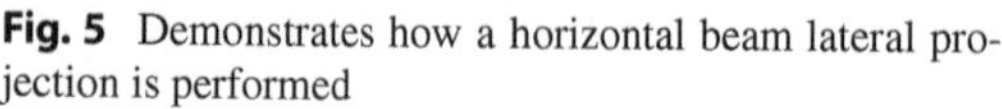

Fig. 5 Demonstrates how a horizontal beam lateral projection is performed

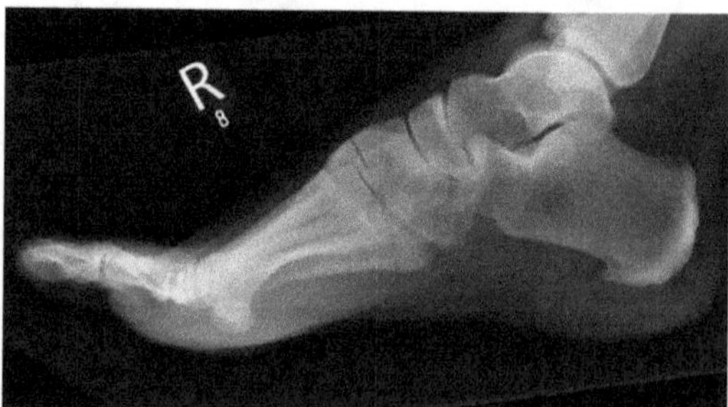

Fig. 6 Horizontal beam lateral projection radiograph

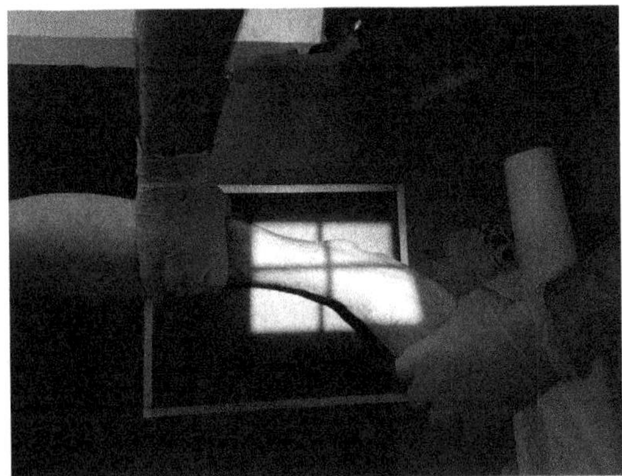

Fig. 7 AP stress projection of ankle

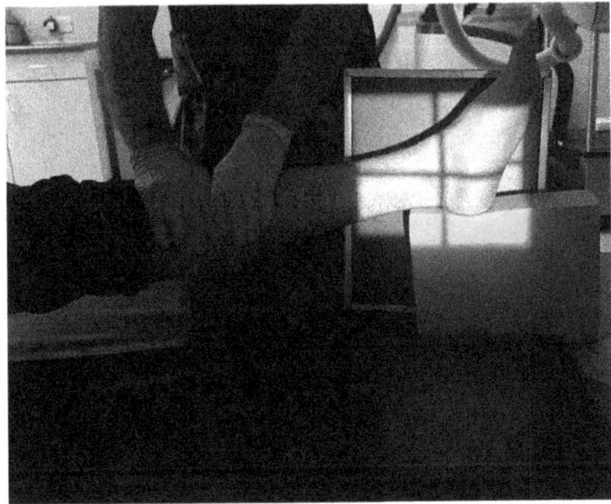

Fig. 8 Lateral stress projection of ankle

foot is placed in a similar position to the basic lateral view; however, a pad is placed under the heel to elevate the leg. The imaging plate is placed behind the lateral or medial aspect of the foot. Pressure is applied by the clinician on the distal leg. The X-rays are centered around the medial or lateral malleoli (Fig. 8).

2.6 Other Radiographic Projections of the Ankle

The anterior posterior (AP) view allows visualization of the proximal talus, proximal fifth metatarsal, and distal fibula. The foot is placed in a dorsiflexed position similar to the mortise view; however, it is not internally rotated. This is less commonly encountered in clinical practice and is often superseded by the mortise view.

3 Anatomy of the Foot

The foot is divided into three components, the hindfoot, midfoot, and forefoot. The hindfoot contains two of the seven tarsal bones; these are the talus and calcaneus. The midfoot consists of the remaining five of the seven tarsal bones; these are the navicular, cuboid, medial, intermediate, and lateral cuneiform bones. The forefoot consists of five metatarsal bones and a set of proximal, middle, and distal phalanges (first toe is exception and consists of proximal and distal phalanx). Indications for an undertaking of a foot radiograph series include traumatic and nontraumatic foot pain.

4 Foot Radiograph

The foot series consists of three views. These are the dorsoplantar (DP), medial oblique, and lateral. The DP and lateral views can be taken in weight-bearing and non-weight-bearing positions. Weight-bearing radiographs allow for better assessment of the foot under stress and can be crucial in identifying any pathology (e.g., Lisfranc injury).

4.1 Dorsoplantar (DP) Projection

This radiograph images the whole foot stretching from the distal end of the tibia and fibula to the toes. It allows for assessment of all structures within the foot. The imaging plate is placed on the plantar aspect of the foot. The central beam of the X-ray is placed over the cuboid-navicular joint (Whitley et al. 2005). Figure 9 demonstrates the dorsoplantar projection when taking weight-bearing radiograph. The tarsal and tarsometatarsal joints should be clearly demonstrated in the image (Fig. 10).

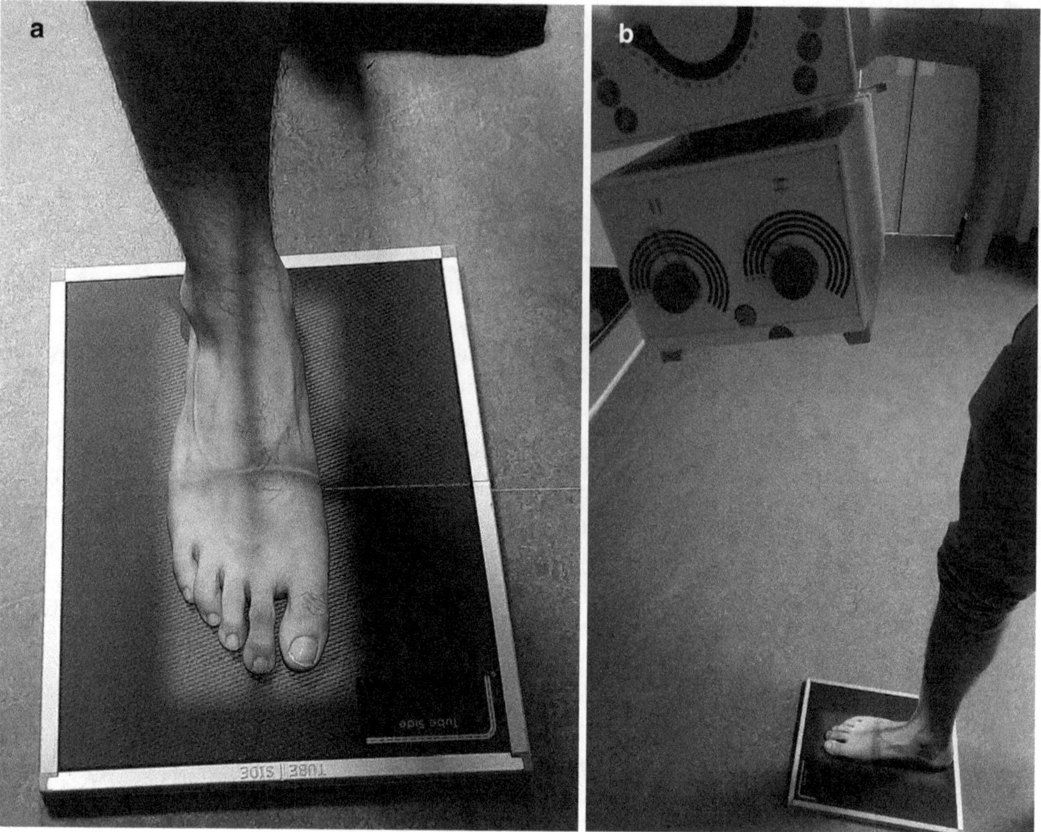

Fig. 9 (**a**, **b**) Demonstrate weight-bearing DP projections of the foot

4.2 Dorsoplantar (DP) Oblique Projection

This projection is obtained with the foot tilted medially, creating a 30–45° angle between the imaging plate and plantar surface of the foot. A pad may be used to support the foot in this position. Similar to the DP view, the central X-ray beam is placed over the cuboid-navicular joint (Whitley et al. 2005). Figure 11 demonstrates the positioning of the foot when obtaining this projection. This radiograph is good for evaluating the alignment of the metatarsal and tarsal bones. Figure 12 shows a dorsoplantar oblique radiograph of a normal foot.

4.3 Lateral Projection

The detector plate is placed behind the foot as shown in Fig. 13. The vertical central X-ray is placed over the navicular cuneiform joint and horizontal central X-ray over the tubercle of the fifth metatarsal (Whitley et al. 2005). This projection allows better assessment of the tarsal and metatarsal bones. It can be obtained in a weight-bearing and non-weight-bearing position. Weight-bearing projections are useful for assessing conditions affecting the longitudinal arches of the foot. Figure 14 shows an annotated lateral projection of the foot in a weight-bearing position.

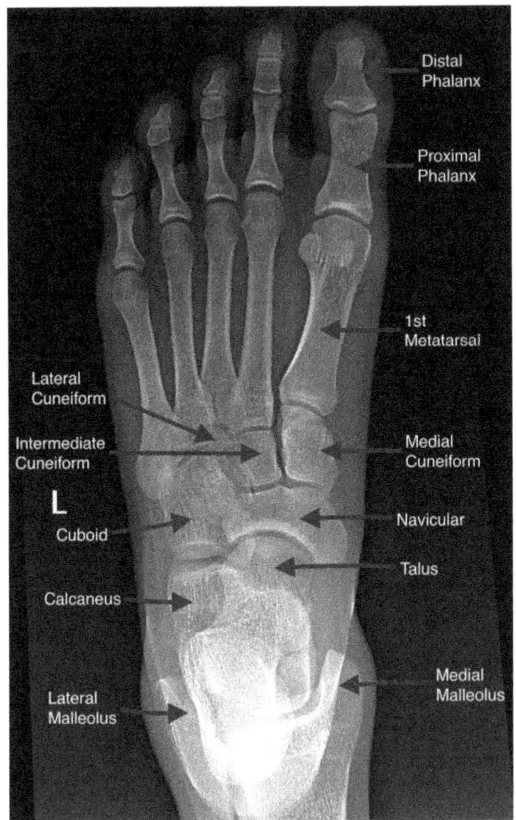

Fig. 10 DP projection foot radiograph

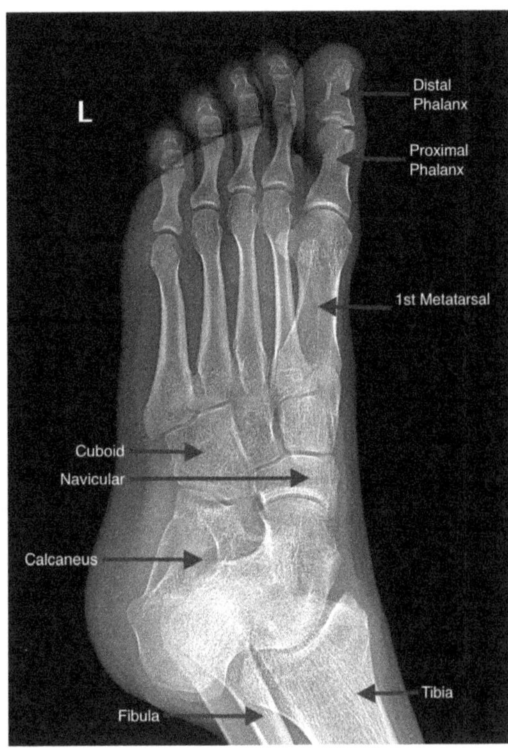

Fig. 12 DP oblique projection of normal foot

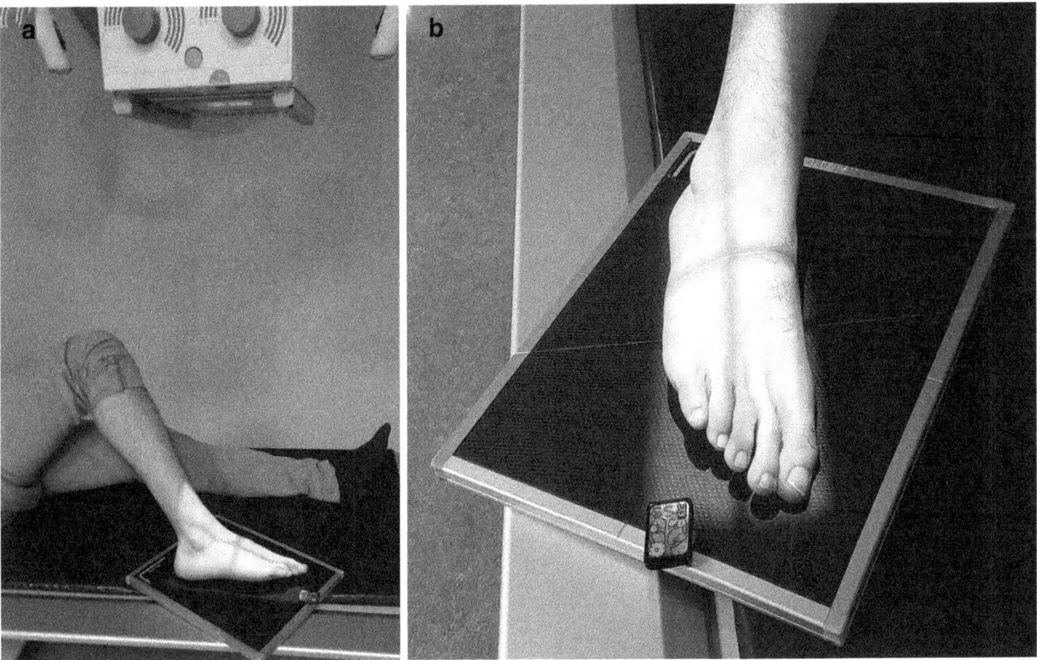

Fig. 11 (**a**, **b**) Demonstrate how a DP oblique projection is obtained

4.4 Calcaneal Projections

These consist of a lateral and axial view. The lateral projection is obtained by placing the patient in a lateral recumbent position. The lateral surface of the foot should be touching the imaging plate; both malleoli should align vertically. The imaging plate is placed beneath the foot. Collimation extends from the anterior part of the hindfoot to the posterior surface of the foot and from the talocrural joint superiorly to the plantar surface of the foot inferiorly. The X-ray beam is centered approximately 2.5 cm distal to the medial malleolus (Whitley et al. 2005). Figure 15 demonstrates a lateral projection of the calcaneus.

The axial projection is done by placing the foot in a dorsiflexed position with support from a band often held by the patient. The X-ray beam is centered around the plantar aspect of the heel (Whitley et al. 2005). Collimation includes medial to lateral skin margins and the skin of the heel to the distal third of the foot. The ideal image should demonstrate the subtalar joint. This projection is good for assessing fractures resulting in medial or lateral displacement of the foot. Figure 16 demonstrates how an axial projection of the calcaneus is taken. Figure 17 shows a normal axial calcaneal projection.

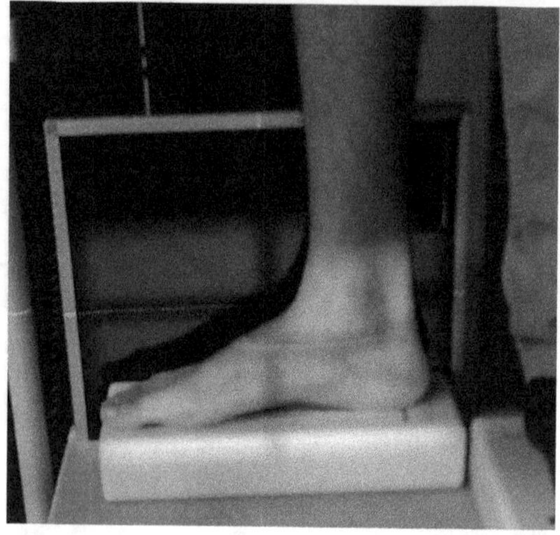

Fig. 13 Picture demonstrates a weight-bearing lateral projection of the foot

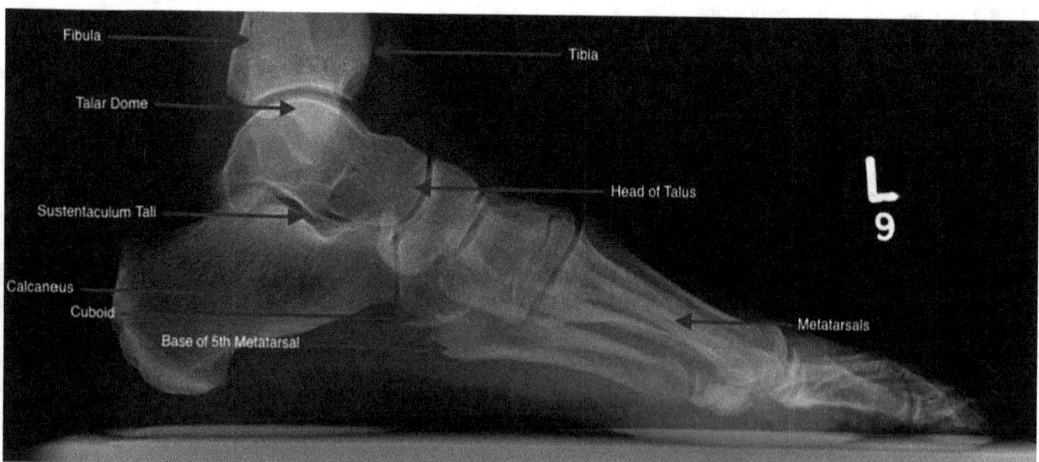

Fig. 14 Weight-bearing lateral projection of a normal foot

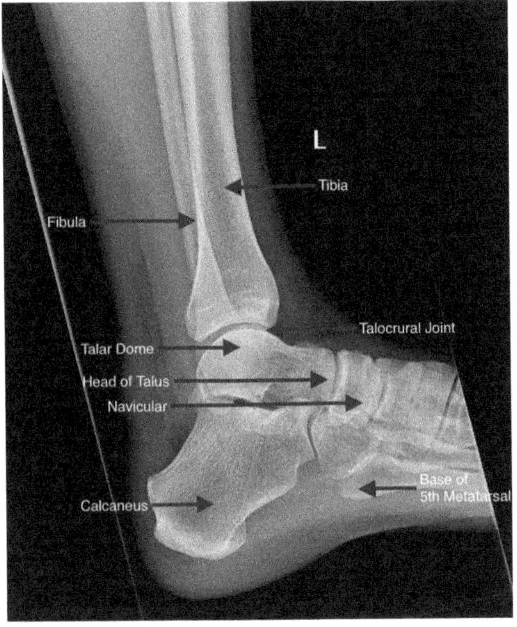

Fig. 15 Lateral calcaneal projection radiograph

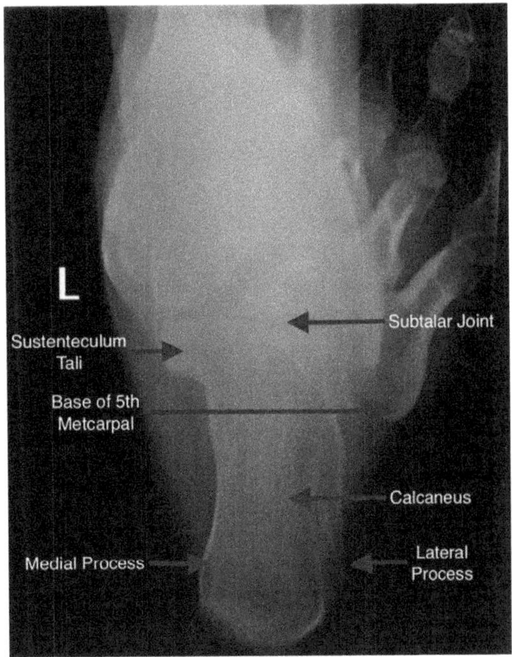

Fig. 17 Axial projection of calcaneus

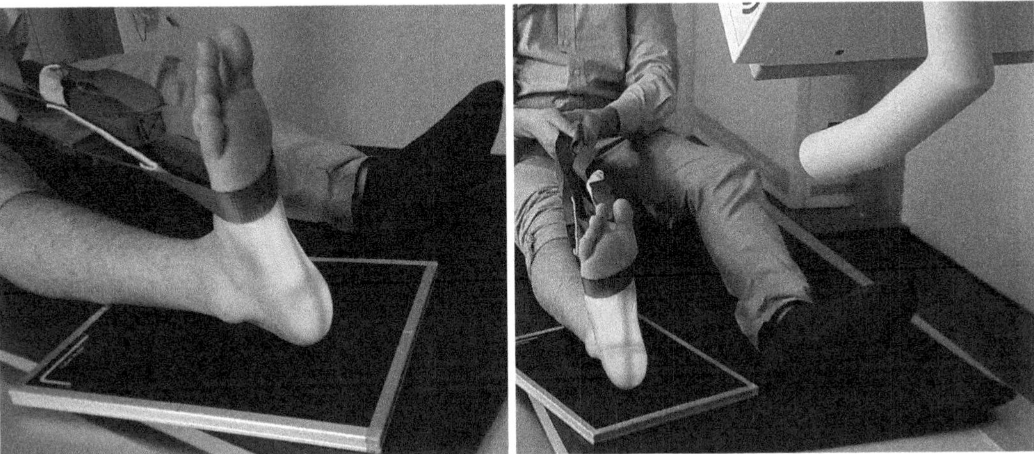

Fig. 16 Foot is held in dorsiflexed position with aid from band. Detector plate is placed beneath the foot

5 Toe Radiograph

5.1 DP Projection

The foot is placed with the plantar surface touching the imaging plate. This is similar to the DP projection of the whole foot; however, the collimation is adjusted to include the toe of interest as well as the adjacent toes. The X-rays are centered along the metatarsophalangeal joint of the respective toe (Whitley et al. 2005). This projection allows assessment of the metatarsals, phalanges, and joints of the toe. It is ideal for assessing foreign bodies as well as acute fractures (Figs. 18 and 19).

5.2 Lateral Projection

The foot is placed with the medial aspect touching the imaging plate. A band is used to move the remaining toes out of view (demonstrated in Fig. 20). Similar to the DP projection, the X-rays are centered around the metatarsophalangeal joint of the toe (Whitley et al. 2005). This projection is ideal for assessing dislocations of the joints of the distal toe alongside fractures (Fig. 21).

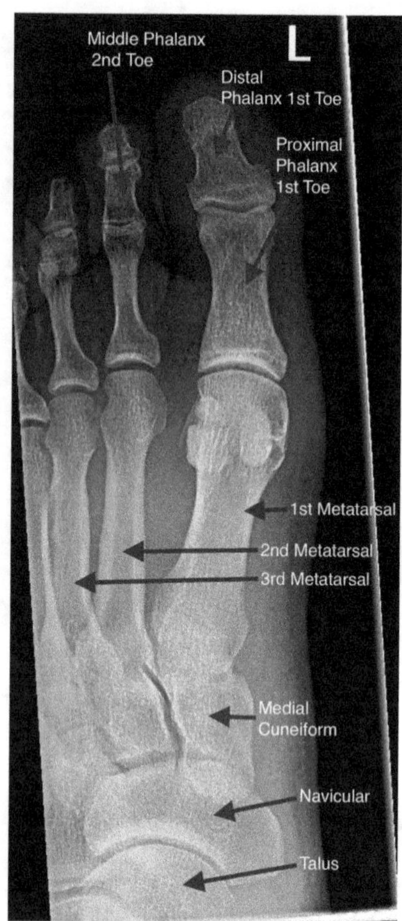

Fig. 19 DP projection for the great toe

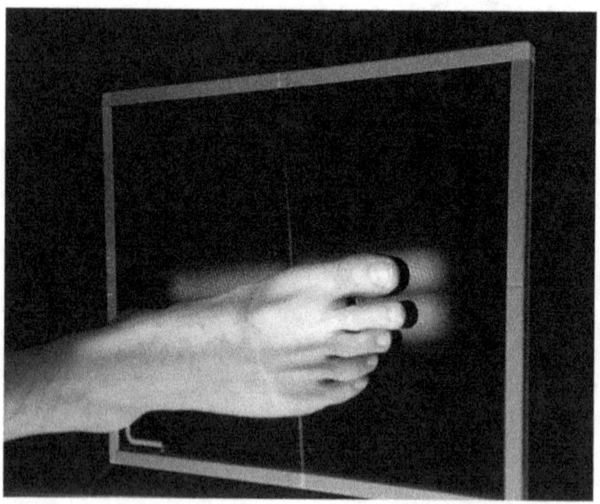

Fig. 18 DP projection for the great toe. The collimation is represented by the white light, which has been adjusted to include the area of interest

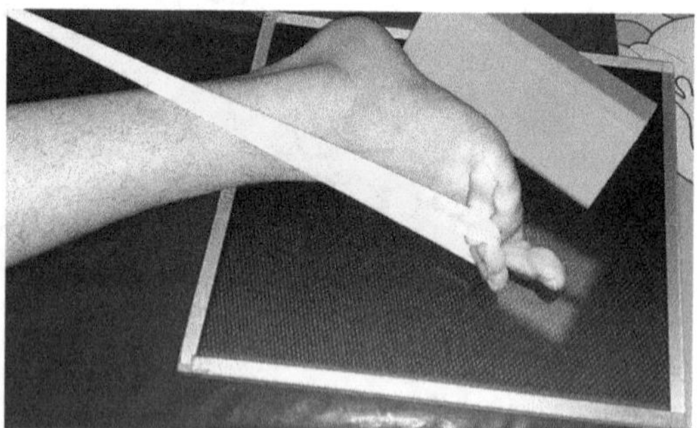

Fig. 20 Lateral projection for the great toe. A band is used to remove the other toes and is often held by the patient

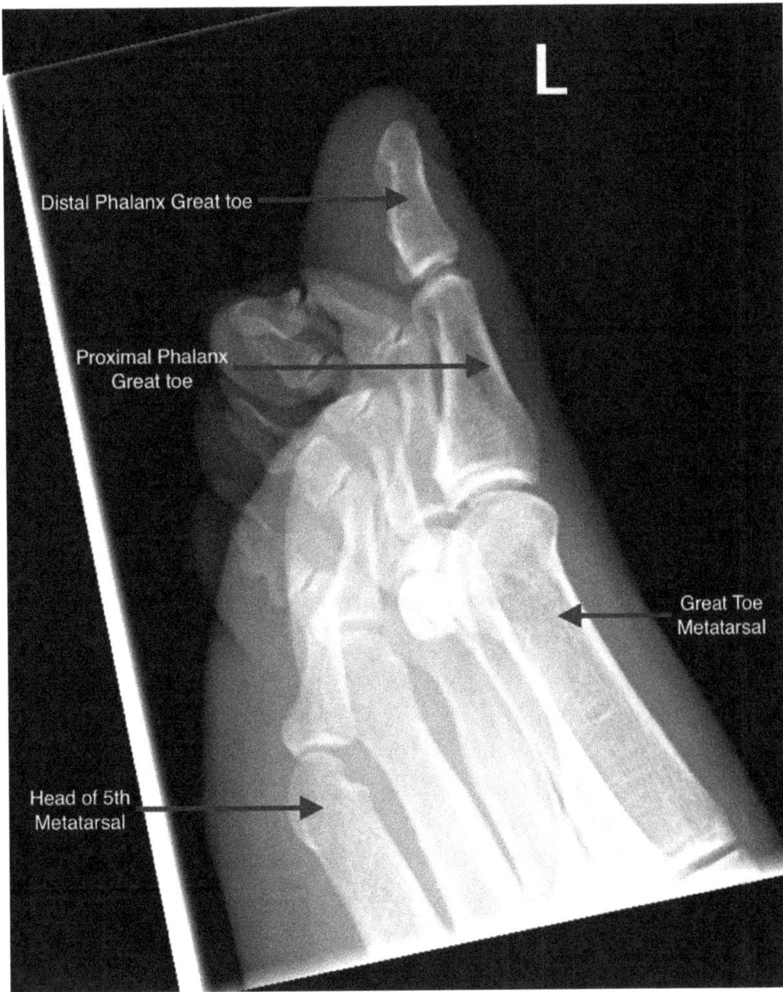

Fig. 21 Lateral projection for the great toe

5.3 Dorsoplantar Oblique Projection

The foot is tilted medially at an angle of 45°. A pad may be used to support the foot in this position. Similar to the DP and lateral, the X-rays are centered over the metatarsophalangeal joint of the toe (Whitley et al. 2005). The adjacent toes to the one being imaged are included. This projection allows further assessment of fractures and dislocations (Figs. 22 and 23).

5.4 Sesamoid Projections

These include a lateral and an axial view. The lateral view is taken by placing the medial aspect of the foot on the imaging plate. A band is used to dorsiflex the hallux. This allows the sesamoid bones to be visualized with minimal artifact from the superimposing structures. The X-rays are centered tangentially over the first metatarsophalangeal joint (Whitley et al. 2005). The axial sesamoid view can be obtained in two different ways. The first involves placing the foot laterally with the imaging plate located behind the heel of the foot. The X-ray source is placed adjacent to the toes opposite the imaging plate. A band is used to dorsiflex the hallux. The second method involves holding the foot in a dorsiflexed position (toes pointing toward the ceiling) with the imaging pate placed into the palmar arch. This is followed by using a band to dorsiflex the hallux (Fig. 24).

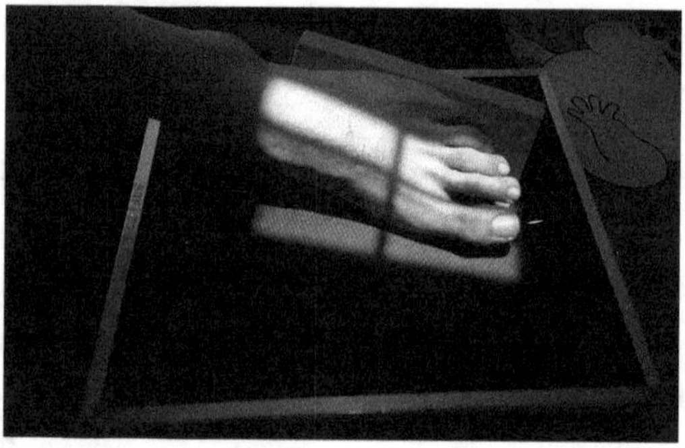

Fig. 22 DP oblique projection for the great toe

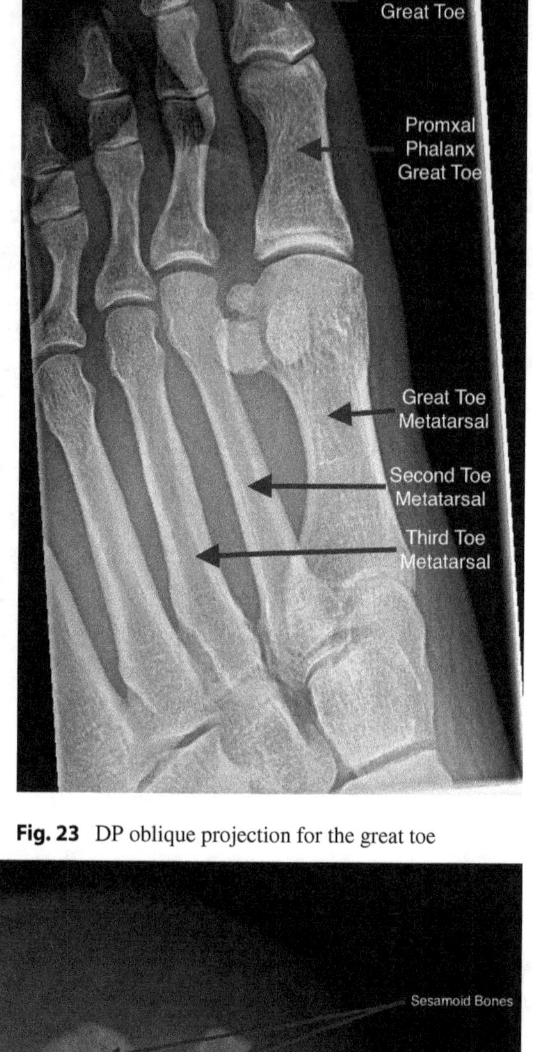

Fig. 23 DP oblique projection for the great toe

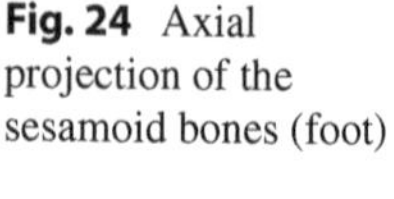

Fig. 24 Axial projection of the sesamoid bones (foot)

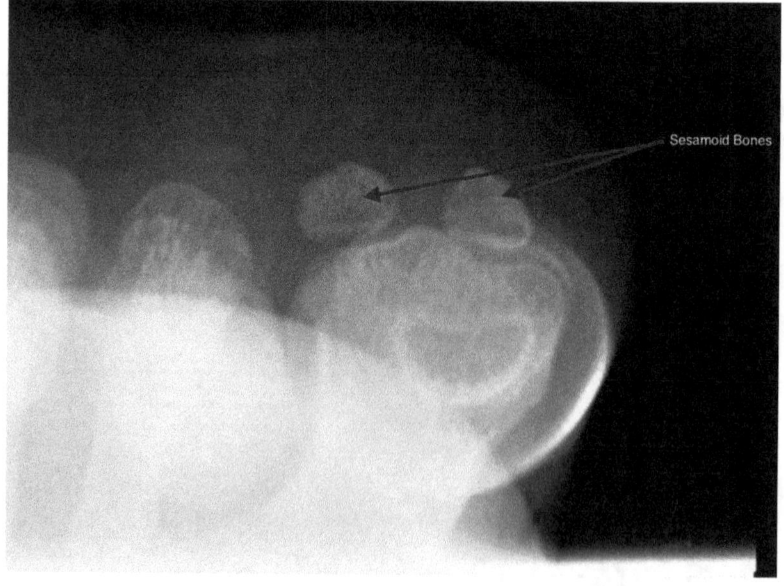

Acknowledgments We would like to thank Sylwia Stanek and Germana Sallemi who have kindly provided their valuable support, time, and advice in helping to prepare this chapter.

References

Croft S, Furey A, Stone C, Moores C, Wilson R (2015) Radiographic evaluation of the ankle syndesmosis. Can J Surg 58(1):58–62

Lau B, Allahabadi S, Palanca A, Oji D (2021) Understanding radiographic measurements used in foot and ankle surgery. J Am Acad Orthop Surg 30(2):e139–e154

Resnick D (2002) Diagnosis of bone and joint disorders. Saunders, Philadelphia

Stiell I, Wells G, Laupacis A, Brison R, Verbeek R, Vandemheen K et al (1995) Multicentre trial to introduce the Ottawa ankle rules for use of radiography in acute ankle injuries. BMJ 311(7005):594–597

Whitley A, Sloane C, Hoadley G, Moore A, Alsop C (2005) Clark's positioning in radiography, 12th edn. Hodder Arnold

CT Arthrography of the Ankle: Technique, Indications, Advantages, and Disadvantages

George A. Kakkos, Michail E. Klontzas, Evangelia E. Vassalou, and Apostolos H. Karantanas

Contents

Abstract

CT is a crucial imaging modality in evaluation of pathologies of foot and ankle. CT provides three-dimensional imaging of the foot and ankle with increased spatial resolution. This is extremely helpful in evaluation of fractures and assessment of arthrodesis. CT arthrography (CTA) is a well-established method in evaluating the articular cartilage of the ankle joint. The application of CTA requires knowledge of indications and limitations as well as the safe injection techniques by the supervising radiologist. CTA is indicated mostly in patients with MR imaging contraindications and in the postoperative painful syndrome where metallic artifacts may downgrade the quality of the images. In addition, CTA is better in showing small cartilage defects due to its higher image resolution. Fluoroscopic guided joint puncture is still the most commonly used image guidance method, but the role of ultrasound is constantly increasing.

1 Introduction

Rapid technological advancements over the previous decade have provided high-resolution magnetic resonance imaging (MRI) and computed tomography (CT) techniques for the evaluation of the ankle. MRI can be invaluable for the evaluation of soft tis-

G. A. Kakkos · E. E. Vassalou
Department of Medical Imaging, University Hospital of Heraklion, Heraklion, Crete, Greece

M. E. Klontzas · A. H. Karantanas (✉)
Department of Medical Imaging, University Hospital of Heraklion, Heraklion, Crete, Greece

Department of Radiology, School of Medicine, University of Crete, Heraklion, Crete, Greece
e-mail: akarantanas@gmail.com

Med Radiol Diagn Imaging (2023)
https://doi.org/10.1007/174_2023_386,
Published Online: 18 April 2023

sue and bone marrow lesions whereas thin-slice multidetector CT (MDCT) can provide a high-resolution evaluation of the osseous structures. Plain CT has been proved to be a valuable adjunct to plain radiographs, regarding infection, early onset osteoarthritis, neoplasia, and trauma of the ankle and foot. Ankle trauma is commonly associated with chondral and osteochondral lesions which are usually occult on plain radiographs and are a significant undiagnosed cause of acute and chronic ankle pain, ultimately leading to osteoarthritis. Reliable detection of such lesions can be achieved by means of CT or MR arthrography. The aim of this chapter is to present the injection and acquisition techniques, the indications, and the advantages and disadvantages of CT arthrography (CTA).

2 Plain CT

CT has been widely applied for the preoperative planning in trauma patients with complex distal tibial fractures, tarsal fractures, and Lisfranc fracture-dislocations (Fig. 1). The advantage of CT over radiographs is its ability to detect and characterize occult fracture displacement or comminution, and articular involvement with accurate measurement of the step-off. Intra-articular or extra-articular osseous fragments are also well seen on CT (Fig. 1). CT scan in trauma patients is performed using thin (0.6–1.0 mm) multidetector scanning with sagittal and coronal reformations. A soft tissue algorithm should be obtained in addition to bone algorithm to allow diagnosis of tendinous injuries, which are often associated with ankle fractures. 3D CT scan is popular in the Orthopedic community but rarely can contribute in understanding complex fracture patterns.

CT has been shown clinical efficiency in assessing bone tumors by adding information on the matrix of the lesion, the type of periosteal reaction, and the best path for biopsy (Fig. 2). In some patients, CT may be useful in assessing infection when MR imaging is contraindicated (Fig. 3).

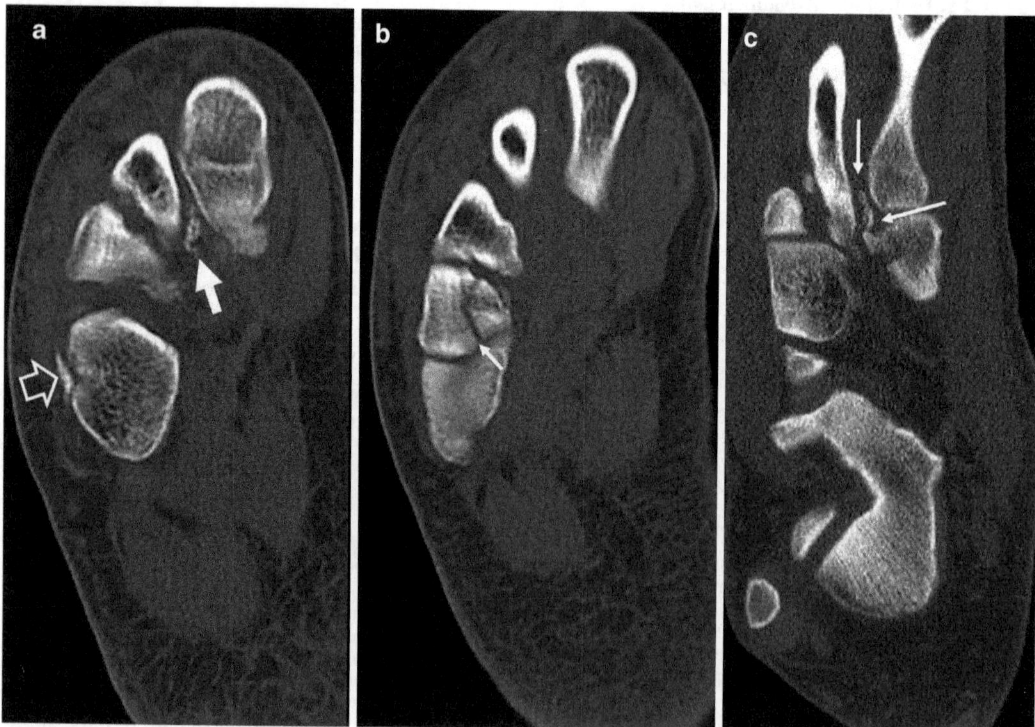

Fig. 1 A 37-year-old male patient involved in a motorbike accident. The axial (**a**, **b**) and oblique axial (**c**) CT images show the Lisfranc (thick arrow in a, thin arrows in c), cuboid (open arrow), and 5th metatarsal base (arrow in b) fractures. Small osseous fragments are also shown

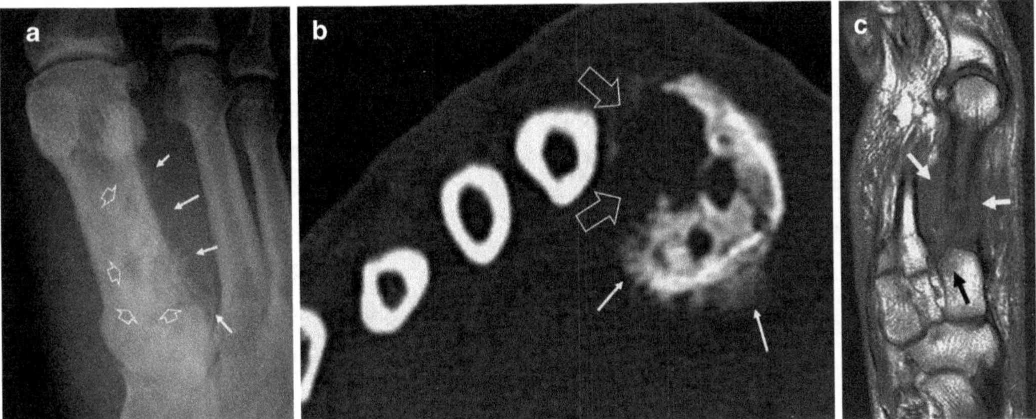

Fig. 2 (**a**) A 63-year-old male patient with a history of pain and swelling in the forefoot. The radiograph shows a mixed sclerotic and lytic lesion (open arrows) with an aggressive periosteal reaction demonstrated with a Codman's triangle anteriorly and hair-on-end posteriorly (arrows). (**b**) The coronal CT reconstruction demonstrates the lysis (open arrows), the abnormal matrix and the periosteal reaction (arrows). (**c**) The axial T1W MR image shows the soft tissue extension of the lesion (arrows) and the extension of the medial cuneiform (black arrow). Histology following surgical excision showed osteosarcoma

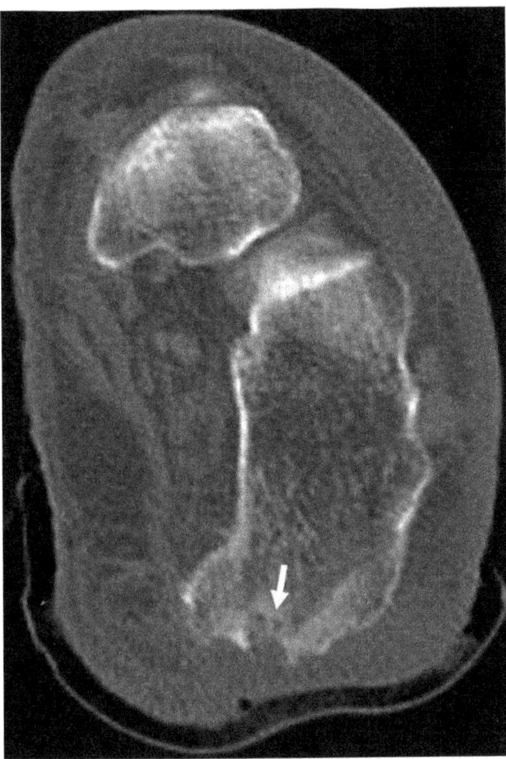

Fig. 3 A 75-year-old male diabetic patient with a skin ulcer posterior to the calcaneus. He was unable to undergo MR imaging due to the presence of a pacemaker and claustrophobia. CT (bone window) shows cortical disruption and osteolysis (arrow) suggesting osteomyelitis. This was confirmed surgically

Dual-energy computed tomography (DECT) or spectral imaging has expanded its clinical applications during the last decade. Regardless of the technology used to achieve spectral imaging, there are now many clinical indications which have highlighted the role of CT. The most important of them are crystal deposition disease such as gout, hydroxyapatite or calcium pyrophosphate dihydrate (Chou et al. 2017), metal artifact reduction (Sverzut et al. 2015), tendon and ligament imaging, and bone marrow evaluation. The latter has shown accuracy in detecting bone marrow edema, as in bone bruise resulting from trauma (Fig. 4), multiple myeloma detection (Thomas et al. 2015), and vertebral fractures (Wang et al. 2013).

A novel application of CT is the weight-bearing (WBCT) for lower limb imaging aiming at better evaluation of the 3D components of a deformity and the joint space morphology under loading (Tuominen et al. 2013; Barg et al. 2018). WBCT relies on cone-beam technology and has been investigated with promising results in various hindfoot deformities (Bernasconi et al. 2021; Lintz et al. 2021; Conti and Ellis 2020). WBCT may reveal occult, on plain/unloaded CT, disorders such as malalignment, instability, joint space narrowing in

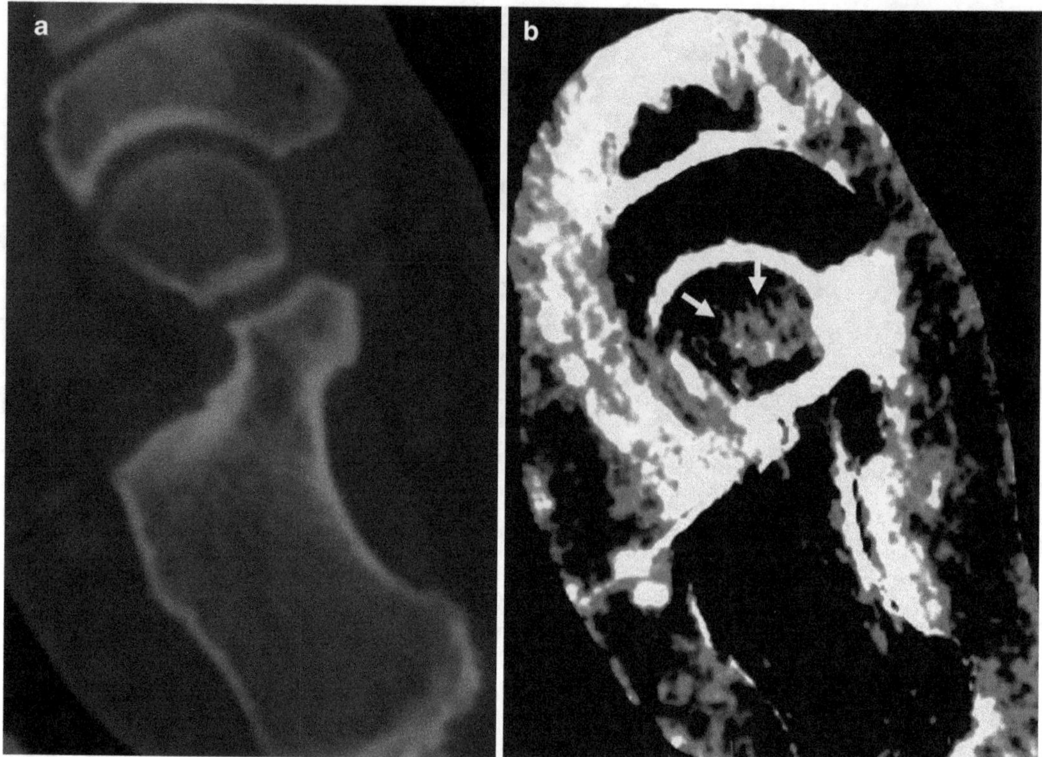

Fig. 4 Dual-energy CT of the ankle of a 30-year-old male following trauma. Monochromatic images (**a**) with a slice thickness of 0.625 mm did not reveal any fracture whereas the superimposed color map (**b**) revealed extensive bone marrow edema of the talar head and neck as well as edema/hemorrhagic infiltration of the surrounding soft tissues (orange)

the context of early onset osteoarthritis, and various impingement syndromes.

The combination of multidetector CT and SPECT provides both morphological and functional imaging. Among other clinical indications under investigation, SPECT/CT has been useful in assessing patients presenting with postoperative foot and ankle pain (Kampen et al. 2018).

3 CT Arthrography

3.1 Contrast Material

Ankle arthrography is a simple procedure that can be performed using either a *single* (iodine) or *double*-contrast (iodine and air) technique (Buckwalter 2006). In the era of MDCT, submillimeter section acquisition enables the production of high-quality multiplanar reconstructions (Lecouvet et al. 2008). Currently, the *single-contrast* technique is used, which is easier to perform, less painful, and more accurate because fluid penetrates better than air into cartilage lesions (Omoumi et al. 2009).

Iodinated contrast material should be diluted with saline and local anesthetic in order to limit or even to avoid the beam hardening artifacts. In one study (Anderson et al. 2008), higher contrast agent concentrations caused the cartilage depicted on the CT images to appear thinner than the reference thickness; thus, the use of a lower contrast agent concentration is likely to reduce the amount of volumetric averaging between actual cartilage and contrast agent. If a joint effusion is present, it should be aspirated to avoid significant dilution of the contrast material.

It has been shown that intra-articular anesthesia may significantly reduce peri-procedural (Fox et al. 2012) as well as post-arthrographic pain. Long-acting local anesthetics such as bupivacaine seem to be more effective than lidocaine to reduce pain (Mosimann et al. 2012). However, due to reported chondrotoxic effects of local anesthetics, lidocaine should be avoided. Low concentrations of long-acting local anesthetics are safer to use (Kreuz et al. 2018). In our practice, we use non-ionic iodinated contrast (300 mg/mL) diluted 1:1 with saline along with 2–3 mL ropivacaine 0.5%. When simultaneous direct CT and MR arthrography is planned, a mixture of 1.25 mmol/L gadolinium and 25% iodinated contrast agent was found to be the optimal mixture ratio (Choi et al. 2008). Once injected in the joint, the concentration of contrast declines and thus the CT scan should be performed within 15–30 min after the injection (Obermann et al. 1989).

3.2 Volume of Contrast Material

Maximal average ankle joint volume varies considerably (Draeger et al. 2009). A 10 mL syringe is typically used, and injection of 6–8 mL is adequate to distend the joint capsule (Rastogi et al. 2016). Sufficient distention is indicated by increased resistance to injection. If pain is generated, the injection should be stopped.

3.3 Pre-injection Procedure

Prior to injection, contraindications such as pregnancy, history of allergic reactions to contrast material or anesthetics, skin infection, and coagulation disorders have to be ruled out. Through the consent process, it is a standard procedure to discuss with the patient the (low) likelihood of bleeding, infection, and injury to adjacent neurovascular structures in addition to the possibility of a vasovagal reaction, allergic response, and post-arthrographic pain.

One of the inherent limitations of CTA is that intra-articular contrast has attenuation similar to that of bone. Thus, intra-articular synthetic materials such as cement or suture anchors, intra-articular osseous loose bodies, hardware, chondrocalcinosis, and other calcific densities such as calcium hydroxyapatite, can be masked on CTA. Radiographs prior to the arthrogram may help to clarify these findings in the subsequent CTA study. However, newer techniques like dual-energy CT may be valuable as it can separate different materials based on their composition rather than on their attenuation (Sandhu et al. 2021).

3.4 Injection Techniques

The diluted contrast material can be injected into the ankle joint space using different approaches: under palpation using anatomic landmarks or using imaging guidance, such as fluoroscopy, CT, or ultrasound (US). Fluoroscopy being a low-cost, efficient, and easy technique is used in most institutions, but it exposes both patient and operator to ionizing radiation. Currently, US guidance is favored over fluoroscopy. The significant advantages of US are the absence of ionizing radiation, low cost, portability, and the possibility of imaging all the soft tissues surrounding the joint with avoidance of any critical structures in the path of the needle (Messina et al. 2016). CT guidance is generally avoided due to higher radiation doses compared to fluoroscopy; however, it may be the technique of choice in cases of disordered anatomy due to significant degenerative changes (Saifuddin et al. 2005).

A blind joint puncture can be performed in the CT imaging suite, using anatomic landmarks. This is primarily applied when there is limited access to a fluoroscopic suite or an US machine. The puncture site is located just medial to the tibialis anterior tendon at the level of the antero-medial ankle joint and about 5 mm proximal to the medial malleolus (Cerezal et al. 2005). This approach is limited by the high rate of extra-articular injection.

In the fluoroscopy suite, the patient is placed in a lateral decubitus position with the ankle positioned in slight plantar flexion and the front of the ankle facing the examiner. The course of the dorsalis pedis artery is palpated and marked to avoid its puncture. Sterile preparation of the overlying skin at the site of access is the next step. We do not normally apply local anesthesia because the needles used are very thin. The ideal needle entry point is located just lateral or medial to the tibialis anterior tendon (Cerezal et al. 2008). When the radiological joint space of the ankle is directly targeted, there is a risk of hitting the distal anterior edge of the tibia. Instead, the anterior recess must be targeted just below the joint line with the needle placed with slight cranial angulation (Fig. 5). This approach facilitates articular injection when the joint space is obscured, by severe degenerative changes (Lungu and Moser 2015). Alternatively, the lateral mortise approach may be used (Wright et al. 2014). A 4 cm 23 or 25-gauge needle is inserted, and the intra-articular position is confirmed when a small amount of contrast medium is injected with little resistance and flows freely into the joint recesses instead of clustering around the needle tip (Rastogi et al. 2016). An amount of 6–8 mL of contrast is usually injected until firm resistance. The patient is then immediately transferred to the CT suite for completion of the examination.

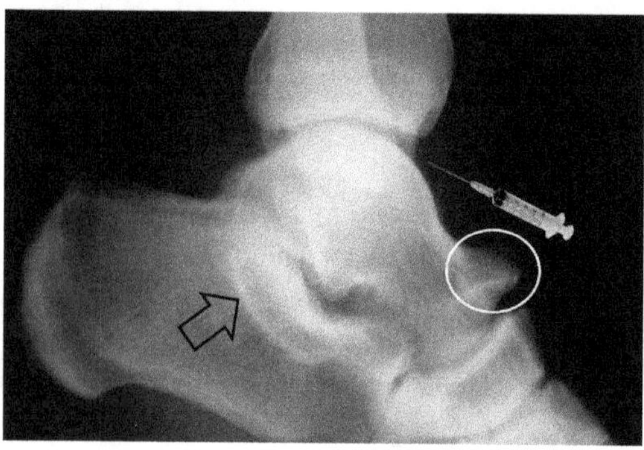

Fig. 5 The injection technique under fluoroscopic guidance is shown on a lateral radiograph with patients in the lateral decubitus position and the ankle slightly plantar flexed. The needle has an upward angulation of 30° in order to avoid the overhanding anterior tip of the tibia where osteophytes often exist. Coexistence of talocalcaneal coalition, "C" shaped sign (open arrow), and anterior new bone formation in the distal talus (circle) are shown

For injection of the contrast material under US, the patient is placed supine on the table with the knee flexed at about 90° and the foot slightly internally rotated. The anterior tibiotalar recess can be assessed by performing a longitudinal scan on the anteromedial aspect of the ankle between the extensor hallucis longus and the tibialis anterior tendon. Power Doppler can be used in order to avoid injury of the dorsalis pedis artery. The recess appears like a triangular hyperechoic area when not distended by fluid, and a thin layer of cartilage is seen over the talus. With the articular joint centered in the middle of the screen, a 23–25 gauge needle is inserted parallel to the distal end of the probe with a caudal-cranial direction around 30° (Fig. 6). The whole length of the needle can be followed on its long axis, and the needle tip can be seen entering the joint space confirming the intra-articular position. The injected contrast material is seen flowing out of

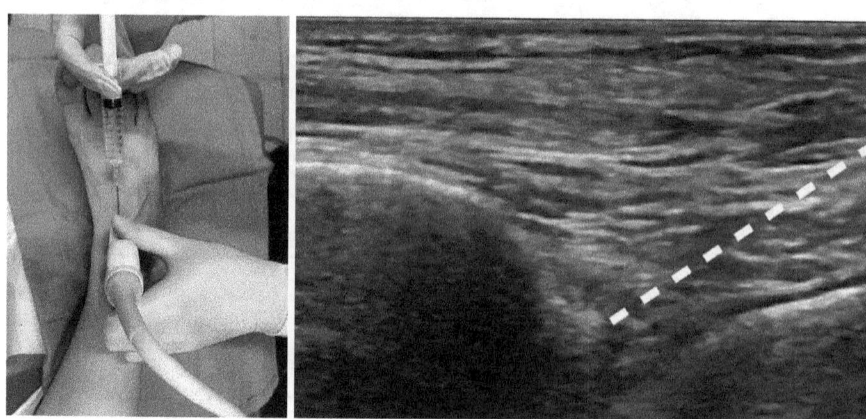

Fig. 6 US-guided injection. The anterior approach (left) and the needle path (dashed line, right) are shown

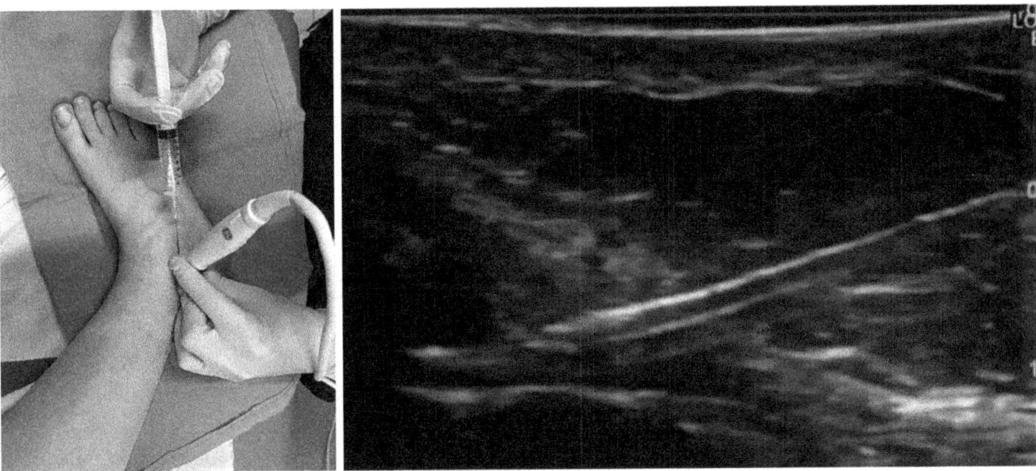

Fig. 7 US-guided injection. The anterolateral approach (left) and the needle insertion into the gutter (right) are shown

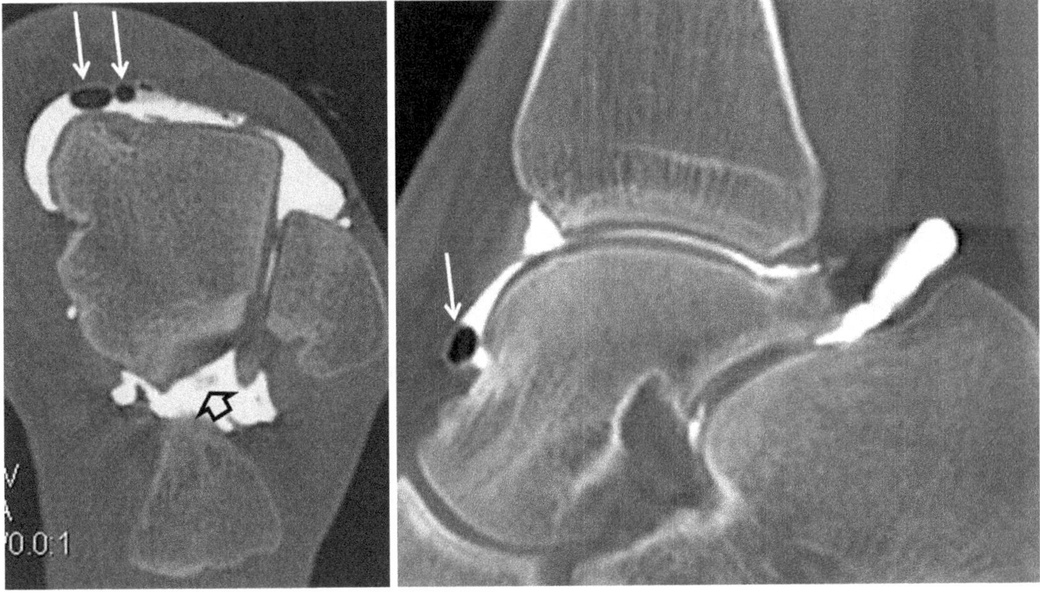

Fig. 8 CT arthrographic images in axial (left) and sagittal (right) planes. Air bubbles injected with the contrast are easily depicted (arrows). A small chondral loose body is shown in the posterior recess (open arrow)

the needle distending the joint capsule until firm resistance. Alternatively, a lateral trans-ligamentous approach through the talofibular ligament may be applied (Fig. 7) (Obradov and Gielen 2018).

Regardless of the method used for injecting the contrast, care should be taken to remove the air bubbles from the dilution. The latter usually are easily recognized on CTA but in the inexperienced radiologists they may be reported as loose bodies (Fig. 8).

3.5 CTA Technique

The patients are scanned in the supine position using high-resolution bone algorithm (Kernel 60–70), thin beam collimation (~0.6 mm), small field of view (~140 mm), and exposure parameters of 120 kVp and 200 mAs. The acquisition volume extends from ~2 cm cranial to the tibiotalar joint down to the bottom of the calcaneus. Post-processing includes reformatting images in four planes, with a reconstruction increment of 2.0 mm and overlaps ~50%, a window center or 450–550 HU, and a window width of 2200–2500 HU. The multiplanar reconstructions should be performed as follows: perpendicular to the distal tibia and parallel to the tibiotalar joint for the axial images, parallel to the malleolar axis for the coronal images, perpendicular to the malleolar axis for the sagittal images, and perpendicular to the posterior facet of the calcaneus for the axial oblique images.

4 CTA: Indications, Advantages, and Disadvantages

Initial evaluation of the painful ankle should start with plain radiographs in frontal, lateral, and mortise views (Chang et al. 2018). Classic radiographic findings of osteoarthritis can be demonstrated in the post-traumatic ankle including joint space narrowing, osteophyte and cyst formation, and subchondral sclerotic changes in addition to fractures and mal-alignments (Gorbachova et al. 2021). In the great majority of cases, chondral and osteochondral lesions are accompanied by non-specific symptoms and as a rule, plain radiographic evaluation yields no significant findings (Schmid et al. 2003). According to the ACR appropriateness criteria for chronic ankle pain in case of unremarkable radiographs but a high suspicion of osteochondral lesions, MRI without use of intravenous gadolinium is indicated as the next diagnostic step (Chang et al. 2018). MRI has the ability to indicate osteochondral lesion instability by revealing a high signal line or cyst formation in fluid-sensitive sequences at the interface between with the surrounding bone. MRI is not as accurate as MR arthrography or CTA in revealing chondral lesions (De Smet et al. 1996). MRI can in addition assess the bone marrow and the surrounding soft-tissue structures. Lesions of the latter may lead to ankle instability and may require surgical repair. US examination with high-frequency probes can also assess reliably the superficial soft-tissue structures around the ankle.

CTA has an excellent spatial resolution and is able to demonstrate radiographically occult lesions in the post-traumatic ankle especially after open reduction and internal fixation, where magnetic susceptibility artifacts can reduce the diagnostic accuracy of MRI (Figs. 9, 10, 11, and 12) (Kraniotis et al. 2012). A great load of literature has demonstrated the superiority of CTA compared to non-arthrographic techniques (conventional MRI and CT) and MR arthrography for the detection of chondral and osteochondral lesions. Conventional MRI has been shown to reveal 54% of the osteochondral lesions that can be detected with CTA (Kirschke et al. 2016). The additional findings revealed by CTA have been shown to change the clinical management of the patients in 15.4% of the cases (Kirschke et al. 2016). In cadaveric studies, CTA has been found to be more accurate in measuring the depth of talar osteochondral lesions (Pohler et al. 2021). The morphology of the lesions and the filling of microfractures with repair tissue can also be demonstrated with the use of CTA (Jung et al. 2018). Small loose bodies can be easily depicted by CTA (Figs. 8 and 12). Apart from the evaluation of chondral and osteochondral lesions, CTA has other applications in the evaluation of the ankle. It can reliably demonstrate the communication of the joint with ganglion cysts that may compress the tarsal tunnel or other subarticular cysts (Fig. 13). In these cases, delayed acquisition 90 min after contrast injection can demonstrate the communication between the cysts and the joint which is not evident in US and conventional MRI (Omoumi et al. 2010). A communication between the ankle joint and the flexor hallucis longus tendon sheath can be identified by CTA in ¼ of the normal population (Ogul et al. 2021). CTA has been also shown to accurately demonstrate anterolateral ankle impingement with a sensitivity and specificity of 97% and 71.4%, respectively, which is significantly higher than the

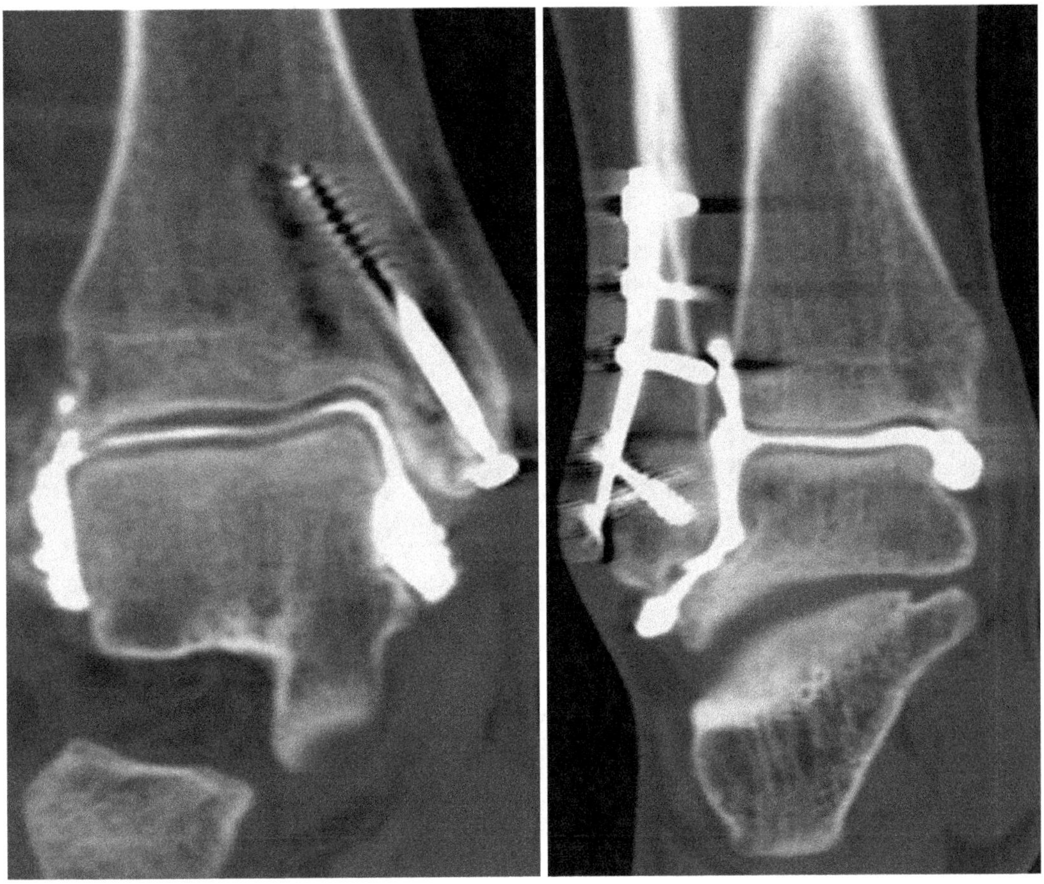

Fig. 9 A 35-year-old man with a bimalleolar fracture due to a motor vehicle accident and mild pain following an ORIF reconstruction. Note that the metal artifacts do not downgrade the quality of the CT arthrographic images. The articular cartilage is intact

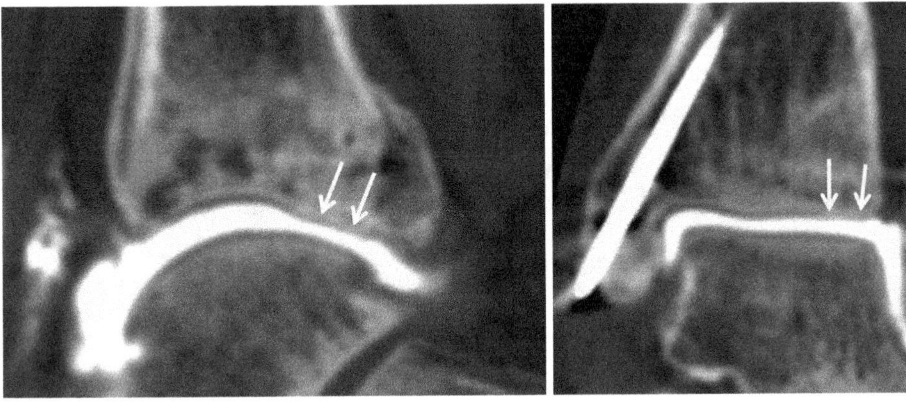

Fig. 10 A 42-year-old female with a trimalleolar fracture after fall from height. Clinically she has persistent pain following an ORIF reconstruction. Note that the metal artifacts do not downgrade the quality of the images. The tibial articular cartilage is severely eroded (arrows)

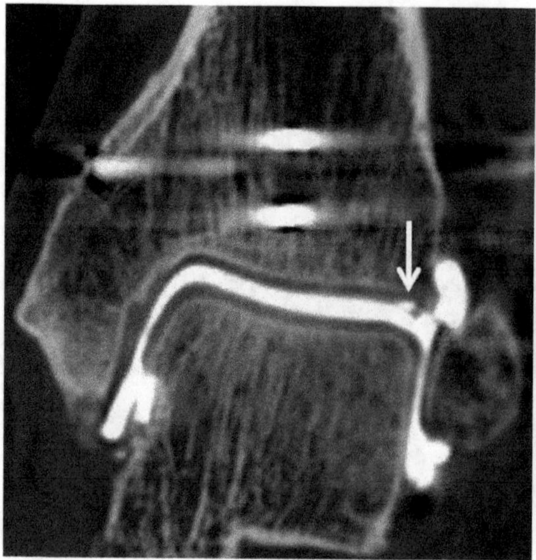

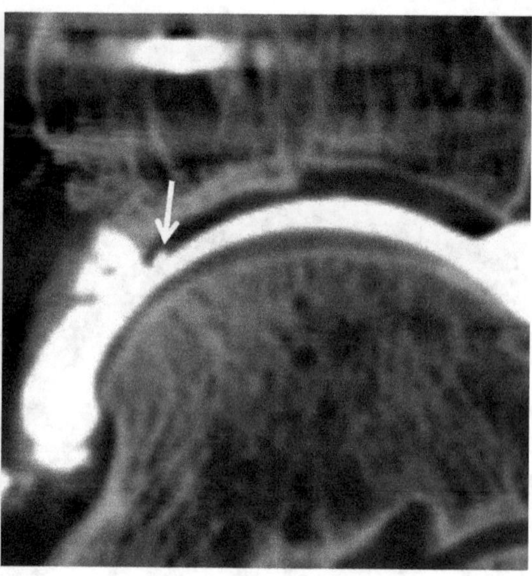

Fig. 11 A 48-year-old man with a bimalleolar fracture due to a motor vehicle accident and mild pain following an ORIF reconstruction. Note that the metal artifacts do not downgrade the quality of the images regarding the joint space. The articular cartilage shows small defects which probably are not symptomatic (arrows)

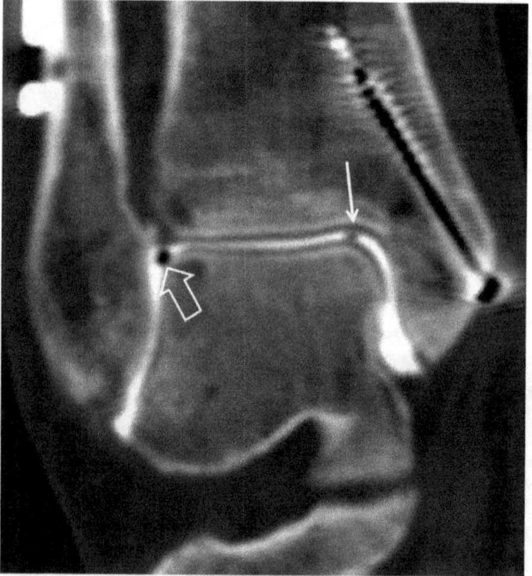

Fig. 12 A 62-year-old male patient who had ORIF for bimalleolar fracture. The coronal CT arthrographic image shows a small cartilaginous loose body (arrow) and a small air bubble injected with the contrast (open arrow)

performance of US which had a sensitivity of 76.5% and a specificity of 57.1% (Cochet et al. 2010). Anterolateral impingement is revealed by examining the anterolateral area proximal to the anterior talofibular ligament and demonstrating irregularity of the lateral groove edges (Hauger et al. 1999). Aside from the aforementioned diagnostic advantages of CTA, it affords other non-diagnostic advantages which can prove extremely valuable in everyday clinical practice. These include the ability to facilitate claustrophobic patients who cannot tolerate MR imaging and the ability to image patients for which MR imaging is contraindicated (Tsai et al. 2015). The cost of the examination is also significantly lower, and the duration of the examination is shorter than MRI or MR arthrography.

Nonetheless, the use of CTA has certain limitations. As in the evaluation of other joints, CTA cannot depict intrasubstance cartilage lesions, since it relies on the passage of iodinated contrast inside cartilage fissures erosions. Finally, the radiation burden is a disadvantage compared to MRI and US. Modern CTA delivers a mean dose of 47.2 mGy (Chemouni et al. 2014), which can be further reduced to ~50% in multislice scanners with the use of lower kV (80–100 kV) and the use of adaptive iterative dose reduction techniques (Gervaise et al. 2013).

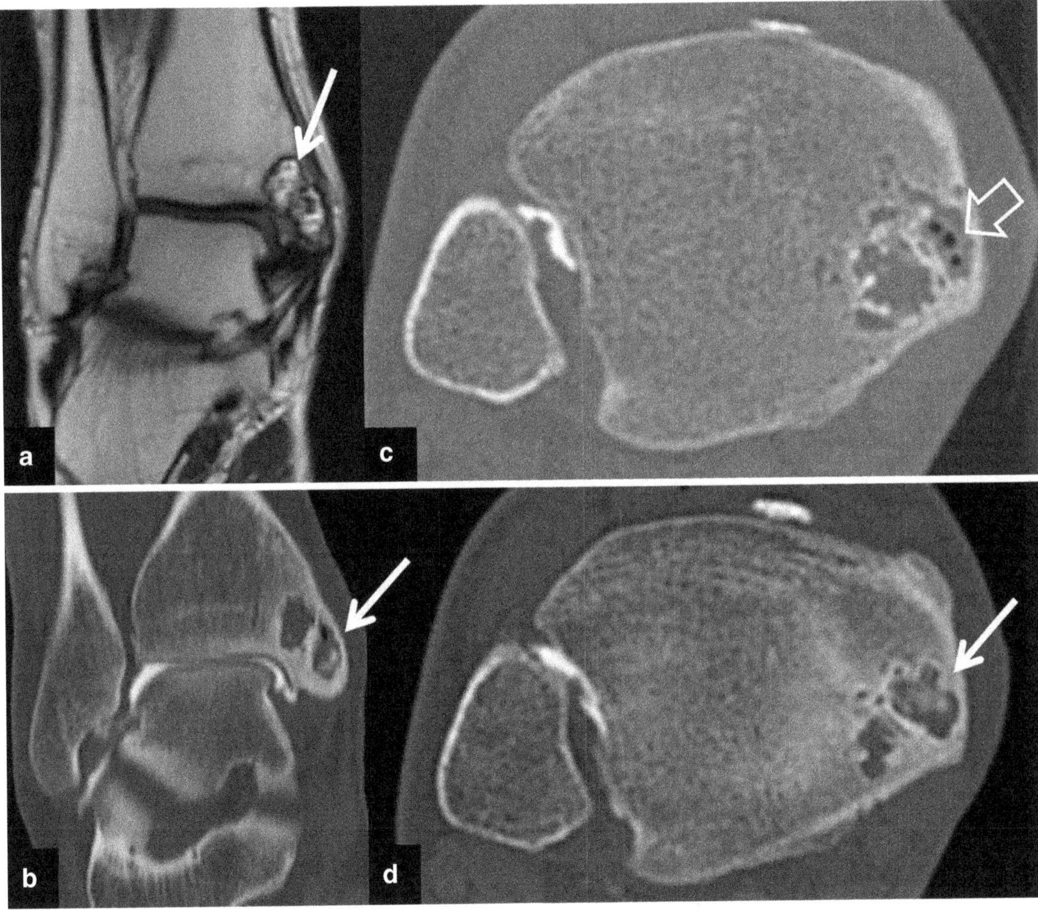

Fig. 13 A 40-year-old man with pain in the medial ankle joint and a radiograph depicting an osteolytic lesion (not shown). A CT arthrogram was performed for preoperative planning. (**a**) The coronal T2W MR image shows the intraosseous cystic lesion in the medial malleolus (arrow). The coronal (**b**) and axial (**c**, **d**) CT arthrographic images show communication of the lesion with the joint with air (thin arrows) and contrast (arrows) depicted in the matrix

References

Anderson AE, Ellis BJ, Peters CL, Weiss JA (2008) Cartilage thickness: factors influencing multidetector CT measurements in a phantom study. Radiology 246(1):133–141

Barg A, Bailey T, Richter M, de Cesar NC, Lintz F, Burssens A et al (2018) Weight bearing computed tomography of the foot and ankle: emerging technology topical review. Foot Ankle Int 39:376–386

Bernasconi A, De Cesar NC, Siegler S, Jepsen M, Lintz F (2021) Weightbearing CT assessment of foot and ankle joints in Pes Planovalgus using distance mapping. Foot Ankle Surg. https://doi.org/10.1016/j.fas.2021.10.004

Buckwalter KA (2006) CT arthrography. Clin Sports Med 25(4):899–915

Cerezal L, Abascal F, García-Valtuille R, Canga A (2005) Ankle MR arthrography: how, why, when. Radiol Clin North Am 43(4):693–707

Cerezal L, Llopis E, Canga A, Rolón A (2008) MR arthrography of the ankle: indications and technique. Radiol Clin North Am 46(6):973–994

Chang EY, Tadros AS, Amini B et al (2018) ACR Appropriateness Criteria® chronic ankle pain. J Am Coll Radiol 15(5):S26–S38

Chemouni D, Champsaur P, Guenoun D, Desrousseaux J, Pauly V, Le Corroller T (2014) Diagnostic performance of flat-panel CT arthrography for cartilage defect detection in the ankle joint: comparison with MDCT arthrography with gross anatomy as the reference standard. AJR Am J Roentgenol 203(5):1069–1074

Choi JY, Heung SK, Sung HH et al (2008) Optimization of the contrast mixture ratio for simultaneous direct MR and CT arthrography: an in vitro study. Korean J Radiol 9(6):520–525

Chou H, Chin TY, Peh WC (2017) Dual-energy CT in gout – a review of current concepts and applications. J Med Radiat Sci 64:41–51

Cochet H, Pelé E, Amoretti N, Brunot S, Lafenêtre O, Hauger O (2010) Anterolateral ankle impingement: diagnostic performance of MDCT arthrography and sonography. AJR Am J Roentgenol 194(6):1575–1580

Conti MS, Ellis SJ (2020) Weight-bearing CT scans in foot and ankle surgery. J Am Acad Orthop Surg 28:e595–e603

De Smet AA, Ilahi OA, Graf BK (1996) Reassessment of the MR criteria for stability of osteochondritis dissecans in the knee and ankle. Skeletal Radiol 25(2):159–163

Draeger RW, Singh B, Parekh SG (2009) Quantifying normal ankle joint volume: an anatomic study. Indian J Orthop 43(1):72–75

Fox MG, Petrey WB, Alford B, Huynh BH, Patrie JT, Anderson MW (2012) Shoulder MR arthrography: intraarticular anesthetic reduces periprocedural pain and major motion artifacts but does not decrease imaging time. Radiology 262(2):576–583

Gervaise A, Teixeira P, Villani N, Lecocq S, Louis M, Blum A (2013) CT dose optimisation and reduction in osteoarticular disease. Diagn Interv Imaging 94(4):371–388

Gorbachova T, Melenevsky YV, Latt LD, Weaver JS, Taljanovic MS (2021) Imaging and treatment of post-traumatic ankle and hindfoot osteoarthritis. J Clin Med 10(24):5848

Hauger O, Moinard M, Lasalarie JC, Chauveaux D, Diard F (1999) Anterolateral compartment of the ankle in the lateral impingement syndrome: appearance on CT arthrography. AJR Am J Roentgenol 173:685–690

Jung HG, Kim NR, Jeon JY et al (2018) CT arthrography visualizes tissue growth of osteochondral defects of the talus after microfracture. Knee Surg Sports Traumatol Arthrosc 26(7):2123–2130

Kampen WU, Westphal F, Van den Wyngaert T et al (2018) SPECT/CT in postoperative foot and ankle pain. Semin Nucl Med 48:454–468

Kirschke JS, Braun S, Baum T et al (2016) Diagnostic value of CT arthrography for evaluation of osteochondral lesions at the ankle. Biomed Res Int 2016:12–16

Kraniotis P, Maragkos S, Tyllianakis M, Petsas T, Karantanas AH (2012) Ankle post-traumatic osteoarthritis: a CT arthrography study in patients with bi- and trimalleolar fractures. Skeletal Radiol 41(7):803–809

Kreuz PC, Steinwachs M, Angele P (2018) Single-dose local anesthetics exhibit a type-, dose-, and time-dependent chondrotoxic effect on chondrocytes and cartilage: a systematic review of the current literature. Knee Surg Sports Traumatol Arthrosc 26(3):819–830

Lecouvet FE, Simoni P, Koutaïssoff S, Vande Berg BC, Malghem J, Dubuc JE (2008) Multidetector spiral CT arthrography of the shoulder. Clinical applications and limits, with MR arthrography and arthroscopic correlations. Eur J Radiol 68(1):120–136

Lintz F, Beaudet P, Richardi G, Brilhault J (2021) Weight-bearing CT in foot and ankle pathology. Orthop Traumatol Surg Res 107(1S):102772. https://doi.org/10.1016/j.otsr.2020.102772

Lungu E, Moser TP (2015) A practical guide for performing arthrography under fluoroscopic or ultrasound guidance. Insights Imaging 6(6):601–610

Messina C, Banfi G, Aliprandi A et al (2016) Ultrasound guidance to perform intra-articular injection of gadolinium-based contrast material for magnetic resonance arthrography as an alternative to fluoroscopy: the time is now. Eur Radiol 26(5):1221–1225

Mosimann PJ, Richarme D, Becce F et al (2012) Usefulness of intra-articular bupivacain and lidocain adjunction in MR or CT arthrography: a prospective study in 148 patients. Eur J Radiol 81(9):e957–e961

Obermann WR, Bioem JL, Hermans J (1989) Knee arthrography: comparison of iotrolan and ioxaglate sodium meglumine. Radiology 173(1):197–201

Obradov M, Gielen JLMA (2018) Image-guided intra- and extra-articular musculoskeletal interventions. Springer International, Cham, Switzerland

Ogul H, Cankaya B, Kantarci M (2021) The distribution in joint recesses and adjacent synovial compartments of loose bodies determined on MR and CT arthrographies of ankle joint. Br J Radiol 94:20201239

Omoumi P, Mercier GA, Lecouvet F, Simoni P, Vande Berg BC (2009) CT arthrography, MR arthrography, PET, and scintigraphy in osteoarthritis. Radiol Clin North Am 47(4):595–615

Omoumi P, De Gheldere A, Leemrijse T et al (2010) Value of computed tomography arthrography with delayed acquisitions in the work-up of ganglion cysts of the tarsal tunnel: report of three cases. Skeletal Radiol 39(4):381–386

Pohler GH, Sonnow L, Ettinger S et al (2021) High resolution flat-panel CT arthrography vs. MR arthrography of artificially created osteochondral defects in ex vivo upper ankle joints. PloS One 16(8 August):1–14

Rastogi AK, Davis KW, Ross A, Rosas HG (2016) Fundamentals of joint injection. AJR Am J Roentgenol 207(3):484–494

Saifuddin A, Abdus-Samee M, Mann C, Singh D, Angel JC (2005) CT guided diagnostic foot injections. Clin Radiol 60(2):191–195

Sandhu R, Aslan M, Obuchowski N, Primak A, Karim W, Subhas N (2021) Dual-energy CT arthrography: a feasibility study. Skeletal Radiol 50(4):693–703

Schmid MR, Pfirrmann CWA, Hodler J, Vienne P, Zanetti M (2003) Cartilage lesions in the ankle joint: comparison of MR arthrography and CT arthrography. Skeletal Radiol 32(5):259–265

Sverzut J, Campagna R, Guerini H, Feydy A, Drapé J, Pessis E (2015) Reduction of metal artifact with dual-energy CT: virtual monospectral imaging with fast kilovoltage switching and metal artifact reduction software. Semin Musculoskelet Radiol 19:446–455

Thomas C, Schabel C, Krauss B, Weisel K, Bongers M, Claussen CD (2015) Dual-energy CT: virtual calcium subtraction for assessment of bone marrow involvement of the spine in multiple myeloma. AJR Am J Roentgenol 204:W324–W331

Tsai LL, Grant AK, Mortele KJ, Kung JW, Smith MP (2015) A practical guide to MR imaging safety: what radiologists need to know. Radiographics 35(6):1722–1737

Tuominen EKJ, Kankare J, Koskinen SK, Mattila KT (2013) Weight-bearing CT imaging of the lower extremity. AJR Am J Roentgenol 200(1):146–148

Wang CK, Tsai JM, Chuang MT, Wang MT, Huang KY, Lin RM (2013) Bone marrow edema in vertebral compression fractures: detection with dual-energy CT. Radiology 269:525–533

Wright PR, Fox MG, Alford B, Patrie JT, Anderson MW (2014) An alternative injection technique for performing MR ankle arthrography: the lateral mortise approach. Skeletal Radiol 43(1):27–33

MRI and MRI Arthrography of Ankle and Foot

Simranjeet Kaur and Radhesh Lalam

Contents

S. Kaur · R. Lalam (✉)
Department of Radiology, Robert Jones and Agnes Hunt Orthopaedic Hospital, NHS, Oswestry, UK
e-mail: radhesh.lalam@nhs.net

1 Introduction

The advancements in MRI in the recent years have widened our horizons in the diagnosis and treatment of musculoskeletal conditions of the foot and ankle. MRI has superb soft tissue contrast resolution, multiplanar imaging capability, and noninvasive nature, which makes it an important investigative tool for the disorders of foot and ankle (Rosenberg et al. 2000). It helps in the detection of soft tissue and osseous abnormalities, which are difficult to diagnose with alternative imaging modalities and provide insight into the diagnosis of pathological conditions of articular cartilage and bone marrow. However, due to its complex anatomy and a very wide spectrum of normal variants and pathological conditions, MRI of the foot and ankle offers an additional challenge for interpretation. This chapter deals with the basics of MRI imaging of foot and ankle along with a brief review of pertinent normal MRI anatomy.

The anatomical regions in foot and ankle consist of the ankle joint, hindfoot (which includes talus and calcaneus), midfoot (consisting of cuboid, navicular, and cuneiform bones), and forefoot (including metatarsals and toes). There are two joints between the talus and calcaneum—posterior talocalcaneal or posterior subtalar joint and talocalcaneonavicular joint, also known as the anterior subtalar joint. The Chopart joint is the joint between the hindfoot and the midfoot, and the Lisfranc joint is between the midfoot and

Med Radiol Diagn Imaging (2023)
https://doi.org/10.1007/174_2023_399,

Published Online: 06 April 2023

the forefoot. The complex anatomy of the foot and ankle can be daunting to the uninitiated. In this chapter, the relevant technique and principles of MRI imaging are expounded followed by a review of the regional anatomy.

2 Routine MRI Protocol

The MRI protocol must be tailored for the three examination zones—ankle and hindfoot, midfoot, and forefoot depending on the clinical question (Gorbachova 2020). The midfoot is usually adequately imaged with either ankle or forefoot. High magnetic field strength and dedicated extremity coils provide a very high signal-to-noise ratio and a very high spatial resolution for the proper imaging of the complex anatomy of ankle and foot.

There are various challenges for the imaging of ankle beyond the complex anatomy. Ankle is the transition between the distal leg and foot, which are orientated perpendicular to each other (Siriwanarangsun et al. 2017). As a result of this transition, imaging at or near magic angle is unavoidable posing problems in the diagnosis of various tendon pathologies.

Imaging at the isocenter of the magnet is imperative for homogeneous field strengths and gradients. This cannot be stressed enough in case of imaging of foot and ankle because of its peripheral position. Use of dedicated surface extremity coils is important for magnetic field homogeneity and better spatial resolution and to optimize signal-to-noise ratio, while imaging small peripheral joints (Rivera et al. 1998). New multichannel coils have improved imaging times and signal-to-noise ratio and allow for parallel imaging techniques (Pruessmann 2004).

There are several advantages of imaging ankle on a 3T MRI scanner as the increase in magnetic field strength increases the SNR, which increases the spatial resolution and reduces the imaging time. However, imaging at high strengths comes with its own set of issues and disadvantages. With the increase in magnetic field strength, the magnetic susceptibility increases resulting in more geometric distortion, inhomogeneous fat suppression, and greater signal loss. The relaxation times are affected by field strength, thereby necessitating changing the pulse sequence parameters, affecting T1 times more than T2 (Ramnath 2006).

Routine MRI ankle is performed in all three planes: axial, coronal, and sagittal parallel to the tabletop (Fig. 1). The patient is supine with foot in approximately 20° plantar flexion. Plantar flexion accentuates the fat plane around the peroneal tendons and allows for better evaluation of the calcaneofibular ligament (Rosenberg et al. 2000).

MRI imaging specially in MSK is a fine balance between fluid sensitivity and spatial contrast resolution. The better the spatial contrast resolution, the better the anatomic detail. Also, in most pathologies, the water content increases; thereby, sequences with best fluid sensitivity will help in better detection of the pathological conditions. Unenhanced FSE proton density and intermediate-density images are most used in imaging of the ankle and foot (Sofka 2017). The intermediate-density images (having TE between the normal PD and the T2-weighted sequences) provide a good balance between the fluid sensitivity and the anatomic detail. These intermediate-density images produce an image with arthrogram effect having excellent contrast between the fatty bone marrow, subchondral bone, overlying articular cartilage, and joint fluid (Siriwanarangsun et al. 2017).

Magic angle effect plays an important role in imaging of the ankle because of the course taken by the tendons toward their insertion onto the foot. The densely packed collagen fibers noted in the tendons have restricted water molecules, thus having short T2 times, resulting in lack of signal. However, when these are oriented at 55° to the magnetic field (54.74° to be precise), the T2 decay time increases. As a result, when they are

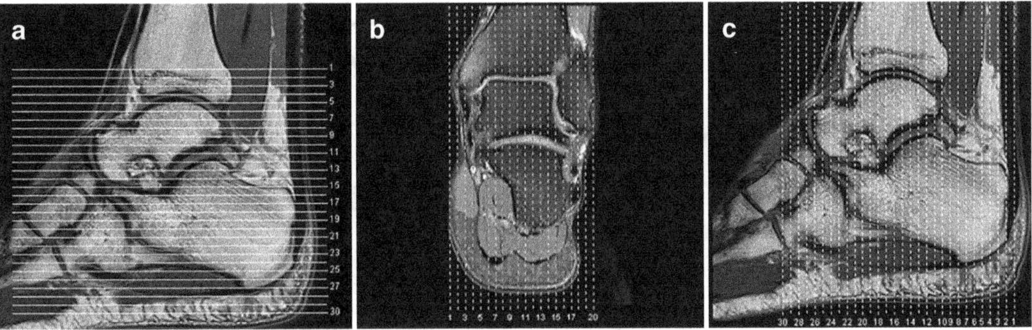

Fig. 1 (**a–c**) Pilot image depicting the alignment/plane of imaging for axial, sagittal, and coronal images

imaged using short TE sequences (PD, T1, and gradient echo), the T2 signal does not decay resulting in increased signal, which can be misinterpreted as pathological. This can be negated using long TE sequences for imaging because by the time the scanner picks up the signal, the T2 signal has already decayed.

The best sequences for marrow abnormalities are fat-suppressed fluid-sensitive sequences like fat-suppressed PD FSE or STIR sequences. The PD FS sequences are more susceptible to magnetic field inhomogeneity, resulting in heterogenous fat suppression and making this sequence suboptimal as compared to STIR.

Unenhanced T1-weighted image provides the best anatomic evaluation but does not have the benefit of fluid sensitivity. The standard MRI protocol thus includes a T1-weighted image in one plane along with one short tau inversion recovery sequence to compensate for the heterogeneous and incomplete fat suppression. Nonfat-suppressed and fat-suppressed T2- and PD-weighted sequences are also commonly used for routine imaging.

In most cases, the standard MRI imaging protocol yields sufficient images for diagnosing and detecting various pathologies. However, sometimes additional sequences and specialized imaging planes are needed to address specific clinical question. Interpretation of the increased signal within the peroneal tendons is one of the difficult areas in ankle imaging as they undergo a 90° directional change during their course from the ankle toward their insertion onto the foot. Imaging in 20° plantar flexion helps to reduce the magic angle (Gyftopoulos and Bencardino 2010). In addition, a peroneal view has been described which is a sagittal oblique view acquired at 2 mm intervals in a plane parallel to a line joining the lateral border of posterior calcaneum and lateral margin of the peroneal tubercle at the mid-calcaneal level (Park et al. 2016). This provides a profile view of the peroneal tendons as they undergo the 90° directional change (Fig. 2).

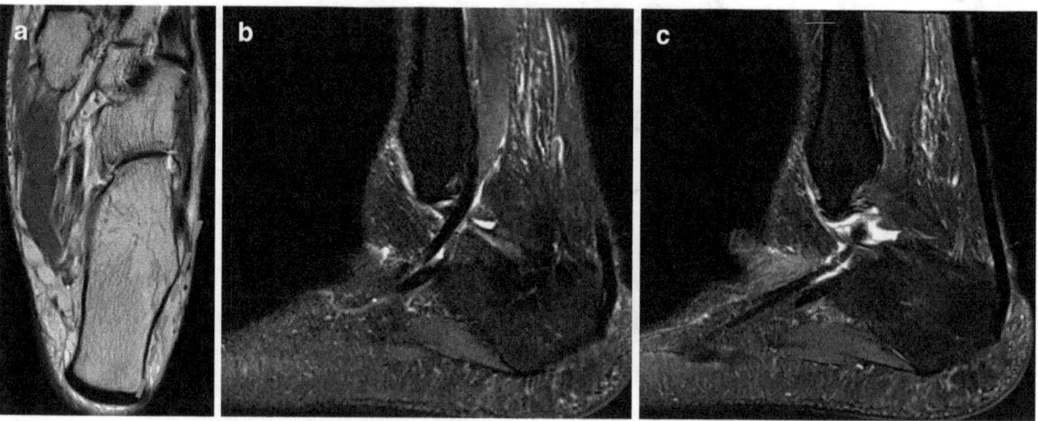

Fig. 2 (**a**) T1-weighted planning image for peroneal view—sagittal oblique view parallel to a line joining the lateral border of posterior calcaneum and lateral margin of the peroneal tubercle at the mid-calcaneal level. PD FS (**b**), (**c**) depicts the peroneal tendons imaged in profile as they undergo the 90° directional change as prescribed from (**a**)

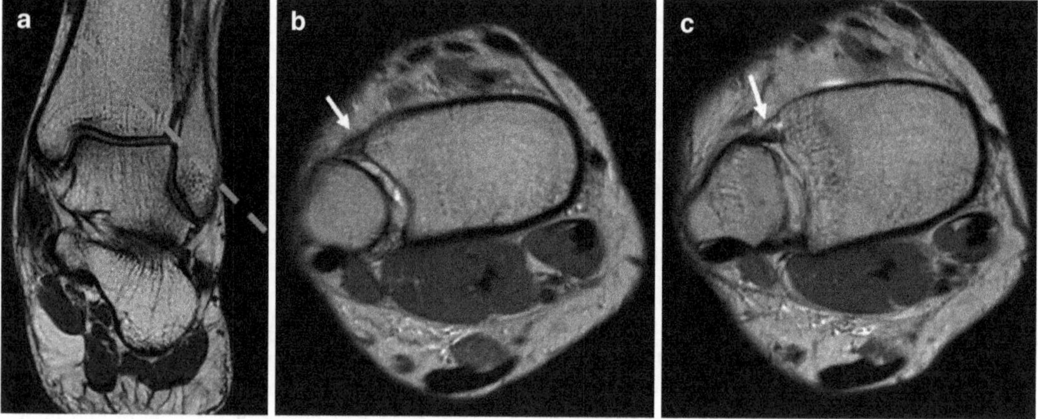

Fig. 3 (**a**) Coronal image depicting the alignment for syndesmotic view. (**b**), (**c**) Axial oblique images orthogonal to the syndesmotic ligament that improves the detection of ligament continuity and contour

The anterior and posterior syndesmotic ligaments and the calcaneofibular ligament run obliquely to the conventional imaging planes. As a result, additional oblique imaging planes are often acquired to increase the sensitivity and detect ligament injuries. Syndesmotic injuries are seen in 11% of ankle sprains, and the frequency can increase to 40% in contact sports (Hopkinson et al. 1990). A syndesmotic view which is an oblique axial view orthogonal to the ligament course has been proposed by Herman et al. improving the detection of ligament continuity and contour (Hermans et al. 2011) (Fig. 3).

Calcaneofibular ligament also has an oblique course having an angle of 13° between the ligament and the calcaneal axis. A coronal oblique imaging plane has been described for proper evaluation of the calcaneofibular ligament (Fig. 4). Park et al. evaluated the diagnostic accuracy of this imaging plane and concluded that it increases the sensitivity and diagnostic accuracy (Park et al. 2015).

In imaging of the foot, the protocol must be tailored to the specific clinical question. For examination for the forefoot, the imaging planes are relative to the axis of the second or third metatarsal bones. The foot is routinely imaged in oblique

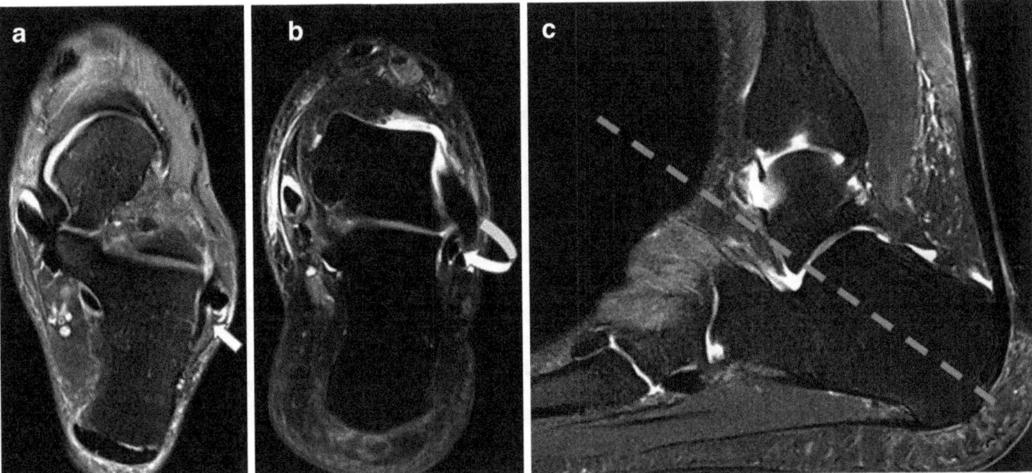

Fig. 4 (**a**) Axial PD FS image showing the intact calcaneofibular ligament forming the floor of peroneal tendons. (**b**) Coronal oblique image showing the ligament in its entirety. (**c**) Sagittal PD FS image shows the plane used for the coronal oblique image in (**b**)

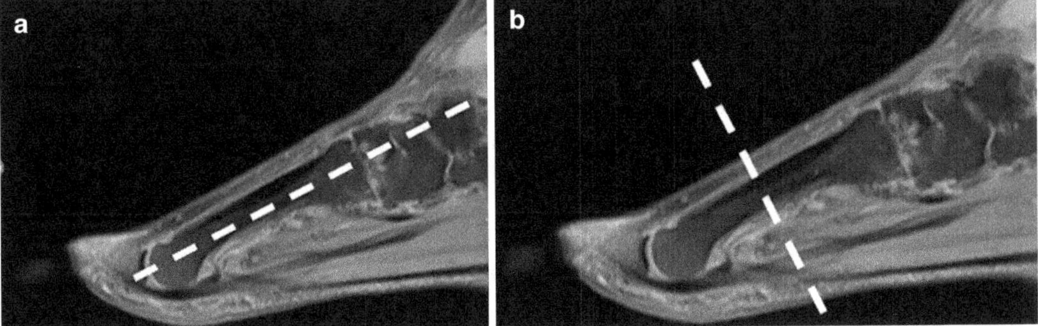

Fig. 5 (**a**) Depicts the oblique axial plane which is parallel to the long axis of the second metatarsal. (**b**) Depicts the orientation for the coronal oblique plane perpendicular to the long axis of the metatarsal

axial plane (parallel to the long axis of the second metatarsal), oblique coronal plane (perpendicular to the long axis of the metatarsal), and oblique sagittal plane (Fig. 5). The axial (long axis) plane is essential for evaluation of the Lisfranc ligament and stress fractures of the metatarsals. The coronal oblique (short axis) is particularly useful for evaluation of Morton's neuroma, plantar plates, and sesamoid bones. For the midfoot and hindfoot, a 12–14 cm field of view is used, whereas for the forefoot, a 10–12 cm field of view is used to improve the soft tissue contrast resolution to image the small peripheral joints in detail. The routine sequences include T1-weighted sequence in coronal and axial planes, STIR in coronal and sagittal or axial planes, and T2-weighted sequence in the coronal plane. Nonfat-suppressed T1-weighted images are acquired in at least one plane. These are very beneficial in imaging of the forefoot for Morton's neuroma. T1-weighted imaging is also very important to look for malignant marrow infiltration and in suspicious case of fractures and osteomyelitis. In cases of fractures, sometimes the fracture line is obscured by the surrounding bone marrow edema, and T1-weighted images are particularly helpful in these to identify the fracture line. T1-weighted images also help to differentiate between bone marrow edema and bone marrow infiltration by an underlying pathological process.

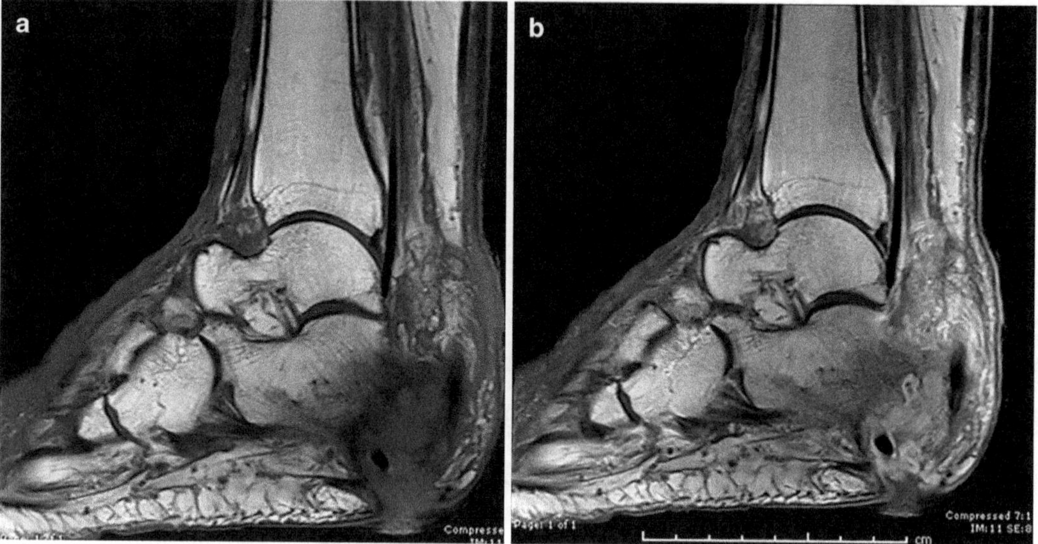

Fig. 6 (**a**) Sagittal T1- and (**b**) postcontrast T1-weighted images in a patient with diabetes demonstrate extensive inflammation and edema in the calcaneum s/o osteomyelitis with overlying skin ulceration and sinus formation

Intravenous gadolinium is administered in suspected infection, synovitis, or a soft tissue lesion to differentiate between a true cystic or a solid mass. There are specific etiologies encountered more frequently in foot and ankle needing contrast administration like cellulitis, diabetic foot, abscess, osteomyelitis, plantar fibroma, and Morton's neuroma. If contrast administration is needed, it is prudent to compare like to like; so, a precontrast T1- or FS T1-weighted image should be acquired followed by postcontrast T1 or T1 FS images depending upon the precontrast image (Fig. 6).

3 New Techniques

3.1 Isotropic 3D Fast Spin-Echo Imaging

The isotropic submillimeter acquisition and the tissue contrast almost approaching that of a 2D FSE acquisition allow for imaging in one plane and then reformation in different planes from the dataset (Kijowski et al. 2009). Radzi et al. used 3D MRI for assessment of postoperative alignment in patients with pilon fracture and found comparative performance of 3D MRI to that of 3D CT reconstructions (Radzi et al. 2016). 3D fast spin-echo imaging helps in the evaluation of complex trauma, osseous alignment, and articular surface, thus providing a one-stop shop avoiding the need for additional imaging study.

3.2 Ultrashort Echo Time MRI (UTE MRI)

The MRI signal characteristic acquired from a tissue depends on a lot of factors including the transverse relaxation time, which in turn depends on the structure and composition of the tissue. Tissues with short relaxation times do not return any signal as they have undergone complete relaxation before the signal can be acquired. Tissues can be divided on the basis of their relaxation times: <0.1 ms—super short, 0.1–1 ms—ultrashort, 1–10 ms—short, and more than 10 ms—long (Chang et al. 2015). The subchondral bone, calcified layer of cartilage, tendon, and ligaments fall into short and ultrashort T2 tissues (Siriwanarangsun et al. 2017). This technique allows for acquisition of signal from tissues with short or ultrashort TE.

The UTE sequences are used in the ankle for evaluation of calcified layer of cartilage in talar dome injuries, tendon, and entheseal abnormalities. It is important to understand the appearance of these structures on the UTE sequences to detect pathological conditions.

The osteochondral junction comprises the hyaline cartilage, deep layer of calcified cartilage, and subchondral bone. Assessment of this layer is important in osteochondral injuries as it has been implicated in mechanisms of development of osteoarthritis. After trauma, this layer may be absent, whereas in case of degeneration, this layer shows increased thickness.

Enthesis has a complex structural composition primarily to reduce the mechanical stress between the tensile tendon and the osseous site of attachment. Robson et al. found that UTE sequences depicted the fascicular pattern of the tendons and the complex structure of the enthesis (Robson et al. 2004). Enthesis was also found to have a fibrocartilaginous nodule within the tendon and at the tendon-bone interface (Siriwanarangsun et al. 2017). The entheseal tendon has received a great clinical interest as some studies have shown that patients with seronegative spondyloarthropathy have subclinical disease involving the lower limb enthesis (Bandinelli et al. 2011). T2* mapping has been used for quantitative evaluation of Achilles tendon. Studies have shown that T2* mapping is more sensitive to early structural changes in tissues with short and ultrashort echo times as compared to long TE tissues.

4 Indications

Ankle injuries are very common among high performing professional athletes as well as the general population, accounting for 10% of A and E visits (Meehan et al. 2017). Ankle sprain is the most frequent injury in a lot of sporting individuals. With the advent of MRI, osteochondral injuries are increasingly being recognized as one of the more common acute sport-related injuries (O'Loughlin et al. 2009).

Trauma and sports injuries are one of the most common clinical indications for imaging of the ankle. There can be an acute traumatic event or chronic repetitive injury resulting in secondary degeneration. It is important to understand the MRI terminology for osseous or osteochondral injuries. Bone marrow edema is an ill-defined area of increased signal intensity on the fluid-sensitive sequences with preserved bone marrow fat signal on the T1-weighted sequences (Gorbachova 2020). T1-weighted images are the best to differentiate between bone marrow edema and infiltration; replacement of the normal fatty marrow signal on T1-weighted images is suggestive of pathological process with marrow infiltration. A subchondral fracture is seen as a linear or curvilinear low signal intensity fracture line representing the impacted trabeculae in the subchondral location without breaching the articular surface. The fracture line is best appreciated on the T1-weighted sequences and can be masked sometimes by surrounding edema on the fluid-sensitive sequences (Fig. 7). An osteochondral injury is defined as an injury when the fracture line disrupts the articular cartilage and the subchondral bone plate. This can be stable or unstable. Presence of a fluid cleft beneath an osteochondral fragment is suggestive of the unstable nature of the defect and often needs surgical intervention (Fig. 8). Ill-defined edema like signal without any fracture line or articular damage is suggestive of bone contusion. The bone marrow edema is always more in case of impaction injuries where compressive forces are at play. Distraction or avulsion injuries do not produce much edema because of the distractive or tensile nature of the forces (Palmer et al. 1997). This should be kept in mind in evaluating a patient with acute traumatic ankle injury as an avulsion fracture can be missed on MRI because of the lack of bone marrow edema or extensive surrounding soft tissue edema engulfing the small fracture fragments (Gorbachova 2020). CT is particularly important for the assessment of such injuries.

Stress injuries are secondary to chronic repetitive microtrauma and are classified as insufficiency fractures or fatigue fractures. Insufficiency fractures result from normal physiological forces applied on a weakened bone, whereas fatigue fractures occur from excessive repetitive stress to a physiologically normal bone. The most com-

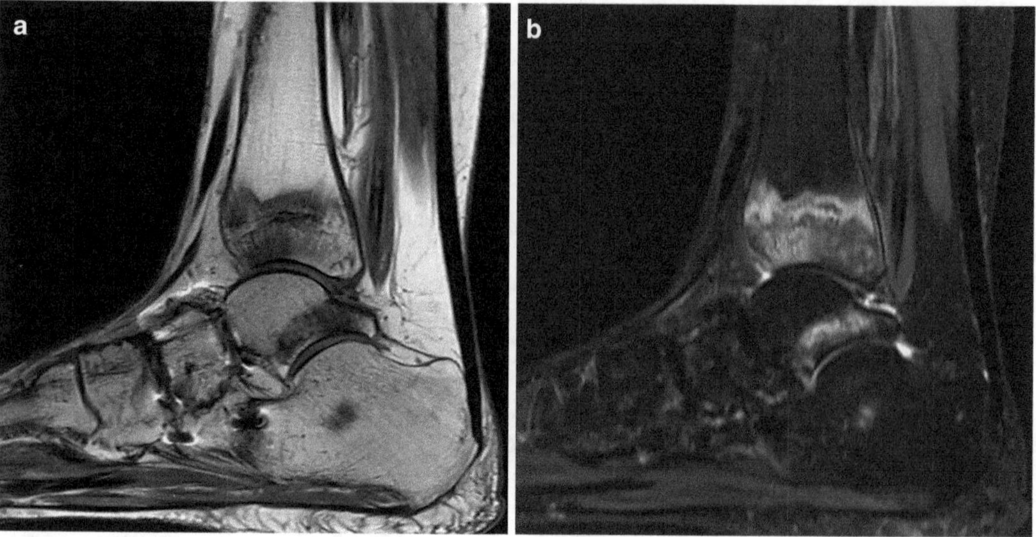

Fig. 7 (**a**) Sagittal T1-weighted image depicting the linear and curvilinear low signal intensity lines representing the impacted trabeculae in a patient with insufficiency fractures in both distal tibia and talus. (**b**) Sagittal PD FS image demonstrates associated surrounding bone marrow edema

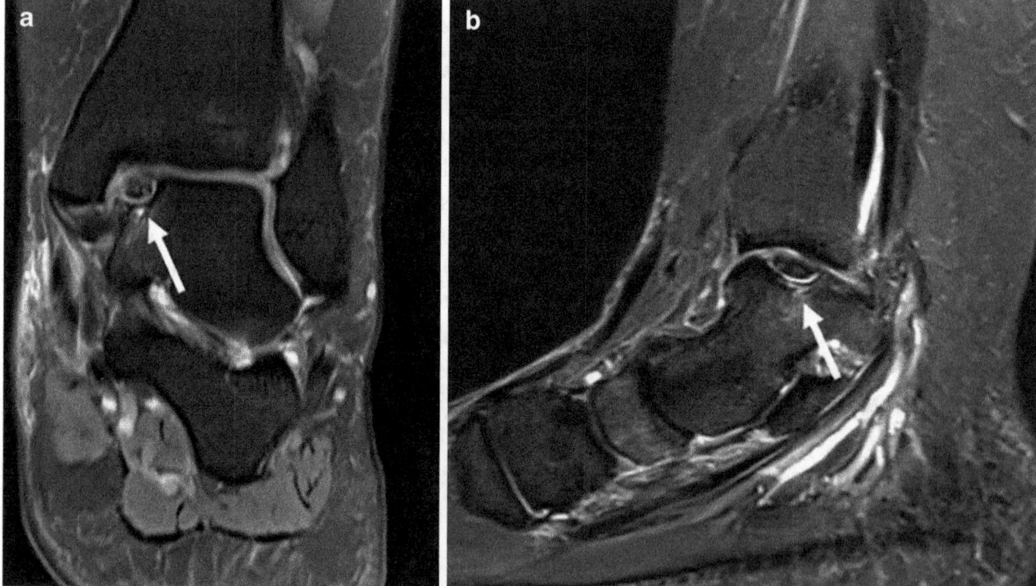

Fig. 8 (**a**) Coronal and (**b**) sagittal PD FS images depicting an unstable osteochondral lesion medial talar dome with fluid signal at the interface

mon sites are posteromedial distal tibia, calcaneus, and metatarsals (Mandell et al. 2017). The fractures located at the concentration of tensile forces and regions of reduced vascularity are high-risk fractures and are at an increased risk of nonunion or delayed union. These are situated at anterior tibial cortex, medial malleolus, talus, navicular, base of second metatarsal, proximal fifth metatarsal, and hallux sesamoids (Mandell et al. 2017).

5 Ankle Ligaments

The ligaments around the ankle are classified into three groups—syndesmotic, lateral, and medial group (Perrich et al. 2009). The syndesmotic ligaments consist of anteroinferior tibiofibular and posteroinferior tibiofibular ligaments, the interosseous ligament which is the thickening of the distal interosseous membrane, and the inferior transverse ligament which is located distal to the posterior tibiofibular ligament. The tibiofibular ligaments appear striated and discontinuous due to fat interposed between the fascicles and the oblique downward course of ligaments toward their insertion on the fibula. Injuries of the syndesmotic ligaments, known as high ankle sprain, are less common than the lateral ligament complex injuries but much more debilitating (Hunt et al. 2015).

The lateral ligament complex consists of anterior talofibular, calcaneofibular, and posterior talofibular ligament, which get injured in the same order. ATFL is the most common ligament to get injured in ankle sprains.

The morphological appearance of the talus and distal fibula is used as a reference point for ligament identification and helps distinguish between the tibiofibular and talofibular ligaments (Rosenberg et al. 2000). A square-shaped talar dome is visible at the level of fibular attachment of anterior tibiofibular ligament. The tibiofibular ligaments attach at the fibula above the level of malleolar fossa, and the cross section of distal fibula is round at this level. The talar body and head are shaped like a snowman or have an oblong shape at the site of attachment of talofibular ligaments (Fig. 9). The sinus tarsi is partially visualized at this level. Also, the distal fibula has a medial indentation, the malleolar fossa at the level of talofibular ligaments (Rosenberg et al. 2000). The calcaneofibular ligament is visualized deep to the peroneal tendons in between the calcaneus and the tendons. The ATFL and PTFL are seen on a single axial section distal to the syndesmotic ligaments. The PTFL has a broad fan-shaped insertion on the fibula and often demonstrates thickening and heterogeneity, which should not be interpreted as a tear.

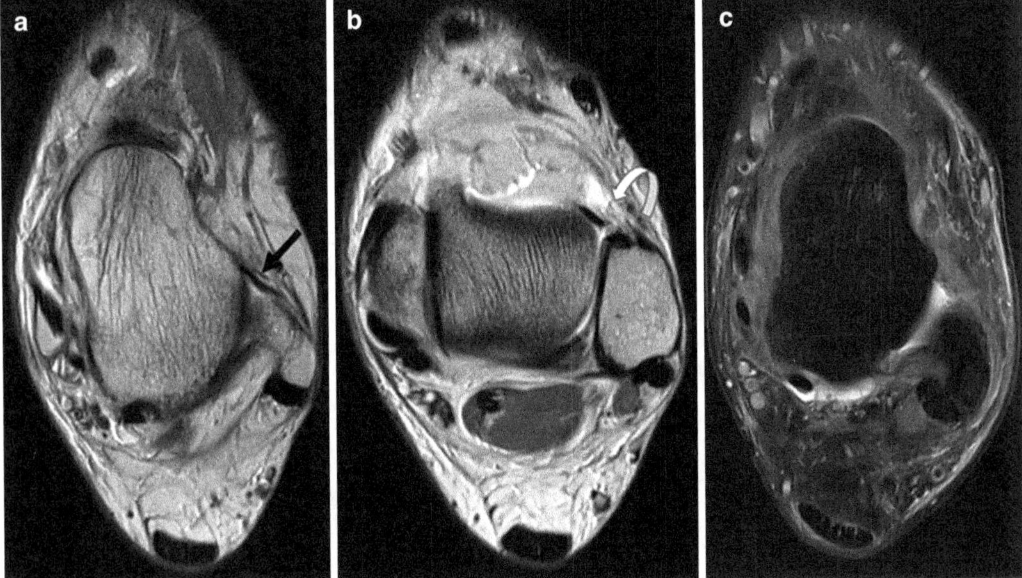

Fig. 9 (**a**) The talar head and body are shaped like a snowman at the level of ATFL as shown in this axial PD non-FS image. (**b**) A square-shaped talar dome is visible at the level of fibular attachment of the syndesmotic ligament. The shape of distal fibula also helps in differentiating as it is round at the level of tibiofibular ligaments and has a medial indentation, the malleolar fossa at the level of the ATFL. (**c**) Axial PD FS demonstrates diffusely thickened and hyperintense ATFL ligament with no normal-appearing fibers suggestive of a high-grade injury

Medial ligament complex is composed of deltoid complex, which has a superficial and deep layer (Mengiardi et al. 2007). The deep layer consists of short ligaments that cross the ankle joint—anterior and posterior tibiotalar ligaments. The posterior tibiotalar ligament is the strongest and thickest component (Gorbachova 2020). The superficial layer is delta/fan shaped with a small attachment at the medial malleolus and a broad fan-shaped attachment at the navicular, spring ligament, and calcaneum. These components are names according to the site of attachment.

The spring ligament complex runs between the navicular and calcaneus at the superomedial and plantar aspects of the foot. It is closely related to the superficial layer of the deltoid ligament. There are three components of the spring ligament—superomedial calcaneonavicular, medioplantar oblique calcaneonavicular, and inferoplantar longitudinal calcaneonavicular ligament (Fig. 10). The tibiospring component of deltoid forms a confluence with the superomedial calcaneonavicular ligament that stabilizes the medial ankle joint and supports the talar head like a hammock. Abnormalities of the spring ligament along with tibialis posterior tendon dysfunction are often seen in the setting of acquired pes planus deformity in adults. There can be thickening,

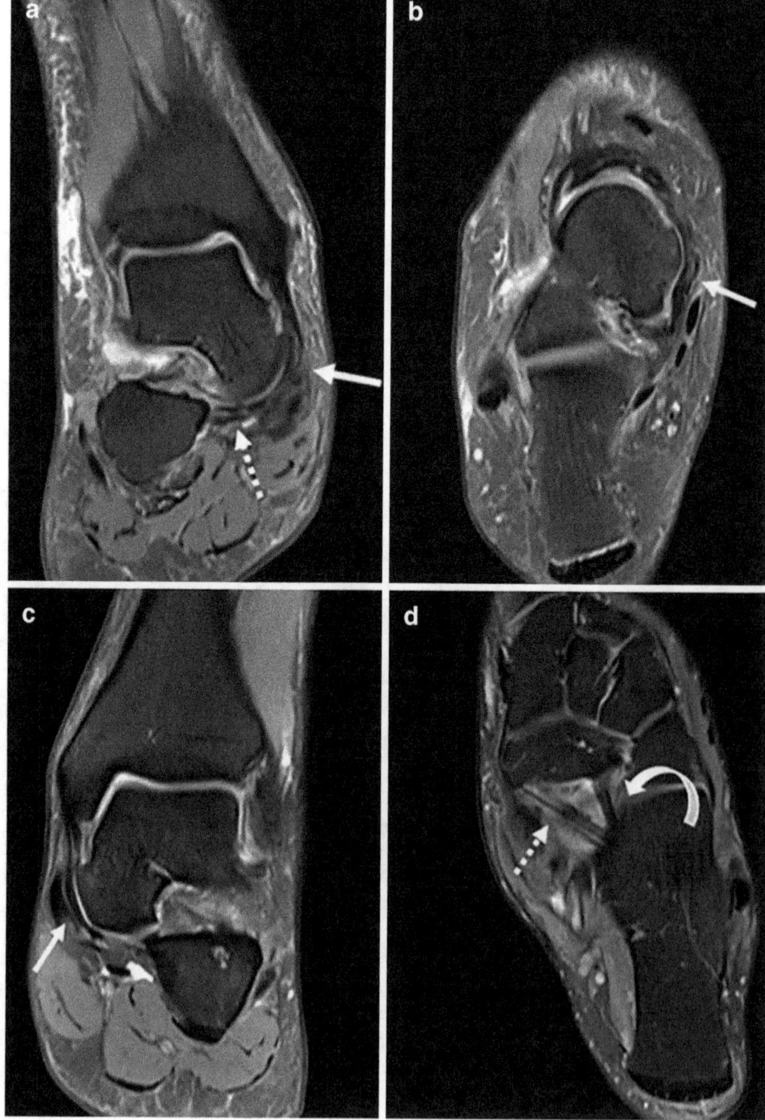

Fig. 10 (**a**) Coronal PD FS demonstrates the superomedial (white arrow) and the inferolateral (dashed arrow) components of spring ligament, which appears intact. The superomedial spring ligament is also seen on the (**b**) axial PD FS image lying deep to the tibialis posterior tendon. (**c**) Coronal PD FS image depicts the superomedial spring ligament merging with the tibiospring ligament forming a hammock for talar head. The other two components of the spring ligament are best seen on the axial image (**d**), which depicts both medioplantar (dashed arrow) and inferoplantar (curved arrow) longitudinal calcaneonavicular ligament

attenuation, or full-thickness rupture of the ligament.

6 Tendons

The tendons around the ankle are divided into four groups—anterior, posterior, medial, and lateral.

6.1 Anterior

There are three tendons in the anterior/extensor compartment of the ankle. From medial to lateral, they are tibialis anterior, extensor hallucis longus, extensor digitorum longus, and peroneus tertius. The tibialis anterior muscle originates from the proximal tibia, and its tendon inserts onto the medial cuneiform and the base of the first metatarsal. It acts as a strong dorsiflexor and invertor of the foot. The tibialis anterior is the largest anterior tendon; tear is often partial and goes unrecognized clinically. The extensor hallucis muscle lies deep to extensor digitorum longus and tibialis anterior, arising from the mid-part of the fibula and adjacent interosseous ligament. Its tendon inserts onto the dorsal base of the distal phalanx of the great toe, and it acts as an extensor of the great toe, weak invertor, and dorsiflexor of the foot. The extensor digitorum longus muscle arises from the lateral tibial condyle, anterior fibula, and interosseous membrane. It has four tendon slips in a common sheath to insert onto the middle and distal phalanges of the second to the fifth ray. All three anterior tendons pass deep to the extensor retinacula, being innervated by the deep peroneal nerve and supplied by the anterior tibial artery. The dorsalis pedis artery and veins and deep peroneal nerve pass deep and parallel to the extensor hallucis longus muscle and tendon.

6.2 Posterior Tendons

Achilles tendon, which is the longest and the thickest tendon in the body, constitutes the posterior group. The tendoachilles is a conjoint tendon made of soleus and gastrocnemius. Anteriorly, the muscle fibers of the soleus muscle extend almost to the distal insertion of the Achilles. The tendon fibers spiral through 90° with the medial fibers becoming more posterior. It does not have a tendon sheath; instead, it has a paratenon which allows for the free gliding of the tendon. It returns a low signal on all sequences and has a straight course on sagittal and coronal planes. Occasionally, there is a solitary vertical line of high signal in the mid-substance of the Achilles tendon, which is thought to be the site of the junction of the soleus and gastrocnemius tendons, or possibly a vascular channel. On axial images, the tendon has a concave anterior margin which is replaced by a convex/bulging margin in case of tendinosis. The most common site of tendinopathy and traumatic tears is 2–6 cm proximal to the calcaneal insertion, which is an avascular zone also known as critical zone. A true synovial lined bursa known as retrocalcaneal bursa is interposed between the posterior surface of calcaneum and the Achilles tendon and allows for smooth movement. This bursa is further bordered anteriorly by the Kager's fat pad. There is an adventitial bursa superficial to the Achilles tendon known as the retro-Achilles bursa. Haglund's syndrome is a painful condition characterized by posterior heel pain and swelling at the site of Achilles insertion. It is characterized by swelling of Achilles tendon at the site of attachment resulting in insertional tendinopathy along with distension of the retrocalcaneal and retro-Achilles bursa. It is associated with pump-style shoes and certain type of athletic footwear. There is an association with prominent dorsal convex calcaneal projection, and chronic irritation results in bone production and overgrowth resulting in a vicious cycle.

Plantaris tendon can also be seen in most people distinct from the Achilles inserting onto the superomedial calcaneal tuberosity. It is absent in only 7–20% of cases (Simpson et al. 1991). The plantaris tendon is the longest tendon in the human body and has little functional significance, being a weak knee flexor with its muscle origin from the posterior femur. It inserts onto the calcaneum, Achilles tendon, or flexor retinaculum and can be used as an autologous graft for a lateral ligament reconstruction. It should not be mistaken for a partially torn Achilles tendon.

6.3 Medial

The medial tendon group is made of tibialis posterior, flexor digitorum longus, and flexor hallucis longus. The tibialis posterior is the largest and functionally most important tendon medially. It is almost twice the size of flexor digitorum and flexor hallucis longus (Fig. 11). If the flexor tendons are of the same size or larger than PTT, it signifies thickening of the flexor tendons suggestive of tendinosis. At the level of the ankle, it is the most anteriorly situated medial tendon, situated just behind the medial malleolus. In the foot, it has a very broad fan-shaped insertion, majorly inserting on the navicular bone but giving slips to the cuneiform, cuboid, and bases of second to fourth metatarsals. An accessory navicular bone is a large accessory ossicle present posteromedial to the navicular bone, and tibialis posterior often inserts onto this ossicle. It is classified into three types. Type 1 is a sesamoid bone embedded within the tibialis posterior tendon. Type 2 accounts for 55% and is typically connected to the underlying navicular tuberosity by a thin layer of cartilage. Type 3 represents an unusually prominent navicular tuberosity, and it is thought to represent fused type 2. It is generally asymptomatic but can give rise to medial foot pain in case of traction between the ossicle and navicular bone (Fig. 12). Tibialis posterior adducts, flexes, and supinates the foot. Tibialis posterior along with the spring ligament supports the talar head. PTT dysfunction is often seen in conjunction with dysfunction or abnormalities of spring ligament. Failure of this tendon results in collapse of the longitudinal arch with plantar flexion of talus resulting in pes planus deformity. This is initially flexible; however, with chronic dysfunction, tendinosis, and degeneration, it becomes fixed. There is uncovering of the talar head with loss of osseous support provided by the navicular bone. Forefoot abduction and hindfoot valgus are also

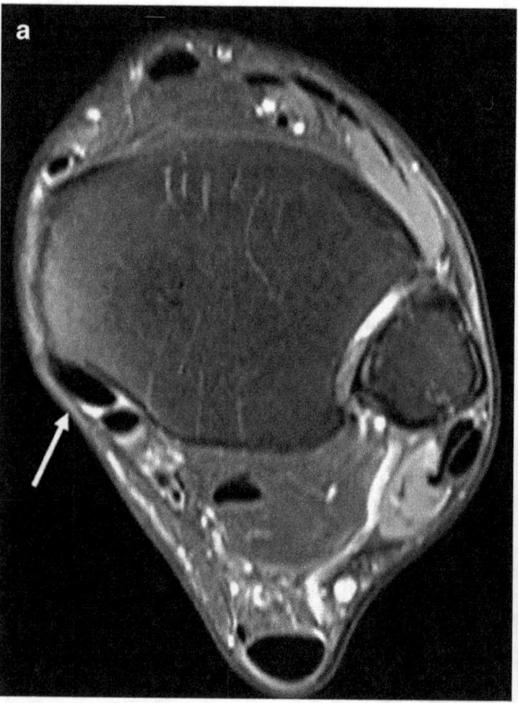

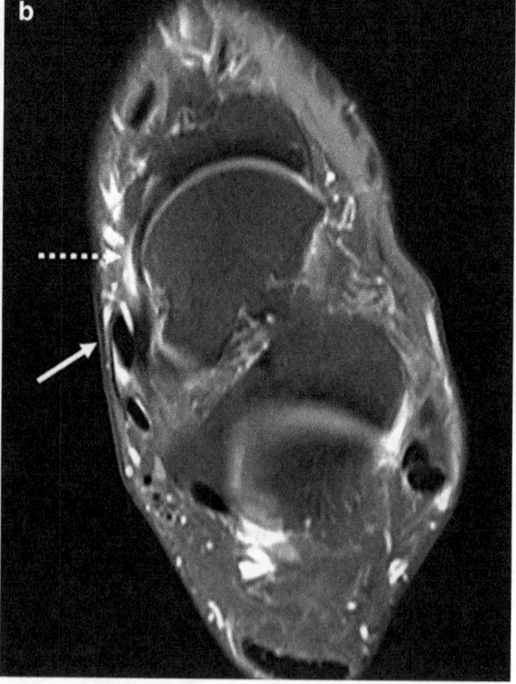

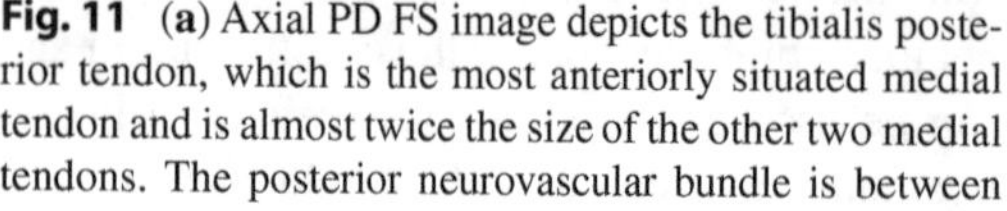

Fig. 11 (**a**) Axial PD FS image depicts the tibialis posterior tendon, which is the most anteriorly situated medial tendon and is almost twice the size of the other two medial tendons. The posterior neurovascular bundle is between FDL and FHL. (**b**) Further distally, the tibialis posterior tendon can be seen superficial to the spring ligament and together these support the talar head and their dysfunction results in pes planus deformity

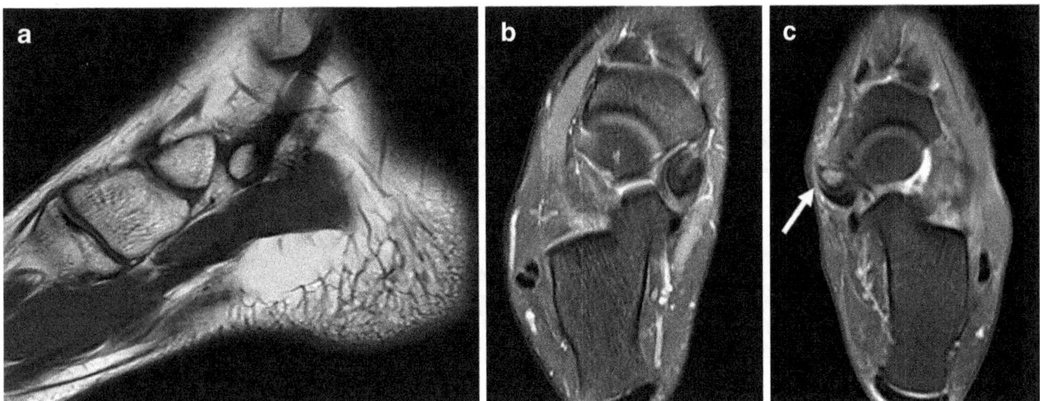

Fig. 12 (**a**) Sagittal T1 and (**b**) axial PD FS image demonstrates the os naviculare within the distal tibialis posterior tendon. (**c**) Axial PD FS image in another patient depicts edema within the accessory navicular with thickening of the tibialis posterior tendon

seen in PTT dysfunction resulting in lateral hindfoot impingement. The lateral hindfoot impingement as a result of tibiotalar valgus results in degeneration and secondary osteoarthritis.

Isolated spring ligament abnormalities are rare, and it is mostly secondary to PTT dysfunction. The MRI criteria for spring ligament injury, predominantly the superomedial calcaneonavicular ligament, are increased signal on PD or T2-weighted sequences with thickening (>5 mm), thinning (<2 mm), and partial or complete discontinuity (Mengiardi et al. 2016).

The flexor digitorum longus muscle originates from the posterior surface of the tibia, and its tendon inserts onto the plantar aspects of the bases of the distal phalanges of the second to the fifth digits. It acts as a flexor of the toes and supinator of the ankle.

Flexor hallucis longus is the closest to the midline of the other medial muscles and tendons, originating from the posterior mid-third aspect of the fibula and inserting onto the base of the distal phalanx of the great toe between the sesamoid bones. Fluid is commonly seen within the flexor hallucis longus tendon sheath in the presence of an effusion of the ankle joint as the tendon sheath communicates with the joint in approximately a fifth of normal individuals. A disproportionate amount of fluid within the tendon sheath relative to the joint is abnormal in keeping with tenosynovitis. It acts as a flexor of the great toe and ankle.

6.4 Tarsal Tunnel

The three medial tendons with the posterior tibial neurovascular bundle traverse in the tarsal tunnel and are isolated in their separate fibrous connective tissue tunnels. The proximal and distal boundaries of the tunnel are imprecise, but generally it is considered to extend from the level of the medial malleolus to the navicular. The roof of the tarsal tunnel is formed by the flexor retinaculum, with the floor represented by the talus and calcaneum. The fibrous connective tissue (septa), which forms the separate tunnels, connects the undersurface of the flexor retinaculum and medial malleolus. Some of the septa are attached to the neurovascular bundle, rendering it relatively immobile and therefore susceptible to traction injury or compression by an adjacent mass lesion. Either of these events may produce the sensory symptoms referred to as tarsal tunnel syndrome (an entrapment neuropathy).

6.5 Lateral

The peroneus brevis and longus muscles form the lateral compartment of the lower leg arising from the superolateral surface of the fibula. The peroneus longus muscle is superior and superficial to brevis. They are supplied by the peroneal artery

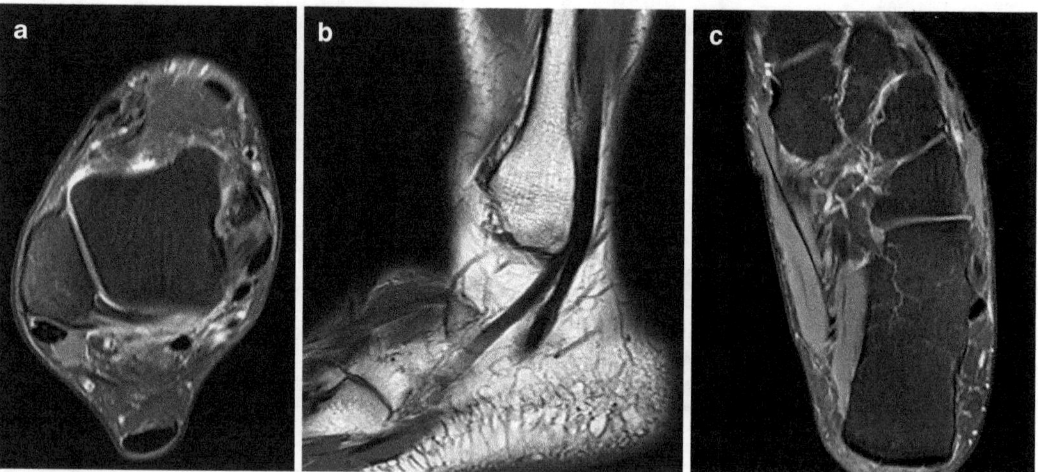

Fig. 13 (**a**) Axial PD FS image demonstrates the retromalleolar location of the peroneal tendons; the peroneus brevis is situated anteromedial to the tendon of peroneus brevis, and both these tendons are contained within the superior peroneal retinaculum. (**b**) Sagittal T1 image demonstrates the relation between the peroneal tendons and their course. (**c**) Axial PD FS further distally demonstrates the anteriorly located peroneus brevis tendon separated from the peroneus longus by the peroneal tubercle

(a branch of the posterior tibial artery) and innervated by the superficial peroneal nerve, also with a branch from the deep peroneal nerve to peroneus longus. They act as evertors of the foot and weak plantar flexors of the ankle.

Peroneus brevis and peroneus longus tendon make up the lateral tendon group. The diameter of both these tendons combined equals the diameter of tibialis posterior tendon. At the level of distal fibula, these tendons are situated in the retro-malleolar groove and are contained by the superior peroneal retinaculum. The peroneus brevis is situated anteromedial to the peroneus longus at this level. Further distally, they run in a very shallow groove between the lateral calcaneum and inferior peroneal retinaculum (Fig. 13). Peroneus brevis is anteriorly separated from the peroneus longus by the peroneal tubercle. The peroneus brevis inserts on the lateral aspect of the base of fifth metatarsal. The peroneus longus takes an acute almost right-angled turn at the level of calcaneocuboid joint and runs in the cuboid tunnel to insert on the plantar aspect of the base of the first metatarsal and medial cuneiform and gives slips that stabilize first TMT and Lisfranc joint (Fig. 14). This cuboid tunnel is a functional variant of enthesis, and often bone marrow edema in the tunnel can be the first clue to an underlying inflammatory arthropathy in patients. The retro-malleolar groove is the most common site of tendinopathy/tendon tear in peroneus brevis. The most common type is an interstitial split tear with distal reconstitution at the level of peroneal tubercle (Taljanovi et al. 2015). Cuboid tunnel is the most common site of tear/rupture of peroneus longus because of high sheer strain as a result of the sharp 90° tendon turn (Hallinan et al. 2019). Os peroneum is a sesamoid bone found within the peroneus longus at the level of calcaneocuboid joint (Fig. 15). Painful os peroneum syndrome is a condition characterized by lateral foot pain. There can be tendinosis, tendon degeneration, and attrition of even full rupture of peroneus longus tendon along with bone marrow edema within the os.

7 Accessory Muscles and Tendons

There are several accessory muscles and tendons, which are encountered as incidental findings while reporting MRI of foot and ankle. A knowledge of these normal variants is important because though mostly asymptomatic, some-

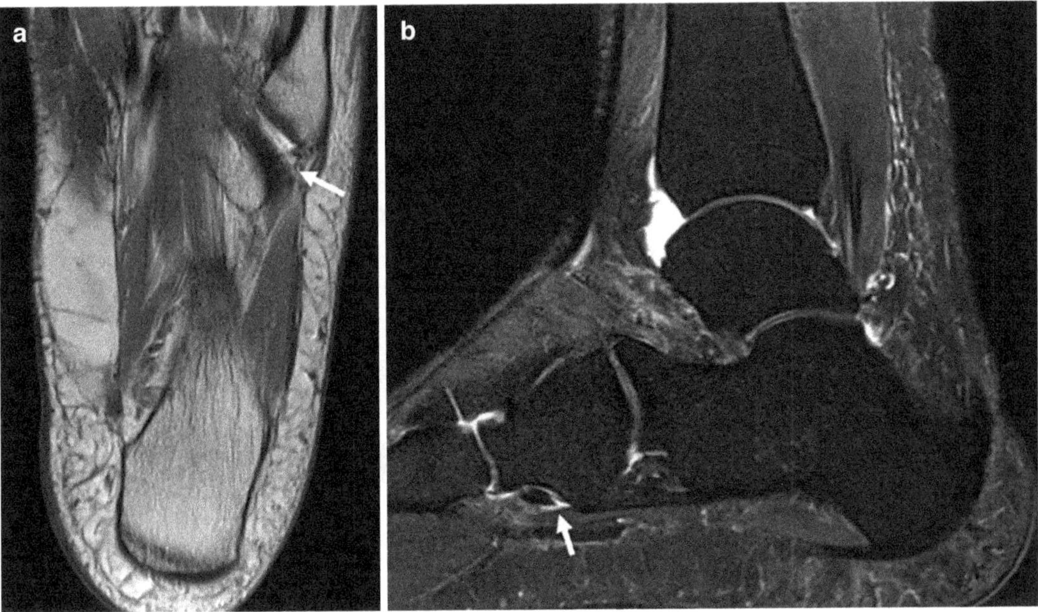

Fig. 14 (**a**) Axial T1 and (**b**) sagittal PD FS image demonstrates the sharp 90° turn of the peroneus longus tendon, at the level of cuboid tunnel, which is the most common site of tendon tear/rupture

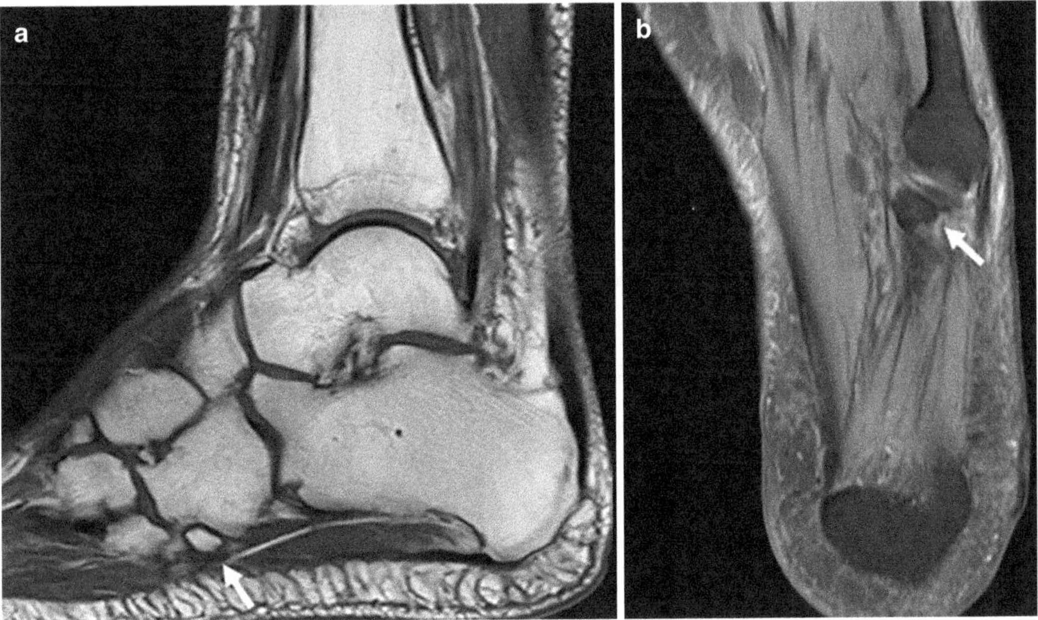

Fig. 15 (**a**) Sagittal T1 and (**b**) axial PD FS image demonstrates os peroneum, which is a sesamoid bone within the peroneus longus tendon

times they can be associated with symptoms of impingement such as in the tarsal tunnel or can present as a lump or mass lesion.

Peroneus tertius is an accessory muscle in the anterior compartment frequently originating from the distal fibula or the extensor digitorum tendon (Sookur et al. 2008). It passes deep to the extensor retinaculum and inserts on the base and dorsal surface of the fifth metatarsal (Fig. 16).

Peroneus quartus is seen in the lateral compartment and mimics the longitudinal split of peroneal tendons (Fig. 17). It arises from the dorsal surface of fibula, peroneus brevis, or longus tendon and most commonly inserts at the retro-trochlear eminence at the lateral aspect of calcaneum posterior to the peroneal tubercle (Cheung et al. 1997). There are several variations of the insertion. It can be associated with crowding of the peroneal tendons beneath the superior peroneal retinaculum predisposing them to tendinopathy, tendon tears, and tenosynovitis (Wang et al. 2005).

There are four accessory muscles in the posteromedial ankle. The most common is flexor digitorum accessorius longus, which is situated deep to the deep aponeurosis within the tarsal

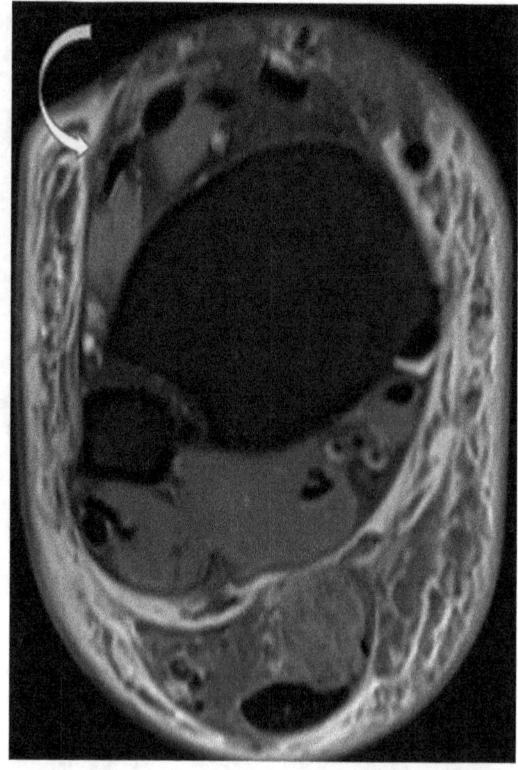

Fig. 16 Axial PD FS image demonstrates the peroneus tertius muscle in the anterior compartment deep to the extensor retinaculum

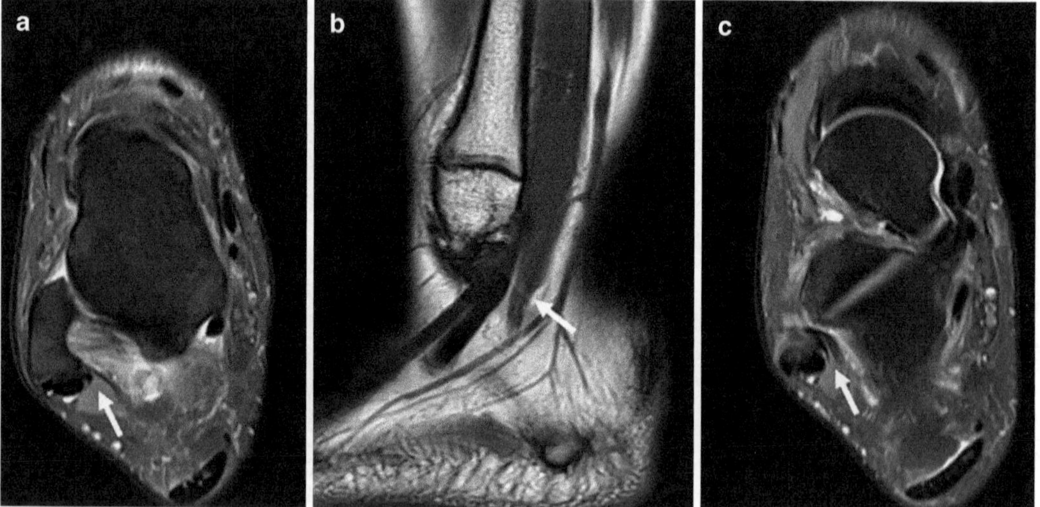

Fig. 17 (**a**) Axial PD FS and (**b**) sagittal T1 image depicting the peroneus quartus muscle, which inserts most commonly at the retro-trochlear eminence. (**c**) Another axial PD FS image clearly demonstrating the three tendons in the lateral compartment with peroneus quartus beneath the peroneal tendons and superficial to the calcaneofibular ligament

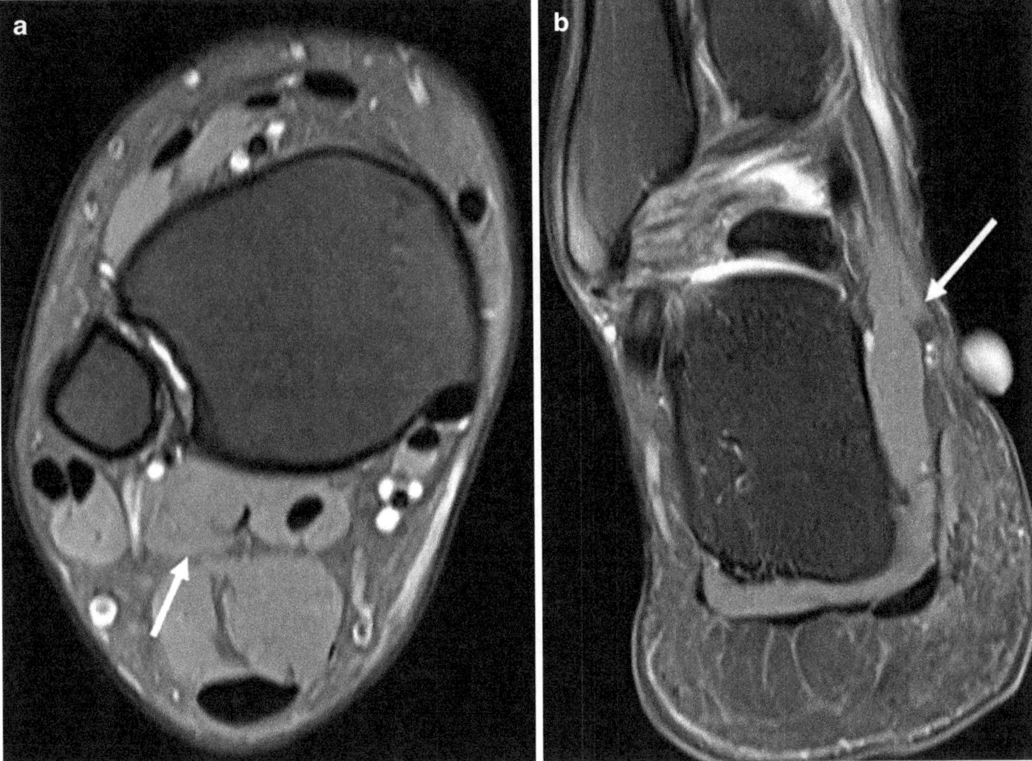

Fig. 18 (**a**) Axial PS FS demonstrates the flexor digitorum accessories longus muscle in the posteromedial ankle within the tarsal tunnel. It inserts on the FDL tendon or quadratus plantae muscle as depicted in the (**b**) coronal PD FS image

tunnel and travels along with the posterior tibial neurovascular bundle, inserting onto the quadratus plantae muscle or FDL tendon (Fig. 18). The presence of FDAL can be associated with tarsal tunnel syndrome.

Accessory soleus is located superficial to the deep aponeurosis outside the tarsal tunnel and inserts at the superior or medial aspect of the calcaneum. When symptomatic, it may present as a painful or painless lump (Fig. 19).

The peroneocalcaneus internus and the tibiocalcaneus internus are much less commonly encountered. The peroneocalcaneus arises from the fibula, traverses lateral to the FHL muscle, and inserts on the base of sustentaculum.

The tibiocalcaneus originates from the tibia, runs posterior to the FHL tendon, and inserts on the medial calcaneus as opposed to the FDAL, which inserts on the FDL tendon or the quadratus plantae (Gorbachova 2020).

8 Foot

The foot can be divided anatomically into the hindfoot, midfoot, and forefoot. Three longitudinal columns—medial, middle, and lateral—have also been described. The medial column comprises the calcaneum, talus, navicular, medial, and intermediate cuneiforms, and the first and second rays. The tibialis posterior tendon and the spring ligament act as supporting slings for the medial longitudinal arch. Loss of the medial longitudinal arch can occur with tibialis posterior tendinopathy.

8.1 Hindfoot

The hindfoot includes the talus and calcaneum and intervening subtalar joints and surrounding soft tissues. The posterior subtalar joint commu-

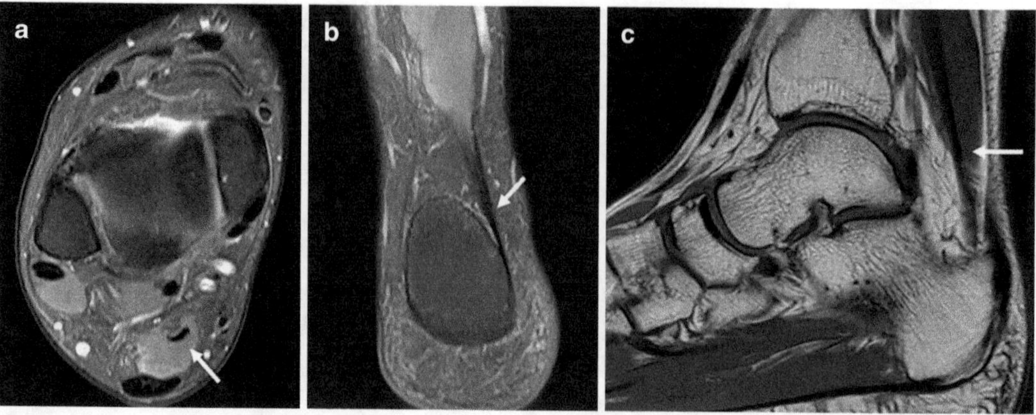

Fig. 19 (**a**) Axial PD FS image demonstrating the accessory soleus muscle located superficial to the deep aponeurosis and tarsal tunnel. (**b**) Coronal PD FS image shows the insertion of the accessory muscle into the medial aspect of the calcaneum. (**c**) Sagittal T1 image once again depicts the myotendinous junction of the accessory soleus muscle located deep to the Achilles tendon

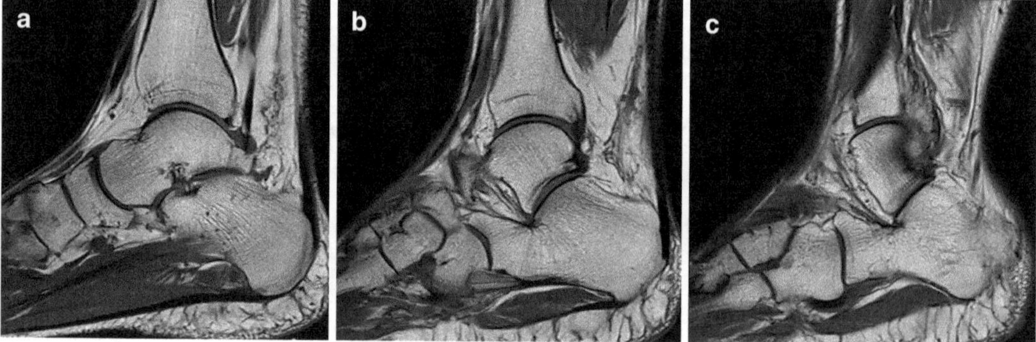

Fig. 20 Sagittal T1 demonstrating the normal fat and neurovascular contents of the sinus tarsi along with the ligaments. The medial bundle has only one band as seen on image (**a**), whereas laterally there are anterior and posterior bands (**b**). Further laterally in the parasagittal plane, (**c**) lateral extensor retinaculum can be seen

nicates with the tibiotalar joint in 10% of individuals. The anterior subtalar joint may communicate with the talonavicular or talocalcaneonavicular joint. The sinus tarsi (or tarsal sinus) is an anatomical space immediately anterior to the posterior subtalar joint between the inferior aspect of the talus (roof) and the superior aspect of the calcaneum (floor). The bony margins of the sinus are irregular. The space is cone shaped with a narrow end medially posterior to the sustentaculum tali and inferior to the medial malleolus. Laterally, the sinus widens to below the lateral malleolus. It contains fat, ligamentous structures, a neurovascular bundle (branch of the posterior tibial artery), and an outpouching synovial bursa from the posterior subtalar joint. Nerve endings in the sinus provide proprioception for the hindfoot, with stability partly maintained by the interosseous ligament. The main ligament in the sinus is the talocalcaneal (or interosseous) ligament, which is composed of a single medial bundle with anterior and posterior bands laterally. The anterior band of the ligament forms the cervical ligament. The lateral extensor retinaculum forms the most lateral portion of the sinus tarsi ligaments (Fig. 20).

The MR anatomy of the sinus tarsi can be well demonstrated on sagittal and coronal imaging, the low-signal ligaments contrasting against the surrounding higher signal from fat. Inflammation and trauma can involve the sinus with loss of the ligaments and normal fat, producing a sinus tarsi syndrome with pain associated with hindfoot instability. It should be noted that MR imaging does not consistently identify the ligaments of the sinus tarsi even if intact, so the absence of the ligaments alone does not justify the diagnosis. It is important to look for any lateral ankle ligament damage and chronic tibialis posterior tendon tears, which are the associated features of a sinus tarsi syndrome.

The plantar fascia, otherwise termed plantar aponeurosis, is a thick, multilayered condensation of fibrous tissue comprised of three components (Theodorou et al. 2000). The larger central layer arises from the inferior part of the calcaneal tuberosity along the plantar surface of the flexor digitorum brevis and attaches distally to the plantar surface of the proximal phalanges and the skin. The central layer is cord-like, measuring 4 mm in normal thickness at the level of its attachment to the calcaneum. The medial and lateral portions of the aponeurosis are membrane sheets with the former being the fascia of abductor hallucis, and the latter arising from the lateral margin of the medial calcaneal tubercle close to the origin of the abductor digiti minimi (Kier 1994). The plantar fascia is easily visualized on sagittal and coronal MR imaging, being of low signal on all sequences (Fig. 21).

8.2 Midfoot

The midfoot compartment comprises the navicular, cuboid, and three cuneiform bones and is bounded proximally by the talonavicular and calcaneocuboid joints (Chopart joint) and distally by the tarsometatarsal joints (Lisfranc joint). The navicular lies on the medial aspect of the foot. It articulates with the talus proximally and with the three cuneiforms distally, occasionally with the cuboid. The cuboid is lateral to the navicular, articulating with the calcaneum proximally and with the fourth and fifth metatarsals distally. The medial side of the cuboid has a facet, which articulates with the lateral cuneiform. There is a groove on the plantar surface of the cuboid for the peroneus longus tendon. The medial cuneiform is the largest of the cuneiforms, articulating with the intermediate cuneiform laterally and the first and second metatarsals distally. The intermediate cuneiform lies between the medial and lateral cuneiforms, articulating with both, and the second metatarsal distally. The lateral cuneiform lies between the intermediate cuneiform and cuboid articulating with both, and the second to the fourth metatarsals distally.

The spring (calcaneonavicular) ligament extends from the calcaneum to the tuberosity of the navicular on the plantar aspect. It is a broad,

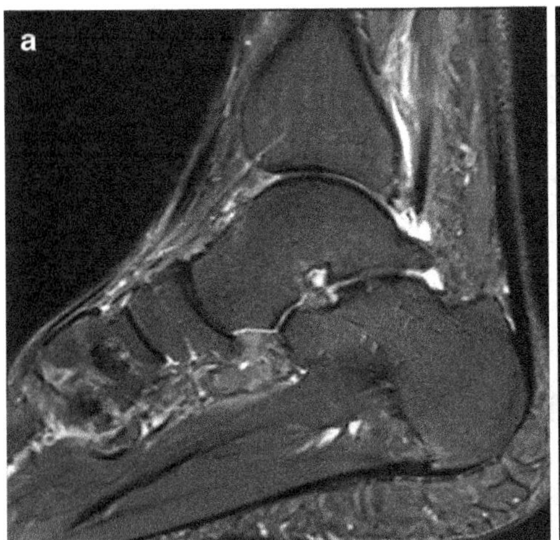

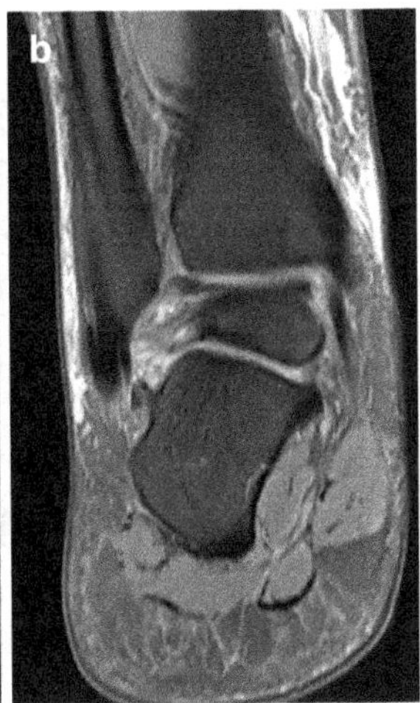

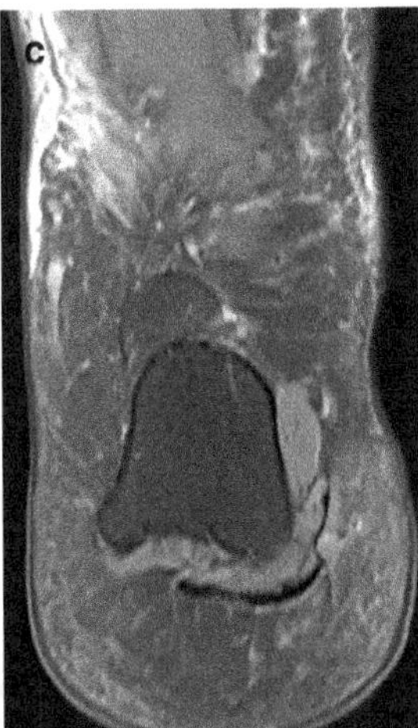

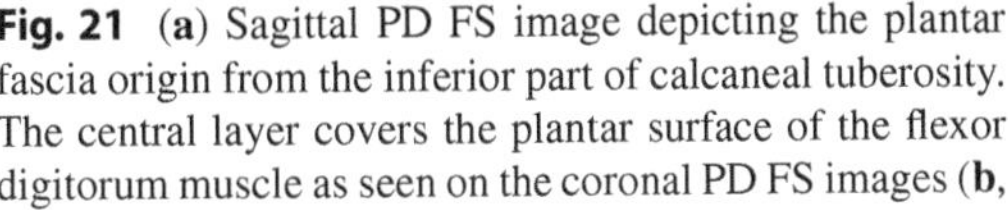
Fig. 21 (**a**) Sagittal PD FS image depicting the plantar fascia origin from the inferior part of calcaneal tuberosity. The central layer covers the plantar surface of the flexor digitorum muscle as seen on the coronal PD FS images (**b**, **c**). The medial and lateral portions merge with the fascia of abductor hallucis and abductor digiti minimi, respectively

thick band connecting the anterior margin of the sustentaculum tali to the plantar surface of the navicular. Both the spring ligament and the tibialis posterior muscle and tendon maintain the medial longitudinal arch. Repair of the spring ligament is a major component of operative intervention in acquired flat foot deformity, but the value of imaging has yet to be established. There are short and long plantar ligaments, which act to maintain the lateral longitudinal arch. The long plantar ligament is the longest ligament of the tarsus, extending from the plantar surface of the calcaneum and its anterior tubercle to the ridge and tuberosity of the cuboid, with superficial fibers extending to insert into the bases of the second to fourth/fifth metatarsals. The short plantar ligament is deeper, being closer to the bone than the long plantar ligament from which it is separated by fatty tissue. It is a strong, short, wide band (Fig. 22).

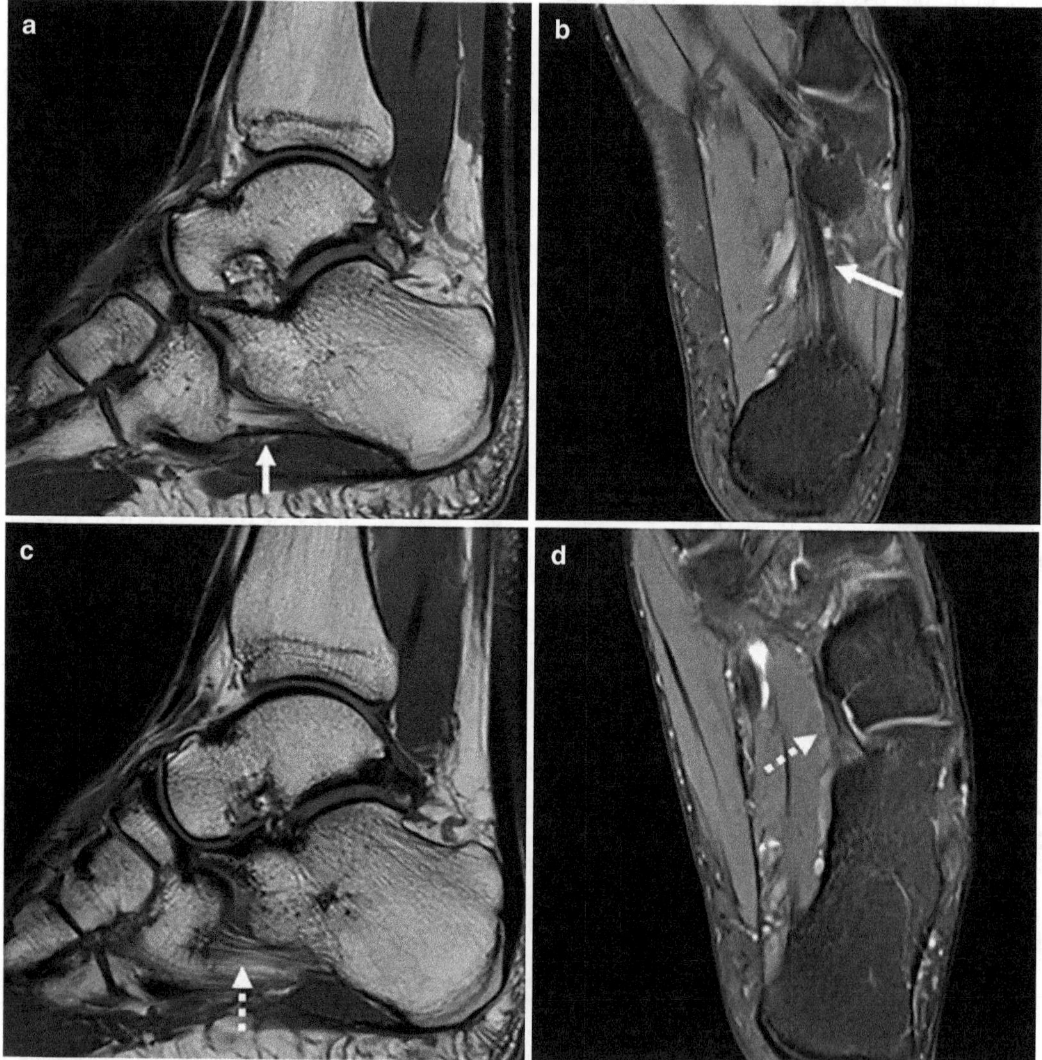

Fig. 22 (**a**) Sagittal T1 and (**b**) axial PD FS demonstrate the long plantar ligament (solid arrow), which originates from the anterior tubercle and plantar surface of calcaneum and inserts onto the cuboid crest and base of 2–4 metatarsals. (**c**) Sagittal T1 and (**d**) PD FS image demonstrates the short plantar ligament (dashed arrow) which is deeper, shorter, and separated from the long plantar ligament by fatty tissue

Although suspected midfoot pathology is an uncommon indication for MR imaging, this area is, however, usually included in MR imaging of the ankle and hindfoot. Unsuspected bone bruising/contusion/fracture and tarsal coalition (calcaneonavicular bar) can be identified.

8.3 Forefoot

This compartment includes the metatarsals and phalanges. The digital nerves arise from the medial and lateral plantar nerves, being derivatives of the posterior tibial nerve. The digital nerves lie on the plantar surface of the deep transverse intermetatarsal ligaments and can become entrapped between the ligament and the plantar surface. The third digital nerve (in the third web space between the heads of the third and fourth metatarsals) is the largest of the digital nerves, being derived from branches of the medial and lateral plantar nerves, and is also, therefore, relatively fixed in position. The third digital nerve is susceptible to entrapment and compression and is the most common one to be involved by a Morton's neuroma.

9 MRI Arthrography Ankle

MRI arthrography can improve the diagnostic accuracy in certain ankle injuries and is useful for a range of clinically suspected intra-articular pathologies. MRI arthrography of the ankle is a two-step procedure involving the intra-articular injection of dilute gadolinium or saline solution followed by MR imaging (Cerezal et al. 2008).

The patient is typically placed in lateral decubitus position with the ankle in lateral position (Cerezal et al. 2005). The dorsalis pedis is palpated and marked to avoid inadvertent puncture. The skin puncture can be at two sites—either immediately medial to the tibialis anterior tendon or medial to the extensor hallucis tendon.

Under fluoroscopic guidance, a 22–23-gauge needle is advanced with a slight cranial tilt to avoid the overhanging margin of distal tibia (Fig. 23). Before the injection of contrast medium, the ankle joint is aspirated to avoid dilution of the contrast. The intra-articular position is confirmed using 1–2 mL of iodinated contrast. If the needle is intra-articular, the contrast flows away from the needle tip and spreads into the capsular recesses. Once the intra-articular position is confirmed, dilute gadolinium is injected till the joint cavity is properly distended (approx. 6–10 mL). The injection is stopped if the patient experiences extreme discomfort or there is severe resistance to the contrast injection to avoid capsular disruption. The contrast solution enters the tendon sheath of the FHL in 25% of cases because of the communication of the tendon sheath with the joint cavity. Patient is then transferred to the MRI suite for further imaging. MRI is ideally performed within 20–30 min of contrast injection to minimize absorption of contrast and have the desired capsular distension. Images are acquired in axial, sagittal, and coronal planes using extremity coil and small field of view, increasing the SNR providing detailed evaluation of the intra-articular structures. T1-weighted spin echo with and without fat suppression should be included along with 3D gradient-echo images and STIR/T2-weighted sequence in one plane. The 3D GRE sequence allows reconstruction in any plane and is useful for the detection of cartilage lesions and loose bodies.

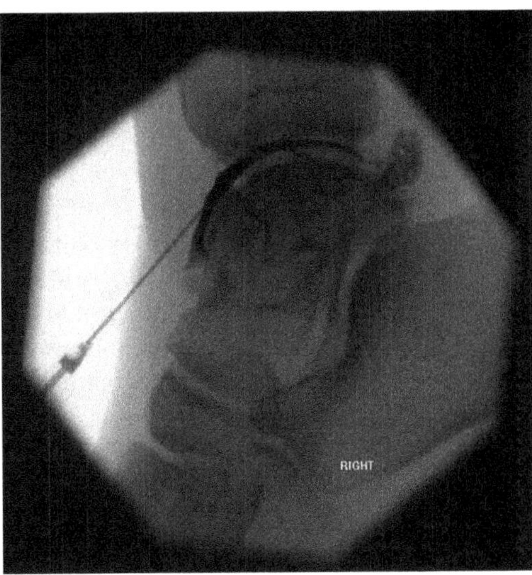

Fig. 23 Fluoroscopic spot image depicting the intra-articular position of needle using iodinated contrast

9.1 Indirect MRI Arthrography

It is a noninvasive alternative to direct MRI arthrography. Imaging after iv administration of standard dose of gadolinium followed by 5–10 min of exercise can produce arthrogram-like images of the ankle joint (Bergin and Schweitzer 2003). The imaging delay is important as it takes time for the contrast agent to diffuse from the blood pool into the joint. However, the degree of enhancement depends on a lot of factors like joint volume, blood concentration of contrast, blood flow, synovial area, inflammation, and permeability. As these variables are difficult to control, the quality of indirect MR arthrogram is often variable and heterogeneous.

9.2 Indications

The most common indication for MRI arthrogram is the evaluation of the osteochondral and chondral lesions of the talus. These injuries are common in ankle and predispose to early development of secondary osteoarthritis. Talus is the third most common site for osteochondral lesions after knee and elbow (Cerezal et al. 2008). The medial aspect of the talar dome is affected in 55%, whereas the lateral aspect of the talar dome is involved in 45% of cases (Cerezal et al. 2008). The lateral lesions tend to involve the anterolateral portion of the dome, whereas the medial lesions are situated over the posteromedial portion.

Berndt and Harty classification scheme is the most widely accepted staging for osteochondral lesions of talus (Berndt and Harty 2004). Stage I represents subchondral impaction fracture. Stage II involves partial detachment of the osteochondral fragment. In stage III, the osteochondral fragment is completely detached but not displaced from the donor site. Stage IV comprises displaced and detached osteochondral fragments.

MRI arthrography is more accurate than conventional MRI for the assessment of chondral damage, determining the stability of the osteochondral lesion and detection of intra-articular loose bodies. It helps in differentiating between stage II and stage III lesions by depicting contrast around the lesion. Because of the joint distension secondary to instillation of the contrast, the fluid is forced underneath the osteochondral defects at the interface with the donor sites. It helps in assessment of the stability of the lesion. On standard non-arthrographic MRI, presence of T2 hyperintensity at the interface between the lesion and the donor site is considered suggestive of instability. However, the T2 hyperintensity can be representative of fibrovascular granulation tissue or fluid. A moderately hyperintense T2 interface is suggestive of fibrovascular granulation tissue, which means the lesion is unstable but can heal with non-weight-bearing (Cerezal et al. 2005). But the presence of contrast undercutting the interface on MRI arthrogram is suggestive of instability, and these lesions need surgery (Fig. 24). MRI arthrography is also helpful in postoperative imaging of osteochondral lesions. It can help in the detection of graft detachment and allows for the differentiation between delamination at the base of the graft and the normal high-signal fibrovascular granulation tissue in the immediate postoperative period.

Intra-articular loose bodies can occur as sequelae of osteochondral defects or other pathologic processes. Brossmann et al. (1996) found MR arthrography to be the most sensitive technique in detecting intra-articular loose bodies when compared with conventional MRI, CT, and CT arthrography (Brossmann et al. 1996). Loose bodies as small as 1 or 2 mm can be detected with MR arthrography (Fig. 25). It is important to distinguish air bubbles introduced during contrast administration from true loose bodies. Loose bodies will have signal characteristics of cartilage or bone. Air bubbles will produce magnetic susceptibility artifact, which will be compounded on gradient-echo images. Air bubbles will typically accumulate in nondependent locations within the ankle joint.

MRI arthrography can also be used in the detection of the ligament tears. Specific patterns of contrast extravasation can be used as secondary signs of lateral ligament tears. These are extravasation of contrast anterior and lateral to the anterior talofibular ligament in ATFL tear, extravasation into the peroneal tendon sheath in CFL tear, and extravasation into the soft tissues posterior to the posterior talofibular ligament in PTFL tear (Fig. 26). Injuries of the ATFL occur

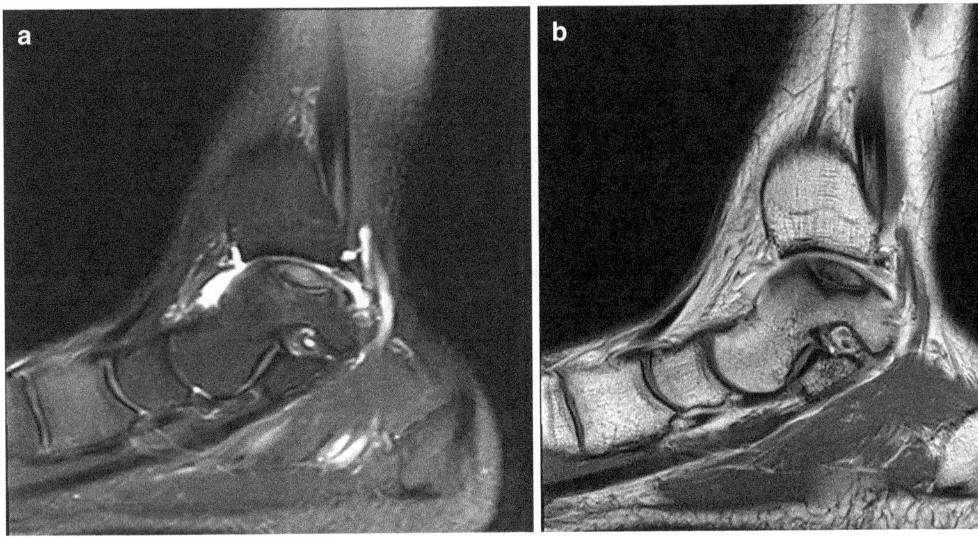

Fig. 24 (**a**) Sagittal T2 FS and (**b**) T1-weighted MRI arthrogram depicts a large osteochondral lesion in the medial talar dome, with T2 hyperintensity at the interface of the defect and the parent bone but no undercutting or extension of intra-articular contrast

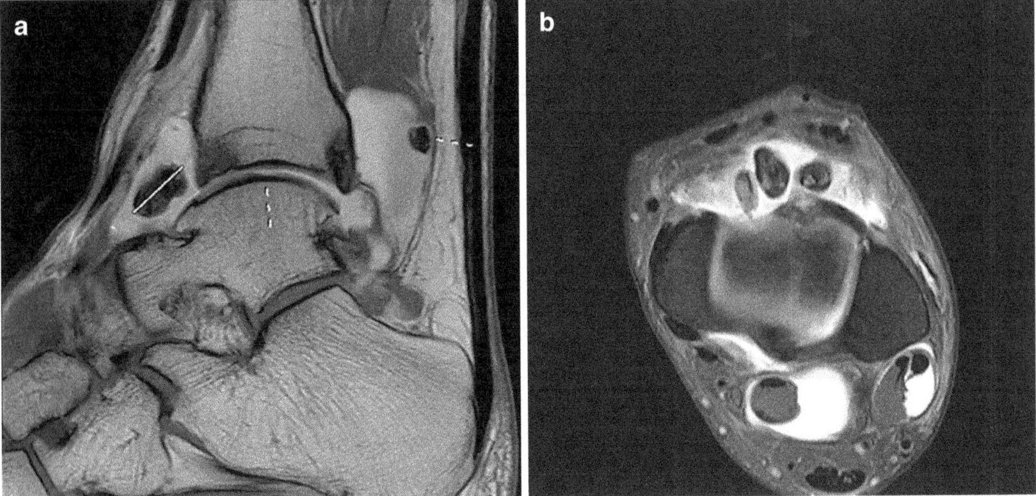

Fig. 25 (**a**) T1 and (**b**) T1 FS MR arthrogram images depicting multiple large intra-articular loose bodies

most frequently, either alone or along with CFL injury, and the PTFL is the least commonly injured ligament (Fig. 27).

Isolated tears of the deltoid ligaments are extremely rare. Tears of thc distal tibiofibular syndesmosis are more common. Syndesmotic injuries are often associated with minimal swelling and may, therefore, be overlooked or underestimated. Syndesmotic sprains have been linked to prolonged disability (Gerber et al. 1998). The components of the syndesmotic ligamentous complex are best seen in the transverse plane cephalad to the ATFL. Tears are identified as discontinuity of these ligaments. Disruption of the interosseous ligament can be diagnosed by contrast extending cephalad into the interosseous space beyond the normal 1 cm synovial recess (Lee et al. 1998).

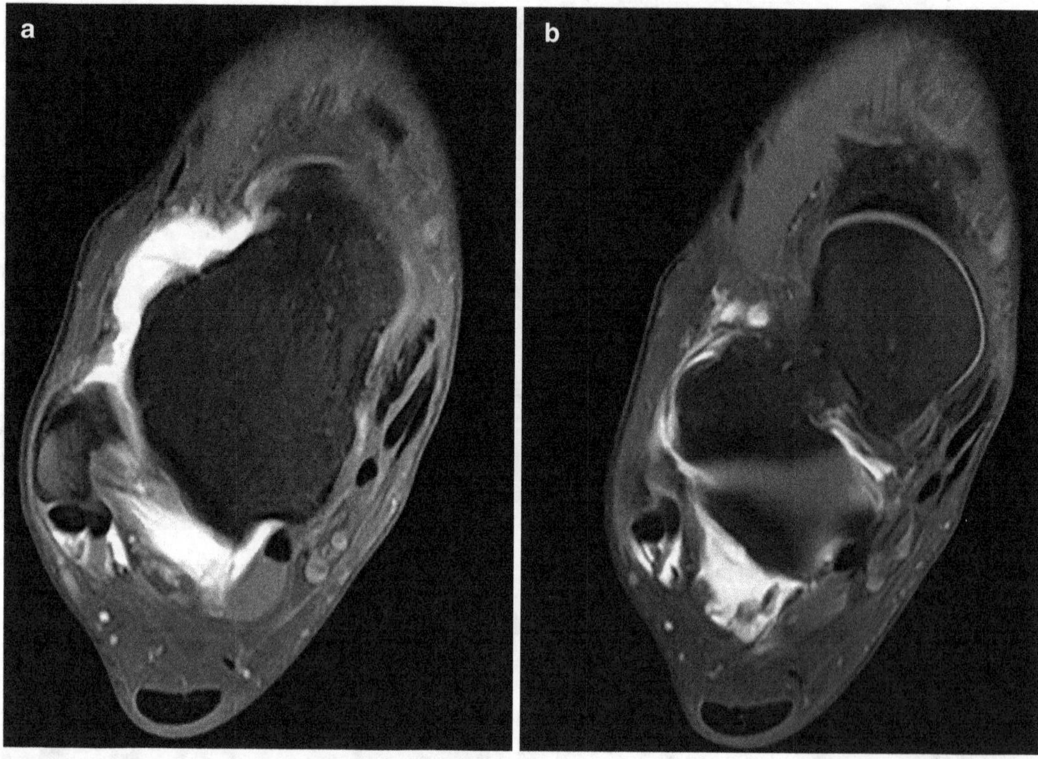

Fig. 26 (**a**) Axial T1 image demonstrates the communication of the intra-articular contrast with the peroneal tendon sheath suspicious for a CFL tear. The ligament itself is imaged in (**b**), which appears thickened and flimsy

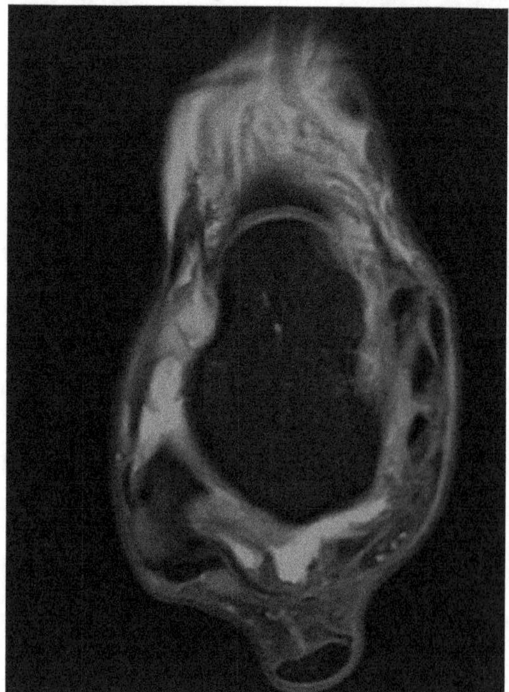

Fig. 27 Axial T1 FS image depicting full-thickness rupture of ATFL with extravasation of intra-articular contrast anterolaterally

Anterolateral impingement is a condition in which soft tissue becomes entrapped in the anterolateral gutter of the ankle. This material can be hypertrophied synovium, fibrotic scar, or part of the ATFL. A soft tissue signal mass is seen in the anterolateral gutter on MRI. Detection of this soft tissue mass is improved when joint fluid is present, as in MR arthrography (Rubin et al. 1997).

10 Conclusion

MR imaging has an unrivaled ability in the assessment and detection of soft tissue abnormalities and some bone lesions in the ankle and foot and is being used more and more often. It is opening new horizons in the diagnosis and treatment of various ankle and foot disorders. A clear understanding of the complex applied anatomy of the ankle and foot, together with a firm grasp of the normal appearances and variants as shown on MR, is vital to the correct interpretation of MR imaging and to an understanding of the various pathologies and syndromes to be expected.

References

Bandinelli F, Milla M, Genise S, Giovannini L, Bagnoli S, Candelieri A, Collaku L, Biagini S, Cerinic MM (2011) Ultrasound discloses entheseal involvement in inactive and low active inflammatory bowel disease without clinical signs and symptoms of spondyloarthropathy. Rheumatology (Oxford) 50(7):1275–1279. https://doi.org/10.1093/RHEUMATOLOGY/KEQ447

Bergin D, Schweitzer ME (2003) Indirect magnetic resonance arthrography. Skelet Radiol 32(10):551–558. https://doi.org/10.1007/S00256-003-0669-2

Berndt AL, Harty M (2004) Transchondral fractures (osteochondritis dissecans) of the talus. J Bone Joint Surg Am 86(6):1336. https://doi.org/10.2106/00004623-200406000-00032

Brossmann J, Preidler KW, Daenen B, Pedowitz RA, Andresen R, Clopton P, Trudell D, Pathria M, Resnick D (1996) Imaging of osseous and cartilaginous intraarticular bodies in the knee: comparison of MR imaging and MR arthrography with CT and CT arthrography in cadavers. Radiology 200(2):509–517. https://doi.org/10.1148/RADIOLOGY.200.2.8685349

Cerezal L, Abascal F, García-Valtuille R, Canga A (2005) Ankle MR arthrography: how, why, when. Radiol Clin N Am 43(4):693–707. https://doi.org/10.1016/J.RCL.2005.01.005

Cerezal L, Llopis E, Canga A, Rolón A (2008) MR arthrography of the ankle: indications and technique. Radiol Clin North Am 46(6):973–994. https://doi.org/10.1016/j.rcl.2008.09.002

Chang EY, Du J, Chung CB (2015) UTE imaging in the musculoskeletal system. J Magn Reson Imaging 41(4):870–883. https://doi.org/10.1002/JMRI.24713

Cheung YY, Rosenberg ZS, Ramsinghani R, Beltran J, Jahss MH (1997) Peroneus quartus muscle: MR imaging features. Radiology 202(3):745–750. https://doi.org/10.1148/RADIOLOGY.202.3.9051029

Gerber JP, Williams GN, Scoville CR, Arciero RA, Taylor DC (1998) Persistent disability associated with ankle sprains: a prospective examination of an athletic population. Foot Ankle Int 19(10):653–660. https://doi.org/10.1177/107110079801901002

Gorbachova T (2020) Magnetic resonance imaging of the ankle and foot. Polish J Radiol 85(1):532–549. https://doi.org/10.5114/pjr.2020.99472

Gyftopoulos S, Bencardino JT (2010) Normal variants and pitfalls in MR imaging of the ankle and foot. Magn Reson Imaging Clin N Am 18(4):691–705. https://doi.org/10.1016/J.MRIC.2010.07.007

Hallinan JTPD, Wang W, Pathria MN, Smitaman E, Huang BK (2019) The peroneus longus muscle and tendon: a review of its anatomy and pathology. Skeletal Radiol 48(9):1329–1344. https://doi.org/10.1007/S00256-019-3168-9

Hermans JJ, Ginai AZ, Wentink N, Hop WCJ, Beumer A (2011) The additional value of an oblique image plane for MRI of the anterior and posterior distal tibiofibular syndesmosis. Skelet Radiol 40(1):75–83. https://doi.org/10.1007/S00256-010-0938-9

Hopkinson WJ, St. Pierre P, Ryan JB, Wheeler JH (1990) Syndesmosis sprains of the ankle. Foot Ankle 10(6):325–330. https://doi.org/10.1177/107110079001000607

Hunt KJ, Phisitkul P, Pirolo J, Amendola A (2015) High ankle sprains and syndesmotic injuries in athletes. J Am Acad Orthop Surg 23(11):661–673. https://doi.org/10.5435/JAAOS-D-13-00135

Kier R (1994) Magnetic resonance imaging of plantar fasciitis and other causes of heel pain. Magn Reson Imaging Clin N Am 2(1):97–107. https://doi.org/10.1016/S1064-9689(21)00329-9

Kijowski R, Davis KW, Woods MA, Lindstrom MJ, de Smet AA, Gold GE, Busse RF (2009) Knee joint: comprehensive assessment with 3D isotropic resolution fast spin-echo MR imaging—diagnostic performance compared with that of conventional MR imaging at 3.0 T. Radiology 252(2):486–495. https://doi.org/10.1148/RADIOL.2523090028

Lee SH, Jacobson J, Trudell D, Resnick D (1998) Ligaments of the ankle: normal anatomy with MR arthrography. J Comput Assist Tomogr 22(5):807–813. https://doi.org/10.1097/00004728-199809000-00027

Mandell JC, Khurana B, Smith SE (2017) Stress fractures of the foot and ankle, Part 2: Site-specific etiology, imaging, and treatment, and differential diagnosis. Skelet Radiol 46(9):1165–1186. https://doi.org/10.1007/S00256-017-2632-7

Meehan TM, Martinez-Salazar EL, Torriani M (2017) Aftermath of ankle inversion injuries: spectrum of MR imaging findings. Magn Reson Imaging Clin N Am 25(1):45–61. https://doi.org/10.1016/J.MRIC.2016.08.012

Mengiardi B, Pfirrmann CWA, Vienne P, Hodler J, Zanetti M (2007) Medial collateral ligament complex of the ankle: MR appearance in asymptomatic subjects. Radiology 242(3):817–824. https://doi.org/10.1148/RADIOL.2423060055

Mengiardi B, Pinto C, Zanetti M (2016) Spring ligament complex and posterior tibial tendon: MR anatomy and findings in acquired adult flatfoot deformity. Semin Musculoskelet Radiol 20(1):104–115. https://doi.org/10.1055/S-0036-1580616/ID/JR00874-39

O'Loughlin PF, Heyworth BE, Kennedy JG (2009) Current concepts in the diagnosis and treatment of osteochondral lesions of the ankle. Am J Sports Med 38(2):392–404. https://doi.org/10.1177/0363546509336336

Palmer WE, Levine SM, Dupuy DE (1997) Knee and shoulder fractures: association of fracture detection and marrow edema on MR images with mechanism of injury. Radiology 204(2):395–401. https://doi.org/10.1148/RADIOLOGY.204.2.9240526

Park HJ, Lee SY, Park NH, Kim E, Chung EC, Kook SH, Lee JW (2015) Usefulness of the oblique coronal plane in ankle MRI of the calcaneofibular ligament.

Clin Radiol 70(4):416–423. https://doi.org/10.1016/J.CRAD.2014.12.008

Park HJ, Lee SY, Kim E, Kim MS, Chung EC, Choi SH, Yun JS (2016) Peroneal tendon pathology evaluation using the oblique sagittal plane in ankle MR imaging. Acta Radiol (Stockholm, Sweden: 1987) 57(5):620–626. https://doi.org/10.1177/0284185115597264

Perrich KD, Goodwin DW, Hecht PJ, Cheung Y (2009) Ankle ligaments on MRI: appearance of normal and injured ligaments. AJR Am J Roentgenol 193(3):687–695. https://doi.org/10.2214/AJR.08.2286

Pruessmann KP (2004) Parallel imaging at high field strength: synergies and joint potential. Top Magn Reson Imaging 15(4):237–244. https://doi.org/10.1097/01.RMR.0000139297.66742.4E

Radzi S, Dlaska CE, Cowin G, Robinson M, Pratap J, Schuetz MA, Mishra S, Schmutz B (2016) Can MRI accurately detect pilon articular malreduction? A quantitative comparison between CT and 3T MRI bone models. Quant Imaging Med Surg 6(6):634–647. https://doi.org/10.21037/QIMS.2016.07.01

Ramnath RR (2006) 3T MR imaging of the musculoskeletal system (Part I): Considerations, coils, and challenges. Magn Reson Imaging Clin N Am 14(1):27–40. https://doi.org/10.1016/J.MRIC.2006.01.001

Rivera M, Vaquero JJ, Santos A, Ruiz-Cabello J, del Pozo F (1998) MRI visualization of small structures using improved surface coils. Magn Reson Imaging 16(2):157–166. https://doi.org/10.1016/S0730-725X(97)00273-7

Robson MD, Benjamin M, Gishen P, Bydder GM (2004) Magnetic resonance imaging of the Achilles tendon using ultrashort TE (UTE) pulse sequences. Clin Radiol 59(8):727–735. https://doi.org/10.1016/j.crad.2003.11.021

Rosenberg ZS, Beltran J, Bencardino JT (2000) From the RSNA refresher courses. MR imaging of the ankle and foot. Radiographics 20 Spec No:S153–S179

Rubin DA, Tishkoff NW, Britton CA, Conti SF, Towers JD (1997) Anterolateral soft-tissue impingement in the ankle: diagnosis using MR imaging. AJR Am J Roentgenol 169(3):829–835. https://doi.org/10.2214/AJR.169.3.9275907

Simpson SL, Hertzog MS, Barja RH (1991) The plantaris tendon graft: an ultrasound study. J Hand Surg Am 16(4):708–711. https://doi.org/10.1016/0363-5023(91)90198-K

Siriwanarangsun P, Bae WC, Statum S, Chung CB (2017) Advanced MRI techniques for the ankle. Am J Roentgenol 209(3):511–524. https://doi.org/10.2214/AJR.17.18057

Sofka CM (2017) Technical considerations: best practices for MR imaging of the foot and ankle. Magn Reson Imaging Clin N Am 25(1):1–10. https://doi.org/10.1016/J.MRIC.2016.08.001

Sookur P, Naraghi A, Bleakney R, Chan O (2008) Accessory muscles: anatomy, symptoms, and radiologic. Radiographics 28(2):481–499

Taljanovi MS, Alcala JN, Gimber LH, Rieke JD, Chilvers MM, Daniel LL (2015) High-resolution US and MR imaging of peroneal tendon injuries. Radiographics 35(1):179–199. https://doi.org/10.1148/RG.351130062

Theodorou DF, Theodorou SJ, Kakitsubata Y, Lektrakul N, Gold GE, Roger B, Resnick D (2000) Plantar fasciitis and fascial rupture: MR imaging findings in 26 patients supplemented with anatomic data in cadavers. Radiographics 20 Spec No:S181–S197. https://doi.org/10.1148/RADIOGRAPHICS.20.SUPPL_1.G00OC01S181

Wang XT, Rosenberg ZS, Mechlin MB, Schweitzer ME (2005) Normal variants and diseases of the peroneal tendons and superior peroneal retinaculum: MR imaging features. Radiographics 25(3):587–602. https://doi.org/10.1148/RG.253045123

Ultrasound Imaging of the Ankle

D. Hoffman, R. Botchu, and S. Bianchi

Contents

1 Introduction

Ultrasound (US) is an excellent modality for the routine assessment of foot and ankle pathologies. In this chapter, a systematic approach to the sonographic evaluation of the ankle is presented.

Currently, there is high-quality evidence supporting the use of US as a first-line advanced imaging modality for assessing pathologies involving the tendons, soft tissues, and ligaments of the ankle (Sconfienza et al. 2018). Furthermore, a growing number of additional US applications have been noted in recent years such as the evaluation of ankle instability (Sconfienza et al. 2018).

The purpose of this chapter is to describe the technique of US examination and to present the normal US anatomy of the ankle.

D. Hoffman
Musculoskeletal Ultrasound Program, Essentia Health, Duluth, MN, USA

R. Botchu
Department of Musculoskeletal Radiology, Royal Orthopedic Hospital, Birmingham, UK

S. Bianchi (✉)
CIM SA, Cabinet d'imagerie médicale, Genève, Switzerland
e-mail: stefanobianchi@bluewin.ch

2 Standard US Examination

A detailed history from the clinician with the indication of the specific structures to be investigated and of the differential diagnosis must be obtained. Focusing on a localized area of the joint not only reduces the time of examination but allows an in-depth, accurate assessment of the structures being examined. US is inferior to MRI or CT scan in the evaluation of intra-articular structures of the ankle. Since the clinician may overlook this limitation, knowledge of the presumptive clinical diagnosis is important to avoid unnecessary examinations. On the other hand, compared with other modalities, US is efficient and economical in the assessment of superficial structures and can be considered the modality of choice in patients with periarticular lesions.

We routinely obtain the patient's history and ask for a recent complete radiographic evaluation

Med Radiol Diagn Imaging (2023)
https://doi.org/10.1007/174_2023_395,
Published Online: 22 April 2023

before starting the US examination. Taking the patient's history is helpful not only in focusing the examination but also in the interpretation of the US findings. The availability of standard radiographs can be essential for understanding US images related to disorders that can be obvious on radiographs. Moreover, radiographs can show coincident bone lesions that cannot be detected by US.

Due to the superficial location of most ankle structures, high-frequency transducers are well suited for the US assessment of the ankle region. Occasionally, in larger joints, lower frequencies may facilitate visualizing deeper structures such as the posterior joint space and the proximal portion of the flexor hallucis longus tendon. Although standard linear probes usually allow adequate evaluation of the ankle region, small footprint transducers (hockey stick) with high resolution are often helpful in negotiating the irregular bony contours of the peri-malleolar regions.

Doppler imaging is useful in the evaluation of vessels, assessment of the vascularity of periarticular masses, and depiction of synovial or tendon hyperemia. The use of extended field of view (EFV) provides a panoramic analysis of the region scanned. Utilization of this technique allows an optimal assessment of the Achilles tendon, which can be imaged from its origin from the triceps surae to its distal insertion onto the calcaneum. Moreover, EFV aids in the interpretation of the US images by the referring physician.

The US examination of the ankle is performed with the patient in the recumbent position. The ability to perform a dynamic examination is a particular advantage of US. Sonograms obtained with different degrees of flexion and extension of the ankle allow filling of the anterior and posterior synovial recesses and facilitate detection of small joint effusions. Ligaments and tendons can be examined at rest and during stress maneuvers or active muscle contraction. Tendons and ligaments are evaluated in positions of slight tension to avoid anisotropy that can occur when in the relaxed state. However, Doppler assessment of these structures should be in the relaxed state to avoid a false-negative result. In the evaluation of intra-articular loose bodies, the displacement of fragments induced by movements of the joint is an important diagnostic criterion (Bianchi and Martinoli 1999). In the assessment of nerve tumors or entrapment neuropathies, US-guided pressure applied with the probe or with the examiner's finger can elicit the patient's symptoms and confirm the neurogenic nature of the lesion (US-guided Tinel's test).

If the normal US anatomy of the ankle is well known, contralateral examination is not routinely performed. However, comparison imaging with the contralateral side can be helpful in selected cases such as patients with congenital anomalies or when potential pathologic findings are subtle.

Standard US examination of the ankle starts with the evaluation of the anterior aspect of the joint, followed by the medial, lateral, and posterior aspects.

2.1 Anterior Aspect

With the patient supine, the anterior aspect of the ankle is evaluated by axial, longitudinal, and oblique sonograms. In this region, US can image the anterior tendons and extensor retinaculum, the anterior tibial vessels and the deep peroneal nerve, the bony cortices of the distal end of the tibia, the anterior portion of the talus and its hyaline cartilage, as well as the anterior capsule and synovial recess (Figs. 1 and 2).

The anterior tendons include, from medial to lateral, tibialis anterior (TA), extensor hallucis longus (EHL), and extensor digitorum longus (EDL). Axial sonograms are initially performed along the full length of the tendon to assess for pathologies of both the tendon and overlying retinaculum. Each tendon should be imaged from myotendinous junction to their insertions in the foot region. The EHL tendon will typically have the most caudal myotendinous junction. Dynamic sonograms obtained during passive movements of the toes can help the inexperienced examiner

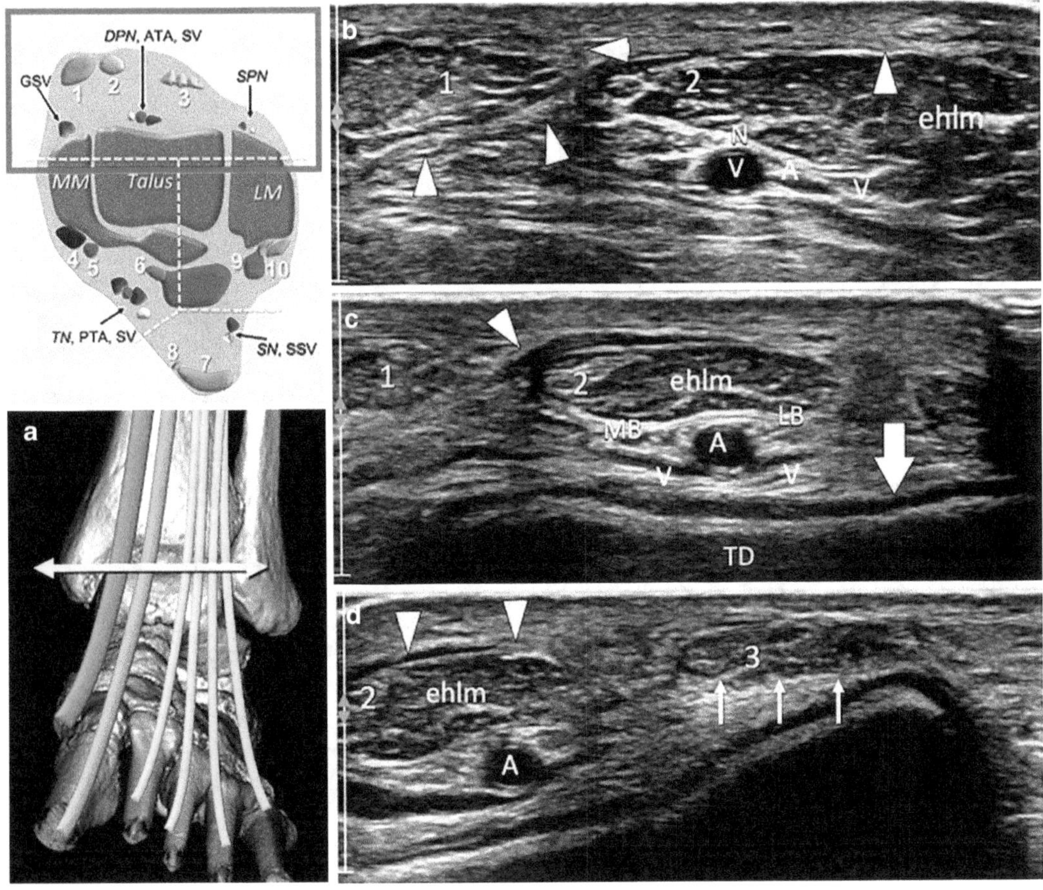

Fig. 1 (**a–d**) Anterior aspect. (**a**) Probe positioning for transverse examination. (**b–d**) Corresponding sonograms obtained from cranial to caudal. (**b**) Cranial sonogram. 1, Tibialis anterior tendon; EHLM, extensor hallucis longus muscle; 2, extensor hallucis longus tendon; V, anterior tibial veins; A, anterior tibial artery; N, deep peroneal nerve; arrowheads, retinaculum. (**c**) Distal sonogram (medial aspect). Arrow, cartilage of the talar dome (TD); MB, medial branch of the deep peroneal nerve; LB, lateral branch of the deep peroneal nerve. (**d**) Distal sonogram (lateral aspect). 3, Extensor digitorum longus tendons (arrows)

distinguish the different tendons. Longitudinal sonograms are then obtained over each tendon to complete the evaluation. High-frequency transducers have increased the ability to assess the internal tendon structure. Longitudinal sonograms show an internal network of many fine, tightly packed parallel echoes which resemble a fibrillar pattern. In the transverse plane, tendons appear as tightly packed echogenic dots contained within a thin bright tendon sheath (Lee and Healy 2005). Tendon evaluation requires careful attention to probe position since they are very susceptible to artifactual hypoechogenicity, or anisotropy. For each tendon, the transducer must be oriented perpendicular to its long axis in transverse scans and parallel to it in longitudinal sonograms. Even a slight obliquity of the angle of incidence of the US beam can result in an artifactual increase in hypoechogenicity and mimic tendon pathology. The anterior ankle tendons are surrounded by a synovial sheath and are held against the bone surfaces by the extensor retinaculum. The synovial sheath is composed of two thin membranes separated by a film of synovial fluid and facilitates smooth tendon gliding. Under normal conditions, the synovial membrane

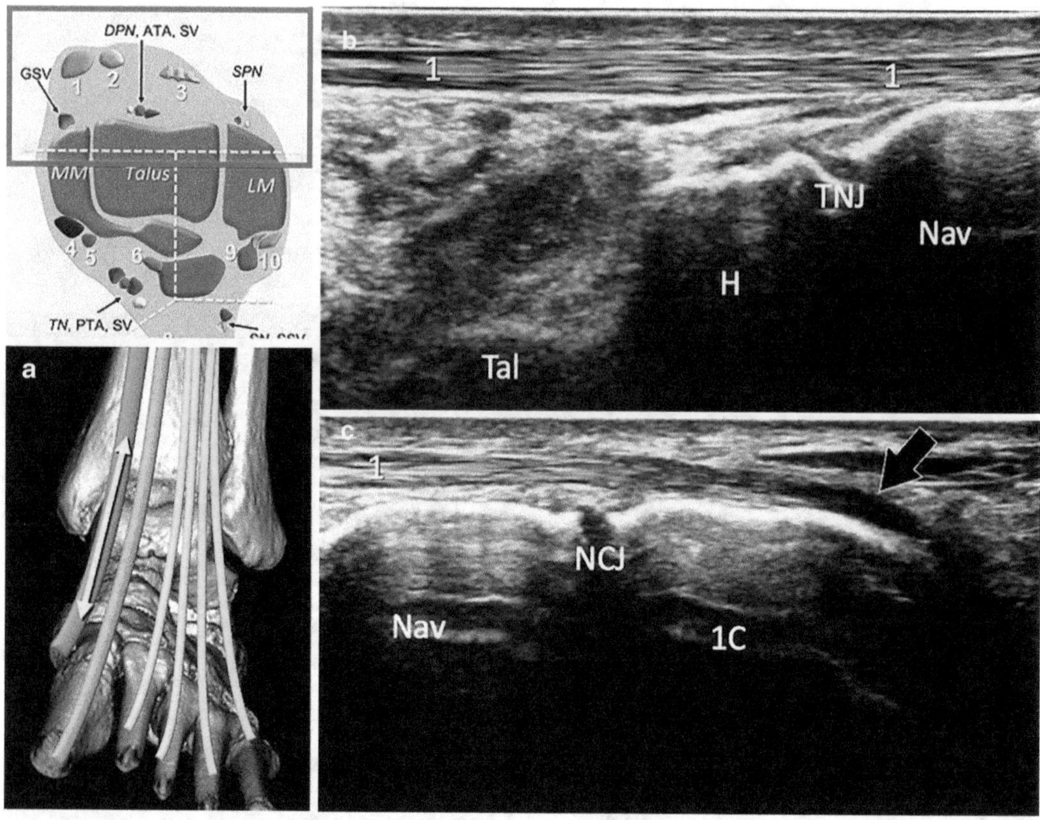

Fig. 2 (**a–c**) Anterior aspect. (**a**) Probe positioning for longitudinal examination of the tibialis anterior tendon. (**b**, **c**) Corresponding proximal and distal sonogram. Tal, talus; H, head of the talus; Nav, navicular bone; 1C, first cuneiform; 1, tibialis anterior tendon. Note anisotropy (arrow) of the distal part of the tendon due to its oblique path. TNJ, talonavicular joint; NCJ, naviculo-cuneiform joint

cannot be detected by US but is often visualized when fluid is present in the tendon sheath. The extensor retinaculum consists of thin fibrous bands that overlie the extensor tendons and provide stability to the tendons during tensile forces created during muscle contraction. The extensor retinaculum is best evaluated in the axial plane and appears as thin hyperechoic bands spanning over the tendons from the cortex of the fibula to the tibia. The extensor retinaculum may split medially to provide a separate tunnel for the anterior tibialis tendon. The extensor retinaculum is generally divided into a superior and inferior component with the inferior fibers having heterogeneity in its morphology (Demondion et al. 2010; Bianchi and Becciolini 2019). Dynamic longitudinal US, which shows smooth gliding of the tendons in normal subjects, is useful in the evaluation of peritendinitis or post-traumatic adhesions. In these conditions, passive movements of the ankle or toes induce displacements of the peritendinous tissue.

The anterior tibial vessels lie in a deep position, between the TA and EHL. The pulsatility of the artery allows its easy detection without the utilization of color Doppler. Arterial wall thickening as well as calcifications are easily assessed by US. The anterior veins are located adjacent to the artery. During their evaluation, attention must be paid to avoid excessive pressure with the probe, which can induce collapse of the veins.

Nerves present a particular appearance on US (Martinoli et al. 2000). Longitudinal sonograms demonstrate a fascicular appearance due to multiple, hypoechoic, parallel but discontinuous linear areas separated by hyperechoic bands. On transverse scans, the hypoechoic areas become rounded, embedded in a hyperechoic background, and have a honeycombed appearance. Histologic correlation demonstrated that the hypoechoic structures correspond to the fascicles and the hyperechoic background to the interfascicular epineurium. Due to its small size, only high-frequency probes can image the deep peroneal nerve. Since the nerve has a close relation with the anterior tibial artery and veins, this acts as a useful landmark in its detection. The superficial peroneal nerve is also readily assessed with US. Careful US scanning of the superficial fascia of the lateral compartment, in a cranial to caudal fashion, allows visualization of the superficial peroneal nerve traversing through the fascia and into the subcutaneous tissue where it splits into terminal sensory branches.

Ultrasound assessment of the talocrural joint is uncomplete due to the limited acoustic window of the bony anatomy. Anterior sagittal sonograms are obtained with the ankle in plantar flexion, which partially uncovers the talar dome and allows visualization of the anterior and midportion of the articular surface of the talus (Kok et al. 2014). US shows, from cranial to caudad, the distal epiphysis of the tibia, anterior portion of dome, neck and head of the talus, and dorsal surfaces of the tarsal bones. The anterior joint capsule can barely be distinguished from the periarticular soft tissue. Under normal conditions, the anterior ankle synovial recess appears as a thin triangular anechoic structure located just anterior to the talocrural joint and posterior to the anterior fat pad (Jacobson et al. 1998). No echogenic material is depicted inside the recess. Since it can be difficult clinically to differentiate fluid from periarticular soft tissue, US has important diagnostic value (Kane et al. 2004). In a study comparing the ability of different techniques in revealing ankle effusions in cadaveric specimens, US was able to detect 2 mL of fluid in the anterior recess. However, care must be exercised in evaluating small amounts of fluid since US can also depict joint, bursal, and tendon sheath effusions in asymptomatic volunteers, thus implying that a detectable effusion does not necessarily indicate underlying abnormalities (Nazarian et al. 1995). Dynamic ankle dorsiflexion can often allow a small effusion to become more conspicuous within the anterior recess. The US diagnosis of a pathological effusion must then be considered only if a large amount of fluid is demonstrated. In doubtful cases, correlation with clinical data and comparison with the contralateral side are helpful. When analysis of the synovial fluid is required for diagnostic purposes, US improves the likelihood of a successful aspiration. Furthermore, US ensures accurate localization for injection (Reach et al. 2009).

2.2 Lateral Aspect

After examination of the anterior ankle, the patient is then asked to rotate the ankle internally to allow evaluation of lateral structures. Structures that are well assessed by US include the small saphenous vein, the sural nerve (Ricci et al. 2010), the superior and inferior peroneal retinaculum, the peroneal tendons, the lateral ligaments, and the lateral aspect of the fibula, talus, and calcaneum (Figs. 3, 4, and 5).

The small saphenous vein is a superficial vein that arises from the lateral aspect of the foot and travels posterior to the lateral malleolus and into the posterior aspect of the lower leg. The sural nerve accompanies the small saphenous vein, and localization of the vein allows for easy detection of the sural nerve. The ability to image the sural nerve with US has clinical importance since iatrogenic injury can occur during surgical procedures involving the lower leg or lateral ankle region.

The peroneal retinaculum is arbitrarily divided into the superior peroneal retinaculum (SPR) and the inferior peroneal retinaculum (IPR) based on its relationship to the lateral malleolus. The superior retinaculum appears as hyperechoic thin laminar bands that overlie the peroneal tendons (PeTs) and insert onto the anterolateral cortex of the lateral malleolus. A hyperechoic triangular structure representing fibrocartilage is viewed at the bony insertion site and serves to reinforce the attachment of the SPR onto the cortex of the lateral malleolus. More distally along the SPR, the fibrocartilage gives way to hyaline cartilage,

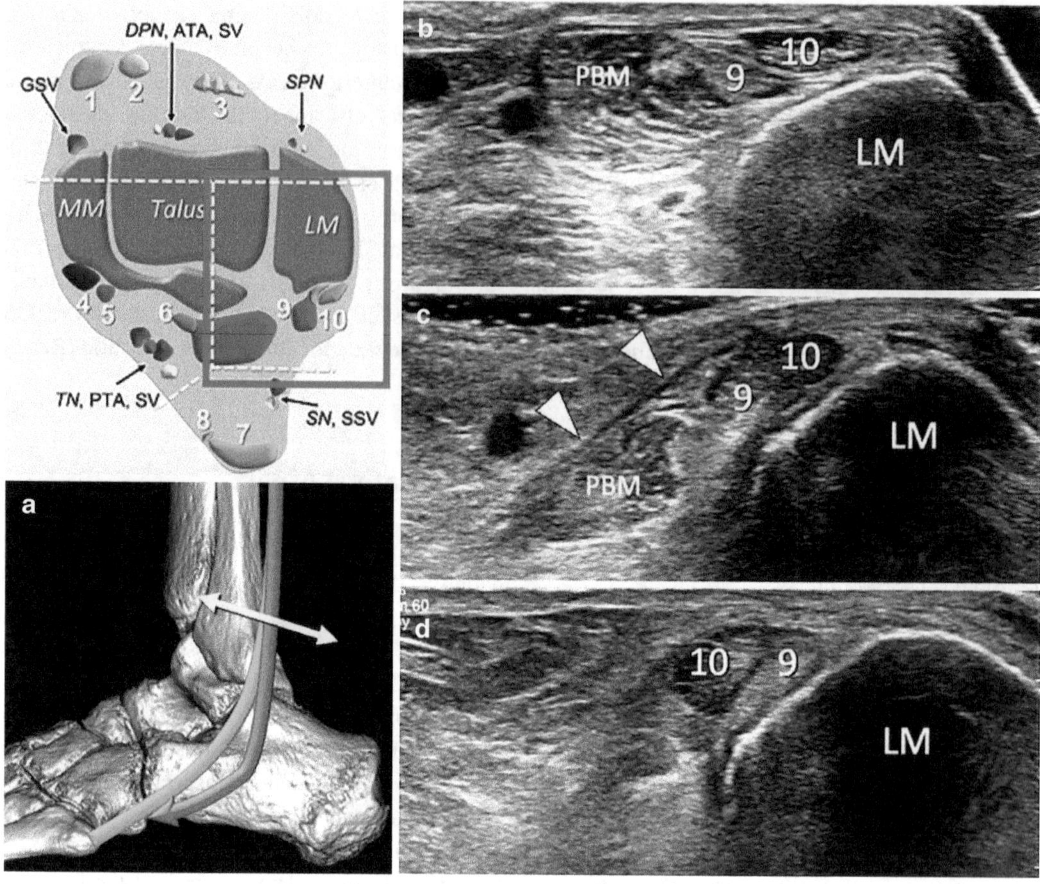

Fig. 3 (**a**–**d**) Lateral aspect. (**a**) Probe positioning for transverse examination of the supramalleolar region. (**b**–**d**) Corresponding sonograms obtained from cranial to caudal. LM, lateral malleolus; PBM, peroneus brevis muscle; 9, peroneus brevis tendon; 10, peroneus longus tendon; arrowheads, retinaculum

which appears hypoechoic. It is important not to mistake this transition from fibrocartilage to hyaline cartilage as an SPR injury. The IPR also appears as thin laminar bands overlying the PeT as they traverse adjacent to the lateral cortex of the calcaneus. Often, a peroneal tubercle is present at this location and separates the more posteriorly positioned peroneus longus (PL) tendon from the anteriorly located peroneus brevis (PB) tendon. The PeTs originate from the peroneal muscles and enter the lateral ankle region posterior to the lateral malleolus in the retro-malleolar groove. The bony morphology of the groove can be evaluated with US and under normal conditions appears concave, which contributes to tendon stability as the tendons curve around the lateral malleolus. In patients with PeT instability, the groove may appear flattened, or even convex, which is an important predisposing factor. US allows accurate evaluation of the PeT throughout their course in the lateral ankle region. Transverse images perpendicular to the long axis of the PeT are particularly useful since they account for the change in planes of the PeT as they course around the lateral malleolus. The PL tendon enters the supramalleolar region in a posterior position in relation to the PB tendon and then moves laterally as it begins to bend around the retro-malleolar groove. As the PB muscle approaches the lateral malleolus, the muscle fibers can be seen inserting in the curvilinear-appearing PB tendon, which is located anteromedial to the PL. At the retro-malleolar groove, the two tendons are closely retained against the lateral malleolus and can be

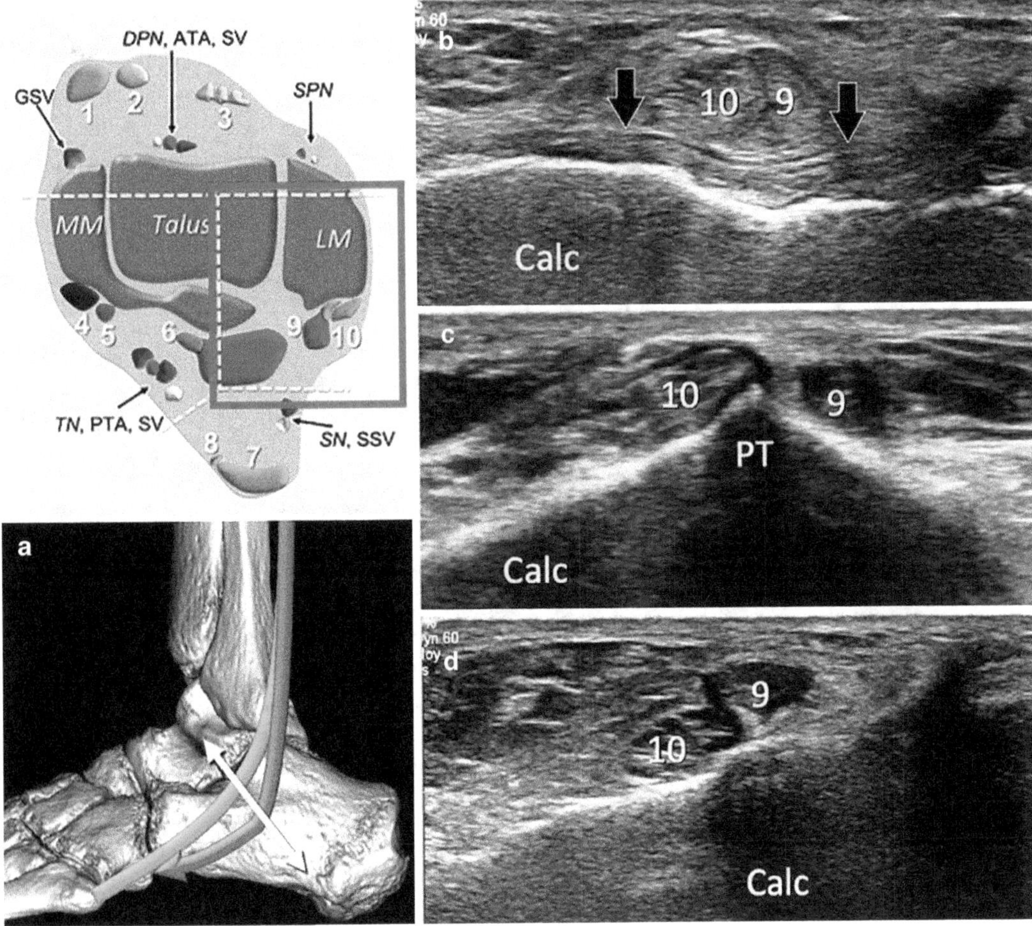

Fig. 4 (**a–d**) Lateral aspect. (**a**) Probe positioning for coronal oblique examination of the infra-malleolar region. (**b–d**) Corresponding sonograms obtained from posterior to anterior. Calc, calcaneum; PT, peroneal tubercle; 9, peroneus brevis tendon; 10, peroneus longus tendon; arrows, peroneocalcaneal ligament

difficult to evaluate. A copious amount of coupling gel and a small footprint transducer can facilitate visualization of the tendons at this location. In the infra-malleolar region, both tendons appear as oval structures that diverge and are separated by the peroneal tubercle of the calcaneum. The PB passes anterior to the tubercle, while PL is located posteriorly. More distally, the PL courses around the cuboid sulcus and into the plantar aspect of the foot to insert onto the base of the first metatarsal. The PB inserts onto the dorsal cortex of the fifth metatarsal tuberosity adjacent to the more laterally oriented insertion of the lateral cord of the plantar fascia. The PeT should also be evaluated with longitudinal images either proximal or distal to the retro-malleolar region where the tendons have a more linear orientation. In the supramalleolar region, the PeTs have a common synovial sheath which splits distally to surround each tendon. Under normal conditions, the tendon sheath and small amount of synovial fluid within the sheath cannot be detected with US. The peroneal tubercle is a bony projection in relation to the lateral aspect of the calcaneum. This can be hypoplastic in some patients. A hypertrophied peroneal tubercle can be associated with stenosing tenosynovitis of peroneal tendons. Dynamic sonograms of the peroneal tendons are achieved by having the patient actively dorsiflex and evert the ankle that can

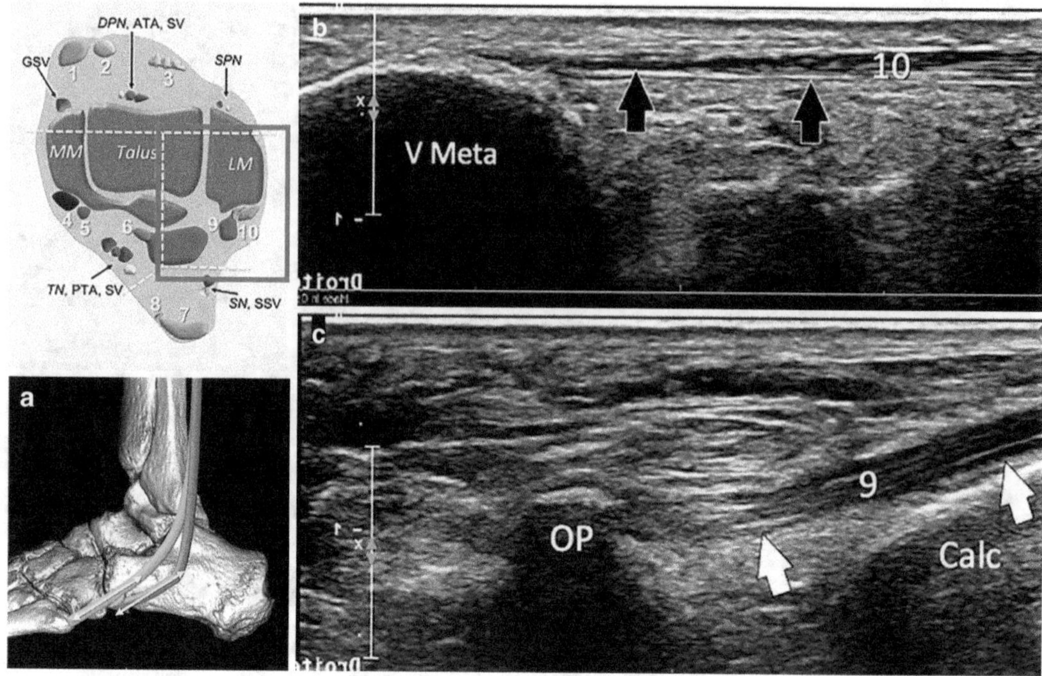

Fig. 5 (**a**, **c**) Lateral aspect. (**a**) Probe positioning for longitudinal examination of peroneus brevis and longus tendon. (**b**, **c**) Corresponding sonogram. V Meta, base of fifth metatarsal; 10, peroneus brevis tendon (black arrows); 9, peroneus longus tendon (white arrows); OP, os peroneum; Calc, calcaneum

demonstrate PeT instabilities (Neustadter et al. 2004). Peroneal tendon instability includes anterior subluxation or dislocation at the lateral malleolus or internal subluxation where the two tendons rotate against each other.

The anterior talofibular (ATFL) and calcaneofibular (CFL) ligaments can be imaged by US on both longitudinal and axial sonograms. A recent meta-analysis comparing US findings with surgical and MRI findings demonstrates that US has high diagnostic performance (Seok et al. 2020). Similar to tendon, ligaments are susceptible to anisotropy and care must be taken to accurately orient the transducer to avoid artifact hypoechogenicity. Ligaments are best evaluated with US when under tension. The ATFL should be imaged with the ankle in plantar flexion and slight inversion, while the CFL is optimally imaged in ankle dorsiflexion and inversion. Ultrasound has the advantage of performing dynamic stress maneuvers, which can increase the detection of tears and help distinguish partial-thickness from full-thickness tears (Campbell et al. 1994). The ATFL appears as a rectilinear hyperechoic band, which joins the anterior aspect of the tip of the malleolus to the neck of the talus. The CFL has a similar echotexture but is more difficult to evaluate because of its curvilinear silhouette. The caudal part of the CFL can be imaged overlying the lateral face of the calcaneum, while the cranial portion is imaged deep to the peroneal tendons.

2.3 Medial Aspect

For the sonographic examination of the medial ankle, the patient externally rotates the ankle to allow full access to medial structures. Structures that are routinely assessed with US include the medial tibiotalar and talocalcaneal joints, flexor retinaculum, flexor tendons, tibial nerve and branches, and posterior tibial artery and vein.

The medial tibiotalar and talocalcaneal joints are best imaged with the transducer in an anatomic coronal plane. Ultrasound can often detect early degenerative changes or bony fragments in the medial tibiotalar joint. Furthermore, US can reveal coalitions of the medial talocalcaneal joint that are difficult to detect without advanced imaging (Bianchi and Hoffman 2013).

The flexor retinaculum is best evaluated with axial sonograms and appears as a thin hyperechoic band encasing the tendons and neurovascular structures within the medial tarsal tunnel. The medial tendons are initially evaluated with axial sonograms and include, from anterior to posterior, the tibialis posterior (TP), flexor digitorum longus (FDL), and flexor hallucis longus (FHL) tendons (Figs. 6, 7, and 8). The TP tendon, the thickest of the medial tendons, appears as an oval hyperechoic structure (Hsu et al. 1997). It lies on the posterolateral aspect of the medial malleolus within an osteofibrous tunnel. The tendon widens distally before its insertion on the tubercle of the navicular (principal insertion). The supplementary insertions (three cuneiforms and bases of second to fourth metatarsals) cannot be visualized with US. Occasionally, US can show a decreased echogenicity of the distal tendon. This may be related to the disparate orientation of collagen fibers in the different tendon portions, which diverge to reach their insertions. Careful examination technique of the distal TP tendon, contralateral comparison, and correlation with the clinical data are helpful to distinguish normal US variation from tendinosis. A small amount of fluid is commonly found in the distal sheath and must not be considered a pathological finding. The FDL is located just posterior and slightly lateral to the TP. Since it is always thinner than the TP tendon, its size can be used as a reference to evaluate TP tendon pathology. The FDL tendon traverses adjacent to the sustentaculum tali and can also serve as a reference location when obtaining comparison images. The FHL tendon is more difficult to evaluate by US due to its deep location. Dynamic examination obtained by passive great hallux

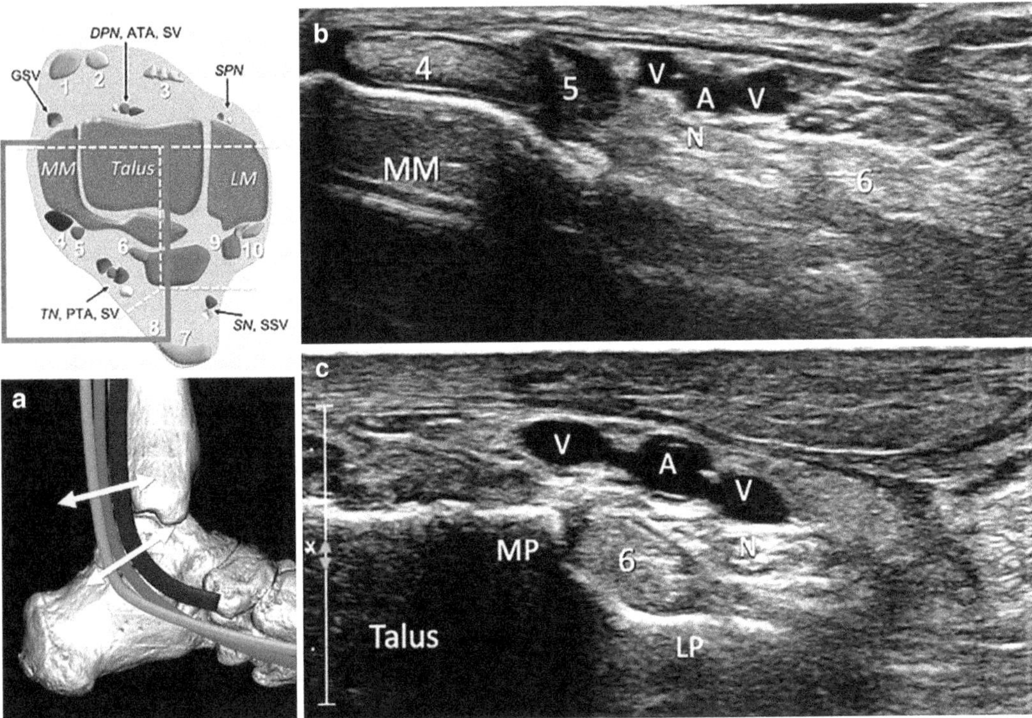

Fig. 6 (**a**–**c**) Medial aspect. (**a**) Probe positioning for transverse examination of the malleolar region. (**b**, **c**) Corresponding sonograms obtained from cranial to caudal. MM, medial malleolus; 4, tibialis posterior tendon; 5, flexor digitorum longus tendon; A, posterior tibial artery; V, posterior tibial veins; N, posterior tibial nerve; MP, medial process of the talus; LP, lateral process of the talus; 6, flexor hallucis longus tendon

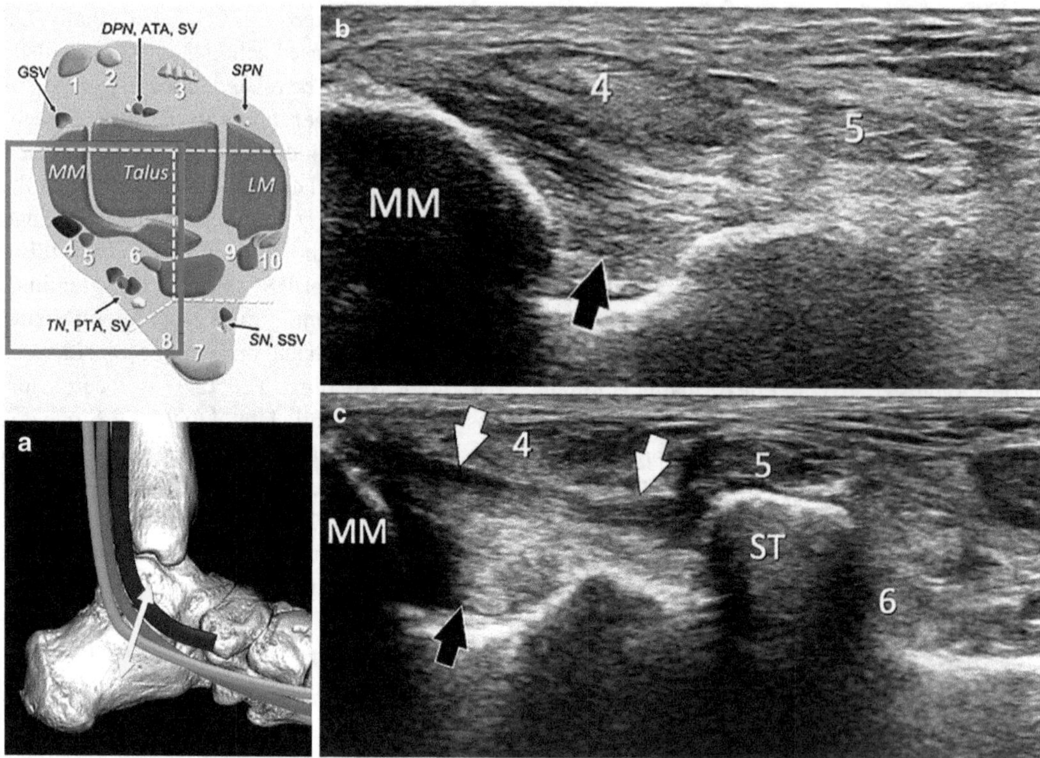

Fig. 7 (**a**–**c**) Medial aspect. (**a**) Probe positioning for coronal examination of the infra-malleolar region. (**b**, **c**) Corresponding sonograms obtained from posterior to anterior. MM, medial malleolus; ST, sustentaculum tali; 4, tibialis posterior tendon; black arrow, deep component of the deltoid ligament; white arrow, superficial component of the deltoid ligament; 5, flexor digitorum longus tendon; 6, flexor hallucis longus tendon

movement can improve conspicuity. A small amount of fluid within the FHL tendon sheath is also a normal finding as the sheath communicates with the talocrural joint in approximately 10–15% of cases. Each of the medial ankle tendons should also be imaged with longitudinal sonograms allowing for a more complete evaluation.

The neurovascular bundle (posterior tibial artery and veins and tibial nerve) is located in a slightly lateral position with respect to the FDL tendon. The artery is differentiated from the adjacent veins by its pulsatility and compressibility. With the utilization of high-frequency transducers, the tibial nerve and its two terminal branches, the medial and lateral plantar nerves, can be visualized. High-frequency probes also allow detection of the medial calcaneal and inferior calcaneal branches. The branching pattern of the tibial nerve is highly variable, and careful axial imaging from proximal to distal will reveal the various branching patterns.

The medial collateral ligament complex, or deltoid ligament (DL), is an important stabilizing structure for the tibiotalar and talocalcaneal joints. While there is variability in the different components of the deltoid ligament, the DL ligament complex has both deep and superficial components that are readily evaluated with US (Martinez-Franco et al. 2022).

2.4 Posterior Aspect

Posterior ankle structures that can be imaged by US include the posterior aspect of the ankle, the Achilles tendon (AT), Kager's fat pad, retrocalcaneal bursa, and plantaris tendon. The patient is examined prone. Because of its superficial location, rectilinear appearance, and high frequency

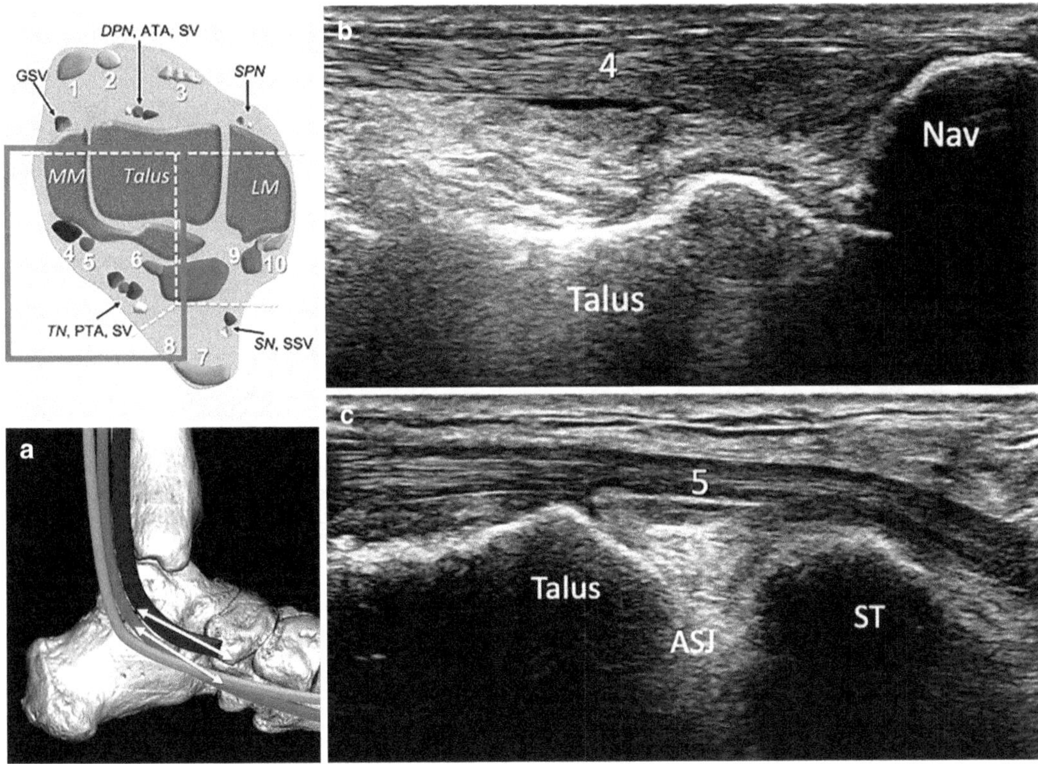

Fig. 8 (**a–c**) Medial aspect. (**a**) Probe positioning for longitudinal examination of the tibialis posterior tendon (4) and flexor digitorum longus tendon (5). (**b, c**) Corresponding sonograms. *Nav* navicular bone, *ST* sustentaculum tali, *fdl* flexor digitorum longus tendon, *ASJ* anterior subtalar joint

of ruptures, the study of the AT was one of the first applications of musculoskeletal US. Thorough sonographic assessment of AT requires both grayscale and Doppler imaging. Grayscale imaging is optimized when the tendon is under slight tension, which is achieved by having the patient slightly dorsiflex at the ankle. Conversely, Doppler imaging is optimized having the patient in slight plantar flexion to avoid a stretch on the tendon and the potential for a false-negative result. The AT should be evaluated in both axial and longitudinal images obtained from the myotendinous junction to the calcaneal insertion (Figs. 9 and 10). Longitudinal images show the AT as a hyperechoic homogeneous fibrillar structure that originates from the triceps surae muscle and inserts on the lower aspect of the posterior tuberosity of the calcaneum. Detailed examination of the proximal tendon reveals two components, a superficial component derived from the gastrocnemius muscle and a deep component derived from the soleus muscle (Bertolotto et al. 1995). Axial sonograms are always performed since they yield accurate evaluation of the most peripheral area, which can be difficult to assess with longitudinal imaging. The tendon has no synovial sheath but is surrounded by a layer of connective tissue, the paratenon, which appears as a thin hyperechoic line. The distal fibers of the AT angle obliquely toward the calcaneus at their insertion and thus are susceptible to anisotropy. It is important to maintain a parallel orientation of the transducer when evaluating the distal fibers to avoid an artifactual increase in hypoechogenicity that can mimic tendinosis. Longitudinal dynamic images obtained during passive flexion and extension of the foot show the smooth gliding of the tendon, which may help in identifying peritendinous adhesions or differentiating a partial-thickness from full-thickness tear. Deep, or

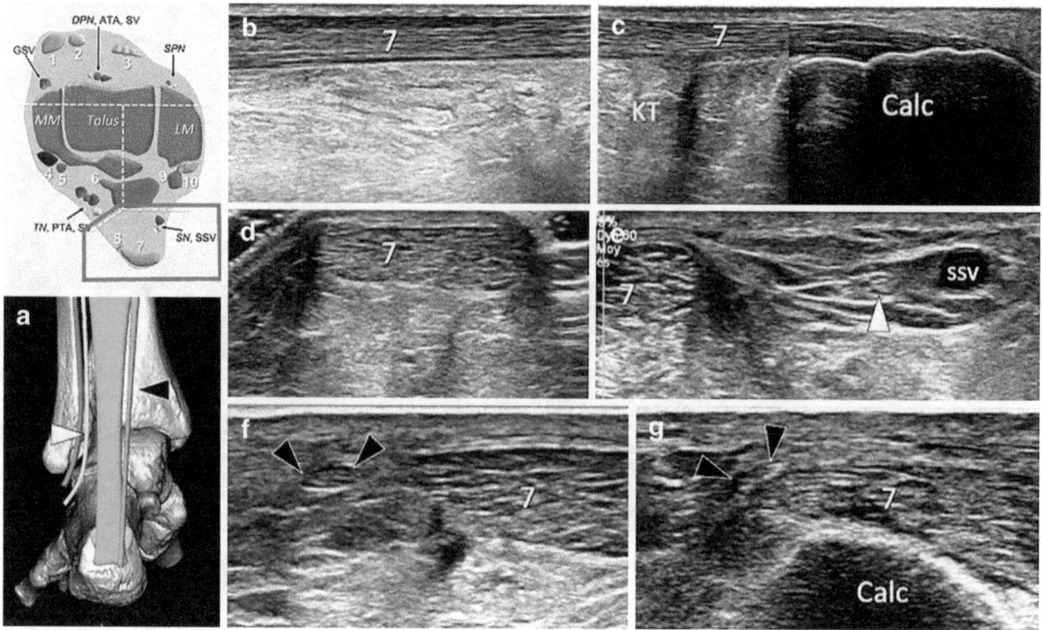

Fig. 9 (**a**–**g**) Posterior aspect. (**a**) Probe positioning for longitudinal and transverse examination of the Achilles tendon region. (**b**–**g**) Proximal to distal corresponding longitudinal (**b**, **c**) and transverse (**d**–**g**) sonograms. 7, Achilles tendon; KT, Kager's triangle; Calc, calcaneus; white arrowhead, sural nerve; SSV, small saphenous vein; black arrowheads, plantaris tendon

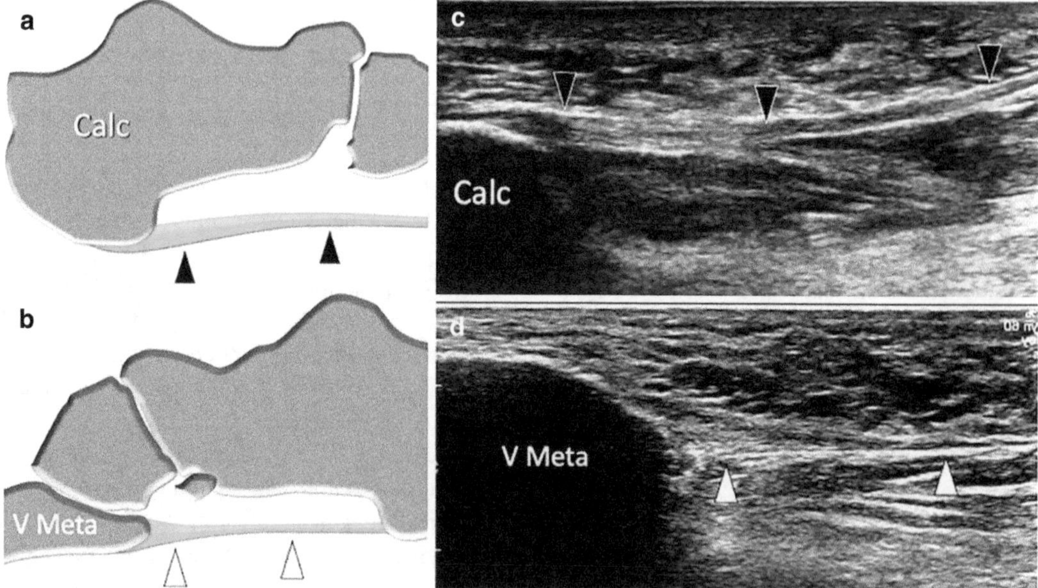

Fig. 10 (**a**–**d**) Inferior aspect. (**a**, **b**) Schematic drawing of the central (**a**) and lateral (**b**) parts of the plantar fascia. (**c**, **d**) Corresponding longitudinal sonograms. Black arrowheads, central part; white arrowheads, lateral part; V Meta, base of fifth metatarsal; Calc, calcaneus

anterior, to the AT is Kager's fat pad which is a mass of adipose tissue occupying Kager's triangle. Kager's fat pad is felt to have an important role in optimal AT function and implicated in Achilles tendinosis and heel pain syndromes (Theobald et al. 2018).

The plantaris tendon can be identified in transverse images either proximally at the musculotendinous junction or distally at its insertion onto the medial aspect of the distal AT. Proximally, the plantaris muscle is readily identified as a triangular shaped muscle located deep to the medial and lateral heads of the gastrocnemius muscle. The muscle gives way to a small, flattened tendon located between the medial head of the gastrocnemius and underlying soleus muscle. The plantaris tendon can be difficult to visualize in the mid-calf region due to its small and flattened morphology. The tendon is often identified in the distal third of the lower leg as a small ovoid tendon at the medial border of the AT. Identification of the plantaris tendon is useful when planning reconstructive surgery that utilizes this tendon as an autologous transplant (Wening et al. 1996). More recently, the plantaris tendon has been implicated as playing a role in chronic midportion Achilles tendinopathy (Masci et al. 2015).

There are two bursae at the distal end of the Achilles tendon. The retrocalcaneal bursa lies anterior to the distal Achilles tendon and distal to Kager's fat pad and may be affected with distal AT disorders or inflammatory arthropathies. The second bursa is a thin adventitial bursa that lies posterior to the distal AT and generally not visible by US in the normal state. It is frequently thickened with distal AT disorders.

An accessory soleus muscle can be found between the AT and the posterior aspect of the ankle (Palaniappan et al. 1999). US demonstrates it as a space-occupying lesion, which presents with a normal muscle structure (Bianchi et al. 1995). The US diagnosis is obvious if this condition is kept in mind.

Deep to Kager's triangle, the myotendinous junction and supramalleolar portion of the flexor hallucis longus tendon as well as the posterior ankle recess can be demonstrated. In evaluating the deep posterior aspect of the ankle joint, care must be taken to adjust the focus of the US beam at the level of the tail of the talus. In larger ankles, a lower frequency probe must be deployed. The posterior ankle recess fills with dorsal flexion of the ankle and is located between the posterior tibial malleolus and the talar queue but is hard to demonstrate in normal ankles. The posterior subtalar recess can be imaged only if distended by pathological effusion; it appears as an anechoic mass located between the talus and the calcaneum.

The retinaculum is the thickening of the crural fascia and is an important stabilizer of tendons of the ankle joint that prevents bowstringing of the tendons. These include the flexor retinaculum, superior extensor retinaculum, inferior extensor retinaculum, superficial peroneal retinaculum, superior peroneal retinaculum, inferior peroneal retinaculum, and deep aponeurosis posteriorly. These are linear hypoechoic on ultrasound that are normally of 1–2 mm thickness. The thickness of retinaculum can be different depending on the location.

References

Bertolotto M, Perrone R, Martinoli C et al (1995) High resolution US anatomy of normal Achilles tendon. Br J Radiol 68:986–991

Bianchi S, Martinoli C (1999) Detection of loose bodies in joints. Radiol Clin N Am 37:679–690

Bianchi S, Abdelwahab IF, Oliveri M et al (1995) Sonographic diagnosis of accessory soleus muscle mimicking a soft tissue tumor. J Ultrasound Med 14:707–709

Bianchi S, Hoffman D (2013) Ultrasound of talocalcaneal coalition: retrospective study of 11 patients. Skeletal Radiol 42(9):1209–14.

Bianchi S, Becciolini M (2019) Ultrasound Features of Ankle Retinacula: Normal Appearance and Pathologic Findings. J Ultrasound Med (12):3321–334

Campbell DG, Menz A, Isaacs J (1994) Dynamic ankle ultrasonography. A new imaging technique for acute ankle ligament injuries. Am J Sports Med 22:855–858

Demondion X, Canella C, Moraux A, Cohen M, Bry R, Cotten A (2010) Retinacular disorders of the ankle and foot. Semin Musculoskelet Radiol 14(3):281–91

Hsu TC, Wang CL, Wang TG et al (1997) Ultrasonographic examination of the posterior tibial tendon. Foot Ankle Int 18:34–38

Jacobson JA, Andresen R, Jaovisidha S et al (1998) Detection of ankle effusions: comparison study in cadavers using radiography, sonography, and MR imaging. AJR Am J Roentgenol 170:1231–1238

Kane D, Grassi W, Sturrock R et al (2004) Musculoskeletal ultrasound—a state of the art review in rheumatology. Part 2: clinical indications for musculoskeletal ultrasound in rheumatology. Rheumatology (Oxford) 43(7):829–838

Kok AC, Terra MP, Muller S, Askeland C, van Dijk CN, Kerkhoffs GM, Tuijthof GJ (2014) Feasibility of ultrasound imaging of osteochondral defects in the ankle: a clinical pilot study. Ultrasound Med Biol 40(10):2530–6.

Lee JC, Healy JC (2005) Normal sonographic anatomy of the wrist and hand. Radiographics 25(6):1577–1590. https://doi.org/10.1148/rg.256055028

Martinez-Franco A, Gijon-Nogueron G, Franco-Romero AG et al (2022) Ultrasound examination of the ligament complex within the medial aspect of the ankle and foot. J Ultrasound Med. https://doi.org/10.1002/jum.15964. Epub ahead of print

Martinoli C, Bianchi S, Gandolfo N et al (2000) US of nerve entrapments in osteofibrous tunnels of the upper and lower limbs. Radiographies 20(Spec No):S199–S217

Masci L, Spang C, van Schie HT et al (2015) Achilles tendinopathy-do plantaris tendon removal and Achilles tendon scraping improve tendon structure? A prospective study using ultrasound tissue characterisation. BMJ Open Sport Exerc Med 1(1):e000005

Nazarian LN, Rawool NM, Martin CE et al (1995) Synovial fluid in the hindfoot and ankle: detection of amount and distribution with US. Radiology 197:275–278

Neustadter J, Raikin SM, Nazarian LN (2004) Dynamic sonographic evaluation of peroneal tendon subluxation. AJR Am J Roentgenol 183(4):985–988

Palaniappan M, Rajesh A, Rickett A et al (1999) Accessory soleus muscle: a case report and review of the literature. Pediatr Radiol 29:610–612

Reach JS, Easley ME, Chuckpaiwong B et al (2009) Accuracy of ultrasound guided injections in the foot and ankle. Foot Ankle Int 30(3):239–242. https://doi.org/10.3113/FAI.2009.0239

Ricci S, Moro L, Antonelli Incalzi R (2010) Ultrasound imaging of the sural nerve: ultrasound anatomy and rationale for investigation. Eur J Vasc Endovasc Surg 39(5):636–641. https://doi.org/10.1016/j.ejvs.2009.11.024

Sconfienza LM, Albano D, Allen G et al (2018) Clinical indications for musculoskeletal ultrasound updated in 2017 by European Society of Musculoskeletal Radiology (ESSR) consensus. Eur Radiol 28(12):5338–5351. https://doi.org/10.1007/s00330-018-5474-3. Epub 2018 Jun 6

Seok H, Lee SH, Yun SJ (2020) Diagnostic performance of ankle ultrasound for diagnosing anterior talofibular and calcaneofibular ligament injuries: a meta-analysis. Acta Radiol 61(5):651–661

Theobald P, Bydder G, Dent C et al (2018) The functional anatomy of Kager's fat pad in relation to retrocalcaneal problems and other hindfoot disorders. J Anat 1:91–97

Wening JV, Katzer A, Phillips F et al (1996) Detection of the tendon of the musculus plantaris longus—diagnostic imaging and anatomic correlate. Unfalkhirurgie 22:30–35

Intra-articular Injections of the Ankle and Foot (Intervention of Foot and Ankle)

Hema N. Choudur and Ari Damla

Contents

1 Introduction

Imaging modalities: Fluoroscopy and ultrasound are the most commonly used modalities for image-guided interventions of the ankle and foot. Fluoroscopy continues to be the modality of choice for injecting the ankle joint, posterior subtalar joint, and small joints of the midfoot, despite the radiation involved with this procedure. This is due to the ease and rapidity of the procedure and due to excellent joint and bone visualization for needle guidance. However, in some centers, these joints are injected under ultrasound guidance as ultrasound is easily accessible. Ultrasound provides excellent resolution of superficial soft tissues, dynamic vision of the soft tissue target, and needle tip localization. It is the modality of choice for soft tissue interventions, be it tendon, ligament, nerve, bursa, or plantar fascia. MR guided perineural injections are uncommon and are undertaken in a few academic centers. The injectables for these procedures include local anesthetics that are utilized for performing diagnostic blocks, intra-articular steroid injections, steroid injections into bursae and perineural areas, autologous blood or PRP injections into joints, tendons, ligaments, neuromas, plantar fascia, hyaluronic acid into joints, and gadolinium injection into the ankle joint for MR arthrography. US-guided soft tissue/bone biopsies and foreign body removal are described briefly, as these techniques are similar to the rest of the body. Each intervention will be dealt with separately for easy comprehension and for day-to-day application by the reader.

2 Types of Interventions

2.1 Joint Injections

1. **Ankle joint**: The tibiotalar joint and small joints of the midfoot can be accessed from the

H. N. Choudur (✉)
MSK Imaging, Department of Radiology, McMaster University, Hamilton General Hospital, HHSC, Hamilton, ON, Canada
e-mail: hnalinic@yahoo.com; choudur@hhsc.ca

A. Damla
MSK Imaging, Department of Radiology, Boston University Chobanian & Avedisian School of Medicine, Boston Medical Center, Boston, MA, USA
e-mail: ari.damla@bmc.org

Med Radiol Diagn Imaging (2023)

https://doi.org/10.1007/174_2023_389,
Published Online: 19 April 2023

dorsal aspect using either fluoroscopy or ultrasound (Fox et al. 2013). For fluoroscopy-guided ankle joint injection, the dorsalis pedis artery pulsations are palpated and the skin needle entry is targeted either medial or lateral to it. A 22 or 25-g needle will suffice, be it for injecting diluted gadolinium injection for MR arthrography or intra-articular injection of local anesthetic, steroid, hyaluronic acid, or PRP. Prior to the injection, 0.5 mL of iodinated contrast is injected to confirm intra-articular location of the needle tip. The iodinated contrast will outline the tibial plafond/talar dome and the joint recesses. For MR arthrography of the ankle, 3–4 mL of diluted gadolinium can be injected into the joint or until resistance is felt to further injection. Three to four milliliter of diluted iodinated contrast is injected for CT arthrography (Fig. 1). If using ultrasound guidance, the dorsalis pedis artery and the overlying tibialis anterior and extensor digitorum tendons are identified with the probe in the short-axis plane to these structures. Thereby, these structures are avoided while marking an entry path into the ankle joint. Thereafter, the US probe can be placed either in the long or short-axis planes to visualize the needle tip dynamically for the injection.

2. **Posterior subtalar joint**: The posterior subtalar joint is injected by a medial or lateral approach (Kirk et al. 2008). It is easier to inject this joint under fluoroscopy than ultrasound as the entire ankle and hind foot are visualized on the fluoroscopic image and the

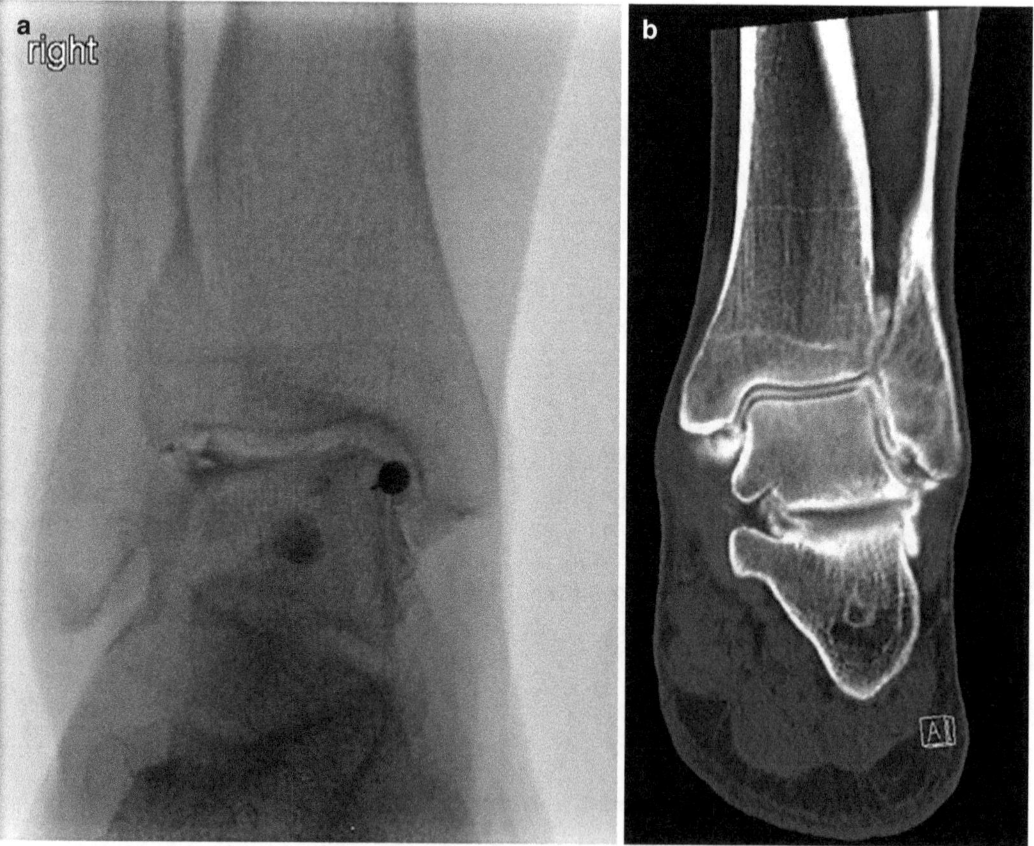

Fig. 1 (**a**) Anterior approach injection of the tibiotalar joint medial to the palpated location of the dorsalis pedis, fluoroscopy confirms intra-articular contrast. (**b**) Intra-articular extension of contrast within the tibiotalar joint on coronal CT

posterior subtalar joint is clearly identified. The lateral approach with the patient lying on his side, opposite knee flexed and out of the field, the injected side supported by a folded towel, is the most comfortable position for the patient and the radiologist (Fig. 2). This is the easiest approach for a new learner. The point of skin entry is made immediately inferior and posterior to the tip of the fibula, thereby avoiding the peroneal tendons. The needle tip is then directed into the posterior subtalar joint under fluoroscopic vision. 0.5 mL of iodinated contrast is injected to confirm intra-articular location of the needle tip, prior to injecting the injectables, which is usually local anesthetic and/or steroid, iodinated contrast for CT arthrography or occasionally, hyaluronic acid, or PRP for arthritis. On ultrasound, visualization of the tibialis posterior tendon during the medial approach and the peroneal tendon during the lateral approach helps to avoid injecting these structures. Ultrasound-guided injection is advantageous over fluoroscopy in cases of severe osteoarthritis wherein the large marginal osteophytes serve as a barrier for needle entry into the joint space.

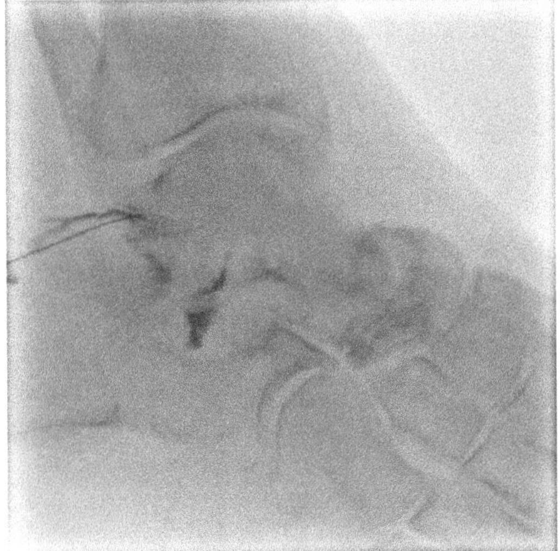

Fig. 2 Lateral approach fluoroscopic subtalar joint injection demonstrating placement of the needle into the posterior aspect of the subtalar joint with intra-articular spread of contrast

3. **Talonavicular, calcaneocuboid joints, and the joints of the mid and forefoot**: These joints are easily injected under fluoroscopy, using a dorsal, dorsomedial, or dorsolateral approach based on the joint injected (Hansford et al. 2019). Iodinated contrast can be used to confirm intra-articular location of the needle tip (Fig. 3). Ultrasound can also be used as an alternative modality to provide image guidance. It demonstrates the joint capsule, and intra-articular passage of the needle tip can be well visualized dynamically.

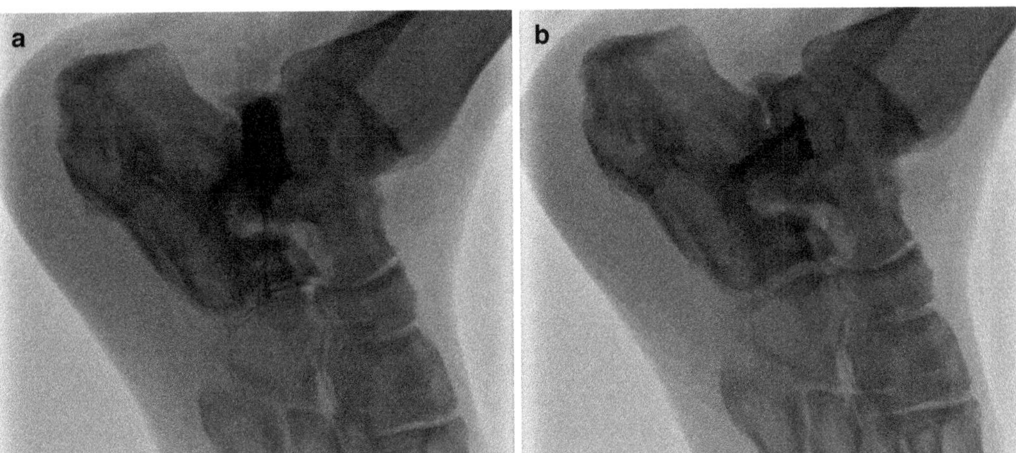

Fig. 3 (**a**) Lateral approach fluoroscopy-guided injection of the calcaneocuboid joint. (**b**) Distension of the calcaneocuboid joint following injection with steroid and local anesthetic

4. **Diagnostic aspiration, synovial biopsy, and MR/CT arthrography of joints of the ankle and foot**: All the above joints can be aspirated using either fluoroscopy or ultrasound. When a dry aspirate is obtained, a saline lavage of the joint can be performed. If a synovial biopsy is necessary, a co-axial method can be utilized utilizing small length needles. MR arthrography wherein gadolinium is injected into the ankle joint is not a popular technique as the PD-T2 fat sat or T2 fat sat sequences provide optimum fluid contrast within the joint. The most common indication for MR or CT arthrography is for the assessment of stability of an osteochondral lesion of the talar dome or for evaluation of intra-articular bodies within the ankle joint. Fluoroscopy-guided diluted iodinated contrast injection prior to performing the CT scan is an alternative to MR arthrography (Wiewiorski et al. 2009). A mixture of 3–4 mL of iodinated contrast in 7–6 mL of sterile saline will provide optimum dilution of iodinated contrast, preventing CT artifacts from dense contrast.

2.2 Tendon Interventions

Achilles tendinopathy and associated tears are a very frequently encountered problem at the ankle. Besides Achilles tendinosis, tendon tears, and tenosynovitis of the foot and ankle are also a common occurrence. Tendinosis is degenerative and can be a result from aging, overuse, and chronic stress. It can also be a result of mechanical factors from altered weight-bearing mechanics. Inflammatory or infective etiology causing tenosynovitis may necessitate image-guided injection/aspiration (Fox et al. 2013).

Due to the high spatial resolution, ultrasound is the modality of choice over MRI to assess tendons of the ankle and foot (Kirk et al. 2008). The normal internal echotexture of tendons comprised of parallel echogenic lines (collagen bundles) with fine intervening hypoechoic bands (connective tissue). In chronic tendinosis, the Achilles tendon loses its normal fibrillary appearance, and hypoechoic areas are seen in the area affected by the tendinosis (from degenerative changes). Doppler hyperemia can be present within these areas of tendinosis (Hansford et al. 2019). The Achilles tendon does not have a tendon sheath. However, peritendinous inflammation of the surrounding connective tissue can occur, termed paratenonitis. Micro or macrotears within the area of tendinosis can occur and are seen as anechoic/echo poor areas. Tendon ruptures can also occur on a background of tendinosis or can occur acutely post-trauma in otherwise normal tendons, as seen in athletes. Tendinosis usually affects the mid and distal thirds of the tendon. Following tendon rupture, the area between the retracted torn ends can be well identified on US, and the distance between the torn ends or between the retracted torn end and the calcaneus (in insertional tears) can be accurately delineated on US. The dynamic assessment for tendon separation can be measured on plantar and dorsiflexion, which helps in clinical decision-making and is a distinct advantage of ultrasound over MRI. Ruptured Achilles tendons are treated conservatively in a boot cast or surgically, based on the extent of separation between the retracted tendon ends and the ankle surgeon's approach. Ultrasound-guided intervention is not undertaken in such cases. Ultrasound-guided interventions are limited to tendinosis and low to moderate grade tears. These are performed to facilitate tendon healing (Asplund and Best 2013; Bianchi and Martinoli 2007).

Achilles tendinosis can be treated with dry needling (tendon fenestration) or with injectables that include autologous blood, PRP injection, or polidocanol (Riley 2008). The patient is positioned prone with the foot resting at the edge of the bed. A high-frequency linear transducer (7–18 MHz) is used. A hockey stick transducer can also be used as it allows more room for accessing the target area and helps in maneuvering the needle tip. After the pathological area within the tendon is identified, doppler US is used to assess the area with maximum flow (neovascularity). The entry point of the needle is marked on the skin, with the probe in the long- or short-axis plane. Using sterile conditions, a 25-to-23-g needle is used for the procedure. After administration of a local anesthetic at the skin entry site, the needle tip is advanced to the surface of the posterior tendon, in either the short- or long-axis planes. A few mL of 0.5% Sensorcaine is injected over the surface of the tendon, and the needle tip is advanced into the area of tendinosis. Using to-and-fro gentle movements of the needle tip, dry needling is performed, maintaining the needle tip within the tendon during the entire procedure, to prevent multiple entries on the surface of the tendon, thereby weakening it. About 15–20 such movements are made by changing the angle of the needle tip within the area of tendinosis, so the entire area of tendinosis is fenestrated (Fig. 4). Following this, if PRP is to be injected, the injection is targeted into the areas of low-grade intratendinous tears. The patient's blood is drawn from a subcutaneous vein at the elbow into the PRP syringe. After using the centrifuge to separate the patient's serum containing the platelets, the PRP solution is ready for use. The needle tip is localized to the tear and 1–2 mL of PRP is injected into the tear until resistance is felt to further injection. The needle tip is then gently withdrawn. In some centers, autologous blood (taken from the patient's vein) is also injected directly if the PRP centrifuge is not available to separate the platelet-rich plasma (James et al. 2007). Prolotherapy using hyperosmolar dextrose is the other injectable, and its efficacy is described in some trials. Polidocanol is injected as a sclerosing agent into the area of neovascularity, identified by color doppler. This serves to reduce the pain from the tendinosis (Riley 2008). High volume saline stripping between the deeper aspect of the Achilles tendon and the Kager's fat pad is another intervention recently described to reduce pain from chronic tendinosis. Peritendinous injection of hyaluronic acid can be used in relieving chronic adhesions, either in the post-trauma situation or following surgical repair of the tendon (Riley 2008).

Chronic inflammation of the paratenon may result in adhesions between the paratenon and the Achilles tendon, leading to paratenonitis. Brisement, also known as paratenon stripping, includes the injection of saline solution into the tendon/peritenon interspace to break up adhesions. Under ultrasound guidance, a needle is placed deep to the paratenon in the short-axis plane and a solution of normal saline, and 1% lidocaine is gently injected. Brisement injections have long been used although there is lack of data in the literature to specifically evaluate this technique.

Extracorporeal shortwave therapy, eccentric loading, and conservative wait-and-watch techniques are other approaches to treat Achilles tendinosis. There is lack of Level 1 evidence regarding the best injectable for treatment for Achilles' tendinosis and tears (Rompe et al. 2007).

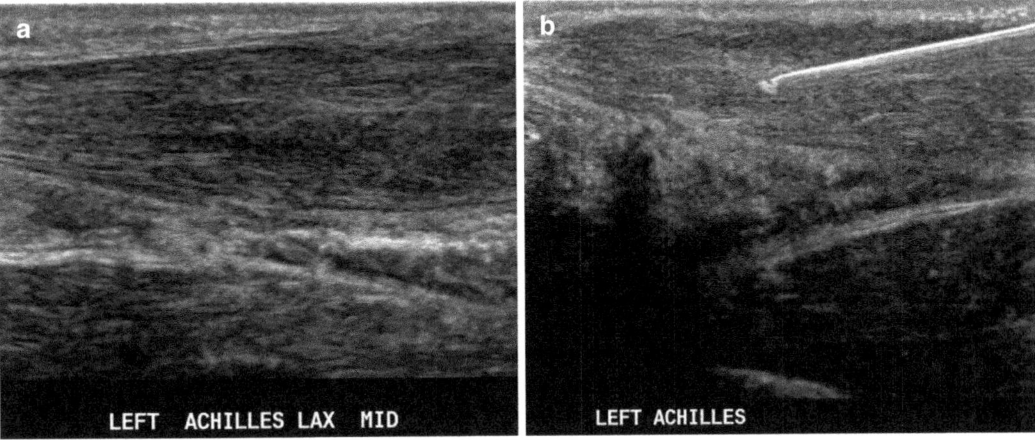

Fig. 4 (**a**) Long-axis ultrasound of the Achilles tendon demonstrates hypoechoic thickened of the tendon compatible with tendinopathy. (**b**) Subsequent fenestration of the tendon with the needle in long axis

2.2.1 Injectables

1. **Steroids**: Traditionally, steroids have been used in the past to treat tendinosis. However, there has been a lot of evidence against the use of steroids for tendinosis as the effect is temporary and not longstanding. Furthermore, there is increased risk of tendon rupture, overlying fat atrophy, and abnormal skin pigmentation (Hansford et al. 2019).
2. **Glyceryl trinitrate**: This injectable has been shown to be of benefit in Achilles tendinosis (Paoloni et al. 2004). The side effect is headache. This injectable is not licensed in many countries like the UK.
3. **Prolotherapy**: Injection of concentrated (hyperosmolar) dextrose causes local inflammatory response at the site of injection in the tendon, thereby promoting healing. Some centers utilize six weekly injections of this injectate into the area of tendinosis (Yelland et al. 2004).
4. **Polidocanol**: The sclerotherapy is performed by injection of polidocanol inside or close to the neovascularity within the area of tendinosis, identified by color doppler. The treatment can be repeated but intervals are not clear (Cole et al. 2018). This is followed by eccentric loading exercises.
5. **PRP or autologous blood therapy**: These injectables were very popular in athletes but recent meta-analysis has shown that these injectables are not as promising as were initially propagated (Ferrero et al. 2012).
6. **Saline stripping:** Injection of small or large volumes of saline (up to 40 mL) with 0.5% Sensorcaine (up to 10 mL) and steroid under ultrasound guidance helps with reduction of pain. This is from stripping of the anterior aspect of the Achilles tendon from the adjacent vessels and nerves (Kakkos et al. 2021).
7. **Tenocyte transplant and stem cell injections**: This is a new method of treatment of tendinosis and is still in the research and experimental phase. It entails in vitro culture of skin derived tenocytes which are then injected into the area of tendinosis under ultrasound guidance. These tenocytes then produce Type 1 collagen aiding with repair of the tendinosis. Stem cell injections are emerging as a form of treatment for Achilles tendinosis. Some trials have shown that allogenic derived stem cells or bone marrow derived stem cell injections led to faster recovery when compared to PRP. However, the potential long-term side effects have not been studied, and these stem cell injections are still in the research phase and are not mainstream treatment options (Lui 2015).

2.2.2 Conservative

Rest and activity modification, orthotics, NSAIDS that inhibit prostaglandin synthesis and inhibit pain, glyceryl trinitrate patch that promotes vasodilatation and reduces pain.

2.2.3 Other Treatments

1. **Laser treatment** acts by suppressing prostaglandin E2 production and other nonspecific cell activities.
2. **Cryotherapy** that reduces cell metabolism and inflammation.
3. **Ultrasound** that stimulates cell activity and blood flow by its thermal effect.
4. **Steroid injection**: Reduces inflammation and has other nonspecific effects by inhibiting protein synthesis.
5. **Autologous blood** acts via the growth factors and aids in promoting tissue repair. The platelet-derived growth factors and growth factors B affect tissue healing.
6. **Platelet-rich plasma** promotes tissue repair and matrix synthesis through the growth factors concentrate (including platelet-derived growth factor and growth factor β).
7. **Sclerosant injection** targets neovascularization by destroying the vascularity and prevents nerve growth and thereby reduces pain.

8. **Eccentric loading** stretching the muscle tendon complex affecting cell activity and restoring normal structure by remodeling the muscle tendon complexes.
9. **ESWL**: Extracorporeal shortwave therapy is using shockwave under ultrasound guidance to overstimulate the area of pain within the tendon. This decreases the pain signals to the brain. This hyperstimulation causes regeneration of tenocytes to produce collagen similar to the effect of dry needling. It also helps to break down intratendinous calcification. The NICE has concluded that this is a safe procedure for treatment of tendinosis, but there is no consensus on overall efficacy (Rasmussen et al. 2008).

2.3 Tenosynovitis

Ultrasound can also be used to inject local anesthetic and steroid into the tendon sheath for treatment of inflammatory tenosynovitis (Kearney et al. 2015). An US-guided aspiration of fluid within the tendon sheath can be performed for infective tenosynovitis of the foot and ankle. The aspirate can be obtained using a 20 g needle if the 22 g aspiration is not successful.

2.4 Bursitis

The bursae in the foot and ankle are fewer than other regional body parts and include the retrocalcaneal bursa, retro-Achilles bursa, intermetatarsal bursa, and adventitious (chronic inflammatory) bursa. These bursae cause pain and tenderness when inflamed and can be injected under ultrasound guidance (Bianchi and Martinoli 2007). The US probe and the injecting needle are placed in the short-axis plane to inject the bursa and less often in the long-axis plane (Fig. 5). For injecting the retrocalcaneal and retro-Achilles bursa, the patient is positioned in the prone position with the foot hanging along the edge of the bed. The intermetatarsal bursa is approached with the foot flat on the table, facilitated by a bent knee. A small towel can be placed under the distal foot to facilitate the injection. The approach to the intermetatarsal bursa is from the dorsal aspect as this causes less pain from the procedure than the planter aspect injection. However, if the latter approach is undertaken, it can be performed with the foot hanging at the edge of the bed with the patient in a prone position. A 22 g needle can be utilized for this procedure. Skin injection with a local anesthetic followed by 1–2 mL Sensorcaine and 1 mL of steroid injection (e.g., Depo-Medrol) are injected into the bursa under dynamic vision.

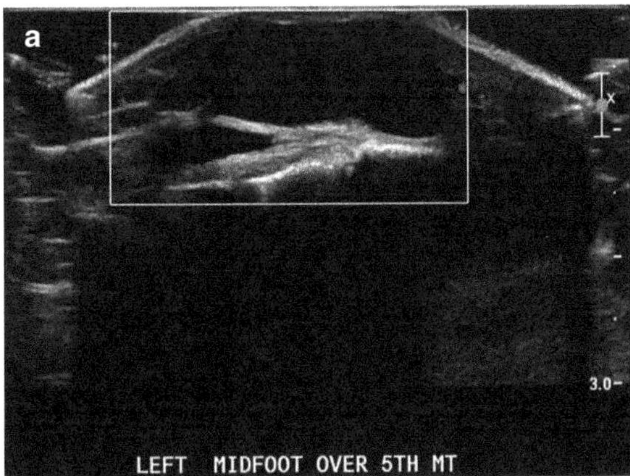

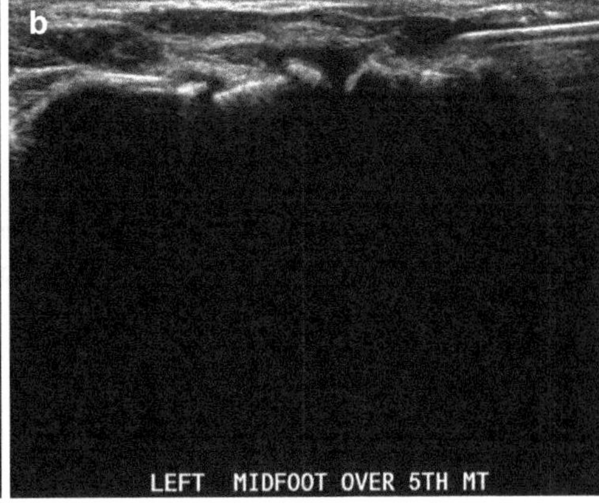

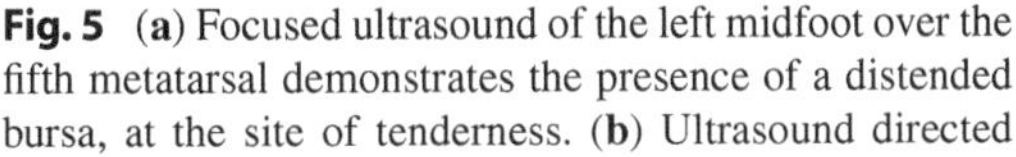

Fig. 5 (**a**) Focused ultrasound of the left midfoot over the fifth metatarsal demonstrates the presence of a distended bursa, at the site of tenderness. (**b**) Ultrasound directed needle aspiration was performed completely collapsing the bursa with subsequent steroid injection

2.5 Morton's Neuroma

Morton's neuroma is fusiform thickening of the digital nerve causing pain and tenderness. The digital nerves are branches of the medial and lateral plantar nerves. The fusiform enlargement of the nerve in the intermetatarsal space occurs deep to the intermetatarsal ligament, from chronic pressure over the nerve. This results in chronic intra and perineural fibrosis (Hassouna and Singh 2005). Therefore, a Morton's neuroma is not a true neuroma. The various causes of a Morton's neuroma include excessive altered weight-bearing mechanics, most commonly from a flat foot (result of collapse of the medial plantar arch). There is resultant forefoot rotation during walking with formation of hallux valgus deformity. The digital nerves are compressed by the overlying intermetatarsal ligament and there could be entrapment of the nerve by the surrounding fibrosis with or without development of intermetatarsal bursitis. This abnormality is more common in females, who wear high heels preferentially affecting the third digital nerve. However, multiple Morton's neuromas can be seen in the other intermetatarsal spaces. Clinical assessment includes the thumb index finger test and the Mulder's click. These are specific and sensitive for Morton's neuroma (Quinn et al. 2000).

Ultrasound and MRI are modalities used for diagnosis of Morton's neuromas. US is quick and accurate with 85% to 100% sensitivity (Xu et al. 2015). On ultrasound, imaging is done in the plane parallel to the metatarsals (long-axis plane) and perpendicular to the metatarsals (short-axis plane). The presence of a fusiform hypoechoic mass in the web space between the metatarsal heads, with the interdigital nerve entering and exiting the lesion, confirms the presence of a Morton's neuroma. The sonographic Mulder's sign is performed by squeezing the metatarsal heads after cupping them between the thumb and fingers. The lesion slides plantar to the metatarsal heads, often with a demonstrable click. Intermetatarsal bursitis can co-exist with the neuroma and will be located dorsal to it. The bursa can be compressed on the Mulder's sign or with probe pressure. The size of neuromas range between 3 and 10 mm. For equivocal lesions, MRI is performed. The lesion is of low signal intensity on T1 and T2 (Xu et al. 2015). Enhancement is variable and can be inhomogeneous. Most neuromas smaller than 5 mm are well seen on MRI. In the coronal plane, the mass has a biconcave shape caused by compression of the adjacent structures. This shape is called the Gingko leaf sign. The differential diagnosis includes intermetatarsal bursitis, ganglionic cyst, giant cell tumor of tendon sheath, rheumatoid nodule, fibroma, schwannoma, or other neoplasms. The Morton's neuromas can be asymptomatic and therefore clinical correlation and clinical provocative tests such as Mulder's sign are necessary to make a confident diagnosis (Quinn et al. 2000).

Conservative treatment with change to appropriate shoes and orthotics is often sufficient. In nonresponsive cases, US-guided injection of local anesthetic, steroid, or alcohol can be undertaken to reduce pain (Morgan et al. 2014) (Fig. 6). US-guided steroid injections are cost effective and can reduce pain for 3–9 months. The effects of the injection last longer if undertaken when the size of the lesion is less than 5 mm (in the mediolateral dimension measured in the short-axis plane) (Morgan et al. 2014). Extravasation of injected steroid can cause adjacent fat necrosis and therefore the intralesional localization of the needle tip is important. For refractory cases, US-guided injection of alcohol and local anesthetic is useful to reduce the pain. Ninety-four percent of patients demonstrate reduced pain in 6 months and 74% at 1-year postinjection. At 6 months, there is 30% reduction in size and can be assessed by US. The complications of alcohol injection include extravasation with tissue necrosis and therefore constant dynamic assessment of the fluid being injected into the neuroma is essential (Morgan et al. 2014). The other ultrasound-guided techniques for ablation of the Morton's neuroma are radiofrequency ablation under local anesthetic cover or injection with botulinum. The reported success rate is 85% at 6 months postinjection with RF ablation (Chuter et al. 2013). There are no high-level studies for assessing response to botulinum injections.

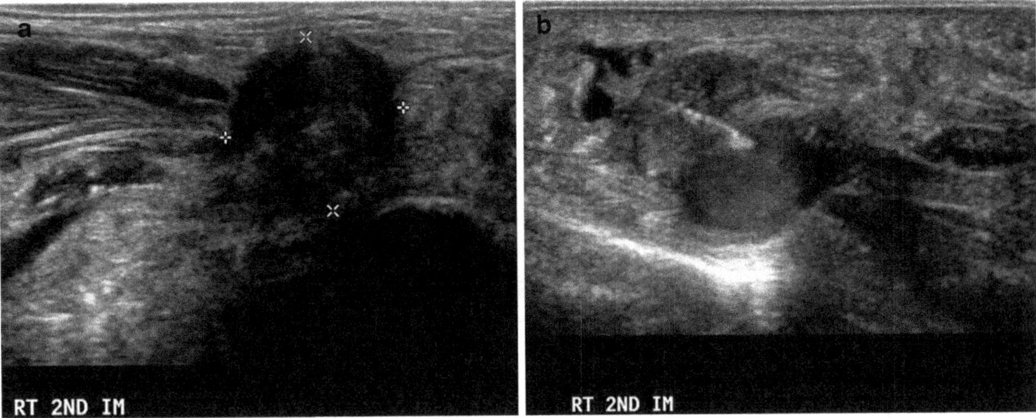

Fig. 6 (**a**) Focused ultrasound at the second intermetatarsal space demonstrates the presence of a Morton's neuroma. (**b**) Subsequent image shows injection of the neuroma with a combination of steroid and local anesthetic

With the patient in the supine position, the Morton's neuroma is injected from the dorsal or plantar aspect at the webspace. The dorsal injection is preferred as it is less painful to enter the skin from this aspect and fat atrophy at the site of injection is avoided if there is any leakage of steroid. Once the lesion is identified with the probe in the long axis of the intermetatarsal space, the needle tip is directed up to the lesion under aseptic technique. A 23 or 25 g needle is used with 1% xylocaine as local anesthesia. One to two milliliter of local anesthetic (bupivacaine) is injected over the surface of the lesion. Under US visualization, the needle tip is directed into the neuroma and the steroid is injected. A 1–1.5 mL mixture of 1 mL of steroid (40 mg mL, e.g., Depo-Medrol) and 0.5% bupivacaine is injected into the Morton's neuroma. One to two milliliter of a similar mixture of steroid and local anesthetic can also be injected into the intermetatarsal bursa if there is bursitis adjacent to the neuroma. The patient is asked to avoid heavy exercises or excessive weight-bearing for a week after the injection and is asked to wear orthotics. A pain diary will help to assess response to the injection. A total of three injections at weekly intervals can be performed, based on the pain response to the steroid injection. The longer acting local anesthetic (bupivacaine) reduces the occurrence of the painful flare response that is occasionally seen with percutaneous steroid injections. There is reduced risk of fat atrophy and skin discoloration with highly soluble steroid (methylprednisolone) which is therefore preferred to larger crystals of steroid (hydrocortisone) (Morgan et al. 2014).

A mixture of 0.1 mL of 100% ethyl alcohol diluted in 0.4 mL of 0.25% bupivacaine (total = 0.5 mL of 20% ethyl alcohol) is used for injection of alcohol into the neuroma under direct ultrasound guidance. The injected material is seen as echogenic filling of the neuroma. Extravasation of alcohol needs to be avoided, and a close watch is necessary while injecting the neuroma, as extravasated alcohol can cause tissue necrosis.

If the Morton's neuroma is unresponsive to the above injections of steroid or local anesthetic, then a surgical excision is often undertaken if the patient is severely symptomatic. Botulinum injection into the Morton's neuroma and radiofrequency ablation are other methods that are now available as an alternative or to non-responding neuromas, before considering surgical excision. Overall, ultrasound is the modality of choice for diagnosis and for image-guided percutaneous ablation of Morton's neuroma.

2.6 Plantar Fasciitis

The commonest cause of heel pain in adults is plantar fasciitis. It affects the plantar fascia at its attachment to the medial tubercle of the calcaneus. Occurrence is similar in males and females and chiefly affects middle aged people, between ages 40 and 60 (Lemont et al. 2003).

The histological diagnosis supports a degenerative rather than inflammatory etiology, with tissue destruction, repair, neovascularity and infiltration of macrophages, plasma cells, and lymphocytes. Altered weight-bearing mechanics including overpronation, flat foot deformity, excessive femoral anteversion, or excessive lateral tibial torsion result in excessive tensile pressure. In athletes, it can occur with overuse. These effects result in chronic thickening with microtears within the fascia, at the medial tubercle attachment, with accompanying enthesophytes commonly seen. The condition is mostly self-limiting lasting 6–12 months. There are a wide variety of treatments for plantar fasciitis. They include conservative treatments such as strengthening and stretching exercise regimens, slowing down activities aggravating the symptoms, using orthotic or in shoe arch supports and night splints. Other forms of treatment include NSAID medications, extracorporeal shock wave therapy, and iontophoresis. Previously steroid injections were undertaken as the etiology of plantar fasciitis was considered to be inflammatory. However, during the past decade, there has been a surge of evidence regarding the interventions and injectables effective for treating plantar fasciitis. Though the quality of the trials is poor, in the few published trials, it was found that steroid injections are effective for the short term, during the first 4 weeks but the symptomatic relief does not persist at 3 months. Moreover, there was lack of consistency in the method of performing this procedure. Some are done blindly by palpating the point of maximum pain and tenderness. Many centers use ultrasound guidance to perform dry needling or PRP injection as treatment for plantar fasciitis (Goff and Crawford 2011). There is lack of evidence on the amount of PRP to be injected, the type of PRP (leucocyte rich or leucocyte poor), the type of centrifuge used for the PRP, volume of injection, and the platelet count. There is some evidence that autologous plasma injection has a good response compared to ESWL. The evidence for botulinum injection is limited. There is no agreement of the most effective surgical method in resistant cases of plantar fasciitis. Under fluoroscopic guidance, fasciotomy can be undertaken. Perineural injection of Baxter's nerve with steroid or radiofrequency are other forms of treatment and can be combined with dry needling and PRP of plantar fasciitis. Drilling or posterior calcaneus osteotomy are the surgical techniques in long standing resistant cases.

The US-guided technique involves identifying the area of plantar fasciitis in the short- or long-axis planes. A linear array or hockey stick can be utilized for the procedure. The entry mark is made on the skin, along the distal most aspect of the heel in the short-axis plane at the level of the thickened abnormal fascia or one finger width distal to the fascial abnormality in the long-axis plane. Taking aseptic precautions, under local anesthesia, a 25-g needle is used for dry needling. One milliliter of 0.5% bupivacaine is injected on the surface of the fascia before needle entry. Using a single point of entry into the fascia, using varying angles, the area of abnormality is fenestrated by gentle to-and-fro movements of the needle tip, under dynamic US guidance (Fig. 7). If PRP is being injected, the needle tip is directed into the area of the tear and then injected. Oftentimes, Baxter's nerve can be tender to palpate and if there are associated neural features, a perineural injection of steroid (1 mL of steroid, e.g., 40 mg/mL Depo-Medrol) can be injected around the nerve immediately deep to the plantar fascia or proximal to its passage deep to the plantar fascia. The post-procedure pain can be reduced if a perineural injection of steroid and local anesthetic is performed. After the dry needling or PRP injection, the patient is informed to avoid vigorous activities using the feet, but all routine tasks can be performed. After 3 weeks, supervised physiotherapy can be undertaken. Hot compresses can be used for post-procedure pain but cold compresses and NSAIDS are avoided as they impede the inflammatory processes which is necessary for healing and regeneration of the plantar fascia.

Injection of steroid around the fascia can result in atrophy of the heel fat and rupture of the

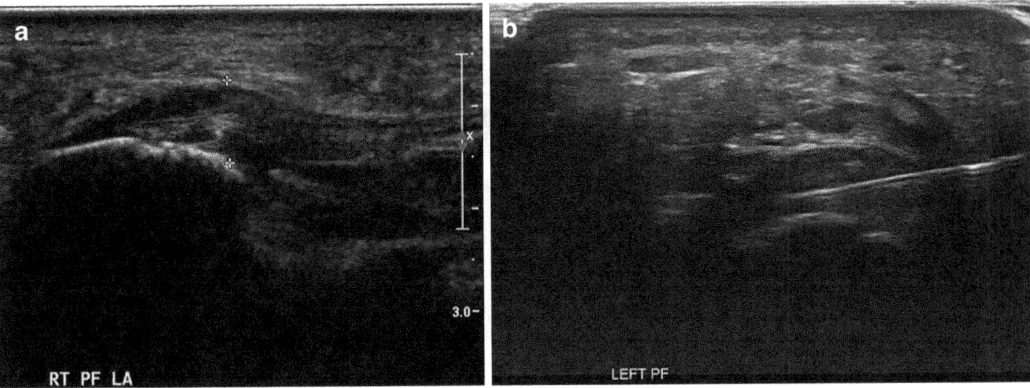

Fig. 7 (**a**) Long-axis ultrasound image demonstrating a thickened and hypoechoic appearance of the plantar fascia in a patient with clinical diagnosis of plantar fasciitis. (**b**) Subsequent image demonstrates ultrasound-guided fenestration of the plantar fascia with needle in long axis

fascia and therefore steroid injections are currently not undertaken, though steroids can provide short-term relief of pain by affecting the inflammatory response.

2.7 Perineural Injections

Ultrasound-guided perineural injections of the foot and ankle are a safe and effective procedure resulting in relief of neural pain from neuritis and relief of nerve entrapment. The common perineural injections include the hallux branch of the medial plantar, sural, superficial and deep peroneal, medial and lateral plantar, posterior tibial, and saphenous nerves.

The structural abnormality is identified using US. The peripheral nerves are clearly visualized in the short access plane as a honeycomb structure with tiny dark dots interspersed between the echogenic connective tissue with an echogenic epineurium. Doppler flow is used to assess vascularity within the nerve and the surrounding echogenic rind of chronic inflammatory perineural area. Nerve impingement by ganglia, hardware, or osteophytes/bony prominences can be easily identified prior to performing the perineural injection. The abnormal nerve will appear thickened, hypoechoic with loss of neurofibrillary appearance and will demonstrate perineural echogenicity (scarring). Once identified, using sterile precautions under local anesthesia, a skin mark is made in the short-axis plane of the nerve, defining the trajectory of the needle. A sterile cover is used with gel overlying the probe, and sterile gel is smeared over the area of the skin surface. High-frequency linear transducers or hockey stick probes are used for the injection. The tip of the 25 g needle is positioned in the immediate vicinity of the nerve under dynamic ultrasound vision. The tip of the needle should be placed adjacent to the echogenic epineurium of the nerve. Short access plane is the best technique for perineural injection. The bevel should face the nerve, and a test injection is performed with a local anesthetic prior to injecting the other injectables. If the patient has pain during the trial injection, the needle tip should be repositioned to obtain optimum injection along the entire surface of the nerve. The injected solution around the nerve is generally a mix of local anesthetic and steroid. A long-acting local anesthetic such as 0.25–0.5% bupivacaine can be used to assess relief of symptoms postinjection. The needle trajectory should be such that the needle is perpendicular to the beam from the transducer for optimum visualization of the needle and its tip. Using sterile saline or local anesthetic, a gentle hydrodissection is performed, using the injectate to separate the surrounding soft tissues from the nerve. The needle tip position can be changed to obtain optimum separation of the nerve from the perineural soft tissues. One mil-

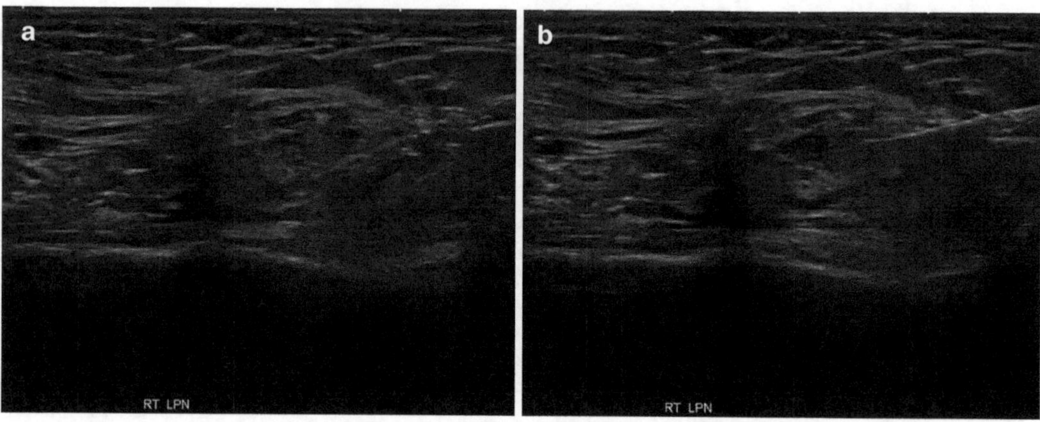

Fig. 8 (**a**) Ultrasound-guided hydrodissection and steroid injection around a thickened and symptomatic lateral plantar nerve with needle direction below (**a**) and above (**b**) the nerve

liliter of steroid can be injected around the nerve (Fig. 8). Alternatively, dextrose can be used for hydrodissection. Perineural PRP injection can also be performed.

The risks from the peripheral nerve injections and the contraindications are similar to other standard MSK interventions. Numbness of the skin is an expected feature postinjection. Weakness is another symptom experienced by patients. However, prolonged nerve blocks and neuropathic symptoms could be related to procedure-related nerve injury and should be dealt with appropriately. Throughout the procedure, entry of the needle tip into the nerve should be avoided to prevent intraneural injection and resultant axonal damage.

Ultrasound has been found to be a very sensitive and specific modality for diagnosis of peripheral neuropathy and for image-guided injection. The use of dynamic imaging techniques, comparison with the opposite side, and using palpation with ultrasound are additional advantages then compared to MRI. Unlike blind injections, targeted injection can be performed around the abnormal nerve and these injections can be easily performed without use of any special needles. The amount of injected material can be optimized and controlled by observing the perineural injection under dynamic ultrasound. A 25-to-27-g needle is most often utilized for the injection. There is still no consensus on whether a circumferential coverage of the nerve with the injected material needs to be obtained. However, this could be easily obtained under ultrasound guidance by gentle needle manipulation.

The various perineural injections in the foot and ankle include injection around the tibial nerve at the tarsal tunnel, medial and lateral plantar nerves, Baxter's nerve, sural nerve, saphenous nerve, and infrequently the deep peroneal nerve. Hydrodissection of these nerves can also be performed in addition to diagnostic and therapeutic blocks (Dellon 1990).

Deep Peroneal Nerve This nerve is best visualized along the anterior aspect of the ankle joint where it is accompanied by the dorsalis pedis artery. Ultrasound-guided injection is used to avoid any vascular injury during the injection. The injection is best performed with the hockey stick probe and the needle in the short-axis plane to the nerve and the artery to enable careful perineural injection around the nerve without injury to the artery (Chang et al. 2020).

Tibial Nerve Entrapment of the tibial nerve within the tarsal tunnel can result in neuropathic symptoms at the medial ankle and the planter foot. This neuropathy could be a result of entrapment from various causes that include scar formation of overlying flexor retinaculum, tenosynovitis, accessory muscles, lipoma, venous engorgement, or ganglionic cyst. If the entrapment is proximal, it could cause neuropathic features of the tibial nerve or affect the medial plantar branch resulting in Jogger's foot. In more distal involvement, the first branch of the lateral plantar nerve (Baxter's nerve) is involved (Chang et al. 2020).

The treatment of tarsal tunnel syndrome could be conservative with anti-inflammatory medication, periods of immobilization, and modification of footwear. Surgical treatment by release of the flexor retinaculum in cases of scar formation or excision of tumors within the tunnel can be undertaken. Aspiration of ganglionic cysts helps relieve compression of the tibial nerve within the tarsal tunnel and is best performed with the nerve and cyst visualized in the short-axis plane on US. The perineural injection of the tibial nerve within the tarsal tunnel is performed with the patient in the lateral decubitus position with the affected side on the table, so the medial aspect of the hindfoot and ankle is accessible. In this position, the nerve is demonstrated posterior to the medial malleolus, posterior to the flexor digitorum longus, and superficial to the flexor hallucis longus tendon. A hockey stick probe is best utilized for this injection, and the needle is constantly visualized during the procedure to avoid injury of the vascular structures. Alternatively, injection can be performed with the patient in the prone position and the foot hanging at the edge of the bed. In this position, the nerve is visualized in the short-axis plane, and the needle entry is from the lateral aspect of the probe. This technique is similar to ultrasound-guided injection of the flexor hallucis longus tendon. Two to three milliliter of injected solution will ensure even spread around the nerve.

If only the medial or lateral plantar nerves are to be injected, these nerves are identified by following the tibial nerve within the proximal tunnel further distally to the bifurcation to identify the individual nerves. The medial plantar nerve is the anterior branch, and the lateral plantar nerve is a posterior branch. The first branch of the lateral plantar nerve is the Baxter's nerve. The injection of these nerves is best undertaken in the short-axis plane using a hockey stick probe.

Sural Nerve Sural neuropathy from entrapment/impingement results in numbness, burning, and pain at the posterolateral aspect of the leg. Causes include trauma from a fibular fracture, following Achilles' tendon repair or total ankle arthroplasty, where there is iatrogenic injury to the nerve. Management can be conservative and includes physiotherapy or image-guided hydrodissection and/or steroid injection. Surgical release of the nerve is undertaken in chronic and recalcitrant cases. The perineural injection could be for diagnostic purposes to assess whether the patient's symptoms respond, to decide on surgical intervention and the hydrodissection can be performed prior to considering open surgical intervention (Tople and Bhuyan 2021). For this purpose, the lateral aspect of the Achilles tendon is evaluated to identify the sural nerve as it courses posterior to the lateral malleolus and posterior to the peroneal tendons. From here it becomes dorsolateral to the foot and is termed the lateral dorsal cutaneous nerve. Identification of the short saphenous vein in the vicinity of the nerve will help to localize the nerve as it is very tiny structure. The patient lies in the lateral decubitus position with the affected site up. Pillows can be used to support the foot and ankle. The nerve is identified in the short-axis plane and under ultrasound vision, the perineural injection is performed using approximately 2 mL of injected solution which could be a combination of steroid and long-acting local anesthetic for therapeutic purposes or a short- and long-acting anesthetic combination for diagnostic purposes.

2.8 Ganglia

Ganglionic cysts are quite common in the foot and are frequently seen along the dorsolateral aspect of the foot arising from the intertarsal and tarsometatarsal joints (Saboeiro and Sofka 2008). The diagnosis is made on ultrasound although the communicating neck with the adjacent joint may not be clearly demonstrated in all cases. Ultrasound-guided aspiration is performed if clinically indicated and for cosmetic purposes. If the cyst cannot be decompressed using a 20–22-g needle, then an 18 g needle can be used for the aspiration as the contents are often too thick and viscous to be aspirated with a small-bore needle. The entry of the needle tip into the ganglionic cyst is well visualized on ultrasound with the probe and the needle in the short- or long-axis planes to the ganglionic cyst. Once it is decompressed, 1 mL of steroid (e.g., Depo-Medrol 40 mg per mL) can be injected into the ganglionic cyst to reduce inflammatory changes within the cyst and adjacent joint. If aspiration is not possible, fenestration of the wall is performed creating multiple holes in the surrounding sheath through which the fluid from the ganglionic cyst can extravasate over time or alternatively, the punctured wall can rupture, discharging its contents into the adjacent soft tissues. The overall management of the ganglionic cyst is similar to other areas in the body, such as the wrist.

2.9 Sinus Tarsi

During moments of inversion and eversion of the hindfoot, the sinus tarsi provides posterior foot stability. It is rich in nerve endings and proprioceptive cells and filled with fat and connective tissue. Sinus tarsi syndrome presents as pain along the anterolateral aspect of the ankle, overlying the entry into the sinus tarsal tunnel (Smith et al. 2015). This pain can be increased with activities such as long periods of standing, running, and walking. There can be associated instability. The exact cause for this syndrome is not understood. The multiple risk factors include traumatic injury with associated ankle ligament tears; 43% of ankle ligament tears were found to be associated with the onset of sinus tarsi syndrome (Saboeiro and Sofka 2008); multiple/repetitive sprains of the ankle and associated ligaments, impingement of the sinus tarsi from the thickened adjacent ligaments or adjacent spurs; generalized joint laxity from hypermobility syndrome or flat feet with pronated foot arch resulting in compression of the sinus tarsi.

Literature has long documented that the gold standard tool used for diagnosis of sinus tarsi syndrome is MRI (Lee et al. 2008). Inflammatory changes are seen on the T2 fat sat sequences within the sinus tarsi with loss of the fat signal within the tunnel on the T1-weighted images. MRI also helps to evaluate the cause for this syndrome by accurately assessing the joints, tendons, and ligaments of the foot for related pathology.

The first treatment approach is generally conservative management. Image-guided injection of steroid and local anesthetic into the sinus tarsi is undertaken if the patient does not respond to conservative treatment. This injection can be performed under fluoroscopy, CT, or ultrasound. Due to the lack of radiation with ultrasound, US-guided injection is gaining more popularity than the other image-guided techniques. Under fluoroscopic vision, direct injection into the sinus tarsi could be followed with injection of 1 mL of steroid and local anesthetic (Fig. 6). The injected solution into this tunnel tracks into the posterior subtalar joint and therefore can be used as an alternative route for injection. Prior to performing the ultrasound-guided injection for this syndrome, the diagnostic ultrasound is performed to detect inflammatory Doppler flow within the tunnel, evaluate for any ganglionic cyst arising from this tunnel, and evaluate for communicating fluid along the entire lateral aspect of the ankle anterior to the lateral malleolus. The fluid could be aspirated before injecting the steroid and local anesthetic. This injection can provide a window for rehabilitation by relieving the pain and facilitating physiotherapy.

The patient lies in a lateral decubitus position, with the side to be injected supported by a pillow. The ultrasound probe is placed anterior to the lateral malleolus. The hockey stick transducer is placed in a coronal oblique plane with the needle entry along the long axis of the transducer. At the point of bulging of the fluid contents from the sinus tarsi, a skin injection using local anesthetic is performed taking strict aseptic precautions. By using out of plane technique and a 22-g needle, the needle tip is tracked into the sinus tarsi. One milliliter of steroid followed by 2 mL of long-acting local anesthetic is injected into the sinus tarsi. The injected material can be seen filling the posterior subtalar joint as this can be used as an alternative technique to inject the posterior subtalar joint, when clinically appropriate.

2.10 Soft Tissue/Bone Biopsies and Foreign Body Removal

This is not dealt with in this chapter as these interventions utilize similar techniques performed at other musculoskeletal bone/soft tissue sites elsewhere in the body.

3 Conclusions

Image-guided musculoskeletal interventions are commonly performed interventions in the Radiology Department. These procedures are most often performed under ultrasound guidance, though some joint injections are undertaken under fluoroscopy. Most procedures are relatively easy to perform with a short learning curve. In this chapter, we have attempted to provide the reader with an overview of most of the musculoskeletal interventions of the foot and ankle. We hope that this will encourage the radiology residents, fellows, new radiologists, and practicing musculoskeletal radiologists to embark on performing these procedures.

References

Asplund CA, Best TM (2013) Achilles tendon disorders. BMJ 346:f1262. https://doi.org/10.1136/bmj.f1262

Bianchi S, Martinoli C (2007) US of the musculoskeletal system. Springer, Berlin

Chang KV, Wu WT, Özçakar L (2020) Ultrasound imaging and guidance in peripheral nerve entrapment: hydrodissection highlighted. Pain Manag 10(2):97–106

Chuter GS, Chua YP, Connell DA, Blackney MC (2013) US-guided radiofrequency ablation in the management of interdigital (Morton's) neuroma. Skeletal Radiol 42:107–111. https://doi.org/10.1007/s00256-012-1527-x

Cole B, Lam P, Hackett L, Murrell G (2018) Ultrasound-guided injections for supraspinatus tendinopathy: corticosteroid versus glucose prolotherapy - a randomized controlled clinical trial. Shoulder Elbow 10(3):170–178. https://doi.org/10.1177/1758573217708199

Dellon AL (1990) Deep peroneal nerve entrapment on the dorsum of the foot. Foot Ankle 11(2):73–80. https://doi.org/10.1177/107110079001100203. PMID: 2265812

Ferrero G, Fabbro E, Orlandi D, Martini C, Lacelli F, Serafini G, Silvestri E, Sconfienza LM (2012) Ultrasound-guided injection of platelet-rich plasma in chronic Achilles and patellar tendinopathy. J Ultrasound 15(4):260–266. https://doi.org/10.1016/j.jus.2012.09.006

Fox MG, Wright PR, Alford B, Patrie JT, Anderson MW (2013) Lateral mortise approach for therapeutic ankle injection: an alternative to the anteromedial approach. AJR Am J Roentgenol 200:1096–1100. https://doi.org/10.2214/AJR.12.9227

Goff JD, Crawford R (2011) Diagnosis and treatment of plantar fasciitis. Am Fam Physician 84:676–682

Hansford BG, Mills MK, Hanrahan CJ, Yablon CM (2019) Pearls and pitfalls of fluoroscopic-guided foot and ankle injections: what the radiologist needs to know. Skeletal Radiol 48(11):1661–1674. https://doi.org/10.1007/s00256-019-03226-9. Epub 2019 May 6. PMID: 31062056

Hassouna H, Singh D (2005) Morton's metatarsalgia: pathogenesis, aetiology and current management. Acta Orthop Belg 71:646–655

James SL, Ali K, Pocock C, Robertson C, Walter J, Bell J et al (2007) US guided dry needling and autologous blood injection for patellar tendinosis. Br J Sports Med 41:518–521.; discussion 522. https://doi.org/10.1136/bjsm.2006.034686

Kakkos GA, Klontzas ME, Koltsakis E, Karantanas AH (2021) US-guided high-volume injection for Achilles tendinopathy. J Ultrason 21(85):e127–e133. https://doi.org/10.15557/JoU.2021.0021

Kearney RS, Parsons N, Metcalfe D, Costa ML (2015) Injection therapies for Achilles tendinopathy. Cochrane Database Syst Rev (5):CD010960. https://doi.org/10.1002/14651858.CD010960.pub2. PMID: 26009861

Kirk KL, Campbell JT, Guyton GP, Schon LC (2008) Accuracy of posterior subtalar joint injection without fluoroscopy. Clin Orthop Relat Res 466:2856–2860. https://doi.org/10.1007/s11999-008-0236-1

Lee KB, Bai LB, Song EK, Jung ST, Kong IK (2008) Subtalar arthroscopy for sinus Tarsi syndrome: arthroscopic findings and clinical outcomes of 33 consecutive cases. Arthroscopy 24(10):1130–1134. https://doi.org/10.1016/j.arthro.2008.05.007

Lemont H, Ammirati KM, Usen N (2003) Plantar fasciitis: a degenerative process (fasciosis) without inflammation. J Am Podiatr Med Assoc 93:234–237. https://doi.org/10.7547/87507315-93-3-234

Lui PP (2015) Stem cell technology for tendon regeneration: current status, challenges, and future research directions. Stem Cells Cloning 8:163–174. https://doi.org/10.2147/SCCAA.S60832

Morgan P, Monaghan W, Richards S (2014) A systematic review of US-guided and non-US-guided therapeutic injections to treat Morton's neuroma. J Am Podiatr Med Assoc 104:337–348. https://doi.org/10.7547/0003-0538-104.4.337

Paoloni JA, Appleyard RC, Nelson J, Murrell GA (2004) Topical glyceryl trinitrate treatment of chronic noninsertional achilles tendinopathy. A randomized, double-blind, placebo-controlled trial. J Bone Joint Surg Am 86-A:916–922

Quinn TJ, Jacobson JA, Craig JG, van Holsbeeck MT (2000) Sonography of Morton's neuromas. AJR Am J Roentgenol 174:1723–1728. https://doi.org/10.2214/ajr.174.6.1741723

Rasmussen S, Christensen M, Mathiesen I, Simonson O (2008) Shockwave therapy for chronic Achilles tendinopathy: a double-blind, randomized clinical trial of efficacy. Acta Orthop 79:249–256. https://doi.org/10.1080/17453670710015058

Riley G (2008) Tendinopathy–from basic science to treatment. Nat Clin Pract Rheumatol 4:82–89. https://doi.org/10.1038/ncprheum0700

Rompe JD, Nafe B, Furia JP, Maffulli N (2007) Eccentric loading, shock-wave treatment, or a wait-and-see policy for tendinopathy of the main body of tendo Achillis: a randomized controlled trial. Am J Sports Med 35:374–383. https://doi.org/10.1177/0363546506295940

Saboeiro GR, Sofka CM (2008) Ultrasound-guided ganglion cyst aspiration. HSS J 4(2):161–163. https://doi.org/10.1007/s11420-008-9079-2

Smith J, Maida E, Murthy NS, Kissin EY, Jacobson JA (2015) Sonographically guided posterior subtalar joint injections via the sinus tarsi approach. J Ultrasound Med 34(1):83–93

Tople J, Bhuyan D (2021) Ultrasound-guided hydrodissection of sural nerve for foot pain-a case report. Authorea Preprints

Wiewiorski M, Valderrabano V, Kretzschmar M, Rasch H, Markus T, Dziergwa S, Kos S, Bilecen D, Jacob AL (2009) CT-guided robotically-assisted infiltration of foot and ankle joints. Minim Invasive Ther Allied Technol 18(5):291–296. https://doi.org/10.1080/13645700903059193. PMID: 19544217

Xu Z, Duan X, Yu X, Wang H, Dong X, Xiang Z (2015) The accuracy of ultrasonography and magnetic resonance imaging for the diagnosis of Morton's neuroma: a systematic review. Clin Radiol 70:351–358. https://doi.org/10.1016/j.crad.2014.10.017

Yelland MJ, Del Mar C, Pirozzo S, Schoene ML (2004) Prolotherapy injections for chronic low back pain: a systematic review. Spine (Phila Pa 1976) 29:2126–2133. https://doi.org/10.1097/01.brs.0000141188.83178.b3

Part II

Clinical Problems

Congenital and Developmental Disorders of the Foot and Ankle

Timothy Shao Ern Tan,
Eu Leong Harvey James Teo,
and Wilfred C. G. Peh

Contents

T. S. E. Tan · E. L. H. J. Teo (✉)
Department of Diagnostic and Interventional Imaging, KK Women's and Children's Hospital, Singapore, Singapore
e-mail: timothy.tan.shao.ern@doctors.org.uk; Harvey.teo.e.l@singhealth.com.sg

W. C. G. Peh
Department of Diagnostic Radiology, Khoo Teck Puat Hospital, Singapore, Singapore
e-mail: Wilfred.peh@gmail.com

Med Radiol Diagn Imaging (2023)
https://doi.org/10.1007/174_2023_400,
Published Online: 12 April 2023

Abstract

Congenital and developmental conditions affecting the foot and ankle are not commonly encountered but can result in significant disabling deformities if not diagnosed and treated in a timely manner. Imaging evaluation of these disorders complements clinical findings and provides critical information to guide orthopedic treatment. Radiographs are frequently performed as the initial imaging modality for pediatric foot and ankle disorders. However, radiographic interpretation can be challenging due to varied imaging presentations at different ages, even between patients of the same age and between males and females. Furthermore, bones of the foot become radiographically visible at different stages of development, confounding evaluation of osseous relationships and alignment. This chapter aims to address these challenges by discussing normal developmental bony anatomy, normal bony variants of the foot, and alignment relationships. Congenital and developmental abnormalities are also discussed, ranging from disorders of foot alignment, such as hindfoot valgus/varus, to structural deformities of the ankle, foot, and toes, including ball-and-socket ankle, clubfoot, cavus deformity, multiple types of flatfoot (including tarsal coalition), and metatarsus adductus. Some important skeletal dysplasias are also described. Where relevant, the role of further cross-sectional imaging evaluation (e.g., computed tomography and magnetic resonance imaging) is highlighted.

1 Introduction

The foot and ankle are affected by a myriad of congenital and developmental disorders, which are not commonly encountered in routine radiological practice. Some of these conditions can result in longstanding disabling deformities which impair normal function and quality of life, such as immobility resulting from rigid flatfoot and untreated clubfoot, as well as limb-length discrepancy and chronic osteoarthrosis resulting from congenital diastasis of the inferior tibiofibular joint and ball-and-socket ankle. Sound knowledge of these conditions will therefore aid in timely diagnosis, and in turn, provide essential information to guide orthopedic treatment.

Radiographs remain the initial imaging modality for evaluating many of these conditions. However, to interpret foot and ankle radiographs accurately, a thorough knowledge of the normal variants affecting this area is also required, with close attention to those that may mimic or obscure pathology. A clear understanding of normal foot and ankle alignment is also useful in the analysis of malalignment deformities. In recent years, advanced cross-sectional imaging has increasingly been utilized to complement radiographs and clinical findings, with magnetic resonance imaging (MRI) being at the forefront of musculoskeletal imaging. These cross-sectional imaging modalities are useful in evaluating soft tissue and chondro-osseous structures to delineate disease extent, complications, and for preoperative planning with the aim of improving patient care. Moreover, as foot and ankle malformations may sometimes be the first presentation of a serious systemic disease, radiologists also play an important role in directing further investigations for definitive diagnosis.

This chapter describes normal development, bony variants, and congenital and developmental disorders related to the foot and ankle in children. The assessment of foot alignment, which can be applied to structural deformities of the foot, including clubfoot, cavus deformity, and types of flatfoot (including tarsal coalition), is also discussed.

2 Bony Anatomy of the Foot and Ankle

The ankle joint consists of the distal tibia, distal fibula, and talus and is stabilized by multiple ligaments and tendons, forming a hinge joint allowing dorsiflexion and plantar flexion. The talocalcaneal articulation comprised of the posterior, middle, and anterior subtalar joints, with the posterior joint being the largest. The sustentaculum tali is a prominent bony projection arising from the medial aspect of the calcaneus which supports the middle talar articular facet. The anterior calcaneal facet may or may not be continuous with the middle facet. The medial and lateral (posterior) tubercles and medial and lateral facets of the talus articulate with the medial and lateral malleoli, respectively. The ankle joint includes anterior and posterior recesses which communicate with the posterior subtalar and talocalcaneonavicular joints.

The foot can be divided into three units: hindfoot, midfoot, and forefoot. Knowledge of the anatomy of these units is essential to understanding foot function, biomechanics, and pathophysiology. The hindfoot is composed of the talus and calcaneus, the forefoot comprised of the metatarsals and phalanges, while the midfoot includes the intervening tarsal bones: the cuneiforms, navicular, and cuboid. The foot performs various biomechanical functions, including weight-bearing, shock absorption, and propulsion during walking and running, as well as accommodating uneven surfaces.

The anatomical relationship of the tarsal bones changes during development. Notably, the talocalcaneal angle gradually decreases with growth as the talus becomes less vertical, as indicated by a decrease in the lateral talocalcaneal angle from 45° on average in the newborn to 33° at the age of 4 years (Vanderwilde et al. 1988). The dorsiflexion-plantar flexion range of the foot also decreases with age, for example, from 76° at birth to 60° at 1 year of age.

3 Ossification of the Foot Bones

The cartilaginous structures that form the bones of the foot typically develop around the seventh to ninth week of gestation. Often, by the fifth intrauterine week, embryological differentiation of the foot occurs where tarsal bone anlage forms and culminates in condensation of the mesenchymal tissue. Following this, tissue differentiation to pre-cartilage and cartilage occurs, and all skeletal elements of the foot begin to chondrify by 7 weeks, except for the distal phalanx of the little toe. Homogenous interzones develop at the ankle and between all tarsal, tarsometatarsal, metatarsophalangeal, and interphalangeal joints. The three-layered interzone develops earliest at the ankle and metatarsophalangeal joints at the end of the embryonic period (8 weeks). Cavitation of the interzone to form vascularized synovial tissue is seen in most joints of the foot at 9–11 weeks, beginning first at the ankle and progresses distally, forming last in the interphalangeal joints. By the end of the embryonic period (8 weeks), the foot resembles that of the adult in most details, and the articular surfaces of the ankle joint and other joints of the foot are highly differentiated before the resorption phase of the interzone (Hammer and Pai 2015).

The foot ossifies in a sequential manner, starting in the forefoot with the metatarsal epiphyses, followed by the metatarsal shafts and subsequently, the proximal, middle, and distal phalanges. The metatarsals grow at both ends from cartilaginous physes but only have epiphyses and secondary ossification centers at one end. The epiphysis of the first metatarsal is at the proximal end of the bone, while those of the second to fifth metatarsals are located distally. An epiphysis is also frequently present at the tubercle of the base of the fifth metatarsal. Ossification of the metatarsal shafts begin around the eighth to tenth week of gestation; with the second and third metatarsals ossifying first, followed by the fourth and fifth metatarsal, and the first metatarsal being the last to ossify. The metatarsal epiphyses ossify in the third to fifth years of life, with the epiphysis of the base of the first metatarsal ossifying first. The metatarsal epiphyses are expected to unite with the shafts between 17 and 20 years of age.

The phalanges are ossified from two centers: a primary one for the shaft and an epiphysis for the base. The phalangeal shaft centers ossify and are radiologically apparent in the fetal period, first in the distal phalanges (8th week), then in the proximal phalanges (between 12th and 16th weeks), and lastly in the middle phalanges (after the 16th week). Epiphyseal centers of the phalanges ossify and become apparent on radiographs in the third to fifth years, and subsequently unite with the shafts at around 17 and 18 years (Shapiro 2019).

The tarsal bones ossify later, around 24–28 weeks of gestation, each from a single center, except the calcaneus which has a posterior epiphysis. The calcaneus is the first tarsal bone to ossify, with the main calcaneal ossification center formed endochondrally, starting from 6 months gestation. The posterior calcaneal apophysis forms between 6 and 10 years of age, fusing by 17 years. Next, intrauterine ossification of the talus occurs via the endochondral mechanism, beginning in males at 7 months. In females, this may occur a few weeks earlier. The ossification center forms near the geometric center of the talus, also known as the centric ossification center. The endochondral center then joins a layer of periosteal bone in the tarsal canal. The cuboid ossifies next from a single nucleus, shortly before birth in females and after birth in males. The other tarsals ossify postnatally: lateral cuneiform in the first year, medial cuneiform in the third year, middle cuneiform in the fourth year, and navicular by the fourth year. Ossification of the sustentaculum tali only begins around the age of 1–2 years and is not fully developed until age of 5 years (Vallejo and Jaramillo 2001) (Fig. 1). Cartilage canals contain blood vessels that are found in the hyaline cartilage prior to the formation of a secondary ossification center. Cartilage canals form first in the talus and calcaneus, followed by other tarsal bones.

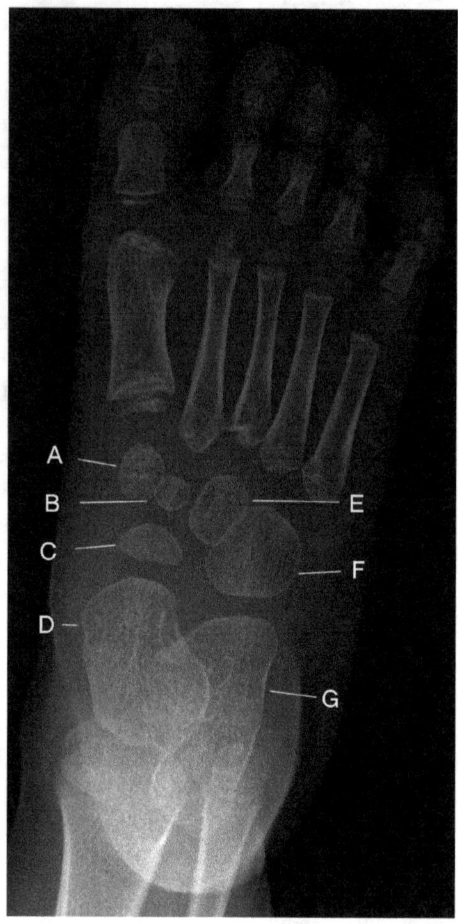

Fig. 1 AP foot radiograph of a 3-year-old boy shows developing ossification centers in the medial (A), middle (B) and lateral (E) cuneiforms, and the navicular (C), talus (D), cuboid (F), and calcaneus (G). The epiphyses of the digits are proximally located in the phalanges. The epiphysis of the first metatarsal is also proximally located but the epiphyses of the second to fifth metatarsals are distally located

Intrauterine feet are proportionally long compared to the whole body, with the foot's length comprising one-third of its final foot length (DiMeglio 2001). From infancy to the age of 5 years, the foot grows rapidly, as much as about 24 mm in length yearly between ages 1 and 3 years, and slowing to about 12 mm in length yearly between ages 3 and 5 years, thereby reaching about one-half its adult size. The primary linear growth then slows further exponentially in both gender to about 8–10 mm in length yearly between ages of 5 and 12 years. During this period, foot length in males is on average 2 mm longer than in females. Growth ceases at about age 12–13 years in girls and 13–15 years in boys, when the foot is considered mature, with the foot length comprising about 15% of body height (Barisch-Fritz and Mauch 2021).

4 Bony Normal Variants of the Foot and Ankle

There are various bony normal variants found in the foot and ankle, including sesamoid bones and accessory ossicles (Mellado et al. 2003). Sesamoid bones arise within a tendon in the metatarsal and phalangeal regions and function by protecting the tendon and providing mechanical advantage to the tendon (Sarin et al. 1999). Common sesamoids in the foot include the hallux sesamoids, lesser metatarsal sesamoids, and interphalangeal sesamoids (Nwawka et al. 2013). Accessory ossicles, also known as supernumerary bones, are usually derived from unfused accessory ossification centers. More than 30 accessory ossicles have been described in this region. The significant ones are discussed below.

Although sesamoids and accessory ossicles are frequently asymptomatic, they can result in degenerative changes, stress, and painful syndromes due to impingement of adjacent soft tissues. They may also simulate fractures, hence recognizing their characteristic appearances and location on imaging helps avoid misdiagnosis of a fracture or other injury. Generally, fracture margins appear poorly corticated, whereas accessory ossicles and their bipartite/multipartite variants are well-corticated. Old avulsion injuries, which appear as well-corticated, round ossific fragments in a similar location, may resemble and be confused with accessory bones and vice versa. In doubtful cases, a comparison radiograph of the contralateral foot may be helpful although this can be confounded by variability in bilateralism. Follow-up radiographs may also demonstrate callus formation in fractures. Ultrasonography (US) can be used to identify non-ossified or cartilaginous accessory bones and to evaluate associated soft tissue inflammation or injury (Nwawka et al. 2013). Computed tomography (CT) is useful for delineating fractures, especially in cases where early surgical management is crucial (Yan et al. 2016). MRI provides additional information such as marrow edema and associated soft tissue injuries. Technetium (Tc)-99m bone scan shows radioisotope uptake within 24 h of a fracture and is a highly sensitive but not specific modality.

The more common accessory ossicles in the foot and ankle are the (1) os trigonum, (2) os supranaviculare, (3) os peroneum, (4) os tibiale externum, now commonly known as the accessory navicular, and (5) os intermetatarseum, which are discussed in further detail below. Other less encountered accessory ossicles include the os calcaneus secundarius, adjacent to the anterior calcaneal process; os subfibulare, distal to the tip of the lateral malleolus; os subtibiale, inferior to the medial malleolus; os vesalianum, in close contact with the inferolateral border of the fifth metatarsal base; and the os intercuneiform, located in between the medial and intermediate cuneiforms, anterior to the navicular bone.

The growth plates or physes of the distal tibia and fibula often appear irregular and fragmented, manifesting as discrete ossific densities adjacent to the physis (Love et al. 1990). They are likely to be due to irregularity at the zone of provisional calcification. This appearance has been described as a fibular ossicle and should not be mistaken as a fracture in the absence of a radiographically apparent joint effusion (Fig. 2). A focal superiorly oriented notch at the medial aspect of the distal tibial physis is normal and is known as Kump's bump.

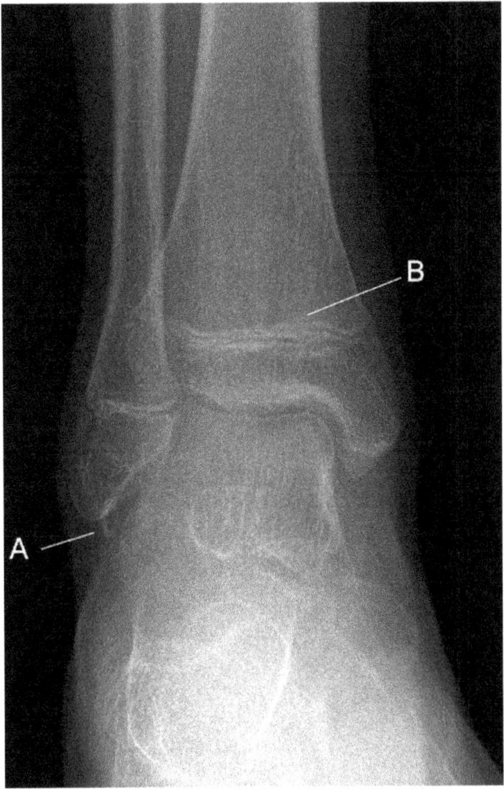

Fig. 2 AP ankle radiograph of a 13-year-old boy shows a small rounded corticated density distal to the tip of the lateral malleolus; os subfibulare (A) and a superiorly oriented notch at the medial distal tibial physis; Kump's bump (B)

4.1 Sesamoids

The two sesamoids at the plantar surface of the first metatarsal head are present in almost all individuals, while single sesamoid bones at the other four metatarsal heads are very rare. The most common variation of the hallux sesamoid complex is the bipartite hallux sesamoid with a prevalence of 16.5% (Karadaglis and Grace 2003) (Fig. 3). The medial hallux sesamoid is more commonly injured due to its position directly plantar to the first metatarsal head (Biedert and Hintermann 2003). Fractures of the hallux sesamoids can closely mimic appearances of normal bipartite/multipartite variations but can be distinguished from normal variants by its irregular edges, increased separation of the parts, or evidence of comminution (Boike et al. 2011).

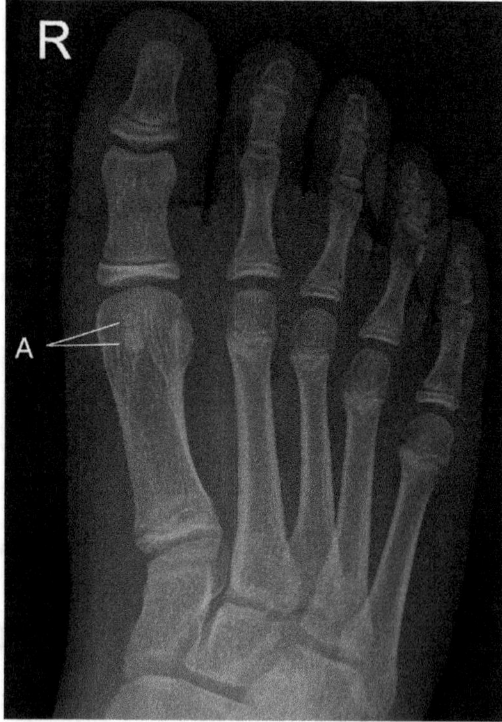

Fig. 3 AP foot radiograph of a 12-year-old boy shows two sesamoids at the plantar surface of the first metatarsal head, consistent with a bipartite medial hallux sesamoid (A). Note the smooth well-corticated margins of both components

4.2 Os Trigonum

The posterior tubercle of the talus is sometimes ossified from an independent center and may remain connected to the rest of the bone by cartilage, termed as the os trigonum. This is the most common accessory ossicle with a prevalence of up to 25% and is seen close to the posterior inferior border of the talus on lateral radiographs (Kose et al. 2006). The os trigonum syndrome refers to acute or chronic pain centered on the os trigonum that is usually caused by forced plantar hyperflexion, occurring in individuals who participate in intense physical activities such as downhill running (Escobedo et al. 2006). Soft tissue swelling and fat stranding surrounding the os trigonum on lateral radiographs are suggestive of the syndrome and may be accompanied with bony hypertrophy of the os trigonum after repeated trauma (Karasick and Schweitzer 1996). Cross-sectional imaging is useful in delineating fractures of the os trigonum, as well as degeneration at the synchondrosis and associated joint synovitis and/or features of flexor hallucis longus (FHL) tenosynovitis (Wong and Tan 2016) (Fig. 4). MRI is the single most useful imaging modality in evaluating for the os trigonum syndrome, evidenced by the presence of bone marrow edema around the synchondrosis, fluid within or joint effusion, or signs of soft tissue involvement, such as edema in surrounding structures or presence of FHL tenosynovitis. A bipartite os trigonum, os trigonum fracture, and posterior talar process fracture may appear very similar on radiographs, and distinction needs to be made between these entities as the fracture may require surgical intervention.

4.3 Accessory Navicular

The accessory navicular (os naviculare) ossifies around the age of 7–11 years (Miller et al. 1995) and appears radiographically as a pea-sized accessory bone adjacent to the medial border of the navicular bone, often at the tibialis posterior muscle tendon insertion site. It is the second most common accessory ossicle with a prevalence of

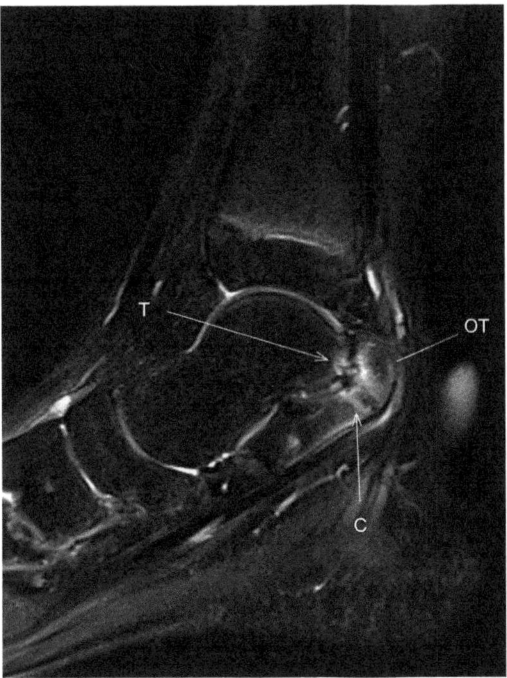

Fig. 4 Sagittal fat-suppressed T2-weighted MR image of a 7-year-old boy shows hyperintense marrow signal within the os trigonum (OT) and around the synchondrosis involving the talus (T) and calcaneum (C). Along with focal tenderness in this region, findings are in keeping with the os trigonum syndrome

4–21% (Mellado et al. 2003), and 50–90% are found bilaterally (Nwawka et al. 2013).

Three subtypes are recognized based on the configuration. The type 1 accessory navicular, also known as os tibiale externum or naviculare secundarium, is a 2–6 mm round or oval ossicle that is separate from and positioned about 2–5 mm proximal to the navicular body, representing a sesamoid bone within the posterior tibial tendon. It accounts for about 30% of accessory naviculars and is often asymptomatic (Hammer and Pai 2015). The type 2 accessory navicular is referred to as the pre-hallux or bifurcated hallux and accounts for up to 70% of accessory naviculars (Fig. 5). It is larger than the type 1 accessory navicular and forms a facet with the medial proximal navicular tubercle, giving rise to a triangular ossicle. Injury to the type 2 accessory navicular can result in fracture and secondary pseudarthrosis of the synchondrosis, or painful tendinosis or synovitis in older children, also known as the accessory navicular syndrome (Bennett et al. 1990). These injuries are difficult to diagnose on radiographs and are better evaluated on MRI, where there is abnormal marrow edema within the accessory navicular and navicular tubercle (with increased fluid signal in the synchondrosis), soft tissue changes, and distal posterior tibialis tendinosis. The type 3 accessory navicular or cornuate navicular is a prominent tuberosity contiguous with the medial margin of the navicular, which may result from osseous bridging of a previously separate center (Nwawka et al. 2013), it occasionally causes symptoms as a result of painful bunion formation over the bony protuberance.

4.4 Os Supranaviculare

The os supranaviculare appears as a well-corticated bony fragment at the proximal dorsal aspect of the navicular with an estimated prevalence of up to 3.5%. It typically fuses by about 5 years of age (Guo et al. 2019) (Fig. 6). The os supranaviculare can be misdiagnosed as an avulsion fracture of the navicular or talar head, in the context of trauma. Appearance of a thin flake of bone with adjacent soft tissue swelling favors a diagnosis of fracture. Rarely, the os supranaviculare can cause dorsal foot pain, requiring surgical resection (Mellado et al. 2003).

4.5 Os Peroneum

The os peroneum is radiographically evident in its ossified form in up to 9% of the population. It lies within the peroneus longus tendon, posterior to the base of the fifth metatarsal and underneath the cuboid. About 30% are bipartite, and 60% present bilaterally (Guo et al. 2019) (Fig. 7). A bipartite os peroneum can simulate a fracture with its slight irregular appearance. The os peroneum can cause lateral pain and tenderness along the peroneus longus tendon course, particularly with resisted plantar flexion (Oh et al. 2012) and is also known as the os peroneum syndrome. Acute pain may result from rupture of the pero-

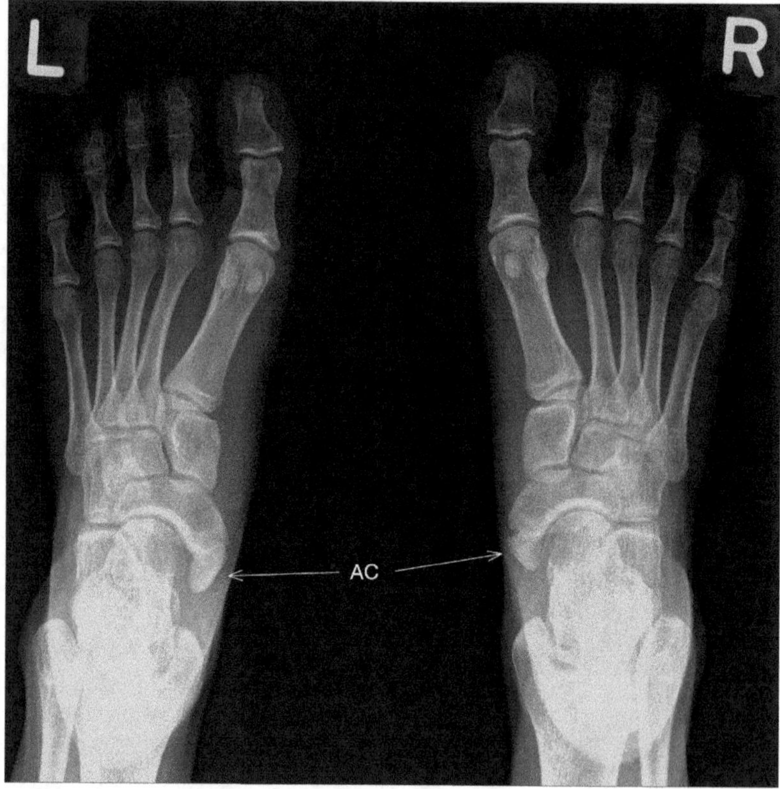

Fig. 5 Bilateral AP foot radiograph of a 15-year-old boy shows bilateral symmetrical triangular ossicles forming a facet with the medial proximal navicular tubercles, consistent with bilateral type 2 accessory naviculars (AC)

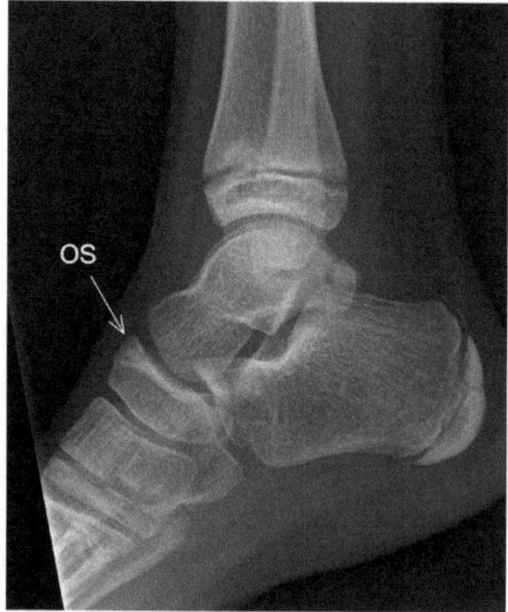

Fig. 6 Lateral ankle radiograph of a 11-year-old girl shows a corticated bony fragment at the proximal dorsal aspect of the navicular, consistent with os supranaviculare (OS)

neus longus tendon or os peroneum fracture, while chronic pain may be caused by attrition of the peroneus longus tendon or diastasis of a multipartite os peroneum (Chagas-Neto et al. 2016).

4.6 Os Intermetatarseum

The os intermetatarseum is commonly located between the bases of the first and second metatarsals, with an estimated prevalence of 1.2–10% (Mellado et al. 2003). On radiographs, it can appear ovoid, round, or spindle-shaped, and may either be seen as a completely independent ossicle, forming a synovial joint with the first or second metatarsal or medial cuneiform, or fused with adjacent bones, forming a bony spur (Fig. 8). The os intermetatarseum may be fractured during injury or compress the superficial or deep peroneal nerves, causing dorsal midfoot pain at the first intermetatarsal space (Miller 2002). An os intermetatarseum may be distinguished from second metatarsal base fractures as seen in Lisfranc

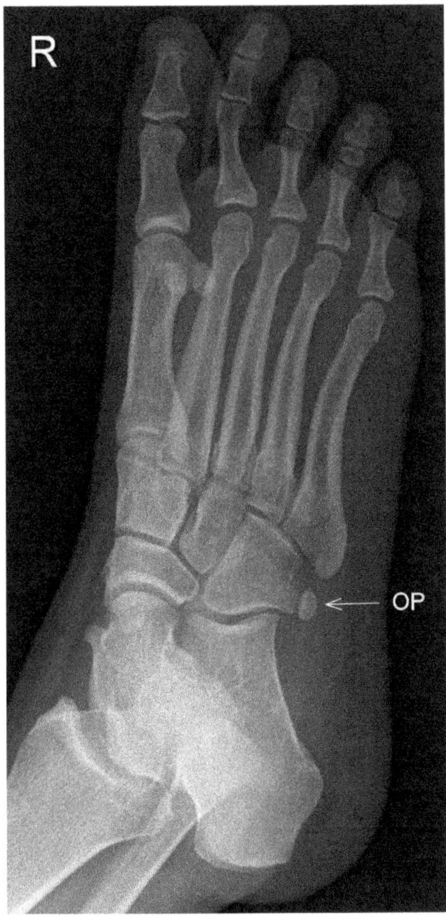

Fig. 7 Oblique foot radiograph of a 15-year-old boy shows a bean-shaped corticated density located posterior to the base of the fifth metatarsal and underneath the cuboid, consistent with os peroneum (OP)

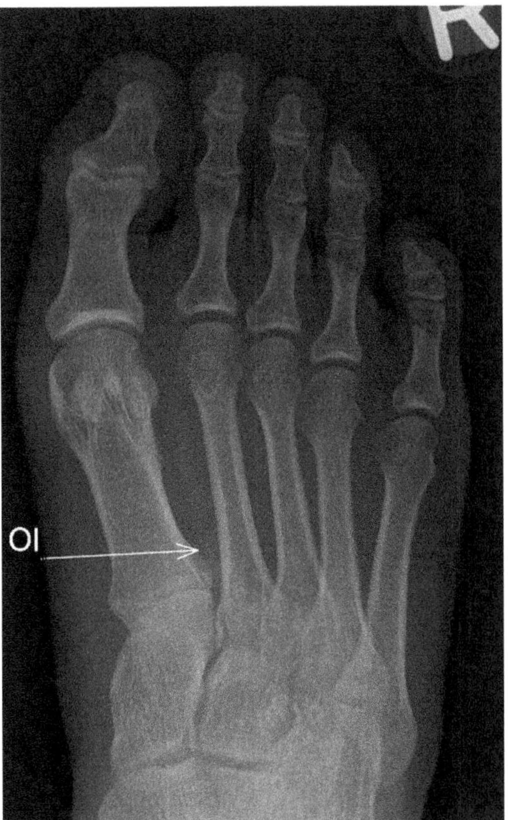

Fig. 8 AP foot radiograph of a 17-year-old boy shows a spindle-shaped corticated density located between the first and second metatarsal bases, consistent with an os intermetatarseum (OI)

injuries by the presence of bony malalignment and soft tissue swelling in the latter (Nwawka et al. 2013).

4.7 Calcaneal Apophysis

The calcaneal apophysis is the insertion site for the Achilles tendon and serves as an origin for the plantar aponeurosis and short intrinsic foot muscles. The apophysis acts as a pivot for combined tractional and compressional forces during gait. The posterior cortical margin of the calcaneus initially appears smooth in infants and young children and eventually becomes irregular with a sawtooth outline before ossification centers for the apophysis appear. The calcaneal apophyseal centers appear between 4 and 7 years of age in girls and between 7 and 10 years in boys. Often, the normal ossification centers are dense and more sclerotic than the calcaneal body on lateral radiographs (Fig. 9). Adolescents may encounter heel pain during rapid growth of the calcaneal tubercle, where a sclerotic and irregular calcaneal apophysis may be seen on radiographs, possibly in response to weight-bearing. The apophysis fuses at the age of 12–15 years, and the posterior calcaneal margin becomes isodense to the rest of the bone (Hammer and Pai 2015).

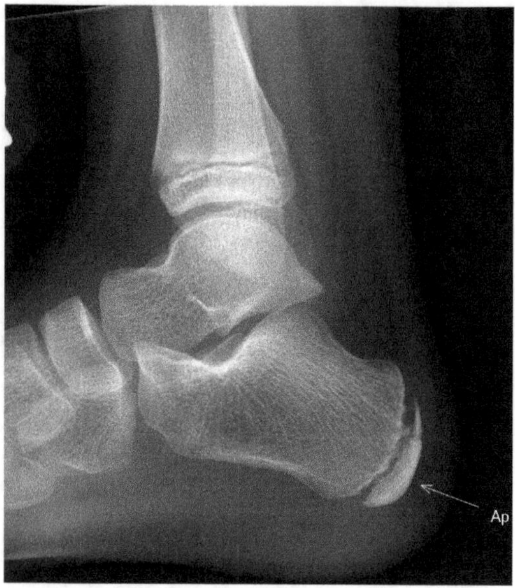

Fig. 9 Lateral radiograph of an 8-year-old boy shows the calcaneal apophysis (Ap) and its normal ossification center, characteristically appearing more sclerotic than the calcaneal body

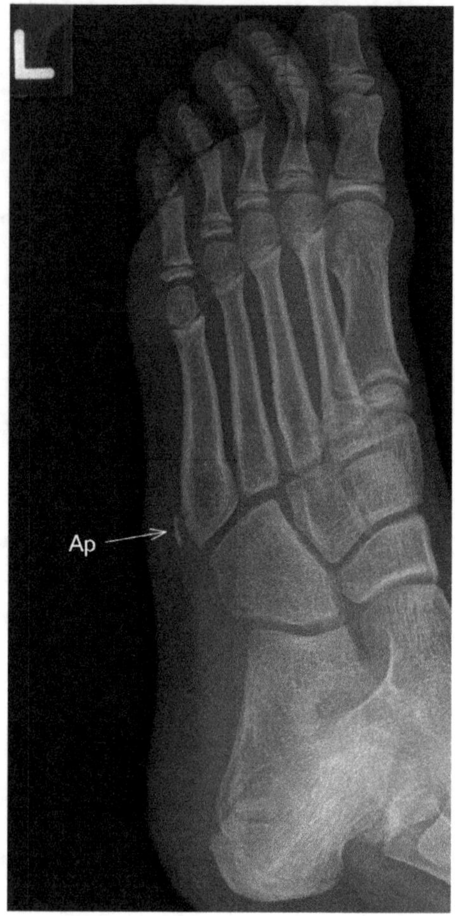

Fig. 10 Oblique foot radiograph of a 12-year-old boy shows a fifth metatarsal base apophysis (Ap). It is recognized by its longitudinal and parallel orientation to the axis of the metatarsal, differentiating it from a fracture, which shows a transverse or oblique orientation

4.8 Fifth Metatarsal Base Apophysis

This secondary ossification center develops at about 12 years of age and usually parallels the lateral cortex of the fifth metatarsal. Normally, it fuses by the age of 16 years, but can continue into adulthood as a persistent apophysis or os vesalianum. On radiographs, the fifth metatarsal base apophysis is present bilaterally and appears symmetrical. It can be differentiated from base of fifth metatarsal fractures, as the apophysis or os vesalianum is always aligned longitudinally and parallel to the axis of the metatarsal (Strayer et al. 1999) (Fig. 10), whereas most fractures are oriented in a transverse or oblique direction. Identifying the apophysis on the contralateral foot can also be helpful in distinguishing a persistent apophysis from a fracture.

4.9 Epiphyseal Variants

In about half of the general population, there is fusion of the distal interphalangeal joint of the fifth toe, resulting in two phalanges. The epiphyses of the proximal phalanges are frequently cone-shaped, possibly attributed to premature closure of the central physis (Fig. 11a). A bifid epiphysis may appear at the proximal phalanx of the first toe due to incomplete ossification. The proximal epiphyses of other toes may also be affected. Pseudoepiphyses may be seen at the metatarsal bases and at the distal aspects of the phalanges (Fig. 11b).

A longitudinal epiphyseal bracket is a rare entity where the normally transverse epiphysis is C-shaped and oriented along the longitudinal edge of the bone, due to abnormal fusion of the proximal and distal epiphyses (Fig. 11c). In turn, this causes abnormal transverse growth, phalan-

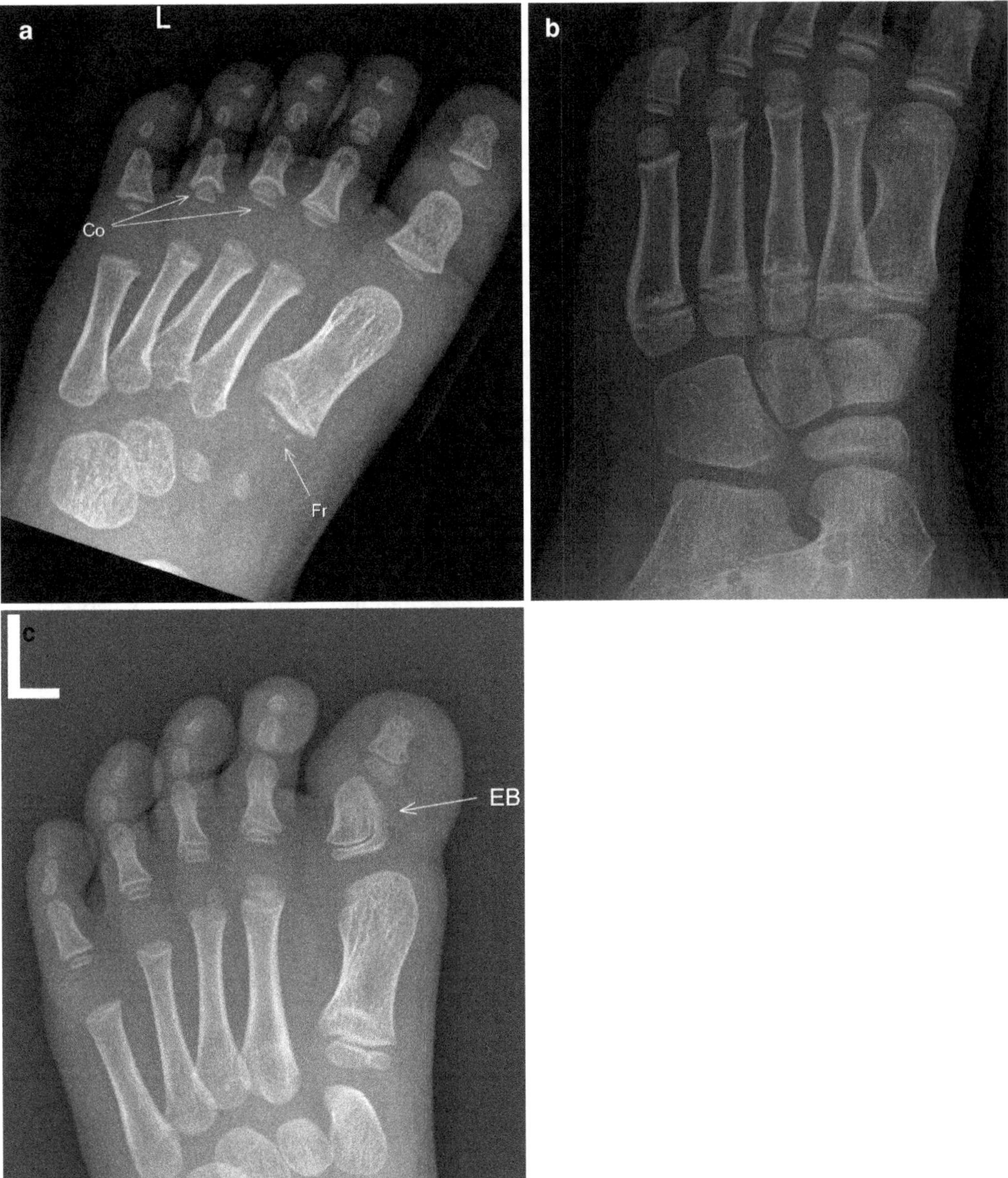

Fig. 11 (**a**) AP foot radiograph of a 2-year-old boy shows cone-shaped epiphysis in the proximal phalanges of the third and fourth toes (Co). The epiphysis of the first metatarsal appears fragmented which is a normal appearance in the initial stages of epiphyseal ossification (Fr). (**b**) Oblique foot radiograph in another patient shows pseudo-epiphyses in the second to fifth metatarsal bases. (**c**) AP foot radiograph of a 2-year-old boy shows a longitudinal epiphyseal bracket (EB), whereby the normally transverse epiphysis is C-shaped and oriented along the longitudinal edge of the bone

geal shortening, and angular deformity. About 11% of cases involve the first toe (Schreck 2006). Surgical resection is often required (Mahboubi and Davidson 1999).

5 Alignment of the Foot and Ankle

The alignment of the ankle, hindfoot, midfoot, and forefoot is best evaluated separately, although they are intimately related, both anatomically and functionally. Varus and valgus deformities may occur at the hindfoot, while cavus and planus deformities occur at the midfoot. Forefoot deformities are related to adduction and abduction. Inversion and eversion are complex motions involving most of the foot around a stationary talus and usually occur at the intertarsal joints. Normal angular relationships for the hindfoot and forefoot are presented in Table 1.

5.1 Hindfoot

Hindfoot alignment may be assessed by analyzing the talocalcaneal relationship on standard anteroposterior (AP) and lateral foot radiographs. Lines are drawn along the central axes of the talus and calcaneus, and the intersection of these lines forms the talocalcaneal angle, which should be between 30° and 45° on weight-bearing radiographs and decreases with age and development. In a normally aligned foot, the long axis of the calcaneus should intersect through the fourth metatarsal base and the talar long axis should pass through or slightly medial to the first metatarsal base on the AP radiograph while a line drawn along the long axis of the talus on a lateral radiograph should align with the long axis of the first metatarsal (the Meary's angle).

5.2 Midfoot

There are ligamentous connections between the midfoot bones and the calcaneus but not between the midfoot bones and the talus. As such, an abnormal calcaneal position relative to the talus would be evident by a change in the relation of the midfoot bones to those of the hindfoot. The navicular, when ossified, is commonly seen immediately distal to the middle portion of the talar head on both AP and lateral projections. Any change in position would indicate an abnormal

Table 1 Normal angular relationships for the hindfoot and forefoot measured on radiographs

Angle	Newborn	2 years	4 years	6 years	9 years
AP view					
Talocalcaneal	42° (27–56)°	40° (27–50)°	34° (24–45)°	30° (20–40)°	18° (5–35)°
Calcaneal-fifth MT	3° (−9 to +14)°	0° (−10 to +10)°	−1° (−10 to +8)°	0° (−10 to +8)°	3° (−8 to +15)°
Talar-first MT	20° (+12 to +31)°	15° (+2 to +27)°	10° (−4 to +23)°	7° (−7 to +20)°	4° (−9 to +17)°
Lateral view					
Talocalcaneal	39° (23–55)°	41° (27–56)°	44° (31–57)°	44° (33–56)°	40° (28–52)°
Talocalcaneal in dorsiflexion	45° (35–56)°	44° (33–54)°	43° (32–52)°	42° (31–51)°	41° (31–51)°
Tibiocalcaneal	77° (60–95)°	72° (57–87)°	68° (56–81)°	67° (58–76)°	68° (63–74)°
Tibiocalcaneal in dorsiflexion	42° (25–60)°	48° (27–68)°	50° (30–72)°	51° (33–71)°	50° (33–71)°
Tibiotalar	115° (86–145)°	114° (95–130)°	113° (100–122)°	111° (101–118)°	108° (89–123)°
Talar-first MT (Meary's angle)	18° (−2 to +44)°	12° (−4 to +28)°	8° (−5 to +22)°	7° (−5 to +18)°	7° (−7 to +20)°
Talar-horizontal	34° (14–55)°	32° (18–45)°	30° (20–40)°	26° (20–36)°	25° (13–35)°

Adapted from Vanderwilde et al. (1988) and Hammer and Pai (2015)

[a] *MT* metatarsal

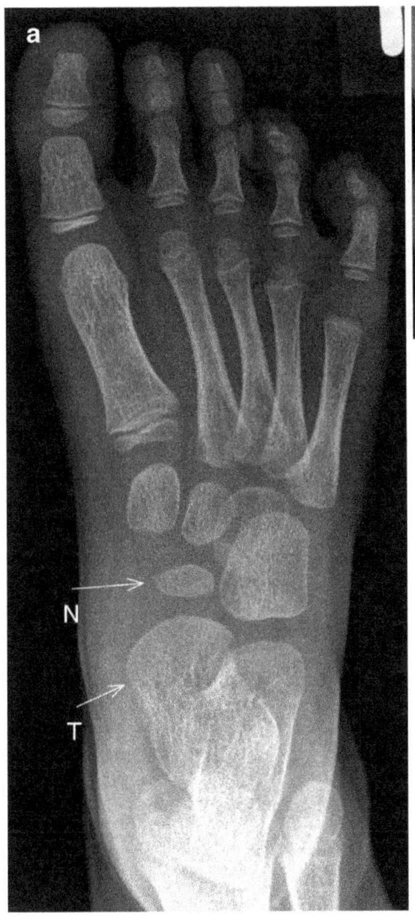

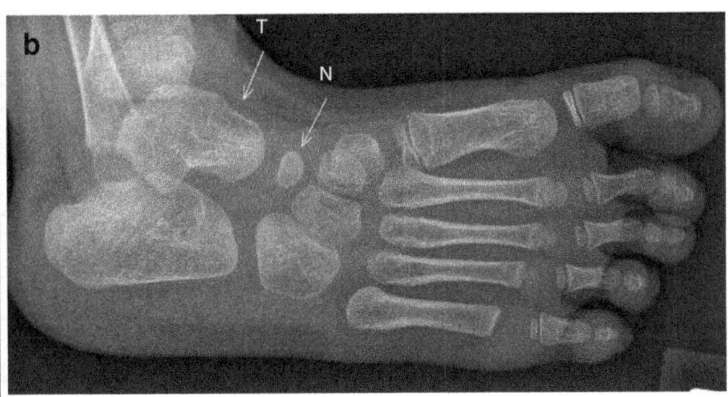

Fig. 12 (**a**) AP and (**b**) lateral foot radiographs of a 3-year-old boy show normal alignment of the navicular bone (N) immediately distal to the middle portion of the head of the talus (T) on both views

relationship between the midfoot and the hindfoot (Fig. 12). If the navicular is not yet ossified, assessment of alignment depends on the metatarsal bases. The lateral cuneiform, when ossified, may also help indicate midfoot and hindfoot deformity, where there is a slight overlap or convergence of the bases of the metatarsals on the AP radiograph.

5.3 Forefoot

Although the forefoot comprises the metatarsals and phalanges, the metatarsals are generally only analyzed in forefoot alignment, where the metatarsal bases have a constant relationship to the distal tarsal row. However, analysis of metatarsal shaft alignment may not be reliable due to forefoot flexibility, which can alter metatarsal alignment with variable degrees of weight-bearing and foot straightening.

5.3.1 Inversion and Eversion

Inversion and eversion are complex deformities of the entire foot. The sole of the foot faces medially during inversion, whereas it faces laterally during eversion; typically occurring at the subtalar and transverse tarsal joints. Inversion and eversion comprise three specific motions, namely supination or pronation, followed by abduction or adduction, and lastly dorsiflexion or plantar flexion. Inversion results from increased activity of the tibialis posterior and anterior muscles, combining supination, adduction, and plantar

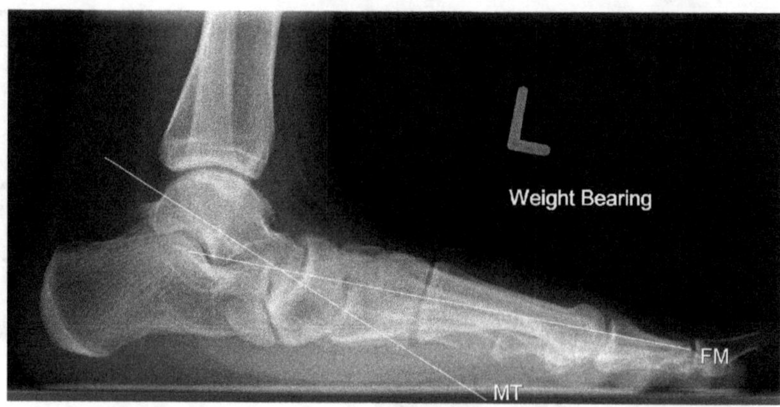

Fig. 13 Lateral weight-bearing foot radiograph of a 15-year-old girl shows the Meary's angle (angle between the mid-talar axis [MT] and the first metatarsal axis [FM]) to be convex down consistent with pes planus. The normal Meary's angle is 0°

flexion. Eversion results from increased activity from the peroneal and extensor digitorum longus muscles and combines pronation, abduction, and dorsiflexion. Supination and pronation refer to medial and lateral rotation of the foot about an AP axis. Abduction and adduction describe motion of the anterior portion of the foot about a vertical axis, where the metatarsals move as a unit away from (abduction) or toward (adduction) the midline, pivoting at their bases.

On AP radiographs, forefoot inversion classically presents with deviation of the metatarsals toward the midline (adduction) and increased overlap of the metatarsal bases and forefoot narrowing (supination). On lateral radiographs, the fifth metatarsal appears more plantar than the first; and a ladder-like array is seen, with the first metatarsal appearing most dorsal. Eversion can be difficult to identify on radiographs. On AP radiographs, the metatarsal bases appear separated, and the metatarsal shafts are more parallel and less divergent than normal. On lateral radiographs, the first metatarsal is the most plantar, with the fifth metatarsal most dorsal, and a step-ladder appearance may be seen reversed from that with inversion.

5.4 Plantar Arch

The plantar arch is best assessed on the lateral radiograph by measuring the alignment of the hindfoot and metatarsals with the lateral talar-first metatarsal angle, or the angle of Meary (Fig. 13). This angle is formed between a line drawn along the central talus and a line drawn along the first metatarsal shaft (shortest and widest metatarsal) and should be near zero. Normal values vary and generally decrease slightly with age. An angle greater than 8° convex upward results in an exaggerated arch and pes cavus, while an angle greater than 4° convex downward results in pes planus or flattening of the plantar arch.

6 Deformities of Foot and Ankle

6.1 Hindfoot Valgus and Hindfoot Varus

When there is valgus and varus motion of the hindfoot, the position of the calcaneus is described in relation to the talus. With hindfoot valgus, the calcaneus rotates laterally under the talus so that its anterior part is lateral to the talus, resulting in loss of its medial support. The long axis of the talus is medially deviated relative to the midline on the AP radiograph and becomes more vertically oriented than normal, pointing more plantar compared to the long axis of the first metatarsal on the lateral radiograph. As such, the calcaneus and talus appear divergent on both views (Fig. 14). The talocalcaneal angle is consequently increased greater than 45°. The navicular

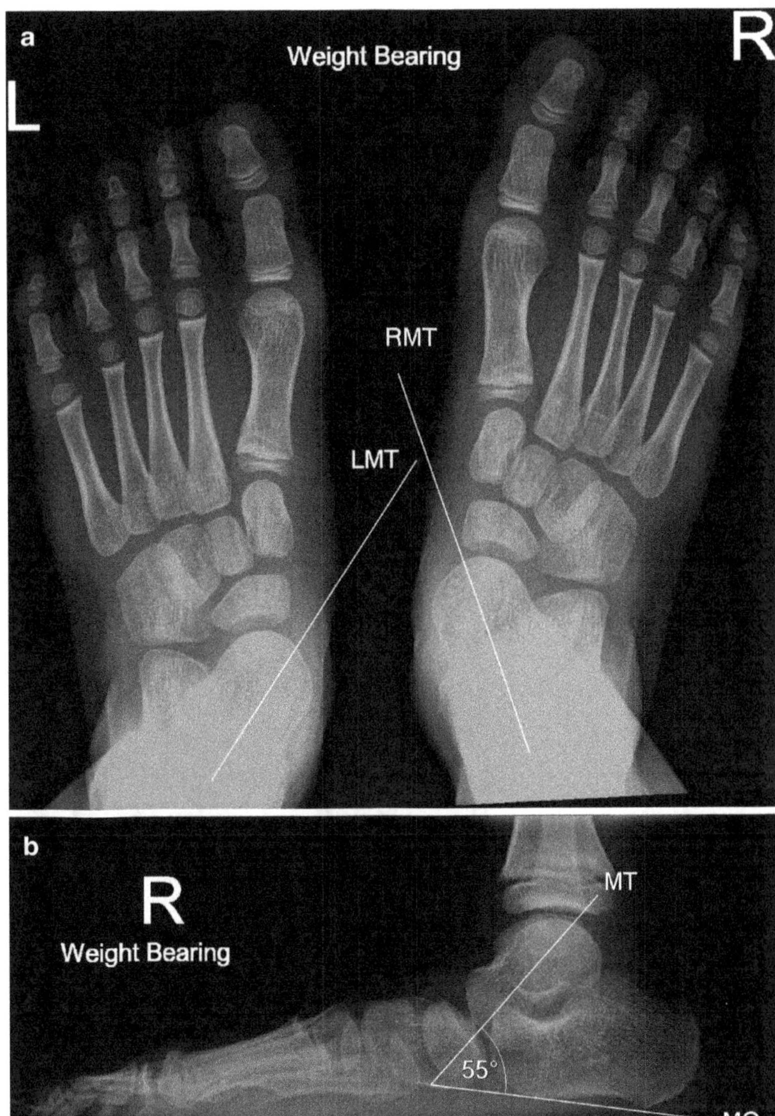

Fig. 14 (**a**) AP radiograph of both feet and (**b**) lateral radiograph of the right foot in a 5-year-old boy show bilateral hindfoot valgus. In the AP view, both the left and right mid-tarsal lines (LMT and RMT, respectively) pass medial to the base of their respective first metatarsals which is abnormal. In the lateral image of the right foot, the tarsal bone is more vertical than normal and mid-tarsal line (MT) does not pass through the base of the first metatarsal. The talocalcaneal angle is also increased (angle between lines MT and MC is >45° which is abnormal). These findings are consistent with hindfoot valgus

may be displaced laterally to the talar head. Hindfoot valgus occurs in congenital and neurogenic deformities of the foot including flatfoot, skewfoot, congenital vertical talus, and cerebral palsy.

In hindfoot varus, the calcaneus is medially rotated under the talus, reducing the normal plantar angulation of the talus. On AP radiographs, there is lateral deviation of the long axis of the talus relative to midline. On lateral radiographs, the talar long axis appears dorsal to that of the long axis of the first metatarsal. The talus assumes are more parallel position relative to the calcaneus with a decreased talocalcaneal angle of less than 30° (Fig. 15). The navicular is displaced medial to the talar head. Varus deformity is observed in congenital clubfoot deformity and in peripheral neuropathies.

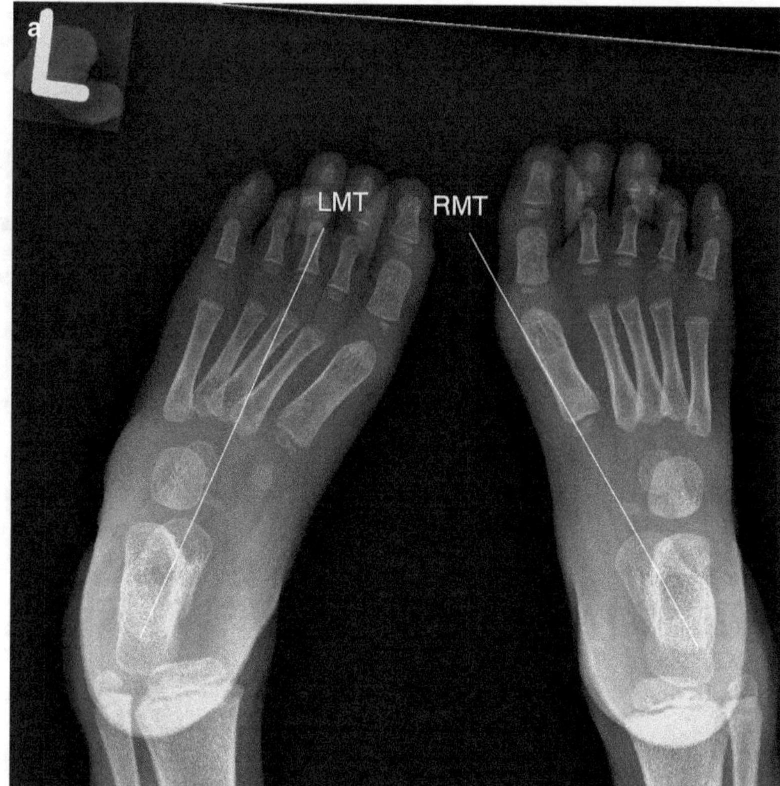

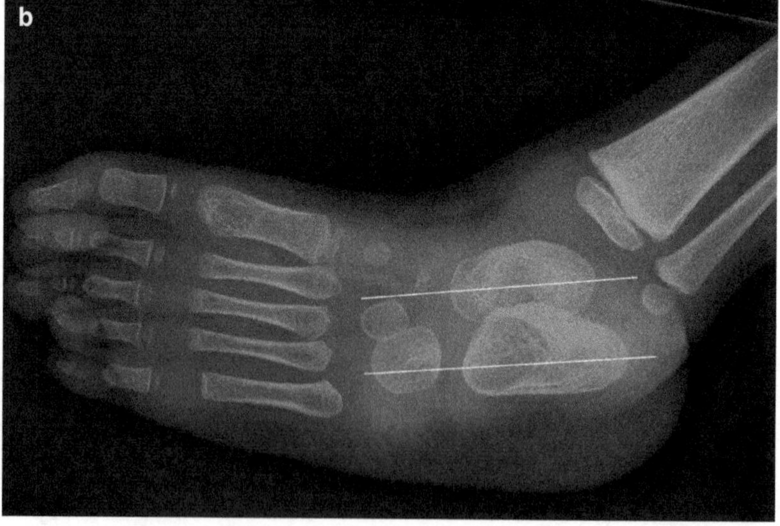

Fig. 15 (**a**) AP radiograph of both feet and (**b**) lateral radiograph of the left foot in a 4-year-old boy with an intra-spinal lipoma show left hindfoot varus. In the AP view, the left mid-tarsal line (LMT) passes lateral to the base of the first metatarsal which is abnormal. The right mid-tarsal line (RMT) passes through the base of the first metatarsal which is normal. In the lateral view, the talocalcaneal angle is reduced and almost parallel. These findings are consistent with hindfoot varus deformity

6.2 Metatarsals

6.2.1 Metatarsus Adductus or Varus

Metatarsus adductus (also referred to as metatarsus varus) is a foot deformity where there is medial deviation of the forefoot (adduction) relative to the midfoot and hindfoot. This results in a concave medial border and a convex lateral border of the foot with high arch. The distal medial cuneiform may be wedged, resulting in malalignment of the tarsometatarsal articulations or medial deviation/adduction of the talar neck (Knörr et al. 2014). Associated variable forefoot inversion and varus, as well as internal tibial torsion, may be present. This deformity may be idiopathic or congenital and can also be inherited. Idiopathic metatarsus adductus is the most common pediatric foot deformity (Widhe 1997) and is more common than congenital clubfoot.

Metatarsus adductus is recognized at birth in two-thirds of patients and manifests during the first year of life when a child starts to walk in the remaining cases. The etiology is unknown, but muscle imbalance may play a role. Idiopathic metatarsus adductus can resemble clubfoot after Ponseti treatment. On AP foot radiographs, forefoot adduction relative to the midfoot is seen (Fig. 16). In true metatarsus adductus, the hindfoot alignment is normal. Varying degrees of inversion may be assessed on lateral radiographs by examining the alignment of the metatarsals and looking for the stepladder deformity with the first metatarsal seen most dorsally.

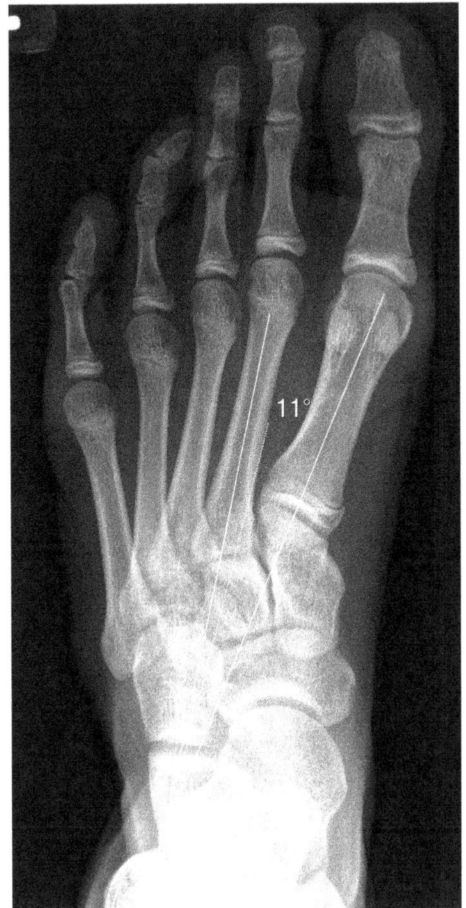

Fig. 16 AP foot radiograph in a 13-year-old boy shows an increased intermetatarsal angle of 11° (normal is less than 9°) with overall forefoot adduction relative to the midfoot, consistent with mild metatarsus adductus with resultant concave medial border of the foot

Severe metatarsus adductus is referred to as skewfoot, metatarsus adductovarus, or pes adductus. It is a rare distinct entity often encountered in otherwise normal children but can be present in patients with severe cerebral palsy, in the setting of incompletely treated clubfoot and certain syndromes such as the Larsen, Proteus, and Ehlers-Danlos syndromes (Hagmann et al. 2009). On radiographs, there is hindfoot valgus with an increased talocalcaneal angle (opposed to metatarsus adductus where hindfoot alignment is normal), forefoot adduction, and divergent appearance of the talus and calcaneus on both frontal and lateral views. The navicular is shifted lateral to the talar head. Connecting lines drawn along the talar head and first metatarsal base give rise to a "zig-zag" or "Z" configuration.

Before 1 year of age, the deformity is flexible and correctable with eversion. Beyond this age group, the deformity can persist with bony remodeling of the growing adducted metatarsals and tarsometatarsal joints. Serial casting is often sufficient. Surgical intervention is reserved for severe or late-presenting cases (Knörr et al. 2014).

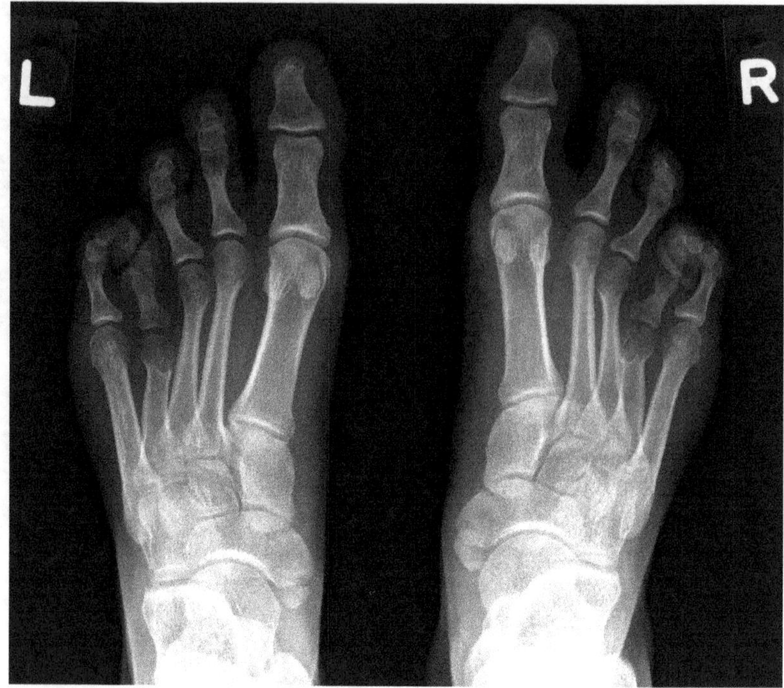

Fig. 17 Bilateral AP foot radiograph of a 16-year-old girl shows symmetrical shortening of both fourth toe metatarsal shafts. There was no known cause, and the child was well other than presenting with bilateral fourth toe deformities

6.2.2 Metatarsal Shortening

Also known as brachymetatarsia, metatarsal shortening is rare condition developing from premature closure of the growth plate and is seen almost exclusively in females (Schimizzi and Brage 2004). It typically affects the fourth ray and may involve more than one metatarsal bone. Metatarsal shortening has been associated several syndromes such as Trisomy 21, Turner syndrome, and conditions such as pseudohypoparathyroidism, pseudopseudohypoparathyroidism, and McCune-Albright syndrome (Fig. 17). Mild cases are managed conservatively with footwear modifications. Surgical metatarsal lengthening may be indicated in patients with persistent pain with footwear (Kim et al. 2003).

6.3 Pes Planus and Rocker Bottom Deformity

Pes planus refers to flat foot or flattening of the plantar arch, which may occur at the talonavicular joint, naviculocuneiform or cuneiform-metatarsal joints. On weight-bearing lateral radiographs, the calcaneus appears horizontal, and the long axis of the talus is *angled plantarward in relation to the first metatarsal* (i.e., the Meary's angle) (Fig. 13). Lateral radiographs taken with maximum dorsiflexion and plantar flexion can help assess for hypermobility through the midfoot or stiffness at the hindfoot. The etiology of flat foot (pes planus) can be derived from knowledge of age of onset (congenital versus acquired) and correctability (rigid and immobile versus flexible and correctable by manipulation), which are discussed below.

The rocker bottom deformity is a severe form of pes planus where the plantar arch is convex, rather than concave, as the calcaneus is in equinus position and the metatarsals are dorsiflexed. This deformity can be present in congenital vertical talus (Fig. 18), severe cerebral palsy with hindfoot valgus, or overcorrected clubfoot.

6.4 Flexible Flat Foot Deformities

6.4.1 Congenital Calcaneovalgus Foot

Congenital calcaneovalgus foot deformity is present in up to half of newborns and is often bilateral (Sullivan 1999). It is postulated to be

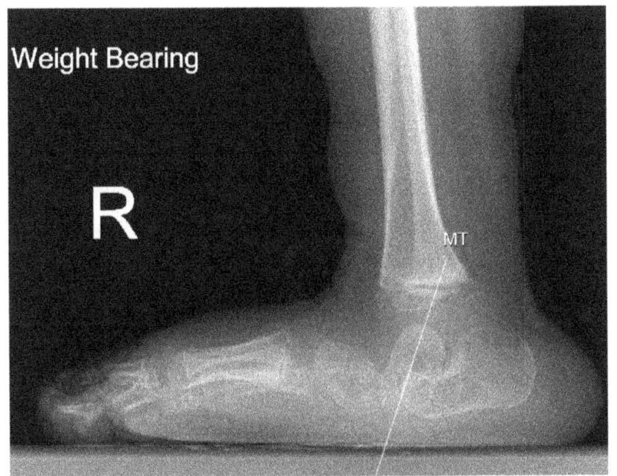

Fig. 18 Lateral weight-bearing foot radiograph of a 3-year-old girl shows marked plantar flexion of the talus (MT) consistent with a vertical talus. The calcaneum is in equinus, and the plantar arch is convex shaped. Overall findings are typical of a rocker bottom foot

related to in-utero dorsiflexion and eversion of the foot with forefoot abduction. The heel and hindfoot adopt a valgus configuration with a plantar-flexed talus and slight flattening of the arch. This deformity is flexible and often resolves without treatment, rarely requiring corrective casting or surgical management (Yu and Hladik 1994). Diagnosis is usually made clinically with little role for imaging.

6.4.2 Acquired Planovalgus (Common Flat Foot)

This is the most common of the flat foot deformities. Plantar arch flattening is considered normal under 5 years of age. The prevalence of flat foot markedly decreases thereafter, with about 4% of 10-year-olds having flat foot (Rao and Joseph 1992). While the cause of persistent flat foot is not well established, it is suggested that abnormal ligamentous support structures are the main contributory factor (Basmajian and Stecko 1963). Imaging plays a role in painful flat foot to exclude other etiologies and look for complications, such as synovitis or tendinosis, which can cause pain. Imaging can also be useful in assessing lower extremity alignment abnormalities, such as genu valgum or increased femoral anteversion, which can worsen symptoms (Villarroya et al. 2009). Treatment typically involves supportive footwear, while surgical management is reserved for symptomatic feet that have failed non-operative measures. Patients with cerebral palsy may develop hindfoot valgus with a stiff pronated flatfoot, resembling common flat foot. This is often accompanied with extreme forefoot abduction and hallux valgus, and a vertical talus with preserved talonavicular relationship.

6.5 Rigid Flat Foot Deformities

6.5.1 Congenital Vertical Talus (Congenital Convex Pes Valgus)

Congenital vertical talus is characterized by an abnormally vertically oriented talus with fixed dorsal subluxation of the navicular relative to the talus (Bosker et al. 2007). Hindfoot varus may be present. About half of cases have a syndromic association and are also seen in conditions such as cranio-carpo-tarsal dysplasia (Freeman-Sheldon syndrome), trisomies (Hammer and Pai 2015), cerebral palsy, myelomeningocele, arthrogryposis, and neurofibromatosis. Proposed mechanisms include arrested normal rotational development of the foot during early fetal life and muscle imbalance.

The vertical talus points medially and does not align with the metatarsals (Fig. 18), instead often seen parallel to the long axis of the tibia on lateral radiographs. The calcaneus is in equinus, due to a short Achilles tendon, and this results in the rocker bottom deformity. The navicular is dorsally displaced toward the talar neck but articulates normally with the midfoot bones. The foot may be everted. Late radiographic changes include hour-glass deformity of the talus, wedging of the navicular, and secondary avascular necrosis. Treatment combines manipulation and casting, followed by talonavicular reduction and pinning, along with Achilles tenotomy (Dobbs et al. 2006). Early treatment during infancy is preferred.

Oblique talus is a flexible deformity which is managed non-operatively and can mimic congenital vertical talus clinically. The ability to reduce talonavicular dislocation during plantar flexion on US confirms the presence of an oblique, rather than vertical, talus (Supakul et al. 2013). Hindfoot valgus deformity following clubfoot correction may also resemble congenital vertical talus but is differentiated by clinical history and lack of talonavicular dislocation in the former.

6.5.2 Tarsal Coalition

Tarsal coalition is a developmental abnormality where there is union of two tarsal bones by bony (synostosis), cartilaginous (synchondrosis) or rarely, fibrous (syndesmosis) connections. Talocalcaneal coalition almost exclusively involves the middle talar articular facet, talus, and sustentaculum tali, with occasional involvement of the anterior or posterior facets (Lee et al. 1989). Talocalcaneal coalition has a male predilection, with about half of cases having bilateral involvement. There is late onset of symptoms, usually between the ages of 12 and 16 years.

On lateral weight-bearing radiographs, talocalcaneal coalition presents as flattening of the longitudinal arch with non-visualization of the subtalar joint spaces. Talar beaking is seen on the lateral radiograph as an osseous beak arising from the talar ridge and projects dorsally at the talonavicular joint (Fig. 19). Abnormal subtalar rigidity restricts movement in patients with coalition, causing dorsal subluxation and impaction of the navicular on the talus. In turn, this causes elevation of the talonavicular ligament and periosteum, thus forming the talar beak. A prominent proximal talar ridge can mimic the talar beak and can be distinguished by its location about 7–14 mm anterior to the trochlear articular surface, which are attachment sites of the tibiotalar joint capsule and talonavicular ligament (Resnick 1984). Other radiographic signs include apparent posterior subtalar joint narrowing, as well as broadening and rounding of the lateral talar process occurring from stresses due to valgus position of the calcaneus. The undersurface of the talar neck can also appear short and concave.

The lateral radiographic C-sign is often associated with talocalcaneal coalition but has low sensitivity as it can be present in other coalitions and flatfoot. It appears as a contiguous osseous structure outlining the medial talar dome and inferior sustentaculum tali indicative of bridging (Lateur et al. 1994) (Fig. 20). CT and MRI aid in operative planning by delineating the extent of fusion. If the coalition involves more than one-third of the total joint surface area, it may not

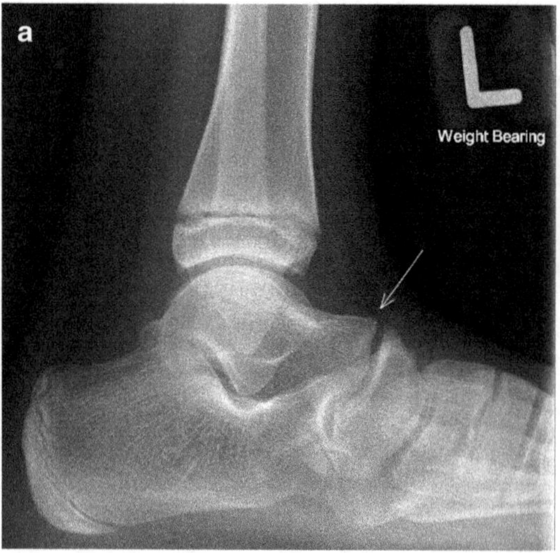

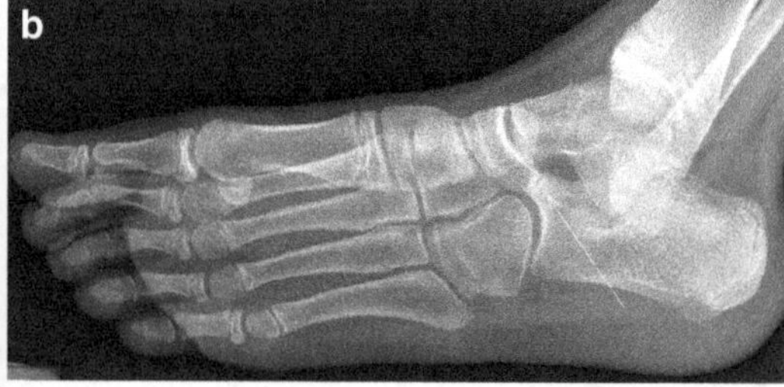

Fig. 19 (**a**) Lateral ankle radiograph of a 10-year-old girl shows an osseous beak arising from the talar ridge, projecting dorsally at the talonavicular joint, consistent with a talar beak (arrow). (**b**) Oblique foot radiograph in the same patient shows abnormal articulation with irregular sclerotic surfaces between a tubular elongated calcaneal anterior process and the navicular (anteater nose sign), consistent with non-osseous calcaneonavicular coalition (arrow), which is the cause of the talar beak

respond well to surgical intervention (Comfort and Johnson 1998) (Fig. 21).

Calcaneonavicular coalition has an autosomal dominant inheritance in most patients and is often asymptomatic. Some patients may experience a rigid foot. The osseous bar of a calcaneonavicular coalition is best demonstrated on oblique foot radiographs and usually becomes apparent around 8–12 years of age. In non-osseous coalition, abnormal articulation with irregular sclerotic surfaces as well as a flattened and wide anteromedial calcaneus may be seen (Fig. 19b). Elongation of the anterior dorsal calcaneus with a slightly diminutive talar head may be seen on lateral radiographs. Further imaging is usually not warranted.

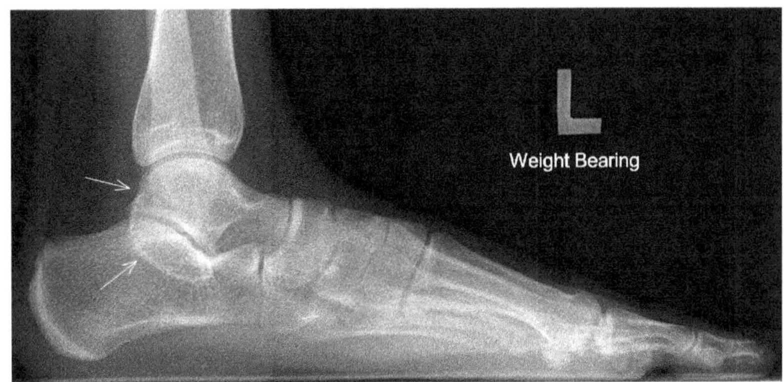

Fig. 20 Lateral foot radiograph of a 15-year-old girl shows a continuous osseous C-shaped arc (arrows) formed by the medial outline of the talar dome and the posteroinferior aspect of the sustentaculum tali of the calcaneum due to the talocalcaneal coalition

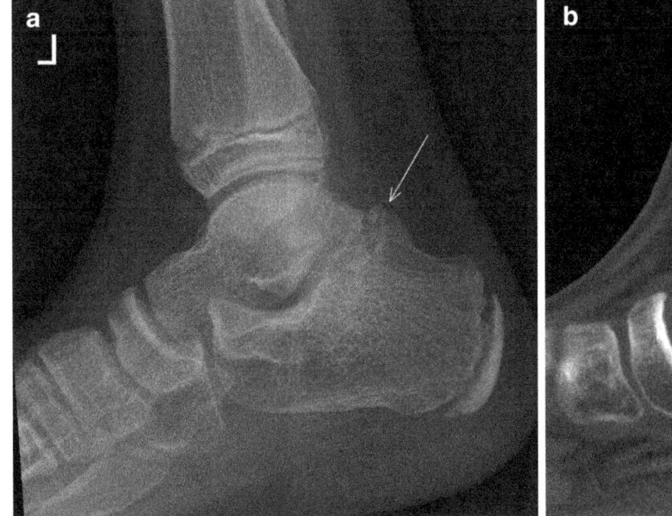

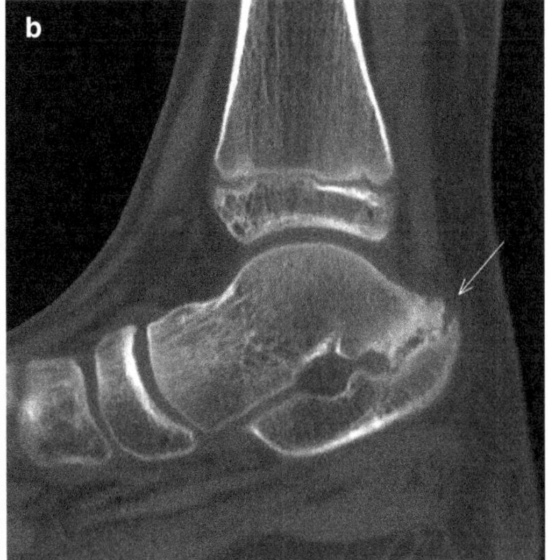

Fig. 21 A 13-year-old boy with posterior talocalcaneal coalition. (**a**) Lateral radiograph shows a humpback superior calcaneal tuberosity (arrow) and irregularity of the posterior talocalcaneal joint. Reformatted (**b**) sagittal and (**c**) coronal CT images show osseous coalition of the posterior subtalar joint (arrows). Narrowing, sclerosis, and subchondral irregularities are also noted indicating that fibrous coalition is also present. (**d**) Sagittal and (**e**) coronal fat-suppressed T2-weighted MR images show the osseous and fibrous coalition (arrows) with bone edema noted in the talus (T) and calcaneus (C)

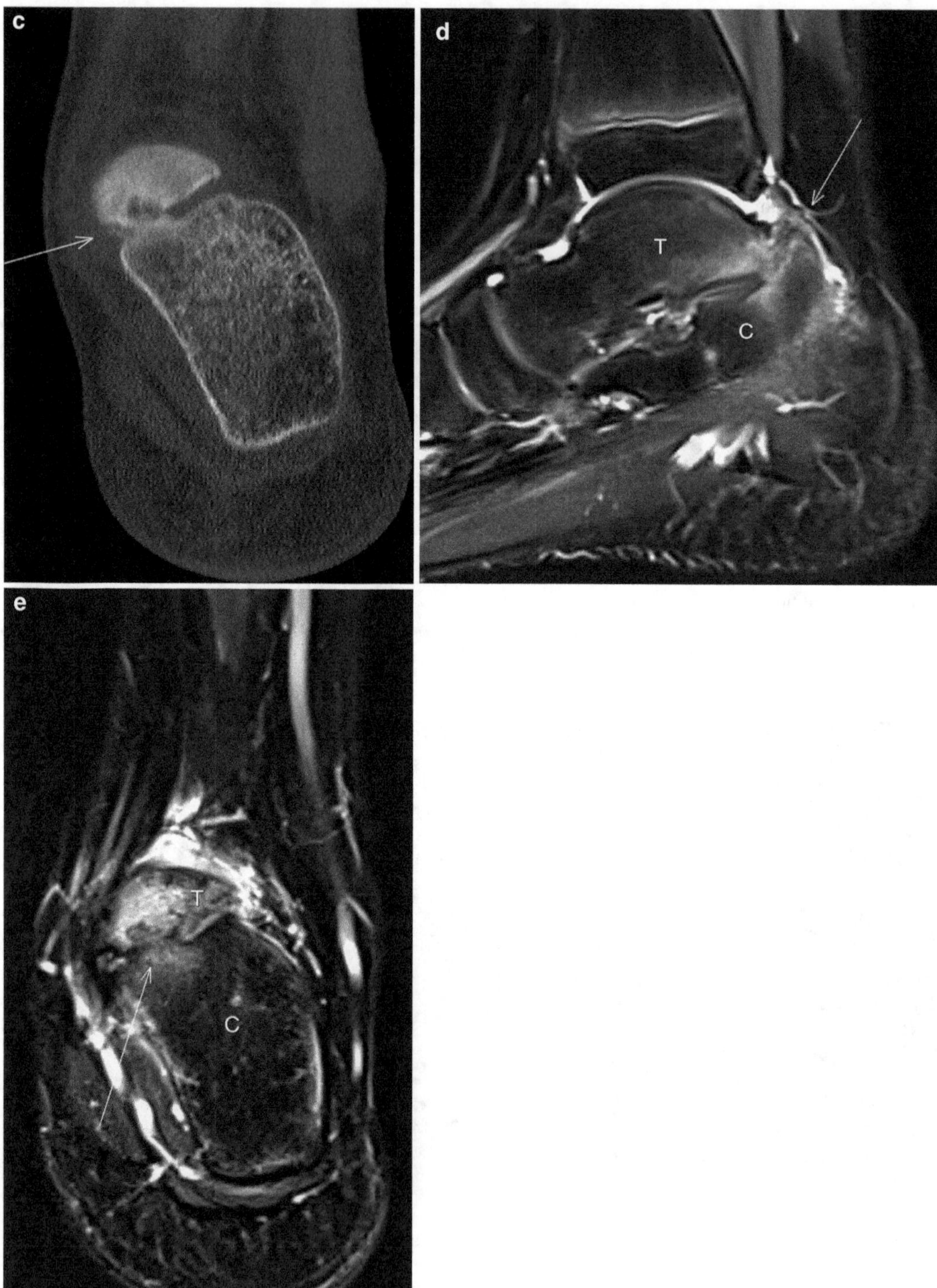

Fig. 21 (continued)

6.6 Pes Cavus

Pes cavus or an abnormally high plantar arch forms part of several foot deformities and can be idiopathic or congenital (Barenfeld et al. 1971). Cavoadductus foot is the commonest type of idiopathic pes, where there is skewfoot deformity. The congenital forms are milder and present later than those associated with underlying neuromuscular conditions. Cavovarus, which is more common, is often present with Charcot-Marie-Tooth disease, cerebral palsy, and poliomyelitis, where the posterior tibialis muscle is stronger than the peroneal muscles (Nagai et al. 2006). Incomplete clubfoot correction may also lead to cavovarus. In contrast, calcaneocavus deformity has been associated with poliomyelitis, Friedreich ataxia, sacral myelomeningocele, and peripheral neuropathy where there are weak plantar flexors and strong toe extensors (Schwend and Drennan 2003). Cavus foot with forefoot adduction may cause in-toeing, characterized by internal rotation of the long axis of the foot (Harris 2013).

On lateral radiographs, there is increased dorsiflexion of the anterior calcaneus, which also has a square contour, due to varus position of the foot. Simultaneous metatarsal plantar flexion gives rise to a deep plantar arch (Fig. 22). The Hibbs angle quantifies the extent of cavus, formed by intersecting lines annotated along the long axis of the calcaneus and the first metatarsal, and is narrowed to less than 150° in pes cavus (Weseley et al. 1982). Adventitious bursa may form along the plantar aspect of the foot, and this is best evaluated on US or MRI. Management of the pes cavus is directed at the underlying causes. To achieve good functional and anatomic results, the majority of cases require surgical intervention through soft tissue release, tendon transfers, osteotomies and sometimes, arthrodesis. Correction of associated toe deformities is sometimes necessary. Non-operative supportive foot orthotics is reserved for mild non-progressive deformities.

6.7 Talipes Equinovarus (Clubfoot)

Clubfoot deformity is characterized by ankle plantar flexion (equinus) with hindfoot varus, forefoot adduction, and foot inversion. It may be positional, congenital (isolated), or part of a syndrome. Clubfoot has an incidence of about 0.5–1.25 per 1000 births, more commonly affecting males with bilateral foot involvement. Approximately 25% of pediatric clubfoot deformities have a known family history. To date, no specific cause has been identified. However, it has been postulated that a polygenetic threshold model with transcription pathway mutations is implicated in clubfoot (Dobbs and Gurnett 2012).

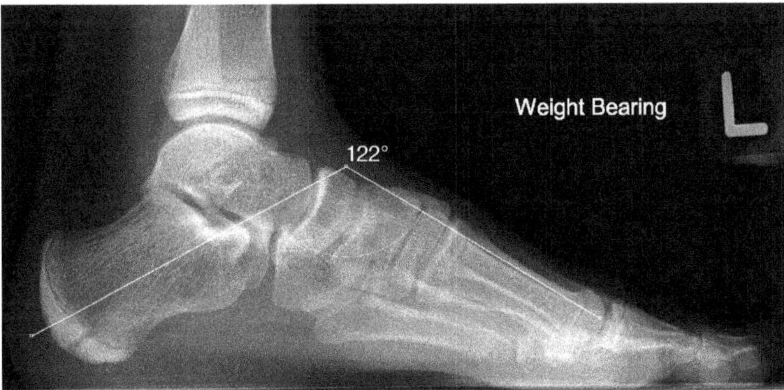

Fig. 22 Lateral weight-bearing foot radiograph of a 13-year-old girl with pes cavus shows the Hibbs angle, formed by intersecting lines drawn along the long axis of the calcaneus and the first metatarsal, to be approximately 122°. Along with increased dorsiflexion of the anterior calcaneus and simultaneous metatarsal plantar flexion, these findings are consistent with the diagnosis of pes cavus. The normal Hibbs angle is at least 150°

Other suggested mechanisms include tarsal developmental anomalies, muscle imbalance or neuromuscular abnormalities, intrauterine positioning deformity, arrested fetal development, and ligamentous laxity in the setting of connective tissue disease (e.g., diastrophic dysplasia) (Shapiro 2019).

In idiopathic clubfoot, there is isolated unilateral or bilateral deformity without any clinical or pathophysiologic evidence of an underlying neuromuscular disorder. Non-idiopathic causes of clubfoot result from mechanical factors with disorders such as myelomeningocele (present in-utero), arthrogryposis (multiple joint contractures), and tibial longitudinal deficiency. For a diagnosis of clubfoot with arthrogryposis to be made, at least one other joint should be affected.

Postnatal neuromuscular clubfoot is often attributed to an underlying neurogenic or myopathic cause, more commonly seen with spasticity disorders of cerebral palsy or peripheral neuropathies (e.g., Charcot-Marie-Tooth disease), as well as diastematomyelia and tethered cord syndromes. There is associated muscle imbalance where the plantar flexors (gastrocsoleus) and invertors (tibialis anterior and tibialis posterior) are stronger than the dorsiflexors (extensor hallucis and digitorum longus) and evertors (peroneus longus and brevis). Talipes, referring to ankle (talus) and foot (pes), is also applied to other congenital abnormalities of the foot, such as talipes varus, talipes calcaneovalgus, talipes equinovalgus, and talipes calcaneovarus.

6.7.1 Clinical Grading of Clubfoot

Clinical assessment of clubfoot is often made at birth to initiate casting or splinting treatment.

To date, several classifications are used to help treat and assess clubfoot deformities. Currently, the classifications by Dimeglio et al. and Pirani et al. are more widely applied in clinical practice. The classification system by Diméglio et al. (1995) assesses deformity by determining the relative degrees of equinus, varus tilt, forefoot adduction, and inversion of the subtalar and talocalcaneal-navicular joint as well as assessing posterior crease, medial crease, cavus deformity, and muscle condition. Scores range from 0 (normal) to 20 (severe clubfoot), with four categories of clubfoot graded as benign (grade I), moderate (grade II), severe (grade III), and very severe (grade IV). This classification is reliable in providing a semiquantitative indication of the extent of deformity to help evaluate treatment progress.

Pirani et al. (Dyer and Davis 2006) uses a 6-point clinical classification system for assessing the severity of each of the components of a clubfoot. It is based on three signs related to the midfoot (curvature of the lateral border, severity of the medial crease, position of the lateral part of the talar head) and three signs related to the hindfoot (severity of the posterior crease, emptiness of the heel, rigidity of equinus). Scoring for each parameter is as follows: 0 for no abnormality, 0.5 for moderate abnormality, and 1.0 for severe abnormality. Each foot is scored between 0 and 6. Several studies have reported that these newer grading systems are useful in projecting the number of casts needed for correction, likelihood of the need for tenotomy, and prognostication (Wainwright et al. 2002; Dyer and Davis 2006). In general, the higher the scores, or the stiffer the deformity, the higher the likelihood for surgical intervention as well as subsequent relapse after treatment.

6.7.2 Imaging of Clubfoot

In untreated clubfoot, there is hindfoot varus, resulting in lateral deviation of the long axis of the talus from midline on the frontal radiograph. The talocalcaneal angle is narrowed, and the talus and calcaneus are parallel on both AP and lateral radiographs. On the lateral radiograph, the calcaneus is in equinus. The forefoot is adducted and the foot inverted, giving rise to a ladder-like array of the metatarsals with the fifth metatarsal being the most plantar on the lateral radiograph (Figs. 23 and 24). Additional findings include small talus and calcaneus, medial and plantar deviation of the talar neck, as well as reduced convexity of talar dome. The ossified navicular is also displaced medially (Thometz and Simons 1993). In longstanding severe untreated clubfoot, abnormal weight-bearing on the lateral foot may lead to periosteal reaction, sclerosis, and stress fractures of the lateral metatarsals.

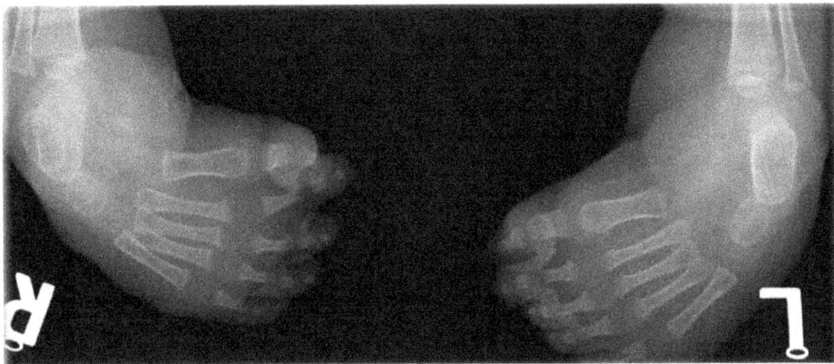

Fig. 23 A 1-year-old boy with untreated severe talipes equinovarus. AP radiograph shows ankle plantar flexion (equinus) with hindfoot varus, forefoot adduction, and foot inversion. The talocalcaneal angle is narrowed, and the talus and calcaneus are parallel to each other

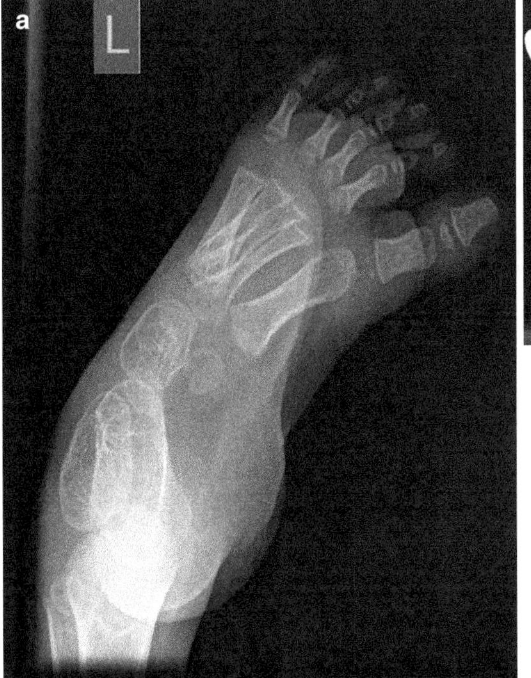

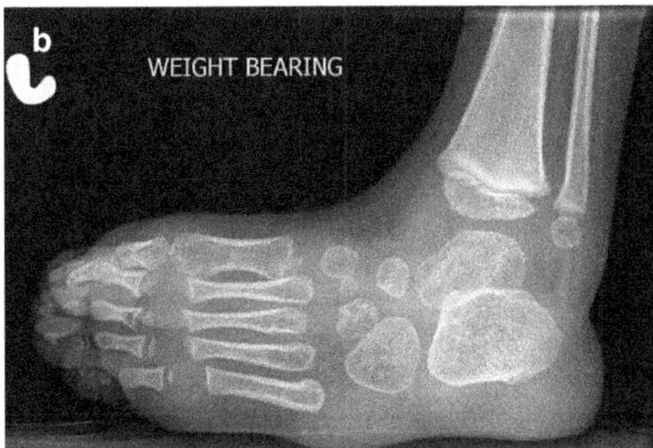

Fig. 24 A 3-year-old boy with untreated clubfoot. (**a**) AP foot radiograph shows superimposition of the talus and calcaneus, with loss of the normal angle between them. The axis of the talus is far lateral to the first metatarsal base. (**b**) Lateral weight-bearing radiograph shows the talus and calcaneus to be parallel to one another and plantar-flexed into equinus. There is a ladder-like array of the metatarsals with the fifth metatarsal appearing the most plantar

Incompletely corrected calcaneal equinus or relapsed clubfoot demonstrates an abnormally horizonal calcaneus with persistent increased talar and calcaneal parallelism seen on lateral radiographs. Correction of the tibialcalcaneal angle in calcaneal equinus often results in improved ankle dorsiflexion after treatment, particularly post-Achilles tenotomy (Radler et al. 2007; Radler 2013). The plantar arch may remain abnormal after treatment. A convex plantar (rocker bottom) arch may develop due to premature application of dorsiflexion before the equinus and varus have been corrected, while a cavus arch deformity may result from incomplete correction of the midfoot deformity and/or overcorrection of the calcaneal position. The sequelae of successfully treated clubfeet include a flattened talar dome, wedge-shaped talar head, deformed posterior navicular articular surface, distorted subtalar joints, and residual calcaneal supination with resulting sustentacular hypoplasia.

Pre-natal US can detect up to 80% of clubfeet from as early as 12 weeks of gestation onwards (Shapiro 2019). As clubfoot can be associated with anomalous karyotypes or other limb abnormalities (Shipp and Benacerraf 1998), pre-natal diagnosis may play a role in further work-up with karyotypic studies via amniocentesis. Postnatal US is more widely used in the diagnosis of clubfoot, its severity and evaluating treatment by demonstrating cartilaginous structures and their relationships (Aurell et al. 2002; Suda et al. 2006). For example, if the navicular bone is displaced medially, the distance between the cartilaginous medial malleolus and the navicular is decreased (Desai et al. 2008). The ability to assess the medial malleolar-navicular distance dynamically during simulated Ponseti maneuvers aids in treatment planning (Kuhns et al. 2003). MRI is superior in making a global assessment of foot alignment, as well as evaluating foot chondro-osseous abnormalities. Post-treatment evaluation MRI has also been found to demonstrate long-term differences in the talonavicular angle between patients who underwent posteromedial release and those who had posterior release or casting only (Moritani et al. 2000). MRI is however often limited by the need for sedation in pediatric patients and relatively long scan times.

6.7.3 Treatment of Clubfoot

The mainstay of clubfoot treatment revolves around the Ponseti method of serial casting until forefoot and midfoot alignment is corrected (Ponseti 1992), followed by Achilles tenotomy to correct residual foot equinus. Long-term foot bracing helps prevent recurrent malalignment (Dobbs et al. 2004). Dynamic supination is an unintended outcome of the Ponseti treatment in which some children experience over-pull of the tibialis anterior accompanied by flexible adduction. Complex surgery involving soft tissue release, tendon transfers, and osteotomies are reserved for refractory cases to alter the mechanics of the supporting structures (Park et al. 2009). If these measures fail, more invasive procedures, such as lateral column shortening, may be attempted. If an associated systemic neuromuscular or connective tissue disorder is present, non-operative treatment will be less effective than in otherwise isolated or idiopathic congenital clubfoot.

6.8 Deformities of the Big Toe

6.8.1 Hallux Valgus

The hallux valgus deformity comprised of adduction of the first metatarsal and valgus angulation at the first metatarsophalangeal joint, with resultant lateral deviation of the big toe proximal and distal phalanges (Thompson 1996). Children are affected as early as 8 years of age, and there is usually bilateral involvement with a female preponderance. Affected children often present with difficulty fitting shoes and parental concerns of foot appearance. Pain is rarely a primary presenting symptom in this age group. The disorder may also be referred to in the childhood years as metatarsus primus varus, defined as an abnormally increased angle between the first and second metatarsals (Davids et al. 2007). The etiology of isolated hallux valgus is thought to result from a primary change in the first metatarsophalangeal joint or due to abnormal angulation of the first and second metatarsals. Hallux valgus may also be present in patients with cerebral palsy, likely due to muscle imbalance and increased spasticity of the adductor hallucis.

On radiographs, hallux valgus is seen as an adducted first metatarsal that is shorter than the second metatarsal, with an increase of the intermetatarsal angle greater than 10 (about 25) degrees and of the first metatarsophalangeal angle (hallux valgus angle) greater than 15 (about 45) degrees. The intermetatarsal angle is measured at the intersection between a line drawn along the first metatarsal proximal articular surface and base and similar line drawn along the second metatarsal. An increased metatarsophalangeal angle associated with uncovering of the medial part of the first metatarsal head is considered abnormal and could progress to frank subluxation (Fig. 25). Additionally, the hallux sesamoids are often laterally displaced. The relationship of the long axis of the metatarsal to the orientation of the distal metatarsal articular surface is assessed with distal metatarsal articular angle, where the slope of the distal first metatarsal articular surface is measured in relation to the long axis of the first metatarsal shaft (normal angle is 8° or less). These angles are part of presurgical assessment (Karasick and Wapner 1990).

Surgical correction is often reserved for cases of worsening discomfort, or for progressive or severe deformity at or near the time of skeletal maturity. This is usually achieved with opening wedge proximal valgus osteotomy (Trethowan procedure), minimal trimming of the medial bone prominence of the metatarsal head, capsulorrhaphy to tighten and shorten the medial first metatarsophalangeal capsule, and a medial closing wedge varus osteotomy of the proximal phalanx, with care being taken not to injure the proximal physis (Shapiro 2019).

6.8.2 Hallux Varus

Congenital hallux varus is rare and is characterized by a shortened, thickened, globular-shaped first metatarsal with medial deviation of the hallux at the metatarsophalangeal joint, often with bilateral involvement (Fig. 26). This disorder may be associated with an accessory hallux at the medial

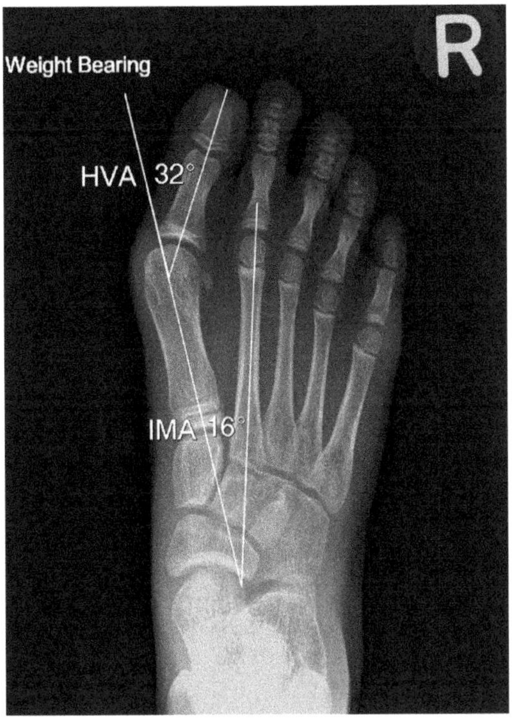

Fig. 25 A 9-year-old girl with hallux valgus. AP weight-bearing foot radiograph shows an adducted first metatarsal with the hallux valgus angle (HVA) to be 32° and the intermetatarsal angle (IMA) to be 16° (normal values are less than 10° and 15°, respectively). Uncovering of the medial part of the first metatarsal head is also present

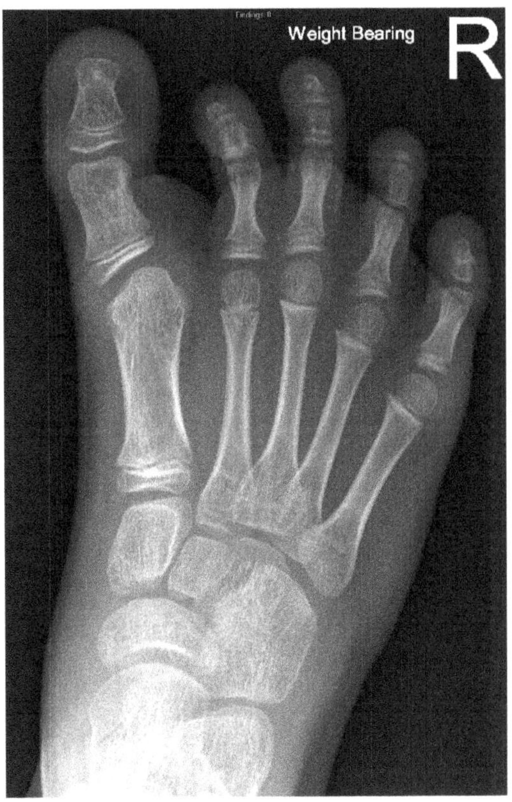

Fig. 26 AP foot radiograph of a 7-year-old boy shows a thickened, globular-shaped first metatarsal with medial deviation of the hallux at the metatarsophalangeal joint, consistent with congenital hallux varus

metatarsophalangeal joint, syndactyly, hypoplastic phalanges, or longitudinal epiphyseal bracket. Rarely, congenital hallux varus is an early associated sign of fibrodysplasia ossificans progressiva. Surgical correction is warranted to enable normal footwear use, accomplished by a medial metatarsophalangeal capsular release with a lateral capsule distally based flap which is reinforced by the extensor hallucis brevis tendon. Syndactylism is created between the great and second toes to hold the repair. A rotation skin flap might be needed for medial coverage, depending on the extent of correction needed (Shapiro 2019).

6.9 Other Toe Deformities

6.9.1 Overlapping Toes

Overlapping toes more commonly occur with severe hallux valgus, where there is plantar flexion and coverage of its dorsal second toe by the overlying big toe. Occasionally, the big toe is normal, but the third toe overlaps the second toe. Overlapping fourth and fifth toes may interfere with footwear usage. Surgical intervention is rarely needed. However, if overlapping toes becomes bothersome, correction of the hallux valgus or third toe followed by the second toe by dorsal capsular tightening or extensor digitorum longus shortening may be performed.

6.9.2 Syndactyly

Syndactyly refers to fusion between two adjacent toes and most commonly affects the second and third toes, often involving soft tissue components, although bone fusions may also occur (Fig. 27). The osseous integrity of the fused toes is usually preserved. Fusion or webbing may be complete or partial. It may be isolated or syndromic, e.g., a feature of both Poland and Apert syndromes. Indications for surgical separation are often cosmetic rather than for functional purposes.

6.9.3 Polysyndactyly and Polydactyly

Polysyndactyly refers to duplication with syndactyly of the digit, often involving the fifth toe. The fourth toe is occasionally also involved and fused with the duplicate fifth toe. The most lateral extra toe is usually excised around 1 year of age with skin grafting for closure. Polydactyly can be classified into preaxial (extra digit medial to the hallux) (Fig. 28), post-axial (extra digit lateral to the little toe) (Fig. 29), or central (middle three digits involved) subtypes. The accessory toe can vary, ranging from a spicule of phalangeal bone and vestigial nail to rudimentary phalanges articulating with the distal fifth metatarsal.

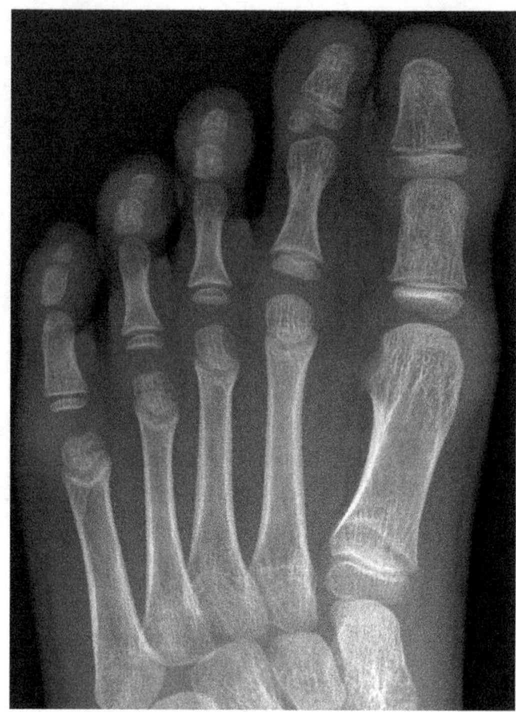

Fig. 27 AP forefoot radiograph of an 8-year-old boy shows soft tissue syndactyly between the first and second toes without osseous involvement. The middle phalanx of the second toe is also deformed

Post-axial polydactyly is the commonest form, occurring in up to 79% of a study of 194 supernumerary toes (Phelps and Grogan 1985). Preaxial (great) toes are only seen in 15%, while central duplications of the second, third, and fourth toes are very rare. Extra toes either articulate with the corresponding metatarsal or can be rudimentary without articulation, while adjacent metatarsals are either normal, block, Y-shaped, or T-shaped with a wide head (Venn-Watson 1976). The majority of polydactylies are isolated but may be associated with skeletal dysplasias such

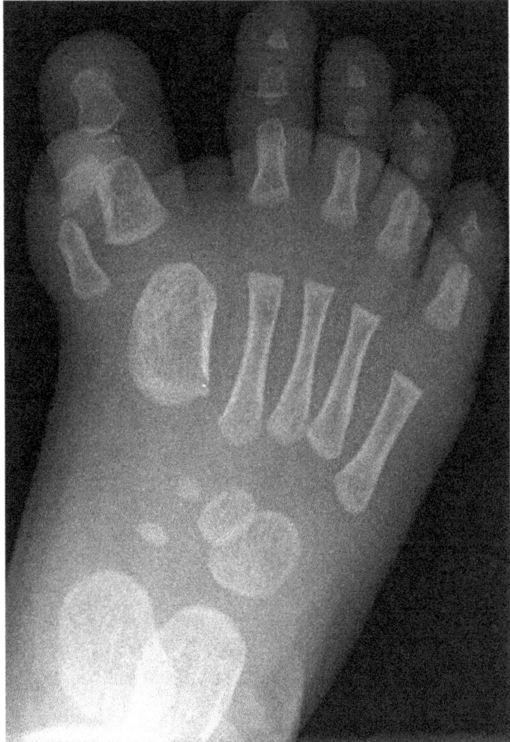

Fig. 28 AP foot radiograph shows an extra digit medial to the hallux, typical of preaxial polydactyly. This digit comprises well-formed proximal and distal phalanges

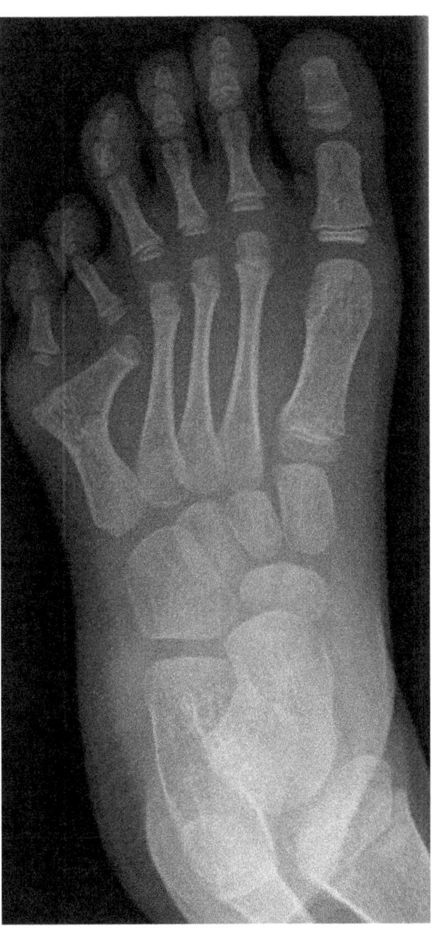

Fig. 29 AP foot radiograph of a 5-year-old child shows an extra digit lateral to the little toe, typical of post-axial polydactyly. The fifth metatarsal is Y-shaped with a large head which articulates with both the fifth and the extra digit

as chondroectodermal dysplasia and trisomies 13 and 21. Surgical removal is warranted before a child starts walking.

6.9.4 Macrodactyly

Macrodactyly is characterized by localized enlargement of a digit involving all mesenchymal tissues, due to excessive overgrowth of adipose tissue within a fibrous stroma. Its etiology is not well understood, but some studies have postulated that it is related to hyperstimulation of a neurotrophic mechanism responsible for normal pedal growth. Macrodactyly is more common in the upper extremities, where there is hypertrophy of digital nerves in the hands. In contrast, the foot tendons and nerves are usually spared. However, in the foot, the second and third digits are affected most often (Bazarov and Williams 2020) (Fig. 30). Generally, it affects one ray, although adjacent rays can be involved to a lesser degree with occasional syndactyly (Shapiro 2019).

Primary macrodactyly of the foot should be distinguished from localized enlargement from other disorders such as hemangioma, lymphangioma, enchondroma, or neurofibromatosis. On clinical and radiological examination, the affected foot or digit appears wider and longer compared to the unaffected one. Dorsal subluxation with medial or lateral deviation of the affected digit may be present. MRI is useful in assessing soft tissue structural variation in macrodactyly (Mahmood and Mahmood 2015). Surgical treatment is aimed at enabling normal footwear, which involves size reduction of the affected ray. Ray resection is preferred as it

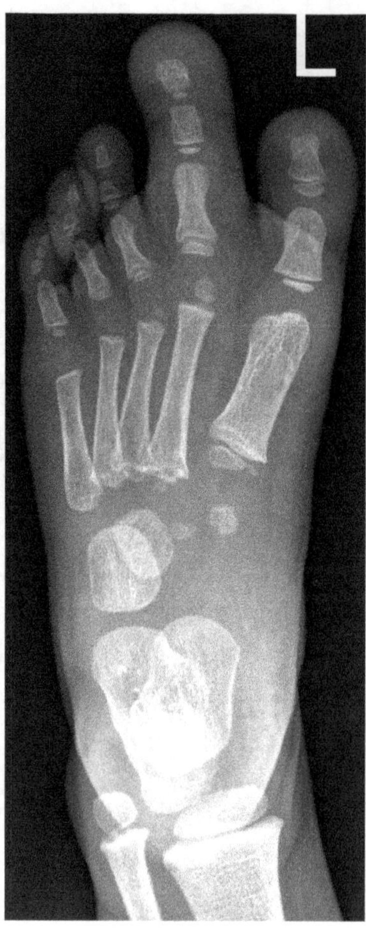

Fig. 30 AP foot radiograph of a 3-year-old child shows generalized macrodactyly of the second ray involving bone and soft tissue

decreases intermetatarsal width and forefoot bulk (Chang et al. 2002; Kim et al. 2015). Other approaches include osteotomy for ray straightening or shortening.

6.9.5 Claw Toe, Hammer Toe, Curly Toe, and Mallet Toe

Claw toe is an extension deformity at the metatarsophalangeal joint and flexion at the proximal and distal interphalangeal joints. It involves some or all the lateral four toes and may be flexible or rigid. Common associations include peripheral neuropathies, neuromuscular diseases (e.g., multiple sclerosis and cerebral palsy) and metabolic diseases (e.g., diabetes mellitus) (Federer et al. 2018).

Hammer toe is a flexion deformity of the proximal interphalangeal joint with extension of the distal interphalangeal and metatarsophalangeal joints. Ill-fitting footwear is often the cause of this deformity.

Curly or underlapping toe is a congenital digital deformity characterized by plantar flexion, medial deviation, and varus rotation of the toe at the interphalangeal joints, commonly affecting the third, fourth, and fifth toes. The metatarsophalangeal joint is preserved. The condition is often hereditary, with positive family history and demonstrates an autosomal dominant pattern of inheritance. Its etiology is not well understood, but curly toe is more frequently observed in cases of flexible pes planus and metatarsal adductus, suggesting impairment of flexor stabilization mechanism (Bazarov and Williams 2020).

Mallet toe is a hyperflexion deformity of the distal interphalangeal joint and may be caused by trauma or inappropriate footwear, potentially leading to a tightened flexor digitorum longus tendon, callus formation, and nail deformities.

Non-operative treatment of these toe deformities can involve orthotics, toe strapping/protectors, while surgical treatment is reserved for patients with persistent symptomatic deformity.

6.10 Congenital Diastasis of the Inferior Tibiofibular Joint

This condition is a very rare, severe deformity that forms part of a spectrum of distal tibial dysplasia with an intact fibula (Jones et al. 1978) and can resemble clubfoot (Skolan et al. 2013). Diastasis of the distal tibia and fibula results in superior talar migration with posteromedial displacement of the medial malleolus and distal fibular dislocation. Other congenital anomalies such as clubfoot and congenital heart disease can be associated with this condition. Management is aimed at ankle stabilization and correcting leg length discrepancies.

6.11 Ball-and-Socket Ankle

The ball-and-socket ankle is characterized by a hemispheric configuration of the talar articular surface with corresponding concavity of the distal tibial articular surface, which has been observed as early as 6 weeks of gestational age. It is associated with varying degrees of leg length discrepancy and other anomalies of the forefoot rays. Up to 60% of patients with ball-and-socket ankle can have talonavicular or calcaneocuboid coalition and fusion of the hindfoot and midfoot structures (Pistoia et al. 1987). Congenital etiologies of the ball-and-socket ankle include short extremities, tarsal coalition, absent/fused rays, hypoplastic fibula, clubfoot, and acrocephalosyndactyly, while acquired etiologies include tarsal coalitions, polio (post-surgical arthrodesis), myelomeningocele, and hyperlaxity (Ilyas et al. 2009).

It has been hypothesized that the ball-and-socket ankle occurs due to secondary adaptation to allow ankle inversion and eversion in the setting of congenital tarsal fusions. During development, there is delayed ossification of the abnormal talus with abnormal morphology, which may be detected on radiographs before 1 year of age, with the ankle articulation achieving a congruent hemisphere by the age of 5 or 6 years (Takakura et al. 1999). Surgical correction in the setting of the ball-and-socket ankle is usually reserved for limb-length discrepancies and malalignment to prevent chronic osteoarthrosis and pain (Stevens et al. 2006).

7 Bone Dysplasias

7.1 Achondroplasia, Pseudoachondroplasia, and Hypochondroplasia

Achondroplasia is commonest form of skeletal dysplasia associated with rhizomelic dwarfism. It is nonlethal and caused by gain-of-function mutations in the *FGFR3* gene, in turn causing impairment of endochondral bone formation (Bellus et al. 1995). Inheritance is autosomal dominant, though most cases are spontaneous mutations. The changes in the foot are less pronounced than in the hand. The great toe metatarsal is broad, while the third metatarsal is the longest. The fourth and fifth metatarsals are slightly shorter than the third metatarsal. All the metatarsals are relatively, but not severely, shortened (Fig. 31). The phalanges are spared. No trident deformity is present in the foot as opposed to in the hand, where there is inability to oppose the third and fourth fingers. Main radiological findings include a combination of impaired endo-

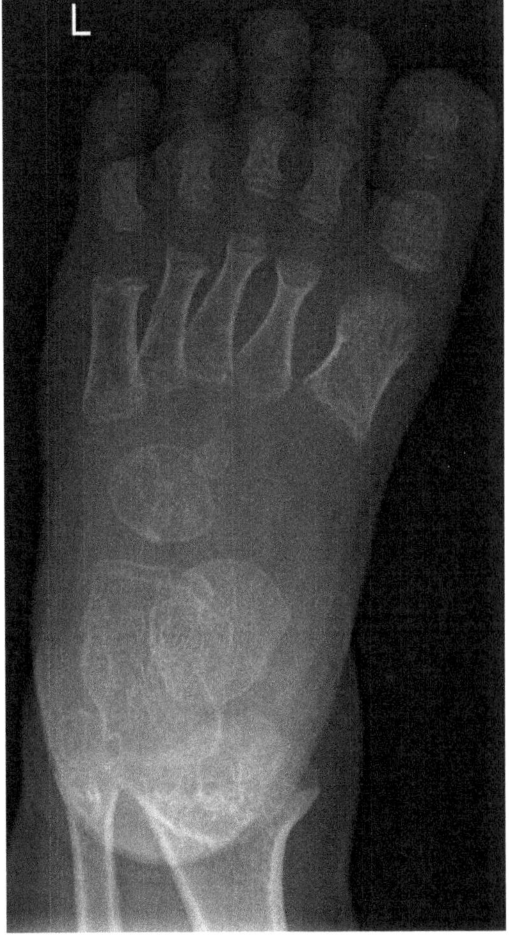

Fig. 31 AP foot radiograph of a 6-year-old boy shows short and broad toe metatarsals, with generalized flaring of their metaphyses, consistent with achondroplasia. The phalanges are spared. Unlike in the hand, the trident deformity is absent

chondral bone formation and preserved intramembranous ossification. The presence of proximal femoral radiolucency in neonates and infants is pathognomonic of achondroplasia (Handa et al. 2022).

Pseudoachondroplasia exists in autosomal dominant and recessive forms, which may be either mild or severe with major deformities. The major tubular bones are short and bowed with flared metaphyses; and the epiphyses are small and irregular. In the feet, the tubular bones are short and broad, as they are in achondroplasia, while the tarsal bones are hypoplastic. The interpedicular distances are normal in the lumbar spine. In severe cases, major spinal deformity is seen.

Hypochondroplasia is an autosomal dominant skeletal dysplasia where the skull is normal and there is narrowing of the interpedicular distances in the lumbar spine distally. The fibula is characteristically long. The feet show cone-shaped epiphyses at the phalangeal bases.

7.2 The Mucopolysaccharidoses (Dysostosis Multiplex)

Dysostosis multiplex encompasses skeletal phenotypes in mucopolysaccharidoses (MPS) and lysosomal storage diseases with absent or faulty enzymes required for the breakdown of glycosaminoglycans (e.g., Hurler syndrome) (Handa et al. 2022).

7.2.1 MPS I to II (Hurler Syndrome)

The Hurler syndrome is inherited as an autosomal recessive condition and is usually apparent shortly after birth. There is mental retardation. Radiologically, there is macrocephaly, craniosynostosis, and a J-shaped sella. The ribs appear paddle-shaped and widened anteriorly. Vertebral bodies show posterior scalloping. Coxa valga, acetabular hypoplasia, and a tibiotalar slant in the ankle are present (Fig. 32). Skeletal retardation is present in the hands and feet. The metatarsals are demineralized and shortened, with pointed proxi-

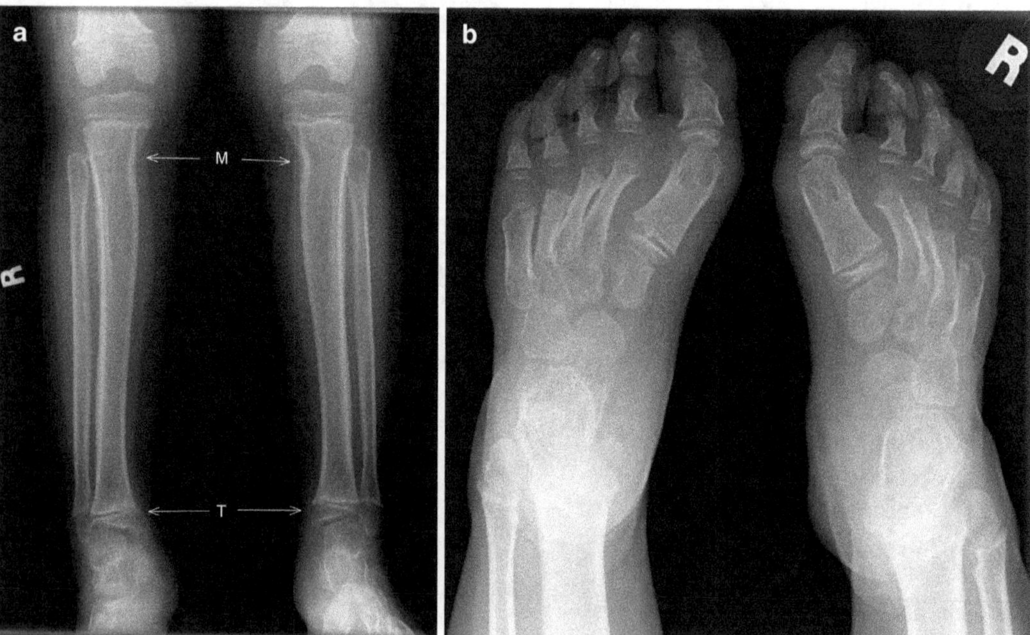

Fig. 32 A 9-year-old girl with Hurler syndrome. (**a**) AP radiograph of both tibiae and ankle joints shows tibial metaphyseal narrowing (M) resulting in relative diaphyseal widening. A tibiotalar slant is also noted due to the wedge-shaped distal tibial epiphysis (T). (**b**) AP radiograph of both feet shows subtle diaphyseal broadening and metaphyseal constriction of the metatarsals and phalanges. There is also fixed flexion deformity of the distal interphalangeal joints and bilateral pes abductovalgus

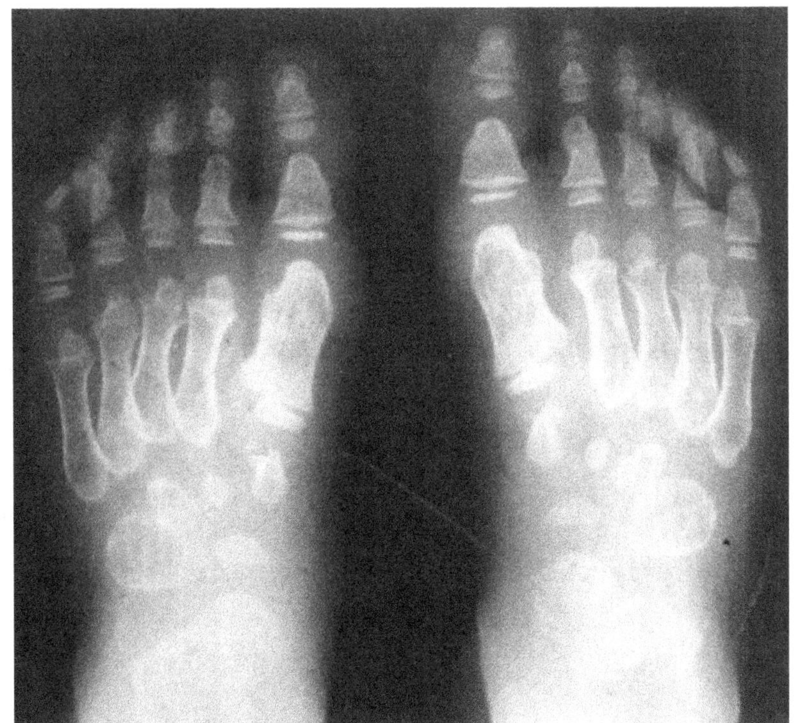

Fig. 33 Patient with Morquio-Brailsford syndrome (MPS IV). Here, the appearances are not as severe as those of Hurler syndrome, but the features are still those of a mucopolysaccharidosis. There is pointing of the metatarsal bases and irregularity of the tarsus. The phalanges are broadened

mal ends. The phalanges are bullet shaped, with pointed distal ends. There is diaphyseal broadening and metaphyseal constriction of the long bones, proximal pointing of the metacarpals, as well as bullet-shaped metatarsals and phalanges (Kennedy et al. 2013).

7.2.2 MPS IV (Morquio-Brailsford Syndrome)

The Morquio-Brailsford syndrome is inherited as an autosomal recessive condition, manifesting as short spine dwarfism with no mental deficit. In the spine, central beaking of many vertebral bodies is present. Initially, the major epiphyses appear normal, but become progressively flattened, irregular, and sclerotic. A tibiotalar slant is seen. Metatarsals are short, broad and have pointed proximal ends. Phalanges are broadened (Fig. 33).

7.3 Skeletal Dysplasias with Disorganized Development of Bone

7.3.1 Dysplasia Epiphysealis Hemimelica (Trevor Disease)

Dysplasia epiphysealis hemimelica is a rare condition characterized by asymmetric overgrowth of the epiphyseal cartilage, leading to progressive deformity of the involved joints, most commonly affecting the lower limb in males (Trevor 1950). The main imaging feature is focal osseous overgrowth at the affected epiphysis, more commonly involving the medial side, which can later result in a larger-than-normal epiphysis (Fig. 34). Changes in the feet comprise irregular exostoses on the articular surfaces, especially at the talar dome, and osseous overgrowth.

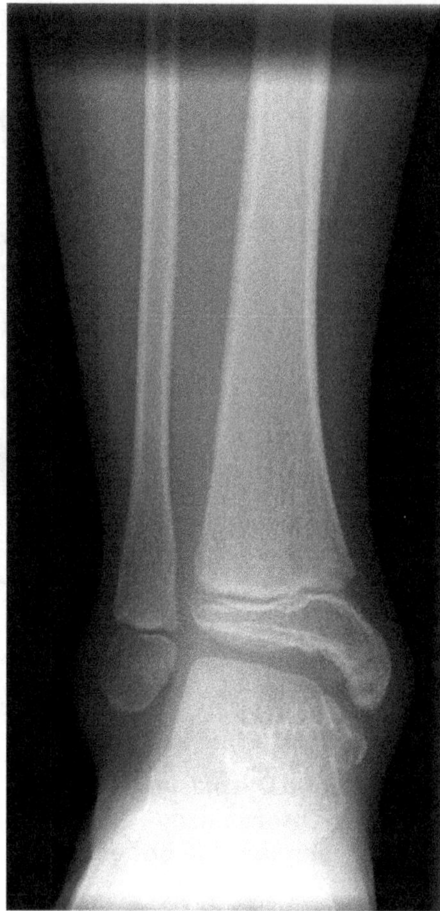

Fig. 34 AP ankle radiograph of a 5-year-old boy shows focal irregular osseous overgrowth on the medial aspects of the epiphysis of the distal tibia and talar dome consistent with dysplasia epiphysealis hemimelica (Trevor disease)

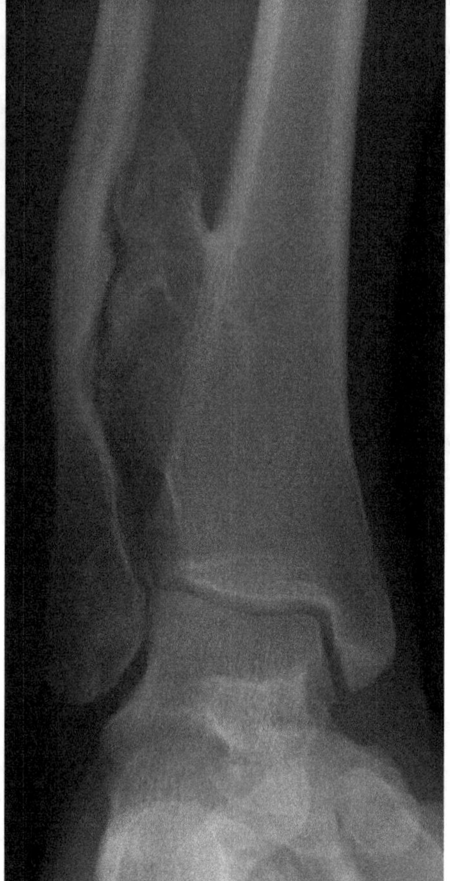

Fig. 35 AP ankle radiograph of a 12-year-old boy with diaphyseal aclasia shows a sessile osseous protrusion along the lateral aspect of the distal tibial diaphysis, consistent with a bony exostosis, causing pressure deformity of the adjacent distal fibula

7.3.2 Diaphyseal Aclasia (Hereditary Multiple Exostoses)

Diaphyseal aclasia is an autosomal dominant condition related to *EXT1* or *EXT2* mutation with a male preponderance. The hallmark of this condition is multiple osteochondromas, which are osseous exostoses arising from the ends of tubular bones, ribs, and cartilaginous parts of the axial skeleton, pointing away from the joint (Raskind et al. 1995; Murphey et al. 2000). The bony exostoses may result in nerve compression, tendon irritation, or vascular compromise. On imaging, these lesions manifest as sessile or pedunculated osseous protrusions with corticomedullary continuity with the underlying bone (Fig. 35).

The osteochondromas may impair tubulation (metaphyseal broadening) or bone growth. There is an incidence of 1–3% of malignant transformation to chondrosarcoma, which is generally suspected when the cartilage cap is thicker than 1.5 cm. This is often best evaluated on MRI. Other features worrisome for malignant change include continued growth after skeletal maturity, rapid size increase, underlying bone destruction, variegated appearance, or new onset of pain.

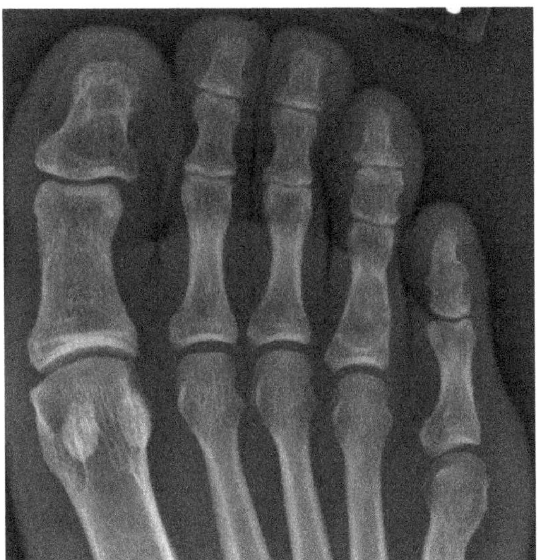

Fig. 36 AP forefoot radiograph of a young adult shows a well-defined ovoid osteolytic lesion in the proximal phalanx of the fourth toe. There is stippled calcification within this lesion, typical of an enchondroma

7.3.3 Enchondromatosis (Ollier Disease)

Enchondromatosis is characterized by multiple circumscribed lesions containing chondroid matrix with "ring and arcs" calcifications, predominantly in the metaphyses, usually unilateral and mostly sporadic (Fig. 36). In the foot, it usually involves the tarsal bones, metatarsals, and phalanges (Handa et al. 2022). Pathological fractures may occur. Like osteochondromas, enchondromas can impair growth and cause limb asymmetry. Maffucci syndrome comprises co-existing enchondromatosis and multiple hemangiomas. Malignant transformation to chondrosarcoma should be suspected when "new growth" of an enchondroma is seen in adulthood.

7.4 Dysplasias with Abnormality of Bone Density

7.4.1 Osteogenesis Imperfecta

Osteogenesis imperfecta (OI) is a group of congenital, non-sex-linked, genetic syndromes characterized by abnormal synthesis of collagen type I in connective tissues and bones (Renaud et al. 2013; Forlino and Marini 2016). Most cases are autosomal dominant and result from heterozygous mutations in *COL1A1* or *COL1A2*. Common features of OI include osteoporosis, bone, dental and soft tissue fragility, blue sclera, and hearing loss. OI is mainly categorized into four subtypes using Sillence's classification, which is based on severity (Sillence and Rimoin 1978).

Mild forms of OI often manifest with recurrent fractures following minor trauma, while severe forms present with multifocal fractures and deformity/bowing of the limbs in-utero. General radiological features of OI include diffuse osteoporosis, bowing of the bones, and multiple fractures (Fig. 37). Multiple wormian bones and widely opened fontanelles may be seen in defective calvarial ossification. OI must be differentiated from non-accidental injury, which can often be challenging. Radiological features suggesting non-accidental injury include classic metaphyseal lesions, complex skull fractures, and posterior rib fractures.

7.4.2 Osteopetrosis (Albers-Schonberg Disease)

Osteopetrosis is characterized by diffuse bony sclerosis due to osteoclast dysfunction and impaired absorption of immature bone (Sobacchi et al. 2013), resulting in abundant immature bone which are dense but brittle with obliterated bone marrow. Osteopetrosis is classified into three groups based on the age of onset: infantile, intermediate (autosomal recessive), and late-onset (autosomal dominant) forms. Clinical features vary between the three groups.

Key radiological findings include generalized increased bone density with poor corticomedullary differentiation and indiscernible bone trabecular pattern, particularly in the infantile form (Ihde et al. 2011) (Fig. 38). Sclerosis may be uniform or the cyclical nature of impaired immature bone resorption may give rise to the classical "bone-in-bone" appearance and "sandwich" vertebrae (sclerotic endplates). Infantile and intermediate forms are associated with modeling failure with resultant bone undertubulation or "Erlenmeyer flask" deformity.

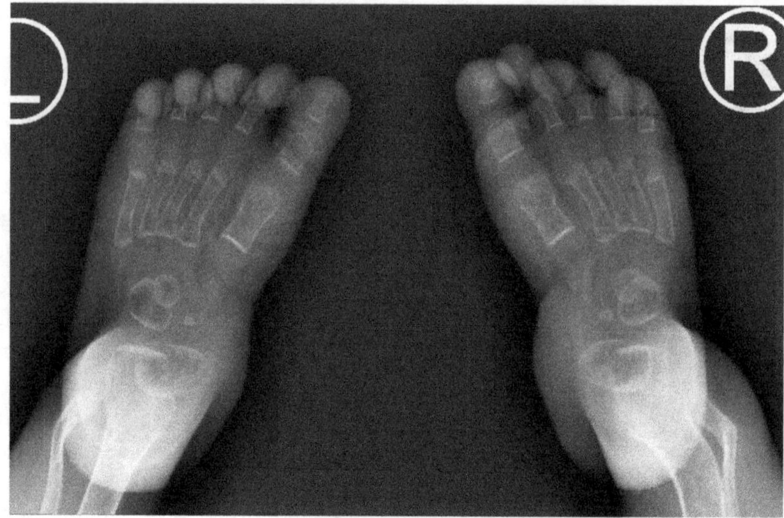

Fig. 37 A 2-year-old child with osteogenesis imperfecta. AP radiograph of both feet shows diffuse osteopenia. The imaged bilateral distal tibia and fibula appear gracile with bilateral bowing. Diffuse cortical thinning is also present. Overall findings are consistent with bone softening

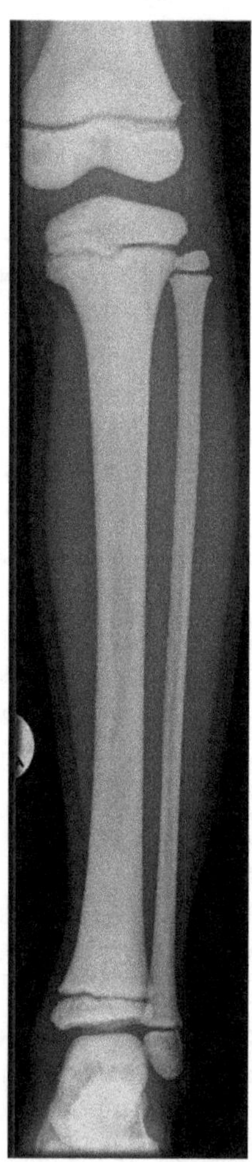

Fig. 38 AP radiograph of a 14-year-old boy shows uniform sclerosis of the distal femur, tibia and fibula, typical of osteopetrosis

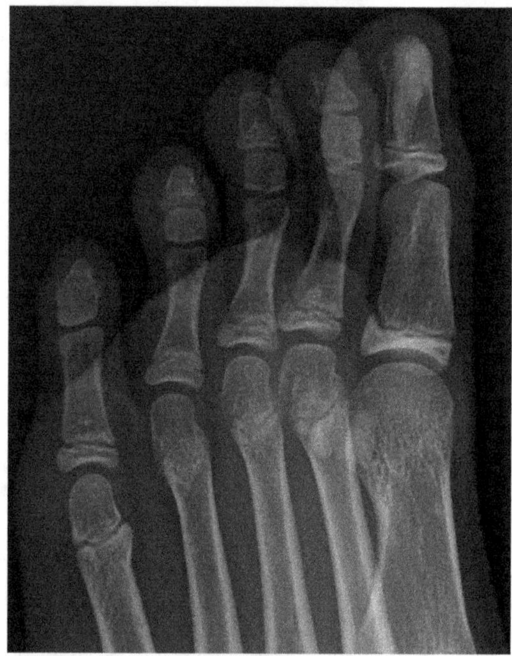

Fig. 39 Oblique radiograph of the forefoot shows focal cortical thickening with patchy sclerosis of the distal phalanx of the big toe, presumed to be monostotic melorheostosis

7.4.3 Melorheostosis

This condition is characterized by cortical hyperostosis resembling "dripping candle wax" and is named after the appearance (*melos*: limb; *rhein*: to flow; *ostos*: bone) in Greek, often affecting a single bone, limb, or unilateral body side and following a sclerotome pattern (neural innervation of bone) (Freyschmidt 2001) (Fig. 39). Other clinical

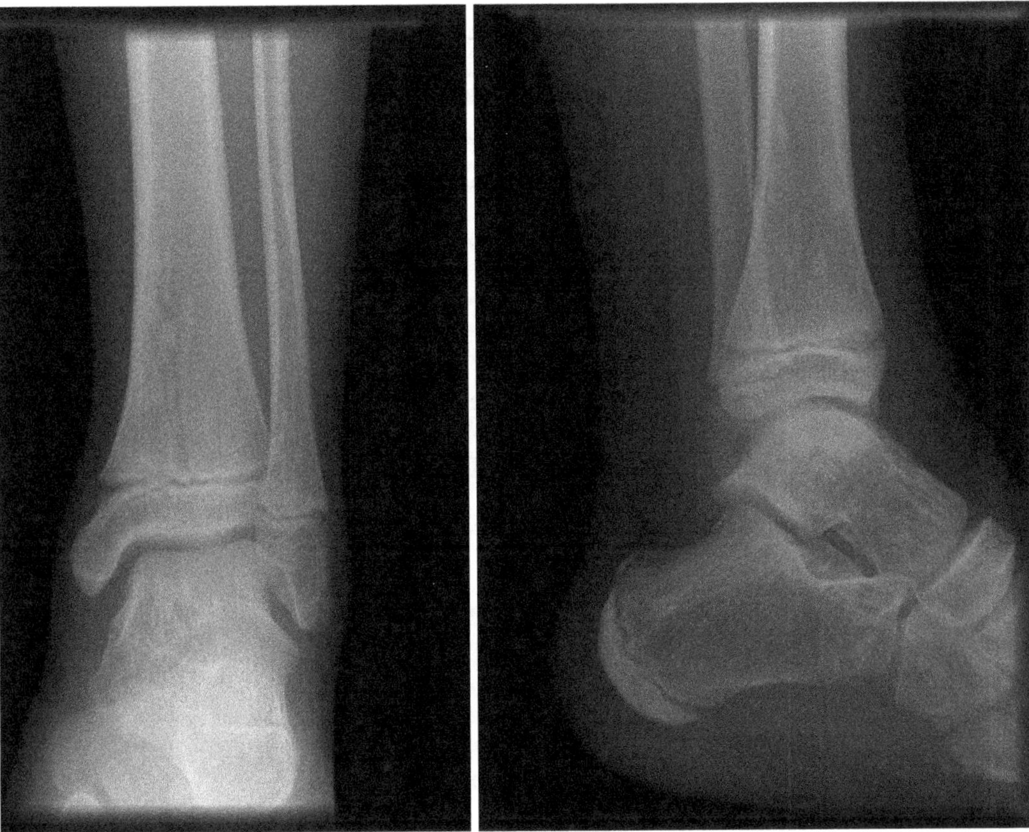

Fig. 40 AP (left) and lateral (right) ankle radiographs of a 13-year-old boy show multiple small rounded sclerotic foci aligned parallel to adjoining bone trabeculae in the distal tibia, fibula, and visualized bones of the foot, consistent with osteopoikilosis

features include limb-length discrepancy, joint contracture, muscular atrophy, and erythematous skin changes. Melorheostosis can occur together with osteopoikilosis and osteopathia striata, also termed as mixed sclerosing bone dysplasia. Soft tissue ossification occurs around affected joints in about 25% of cases. Soft tissue hemangiomas and enlarged superficial blood vessels may accompany the overgrown bones.

7.4.4 Osteopoikilosis

Osteopoikilosis is an autosomal dominant condition related to *LEMD3* mutation and is characterized by numerous small sclerotic foci at the epi-metaphyses of the long bones, resembling bone islands (Hellemans et al. 2004) (Fig. 40). The diaphyses are spared. The sclerotic foci are aligned parallel to adjoining bone trabeculae and typically do not show temporal change in size. Affected individuals are often asymptomatic. Histopathological findings are identical to benign bone islands.

7.4.5 Osteopathia Striata

Osteopathia striata is characterized by longitudinal sclerotic striations in the long bone metaphyses extending to the joint and is often asymptomatic (Handa et al. 2022) (Fig. 41). If cranial sclerosis is present, this is termed as osteopathia striata–cranial sclerosis (OS–CS), which is a X-linked dominant disorder with male lethality (Jenkins et al. 2009). Osteopathia striata may be associated with Goltz syndrome.

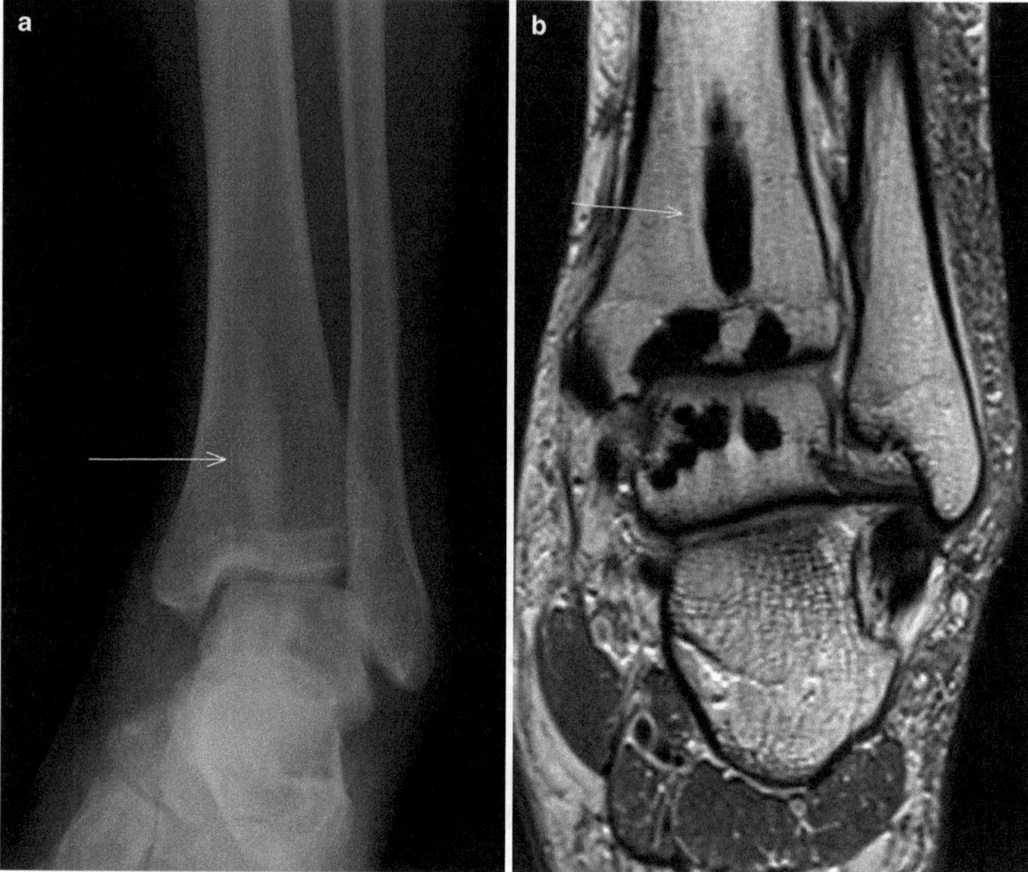

Fig. 41 A 17-year-old boy with osteopathia striata. (**a**) AP radiograph of the left ankle shows a longitudinal sclerotic striation in the distal tibial metaphysis extending to the ankle joint (arrow). Similar sclerotic striations are seen in the talar bone. (**b**) Coronal proton density MR image shows multiple sclerotic striations as areas of signal hypointensity in the distal tibia (arrow) as well as the talus

8 Conclusion

Timely diagnosis and treatment of congenital and developmental conditions affecting the foot and ankle rely heavily on robust clinical assessment and knowledge of the wide spectrum of imaging features. Accurate interpretation of imaging studies, particularly radiographs, is crucial in assessing the foot and ankle structures and relationships. This helps guide orthopedic treatment, which aims at preventing disabling deformities. As many congenital foot and ankle disorders are also associated with an underlying neuromuscular or genetic disease or skeletal dysplasia, radiologists play an essential role in directing further investigations for definitive diagnosis. MRI complements radiographs and is the current modality of choice for evaluating soft tissue and chondro-osseous structures, as well as disease extent and complications. MRI is also useful in preoperative planning for conditions such as tarsal coalition and clubfoot.

References

Aurell Y, Johansson A, Hansson G, Jonsson K (2002) Ultrasound anatomy in the neonatal clubfoot. Eur Radiol 12:2509–2517

Barenfeld PA, Weseley MS, Shea JM (1971) The congenital cavus foot. Clin Orthop Relat Res 79:119–126

Barisch-Fritz B, Mauch M (2021) Foot growth. In: Luximon A (ed) Handbook of footwear design and manufacture, 2nd edn. Woodhead Publishing, Elsevier, Cambridge, pp 105–126

Basmajian JV, Stecko G (1963) The role of muscles in arch support of the foot. J Bone Joint Surg Am 45:1184–1190

Bazarov I, Williams ML (2020) Digital deformities of the pediatric foot. In: Butterworth M, Marcoux J (eds) The pediatric foot and ankle. Springer, Cham, pp 95–106

Bellus GA, Hefferon TW, Ortiz de Luna RI et al (1995) Achondroplasia is defined by recurrent G380R mutations of FGFR3. Am J Hum Genet 56:368–373

Bennett GL, Weiner DS, Leighley B (1990) Surgical treatment of symptomatic accessory tarsal navicular. J Pediatr Orthop 10:445–449

Biedert R, Hintermann B (2003) Stress fractures of the medial great toe sesamoids in athletes. Foot Ankle Int 24:137–141

Boike A, Schnirring-Judge M, McMillin S (2011) Sesamoid disorders of the first metatarsophalangeal joint. Clin Podiatr Med Surg 28:269–vii

Bosker BH, Goosen JH, Castelein RM, Mostert AK (2007) Congenital convex pes valgus (congenital vertical talus). The condition and its treatment: a review of the literature. Acta Orthop Belg 73:366–372

Chagas-Neto FA, de Souza BN, Nogueira-Barbosa MH (2016) Painful Os Peroneum Syndrome: Underdiagnosed Condition in the Lateral Midfoot Pain. Case Rep Radiol 2016:8739362

Chang CH, Kumar SJ, Riddle EC, Glutting J (2002) Macrodactyly of the foot. J Bone Joint Surg Am 84:1189–1194

Comfort TK, Johnson LO (1998) Resection for symptomatic talocalcaneal coalition. J Pediatr Orthop 18:283–288

Davids JR, McBrayer D, Blackhurst DW (2007) Juvenile hallux valgus deformity: surgical management by lateral hemiepiphysiodesis of the great toe metatarsal. J Pediatr Orthop 27:826–830

Desai S, Aroojis A, Mehta R (2008) Ultrasound evaluation of clubfoot correction during Ponseti treatment: a preliminary report. J Pediatr Orthop 28:53–59

DiMeglio A (2001) Growth in pediatric orthopaedics. J Pediatr Orthop 21:549–555

Diméglio A, Bensahel H, Souchet P, Mazeau P, Bonnet F (1995) Classification of clubfoot. J Pediatr Orthop B 4:129–136

Dobbs MB, Gurnett CA (2012) Genetics of clubfoot. J Pediatr Orthop B 21:7–9

Dobbs MB, Rudzki JR, Purcell DB, Walton T, Porter KR, Gurnett CA (2004) Factors predictive of outcome after use of the Ponseti method for the treatment of idiopathic clubfeet. J Bone Joint Surg Am 86:22–27

Dobbs MB, Purcell DB, Nunley R, Morcuende JA (2006) Early results of a new method of treatment for idiopathic congenital vertical talus. J Bone Joint Surg Am 88:1192–1200

Dyer PJ, Davis N (2006) The role of the Pirani scoring system in the management of club foot by the Ponseti method. J Bone Joint Surg Br 88:1082–1084

Escobedo EM, MacDonald TL, Hunter JC (2006) Acute fracture of the os trigonum. Emerg Radiol 13:139–141

Federer AE, Tainter DM, Adams SB, Schweitzer KM Jr (2018) Conservative management of metatarsalgia and lesser toe deformities. Foot Ankle Clin 23:9–20

Forlino A, Marini JC (2016) Osteogenesis imperfecta. Lancet 387:1657–1671

Freyschmidt J (2001) Melorheostosis: a review of 23 cases. Eur Radiol 11:474–479

Guo S, Yan YY, Lee SSY, Tan TJ (2019) Accessory ossicles of the foot-an imaging conundrum. Emerg Radiol 26:465–478

Hagmann S, Dreher T, Wenz W (2009) Skewfoot. Foot Ankle Clin 14:409–434

Hammer MR, Pai DR (2015) The foot and ankle: congenital and developmental conditions. In: Stein-Wexler R, Wootton-Gorges S, Ozonoff M (eds) Pediatric orthopedic imaging. Springer, Berlin, pp 463–516

Handa A, Nishimura G, Zhan MX, Bennett DL, El-Khoury GY (2022) A primer on skeletal dysplasias. Jpn J Radiol 40:245–261

Harris E (2013) The intoeing child: etiology, prognosis, and current treatment options. Clin Podiatr Med Surg 30:531–565

Hellemans J, Preobrazhenska O, Willaert A et al (2004) Loss-of-function mutations in LEMD3 result in osteopoikilosis, Buschke-Ollendorff syndrome and melorheostosis. Nat Genet 36:1213–1218

Ihde LL, Forrester DM, Gottsegen CJ et al (2011) Sclerosing bone dysplasias: review and differentiation from other causes of osteosclerosis. Radiographics 31:1865–1882

Ilyas I, Wade WJ, Al Barrag M, Al Hussainan TS, Lotaibi LA, Alssayad M (2009) A rare pentad of foot and ankle deformities in hyperlax children. J Child Orthop 3:115–120

Jenkins ZA, van Kogelenberg M, Morgan T, Jeffs A et al (2009) Germline mutations in WTX cause a sclerosing skeletal dysplasia but do not predispose to tumorigenesis. Nat Genet 41:95–100

Jones D, Barnes J, Lloyd-Roberts GC (1978) Congenital aplasia and dysplasia of the tibia with intact fibula. Classification and management. J Bone Joint Surg Br 60:31–39

Karadaglis D, Grace D (2003) Morphology of the hallux sesamoids. Foot Ankle Surg 9:165–167

Karasick D, Schweitzer ME (1996) The os trigonum syndrome: imaging features. AJR Am J Roentgenol 166:125–129

Karasick D, Wapner KL (1990) Hallux valgus deformity: preoperative radiologic assessment. AJR Am J Roentgenol 155:119–123

Kennedy J, Noel J, O'Meara A, Kelly P (2013) Foot and ankle abnormalities in the Hurler syndrome: additions to the phenotype. J Pediatr Orthop 33:558–562

Kim HT, Lee SH, Yoo CI, Kang JH, Suh JT (2003) The management of brachymetatarsia. J Bone Joint Surg Br 85:683–690

Kim J, Park JW, Hong SW, Jeong JY, Gong HS, Baek GH (2015) Ray amputation for the treatment of foot macrodactyly in children. Bone Joint J 97-B:1364–1369

Knörr J, Soldado F, Pham TT, Torres A, Cahuzac JP, de Gauzy JS (2014) Percutaneous correction of persistent severe metatarsus adductus in children. J Pediatr Orthop 34:447–452

Kose O, Okan AN, Durakbasa MO, Emrem K, Islam NC (2006) Fracture of the os trigonum: a case report. J Orthop Surg (Hong Kong) 14:354–356

Kuhns LR, Koujok K, Hall JM, Craig C (2003) Ultrasound of the navicular during the simulated Ponseti maneuver. J Pediatr Orthop 23:243–245

Lateur LM, Van Hoe LR, Van Ghillewe KV, Gryspeerdt SS, Baert AL, Dereymaeker GE (1994) Subtalar coalition: diagnosis with the C sign on lateral radiographs of the ankle. Radiology 193:847–851

Lee MS, Harcke HT, Kumar SJ, Bassett GS (1989) Subtalar joint coalition in children: new observations. Radiology 172:635–639

Love SM, Ganey T, Ogden JA (1990) Postnatal epiphyseal development: the distal tibia and fibula. J Pediatr Orthop 10:298–305

Mahboubi S, Davidson R (1999) MR imaging in longitudinal epiphyseal bracket in children. Pediatr Radiol 29:259–261

Mahmood A, Mahmood NF (2015) Macrodystrophia lipomatosa: a troubled second big toe. Radiol Case Rep 3:92

Mellado JM, Ramos A, Salvadó E, Camins A, Danús M, Saurí A (2003) Accessory ossicles and sesamoid bones of the ankle and foot: imaging findings, clinical significance and differential diagnosis. Eur Radiol 13(Suppl 6):L164–L177

Miller TT (2002) Painful accessory bones of the foot. Semin Musculoskelet Radiol 6:153–161

Miller TT, Staron RB, Feldman F, Parisien M, Glucksman WJ, Gandolfo LH (1995) The symptomatic accessory tarsal navicular bone: assessment with MR imaging. Radiology 195:849–853

Moritani T, Aihara T, Oguma E, Shimanuki Y, Takano H, Sato M (2000) MR evaluation of talonavicular angle in congenital talipes equinovarus. Clin Imaging 24:243–247

Murphey MD, Choi JJ, Kransdorf MJ, Flemming DJ, Gannon FH (2000) Imaging of osteochondroma: variants and complications with radiologic-pathologic correlation. Radiographics 20:1407–1434

Nagai MK, Chan G, Guille JT, Kumar SJ, Scavina M, Mackenzie WG (2006) Prevalence of Charcot-Marie-Tooth disease in patients who have bilateral cavovarus feet. J Pediatr Orthop 26:438–443

Nwawka OK, Hayashi D, Diaz LE et al (2013) Sesamoids and accessory ossicles of the foot: anatomical variability and related pathology. Insights Imaging 4:581–593

Oh SJ, Kim YH, Kim SK, Kim MW (2012) Painful os peroneum syndrome presenting as lateral plantar foot pain. Ann Rehabil Med 36:163–166

Park SS, Kim SW, Jung BS, Lee HS, Kim JS (2009) Selective soft-tissue release for recurrent or residual deformity after conservative treatment of idiopathic clubfoot. J Bone Joint Surg Br 91:1526–1530

Phelps DA, Grogan DP (1985) Polydactyly of the foot. J Pediatr Orthop 5:446–451

Pistoia F, Ozonoff MB, Wintz P (1987) Ball-and-socket ankle joint. Skeletal Radiol 16:447–451

Ponseti IV (1992) Treatment of congenital club foot. J Bone Joint Surg Am 74:448–454

Radler C (2013) The Ponseti method for the treatment of congenital club foot: review of the current literature and treatment recommendations. Int Orthop 37:1747–1753

Radler C, Manner HM, Suda R, Burghardt R, Herzenberg JE, Ganger R, Grill F (2007) Radiographic evaluation of idiopathic clubfeet undergoing Ponseti treatment. J Bone Joint Surg Am 89:1177–1183

Rao UB, Joseph B (1992) The influence of footwear on the prevalence of flat foot. A survey of 2300 children. J Bone Joint Surg Br 74:525–527

Raskind WH, Conrad EU, Chansky H, Matsushita M (1995) Loss of heterozygosity in chondrosarcomas for markers linked to hereditary multiple exostoses loci on chromosomes 8 and 11. Am J Hum Genet 56:1132–1139

Renaud A, Aucourt J, Weill J et al (2013) Radiographic features of osteogenesis imperfecta. Insights Imaging 4:417–429

Resnick D (1984) Talar ridges, osteophytes, and beaks: a radiologic commentary. Radiology 151:329–332

Sarin VK, Erickson GM, Giori NJ, Bergman AG, Carter DR (1999) Coincident development of sesamoid bones and clues to their evolution. Anat Rec 257:174–180

Schimizzi A, Brage M (2004) Brachymetatarsia. Foot Ankle Clin 9:555–70, ix

Schreck MA (2006) Pediatric longitudinal epiphyseal bracket: review and case presentation. J Foot Ankle Surg 45:342–345

Schwend RM, Drennan JC (2003) Cavus foot deformity in children. J Am Acad Orthop Surg 11:201–211

Shapiro F (2019) Developmental disorders of the foot and ankle, Pediatric orthopedic deformities, vol 2. Springer, Cham, pp 665–797

Shipp TD, Benacerraf BR (1998) The significance of prenatally identified isolated clubfoot: is amniocentesis indicated? Am J Obstet Gynecol 178:600–602

Sillence DO, Rimoin DL (1978) Classification of osteogenesis imperfect. Lancet 1:1041–1042

Skolan V, Šmigovec I, Đapić T, Antičević D (2013) Long-term follow-up of congenital distal tibiofibular diastasis: a report of two female patients. J Pediatr Orthop B 22:464–469

Sobacchi C, Schulz A, Coxon FP, Villa A, Helfrich MH (2013) Osteopetrosis: genetics, treatment and new insights into osteoclast function. Nat Rev Endocrinol 9:522–536

Stevens PM, Aoki S, Olson P (2006) Ball-and-socket ankle. J Pediatr Orthop 26:427–431

Strayer SM, Reece SG, Petrizzi MJ (1999) Fractures of the proximal fifth metatarsal. Am Fam Physician 59:2516–2522

Suda R, Suda AJ, Grill F (2006) Sonographic classification of idiopathic clubfoot according to severity. J Pediatr Orthop B 15:134–140

Sullivan JA (1999) Pediatric flatfoot: evaluation and management. J Am Acad Orthop Surg 7:44–53

Supakul N, Loder RT, Karmazyn B (2013) Dynamic US study in the evaluation of infants with vertical or oblique talus deformities. Pediatr Radiol 43:376–380

Takakura Y, Tanaka Y, Kumai T, Sugimoto K (1999) Development of the ball-and-socket ankle as assessed by radiography and arthrography. A long-term follow-up report. J Bone Joint Surg Br 81:1001–1004

Thometz JG, Simons GW (1993) Deformity of the calcaneocuboid joint in patients who have talipes equinovarus. J Bone Joint Surg Am 75:190–195

Thompson GH (1996) Bunions and deformities of the toes in children and adolescents. Instr Course Lect 45:355–367

Trevor D (1950) Tarso-epiphysial aclasis; a congenital error of epiphysial development. J Bone Joint Surg Br 32-B:204–213

Vallejo JM, Jaramillo D (2001) Normal MR imaging anatomy of the ankle and foot in the pediatric population. Magn Reson Imaging Clin N Am 9:435–46, ix

Vanderwilde R, Staheli LT, Chew DE, Malagon V (1988) Measurements on radiographs of the foot in normal infants and children. J Bone Joint Surg Am 70:407–415

Venn-Watson EA (1976) Problems in polydactyly of the foot. Orthop Clin North Am 7:909–927

Villarroya MA, Esquivel JM, Tomás C, Moreno LA, Buenafé A, Bueno G (2009) Assessment of the medial longitudinal arch in children and adolescents with obesity: footprints and radiographic study. Eur J Pediatr 168:559–567

Wainwright AM, Auld T, Benson MK, Theologis TN (2002) The classification of congenital talipes equinovarus. J Bone Joint Surg Br 84:1020–1024

Weseley MS, Barenfeld PA, Shea JM, Eisenstein AL (1982) The congenital cavus foot. A follow-up report. Bull Hosp Jt Dis Orthop Inst 42:217–229

Widhe T (1997) Foot deformities at birth: a longitudinal prospective study over a 16-year period. J Pediatr Orthop 17:20–24

Wong GNL, Tan TJ (2016) MR imaging as a problem solving tool in posterior ankle pain: a review. Eur J Radiol 85:2238–2256

Yan YY, Mehta KV, Tan TJ (2016) Fracture of the os trigonum: a report of two cases and review of the literature. Foot Ankle Surg 22:e21–e24

Yu GV, Hladik J (1994) Residual calcaneovalgus deformity: review of the literature and case study. J Foot Ankle Surg 33:228–238

Bone Trauma

Sinan Al-Qassab, Prudencia N. M. Tyrrell,
and Victor N. Cassar-Pullicino

Contents

S. Al-Qassab · P. N. M. Tyrrell (✉)
V. N. Cassar-Pullicino
Department of Radiology, The Robert Jones and Agnes Hunt Orthopaedic Hospital, Shropshire, UK
e-mail: prudencia.tyrrell@nhs.net

Abstract

Trauma to the ankle and foot is a common injury at all ages. While the radiograph is typically the first imaging investigation and will detect the majority of bone injuries, subtle fractures can be overlooked on radiographs due to the multiplicity of bones in the midfoot with osseous overlap. Computed tomography (CT) with multiplanar reconstruction is an invaluable adjunct in further evaluation. In more complex injuries, CT acts as a helpful addition for surgical planning. Magnetic resonance imaging (MRI) can detect bone marrow edema and signs of bone bruising/microtrabecular injury in stress and insufficiency fracture scenarios as well as facilitating detail on associated soft tissue injury.

This chapter addresses the spectrum of bone injury at the ankle and foot encompassing the role of radiographs, CT, and MRI and also refers to some commonly used classification systems in use for different injuries.

1 Introduction

Injury to the ankle and foot can be extremely debilitating for the patient and can greatly interfere with mobility. Bone injuries in the foot can

Med Radiol Diagn Imaging (2023)

https://doi.org/10.1007/174_2023_388,
Published Online: 29 April 2023

be very subtle and easily overlooked, due in part to the large number of bones tightly packed together with multiple overlap. Careful scrutiny of radiographs together with use of extra or alternative views can help in the detection of subtle injury. Computed tomography (CT) is particularly valuable in those instances where the radiograph is normal but a high index of suspicion prevails. CT also has a particular role in the evaluation of calcaneal fractures. MRI is superior in detecting bone marrow edema in stress/insufficiency fractures not visible on conventional radiography in addition to its ability to depict ligamentous injuries.

2 Indications for Radiography in Suspected Injury

Trauma to the ankle is a very common injury presenting to the Accident and Emergency (A + E) Department. In the past, an ankle radiographic series was found to be the second most commonly requested musculoskeletal examination in the A + E Department (after a cervical spine series), with more than 90% of such injuries being radiographed (Stiell et al. 1992). The yield of clinically significant fractures (those requiring plaster immobilization or reduction) is less than 15% (Stiell et al. 1993). In an attempt to reduce the number of negative investigations following injury, Stiell introduced a number of clinical criteria, known as the Ottawa Ankle Rules, to determine the need for radiographs of the ankle (Stiell et al. 1994). These criteria included point tenderness over the posterior edge of either the medial or the lateral malleolus (including the distal 6 cm of the tibia and fibula) and inability to bear weight immediately after the injury, or for four consecutive steps in the Emergency Department. Later studies demonstrated that application of the Ottawa Ankle Rules can adequately screen for ankle fractures (Verma et al. 1997).

Although patients may present with symptoms and signs suggestive of an ankle injury, careful perusal of the radiograph at the base of the fifth metatarsal may reveal a clinically unsuspected injury. There are a number of accessory ossicles in relation to the ankle and especially the foot, and these should not be confused with avulsion injuries. An accessory ossicle can usually be identified from a characteristic location and from its well corticated margin (Fig. 1). By comparison, an avulsed fragment will have an irregular margin, and the point from which it was avulsed may be identifiable. There may also be associated soft tissue swelling in the area, and clinical examination may reveal focal tenderness at the site of the avulsed fragment.

However, in the absence of bone injury, soft tissue swelling and tenderness are often indicative of significant soft tissue injury. Such injuries are often referred to as ankle sprains. Since soft tissue injuries about the ankle are almost always treated conservatively, provided the conventional radiograph is negative for bone injury, it is unusual that patients will proceed to further imaging investigation in the form of CT or magnetic resonance imaging (MRI). However, in those centers where ultrasound is readily available, if tendon or ligamentous injury is suspected, transonic examination may often be carried out. Soft tissue injuries are dealt with in more detail in the relevant chapter.

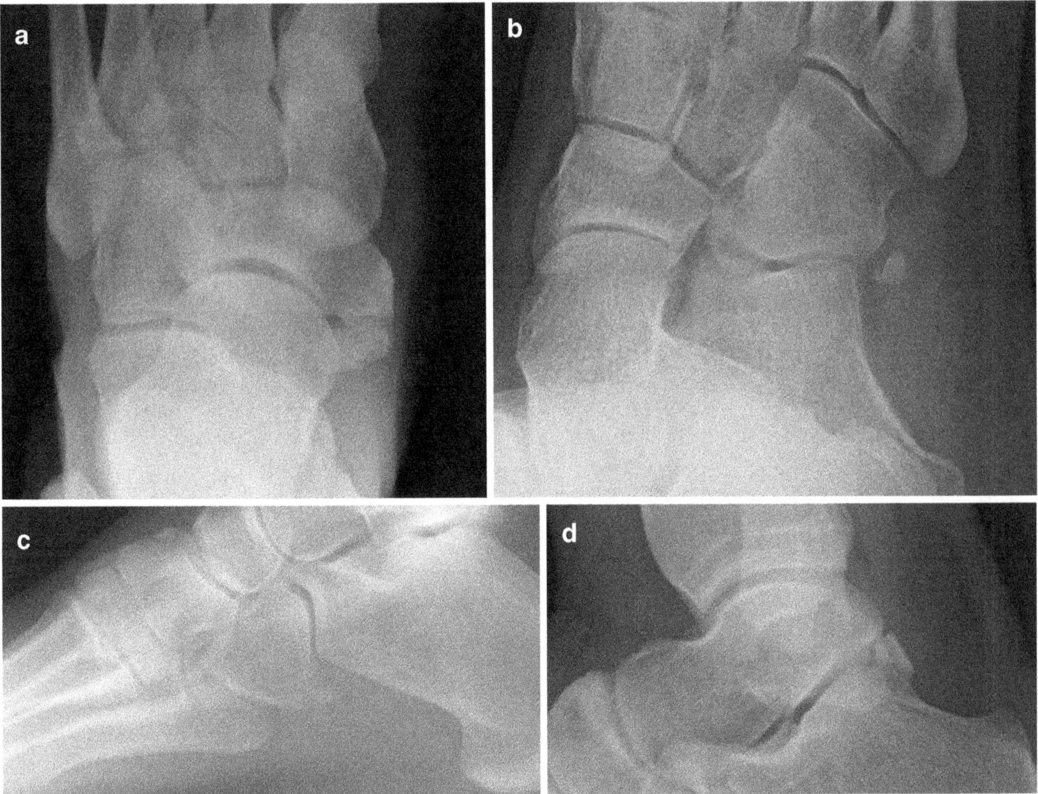

Fig. 1 (**a**) Accessory navicular bone. (**b, c**) os peroneum. (**d**) Accessory ossicle (os trigonum)

3 The Ankle

There are a number of classification systems used in respect of fractures (together with associated ligamentous injuries) at the ankle. The pattern of injury depends on the position of the foot at the time of injury, and the direction, magnitude, and rate of application of the loading forces. Although forces acting on the ankle may be essentially occurring in one direction and hence result in a single type of injury, such as avulsion of a bone fragment from a particular part of the joint, often the injuries are rather more complex involving a combination of movements. The classification systems commonly employed at the ankle are those of Lauge-Hansen (1954) and Danis (1949) and Weber (1972), the latter two being modified in the AO system. Lauge-Hansen (1950, 1954) highlighted the influence that the position of the foot had on the injury pattern and correlated this position with the direction of the deforming forces. In his system of classification, the position of the foot (pronation or supination) at the time of injury is described first, and the direction of the deforming force (abduction, adduction, eversion, and inversion) is described second. Lauge-Hansen found that injuries occurred in a sequential manner.

The Lauge-Hansen classification of injuries is rather complex. However, one advantage of this system is that a particular mechanism of injury is associated with a sequence of injuries, which if recognized can allow one to deduce and assume their presence, even if they are not actually visualized/identified on the radiograph.

The Danis (1949) classification was modified by Weber (1972) (and more recently modified by the AO group). It is based on the level of the fracture of the fibula relative to the syndesmosis and the horizontal portion of the tibiotalar joint. While this system is simpler than the Lauge-Hansen classification, initially it ignored the medial malleolar injuries that were thought biomechanically

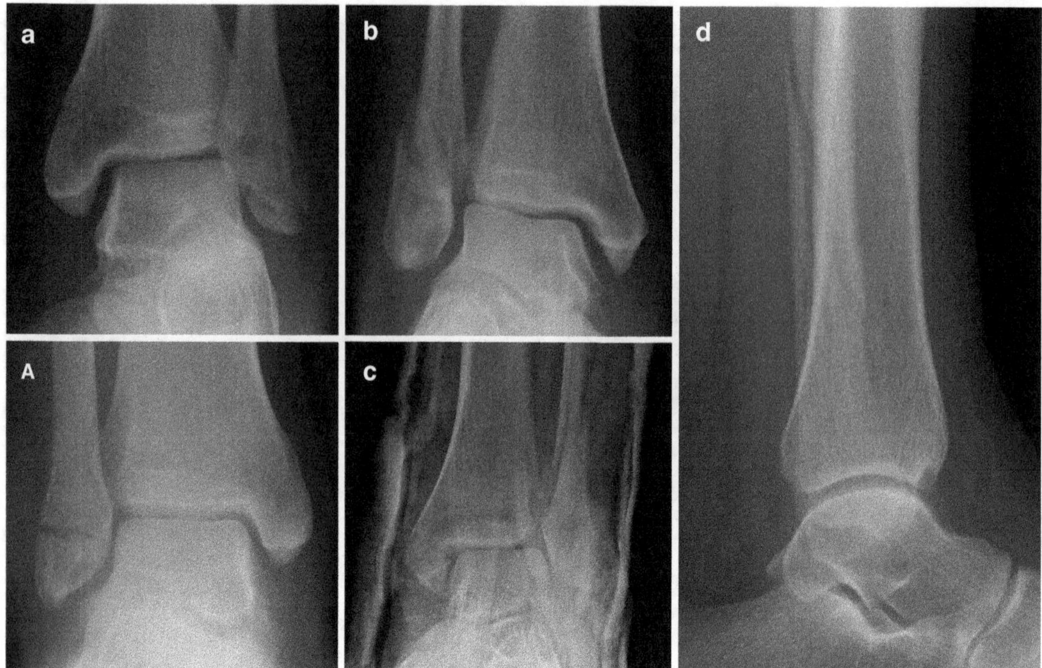

Fig. 2 (**a**, **A**) AP radiograph of the ankle demonstrating a minimally displaced fracture of the lateral malleolus below the level of the joint in two different patients (Weber A). (**b**) AP radiograph of the ankle demonstrating a displaced oblique fracture of the lateral malleolus. Note that the distal extent of the fracture is at the level of the syndesmosis and extends proximally (Weber B). (**c**) AP radiograph of the ankle demonstrating a fracture of the distal fibula above the level of the syndesmosis (Weber C). (**d**) Lateral radiograph of the ankle demonstrating a Weber C fracture of the distal fibula in a different patient

important. Weber's classification has three types of fracture—A, B, and C (Fig. 2). The more proximal the fracture of the fibula, the greater the risk of injury to the syndesmosis and tibiofibular ligaments and the more likely that the ankle mortice will be unstable. Some authors have advocated the expansion of this classification to incorporate the medial injury, and this would almost certainly increase the complexity of the classification (Harper 1992). This is essentially what the AO modification has done.

Henderson (1932) produced a classification system based on radiographic findings that separated injuries into three groups: (1) isolated fractures of the medial, lateral, posterior, or anterior malleolus, (2) bi-malleolar, and (3) tri-malleolar fractures. This is a simple descriptive classification that is sometimes used (Fig. 3).

Vertical loading drives the talus into the distal tibia. The position of the foot and the rate of loading affect the injury pattern which can range from isolated fractures of the anterior or posterior lip of the tibia to complex intra-articular fractures of the distal tibia (pilon fracture) (Fig. 4). The term pilon was first used by Destot in 1911 (Destot 1911). He compared this explosive injury of the talus impacting against the tibia to that of a hammer striking a nail. This fracture involves the tibial plafond of the ankle joint. The injury is associated with high energy, as in falling from a height, and is associated with a large compressive force, significant comminuted disruption of the articular surface, and extensive soft tissue injury (Ayeni 1988; Mainwaring et al. 1988; Ruwe et al. 1993). Due to the complexity of this injury, CT is usually required to understand the configuration of the fracture, carefully assess the orientation of the fractured fragments, and identify tiny avulsion fractures which may indicate associated significant soft tissue injury, like syndesmotic disruption which can be difficult to determine on plain radiographs. Syndesmotic soft tissue injuries will be discussed in the relevant chapter. 3D volume rendered images are usually gener-

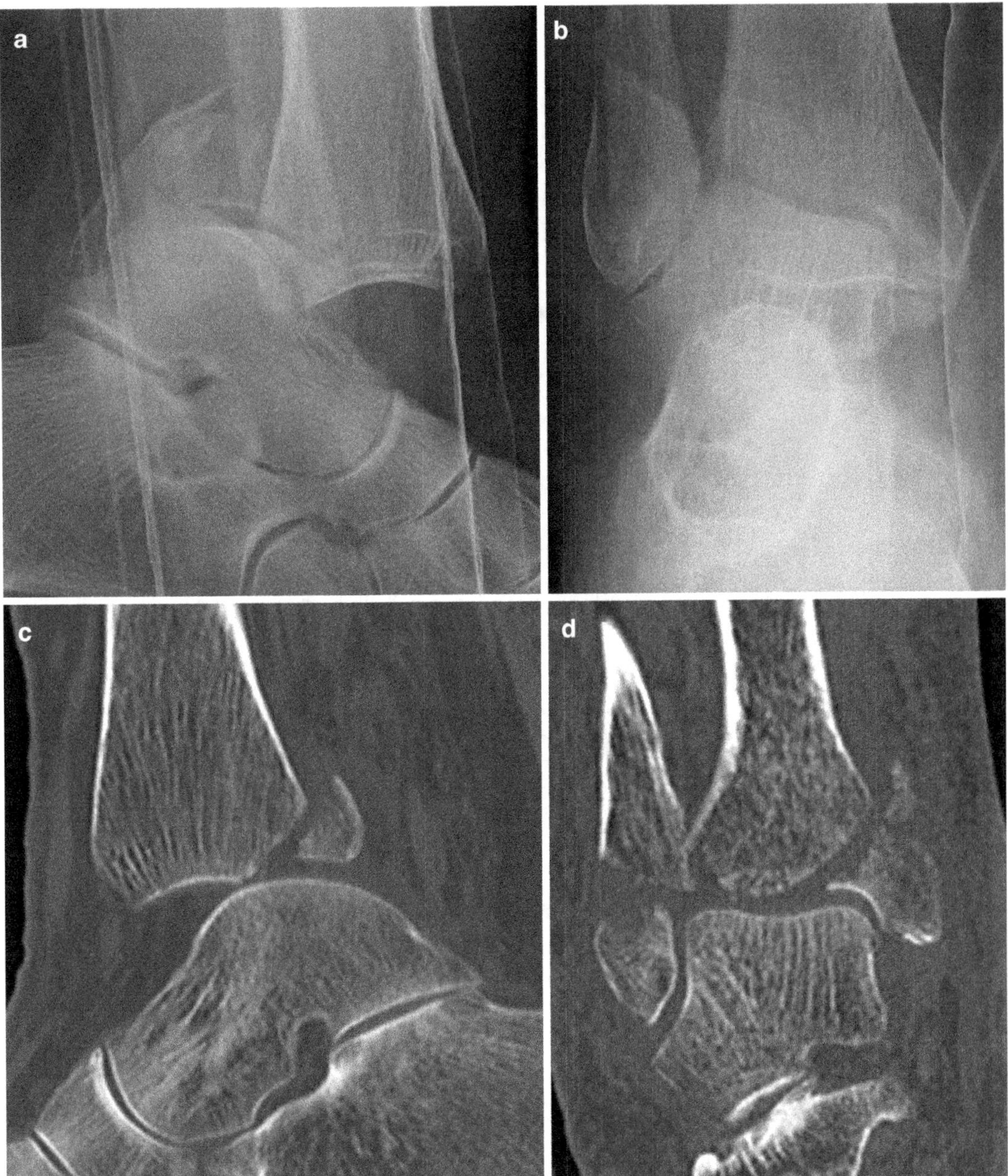

Fig. 3 (**a**, **b**) Lateral and AP radiographs demonstrating a tri-malleolar fracture dislocation of the ankle. (**c**) Sagittal CT image showing the posterior malleolar fracture and the posterior dislocation of the talus. (**d**) Coronal CT image demonstrating the medial and lateral malleolar fractures in the same patient

ated to assist the surgical team in surgical planning (Fig. 5).

Isolated avulsion type fractures at the ankle can occur. Fractures of the medial malleolus may be transverse or oblique. Transverse fractures are the result of tensile forces mediated by the deltoid ligament and may involve the anterior colliculus alone or both the anterior and the posterior colliculi. Oblique fractures usually extend upwards and inwards from the corner of the plafond. These are due to angular forces generated by movement of the talus against the medial malleolus. Fractures of the medial malleolus distal to the corner formed in the ankle mortice within the plafond are more

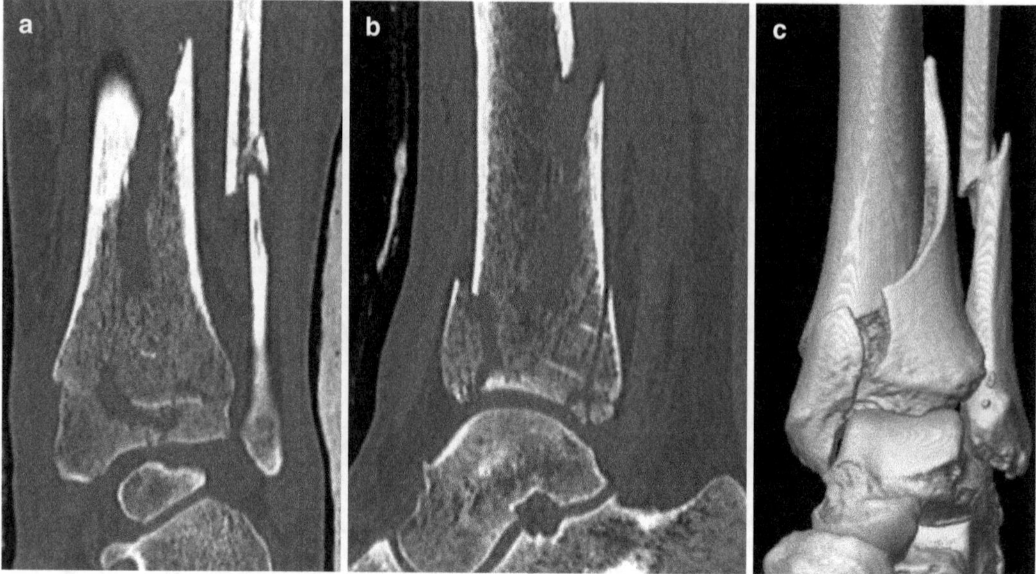

Fig. 4 (**a**, **b**) Coronal and sagittal CT images demonstrating a comminuted intra-articular fracture of the tibial plafond in keeping with a pilon fracture. This fracture usually results from impaction of the talus into the tibial plafond. Note the associated fracture of the distal fibula. (**c**) 3D volume rendering

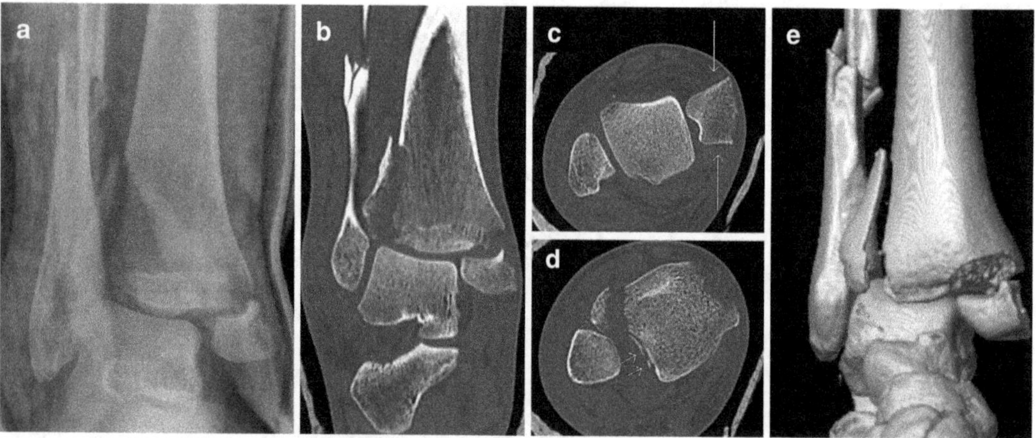

Fig. 5 (**a**) XR demonstrating a comminuted fracture of the distal tibia with intra articular extension and an associated fracture of the distal fibula with the fracture line extending above the joint line. (**b**) Sagittal CT image better demonstrating the fracture configuration. (**c**) Note how the medial malleolar fragment is flipped 90°. (**d**) Note the slender flake of cortical bone (arrows) from the lateral aspect of the distal tibia suggesting syndesmotic injury. (**e**) 3D volume rendering which the surgical team might find helpful

stable than those arising within the plafond, due to the buttressing effect afforded by the medial malleolus. An isolated fracture of the posterior colliculus has been described by Bonnin (1970) and Pankovich and Shivaram (1979) due to avulsion by the deep portion of the deltoid ligament. The fragment extends superiorly and posteriorly and is relatively undisplaced due to the overlying tibialis posterior tendon. It may be seen as a long thin fragment of cortical bone projected just lateral to the cortical contour of the malleolus. It can be difficult to visualize on an anteroposterior radiograph and may be better seen on an external oblique projection.

Classification systems are often employed to facilitate comparisons between different treatment/management regimens. In practical terms, what the orthopedic surgeon wants to know from the radiograph is: what structures are fractured, the degree of separation, displacement, or malalignment, and whether the injury is stable or unstable. Instability is confirmed if under normal loading, abnormal movement or displacement occurs. The answer to these questions largely determines whether conservative or surgical management is required. The appropriate management employed will then hopefully minimize the risk of post-traumatic complications.

Inversion or adduction of the ankle places tension on the lateral collateral ligament resulting either in ligamentous rupture or a transverse fracture of the distal fibula inferior to the level of the tibial plafond. The most common fracture of the lateral malleolus is an oblique or spiral fracture extending from the anteroinferior margin upward and backward to the posterior margin of the shaft of the distal fibula. Fractures may also occur within the distal, mid, or proximal shaft of the fibula. Ankle injuries created by external rotation of the foot can be associated with a fracture of the proximal shaft of the fibula, as described by Maisonneve (1840). This fracture is easily overlooked since patients rarely complain of pain in the region when there are more painful ankle injuries. A Maisonneuve fracture should be suspected, and full-length views of the tibia and fibula obtained when ankle radiographs demonstrate apparent isolated fracture of the posterior lip of the tibia, widening of the medial or lateral clear space, an isolated displaced fracture of the medial malleolus, or when clinically tenderness can be elicited over the syndesmosis or antero-medial aspect of the joint capsule in the absence of obvious underlying injury (Rogers 1992).

Avulsion fractures can occur from the distal tip of the lateral or medial malleolus due to pull of the lateral or medial collateral ligaments. These fractures need to be differentiated from the secondary centers of ossification. An isolated small avulsion fracture of the posterolateral aspect of the lateral malleolus may be associated with dislocation of the peroneal tendons due to the retinaculum which binds down the tendons being avulsed. The fracture flake consists of a small bone fragment 1–2 mm in width but 1–2 cm in length. It lies parallel to the lateral or posterolateral aspect of the lateral malleolus and is best seen on the AP or an internal oblique projection. The injury is not uncommon in skiers and occurs when the peroneal muscles are tensed and the ankle dorsi-flexed. Surgical treatment is required to repair the retinaculum, and the bone fragment is either excised or reattached. A similar small avulsion injury has been identified just proximal and medial to the medial malleolus, associated with rupture of the tibialis posterior tendon. This is associated with either a transverse fracture of the medial malleolus or bi-malleolar fractures of the pronation external rotation variety with the fibular fracture located proximal to the joint line.

Avulsion fracture of the anterior tubercle of the tibia is the result of tension within the antero-inferior tibiofibular ligament and is known as the Tillaux fracture (Cancelmo 1962; Protas and Kornblatt 1981). This is due to external rotation of the foot. The Wagstaffe-Le Fort fracture is an avulsion fracture at the fibular attachment of the anterior tibiofibular ligament. Fractures of the posterior malleolus or posterior lip of the tibia occur as a result of avulsion at the site of attachment of the posterior tibiofibular ligament. These may be small and flake-like or larger and involve some portion of the posterior joint surface of the tibia (Fig. 6). The latter are due to vertical compression of the talus against the tibia. The fracture line is vertically orientated in the coronal plane. Fragments consisting of more than 25% of the articular surface may require surgical fixation. These fractures often occur as part of the tri-malleolar fracture. Dorsiflexion of the foot may result in fractures of the anterior lip of the tibia. Their size determines the need for surgical reduction. If large, they may be associated with a fracture dislocation.

In bi-malleolar fractures, the path of the fracture on the one side is often transverse because of tensile forces, while the other fracture is spiral or oblique. Tri-malleolar fractures involve the posterior lip of the tibia in addition to the malleoli (Fig. 7). Usually these are fracture

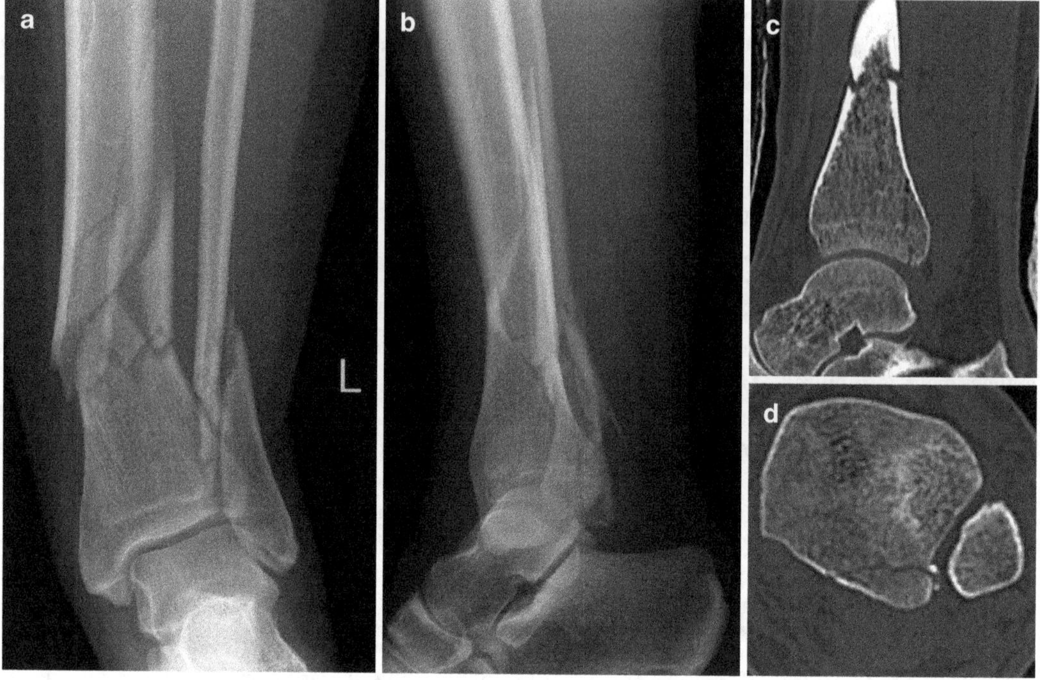

Fig. 6 (**a**, **b**) AP and lateral radiographs of the ankle demonstrating a comminuted distal tibial and fibular fracture with valgus angulation. Also note the posterior malleolar fracture. (**c**) Sagittal CT image demonstrating the intra-articular extension of the posterior malleolar fracture. (**d**) Axial CT image demonstrating the posterior malleolar fracture with widening of the posterior tibiofibular syndesmosis with tiny adjacent bone fragments suggesting a syndesmotic injury

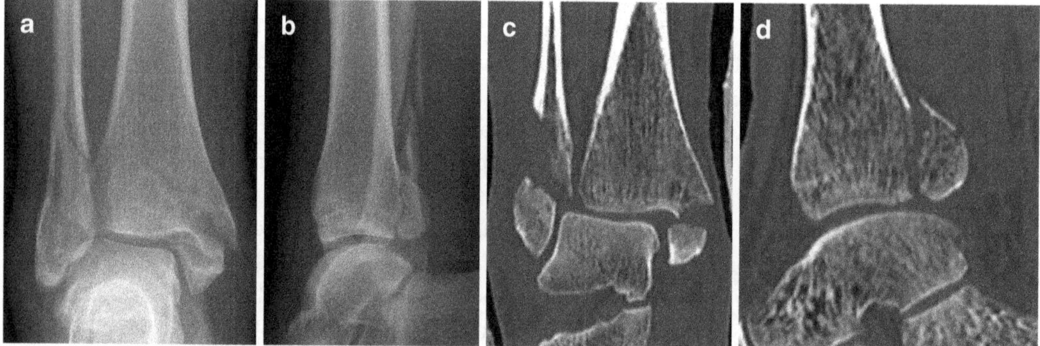

Fig. 7 (**a**, **b**) AP and lateral radiographs demonstrating a tri-malleolar ankle fracture. (**c**) Coronal CT image of the same ankle. Note the lateral talar shift. (**d**) Sagittal CT image demonstrating the minimally displaced posterior malleolar fracture

dislocations. Most are due to external rotation of the foot and therefore are laterally and posteriorly displaced. The lateral collateral ligament remains intact as does the posterior tibiofibular ligament.

4 The Talus

Half of the injuries to the talus consist of fractures, 50% of which are avulsion in nature and the rest consist of vertical or oblique fractures traversing the neck or body in the coronal plane. Twenty-five percent of all injuries are fracture dislocation with fracture of the neck being associated with either subtalar or posterior dislocation of the body. Twenty percent are other forms of dislocation without fracture, and the remaining 5% consist of other fractures including compression fractures of the talus.

Avulsion or chip type fractures occur from the superior aspect of the neck and head of the talus and also from the lateral, medial, and posterior aspect of the body. The most common avulsion fracture is from the antero-superior aspect of the neck at the point of attachment of the capsule (Fig. 8). This fracture needs to be differentiated from an os supratalare. A fracture from the lateral aspect of the body of the talus involves the lateral process that projects laterally beneath the tip of the lateral malleolus (Fig. 9). An avulsion fracture may occur at the attachment of the deltoid ligament medially (Fig. 8), and fractures of the posterior talar surface may occur in extreme plantar flexion. This injury is to be differentiated from the accessory ossicle, the os trigonum (Fig. 1).

Vertical fractures usually occur as a result of a force from below, driving the neck of the talus upward against the anterior lip of the tibia. These are not infrequently seen in road traffic accidents when the sole of the foot is jammed against the brake pedal. They can be associated with dislocation if forces are strong enough. The mechanism of injury is continuation of the dorsiflexion force that produced the fracture of the neck, resulting in rupture of ligamentous structures that bind the talus to the tibia and calcaneum.

Hawkins (1970) proposed a classification of talar fractures: Type I—non-displaced fracture of the neck of the talus without subluxation or dislo-

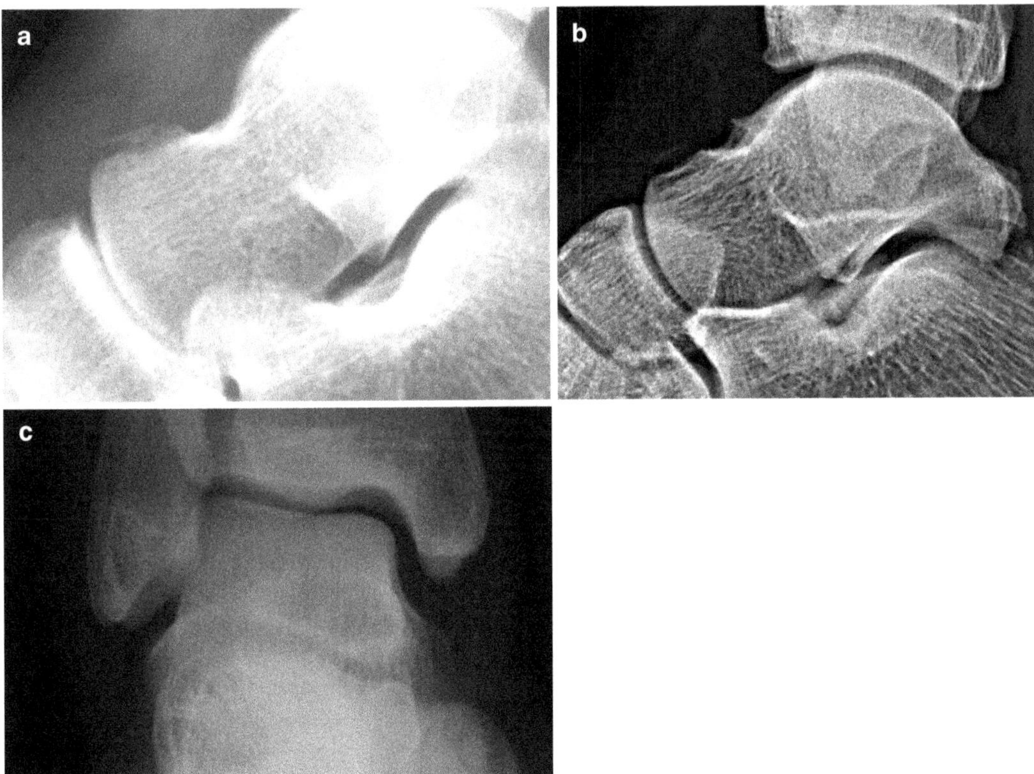

Fig. 8 (**a**) Lateral radiograph of the ankle demonstrating an avulsion fracture of the dorsal aspect of the neck of the talus. (**b**) Lateral radiograph of the ankle of a different patient also demonstrating an avulsion fracture of the dorsal aspect of the neck of talus. (**c**) AP radiograph of the ankle demonstrating a tiny avulsion fracture of the medial aspect of the talus

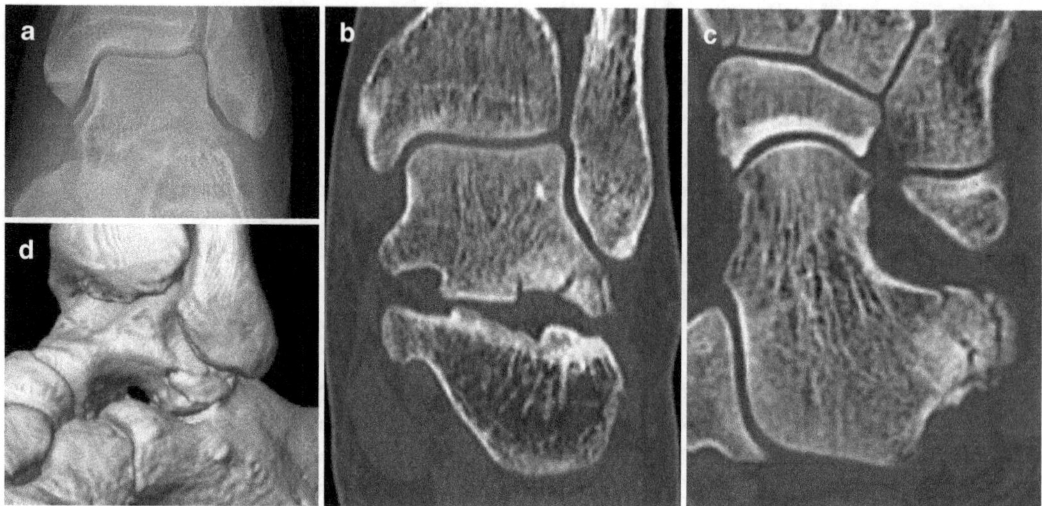

Fig. 9 (**a**) AP radiograph of the ankle demonstrating tiny osseous fragments adjacent to the lateral talus. (**b, c**) Coronal and axial oblique CT images demonstrating the comminuted fracture of the lateral process of the talus. (**d**) 3D volume rendering

cation; Type II—displaced fracture of the talar neck with subluxation/dislocation of the subtalar joint (the ankle joint remains aligned); and Type III—displaced fracture of the talar neck with complete dislocation at the ankle and subtalar joints. Despite posteromedial displacement of the body with most Type II injury, the posterior tibial neurovascular bundle is usually spared. However, in Type III injuries with posteromedial displacement of the body, the neurovascular structures are definitively at risk. Fractures of the neck of the talus can be associated with calcaneal (10%) (Lorentzen et al. 1977) and malleolar fracture (19–28%) (Canale and Kelly Jr 1978; Lorentzen et al. 1977).

Fractures of the body of the talus may involve compression fractures of the talar dome often following a fall from a height. The superior articular surface of the talus only may be involved with disruption of the tibiotalar joint, or the entire body of the talus may fracture with involvement of both the tibiotalar and the subtalar joints. Post-traumatic complications of osteonecrosis and degenerative arthritis can be minimized by anatomical reduction with or without internal fixation. The blood supply of the talus is tenuous, and a vertical fracture of the neck is associated with a risk of avascular necrosis (AVN) of the proximal fragment (Haliburton et al. 1958; Kelly and Sullivan 1963). The risk of disruption of the blood supply and subsequent AVN increases progressively with each type of talar fracture.

5 The Calcaneum

This is the most frequently fractured bone of the tarsus. Approximately 25% of fractures are extra-articular, sparing the subtalar joint, consisting of avulsion of the various processes. Seventy-five percent are intra-articular, involving the subtalar joint and body of the calcaneum. These are invariably due to compression forces such as landing on the feet following a fall from a height. Fractures of the calcaneum are associated with proximal fractures of the tibia and spine in 10–12% of cases. Normally, a dorsi-plantar projection, a lateral and axial calcaneal view will allow identification of most fractures. Oblique projections may be needed for further clarification (Isherwood 1961).

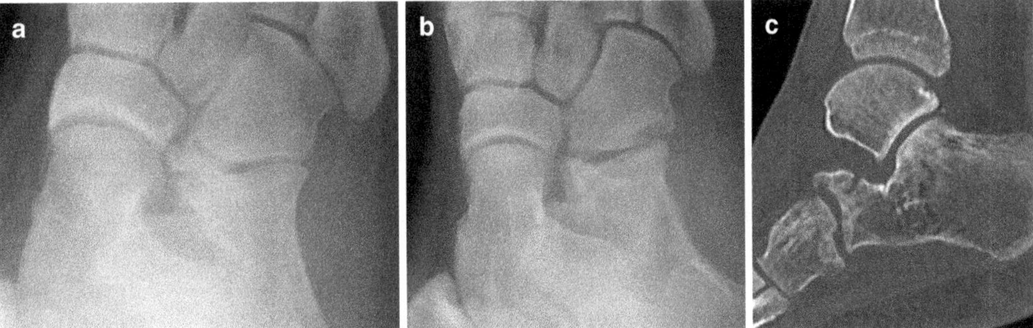

Fig. 10 (**a**) Oblique radiograph of the foot demonstrating a fracture of the anterior process of the calcaneum. (**b**) Oblique radiograph of the right foot of a different patient demonstrating a fracture of the anterior process of the calcaneum. (**c**) CT sagittal reformat of the right foot of the same patient demonstrating the fracture of the anterior process of the calcaneum

5.1 Non-compressive/Avulsive Type Fractures

These involve the anterior process, the sustentaculum tali, the superior portion of the tuberosity, and the medial or lateral surface of the tuberosity (Fig. 10). These fractures spare the subtalar joint. Vertical fractures of the tuberosity may occasionally spare the subtalar joint extending obliquely from the medial to the lateral surfaces of the bone.

A fracture involving the anterior process of the calcaneum needs to be differentiated from an accessory ossicle which can occur adjacent to the antero-superior tip of the calcaneum known as the os calcaneus secundarius.

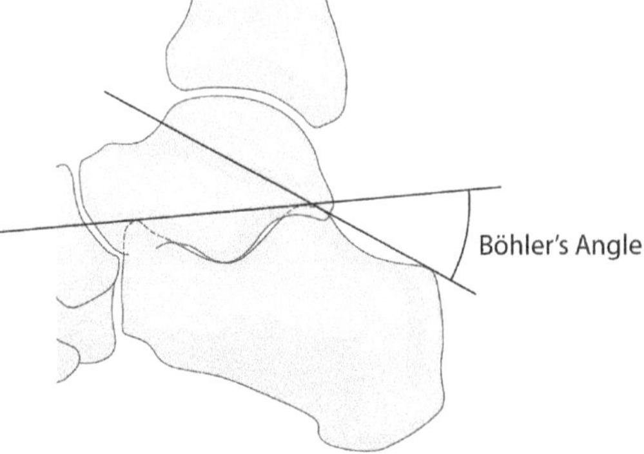

Fig. 11 Bohler's angle is the angle between the line joining the highest point of the anterior process of the calcaneum and the highest point of the posterior articular surface and the line joining the highest point of the posterior articular surface with the highest point of the calcaneal tuberosity. The normal range is 20–45

5.2 Compressive Fractures

Böhler's tuber joint angle is seen on the lateral projection (Fig. 11). It is the complement of the angle formed by two lines; a line drawn between the highest part of the anterior process and the highest part of the posterior articular surface, and a line drawn between the same point on the posterior articular surface and the most superior point of the tuberosity. The angle normally measures between 25° and 40° and is usually similar bilaterally.

The lateral process of the talus is wedge shaped in the lateral projection with its apex directed to the "crucial angle" as originally described by Gissane (Harty 1973). Axial compressive forces impact the talus into the calcaneum, disrupting the subtalar joint and distorting this anatomical angle. The force results in an oblique fracture extending from the apex of the angle, separating the body of the calcaneum. Simultaneously, a vertical split is created within the posterior facet, producing a lateral fragment which is usually larger and contains one half to two thirds of the posterior facet. There is often comminution and depression of the posterior facet from the lateral cortex. The lateral cortex is seen as a thin fragment of cortical bone. The smaller remainder of the facet is attached to a medial fragment containing the sustentaculum tali. Additional forces depress the lateral fragment, containing the majority of the posterior facet, into the body of the calcaneum.

Essex-Lopresti (1952) has defined two principal types of depressed fracture of the calcaneum. In one, the principal fragment of the posterior facet contains the upper portion of the tuberosity. Due to its appearance in the lateral projection, this fragment is designated the "tongue" type. In the second more common form, the principal fragment containing the posterior facet is separated from the tuberosity by a vertical fracture line just posterior to the posterior facet. This type is referred to as the "central lateral" compression type, where central lateral refers to the principal fragment containing the posterior facet, which is laterally situated and depressed into the central portion of the calcaneum. Usually the lateral fragment is depressed downwards and displaced laterally. The vertical split of the posterior facet allows for a variable degree of compression of the medial and lateral fragments.

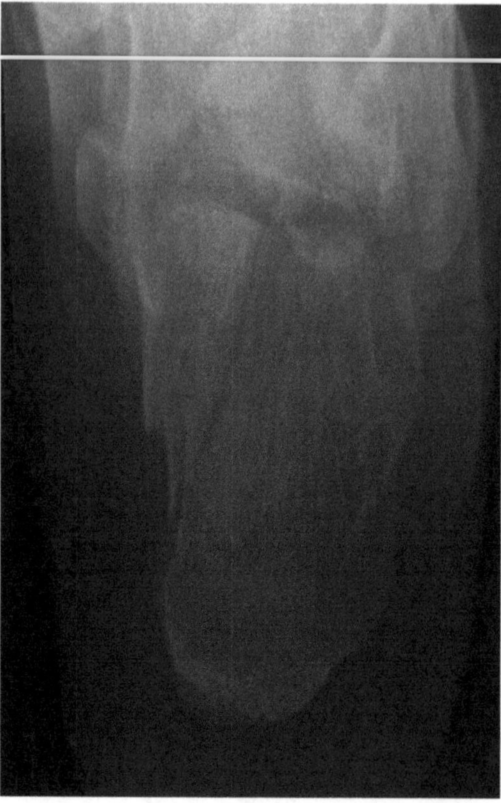

Fig. 12 Axial view of the calcaneum in a different patient demonstrating a comminuted fracture with intra-articular extension anteriorly

A limited degree of information about these injuries can be obtained by conventional radiographs, including the particularly important radiographic sign of reduction of Böhler's angle to less than 25°. A significantly greater amount of information, facilitating a better assessment of the degree and nature of the injury, is obtained by CT (Guyer et al. 1985; Heger et al. 1985; Hindman et al. 1986; Rosenberg et al. 1987) (Figs. 12 and 13). Coronal images give a particularly good assessment of the degree of depression of the posterior facet, the size and number of fragments, the degree of fragment displacement, and calcaneal widening. Sagittal reconstructions will also facilitate three plane evaluation of the injury. 3D rendered images are generated to aid in understanding the configuration of the fracture for surgical planning. In CT of fractures of the calcaneum, not infrequently the peroneal tendons may either be dislocated or impinged between the bone fragments and the inferior most aspect of the fibula. CT is also particularly good in the follow-up evaluation of these fractures and particularly in the assessment of post-traumatic arthritis, a common complication following these injuries.

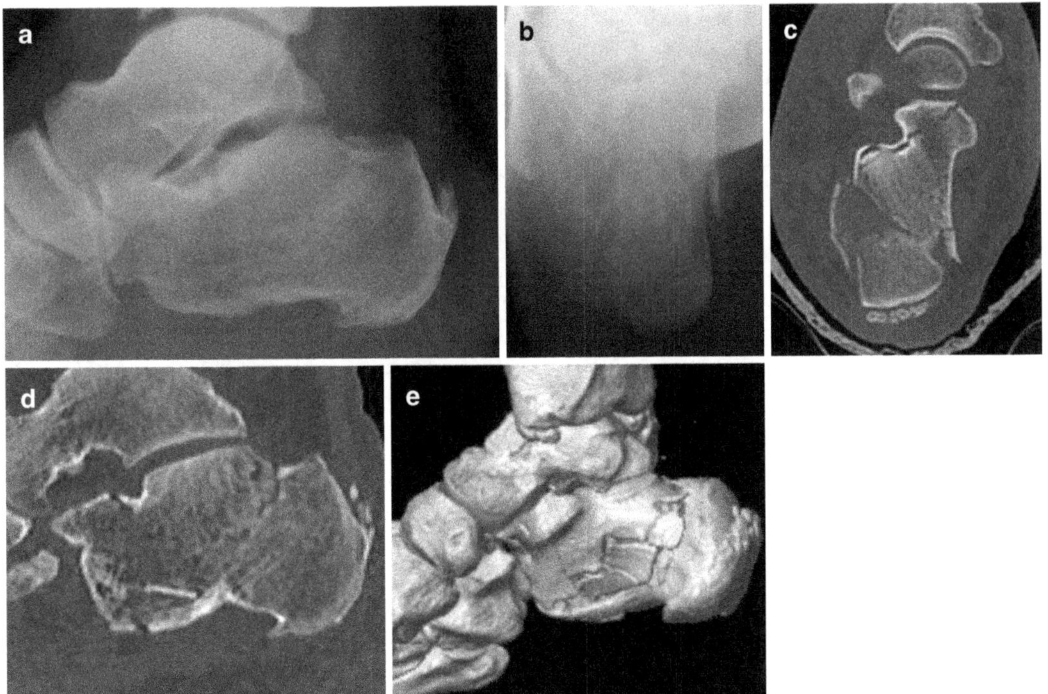

Fig. 13 (**a**, **b**) Lateral and axial radiographs demonstrating a comminuted fracture of the calcaneum. (**c**, **d**) Axial and sagittal CT images demonstrating the intra-articular extension and displacement of the comminuted calcaneal fracture. (**e**) 3D volume rendering which might be useful to the surgical team

6 The Navicular Bone

Fractures of the navicular bone are uncommon. Fractures of the body of the navicular bone occur either in the horizontal or more commonly the vertical plane (Fig. 14). They may be associated with dislocation, particularly the vertical fracture. The vertical fracture will only be visualized in the anteroposterior projection. When associated with dislocation, there is usually medial dislocation of the medial fragment. If a horizontally orientated fracture is associated with dislocation, there is usually dorsal dislocation of the dorsal fragment.

Avulsion fractures are more commonly seen in relation to the navicular bone. The most common of these is from the dorsal aspect of the bone, in the region of the talonavicular joint. This fracture should not be confused with an accessory ossicle, the os supranavicularae. An accessory ossicle can usually be readily differentiated from a fracture fragment by its smooth, well corticated margin. Another site of an avulsion fracture is in relation to the navicular tuberosity. This is the site of attachment of the tibialis posterior tendon. The fracture occurs during abduction of the foot. This fracture is not to be confused with the accessory navicular bone (Fig. 1). This is often a moderately large sized ossicle, attached to the body of the navicular by a synchondrosis. With abduction injuries of the foot, although an actual fracture may not occur, there may be some disruption of the synchondrosis and this is manifest by slight widening of the synchondrosis. If such injury is suspected and MRI is performed, it may show bone marrow edema in both the ossicle and the parent bone and within adjacent soft

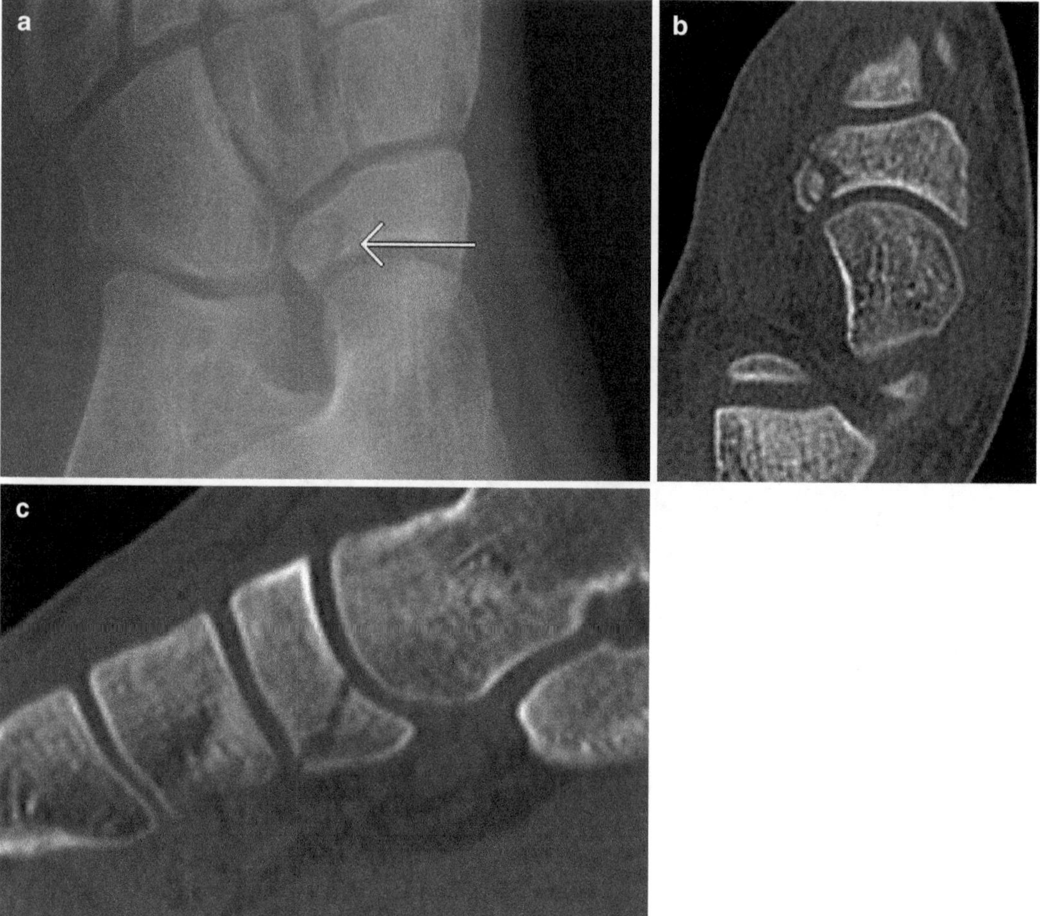

Fig. 14 (**a**) Oblique radiograph of the left foot of a skeletally immature person showing a radiolucent line through the lateral aspect of the navicular bone. (**b**, **c**) Axial and sagittal CT images confirming the minimally displaced fracture of the lateral aspect of the navicular bone

tissue. The ossicle itself again is differentiated from an acute fracture by its well corticated margin. Occasionally, small ossicles may be seen just proximal to the navicular tuberosity. These lie in the substance of the posterior tibial tendon and are known as the os tibiale externum.

7 The Cuboid and Cuneiform Bones

An avulsion fracture from the lateral aspect of the cuboid bone can occur with adduction injuries. This small bone fragment is also not be confused with accessory ossicles along the lateral aspect of the foot, namely the os peroneum and the os vesalianum (Fig. 1). Compression fractures of the cuboid bone or anterior process of the calcaneum may be associated with fracture of the tuberosity of the navicular bone.

Isolated fractures of the cuneiform bones are extremely unusual. If such a fracture is identified, the possibility of tarsometatarsal dislocation (Lisfranc) should be strongly suspected (Fig. 15). In this instance, further radiographic views or alternatively a CT scan should be obtained.

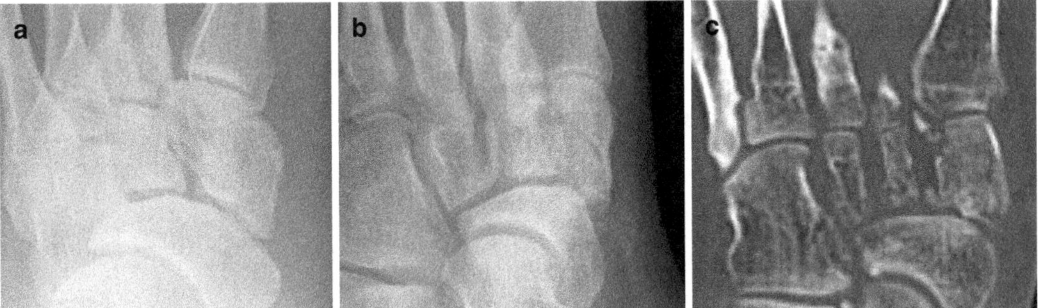

Fig. 15 (**a**) DP radiograph of the midfoot demonstrating ill-defined lucency of the lateral cortex of the medial cuneiform. (**b**) Oblique radiograph demonstrating a radiolucent line across the medial cuneiform. The midfoot can be difficult to assess due to the projection overlap of the tarsal bones and CT is usually required for further assessment. (**c**) CT confirming the presence of a comminuted fracture of the medial cuneiform. Note the tiny osseous fragment between the bases of the first and second metatarsals with irregularity of the medial corner of the base of the second metatarsals suggestive of a Lisfranc injury

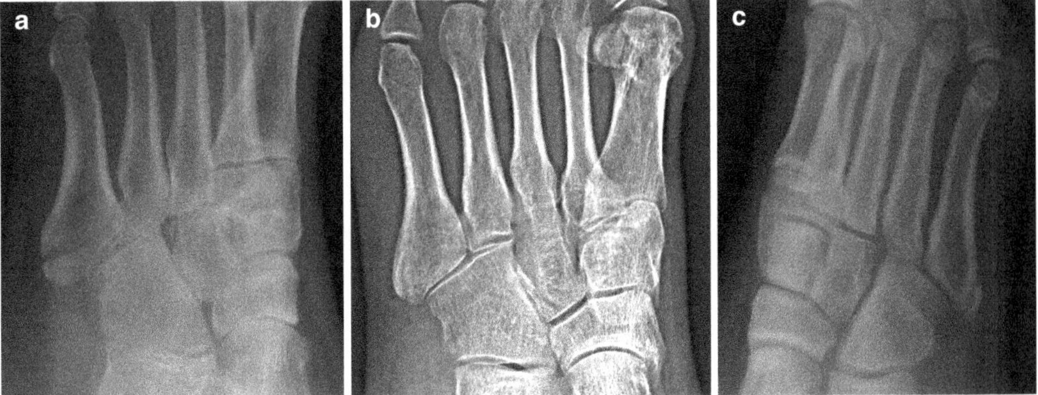

Fig. 16 (**a**) Oblique radiograph of the left foot demonstrating a minimally displaced fracture of the base of the fifth metatarsal. Note the horizontal orientation of the fracture line. (**b**) Oblique radiograph of the left foot of a different patient demonstrating an undisplaced fracture of the base of fifth metatarsal. Again note the horizontal orientation of the fracture line. (**c**) Oblique radiograph of the right foot of a skeletally immature person. Note the vertical orientation of the normal apophysis at the base of the fifth metatarsal

8 The Metatarsals

Fractures at the base of the fifth metatarsal are not uncommon (Dameron Jr. 1975; Torg et al. 1984). These tend to be transverse fractures. There are two distinct types, both of which are due to inversion of the foot. One is an avulsion fracture from the tip of the tuberosity, and the other a transverse fracture of the proximal shaft located approximately 1.5–2 cm distal to the tip of the tuberosity, just distal to the tarsometatarsal joint. This fracture is commonly known as the Jones's fracture, originally described by Sir Robert Jones in 1902 (Jones 1902). The avulsion fracture from the proximal most tip of the fifth metatarsal occurs at the site of insertion of the peroneus brevis tendon. Both of these fractures should be differentiated from the presence of a normally occurring apophysis just lateral to the base of the metatarsal (Fig. 16). The differentiating feature is that the apophysis lies in a longitudinal orientation and the radiographic

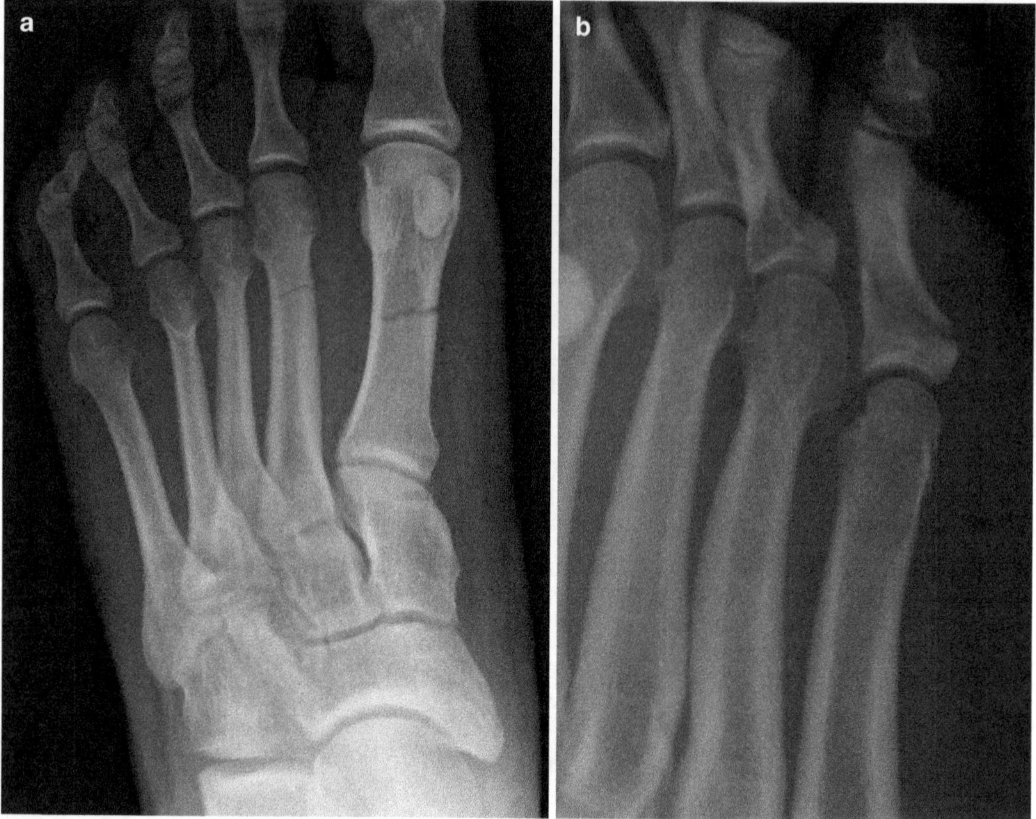

Fig. 17 (**a**) Undisplaced fractures if the first and second metatarsals. (**b**) Oblique radiograph demonstrating a fracture of the proximal phalanx of the little toe in a different patient

space between it and the parent bone is directed longitudinally. Both of the afore mentioned fractures are transverse. On occasion, both a transverse and a longitudinal lucency can be identified, this simply representing a transverse fracture in the presence of an unfused apophysis.

Fractures of the metatarsal shafts and phalanges can occur often due to direct trauma to the foot such as a heavy load falling on the foot or a stamping sports injury (Fig. 17). The metatarsal shafts are common sites of stress fractures (see below).

Freiberg's disease is avascular necrosis of the head of a metatarsal, usually the second, and should not be confused with an acute fracture (Helal and Gibb 1987). There is often a modeling anomaly with slight flattening of the metatarsal head. There may be a cortical infraction but there is usually altered density of the bone, and the combined radiological features allow differentiation from an acute injury.

9 Stress Fractures

A stress fracture occurs as a result of repetitive abnormal stress on physiologically normal bone. This is to be differentiated from an insufficiency fracture which occurs as a result of a normal stress on abnormal bone, usually due to metabolic bone disease (Figs. 18 and 19). There are multiple characteristic sites of these fractures in the bones of the foot (Eisele and Sammarco 1993). The most common is the "March" fracture,

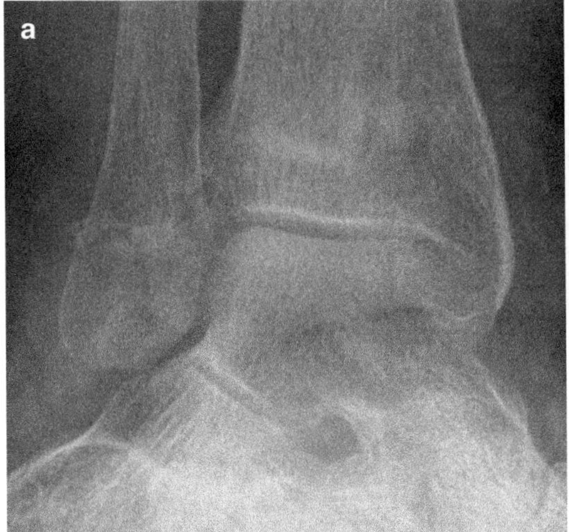

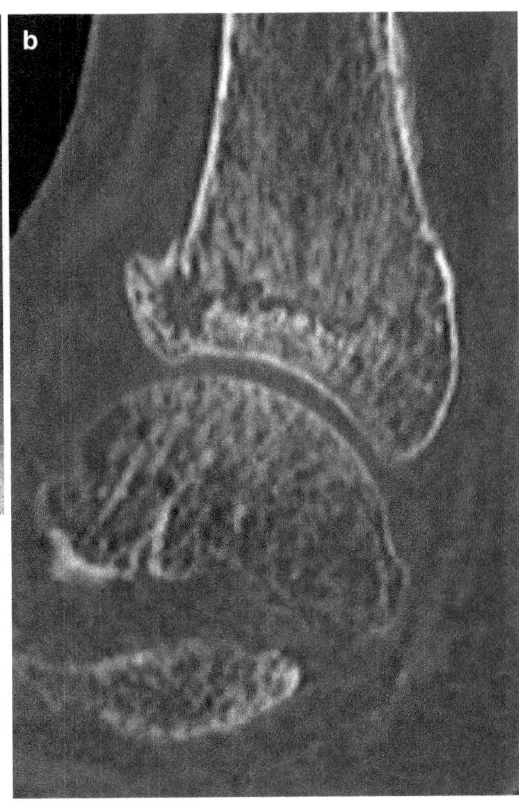

Fig. 18 A 76-year-old female with history of RA and on steroid therapy. (**a**) AP radiograph of the right ankle. Note the sclerotic horizontal line in the distal tibia on the background of diffuse osteopenia. Also note the transverse fracture of the distal fibula with associated periosteal reaction. (**b**) Sagittal CT image confirming the distal tibial fracture on the background of osteopenia in keeping with an insufficiency fracture

occurring in the mid shafts of one or more metatarsals, a commonly found injury in soldiers and occasionally in long distance runners. These fractures present with pain, but the fracture may not be visible on initial radiography. Repeat radiographs 3–4 weeks later usually show evidence of a fracture. Even if a discrete fracture line is not observed, there may be a very subtle periosteal reaction consistent with the injury. If the 3–4 weeks follow-up, radiograph does not show evidence of a fracture and there remains clinical suspicion, MRI would be the next modality of choice. It will show evidence of periosteal and/or marrow edema with intracortical signal change. There may be edema in the surrounding soft tissues. A fracture line visible as a low intramedullary linear signal is a late manifestation on MRI (Mandell et al. 2017).

Importantly, in daily practice, stress/insufficiency fractures may be incidentally picked up on MRI scans being done for foot and ankle pain or other reasons. However, the radiologist should be aware of potential differential diagnoses such as osteoid osteoma, osteomyelitis, and bone forming neoplastic lesions such as Ewing's sarcoma. CT may be used for problem solving in these cases to assess the osseous architecture, presence of osseous destruction, nidus, or a fracture line.

Occasionally, stress fractures may be picked up on ultrasound of the foot which may demonstrate focal buckling of the cortex and surrounding hypoechoic callus (Wall and Feller 2006).

Radionuclide bone scan has been used previously when the radiograph is negative. Stress fractures of the navicular bone are not uncommon but such fractures can occur in almost

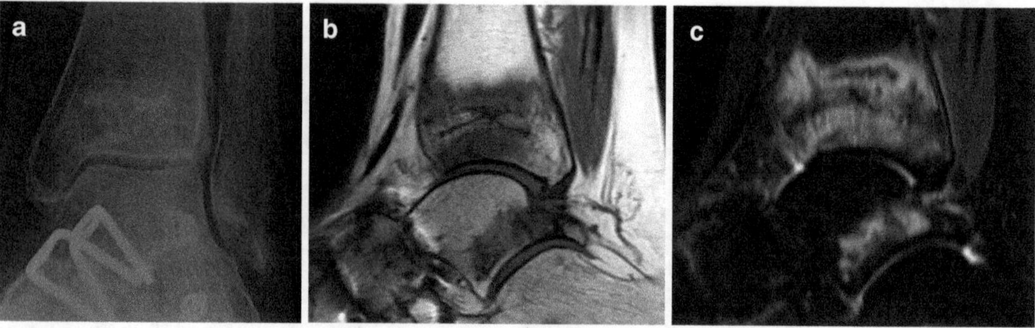

Fig. 19 (**a**) AP radiograph of the ankle. Note the transverse sclerotic line in the distal tibia and also the sclerotic band in the talus on the background of osteopenia. Appearances are suspicious for insufficiency fractures. (**b**, **c**) Sagittal T1 and STIR images of the same patient. Note the transverse low signal lines in the distal tibia and talus. Also note the surrounding marrow edema confirming insufficiency fractures

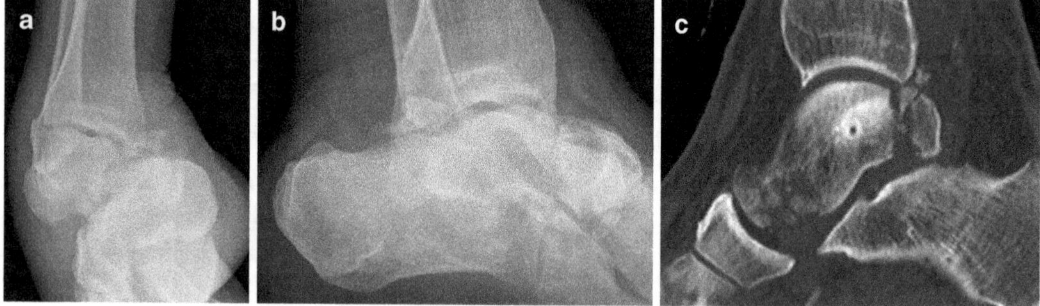

Fig. 20 (**a**, **b**) AP and lateral radiographs demonstrating subtalar fracture dislocation. (**c**) Postreduction sagittal CT image demonstrating the comminuted talus fracture in the same patient

any bone in the foot (Meurman 1981) including the sesamoids (Van Hal et al. 1982). Shelbourne et al. reported stress fractures in the medial malleolus in athletes involved in running and jumping activities (Shelbourne et al. 1988).

Common sites of insufficiency fractures in the foot include the calcaneum and the navicular bone. The presence of pain in a patient whose radiographs demonstrate osteoporosis should raise a strong suspicion of an underlying insufficiency fracture. Again, MRI may demonstrate the marrow edema when the radiograph does not demonstrate any sign of fracture. However, the classic MRI changes of marrow edema can be masked in patients with eating disorders such as anorexia nervosa where there is serous conversion of the marrow resulting in "flip-flop effect" (Tins and Cassar-Pullicino 2006).

10 Dislocation

10.1 Dislocation of the Talus

Subluxation or dislocation of the talus can occur either with or without a talar fracture. Three joints may be involved—the tibiotalar, the subtalar, and the talonavicular. Total talar dislocation involves all three joints. This is usually an open injury. Characteristically the talus is found to lie transversely in front of the lateral malleolus.

The pure form of subtalar dislocation of the foot involves dislocation at the subtalar and talonavicular joints (Fig. 20). Most commonly, the dislocation is medial with the calcaneum and the navicular bone displaced medially, and the head of the talus is dorsolaterally. Less commonly, the subtalar dislocation occurs laterally, with the calcaneum, navicular, and forefoot lying lateral rela-

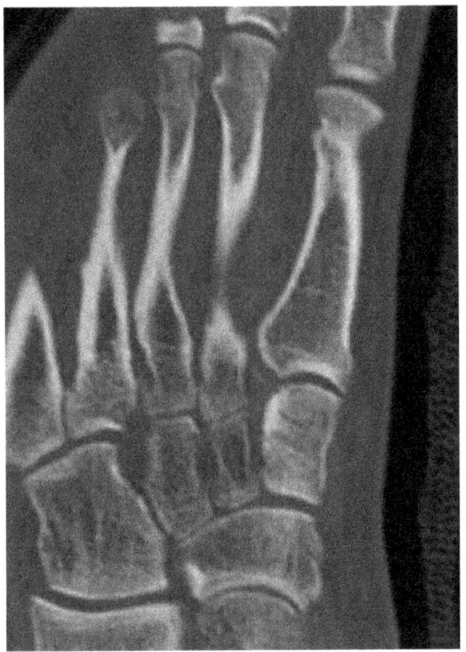

Fig. 21 CT reformatted image demonstrating a subtle undisplaced fracture of the base of the second metatarsal. Note the tiny bone fleck between the bases of the first and second metatarsal suggestive of an avulsion injury. Also note the slight widening of the space between the first and second metatarsals. Appearances are in keeping with a Lisfranc injury

tive to the talus. The diagnosis is best made on the anteroposterior radiographs of the foot and ankle. The tibiotalar and calcaneocuboid joints remain aligned, but medial or lateral displacement of the calcaneum and navicular bones is evident. Such dislocations are often associated with talar or calcaneal osteochondral fracture. CT can be particularly helpful in evaluating these injuries.

On occasion, a dislocation may essentially affect the subtalar joint alone, or alternatively the talonavicular joint alone. The latter is known as a "swivel" dislocation and occurs more commonly medial than lateral. The principal injury is usually apparent but there may be very slight widening of adjacent joint spaces with seemingly satisfactory alignment.

10.2 Mid-Tarsal (Lis Franc) Dislocation

Fracture dislocation in the mid-tarsal region is overlooked in 20% of cases. It can be a difficult region to evaluate on conventional radiographs and careful scrutiny of this area is required (Myerson 1989). If a fracture in the region of tarsometatarsal joints is seen, an associated dislocation should be strongly suspected (Figs. 21 and 22). If it is not

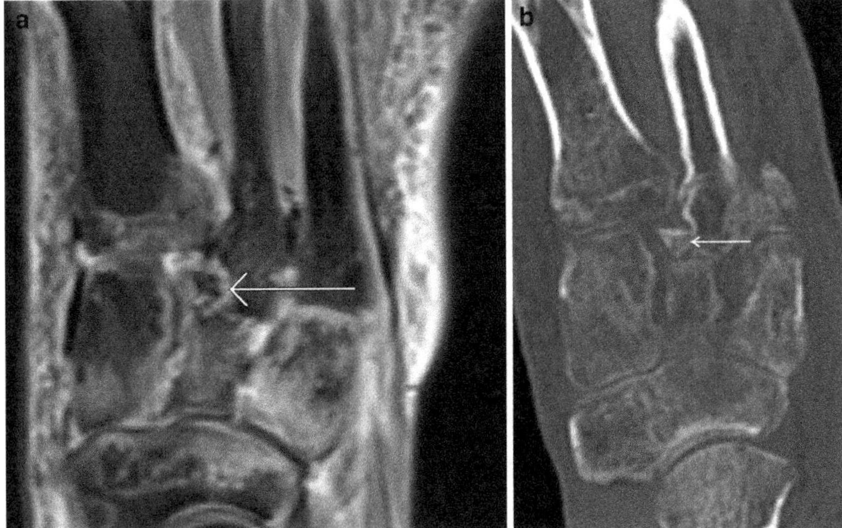

Fig. 22 (**a**) Coronal MRI image of the midfoot demonstrating marked bone and soft tissue edema like signal in the midfoot. Note the small osseous fragment between the bases of the first and second metatarsals (arrows). (**b**) CT confirming the presence of the small osseous fragment adjacent to the base of the second metatarsal (arrow) in keeping with a Lis France avulsion injury

obvious on radiographs, then further imaging with CT is warranted, the coronal plane being particularly valuable in assessment of alignment. MRI is superior in depicting ligamentous injuries and bone marrow edema in case of subtle undisplaced fractures (Gupta et al. 2008).

11 Children

11.1 Fractures of the Distal Tibia and Fibula

The skeletal maturity of the patient determines the resulting bone, ligamentous, or growth plate injury. The growth plate forms a plane of weakness which results in different patterns of injury to those in the adult. The ligaments of children are stronger than the growth plate predisposing to physeal separation in a child. Fractures in children rarely disturb the talotibial relationship (Rang 1983). The distal tibial epiphysis is the second most common site of epiphyseal injury in the entire skeleton, after the distal radius. Tibial epiphyseal injuries often occur in the absence of injury to the fibula indicative of the relative resilience of the fibula in children. As a result of an epiphyseal fracture, the growth plate frequently appears widened. Often there are thin usually metaphyseal flakes of bone representing small avulsion fractures. When the epiphysis is minimally displaced, comparison with the opposite side may be necessary to confirm the diagnosis. The prognosis is dependent on the skeletal maturity of the patient, the severity of the injury, the fracture type, degree of comminution and displacement, and the adequacy of reduction.

11.2 Modified Lauge-Hansen Classification

A classification system of fractures can be anatomical or be related to the mechanism of injury. An anatomical classification such as that used by Salter and Harris (1963) (Fig. 23) is widely used. However, the classification on its own does not make reference to the mechanism of injury. The most widely accepted mechanism of injury classification of ankle fractures in children is that described by Dias and Tachdjian (1978), who modified the adult based Lauge-Hansen classification in their review of 71 fractures.

Classification of childhood ankle fractures is a complex area. Vahvanen and Aalto (1980) compared their ability to classify 310 ankle fractures in children with the Weber (1972), Lauge-Hansen (1954), and Salter and Harris (1963) classification. They found that they were "largely unsuccessful" using the Weber and Lauge-Hansen classifications but could easily classify the fractures using the Salter-Harris system. They suggested that although ankle fractures in children can be extremely complex, they can be roughly divided into avulsion and epiphyseal fractures. Adequately reduced avulsion fractures can be expected to heal well while epiphyseal fractures may give rise to late complications. Spiegel et al. (1978) followed 184 of a series of 237 fractures of the distal end of the tibia or fibula in children. Using the Salter-Harris classification, they identified three groups according to the risk of developing subsequent complications including shortening of the leg, angular deformity of the bone, or incongruity of the joint. According to Spiegel, the low-risk group which consisted of 89 patients, 6.7% of whom had complications, included all Type I and Type II fibula fractures, all Type I tibial fractures, Type III and Type IV tibial fractures with less than 2 mm of displacement, and epiphyseal avulsion injuries. The high-risk group consisted of 28 patients, 32% of whom had complications. This group included Type III and Type IV tibial fractures with 2 mm or more of displacement, juvenile Tillaux fractures, triplane fractures, and comminuted tibial epiphyseal fractures (Type V). The third and unpredictable group was made up 66 patients,

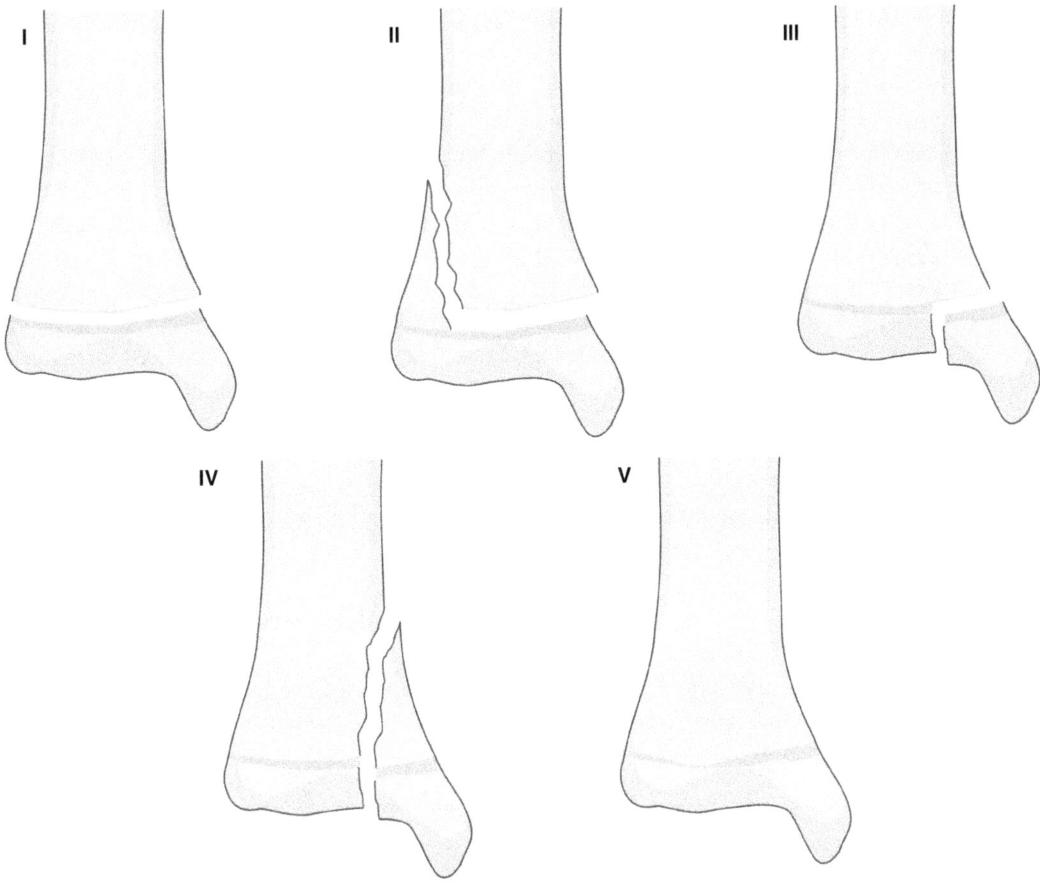

Fig. 23 Salter-Harris Classification

16.7% of them with complications. Only type II tibial fractures were included. Interestingly, in this review, the presence or absence of a fibula fracture in association with a tibial epiphyseal fracture had no prognostic significance as regard the incidence of complications. This is noteworthy, since some classifications systems center around the presence and location of the fracture of the fibula (Weber 1972). In the studies by both Spiegel and Vahvanen and Aalto, different types of fractures tended to occur in different age groups, the data suggesting a relationship between skeletal maturity and the fracture pattern. Vahvanen noted that malleolar and intra-articular tibial fractures occurred at a younger age than those with tibial epiphyseal fractures, two- or triplane fractures. Since the medial part of the distal tibial epiphyseal plate closes before the lateral part (Kleiger and Mankin 1964), this might explain the separation of the lateral part of the tibial epiphysis in triplane fractures and in avulsion fractures of the tibiofibular syndesmosis.

Although there are a number of classification systems available for fractures of the ankle in children, the Salter-Harris classification with its consideration of the involvement of the epiphysis remains very important. Other systems may be helpful as regard management and approach to treatment.

11.3 Salter-Harris Fractures

Distal tibial epiphyseal injuries are usually Salter-Harris Type I. In the more common Salter-Harris Type II injuries, the triangular corner fragment always arises from the side of the metaphysis toward which the epiphysis is displaced (Fig. 24). Salter-Harris Type III epiphyseal separations occur either medially or laterally. Those of the medial portion of the epiphysis occur in adduction injuries, or avulsion by the deltoid ligament when the ankle is injured with the foot in pronation. The medial fragment includes the medial malleolus. Type III fractures involving the lateral half of the epiphysis occur only after the growth plate has started to fuse since closure of the growth plate commences medially. This has been described as a juvenile Tillaux fracture (Kleiger and Mankin 1964). The fracture line extends from the articular surface, traverses the epiphysis, and continues through the physis laterally. A variable sized piece of the anterolateral bony epiphysis is pulled off by the anterior talofibular ligament which is either mildly or moderately displaced.

Salter-Harris Type IV injuries of the distal tibial epiphysis occur as a result of adduction. This type of injury requires open reduction and accurate fixation to prevent growth arrest (Fig. 25). Type V injuries are extremely rare, the radiographs are usually normal initially, and the diagnosis retrospectively made when premature closure is seen on subsequent radiographs.

Most epiphyseal injuries can be adequately reduced by closed means, except the Salter-Harris Type IV adduction injury of the medial portion of the distal tibial epiphysis. Type III injuries are occasionally displaced to such a degree that open reduction is required. Irreducible Salter-Harris Type II separations of the distal tibial epiphysis due to interposition of the anterior tibial tendon and neurovascular bundle have been reported (Grace 1983).

11.4 Triplane Fracture

The triplane fracture described by Marmor in 1970 is an injury unique to the closure of the dis-

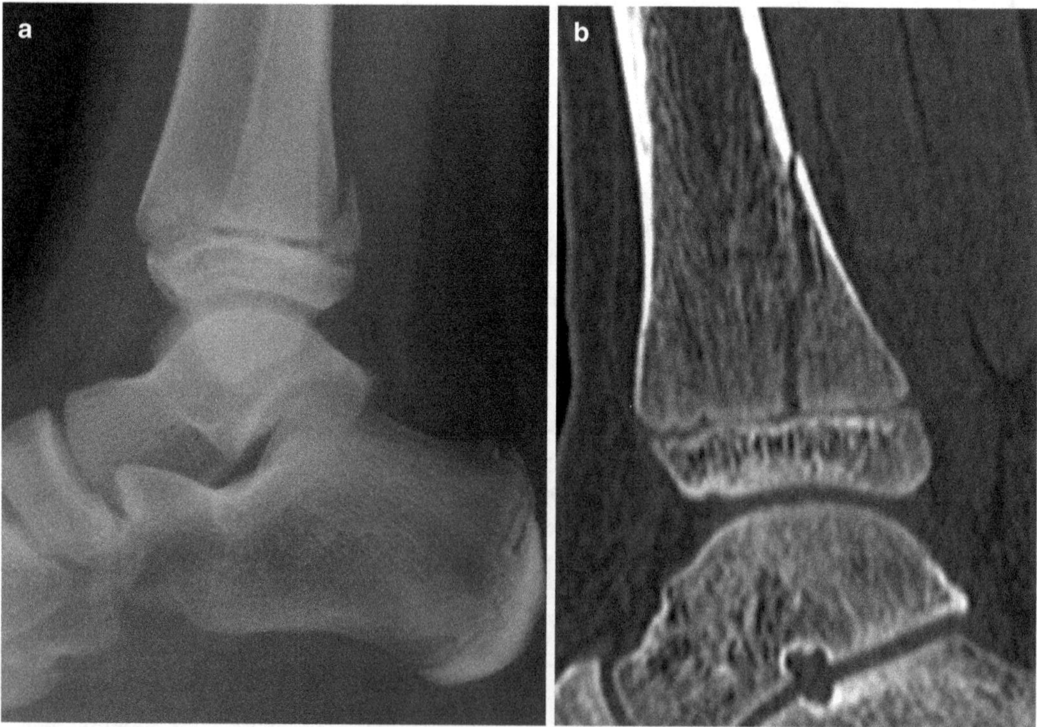

Fig. 24 (**a**, **b**) Lateral radiograph and sagittal CT of the ankle of a skeletally immature individual demonstrating a Salter-Harris II fracture of the posterior malleolus. Note that the fracture line extends proximal to the physis

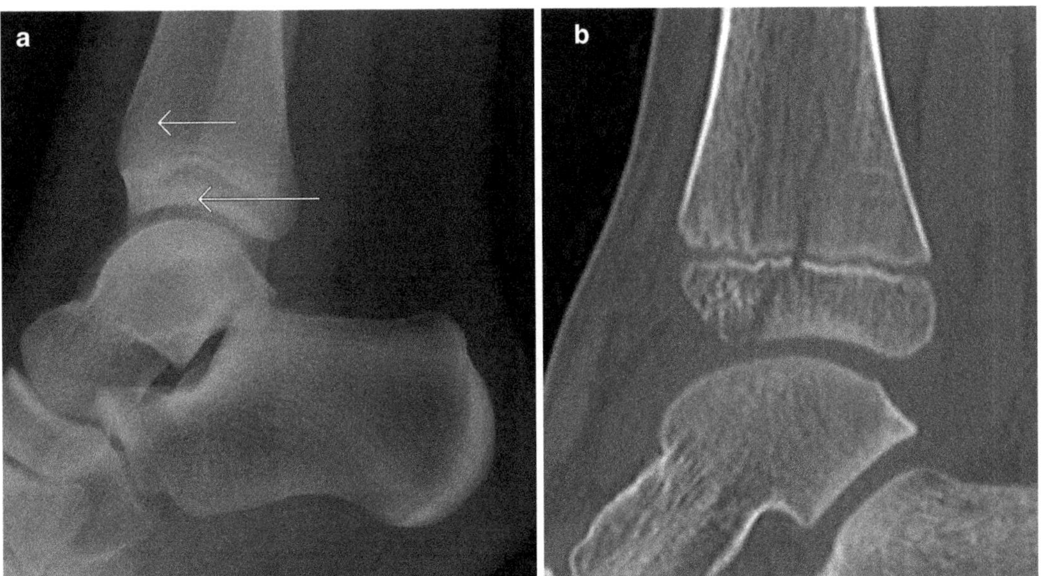

Fig. 25 (**a**, **b**) Lateral radiograph and sagittal CT image of a skeletally immature individual demonstrating a Salter-Harris IV fracture (arrows). Note the fracture line extends from the metaphysis through the physis to the epiphysis

Fig. 26 Line diagram demonstrating the two-part triplane fracture

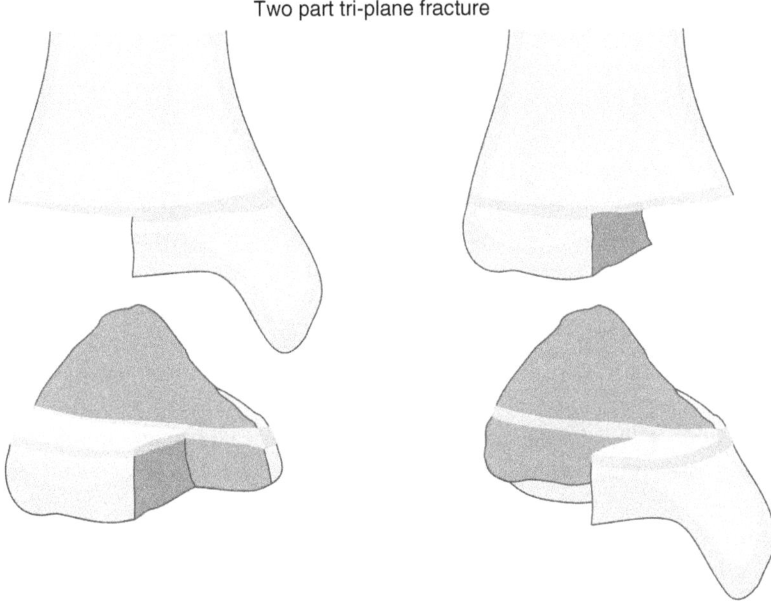

tal tibial physis. This is known as the triplane fracture because there are fracture lines in three planes: a sagittal plane in the epiphysis, a horizontal plane within the physis, and an oblique vertical plane in the posterior distal metaphysis. This produces a multiplanar type IV Salter Harris injury. There are two types of triplane fractures: fractures with two fragments (Fig. 26) and fractures with three fragments (Fig. 27). Both are due to plantar flexion and external rotation and may occur with or without an associated long oblique fracture of the distal fibula. The fracture appears as a Salter-Harris Type III on the AP view and Salter-Harris Type II on the

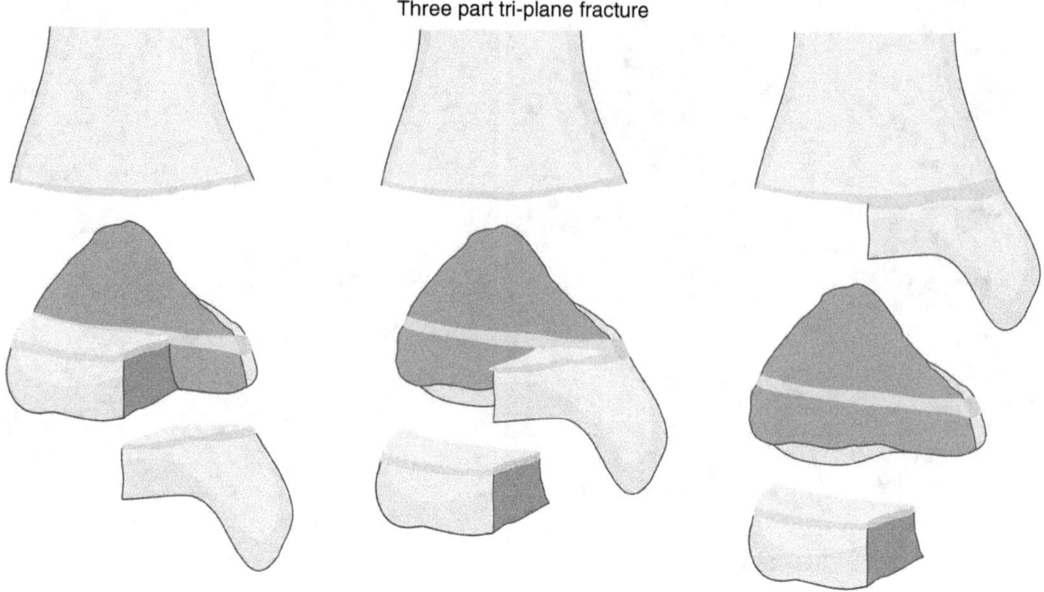

Fig. 27 Line diagram demonstrating the three-part triplane fracture

lateral view. The two-fragment triplane fracture usually occurs after the epiphysis has begun to unite, similar to the juvenile Tillaux fracture. Two subtypes of two-fragment triplane fractures have also been reported, a medial and a lateral. The lateral is the more common, the medial malleolus remaining intact. The three-fragment triplane fractures are less common than the two-fragment fractures and generally occur in younger children before the tibial epiphysis has begun to close (MacNealy et al. 1982; Dias and Giegerich 1983).

Three-part triplane fractures are more likely to require open reduction and internal fixation to restore and preserve the joint. In the three-part fracture, the entire epiphysis is usually displaced posteriorly as opposed to the two-part fracture in which only a portion of the epiphysis is displaced, the other portion remaining attached and properly aligned with the anterior tibial metaphysis. The entire distal tibial epiphysis is also displaced posteriorly in Salter-Harris Type II plantar flexion and external rotational injuries. However, in these latter injuries, the distal tibial epiphysis remains intact without the vertical fracture at the epiphysis found in the triplane fracture.

12 Osteochondral Injuries

This type of injury most commonly affects the talar dome, both its medial and lateral aspect in equal proportions. It usually results from an inversion injury. There is often associated rupture of the lateral ligamentous complex usually involving the anterior talofibular ligament and sometimes also the calcaneofibular ligament. Talar dome injury is often missed (20%) or not visible on conventional radiographs which show evidence of soft tissue lateral ligamentous injury and requires CT or MRI for diagnosis. Injury to the lateral portion of the dome is more common in men. They tend to be symptomatic, shallow and wafer shaped and occur after traumatic inversion with or without dorsiflexion (Fig. 28). Whereas injury to the medial portion of the dome is more common in women. They are usually less symptomatic, deep cup shaped resulting from atraumatic or traumatic plantar flexion, inversion, and lateral rotation (Smitaman and

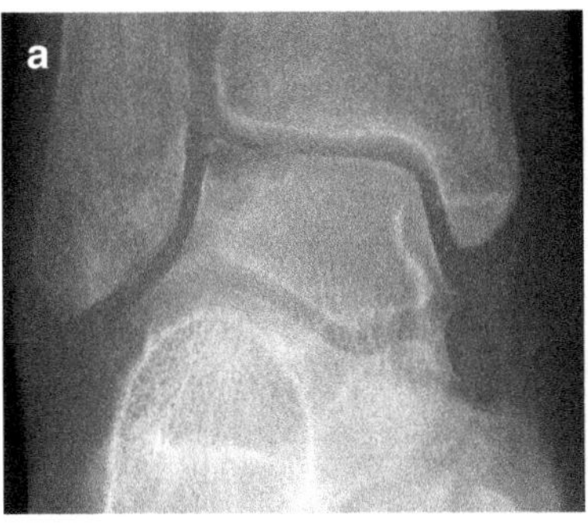

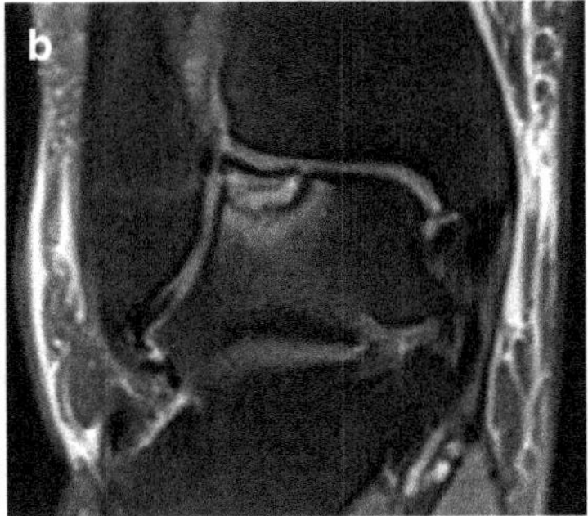

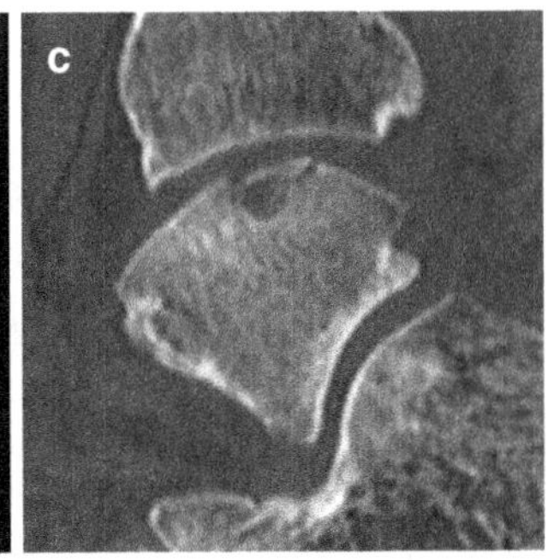

Fig. 28 (**a**) AP radiograph of an ankle of a skeletally mature individual. Note the minimally displaced fracture of the lateral talar dome with subchondral lucency in keeping with an osteochondral fracture. (**b**) Coronal PD FS demonstrating the displaced osteochondral fragment from the lateral talar dome. Note the high signal surrounding the fragment suggesting instability. Also note the subchondral marrow edema. (**c**) Sagittal CT image 9 months post injury demonstrating the non-united osteochondral fracture. Note the subchondral cystic changes and subtle surrounding sclerosis

Davis 2022). The lesion varies from indentation of the dome to partial detachment of the fragment, complete detachment without displacement, and complete detachment with displacement. The radiographic features are best demonstrated on an AP and internal oblique projection. The osteochondral fragment is seen as a fine flake of bone at the lateral or medial edge of the talus. Where the fragment is not visible, further imaging with MRI or CT arthrography may be employed. Very subtle osteochondral abnormalities can also be beautifully demonstrated by MRI (Bohndorf 1999).

13 Complications of Bone Injuries

Complications of bone injuries at the ankle are varied. The most common is post-traumatic osteoarthritis. Close attention to good reduction of fractures at the ankle can help to minimize this complication. It is a frequent problem following compressive fractures of the calcaneum largely as a result of the complex nature of these injuries and the difficulties involved in achieving satisfactory re-alignment of all fragments.

Avascular necrosis is a particular complication associated with vertical fractures through the neck of the talus. The majority of the arterial supply enters through the anterolateral portion of the neck of the talus, through the foramina in the sinus tarsi and tarsal canal and through the foramina in the medial surface of the body (Haliburton et al. 1958; Kelly and Sullivan 1963). When the neck of the talus is fractured, the blood supply is easily disrupted and the body is susceptible to avascular necrosis. This can also occur following dislocation associated with fracture of the neck. Radiologically, the appearances of avascular necrosis of the talus are similar to those elsewhere in the body. There is a geographical demarcation of increased density compared to adjacent bone (which is of normal or reduced density). This pattern can also be readily detected with CT or MRI. The body and talar dome can ultimately collapse with progression to arthritis.

CRPS type I, previously known as "Reflex sympathetic dystrophy (RSD)" is a potential complication of any injury at the ankle. It is manifest clinically by pain, soft tissue swelling, and reduced movement. It remains a clinical diagnosis based on the modified Budapest criteria implemented in 2012 by the International Association of the Study of Pain. Imaging is usually requested as part of the patient's work up and may demonstrate some nonspecific findings. Radiographically there may be soft tissue swelling and osteoporosis. The value of MRI in the diagnosis of CRPS is controversial. It may demonstrate features such as patchy marrow edema, usually of subcortical distribution, edema, and enhancement of the soft tissues and soft tissue thickening. Agten et al. in a review of 50 patients with suspected CRPS of the foot who underwent MRI scan concluded that MRI cannot distinguish between CRPS and non CRPS patients when measured against the gold standard: Budapest criteria (Agten et al. 2020). The radionuclide bone scan has been used on its own or in combination with MRI and shows diffuse increased uptake on both the vascular (diffusion) and static (delayed) phases.

Ankle injury in the child and adolescent, where the growth plate has been disturbed may be complicated by tethering (premature partial or complete fusion) across the growth plate with subsequent angular deformity secondary to asymmetric arrest. It can also rarely be secondary to malunion. Growth problems can lead to leg length discrepancy which accounts for about 20% of the indications for leg lengthening procedures. Distal tibial fractures in skeletally immature individuals may result in osteonecrosis due to disruption of the nutrient vessels (Bhattacharjee et al. 2015).

14 Summary

Bone injury affecting the ankle joint can be complex and difficult to classify. A classification system is usually used in order to facilitate comparison between different modes of management, but can also sometimes help in directing the search for other associated or expected injuries. Not all injuries will fit neatly into a classification system. Furthermore, an injury classified on the basis of conventional radiographs is commonly re-classified when CT is employed.

In the midfoot, where there are many bones tightly packed together and there are many overlapping shadows, a high index of suspicion of a possible Lis Franc fracture dislocation is essential to reduce the risk of overlooking this injury.

This chapter has dealt principally with the radiograph in bone and joint injury, with emphasis on the value of CT particularly in hind and midfoot injuries. MRI will detect occult bone injury, marrow edema, and osteochondral injury but will have its main role in the assessment of soft tissue injury.

Acknowledgment The authors would like to thank the Medical Photography Department in the Robert Jones and Agnes Hunt Orthopaedic Hospital, Oswestry, UK.

References

Agten CA, Kobe A, Barnaure I, Galley J, Pfirrmann CW, Brunner F (2020) MRI of complex regional pain syndrome. Eur J Radiol 129:109044

Ayeni JP (1988) Pilon fractures of the tibia: a study based on 19 cases. Injury 19:109–114

Bhattacharjee A, Singh J, Mangham DC, Freeman R (2015) Osteonecrosis of the distal tibial metaphysis after Salter-Harris type II injury: a case report. J Pediatr Orthop B 24(4):366–369

Bohndorf K (1999) Skeletal Radiol 28(10):545–560

Bonnin JG (1970) Injuries to the ankle. Hafner Publishing Co, New York

Canale ST, Kelly FB Jr (1978) Fractures of the neck of the talus: long-term evaluation of seventy one cases. J Bone Joint Surg Am 60A:143–156

Cancelmo RP (1962) Isolated fracture of the anterior tibial tubercle. AJR Am J Roentgenol 87: 1064–1066

Dameron TB Jr (1975) Fractures and anatomical variations of the proximal portion of the fifth metatarsal. J Bone Joint Surg Am 57A:788–792

Danis R (1949) Les Fractures Malleolaires. In: Danis R (ed) Theorie et Pratique de L'osteosynthese. Masson et Cie, Paris, pp 133–165

Destot E (1911) Traumatismes du Pied et Rayons: X Malleoles, Astragale, Calcaneum Avantpied. Masson, Paris, pp 1–10

Dias LS, Giegerich CR (1983) Fractures of the distal tibial epiphysis in adolescence. J Bone Joint Surg Am 65A:438–443

Dias LS, Tachdjian MO (1978) Physeal injuries of the ankle in children classification. Clin Orthop 136:230–233

Eisele SA, Sammarco GJ (1993) Fatigue fractures of the foot and ankle in the athlete (review). J Bone Joint Surg 75A:290–298

Essex-Lopresti P (1952) The mechanism, reduction technique, and results in fractures of the Os Calcis. Br J Surg 39:395–419

Grace DL (1983) Irreducible fracture-separations of the distal tibial epiphysis. J Bone Joint Surg Am 65B:160–162
Gupta RT, Wadhwa RP, Learch TJ, Herwock SM (2008) Lisfranc injury: imaging findings for this important but often missed diagnosis. Curr Probl Diagn Radiol 37:115
Guyer BH, Levinsohn EM, Fredrickson BE, Bailey GL, Formikell M (1985) Computed tomography of calcaneal fractures: anatomy, pathology, dosimetry and clinical relevance. AJR Am J Roentgenol 145: 911–919
Haliburton RA, Sullivan CR, Kelly PJ, Peterson LFA (1958) The extra-osseous and intra-osseous blood supply of the talus. J Bone Joint Surg Am 40A:115–1120
Harper MC (1992) Ankle fracture classification systems; a case for integration of the Lauge-Hansen and AO-Danis-Weber schemes. Foot Ankle 13:404–407
Harty M (1973) Anatomic considerations in injuries of the calcaneus. Orthop Clin North Am 4:179–183
Hawkins LG (1970) Fractures of the neck of the talus. J Bone Joint Surg Am 52A:991–1002
Heger L, Wulff K, Seddiqi MSA (1985) Computed tomography of calcaneal fractures. AJR Am J Roentgenol 145:131–137
Helal B, Gibb P (1987) Freiberg's disease: a suggested pattern of management. Foot Ankle 8:94–102
Henderson MS (1932) Trimalleolar fractures of the ankle. Surg Clin North Am 12:867–872
Hindman BW, Koss SDK, Sowerby MRR (1986) Fractures of the talus and calcaneus: evaluation by computed tomography CT. J Comput Tomogr 10:191–196
Isherwood I (1961) A radiological approach to the subtalar joint. J Bone Joint Surg Am 43B:566–574
Jones R (1902) Fracture of the base of the fifth metatarsal bone by indirect violence. Ann Surg 35:697–700
Kelly PJ, Sullivan CR (1963) Blood supply of the talus. Clin Orthop 30:37–44
Kleiger B, Mankin HJ (1964) Fracture of the lateral portion of the distal tibial epiphysis. J Bone Joint Surg Am 46A:25–32
Lauge-Hansen N (1950) Fractures of the ankle II. Combined experimental-surgical and experimental-Roentgenologic investigations. Arch Surg 60:957–985
Lauge-Hansen N (1954) Fractures of the ankle III. Genetic Roentgenologic diagnosis of fractures of the ankle. AJR Am J Roentgenol 71:456–471
Lorentzen JE, Christensen SB, Krogsoe O, Sneppen O (1977) Fractures of the neck of the talus. Acta Orthop Scand 48:115–120
MacNealy GA, Rogers LF, Hernandez R, Poznanski AK (1982) Injuries of the distal tibial epiphysis : systematic radiographic evaluation. AJR Am J Roentgenol 138:683
Mainwaring BL, Daffner RH, Riemer BL (1988) Pylon fractures of the ankle: a distinct clinical and radiologic entity. Radiology 168:215–218
Maisonneve JGT (1840) Recherches Sur la Fracture du Périoné. Arch Gen Med 7:165
Mandell JC, Khurana B, Smith SE (2017) Stress fractures of the foot and ankle, Part 1: Biomechanics of bone and principles of imaging and treatment. Skeletal Radiol 46:1021–1029
Marmor L (1970) An unusual fracture of the tibial epiphysis. Clin Orthop Relat Res 73:132–135
Meurman KOA (1981) Less common stress fractures in the foot. Br J Radiol 54:1–7
Myerson MS (1989) The diagnosis and treatment of injuries to the Lisfranc joint complex. Orthop Clin North Am 20:655–664
Pankovich AM, Shivaram MS (1979) Anatomical basis of variability in injuries of the medial malleolus and the deltoid ligament. Acta Orthop Scand 50:225
Protas JM, Kornblatt BA (1981) Fractures of the lateral margin of the distal tibia. The Tillaux fracture. Radiology 138:55–57
Rang M (1983) Children's fractures, 2nd edn. JB Lippincott Co., Philadelphia
Rogers L (1992) Chapter 22. The ankle. In: The radiology of skeletal trauma. Churchill Livingstone, Philadelphia, pp 1376–1377
Rosenberg ZS, Feldman F, Singson RD (1987) Intra-articular calcaneal fractures: computed tomographic analysis. Skeletal Radiol 16:105–113
Ruwe PA, Randall RL, Baumgaertner MR (1993) Pilon fractures of the distal tibia. Orthop Rev 22:987–996
Salter RB, Harris WR (1963) Injuries involving the epiphyseal plate. J Bone Joint Surg Am 45A:587–622
Shelbourne KD, Fisher DA, Retting AC, McCarroll JR (1988) Stress fractures of the medial malleolus. Am J Sports Med 16:60–63
Smitaman E, Davis M (2022) Hindfoot fractures: injury patterns and relevant imaging findings. Radiographics 42:661
Spiegel PG, Cooperman DR, Laros GS (1978) Epiphyseal fractures of the distal ends of the tibia and fibula. A retrospective study of 237 cases in children. J Bone Joint Surg Am 60A:1046–1050
Stiell IG, Greenberg GH, McKnight RD, Nair RC, McDowell I, Worthington JR (1992) A study to develop clinical decision rules for the use of radiography in acute ankle injuries. Ann Emerg Med 21:384–390
Stiell IG, Greenberg GH, McKnight RD et al (1993) Decision rules for the use of radiography in acute ankle injuries: refinements and prospective validation. JAMA 269:1127–1132
Stiell IG, McKnight RD, Greenberg GH, McDowell I, Nair RC, Wells GA, Johns C, Worthington JR (1994) Implementation of the Ottawa Ankle Rules. JAMA 271:827–832
Tins B, Cassar-Pullicino V (2006) Marrow changes in anorexia nervosa masking the presence of stress fractures on MR imaging. Skeletal Radiol 35:857–860

Torg JS, Balduini FC, Zelko RR, Pavlov H, Peff TC, Das M (1984) Fractures of the base of the fifth metatarsal distal to the tuberosity. J Bone Joint Surg Am 66A:209–214

Vahvanen V, Aalto K (1980) Classification of ankle fractures in children. Arch Orthop Trauma Surg 97:1–5

Van Hal ME, Keene JS, Lange TA, Clancy WG Jr (1982) Stress fractures of the great toe sesamoids. Am J Sports Med 10:122–128

Verma S, Hamilton K, Hawkins HH, Kothari R, Singal B, Buncher R, Nguyen P, O'Neill M (1997) Clinical application of the Ottawa Ankle Rules for the use of radiography in acute ankle injuries. An independent site assessment. AJR Am J Roentgenol 169: 825–827

Wall J, Feller JF (2006) Imaging of stress fractures in runners. Clin Sports Med 25(4):781–802

Weber BG (1972) Die Verletzungen des Oberen Sprunggelenkes. In: Aktuelle Prpobleme I der Chirugie No 3, 2nd edn. Hans Huber, Bern

Anterior Ankle Pain

Mohsin Hussein, Karthikeyan P. Iyengar,
Stuart A. Metcalfe, and Rajesh Botchu

Contents

1 Introduction

The anterior ankle contains several osseous, soft tissue, tendinous, and neurovascular anatomic structures, which may be affected in the clinical context of anterior ankle pain. A plethora of pathologies including bone and soft tissue neoplasms, ligamentous or osseous trauma and overuse injuries, inflammatory conditions, as well as other distinct entities can cause anterior ankle pain. Pain may also be referred from other parts of the ankle. A thorough radiological assessment supported by a sound clinical history is necessary to achieve the correct diagnosis and plan management.

This chapter focuses on the relevant anatomy, clinical entities, and respective radiological appearances for pathologies, which may present with anterior ankle pain.

2 Anatomy

The ankle (talocrural) joint is a hinge-type synovial joint made up of the distal tibia, fibula, and superior talus. The distal ends of the tibia and fibula form a malleolar mortise to which the talar trochlear fits. The lateral malleolus of the fibula articulates with the lateral trochlea of the talus, whereas the tibia has two articulations: the first inferior tibial plafond with the dome of the talar trochlea and second medial malleolus with the medial talar trochlea. The mortise configuration allows the malleoli to tightly grip the talar trochlear while allowing dorsiflexion and plantar flexion of the foot with some degree of pronation and supination, which primarily occurs at the subtalar joint.

M. Hussein
Department of Radiology, University Hospitals of Leicester, Leicester, UK
e-mail: mohsin.hussein@nhs.net

K. P. Iyengar
Department of Orthopedics, Southport and Ormskirk Hospital NHS Trust, Southport, UK
e-mail: kartikp31@hotmail.com

S. A. Metcalfe
Spire Parkway Hospital, Solihull, UK
e-mail: Footconsultant@gmail.com

R. Botchu (✉)
Department of Musculoskeletal Radiology, Royal Orthopedic Hospital, Birmingham, UK
e-mail: rajesh.botchu@nhs.net

Med Radiol Diagn Imaging (2023)
https://doi.org/10.1007/174_2023_431,
Published Online: 29 April 2023

The joint capsule is thin anteriorly and posteriorly and is reinforced by collateral ligaments. These include the anterior inferior and posterior tibiofibular ligaments and the interosseous tibiofibular ligaments (collectively termed the distal tibiofibular syndesmosis), medial ligaments, lateral ligaments, and tarsal sinus ligaments. A full description of these structures can be found in the respective chapters.

The tendons of the anterior lower leg muscles have the primary function of dorsiflexion at the ankle joint and extension at the toes. They run over the anterior joint surface together with neurovascular structures. From medial to lateral, the structures constitute the tibialis anterior (TA) tendon, dorsalis pedis artery, deep peroneal nerve, extensor hallucis longus (EHL) tendon, and extensor digitorum longus (EDL) tendon (Fig. 1).

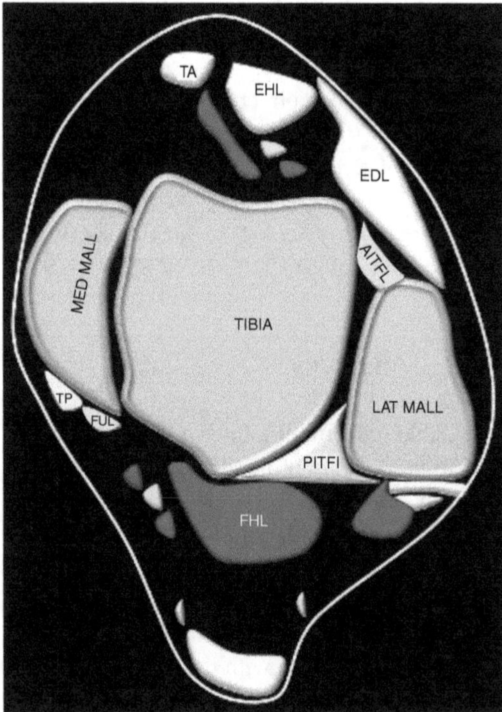

Fig. 1 Anatomy of the ankle. Axial section schematic through the ankle (talocrural) joint. *TA* tibialis anterior, *EHL* extensor hallucis longus, *EDL* extensor digitorum longus, *AITFL* anterior inferior tibiofibular ligament, *PITFL* posteroinferior tibiofibular ligament, *LAT MALL* lateral malleolus, *MED MALL* medial malleolus, *TP* tibialis posterior, *FDL* flexor digitorum longus, *FHL* flexor hallucis longus

The deep peroneal nerve supplies the anterior compartment muscles. It arises at the level of the fibula neck and is one of the two terminal branches of the common peroneal nerve. The dorsalis pedis artery is a continuation of the anterior tibial artery and is formed as it crosses the ankle joint into the foot.

The anterior compartment tendons are tightly bound by a two-part band like thickening of the deep fascia, termed the extensor retinaculum (anterior crural ligament), which prevents bowstringing anteriorly during ankle dorsiflexion (Fig. 2). The superior retinaculum is band shaped and runs from the distal fibula to the tibia, above the level of the malleoli. The inferior retinaculum is Y shaped and runs from the superior calcaneus to the (a) medial malleolus and (b) medial cuneiform.

A variety of normal anatomic bone and tendon variants exist and may sometimes contribute to anterior ankle pain. Tarsal coalition is the osseous or fibrous union of two or more bones of the mid- or hindfoot. They occur in less than 1% of the population, have a male predominance, and commonly occur bilaterally. They are usually encountered in the calcaneonavicular and talocalcaneal

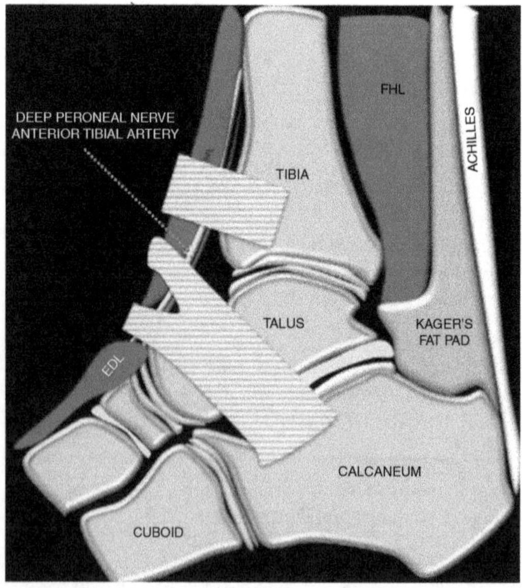

Fig. 2 Anatomy of the ankle. Sagittal section schematic through the ankle (talocrural) joint and midfoot. *EDL* extensor digitorum longus, *FHL* flexor hallucis longus

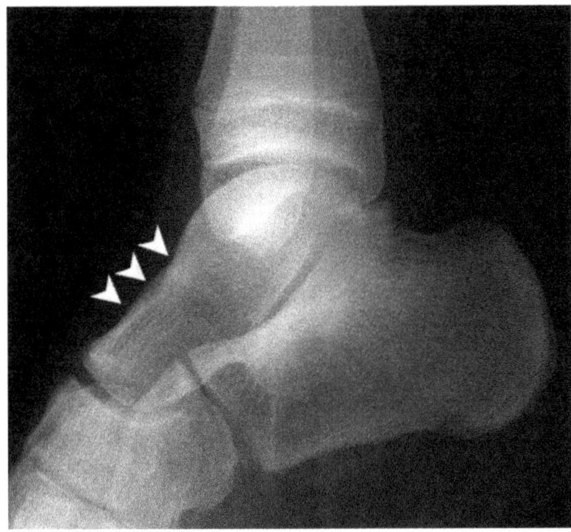

Fig. 3 Lateral radiograph of the ankle showing an osseous coalition (synostosis) of the talonavicular joint

joints, making up 90% of all coalitions, and less commonly in other joints such as the talonavicular (Fig. 3), calcaneocuboid, and cubonavicular joints (Wechsler et al. 1994). Most patients are asymptomatic, but some may present with foot pain.

3 Imaging Tools

Radiographic evaluation of the ankle involves anteroposterior, lateral, and mortise views with additional oblique views in the context of trauma. Computed tomography (CT) may be utilized to better delineate osseous and articular anatomic relationships in the context of trauma or variant anatomy. Magnetic resonance imaging (MRI) is commonly used as it provides excellent soft tissue contrast resolution, allowing for the assessment of ligamentous and tendon injuries. MRI also allows for the depiction of bone marrow signal abnormalities, which may be subclinical and absent on radiographic imaging. It can be vital in the evaluation of hyaline cartilage of the joint as well as in the workup of soft tissue or bone neoplasms. Ultrasound may sometimes be used in evaluating soft tissue neoplasms and ligamentous injuries.

An in-depth discussion on the utility of imaging modalities, MRI sequences, and evaluation of specific anatomic structures has been covered in other sections.

4 Pathologies (Table 1)

4.1 Osseous

4.1.1 Ankle Fractures

Focusing on the anterior ankle, pathologies involving the talus and midfoot may present with anterior ankle pain.

Isolated **navicular fractures** alone are uncommon accounting for approximately 5% of all foot fractures and are commonly missed on conventional radiography. Injuries may be due to acute high-impact trauma or from chronic repetitive stress. In acute trauma, there is impaction of the talar head on the navicular which commonly occurs at the navicular tuberosity or as a dorsal cortical avulsion fracture (Chaturvedi et al. 2020). The navicular tuberosity fracture must be differentiated from an os naviculare, which may occur in a similar place. A CT should be considered if an occult fracture is clinically suspected (Fig. 4). The Sangeorzan classification may be implemented to fractures of the navicular body, which occur in the sagittal and horizontal planes (Rasmussen et al. 2021).

Stress injury of the navicular may occur from repetitive stress, and the diagnosis may be delayed due to vague symptomology, delayed consultation, and normal initial radiographic appearances. Navicular stress injury starts as a navicular stress reaction, which may proceed to navicular stress fracture. Navicular stress reaction occurs when there is mild focal edema within the bone and no discernible fracture line on MR imaging (Fig. 5). In navicular stress fracture, the edema is much more diffuse and a discrete fracture line may be identified (Harris and Harris 2016). MRI is more sensitive than CT in identifying stress injuries (Fig. 6).

Table 1 Osseous, joint, and soft tissue pathologies causing anterior ankle pain

Osseous	Ankle fractures	Navicular fractures
		Navicular stress injury
		Talar fractures
		Talar stress fractures
		Dislocations
	Avascular necrosis	Navicular (Kohler and Mueller-Weiss syndrome)
		Talus
	Infection (osteomyelitis)	
	Neoplasms—benign	Chondroblastoma
		Osteoblastoma
		Osteochondroma
		Trevor disease
		Giant cell tumor
		Aneurysmal bone cyst
	Neoplasm—malignant	Metastases
Joint	Osteoarthritis	
	Inflammatory arthritis	
	Septic arthritis	
	Pigmented villonodular synovitis (PVNS)	
	Synovial osteochondromatosis	
	Ganglion cyst	
	Anterior ankle impingement syndrome	
Soft tissue	Tendinosis, tenosynovitis, and tendon tears	
	Tibialis anterior tendon	
	Giant cell tumor of the tendon sheath (GCTTS)	
	Ganglion cyst of the tendon sheath	
	Extensor hallucis longus and extensor digitorum longus	
	Anterior tarsal tunnel syndrome	
	Tibialis anterior friction syndrome	
	Extensor retinaculum of the ankle	
	Subcutaneous mass lesions—benign	Hematoma
		Peripheral nerve sheath tumor (PNST)
		Soft tissue venous malformation (hemangioma)
	Subcutaneous mass lesions—malignant	Synovial sarcoma
		Myxofibrosarcoma
		Clear cell sarcoma

Talar fractures are another uncommon entity accounting for 3–5% of all foot fractures. They can be further divided into fractures of the neck (most common), head, and body (Melenevsky et al. 2015). Talar fractures occur from high energy trauma and, due to its complex anatomical and functional characteristics, may cause long-term sequala. The modified Hawkins-Canale classification may be used to characterize talar neck fractures to guide management based on prognosis and risk of osteonecrosis (Fig. 7). Talar stress fractures are uncommon but have been reported in physically active individuals such as athletes, military recruits, and dancers (Sormaala et al. 2006). On MRI, they appear as an area of edema within the talar head and neck or without a distinct fracture line paralleling the talonavicular joint (Fig. 8). An association with tarsal coali-

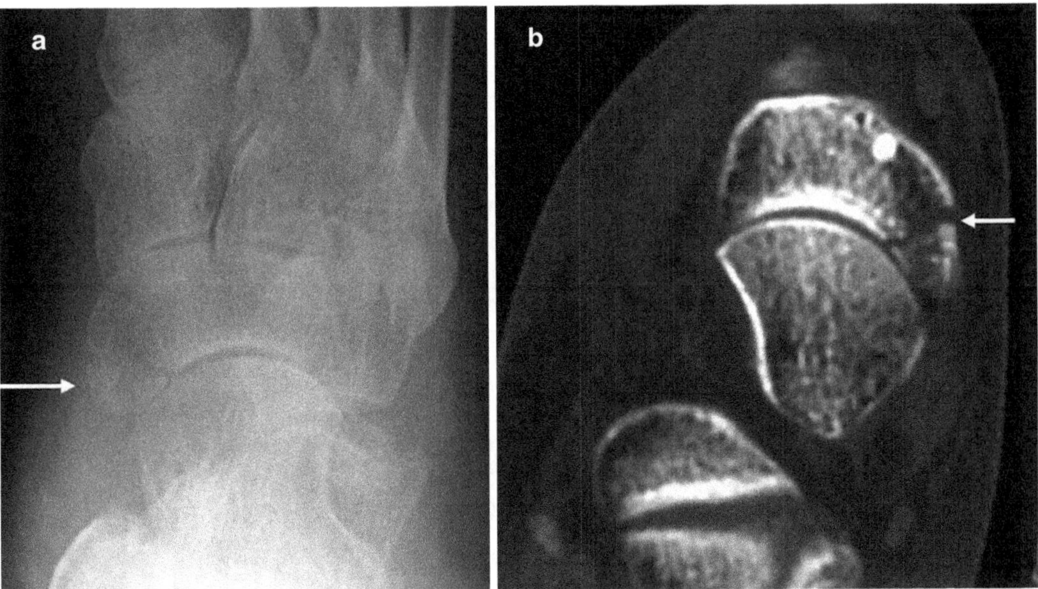

Fig. 4 Dorsoposterior (DP) radiograph (**a**) and CT axial (**b**) showing a fracture of the navicular tuberosity (arrow). Note the sharp cortical interruption and soft tissue swelling differentiating this from an os naviculare

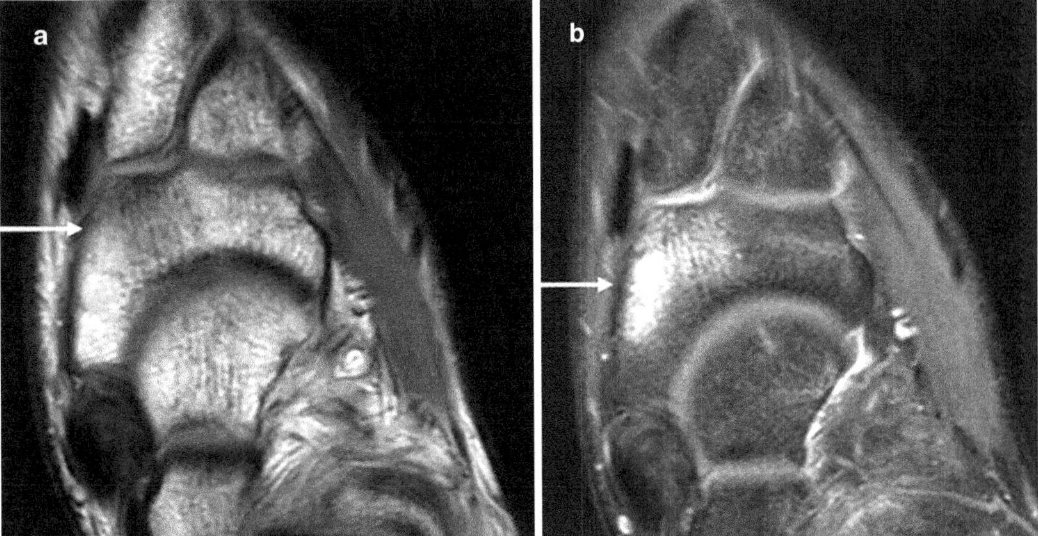

Fig. 5 Navicular stress reaction. Axial T1-weighted image (**a**) showing hypointense signal on the anterolateral navicular and axial proton density-weighted (PDW) image (**b**) showing hyperintense signal in the same area (arrow) consistent with edema

tion has been reported (Long et al. 2012). MR may also be used to identify other uncommon talar insufficiency fractures, which may occur paralleling the tibiotalar joint or at the posteroinferior medial talus. In the case of subchondral fractures, a thin T1 hypointense line may be appreciated adjacent to the chondral surface (Fig. 9).

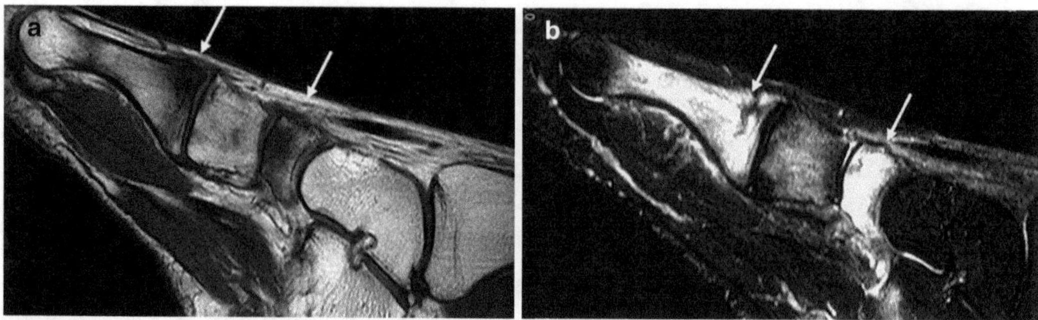

Fig. 6 Navicular stress fracture. Sagittal T1-weighted image (**a**) and sagittal proton density fat-suppressed (PDFS) (**b**) images showing stress fracture of navicular and base of first metatarsal (arrow)

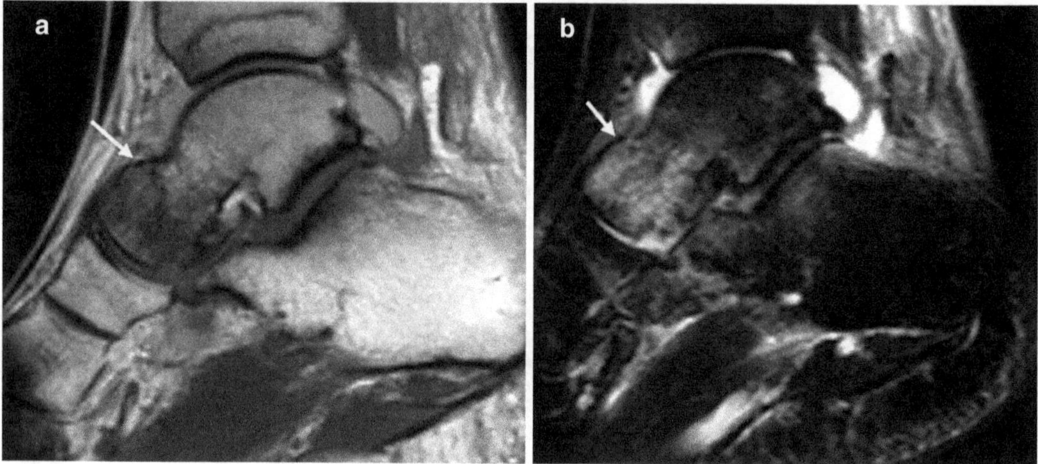

Fig. 7 Talar head fracture. Sagittal T1 (**a**) and STIR (**b**) showing fracture of the talar head with osseous edema (arrow)

Dislocations are less common than fractures of the ankle and foot; the most common dislocation occurs at the tarsometatarsal (TMT) joint complex (the "Lisfranc joint"), the midtarsal joint (Chopart joint), and the subtalar joint (Court-Brown and Caesar 2006). The Myerson classification may be used to divide Lisfranc joint injuries into isolated, divergent, and homolateral subtypes (Myerson et al. 1986). Stress or standing views may make the abnormality more obvious. Associated fractures may occur in the second metatarsal base and less commonly in the third metatarsal, medial and intermediate cuneiforms. A rare subtype is the involvement of the entire medial column of the mid/forefoot extending up to the cuneonavicular joint, which can be seen in severe injuries (Schepers et al. 2014) (Fig. 10).

4.1.2 Avascular Necrosis

Avascular necrosis is bone death due to ischemia from alteration in the vascular supply. In the context of anterior ankle pain, avascular necrosis of the talus and navicular is an important clinical entity. Both traumatic and atraumatic causes exist, including corticosteroids, autoimmune disorders, sickle cell anemia, and bisphosphonate use.

The blood supply to the talus is from the posterior tibial, dorsalis pedis, and perforating peroneal arteries. Injury to these arteries most commonly occurs following fractures of the talar neck with Hawkins-Canale type III and IV carrying the highest risk (Whitaker et al. 2018). Radiographs may appear normal during the initial stage but over time will demonstrate progres-

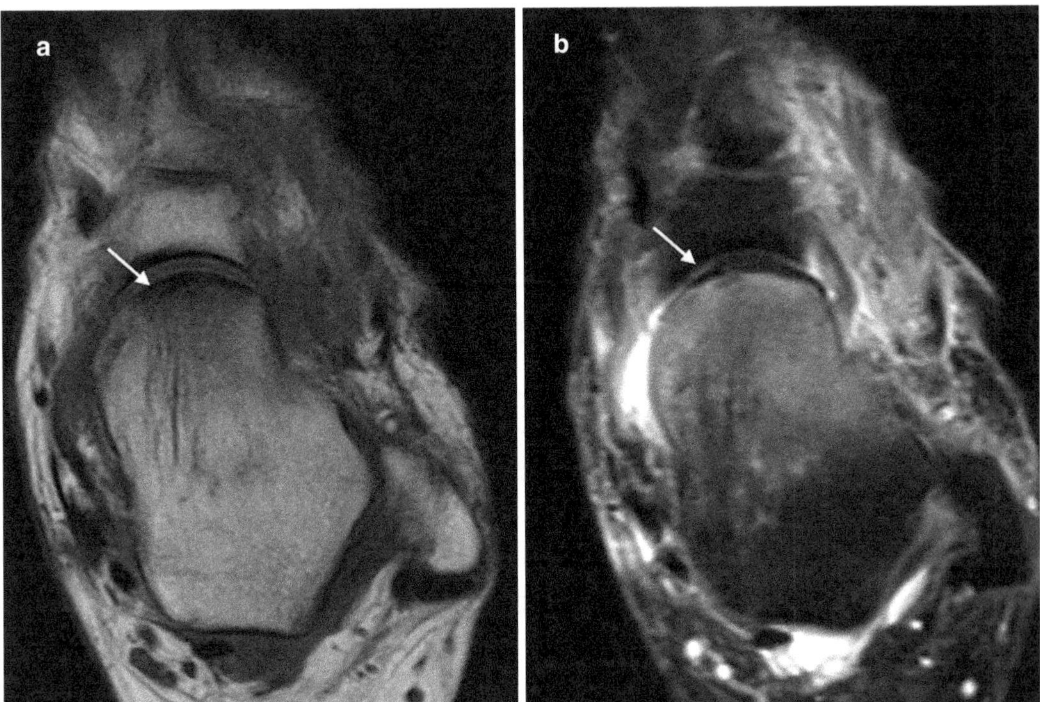

Fig. 8 Subchondral insufficiency fracture of the talus. Axial T1 (**a**) and STIR (**b**) showing subchondral insufficiency fracture of talar head with osseous edema

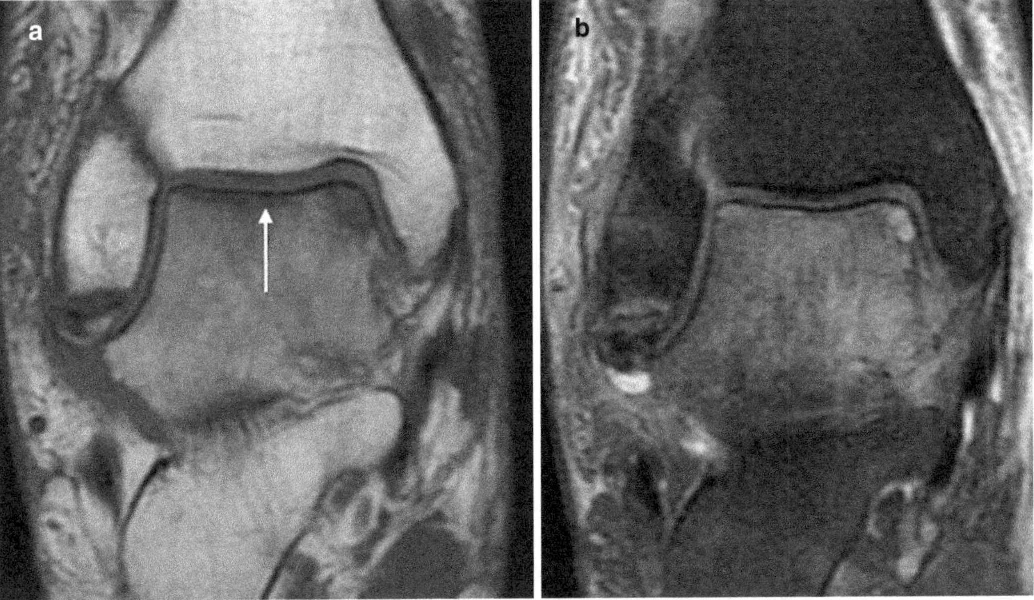

Fig. 9 Talus subchondral insufficiency fracture. Coronal T1 (**a**) and STIR (**b**) showing subchondral insufficiency fracture of body of talus (arrow) with osseous edema. Old fracture of lateral malleolus is also noted

sive sclerosis of the necrotic bone due to an inability to resorb abnormal bone. MR is more sensitive in the early stages (Pearce et al. 2005). If left untreated, the talus will eventually undergo fragmentation and collapse (Fig. 11).

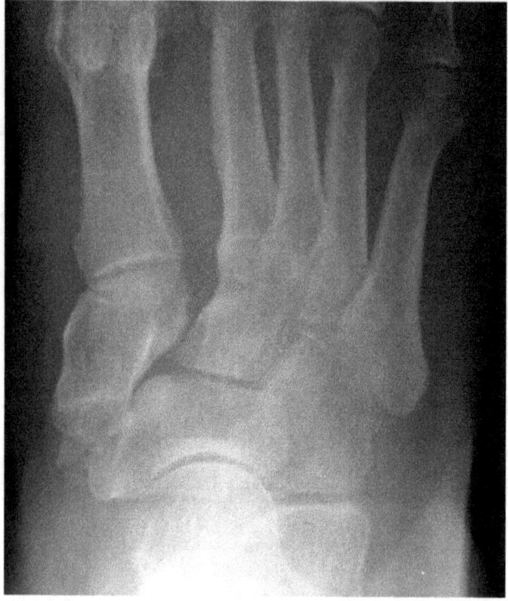

Fig. 10 Dorsoposterior (DP) radiograph of the foot showing fracture subluxation of the cuneonavicular joint and widening of the distance between the medial and intermediate cuneiform as well as the first and second intermetatarsal spaces

Avascular necrosis of the navicular has two eponymous terms; Kohler disease refers to the onset in childhood and Mueller-Weiss syndrome to the adult counterpart. The etiology is unknown, but it may represent a primary osteonecrosis or osteochondrosis or be related to trauma, altered biomechanics, and bone dysplasia. The cause is likely to be multifactorial and secondary to chronic load applied to a suboptimally formed navicular. The central part of the navicular has a watershed vascular distribution making it susceptible to ischemia and osteonecrosis (Samim et al. 2016). In the immature skeleton, radiographic appearance is of a sclerotic, thinned, and fragmented navicular bone (Fig. 12). In adults, the lateral half may preferentially collapse, leading to a "comma" or "hourglass" shape on dorsoplantar radiographs.

4.1.3 Infection

Osteomyelitis refers to infection of the bone, which may be acute or chronic. Early detection is essential to prevent progression to osteonecrosis and septic arthritis. Radiographs have a low sensitivity for detecting acute osteomyelitis as initial radiographs can be normal in up to 80% of patients (Lee et al. 2016). MR imaging is superior in detecting early marrow edema and perios-

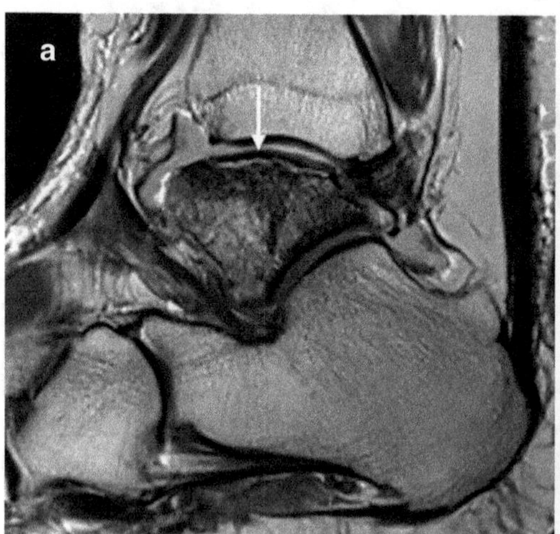

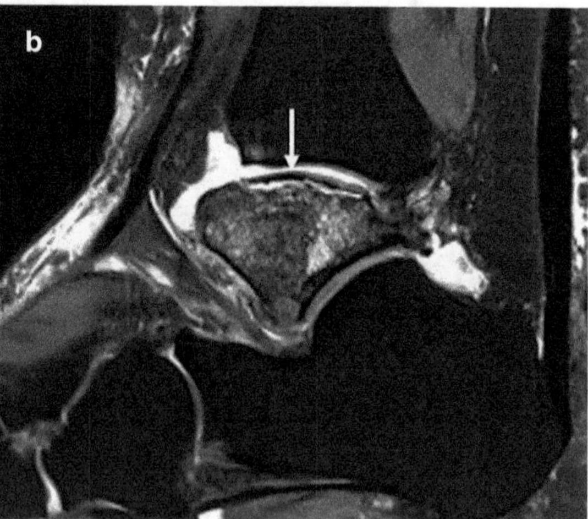

Fig. 11 Avascular necrosis of the talus. Sagittal T1 (**a**) and STIR (**b**) showing diffuse T1 hypointense and T2 hyperintense signal within the talar dome (edema) with areas of matched hypointensity (sclerosis) (arrow). There is collapse of the talar dome with a linear T2 hyperintense area adjacent to the subchondral plate (granulation tissue)

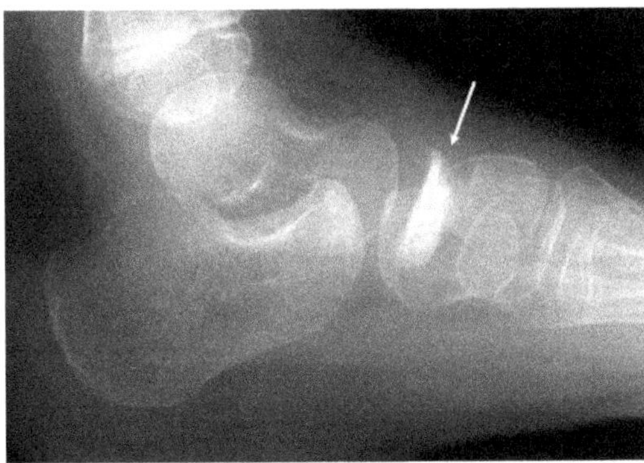

Fig. 12 Avascular necrosis (AVN) of the navicular (Kohler disease). Lateral radiograph of the ankle demonstrates sclerosis and thinning of the navicular bone (arrow)

titis. Two broad routes of spread exist: (a) hematogenous spread which favors the metaphysis owing to its rich vascular supply and most commonly affecting children and (b) contiguous spread from soft tissues or joints, typically in patients with diabetes mellitus, or direct inoculation from trauma and after surgery (Alaia et al. 2021). Other high-risk groups include intravenous drug users and individuals with sickle cell disease.

Subacute and chronic osteomyelitis acts as a smoldering process within the metaphysis with the development of an intra-osseous (Brodie's) abscess (typically in the age group between 18 months and early adulthood where the growth plate is unossified) or extension to the joint in younger and older age groups (Fig. 13). This can present as a clinical dilemma on plain radiograph as it can mimic other tumors such as eosinophilic granuloma. If the infection follows a typical imaging trajectory, expected radiological findings include a sequestrum (central devitalized bone), infected cavity (containing pus), involucrum (surrounding new bone formation), and a cloaca (draining sinus) (Alaia et al. 2021). Several other MR features have been described to support a Brodie's abscess over other entities, and these include the "penumbra" sign and intense peripheral rim enhancement (Fig. 14). In practice, a high index of suspicion is required to achieve the diagnosis early on. Osteomyelitis of the distal tibia and fibula may present with ankle pain.

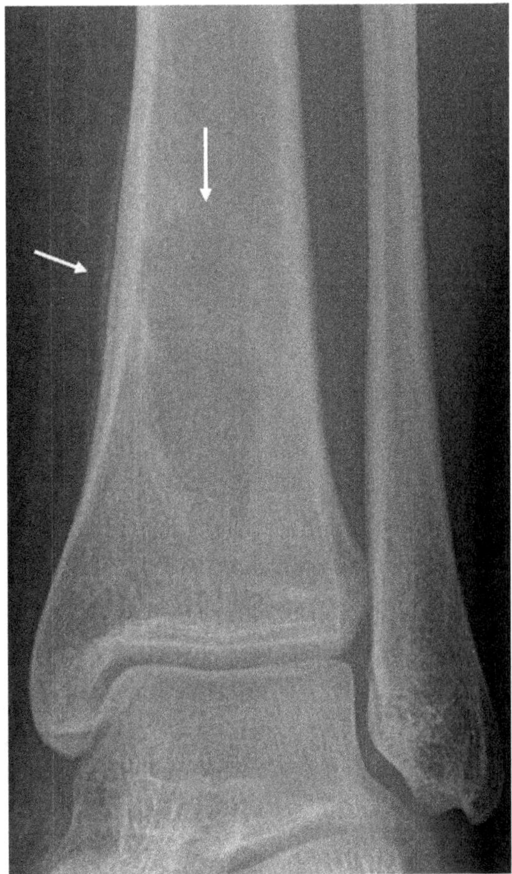

Fig. 13 Subacute pyogenic osteomyelitis manifesting as a bone (Brodie's) abscess. Anteroposterior ankle radiograph demonstrates a lucent lesion within the diametaphyseal region (arrow). Subtle smooth periosteal reaction at the adjacent area to the medial cortex (arrow)

The most common causative organism for pyogenic osteomyelitis is *Staphylococcus aureus*. Others include fungal and tuberculous osteomyelitis which may follow a different clinical and radiological course (Lee et al. 2016). Chronic recurrent multifocal osteomyelitis (CRMO) is a poorly understood subtype affecting children and adolescents. It does not have an infective organism (also termed "aseptic" or nonbacterial osteitis) and presents clinically as repeated episodes of pain and swelling manifesting radiologically as multifocal marrow abnormalities.

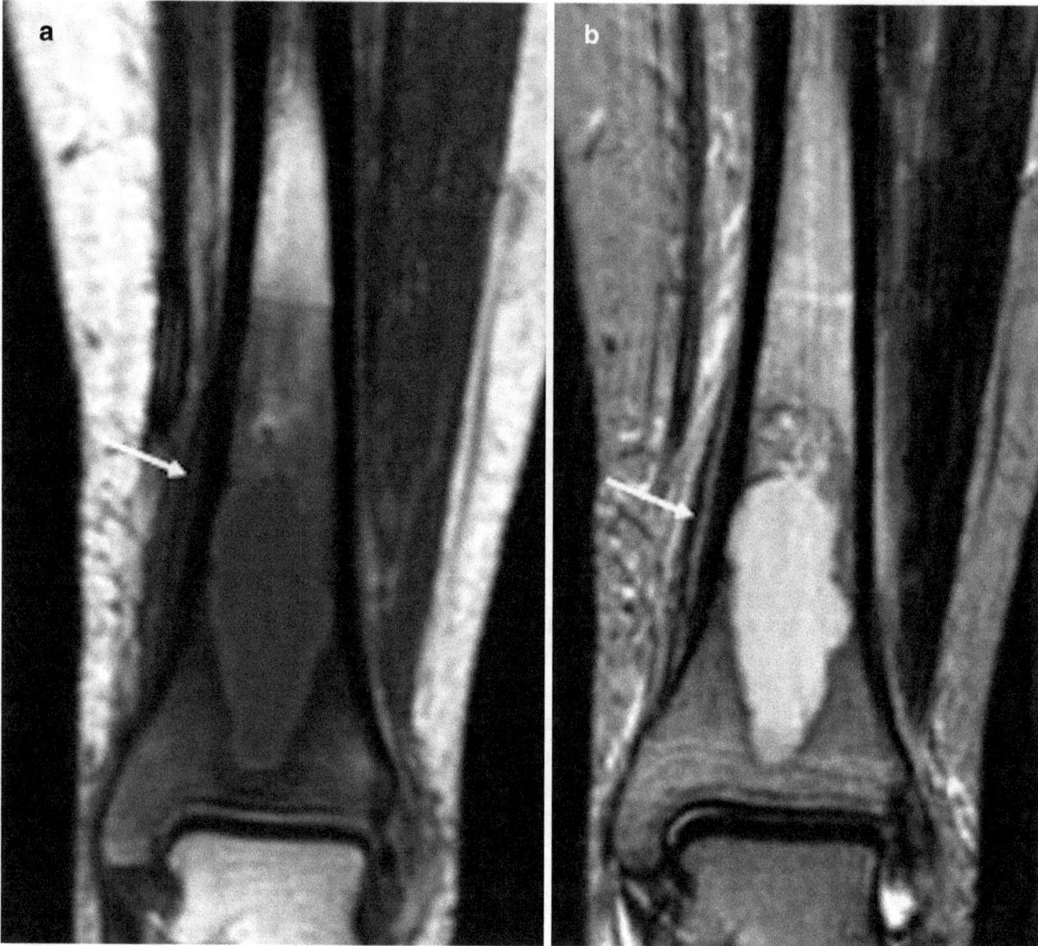

Fig. 14 Subacute pyogenic osteomyelitis manifesting as a bone (Brodie's) abscess. Coronal T1 (**a**) and STIR (**b**) demonstrating Brodie's abscess with a T1 hyperintense rim illustrating the "penumbra" sign (arrow)

4.1.3.1 Neoplasms: Benign

Primary bone neoplasms of the foot and ankle make up only 2–4% of all bone neoplasms. Neoplasms of the hind and midfoot may be asymptomatic, especially if benign and nonaggressive, or may present with anterior ankle pain. Neoplasms typically found in the epiphysis of long bones can also occur in "epiphysial equivalents," which include the tarsal and carpal bones (Boo et al. 2020).

Chondroblastoma is a benign tumor composed of chondroblasts and is one of the most frequent neoplasms affecting the talus in both the pediatric and young adult population. Patients may present with local tenderness and restricted motion. Within the talus, they most commonly occur at the posterior subchondral region (Fink et al. 1997). Radiographically, they appear as lucent lesions and may demonstrate a "fluffy" calcified matrix with expansile growth. On MR imaging, they have a hyperintense signal on proton density and T2-weighted images with a hypointense rim owing to a collagen-rich matrix and sclerotic rim, respectively (Chen and DiFrancesco 2017) (Fig. 15).

Osteoblastoma is another common entity within the benign neoplasms affecting the talus and is most frequently observed in the talar neck (Capanna et al. 1986). It is a bone-forming neoplasm and a larger form (>2 cm) of its counterpart, osteoid osteoma. Classic clinical vignettes are of nocturnal pain relieved by nonsteroidal

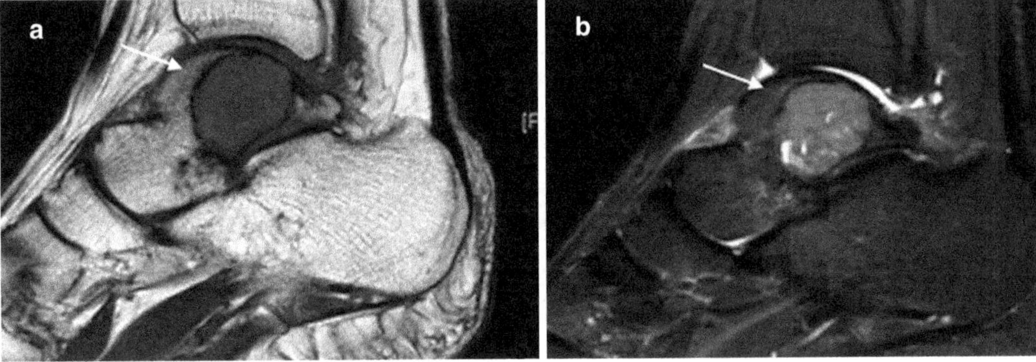

Fig. 15 Chondroblastoma of the talus. Sagittal T1 (**a**) and proton density (PD) fat-suppressed MR (**b**) images demonstrate a well-defined lesion and the posterior talus with predominant PD hyperintense matrix (chondroid) and a hypointense rim (sclerosis) (arrow)

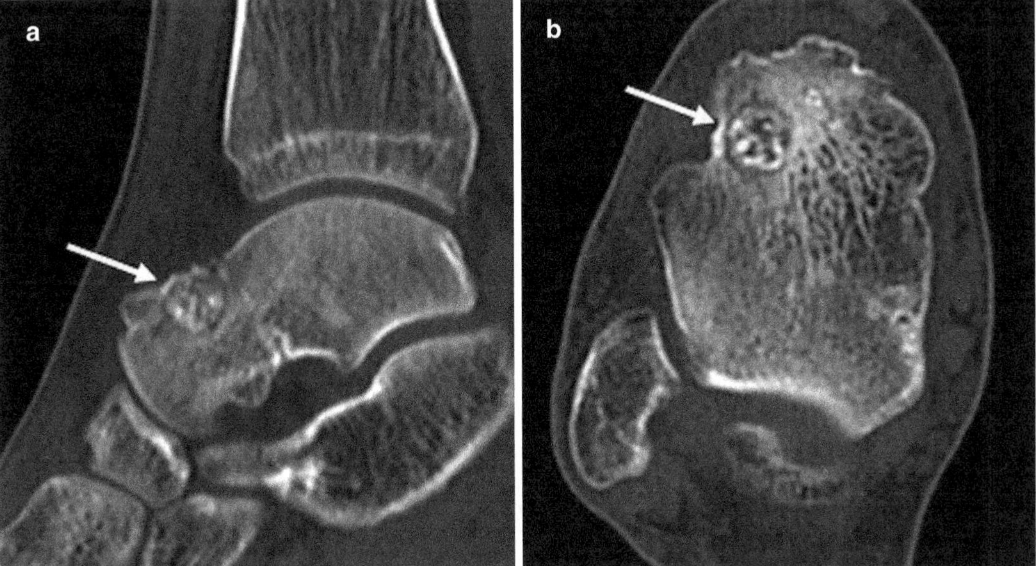

Fig. 16 Osteoblastoma of the talar neck. Sagittal (**a**) and axial (**b**) (CT) images demonstrating a well-defined sclerotic lesion with a calcified matrix (arrow)

anti-inflammatory drugs. On radiograph and computed tomography (CT), they manifest as cortically based lucent lesions with surrounding sclerosis and periostitis. Lesions have an internal calcified matrix and central sclerotic nidus, which is better appreciated on CT (Fig. 16). On MR imaging, they are typically T2 iso-intense with foci of decreased intensity, corresponding to calcification, and extensive surrounding T2 hyperintense signal corresponding to reactive marrow edema (Boo et al. 2020) (Fig. 17).

Osteochondroma is a common benign entity representing osseous protuberances surrounded by a cartilaginous "cap." Radiographically, they are typically incidental findings occurring at the metaphasis of long bones and point away from the articular surface. However, they can occur in any bone. Although asymptomatic, they may present with symptoms of impingement on surrounding structures such as tendons or nerves (Murphey et al. 2000). Malignant degeneration to **chondrosarcoma** is uncommon but may be suspected with the development of pain and an enlarging cartilaginous component. **Trevor disease** (dysplasia epiphysealis hemimelica) is a rare condition characterized by multiple osteochondromas arising from, and with unilateral involvement of, one or more epiphyses (Volders et al. 2011). Radiographically, they appear as irregular ossified masses which may cause deformity of the adjacent bone and disturb local structures (Tyler et al. 2013) (Fig. 18).

Giant cell tumor (osteoclastoma) is a generally benign but locally aggressive neoplasm, which has a rare malignant potential. It is often an incidental finding but may present with pain from local mass effect or with a pathological fracture (Rockberg et al. 2015). Radiographically, it appears in the mature skeleton as a lucent lesion with a non-sclerotic margin, eccentric location, and extension to the subchondral bone (Fig. 19). On MRI, signal intensity may be heterogenous

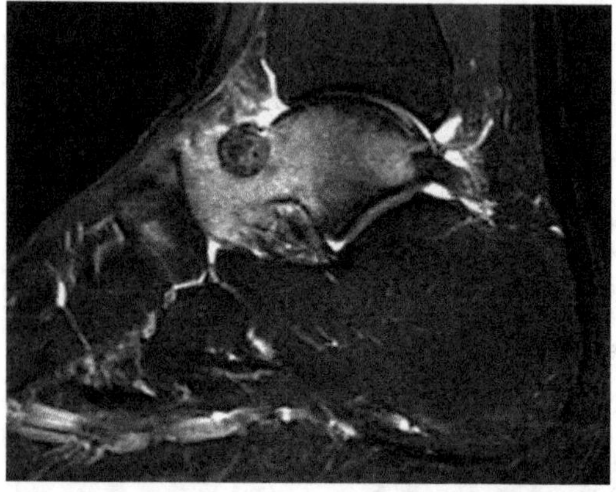

Fig. 17 Osteoblastoma of the talar neck. Sagittal proton density (PD)-weighted fat-suppressed MR image demonstrating a well-defined predominantly iso-intense lesion with hypointense foci corresponding to matrix calcification. There is extensive surrounding hyperintense signal corresponding to reactive edema

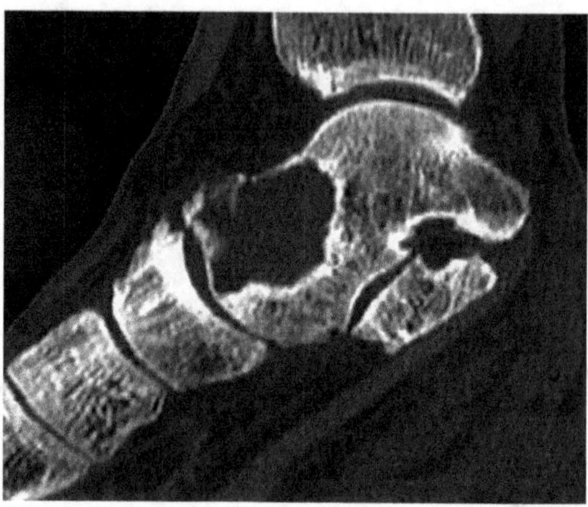

Fig. 19 Giant cell tumor of the talus. Sagittal reconstructed CT image demonstrates a well-defined lytic lesion within the talar neck with thinning of the adjacent cortex

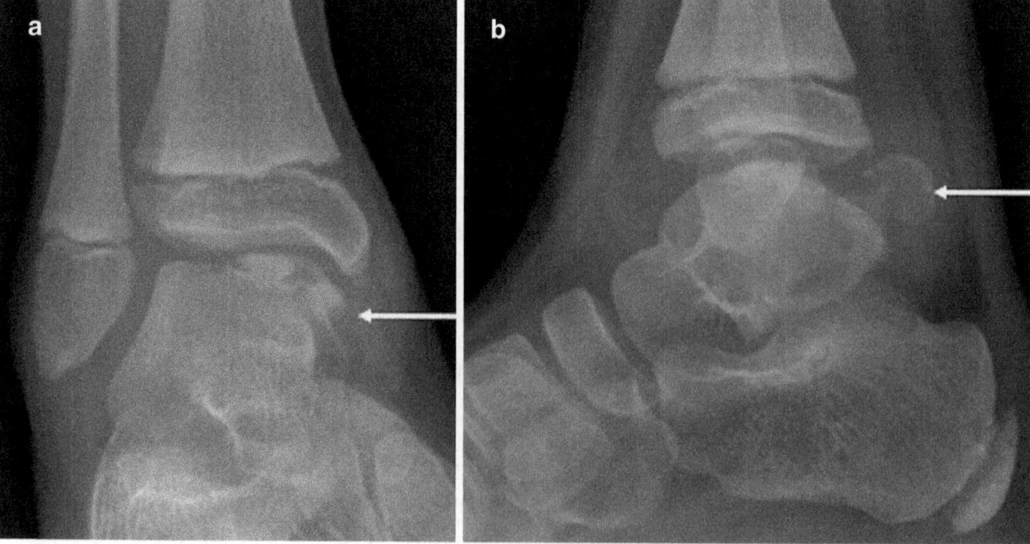

Fig. 18 Trevor disease of the ankle. AP (**a**) and lateral (**b**) radiographs showing multiple well-defined calcified and mass-like lesions adjacent to the medial talus with deformation of the medial talar dome (arrow)

owing to hemorrhagic contents (Fig. 20). GCTs may have secondary **aneurysmal bone cyst (ABC) changes** characterized by expansile osteoclastic cells with blood-filled channels and cystic spaces. On MR, they demonstrate characteristic-dependent fluid-fluid levels (Fig. 21). These neoplasms carry a risk of recurrence following surgical resection.

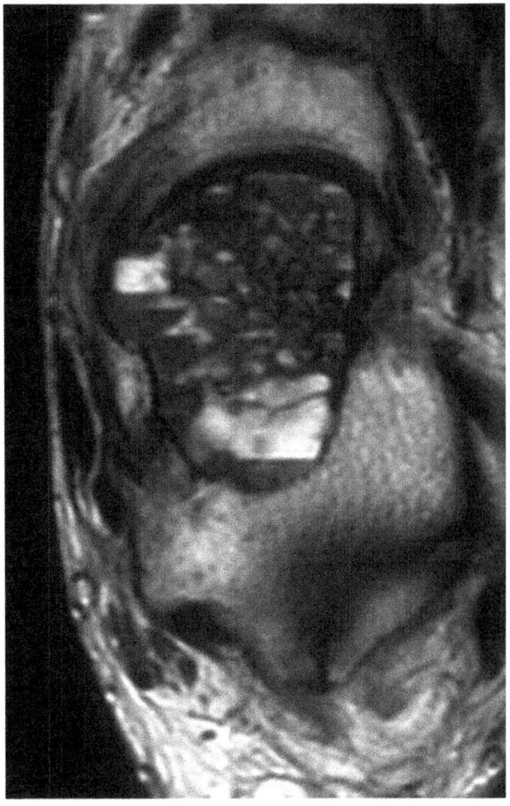

Fig. 21 Giant cell tumor (GCT) with secondary aneurysmal bone cyst. Axial T1-weighted image demonstrates a heterogenous intensity mass within the talus with the development of fluid-fluid levels consistent with secondary ABC

4.1.3.2 Neoplasms: Malignant

Metastases to the bones of the foot are rare and account for 0.01% of all metastatic bone disease. Clinically, patients will present with bone pain and may have a known history of malignancy. Common malignancies which metastasize to bone include prostate, breast, lung, and renal cancer. Radiographically, metastases will appear as either sclerotic or lucent lesions, which are poorly circumscribed and have a wide zone of transition and cortical destruction (Fig. 22). On MR, T1-weighted images demonstrate replacement of the normal hyperintense marrow fat by hypointense soft tissue, which may extend beyond the cortex (Fig. 23). In such cases, a thorough clinical examination and staging CT of the chest, abdomen, and pelvis should ensue (Wu et al. 2020).

The tumors are discussed in detail in the tumor chapter.

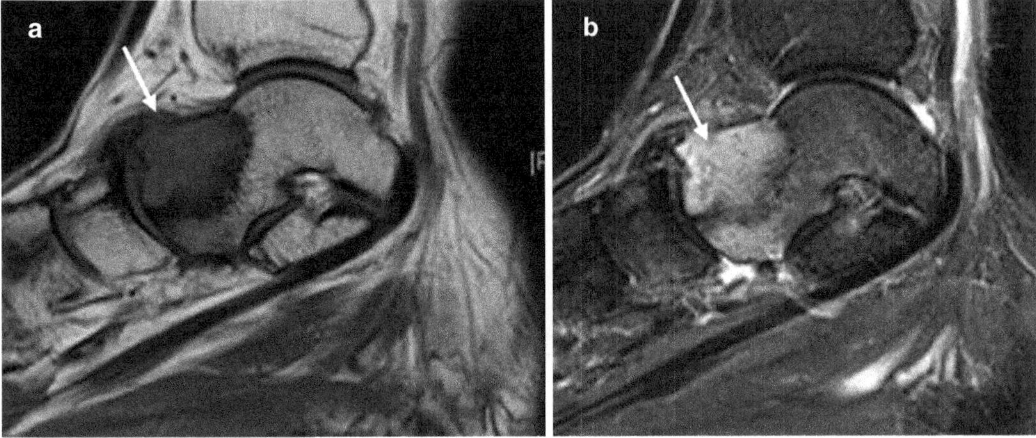

Fig. 20 Giant cell tumor (GCT) of the talus. Sagittal T1 (**a**) and STIR (**b**) demonstrate a well-circumscribed eccentrically located lesion in the talar head and neck (arrow)

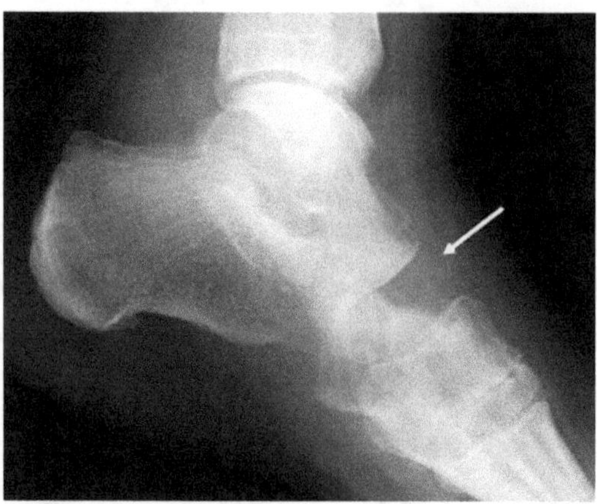

Fig. 22 Navicular metastasis. Lateral radiograph of the foot demonstrates irregular destruction of the dorsal navicular (arrow)

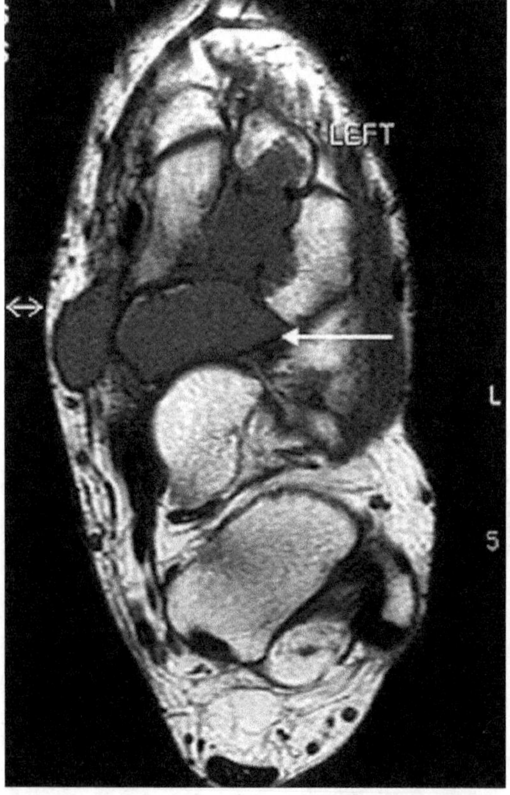

Fig. 23 Tarsal bone metastases. Axial T1 shows T1 hypointense soft tissue masses within the navicular with cortical destruction, soft tissue and transarticular extension to the other tarsal bones (arrow)

4.2 Joint

Osteoarthritis of the ankle joint is uncommon and affects 1% of the world population. Primary osteoarthritis is rare. Previous trauma is the most frequently encountered predisposing factor, and other etiologies include osteochondral lesions, overuse injuries and systemic diseases such as hemochromatosis.

Inflammatory arthritis with involvement of the ankle is more common and can be seen in seronegative spondyloarthropathies, rheumatoid arthritis, and gout (Kiely and Lloyd 2021). Clinically, patients may present with pain, swelling, and synovitis. This manifests radiographically as periarticular erosions, radiolucency, and soft tissue swelling (Fig. 24). MR findings include diffuse synovitis, cartilage loss and inflammatory involvement of tendons and ligaments.

Septic arthritis of the ankle, subtalar, and midfoot joints may be secondary to hematogenous spread from a systemic infection or direct spread from adjacent cellulitis and osteomy-

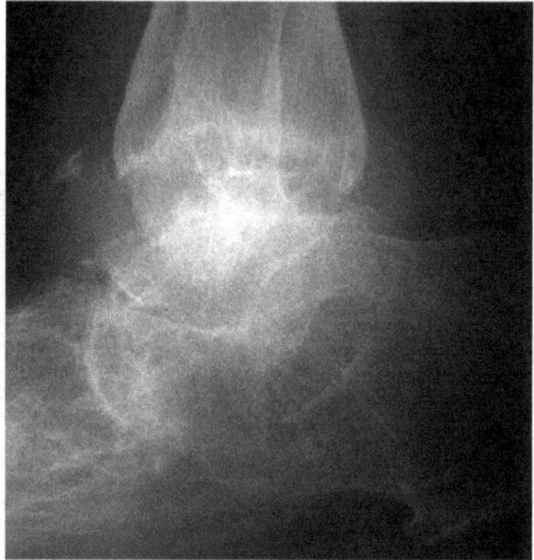

Fig. 24 Rheumatoid arthritis of the ankle joint. Lateral ankle radiograph demonstrates profuse periarticular erosion with secondary bone sclerosis and arthropathy

elitis (please see full description earlier in the chapter). In patients with diabetes mellitus, an important consideration is to differentiate osteomyelitis, occurring at areas of mechanical pressure and skin ulceration, with neuropathic (Charcot) joint arthropathy, which typically involves multiple joints and is independent of focal pressure points. These entities may have overlapping MR findings so a thorough clinical examination and history is essential to reach a diagnosis.

Pigmented villonodular synovitis (PVNS), a diffuse subtype of tenosynovial giant cell tumor (the other being localized tenosynovial GCT of the tendon sheath, described in the next section), is a benign process characterized by synovial proliferation with hemosiderin deposition within joints, bursae, or tendon sheaths (Crim et al. 2021). It typically manifests as a monoarticular process most commonly affecting the knee (60–80%) but can be seen in the ankle (2.5% of cases). MR imaging demonstrates areas of heterogenous intensity synovial proliferation with multi-sequence hypointense foci consistent with hemosiderin staining (Fig. 25). It also demonstrates further signal dropout ("blooming artifact") on gradient recalled echo sequences. Radiographically, the synovial proliferation may erode adjacent cortical bone surfaces, sometimes mimicking an aggressive lesion (Fig. 26). Patients may present with symptoms of ankle impingement due to local mass effect (Morelli et al. 2019).

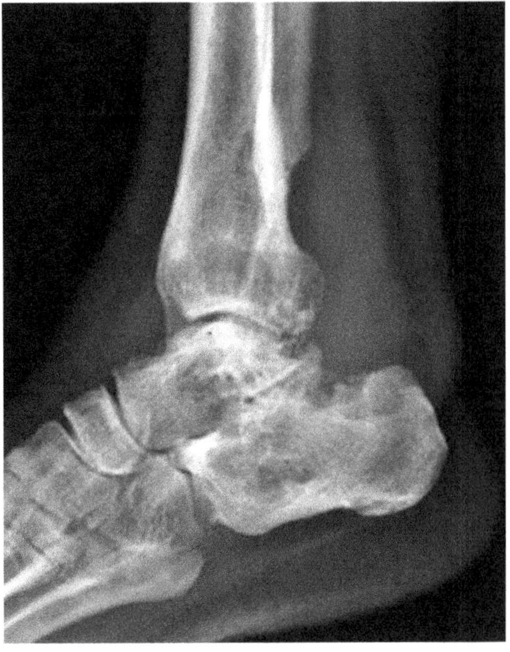

Fig. 26 Pigmented villonodular synovitis (PVNS) of the ankle. Lateral ankle radiograph demonstrates a large soft tissue opacity posterior to the tibia and smaller opacity anterior to the ankle joint. There are multiple cortical erosions of the talus, calcaneus, and posterior tibia at the interface to this opacity

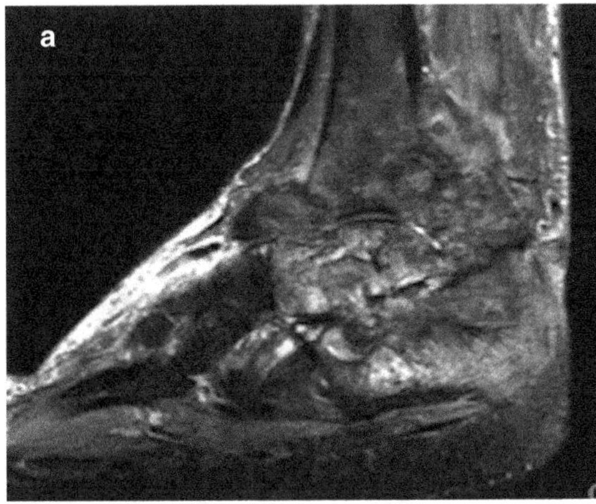

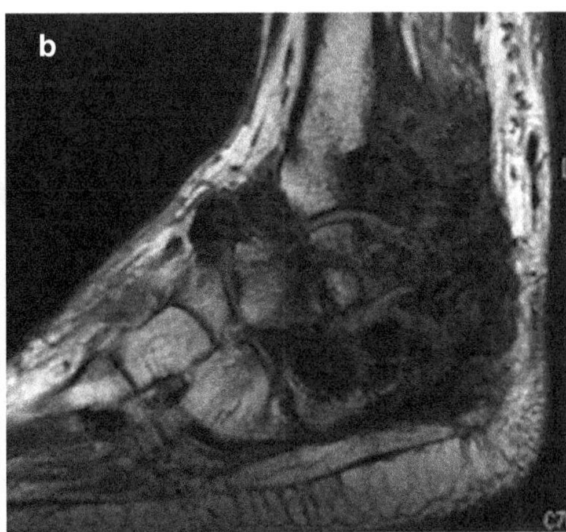

Fig. 25 Pigmented villonodular synovitis (PVNS) of the ankle. Sagittal STIR (**a**) and T2 (**b**) images of the ankle demonstrate diffuse synovial thickening with areas of low signal intensity indicating previous hemorrhage and hemosiderin staining

Synovial chondromatosis is a disorder characterized by multiple loose intra-articular cartilaginous bodies, which may be calcified, resulting in the term "osteochondromatosis" (Figs. 27 and 28). Two main subtypes exist—a primary monoarticular form of unknown etiology and a secondary form caused by a preexisting joint arthropathy, commonly osteoarthritis (Murphey et al. 2007).

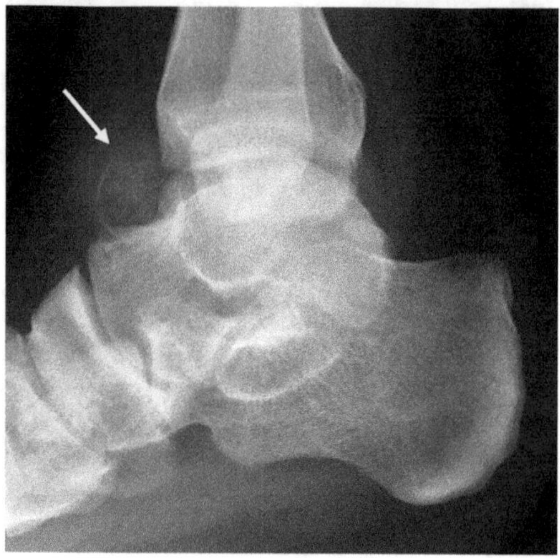

Fig. 27 Synovial osteochondromatosis of the ankle. Lateral radiograph demonstrates an opacity with rim calcification anterior to the ankle joint (arrow)

Ganglion cysts are common benign masses, which may arise from joints, bursae, tendons, and ligaments. They may occur spontaneously or following trauma and surgery. Ganglion cysts of the distal tibiofibular joint (Fig. 29) and anterior ankle joint may present with a swelling with or without associated pain at the anterior ankle.

Anterior ankle impingement syndrome is the result of chronic repetitive trauma of the talar dome against the anterior tibial plafond in the central portion of the ankle recess. It has been commonly reported in soccer players and ballet dancers (Berman et al. 2017). Clinically, patients present with painful and limited dorsiflexion and anterior ankle swelling, although it may be an incidental finding in asymptomatic individuals. Radiographically, small bony spurs are seen originating from the anterior tibial plafond and the anterior talar dome (Fig. 30).

4.3 Soft Tissues

4.3.1 Tendinosis, Tenosynovitis, and Tendon Tears

Pathologies involving the anterior compartment tendons are relatively uncommon as they have a

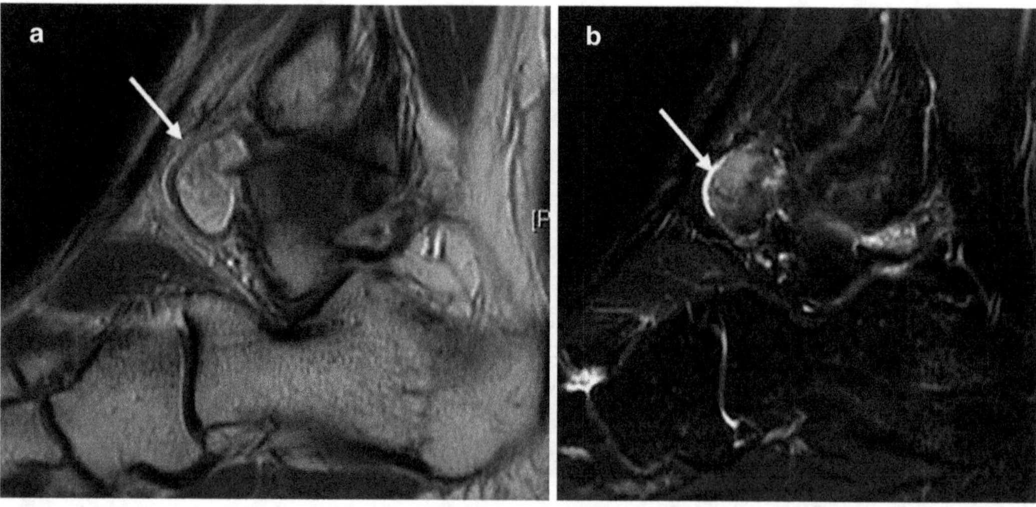

Fig. 28 Synovial osteochondromatosis of the ankle. Sagittal T1 (**a**) and STIR (**b**) showing focus of synovial chondromatosis in the anterior recess of the ankle (arrow)

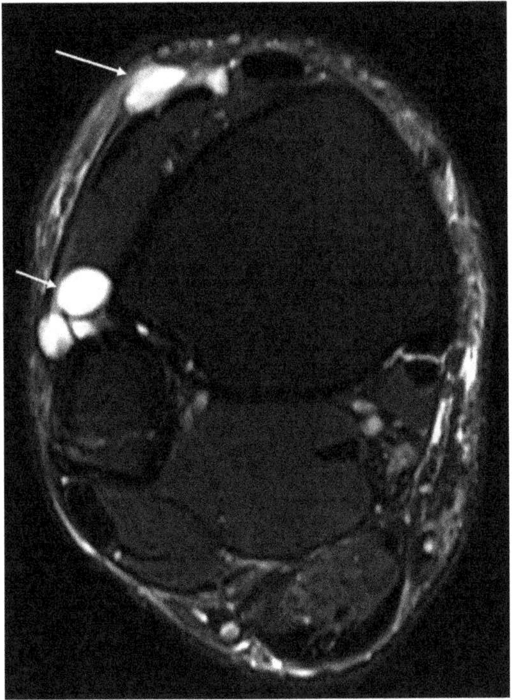

Fig. 29 Axial PDFS of ankle showing ganglion cyst anterior to the ankle joint (long arrow) communicating with the distal tibiofibular joint (short arrow)

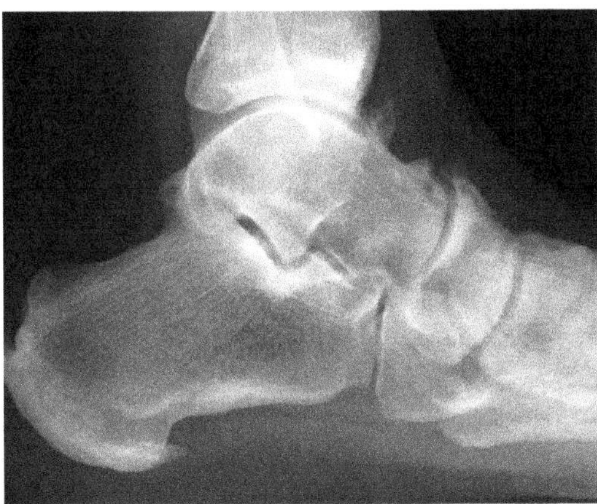

Fig. 30 Anterior ankle impingement syndrome. Lateral radiograph of the ankle demonstrates a large osseous spur originating from the anterior talus

relatively straight course and are exposed to minor mechanical stress under normal circumstances. As such, they are a commonly underreported and overlooked group of disorders (Scheller et al. 1980). They may be associated with depositional diseases such as hydroxyapatite, gout, and amyloidosis; inflammatory conditions such as rheumatoid arthritis and seronegative spondyloarthropathies; and a variety of other systemic diseases such as ochronosis and connective tissue disorders. Patients may present with acute flares in the form of tenosynovitis, which may coexist with tendinopathy. Spontaneous tendon ruptures are rare, and predisposing factors include preexisting tendinopathy, repeat steroid, or direct trauma to the area. Caution must be taken during T1-weighted MR imaging due to false-positive intrasubstance signal change caused by magic angle phenomena (Ng et al. 2013).

1. The **tibialis anterior (TA) tendon** inserts on to the medial cuneiform and performs dorsiflexion of the ankle and inversion of the foot. It is the most common of the extensor tendons to be injured. TA tendinosis refers to tendon degeneration with the formation of fibrous tissue. It may be caused by repetitive strain, depositional disorders, and systemic diseases (Järvinen et al. 1997). On MR imaging, the tendon demonstrates thickening with intrasubstance signal change, which typically occurs at or below the level of the extensor retinaculum (Mengiardi et al. 2005) (Fig. 31). Inflammation of the tendon sheath is termed tenosynovitis and manifests on MR imaging as fluid distension of the tendon sheath (Fig. 32). Tibialis anterior tendon ruptures have been reported in athletes, skiers, and football players and spontaneously in patients with comorbid conditions described above (Stuart 1992). Clinically, patients will present with weakness to dorsiflexion, localized anterior ankle tenderness, and a drop-foot gait. A palpable lump may be felt anterior to the ankle, and this may be visible on radiograph (Fig. 33). Ultrasound and MRI examinations will reveal a retracted tendon with surrounding edema (Varghese and Bianchi 2014) (Figs. 34 and 35).
2. **Giant cell tumor of the tendon sheath (GCTTS)** is a localized form of tenosynovial giant cell tumor. It occurs most commonly in the fingers and less commonly in the ankle

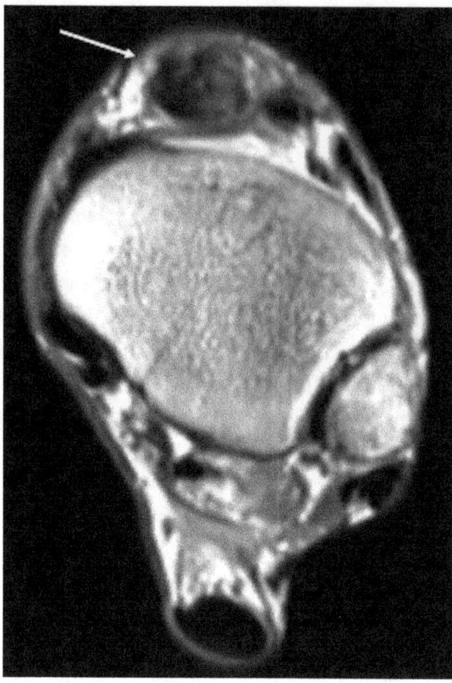

Fig. 31 Tibialis anterior tendinopathy. Axial PD at the level of the distal tibiofibular joint demonstrates intrasubstance iso-intense signal intensity and thickening of the tibialis anterior tendon (arrow)

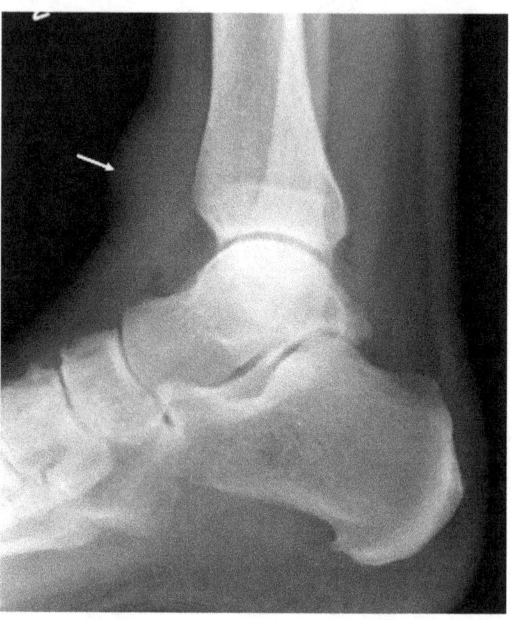

Fig. 33 Tibialis anterior tendon tear. Lateral radiograph of the ankle demonstrates a soft tissue opacity anterior to the distal tibia, which is clinically palpable

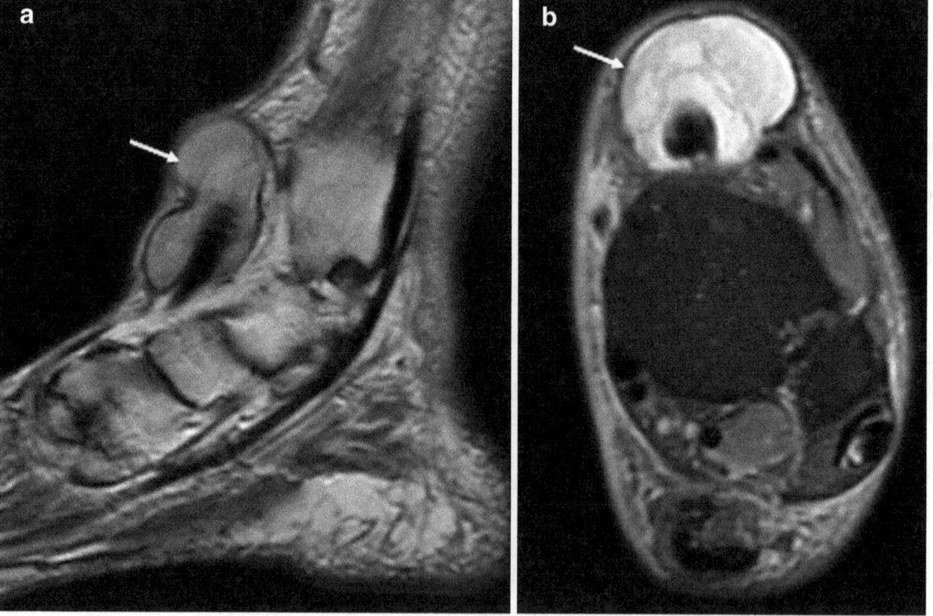

Fig. 32 Tibialis anterior tenosynovitis. Sagittal proton density (PD) (a) and axial PDFS (b) images demonstrate fluid within the tibialis anterior tendon sheath (arrow)

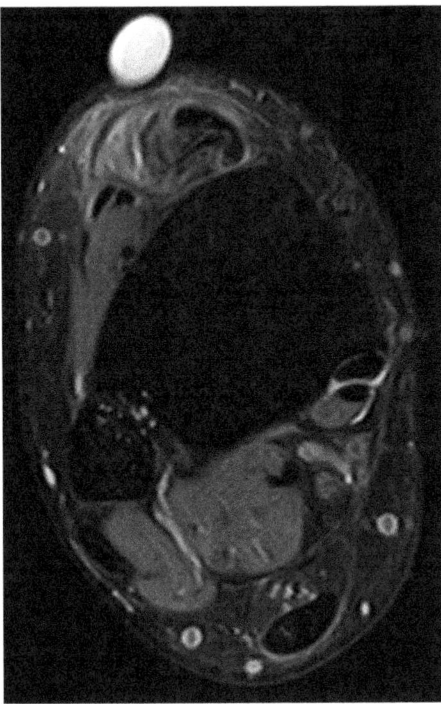

Fig. 34 Tibialis anterior tendon tear. Proton density (PD)-weighted fat-suppressed axial MR image at the distal tibiofibular joint demonstrates heterogenous signal intensity within the tibialis anterior tendon with a swirling appearance from a retracted and torn tendon (marker)

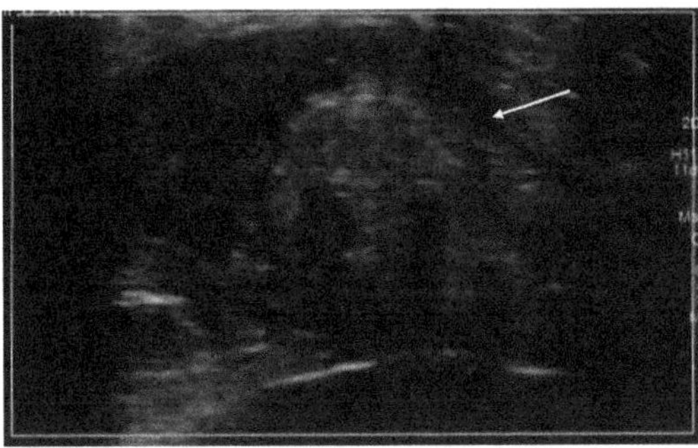

Fig. 35 Tibialis anterior tendon tear. Axial ultrasound image demonstrates a swirled hyperechoic tendon from a retracted and torn tendon (arrow). Additionally, there is diffuse mixed echogenicity peritendinous content with secondary distension of the tendon sheath, likely from hemorrhage

and foot (Crim et al. 2021). It typically presents as a slow-growing painless mass but may cause discomfort owing to footwear and local structures. It may involve any tendon and demonstrates low signal intensity on MR imaging with areas of "blooming" on gradient recalled echo sequences (Fig. 36).

3. **Ganglion cysts** are common benign mass lesions and may involve the tendons of the ankle (Fig. 37).
4. **Extensor hallucis longus and extensor digitorum longus** tendinopathy and tenosynovitis are also infrequently described (Fig. 38). These tendons are susceptible to penetrating trauma due to their superficial location. Tendon rupture may also occur secondary to mechanical overuse and comorbid conditions and has been described in ultramarathon runners. A high clinical suspicion is required to make the diagnosis due to the apparently mild signs of injury on examination of the foot (Ng et al. 2013).
5. **Anterior tarsal tunnel syndrome** refers to entrapment of the deep peroneal nerve as it traverses the inferior extensor retinaculum. Clinically, this presents with anteromedial ankle pain, weakness of the extensor digitorum brevis muscle, and numbness between the first and second digits, owing to their respective nerve supply (Ng et al. 2013).
6. **Tibialis anterior friction syndrome** is a recently described entity occurring in athletes who present with symptoms of tibial stress injury (Kho et al. 2021). The syndrome occurs above the level of the superior retinaculum, different to conventional tendinosis, which occurs at or below the level of the retinacula. It is thought to be due to repetitive rubbing of the tendon between the superior extensor retinaculum and tibia from repetitive dorsiflexion and plantar flexion. The condition has been reported in runners and soccer players. MR imaging demonstrates peritendinous fluid and soft tissue edema surrounding the tibialis anterior tendon (Fig. 39).
7. **Ankle extensor retinacula** injuries are uncommon. However, they have been reported in high-level football players and following traumatic ankle-twisting injuries. Imaging with ultrasound and MR may demonstrate thickening of the extensor retinaculum in both symptomatic and asymptomatic patients alike

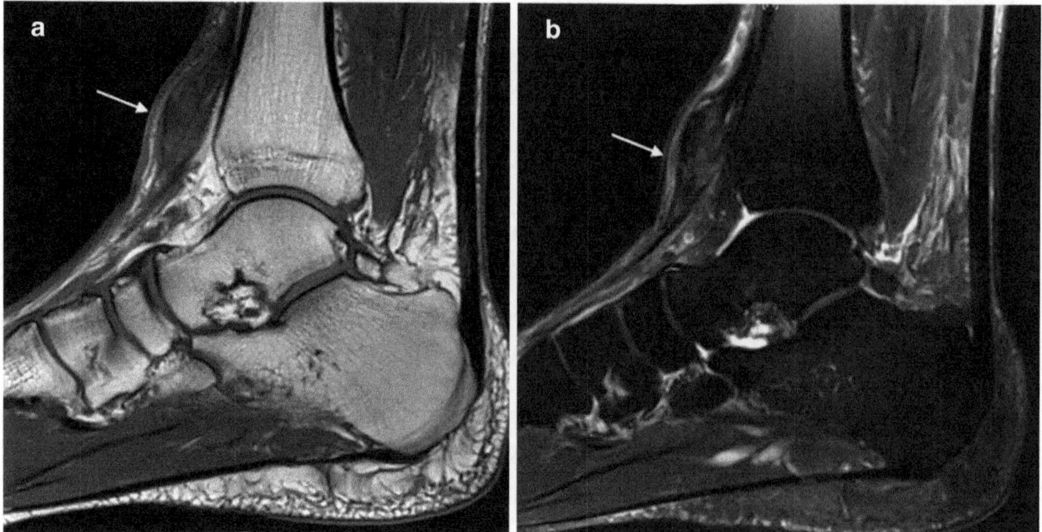

Fig. 36 Tibialis anterior tendon sheath giant cell tumor. Sagittal T1 (**a**) and PD fat-suppressed (**b**) images of the ankle demonstrate lesion within the tibialis anterior tendon consistent with the GCT of tendon sheath (arrow)

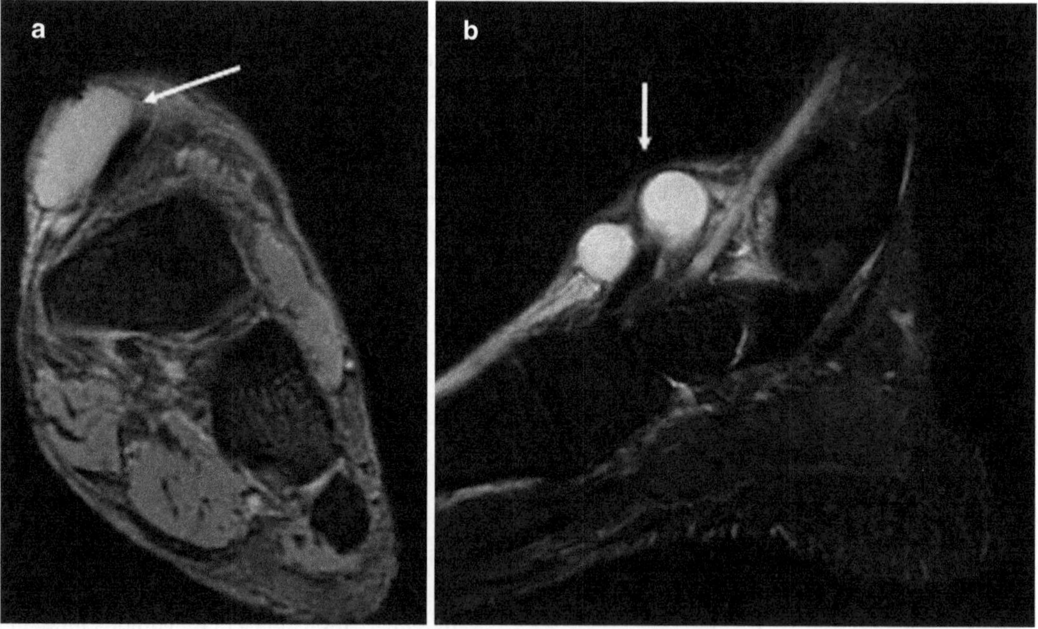

Fig. 37 Tibialis anterior tendon ganglion cyst. Coronal T2* (**a**) and sagittal PD fat-suppressed (**b**) image showing ganglion in relation to tibialis anterior (arrow)

and as such is not a reliable finding alone (Win et al. 2020). Edema on MR imaging surrounding the retinaculum may suggest an acute injury. **Calcific enthesopathy of the extensor retinaculum** is another reported entity, which may present with anteromedial ankle pain. Treatment with barbotage may relieve symptoms (Shah et al. 2022). Although rare, extensor retinacula rupture has also been reported, and clinically patients present with anterior ankle pain, instability, and tendon snapping (Wagner et al. 2016).

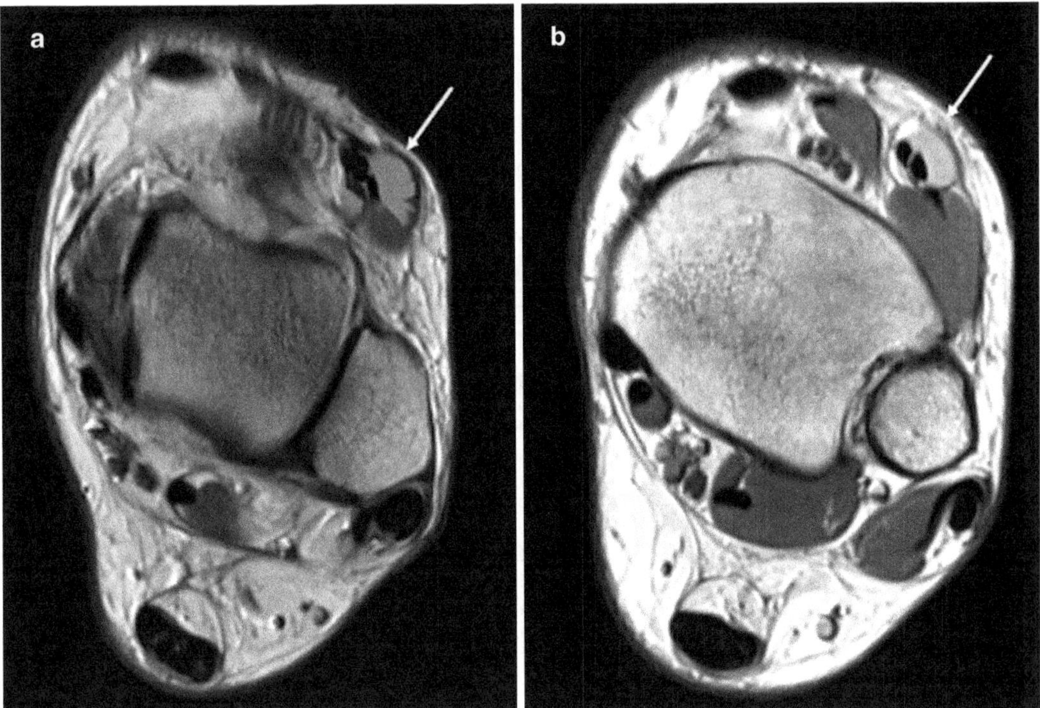

Fig. 38 Extensor digitorum longus tenosynovitis. Axial proton density (PD)-weighted images (**a** and **b**) demonstrating tenosynovitis of EDL (arrow)

Other impingement syndromes may also present with anterior ankle pain and are discussed in other chapters of the book.

4.3.2 Subcutaneous Mass Lesions of the Dorsal Ankle: Benign

The majority of soft tissue lesions of the ankle and foot are benign, but they may pose a diagnostic dilemma due to a considerable overlap in imaging features with malignant lesions. Although ultrasound is often used as an initial screening modality to demonstrate certain benign features, such as a predominant cystic component found in ganglion cysts, MR is a superior tool to characterize lesions and obtain anatomical detail with respect to surrounding structures (Hughes et al. 2019). In practice, these lesions often warrant a multidisciplinary approach consisting of a clinical examination, radiological assessment, and a histological diagnosis, through image-guided or excisional biopsy, to achieve a final diagnosis (Wu and Hochman 2009).

Hematomas may develop following trauma or spontaneously in patients with bleeding diathesis or anticoagulation. Clinically, they appear as a palpable lump with or without discoloration. Although not frequently required, hematomas may be assessed with ultrasound and MR. In the acute stage, MR appears both T1 and T2 hypointense, progressively becoming hyperintense with the conversion of oxyhemoglobin to methemoglobin. This change is usually seen earlier on T1-weighted imaging and may give a distinct T1 hyperintense rim in the subacute stage (Fig. 40). Chronic hematomas appear both T1 and T2 hyperintense and may demonstrate a peripheral hypointense hemosiderin rim. As hematomas can coexist with underlying tumors, follow-up to resolution is required where there is soft tissue nodularity, enhancement, or an absence of antecedent trauma (Wu and Hochman 2009).

Peripheral nerve sheath tumors (PNSTs) comprise schwannomas (neurilemmoma) and neu-

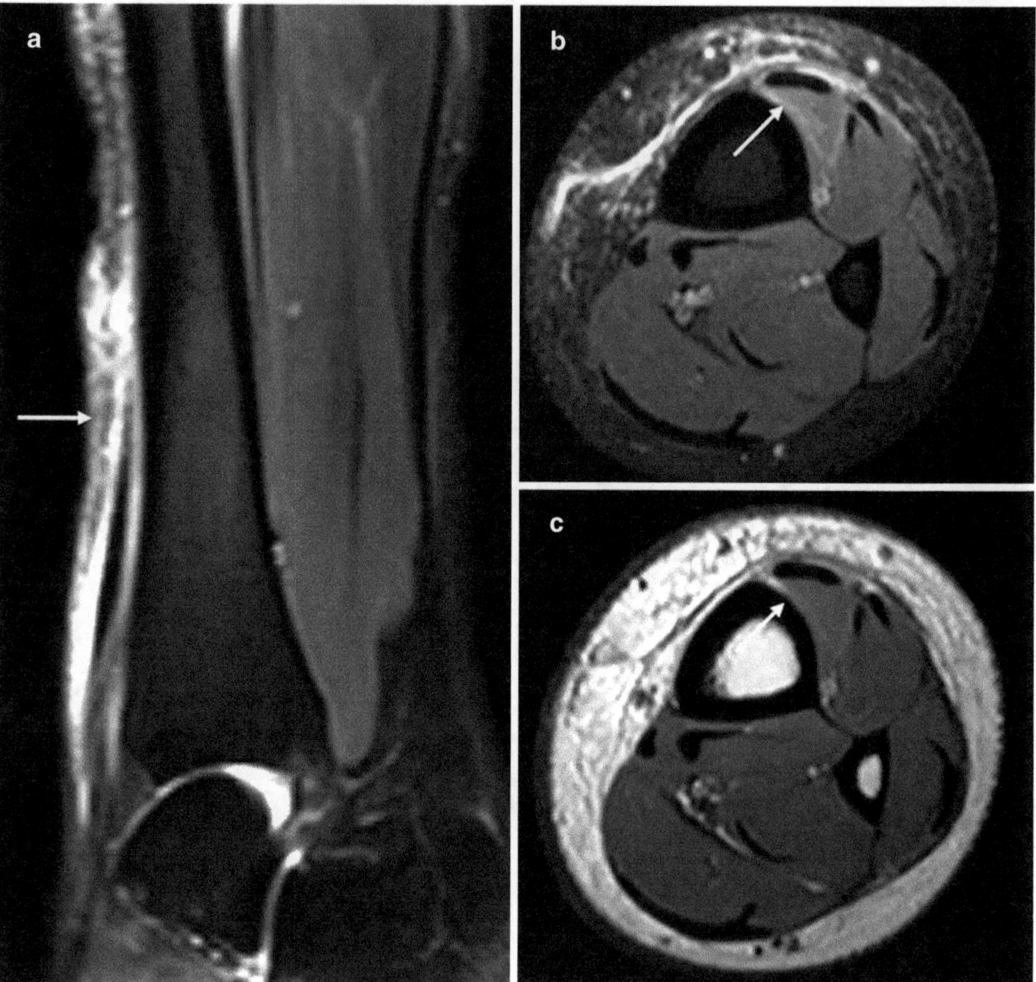

Fig. 39 Tibialis anterior friction syndrome. STIR sag (**a**), PDFS (**b**), and PD (**c**) axial of left leg showing marked edema of the tibialis anterior (arrow) with soft tissue edema

rofibromas. They are benign tumors and 10% occur in the lower limb, most commonly in the tibial and common peroneal nerves. Rarer malignant PNSTs generally occur in the major nerves of the proximal appendicular skeleton. On MR, PNSTs may appear nonspecific with T1 iso-intense and T2 mildly hyperintense signal (Fig. 41). Certain MR findings such as the split-fat sign, nerve entering and exiting sign, and target sign are supportive features demonstrated in 40–60% of lesions (Beaman et al. 2004). Although schwannoma appears eccentric to a nerve compared to neurofibroma which is more central, these features may be less reliable when evaluating smaller nerves.

Soft tissue venous malformations (hemangiomas) are benign vascular soft tissue tumors and may be subdivided according to the International Society of the Study of Vascular Anomalies (ISSVA) classification. Radiographs demonstrate soft tissue swelling and phleboliths. MR characteristics may vary according to whether the lesion has high or low vascular flow. Lesions appear variable on T1 depending on hemorrhage and intrinsic fat. In low-flow areas, they appear T2 hyperintense,

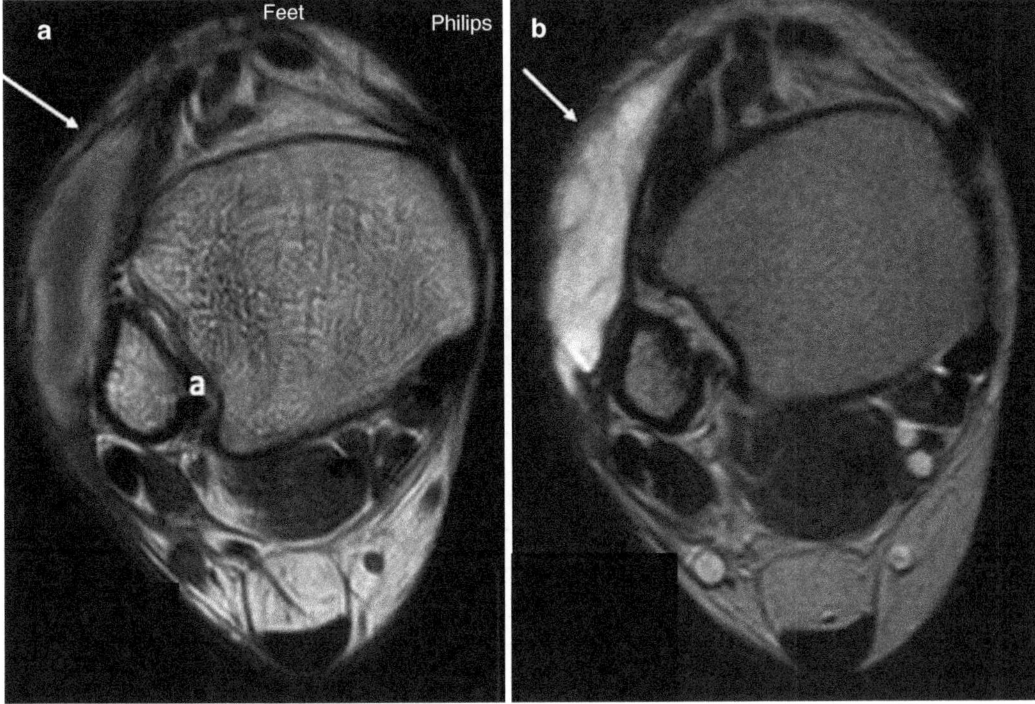

Fig. 40 Subacute hematoma. Axial T1 (**a**) and T2 fat-suppressed (**b**) images illustrating a mass in the anterolateral ankle demonstrating T2 hyperintense lesion with hypointense septa and T1 hypointense lesion with peripheral rim of hyperintensity (arrow)

and in high-flow areas, they demonstrate signal voids. They typically appear well defined and lobulated (Wu and Hochman 2009) (Fig. 42).

4.3.3 Subcutaneous Mass Lesions of the Dorsal Ankle: Malignant

Although T2 hyperintensity attributed to high water content is found in benign masses such as ganglion cysts, certain solid and malignant lesions may demonstrate similar characteristics. A high clinical suspicion with correlation to age and location is key in achieving the correct diagnosis for these malignant neoplasms.

Synovial sarcoma, contrary to the name, occurs close to but does not arise from a joint. It most commonly occurs in the lower extremity in the second to fourth decades (Murphey et al. 2006). On MR, it appears as an aggressive soft tissue neoplasm with destruction of adjacent bone and intense postcontrast enhancement. It may demonstrate a classic "triple sign" consisting of three different signal intensities comprised of fluid, hemorrhage, and a solid component (Fig. 43).

Myxofibrosarcoma, previously known as a myxoid variant of malignant fibrous histiocytoma, is a malignant soft tissue neoplasm. It is most common in the lower limb and typically occurs after the sixth decade, being the most common soft tissue neoplasm to occur in late adulthood (Waters et al. 2007). MR features are variable showing T1 iso- to hypointensity and T2 heterogenous intensity with hyperintense myxoid components (Fig. 44).

Clear cell sarcoma is an extremely rare, slow-growing malignancy, which is commonly found in deep regions of the appendicular skeleton. Ninety-five percent occurs in the

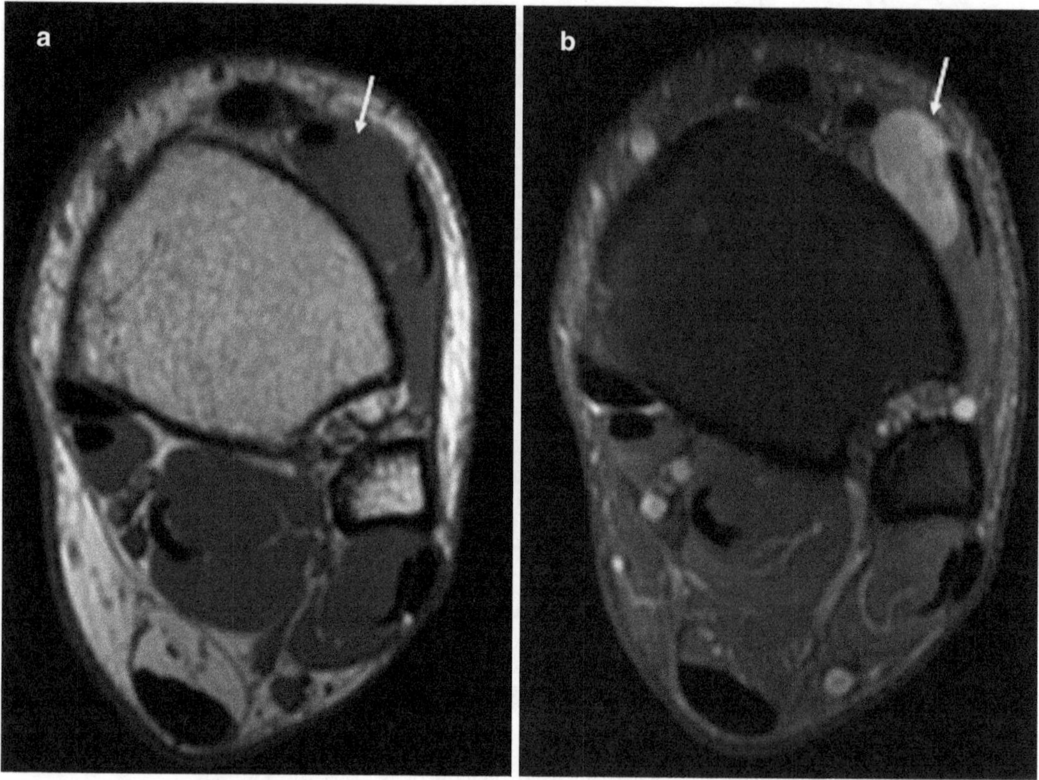

Fig. 41 Peripheral nerve sheath tumor of the deep peroneal nerve. Axial T1 (**a**) and T2 fat-suppressed (**b**) images show a well-circumscribed mass, arising from the deep peroneal nerve at the level of the distal tibiofibular joint, demonstrating T1 iso-intense and T2 hyperintense (with subtle hypointense foci) (arrow)

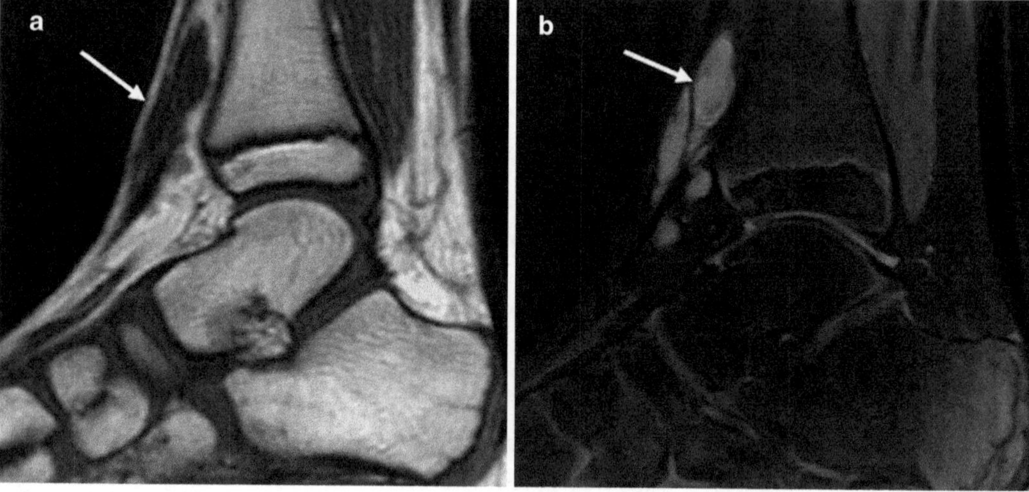

Fig. 42 Soft tissue venous malformation of the anterior ankle. Sagittal T1 (**a**) and STIR (**b**) showing a lobulated mass in the anterior soft tissue of the ankle demonstrating low signal on T1 and high on STIR (arrow)

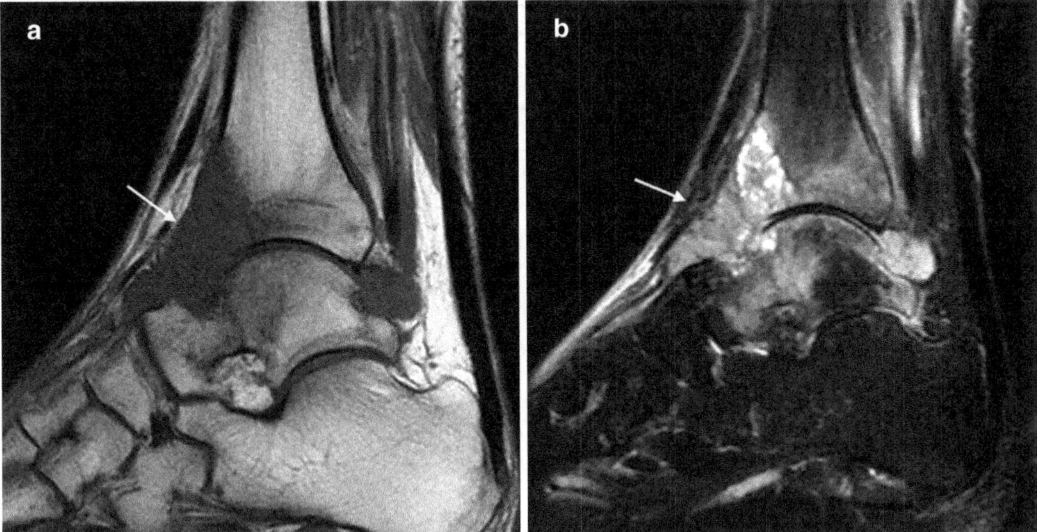

Fig. 43 Synovial sarcoma within the soft tissues of the anterior ankle. Sagittal T1 (**a**) and STIR (**b**) demonstrate an ill-defined T2 heterogenous lesion and T1 iso-intensity with invasion of the adjacent tibia and talus (arrow). A smaller similar area is seen adjacent to the posterior recess of ankle

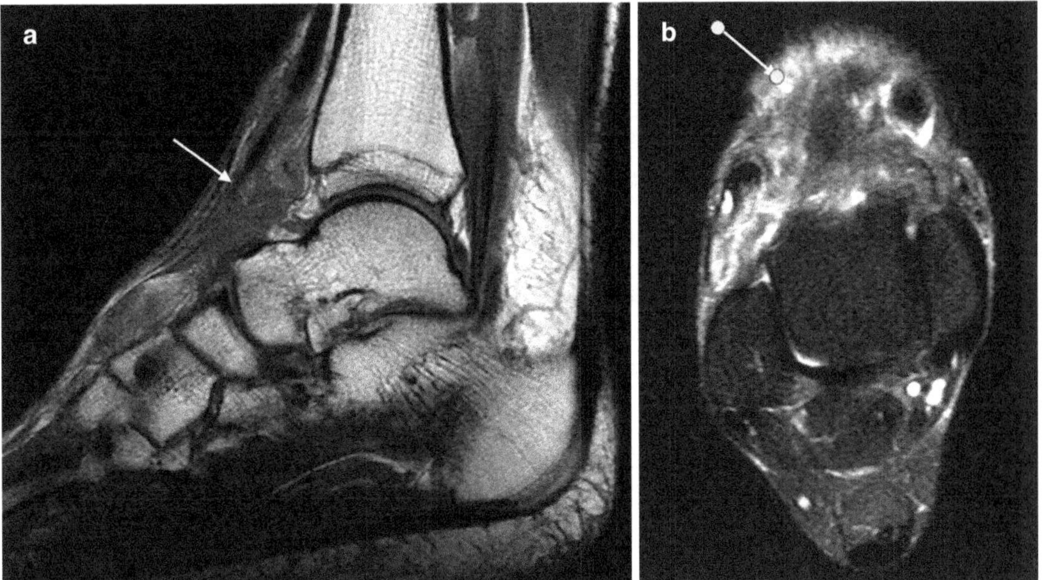

Fig. 44 Myxofibrosarcoma within the soft tissues of the anterior ankle. Sagittal T1 (**a**) and STIR (**b**) demonstrating an ill-defined mass of the anterior ankle, which is T1 iso-intense and T2 heterogenous (arrow)

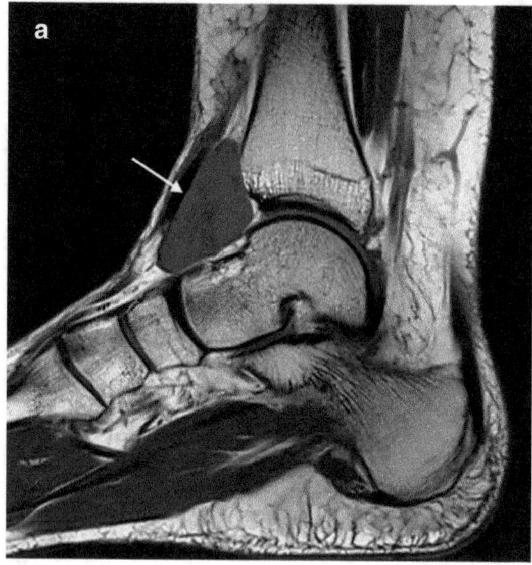

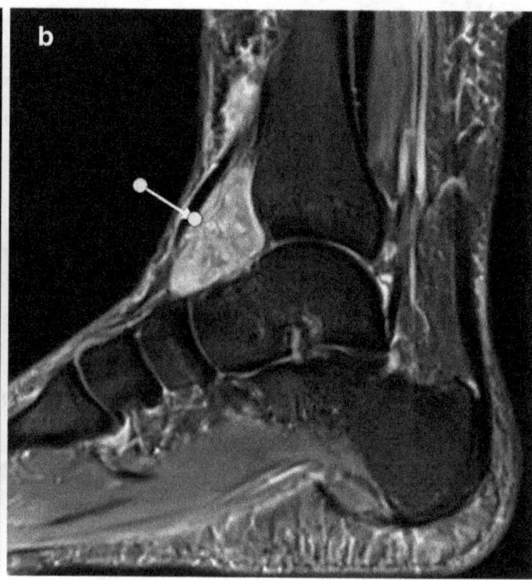

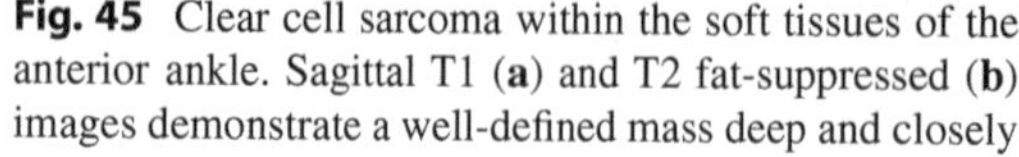

Fig. 45 Clear cell sarcoma within the soft tissues of the anterior ankle. Sagittal T1 (**a**) and T2 fat-suppressed (**b**) images demonstrate a well-defined mass deep and closely related to the extensor tendons. It demonstrates T1 iso-intensity and T2 heterogenous hyperintensity

lower extremity, especially in the ankle and foot, close to tendons and fascial structures and occurs in younger adulthood (Ibrahim et al. 2018). On MR, it appears as a well-defined, relatively homogenously T1 iso-intense and T2 hyperintense with hypointense foci. Consequently, they can be mistaken for a benign lesion and represent a diagnostic difficulty (Fig. 45).

Tumors are discussed in detail in the tumor section of the book.

References

Alaia EF, Chhabra A, Simpfendorfer CS, Cohen M, Mintz DN, Vossen JA et al (2021) MRI nomenclature for musculoskeletal infection. Skeletal Radiol 50(12):2319–2347

Beaman FD, Kransdorf MJ, Menke DM (2004) Schwannoma: radiologic-pathologic correlation. Radiographics 24(5):1477–1481

Berman Z, Tafur M, Ahmed SS, Huang BK, Chang EY (2017) Ankle impingement syndromes: an imaging review. Br J Radiol 90(1070):20160735

Boo SL, Saad A, Murphy J, Botchu R (2020) Tumours of the talus - a pictorial review. J Clin Orthop Trauma 11(3):410–416

Capanna R, Van Horn JR, Ayala A, Picci P, Bettelli G (1986) Osteoid osteoma and osteoblastoma of the talus. A report of 40 cases. Skeletal Radiol 15(5):360–364

Chaturvedi A, Mann L, Cain U, Klionsky NB (2020) Acute fractures and dislocations of the ankle and foot in children. Radiographics 40(3):754–774

Chen W, DiFrancesco LM (2017) Chondroblastoma: an update. Arch Pathol Lab Med 141(6):867–871

Court-Brown CM, Caesar B (2006) Epidemiology of adult fractures: a review. Injury 37(8):691–697

Crim J, Dyroff SL, Stensby JD, Evenski A, Layfield LJ (2021) Limited usefulness of classic MR findings in the diagnosis of tenosynovial giant cell tumor. Skeletal Radiol 50(8):1585–1591

Fink BR, Temple HT, Chiricosta FM, Mizel MS, Murphey MD (1997) Chondroblastoma of the foot. Foot Ankle Int 18(4):236–242

Harris G, Harris C (2016) Imaging of tarsal navicular stress injury with a focus on MRI: a pictorial essay. J Med Imaging Radiat Oncol 60(3):359–364

Hughes P, Miranda R, Doyle AJ (2019) MRI imaging of soft tissue tumours of the foot and ankle. Insights Imaging 10(1):60

Ibrahim RM, Steenstrup Jensen S, Juel J (2018) Clear cell sarcoma-a review. J Orthop 15(4):963–966

Järvinen M, Józsa L, Kannus P, Järvinen TL, Kvist M, Leadbetter W (1997) Histopathological findings in chronic tendon disorders. Scand J Med Sci Sports 7(2):86–95

Kho JSB, Botchu R, Rushton A, James SL (2021) MRI findings of tibialis anterior friction syndrome: a mimic of tibial stress injury. Skeletal Radiol 50(10):2007–2011

Kiely PDW, Lloyd ME (2021) Ankle arthritis - an important signpost in rheumatologic practice. Rheumatology (Oxford) 60(1):23–33

Lee YJ, Sadigh S, Mankad K, Kapse N, Rajeswaran G (2016) The imaging of osteomyelitis. Quant Imaging Med Surg 6(2):184–198

Long NM, Zoga AC, Kier R, Kavanagh EC (2012) Insufficiency and nondisplaced fractures of the talar head: MRI appearances. AJR Am J Roentgenol 199(5):W613–W617

Melenevsky Y, Mackey RA, Abrahams RB, Thomson NB (2015) Talar fractures and dislocations: a radiologist's guide to timely diagnosis and classification. Radiographics 35(3):765–779

Mengiardi B, Pfirrmann CW, Vienne P, Kundert HP, Rippstein PF, Zollinger H et al (2005) Anterior tibial tendon abnormalities: MR imaging findings. Radiology 235(3):977–984

Morelli F, Princi G, Rossato A, Iorio R, Ferretti A (2019) Pigmented villonodular synovitis: a rare case of anterior ankle impingement. J Orthop Case Rep 10(1):16–18

Murphey MD, Choi JJ, Kransdorf MJ, Flemming DJ, Gannon FH (2000) Imaging of osteochondroma: variants and complications with radiologic-pathologic correlation. Radiographics 20(5):1407–1434

Murphey MD, Gibson MS, Jennings BT, Crespo-Rodríguez AM, Fanburg-Smith J, Gajewski DA (2006) From the archives of the AFIP: imaging of synovial sarcoma with radiologic-pathologic correlation. Radiographics 26(5):1543–1565

Murphey MD, Vidal JA, Fanburg-Smith JC, Gajewski DA (2007) Imaging of synovial chondromatosis with radiologic-pathologic correlation. Radiographics 27(5):1465–1488

Myerson MS, Fisher RT, Burgess AR, Kenzora JE (1986) Fracture dislocations of the tarsometatarsal joints: end results correlated with pathology and treatment. Foot Ankle 6(5):225–242

Ng JM, Rosenberg ZS, Bencardino JT, Restrepo-Velez Z, Ciavarra GA, Adler RS (2013) US and MR imaging of the extensor compartment of the ankle. Radiographics 33(7):2047–2064

Pearce DH, Mongiardi CN, Fornasier VL, Daniels TR (2005) Avascular necrosis of the talus: a pictorial essay. Radiographics 25(2):399–410

Rasmussen CG, Jørgensen SB, Larsen P, Horodyskyy M, Kjær IL, Elsoe R (2021) Population-based incidence and epidemiology of 5912 foot fractures. Foot Ankle Surg 27(2):181–185

Rockberg J, Bach BA, Amelio J, Hernandez RK, Sobocki P, Engellau J et al (2015) Incidence trends in the diagnosis of giant cell tumor of bone in Sweden since 1958. J Bone Joint Surg Am 97(21):1756–1766

Samim M, Moukaddam HA, Smitaman E (2016) Imaging of Mueller-Weiss syndrome: a review of clinical presentations and imaging spectrum. AJR Am J Roentgenol 207(2):W8–W18

Scheller AD, Kasser JR, Quigley TB (1980) Tendon injuries about the ankle. Orthop Clin North Am 11(4):801–811

Schepers T, de Jong VM, Luitse JS (2014) Complete medial column dislocation at the cuneonavicular joint: an unusual Lisfranc-like injury. Foot (Edinb) 24(3):135–139

Shah A, Iyengar KP, Hegde G, Ramos J, Botchu R (2022) Calcific enthesopathy of the superior extensor retinaculum - an unusual cause of medial ankle pain. J Ultrason 22(91):e236–e2e9

Sormaala MJ, Niva MH, Kiuru MJ, Mattila VM, Pihlajamäki HK (2006) Bone stress injuries of the talus in military recruits. Bone 39(1):199–204

Stuart MJ (1992) Traumatic disruption of the anterior tibial tendon while cross-country skiing. A case report. Clin Orthop Relat Res 281:193–194

Tyler PA, Rajeswaran G, Saifuddin A (2013) Imaging of dysplasia epiphysealis hemimelica (Trevor's disease). Clin Radiol 68(4):415–421

Varghese A, Bianchi S (2014) Ultrasound of tibialis anterior muscle and tendon: anatomy, technique of examination, normal and pathologic appearance. J Ultrasound 17(2):113–123

Volders D, Vandevenne JE, Van de Casseye W (2011) Trevor's disease and whole-body MRI. Eur J Radiol 79(3):363–364

Wagner E, Ortiz C, Keller A, Zanolli D, Wagner P, Mococain P et al (2016) Case report: Spontaneous rupture of the ankle extensor retinaculum. Clin Res Foot Ankle 4(4). https://doi.org/10.4172/2329-910X.1000216

Waters B, Panicek DM, Lefkowitz RA, Antonescu CR, Healey JH, Athanasian EA et al (2007) Low-grade myxofibrosarcoma: CT and MRI patterns in recurrent disease. AJR Am J Roentgenol 188(2):W193–W198

Wechsler RJ, Schweitzer ME, Deely DM, Horn BD, Pizzutillo PD (1994) Tarsal coalition: depiction and characterization with CT and MR imaging. Radiology 193(2):447–452

Whitaker C, Turvey B, Illical EM (2018) Current concepts in talar neck fracture management. Curr Rev Musculoskelet Med 11(3):456–474

Win K, Gillett R, Botchu R, Suokas AK, Seth A, James SL (2020) Asymptomatic professional footballers: prevalence of ankle retinacula injury with associated lateral ligament and tendon abnormalities. Muscles Ligaments Tendons J 10(3):499–507

Wu JS, Hochman MG (2009) Soft-tissue tumors and tumorlike lesions: a systematic imaging approach. Radiology 253(2):297–316

Wu H, Han R, Zhang Q, Zhao Y, Feng H (2020) Metatarsal metastasis from clear cell renal cell carcinoma: a case report and literature review. BMC Urol 20(1):19

Posterior Ankle Pain

Moomal Rose Haris and Harun Gupta

Contents

1 Introduction

Posterior ankle pain is a common complaint encountered by physicians. It is therefore important to be aware of the several soft tissue and osseous structures within the posterior ankle, which are not only susceptible to traumatic injury and repetitive stress but also impingement. The pain related to posterior ankle impingement is exacerbated during plantar flexion. Athletes, specifically soccer players, fast bowlers (cricket, baseball), and ballet dancers (Baillie et al. 2021), often present with posterior ankle impingement due to the nature in which they perform repeated and/or forced ankle plantar flexion.

This chapter discusses the various causes and associated imaging appearances related to posterior ankle pain.

2 Anatomy

The posterior aspect of the distal tibia at the level of the malleoli and the fibula forms the cranial aspect of the posterior ankle. The inferior tibiofibular joint is stabilized by syndesmotic ligaments including the anterior inferior, posterior inferior tibiofibular ligaments, as well as interosseous membrane. These ligaments and the interosseous membrane help stabilize the distal tibiofibular joint (Ogilvie-Harris et al. 1994). The posterior inferior tibiofibular ligaments are rarely injured in isolation.

The talus and the calcaneus form the hindfoot. The posterior talar process has a medial and lateral tubercle. The lateral tubercle is larger and has its own ossification center. In approximately 24–33% of patients (Batista et al. 2015), this ossification center fails to fuse with the talus resulting in an ossicle at this site known as the os trigonum. Patients with posterior ankle impingement have been found to have a higher prevalence of an os trigonum, and in those without an

M. R. Haris
Calderdale and Huddersfield Foundation Trust, Huddersfield, UK
e-mail: moomalrose@gmail.com

H. Gupta (✉)
Leeds Teaching Hospital Trust, Leeds, UK
e-mail: harungupta@hotmail.com

Med Radiol Diagn Imaging (2023)
https://doi.org/10.1007/174_2023_392,
Published Online: 06 April 2023

os trigonum but with impingement syndrome, an enlarged posterolateral talar tubercle (Stieda process) was observed (Batista et al. 2015).

The tendon of the flexor hallucis longus (FHL) is located within a fibro-osseous tunnel between the posteromedial and posterolateral talar tubercles. This tendon is at risk of impingement and subsequent tendinosis secondary to os trigonum, enlarged posterolateral talar tubercle, and/or repetitive plantar flexion at the ankle (Zwiers et al. 2018).

The Achilles tendon is formed by the medial and lateral gastrocnemius muscles as well as the soleus. These three muscles are collectively known as the triceps surae muscle. Alongside the plantaris muscle, the triceps surae forms the superficial flexor group of the leg and forms the bulk on the back of the calf. The Achilles tendon inserts at the posterosuperior aspect of the calcaneum. Deep to its insertion, there is the retrocalcaneal bursa. The Achilles tendon is unique in that it does not have a synovial tendon sheath but is instead surrounded by a highly vascularized connective tissue-type envelope known as the paratenon. Achilles tendon pathology can include partial- or full-thickness tears as well as inflammation.

The plantar aponeurosis/fascia is a thick triangular layer of fibrous tissue that covers the plantar aspect of the foot. The fascia consists of three parts, a thick central part and thinner medial and lateral parts. The central part arises from the posteroinferior aspect of the calcaneum and attaches distally to the plantar aspect of the proximal phalanges and the skin. The central layer measures approximately 4 mm in normal thickness at the level of its origin at the calcaneum (Abul et al. 2015).

The tibial nerve innervates all the muscles within the posterior compartment of the lower leg. The sural nerve is a cutaneous branch of the tibial nerve, which provides sensory innervation of the posterolateral aspect of the distal third of the leg and lateral aspect of the foot, heel, and ankle (Fig. 1).

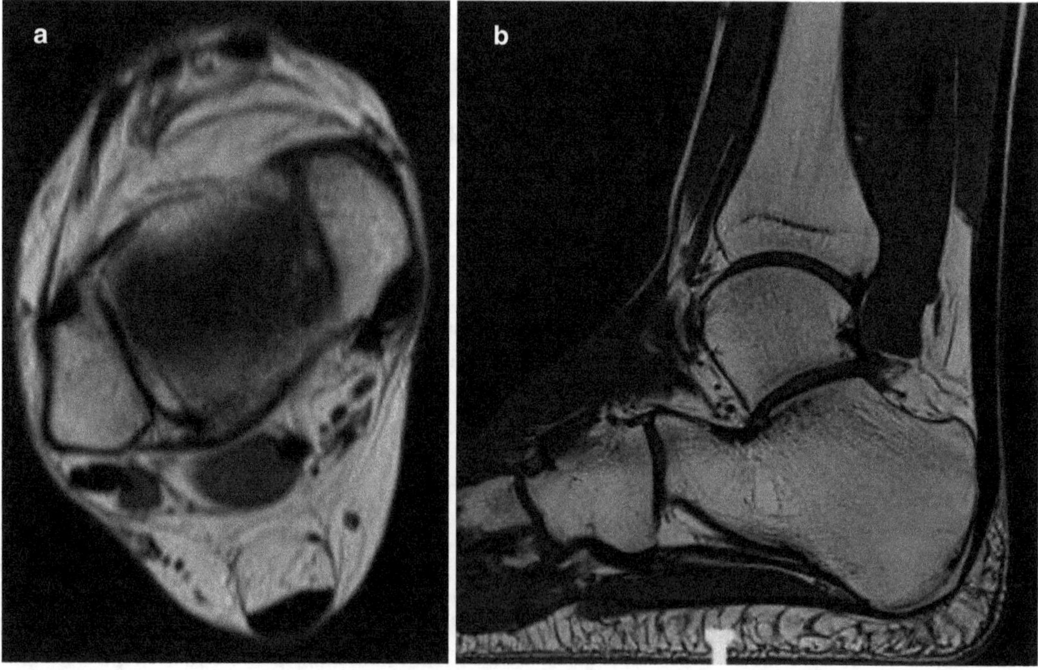

Fig. 1 (**a**) T1-weighted axial MRI at the level of the ankle showing normal anatomy. (**b**) T1-weighted sagittal MRI at the level of the ankle showing normal anatomy

3 Pathology

3.1 Achilles Tendon

Ultrasound and MRI are the most employed imaging modalities for Achilles tendon assessment. Which modality to choose depends on the clinical question, and thus good clinical assessment is important to determine correct imaging modality selection. Ultrasound is generally cheap and readily available and allows dynamic assessment of the tendon, but it is operator dependent. MRI is more expensive and may not be available as a first resource. However, if correct use of foot/ankle coil and protocols are used, MRI will be objective and will be able to look for other pathologies at the same time. Table 1 gives examples of common clinical scenarios and the differences between ultrasound and MRI; as can be noted, there is significant overlap between the two.

The Achilles tendon is composed of three intertwined subtendons (medial and lateral gastrocnemius and soleus) separated by thin septa (Szaro et al. 2021). On MRI, the Achilles tendon should be of low signal; some thin linear high signal may be seen secondary to the septa. This linear high signal is most commonly present in the anterior part of the tendon. This should not be confused for a tear (Szaro et al. 2021), which would be irregular and usually more extensive. The paratenon is not visualized on MRI. On ultrasound, the Achilles tendon should demonstrate a homogenous fibrillar pattern with uniform thickness and echogenicity in the long axis. In the short axis, the Achilles tendon has an oval shape with speckled echogenicity (Szaro et al. 2020). The paratenon is visible on ultrasound as a hyperechoic line seen at the anterior and posterior borders.

The most common abnormality related to the Achilles tendon is non-insertional (mid-substance) tendinosis. Tendinosis refers to a degenerative, noninflammatory process often associated with advancing age (Kannus and Jozsa 1991). Degeneration can be secondary to hypoxia,

Table 1 Imaging indications for Achilles tendon evaluation

Condition	Ultrasound	MRI	Comments
Complete acute tear	Useful to assess the extent of tear and degree of apposition on dynamic assessment	Not often performed in acute setting. MRI will be able to demonstrate an acute tear and the extent	Often a clinical diagnosis imaging not always needed
Partial tear	Can be underestimated	Superior to ultrasound (Ibrahim and Elsaeed 2013)	
Non-insertional tendinosis	Ultrasound is reliable but can overestimate. Better for assessment of hypervascularity and calcific deposits	MRI is reliable and superior to ultrasound if there is additional partial tearing (Shalabi 2004)	
Insertional tendinosis	Ultrasound is reliable	MRI is reliable	
Infection	Ultrasound can be used to assess for peritendinous collections and if drainage needed	MRI is superior as it will show bone and soft tissue involvement simultaneously. Consider IV contrast	
Spondyloarthropathy-related enthesitis	Can demonstrate enthesitis—however may not be able to attribute this to spondyloarthropathy	MRI is superior as able to demonstrate bone marrow edematous changes and erosions. Without erosions, it may be difficult to differentiate from infection. Consider IV contrast. Bone marrow changes known to correlate with HLA-B27 levels (McGonagle et al. 2002)	

calcific, mucoid, and fatty infiltration, or a combination of these. Disruption of the collagen fibers in tendon degeneration can progress to partial- and full-thickness tendon tears. This is most seen with hypoxic and mucoid-type degeneration (Kannus and Jozsa 1991).

Despite its large size, the Achilles tendon is the most frequently torn tendon in the body (Dong and Fessell 2009). This injury tends to occur in a bimodal distribution, with the first peak seen in patients aged between their 20s and 40s, and the second peak occurs in those aged greater than 60. The typical patient is those who are only intermittently active ("weekend warriors"). Tears are often the result of sudden increase in the stress on the Achilles tendon such as running and jumping. Other risk factors include prior intratendinous degeneration, fluoroquinolone use, steroid injections, and inflammatory arthritides (Shamrock and Varacallo 2022). Delay in diagnosis of a full-thickness Achilles tendon tear can result in significant morbidity (Gulati et al. 2015).

The normal thickness of the Achilles tendon ranges between 4 and 7 mm with a mean of 5.2 mm (Kainberger et al. 1990; Mitchell et al. 2009). On ultrasound, tendinosis appears as spindle shaped or fusiform thickening, focal hypoechogenic areas, and neovascularity as demonstrated on Doppler imaging (Mitchell et al. 2009). On MRI, hypoxic degeneration tends to result in tendon enlargement without intrinsic signal change. Mucoid degeneration causes tendon enlargement with increased T2-weighted intrinsic signal reflecting mucoid deposition (Marshall et al. 2002) and interstitial tears. Interstitial tears typically appear as longitudinally orientated linear increased signal on T1-weighted and fluid-sensitive sequences (Schweitzer and Karasick 2000).

Complete tears of the Achilles tendon appear as tendon discontinuity with fluid and/or heterogenous signal hematoma filling the tendon gap. Torn tendon fibers may be seen as distracted or overlapping (Lawrence et al. 2013). Peritendinous hemorrhage and edema are evident with recent tears. As the tear ages, organization of the hematoma, granulation tissue, and scar tissue can make detection of the opposed torn tendon edges difficult (Pierre-Jerome et al. 2010). Chronic ruptures cause muscle atrophy with fatty infiltration, which often represents a poorer prognosis for surgical repair (Pierre-Jerome et al. 2010). Most full-thickness Achilles tendon tears occur at the relatively avascular zone located 2–6 cm from the insertion, which is also known as the "critical zone."

Partial tears of the Achilles tendon can be difficult to differentiate from areas of tendinosis on ultrasound (Alfredson et al. 2011). Partial tears of the Achilles tendons have been described as irregular "wavy" hypoechogenic areas on ultrasound with background tendon thickening. Disruption of the Achilles tendon border particularly at the myotendinous junction is more suggestive of a partial tear than simply tendinosis (Alfredson et al. 2011). On MRI, a partial tear is defined as tendon thickening with hypertense signal on T1-weighted imaging and fluid-sensitive sequences (Syha et al. 2013). A hyperintense area directly located at the tendon border should be interpreted as a partial rupture (Syha et al. 2013; Heyde et al. 2003).

The retrocalcaneal bursa can be secondarily involved with Achilles pathology. On MRI, the asymptomatic retrocalcaneal bursa normally contains detectable high-signal-intensity fluid or synovium or both. A bursa larger than 10 mm anteroposteriorly, 11 mm transversely, or 7 mm craniocaudally is abnormal (Seipel et al. 2005).

Minimally invasive and open surgical repairs of the Achilles tendon are commonplace (Bottger et al. 1998). The postoperative Achilles tendon is larger and wider, surgical material may be seen, and generally the tendon is more vascularized on ultrasound Doppler imaging. Postoperative Achilles tendons are unlikely to regain a normal imaging appearance, and it is important that the reviewing clinician is aware of this so as not to mistake this for new pathology (Bottger et al. 1998) (Figs. 2, 3, 4, and 5).

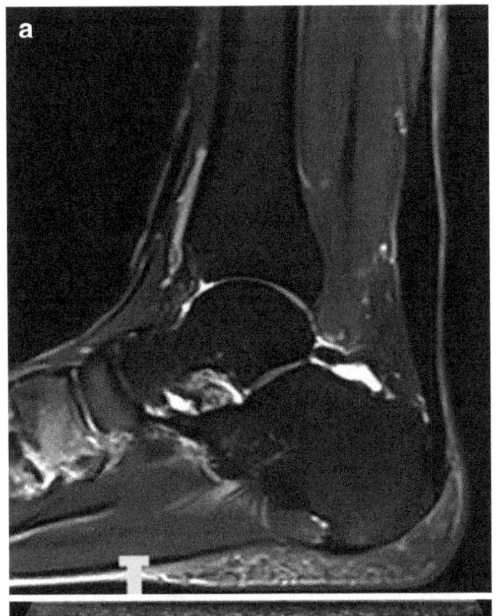

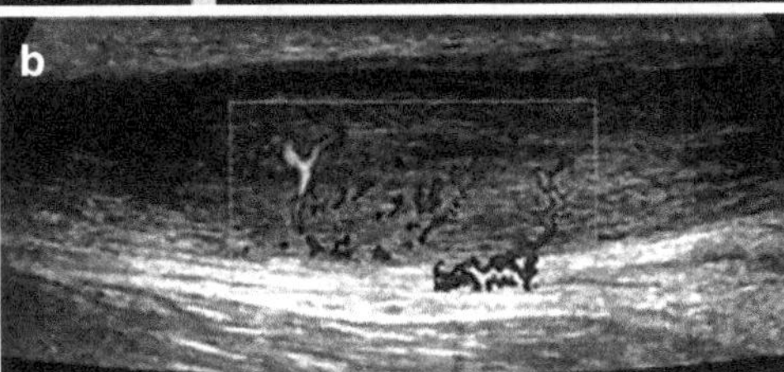

Fig. 2 (**a**) Fluid-sensitive sagittal MRI of the ankle. Thickening of the mid-Achilles tendon is in keeping with non-insertional tendinosis. (**b**) Longitudinal ultrasound of a thickened mid-Achilles tendon with hypervascularity in keeping with non-insertional tendinosis

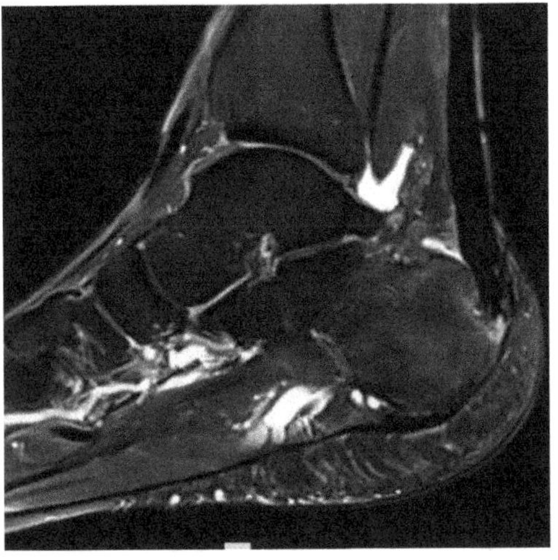

Fig. 3 Fluid-sensitive sagittal MRI of the ankle. Thickening of the distal Achilles tendon at the site of calcaneal insertion. Reactive bone marrow evident within the calcaneum. Appearances are in keeping with insertional Achilles tendinosis

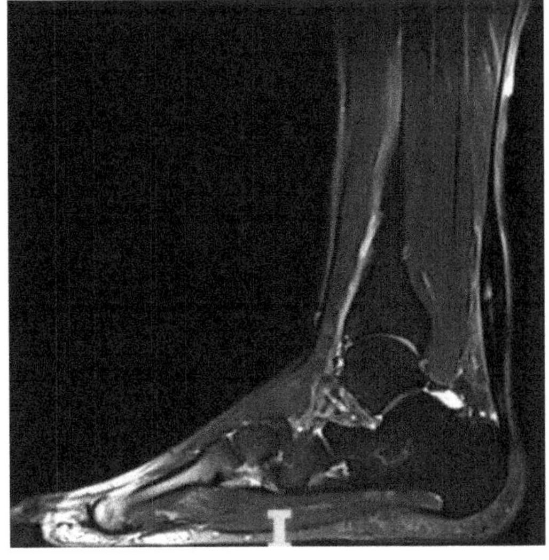

Fig. 4 Fluid-sensitive sagittal MRI of the ankle. Increased signal within the thickened mid-Achilles tendon is in keeping with partial tear of the tendon on a background of tendinosis

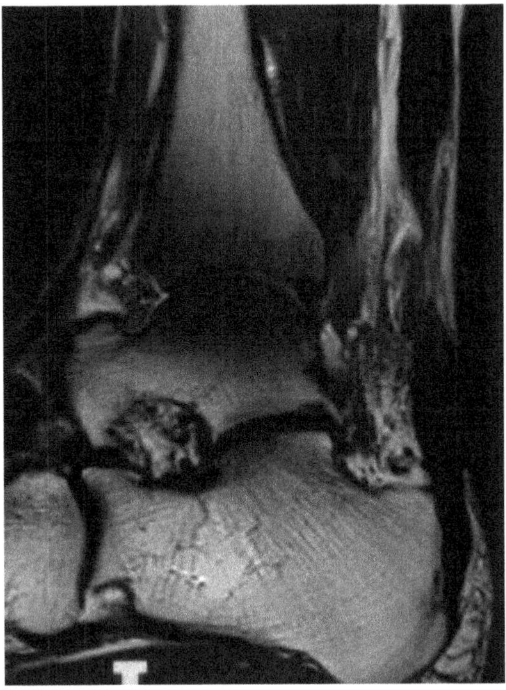

Fig. 5 T1-weighted sagittal MRI of the ankle. Full-thickness tear of the Achilles tendon with blunted retracted tendon

3.2 Soleus Muscle Variation

The soleus accessory muscle is a rare anatomical variation with an estimated prevalence of 0.7–5.5% according to cadaveric studies (Brodie et al. 1997).

Normally, the soleus is positioned in the deep posterior compartment and arises from the proximal fibula, posteromedial tibia, and a fibrous line bridge between the tibia and fibula. The accessory soleus arises from the anterior aspect of the soleus, partially sharing the soleus origin, and descends anteromedially to the Achilles. It lies superficial to the flexor retinaculum, inserting on to the Achilles or the superomedial surface of the calcaneum (Aparisi Gómez et al. 2019).

Accessory solei can be asymptomatic and an incidental finding on imaging (Brodie et al. 1997). They can present as a soft tissue mass in the posteromedial aspect of the ankle. If there is an increase in muscle mass or activity, especially repeated plantar flexion, the soleus muscle will increase in size and can cause a chronic exertional compartment syndrome-type presentation (Romanus et al. 1986; Palaniappan et al. 1999). This exercise-induced pain may be explained by increased intrafascial pressure or insufficient blood supply (Aparisi Gómez et al. 2019; Brodie et al. 1997; Romanus et al. 1986). In some cases, it may cause compression of the posterior tibial nerve with associated tarsal tunnel syndrome where the accessory muscle inserts on to the medial calcaneum.

Limited studies have also demonstrated a high association between accessory soleus muscles and Achilles tendinopathy (Yu and Resnick 1994) (Fig. 6).

3.3 Posterior Ankle Impingement Syndrome (PAIS)

PAIS is a clinical syndrome in which posterior ankle pain occurs in forced ankle plantar flexion (Chianca et al. 2020). PAIS can be further subdivided into posterolateral and posteromedial impingement. Posterolateral impingement is the most frequently encountered, and os trigonum (os trigonum syndrome) and FHL tenosynovitis are the most common causes of this syndrome.

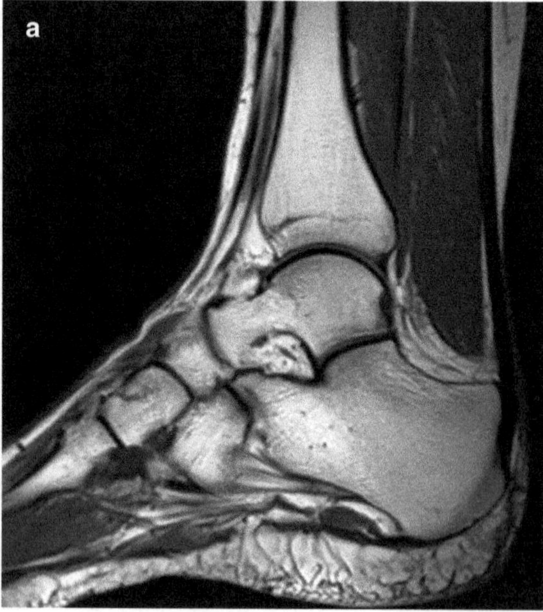

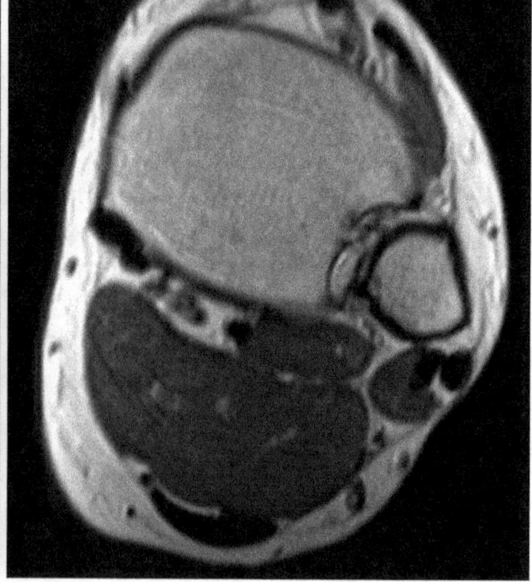

Fig. 6 (**a**) T1-weighted sagittal MRI of the ankle. Accessory soleus muscle evident filling Kager's fat pad. Compare with normal anatomy (Fig. 1b). (**b**) T1-weighted axial MRI of the ankle. Accessory soleus muscle evident filling Kager's fat pad. Compare with normal anatomy (Fig. 1a)

Less common causes can also include ankle osteochondritis, subtalar joint disease, anomalous muscles (Chianca et al. 2020), and fractures (Maquirriain 2005). Patients who repeatedly and forcefully perform plantar flexion such as soccer players, fast bowlers (cricket, baseball), and ballet dancers (Baillie et al. 2021) are most at risk of developing PAIS.

Osseous impingement is related to an os trigonum or enlarged posterolateral talar tubercle (Stieda process). Radiographs can demonstrate the presence of an os trigonum. MRI is the preferred imaging modality for PAIS as it enables the clinician to observe any edema related to the os trigonum and Kager's fat pad, synovitis, as well as FHL tenosynovitis (Kushare et al. 2020).

There are three types of os trigonum based upon the type of connection with the talus. Type I is a single piece of bone not connected to the talus, type II is connected to the talus by hyaline cartilage, and type III is essentially the Stieda process. Type I is the least common type and is generally smaller. Type II ossicles are the largest, and type III are the most common (McAlister and Urooj 2021).

Conservative as well as surgical management which includes both endoscopic and open excision techniques have been described as treatment options for os trigonum syndrome/PAIS (Fu et al. 2019).

Posteromedial ankle impingement occurs in the setting of plantar flexion, inversion, and internal rotational trauma. This can cause synovitis and damage to the posterior tibiotalar ligament (PTTL) of the deltoid ligament with partial encasement of the posterior tibialis tendon (PTT), FHL, and/or the flexor digitorum longus tendon (FDL). Posteromedial ankle impingement is one of the least common ankle impingement syndromes (Giannini et al. 2013; Koulouris et al. 2003). On MRI, pathology of the deltoid ligament, specifically the PTTL, appears as intermediate signal abnormality on fluid-sensitive sequences with loss of the normal fibrillar pattern (Koulouris et al. 2003) (Fig. 7).

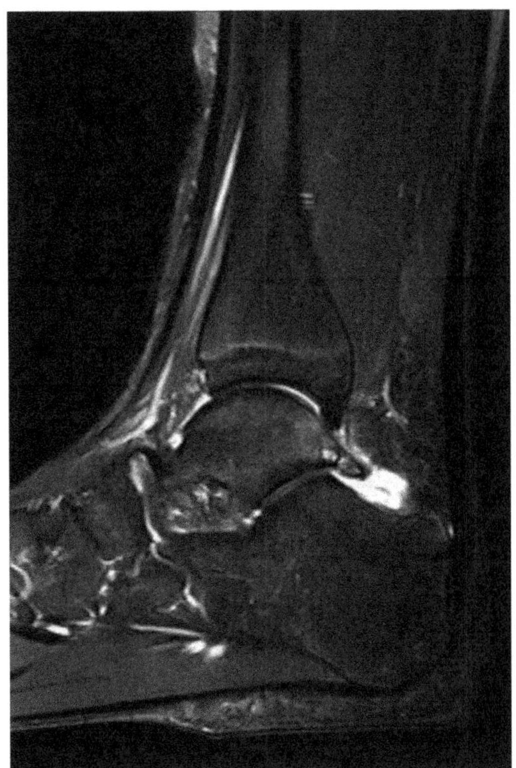

Fig. 7 Fluid-sensitive sagittal MRI of the ankle. Bone marrow edema evident in the os trigonum with increased volume of fluid within the posterior joint recess. Appearances are in keeping with os trigonum syndrome

3.4 Plantar Fascia

Plantar fasciitis is a common cause of heel pain. Thickening of the plantar fascia at the calcaneal origin measuring greater than 5 mm on ultrasound or MRI is suggestive of plantar fasciitis (Karasick and Schweitzer 1996). The plantar fascia appears hyperechoic on ultrasound and is of uniform low signal on all MRI sequences. Heterogenous echogenicity on ultrasound and intermediate signal on MRI with thickening of the plantar fascia, thickened plantar heel fat pad, and plantar calcaneal spurs can all be seen in association with plantar fasciitis (McNally and Shetty 2010). The solitary presence of one of these features does not diagnose plantar fasciitis and patient symptoms, and clinical examination must be considered as well.

Ultrasound is superior to MRI for diagnosis of plantar fibromas. On ultrasound, plantar fibromas or fibromatosis typically appears on the surface of the plantar fascia as long, fusiform, and hypoechoic areas. Lesions greater than 10 mm often demonstrate mixed echogenicity compared to smaller lesions which are hypoechoic (Karasick

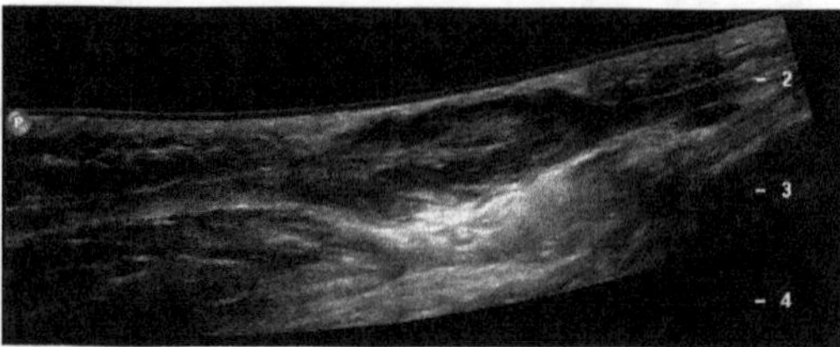

Fig. 8 Longitudinal ultrasound of the plantar fascia demonstrating fusiform thickening of the plantar fascia in keeping with plantar fibromatosis

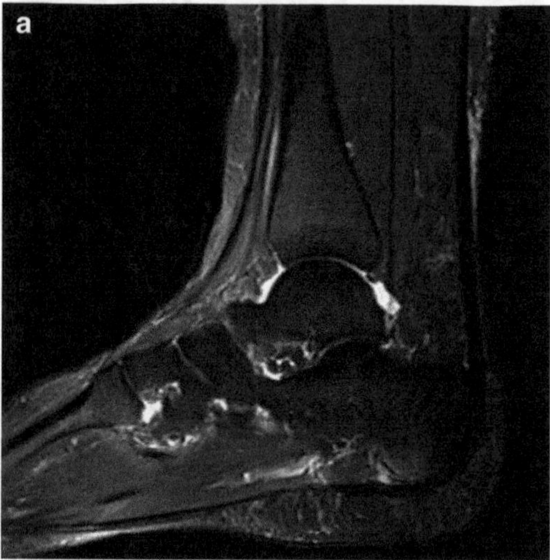

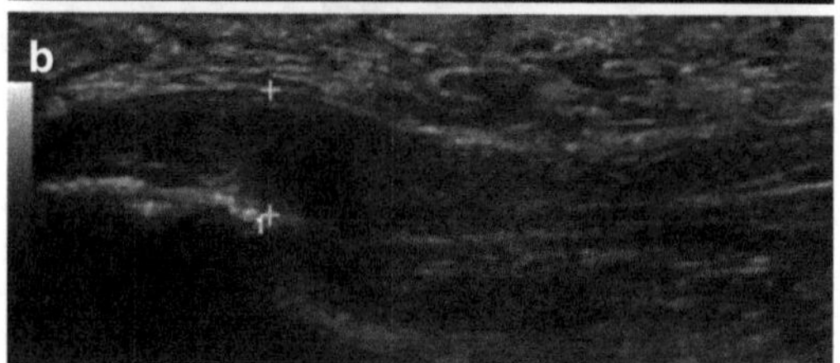

Fig. 9 (**a**) Fluid-sensitive sagittal MRI of the ankle. Thickening of the plantar fascia at the level of the calcaneum with reactive bone marrow edema. Appearances are in keeping with plantar fasciitis. (**b**) Longitudinal ultrasound of the plantar fascia demonstrates thickening at the level of the calcaneum in keeping with plantar fasciitis

and Schweitzer 1996; McNally and Shetty 2010; Drake et al. 2022).

Rupture of the plantar fascia is rare; it can occur spontaneously especially in athletes. However, it is more often seen in patients with plantar fasciitis who had local injections of corticosteroids (Karasick and Schweitzer 1996; McNally and Shetty 2010; Drake et al. 2022).

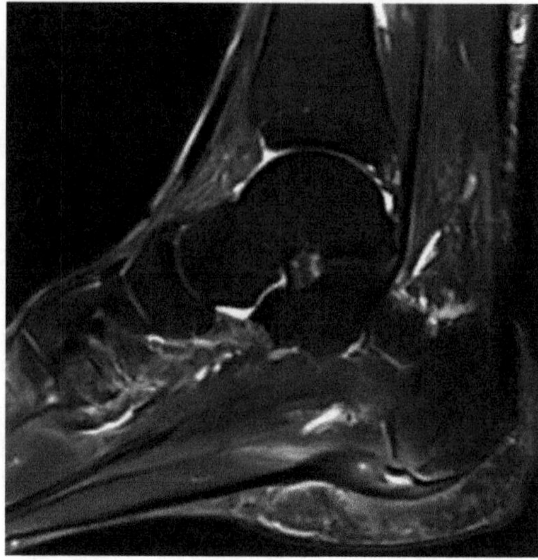

Fig. 10 Fluid-sensitive sagittal MRI of the ankle. Marked thickening of the plantar fascia with intrinsic high signal is in keeping with partial tear of the plantar fascia on a background of fasciitis

Tears of the plantar fascia present with partial or complete fiber interruption on both ultrasound and MRI (Drake et al. 2022; Bedi and Davidson 2001; Mosca et al. 2020; Draghi et al. 2017). Perifascial collections may occasionally be evident (Figs. 8, 9, and 10).

4 Conclusion

This chapter has discussed multiple potential etiologies for posterior ankle pain. However, it is important to know it is beyond the scope of this chapter to discuss every possible etiology for posterior ankle pain. Good clinical history and examination are always the best starting point when determining the etiology of pain, and it is after that the correct imaging modality may be chosen to help confirm or refute the clinician's thoughts.

References

Abul K, Ozer D, Sakizlioglu SS, Buyuk AF, Kaygusuz MA (2015) Detection of normal plantar fascia thickness in adults via the ultrasonographic method. J

Am Podiatr Med Assoc 105(1):8–13. https://doi.org/10.7547/8750-7315-105.1.8

Alfredson H, Masci L, Ohberg L (2011) Partial mid-portion Achilles tendon ruptures: new sonographic findings helpful for diagnosis. Br J Sports Med 45(5):429–432. https://doi.org/10.1136/bjsm.2009.067298. Epub 2009 Nov 27

Aparisi Gómez M, Aparisi F, Bartoloni A et al (2019) Anatomical variation in the ankle and foot: from incidental finding to inductor of pathology. Part I: ankle and hindfoot. Insights Imaging 10:74. https://doi.org/10.1186/s13244-019-0746-2

Baillie P, Cook J, Ferrar K, Smith P, Lam J, Mayes S (2021) Magnetic resonance imaging findings associated with posterior ankle impingement syndrome are prevalent in elite ballet dancers and athletes. Skeletal Radiol 50(12):2423–2431. https://doi.org/10.1007/s00256-021-03811-x. Epub 2021 May 19

Batista JP, Del Vecchio JJ, Golanó P, Vega J (2015) Flexor digitorum accessorius longus: importance of posterior ankle endoscopy. Case Rep Orthop 2015:823107. https://doi.org/10.1155/2015/823107

Bedi DG, Davidson DM (2001) Plantar fibromatosis: most common sonographic appearance and variations. J Clin Ultrasound 29(9):499–505. https://doi.org/10.1002/jcu.10014

Bottger BA, Schweitzer ME, El-Noueam KI, Desai M (1998) MR imaging of the normal and abnormal retrocalcaneal bursae. AJR Am J Roentgenol 170(5):1239–1241. https://doi.org/10.2214/ajr.170.5.9574592

Brodie JT, Dormans JP, Gregg JR, Davidson RS (1997) Accessory soleus muscle. A report of 4 cases and review of literature. Clin Orthop Relat Res 337:180–186. https://doi.org/10.1097/00003086-199704000-00020

Chianca V, Zappia M, Oliva F, Luca B, Maffulli N (2020) Post-operative MRI and US appearance of the Achilles tendons. J Ultrasound 23(3):387–395. https://doi.org/10.1007/s40477-020-00479-2

Dong Q, Fessell DP (2009) Achilles tendon ultrasound technique. AJR Am J Roentgenol 193(3):W173. https://doi.org/10.2214/AJR.09.3111

Draghi F, Gitto S, Bortolotto C, Draghi AG, Ori BG (2017) Imaging of plantar fascia disorders: findings on plain radiography, ultrasound and magnetic resonance imaging. Insights Imaging 8(1):69–78. https://doi.org/10.1007/s13244-016-0533-2. Epub 2016 Dec 12

Drake C, Whittaker GA, Kaminski MR, Chen J, Keenan AM, Rathleff MS, Robinson P, Landorf KB (2022) Medical imaging for plantar heel pain: a systematic review and meta-analysis. J Foot Ankle Res 15(1):4. https://doi.org/10.1186/s13047-021-00507-2

Fu X, Ma L, Zeng Y, He Q, Yu F, Ren L, Luo B, Fu S, Zhang L (2019) Implications of classification of Os trigonum: a study based on computed tomography three-dimensional imaging. Med Sci Monit 25:1423–1428. https://doi.org/10.12659/MSM.914485

Giannini S, Buda R, Mosca M, Parma A, Di Caprio F (2013) Posterior ankle impingement. Foot Ankle Int 34(3):459–465. https://doi.org/10.1177/1071100713477609

Gulati V, Jaggard M, Al-Nammari SS et al (2015) Management of Achilles tendon injury: a current concepts systematic review. World J Orthop 6(4):380–386. Published 2015 May 18. https://doi.org/10.5312/wjo.v6.i4.380

Heyde CE, Kayser R, Jungmichel D, Melzer C (2003) Die Grenzen der Sonographie in der Diagnostik der Achillessehnenteilruptur im Muskelsehnenübergang anhand einer Kasuistik [Limitations of sonography in the diagnosis of partial ruptures of the Achilles tendon in the musculo-tendinous junction: a case report]. Sportverletz Sportschaden 17(1):39–43. German. https://doi.org/10.1055/s-2003-38589

Ibrahim NMA, Elsaeed HH (2013) Lesions of the Achilles tendon: evaluation with ultrasonography and magnetic resonance imaging Egypt. J Radiol Nucl Med 44(3):581–587

Kainberger FM, Engel A, Barton P et al (1990) Injury of the Achilles tendon: diagnosis with sonography. AJR Am J Roentgenol 155:1031–1036

Kannus P, Jozsa L (1991) Histopathological changes preceding spontaneous rupture of a tendon. J Bone Join Surg Am 73(10):1507

Karasick D, Schweitzer ME (1996) The os trigonum syndrome: imaging features. AJR Am J Roentgenol 166(1):125–129. https://doi.org/10.2214/ajr.166.1.8571860

Koulouris G, Connell D, Schneider T, Edwards W (2003) Posterior tibiotalar ligament injury resulting in posteromedial impingement. Foot Ankle Int 24(8):575–583. https://doi.org/10.1177/107110070302400802

Kushare I, Ditzler MG, Jadhav SP (2020) Delayed diagnosis of posterior ankle impingement in pediatric and adolescent patients: does radiology play a role? Pediatr Radiol 50(2):216–223. https://doi.org/10.1007/s00247-019-04547-6. Epub 2019 Nov 9

Lawrence DA, Rolen MF, Abi Morshed K, Moukaddam H, Moukaddam H (2013) MRI of heel pain. AJR 200:845–855. https://doi.org/10.2214/AJR.12.8824

Mitchell AWM, Lee JC, Healy JC (2009) The use of ultrasound in the assessment and treatment of Achilles tendinosis. J Bone Joint Surg Br 91-B:11. Published Online 1 Nov 2009. https://doi.org/10.1302/0301-620X.91B11.23060

Maquirriain J (2005) Posterior ankle impingement syndrome. J Am Acad Orthop Surg 13(6):365–371. https://doi.org/10.5435/00124635-200510000-00001

Marshall H, Larkman DJ, Herlihy AH, Bydder GM (2002) MR imaging of the Achilles tendon, pp 187–192

McAlister JE, Urooj U (2021) Os trigonum syndrome. Clin Podiatr Med Surg 38(2):279–290. https://doi.org/10.1016/j.cpm.2020.12.011. Epub 2021 Feb 13

McGonagle D, MarzoOrtega H, O'Connor P, Gibbon W, Pease C, Reece R, P. (2002) Emery the role of biomechanical factors and HLA-B27 in magnetic resonance imaging-determined bone changes in plantar fascia enthesopathy. Arthritis Rheum 46(2):489–493

McNally EG, Shetty S (2010) Plantar fascia: imaging diagnosis and guided treatment. Semin Musculoskelet

Radiol 14(3):334–343. https://doi.org/10.1055/s--0030-1254522. Epub 2010 Jun 10

Mosca M, Fuiano M, Massimi S, Censoni D, Catanese G, Grassi A, Caravelli S, Zaffagnini S (2020) Ruptures of the plantar fascia: A systematic review of the literature. Foot Ankle Spec 15:272. https://doi.org/10.1177/1938640020974889. Epub ahead of print

Ogilvie-Harris DJ, Reed SC, Hedman TP (1994) Disruption of the ankle syndesmosis: biomechanical study of the ligamentous restraints. Arthroscopy 10(5):558–560. https://doi.org/10.1016/s0749-8063(05)80014-3

Palaniappan M, Rajesh A, Rickett A, Kershaw CJ (1999) Accessory soleus muscle: a case report and review of the literature. Pediatr Radiol 29(8):610–612. https://doi.org/10.1007/s002470050660

Pierre-Jerome C, Moncayo V, Terk MR (2010) MRI of the Achilles tendon: a comprehensive review of the anatomy, biomechanics, and imaging of overuse tendinopathies. Acta Radiol 51(4):438–454

Romanus B, Lindahl S, Stener B (1986) Accessory soleus muscle. A clinical and radiographic presentation of eleven cases. J Bone Joint Surg Am 68(5):731–734

Schweitzer ME, Karasick D (2000) MR imaging of disorders of the Achilles tendon. Am J Roentgenol 175(3):613–625. https://doi.org/10.2214/ajr.175.3.1750613

Seipel R, Linklater J, Pitsis G, Sullivan M (2005) The peroneocalcaneus internus muscle: an unusual cause of posterior ankle impingement. Foot Ankle Int 26(10):890–893. https://doi.org/10.1177/107110070502601016

Shalabi A (2004) Magnetic resonance imaging in chronic Achilles tendinopathy. Acta Radiol Suppl (Stockholm) (432):1–45

Shamrock AG, Varacallo M (2022) Achilles tendon rupture. In: StatPearls. StatPearls Publishing, Treasure Island, FL

Syha R, Springer F, Ketelsen D, Ipach I, Kramer U, Horger M, Schick F, Grosse U (2013) Achillodynia—radiological imaging of acute and chronic overuse injuries of the Achilles tendon. Rofo 185(11):1041–1055. https://doi.org/10.1055/s-0033-1335170. Epub 2013 Jul 25

Szaro P, Ramirez WC, Borkman S, Bengtsson A, Polaczek M, Ciszek B (2020) Distribution of the subtendons in the midportion of the Achilles tendon revealed in vivo on MRI. Sci Rep 10(1):16348

Szaro P, Nilsson-Helander K, Carmont M (2021) MRI of the Achilles tendon—a comprehensive pictorial review. Part one. Eur J Radiol Open 8:100342. ISSN: 2352-0477. https://doi.org/10.1016/j.ejro.2021.100342

Yu JS, Resnick D (1994) MR imaging of the accessory soleus muscle appearance in six patients and a review of the literature. Skeletal Radiol 23(7):525–528. https://doi.org/10.1007/BF00223083

Zwiers R, Baltes TPA, Opdam KTM, Wiegerinck JI, van Dijk CN (2018) Prevalence of os trigonum on CT imaging. Foot Ankle Int 39(3):338–342. https://doi.org/10.1177/1071100717740937. Epub 2017 Dec 22

Medial Ankle Pain

Darshana Sanghvi and Shivika Agrawal

Contents

D. Sanghvi (✉) · S. Agrawal
Department of Radiology, Kokilaben Dhirubhai Ambani Hospital, Mumbai, India
e-mail: sanghvidarshana@gmail.com

Abstract

The medial ankle and adjacent medial midfoot have a complex and unique osseo-ligamentous organization dominated by the posterior tibial tendon and deltoid ligament in conjunction with the tibiotalar, talonavicular joints, and naviculum. Secondary stabilizers include the spring ligament, other flexor tendons, flexor retinaculum, and medial malleolar fascial sleeve. The neurovascular structures of the tarsal tunnel are an additional important anatomical entity in the medial ankle. Medial ankle pain originates from acute trauma, chronic instability, impingement, or malalignment.

MRI allows composite assessment of medial ankle pain. Biplane radiographs are the investigation of choice for assessment of acute fractures and are also useful in evaluation of chronic instability, malalignment, and pes planus. CT may be performed for presurgical planning of complex ankle fractures. USG is sensitive for the assessment of the posterior tibial tendon. USG is also a practical technique for guiding injections for pain relief.

Injuries of the medial soft tissue structures include possible disruptions of four major structures which are the deltoid ligament, posterior tibial tendon, flexor retinaculum, and spring ligament. These injuries are seen in conjunction due to the synergistic nature of

Med Radiol Diagn Imaging (2023)

https://doi.org/10.1007/174_2023_387,
Published Online: 06 April 2023

their function. Additionally, medial ankle pain may emanate from tarsal tunnel syndrome, accessory navicular bones, or coalitions.

1 Introduction

The medial ankle and adjacent medial midfoot have a complex and unique osseo-ligamentous organization dominated by the posterior tibial tendon (PTT) and deltoid ligament complex in conjunction with the tibiotalar and talonavicular joints and navicular tuberosity. Important secondary stabilizers include the spring or calcaneonavicular ligament complex, other flexor tendons, flexor retinaculum, and the medial malleolar fascial sleeve. The neurovascular structures of the tarsal tunnel are an additional important anatomical entity in the medial ankle compartment.

These ligaments and tendons are important reinforcers of the medial longitudinal arch of the foot. Medial ankle pain originates from acute trauma, chronic instability, impingement, or malalignment. The biomechanics of injury most often involve pronation or alternatively supination-external rotation.

2 Imaging Modalities

Magnetic resonance imaging (MRI) allows composite assessment of medial ankle pain. Small field of view, high resolution images in multiple planes are obtained using dedicated foot and ankle coils. Axial and coronal acquisitions are acquired with respect to the talar axis. Standard MRI protocols include fluid sensitive sequences like proton density (PD) with or without fat suppression (FS) in axial, coronal, and sagittal planes, T1-weighted images in at least one plane, and often an additional three-dimensional gradient sequence.

Biplane radiographs are the investigation of choice for assessment of acute fractures and are also useful in evaluation of chronic instability, malalignment, and pes planus. CT may be performed for presurgical planning of more complex ankle fractures. Ultrasonography (USG) is exquisitely sensitive for the assessment of the PTT, superficial deltoid ligament, flexor retinaculum, and the medial malleolar fascial sleeve but is limited by inadequate visualization of the deep deltoid nestled between bony structures. USG is also a practical technique for guiding injections for pain relief.

3 Anatomy and Function

3.1 Deltoid Ligament Complex

The deltoid ligament complex is a central edifice of the medial ankle and consists of two deep components and three superficial components; all originating from various surfaces of the medial malleolus (MM) and extending to attach to different structures in the medial ankle and mid foot (Fig. 1). Thus, the multifascicular deltoid ligament complex has been variously described to have a fan, delta, or cone shape.

The deep deltoid ligament consists of the predominant strong posterior tibiotalar ligament (pTTL) and the delicate anterior tibiotalar ligament or fascicle (aTTL). The main posterior band originates from posterior aspect of anterior colliculus and adjacent posterior colliculus of the medial malleolus and inserts into the fovea at the medial aspect of the body of the talus. On MRI (Fig. 2), the normal and intact pTTL has a striated appearance, akin to the posterior talofibular ligament and anterior cruciate ligament. The smaller and less important aTTL or anterior fascicle inserts in the medial talus at the junction of its neck and body. The aTTL is inconsistently identified on imaging; it is definitively visible on MRI in only approximately 50% of patients (Mengiardi et al. 2007).

The superficial deltoid ligament has three consistently described components (Crim 2017) that

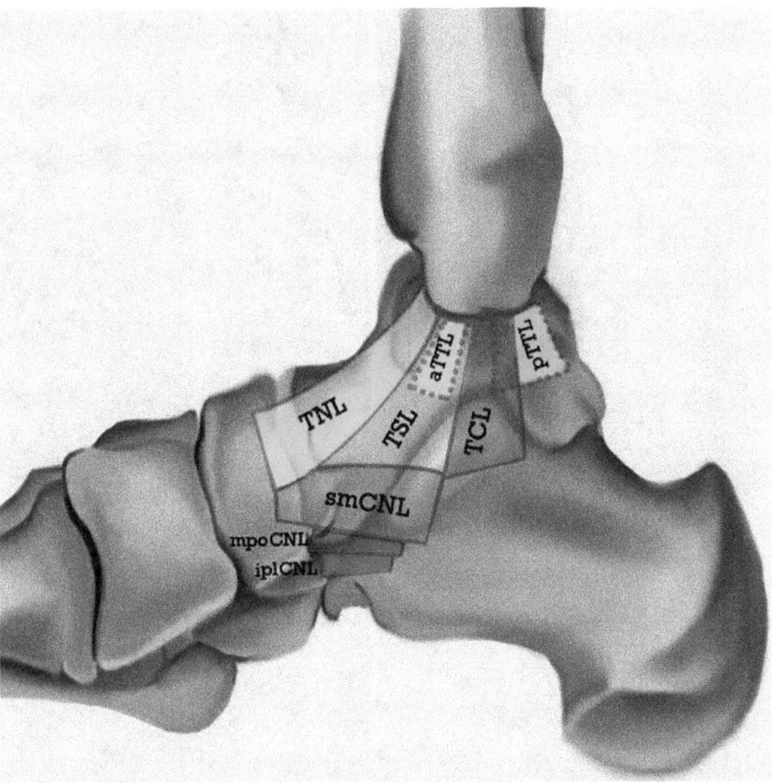

Fig. 1 Normal anatomy of the deltoid and spring ligament complexes. The deltoid ligaments are conveniently named according to their proximal tibial origin and variable distal insertions. The deep deltoid ligament consists of the small anterior tibiotalar ligament (*aTTL*) and the larger, strong posterior tibiotalar ligament (*pTTL*). The superficial deltoid ligament has three components which are the tibionavicular ligament (*TNL*), tibiospring ligament (*TSL*), and tibiocalcaneal ligament (*TCL*). Also seen in the illustration are the three components of the spring ligament which are the superomedial calcaneonavicular ligament (*smCNL*), medioplantar oblique calcaneonavicular ligament (*mpoCNL*) and inferoplantar longitudinal calcaneonavicular ligament (*iplCNL*)

have a common origin at the anterior aspect of the outer surface of MM with variable distal attachments. The nomenclature of the three ligaments conveniently alludes to their common proximal origin and variable distal insertions. From anterior to posterior, the three components are the tibionavicular ligament (TNL), tibiospring ligament (TSL), and tibiocalcaneal ligament (TCL). The tibionavicular ligament is the most anterior ligament of the superficial deltoid complex and extends anteroinferiorly to insert into the naviculum. The tibiospring ligament is the only ligament in the ankle with a distal non-osseous attachment. It originates from the common origin just posterior to the tibionavicular ligament and extends inferiorly to blend with the superomedial calcaneonavicular or spring ligament. The tibiocalcaneal ligament is the strongest of the three superficial deltoid ligaments, originating at the medial malleolus and extending inferiorly to insert on the medial margin of the sustentaculum tali. The superficial deltoid ligaments are best visualized on sequential coronal images (Fig. 3). A fourth component of

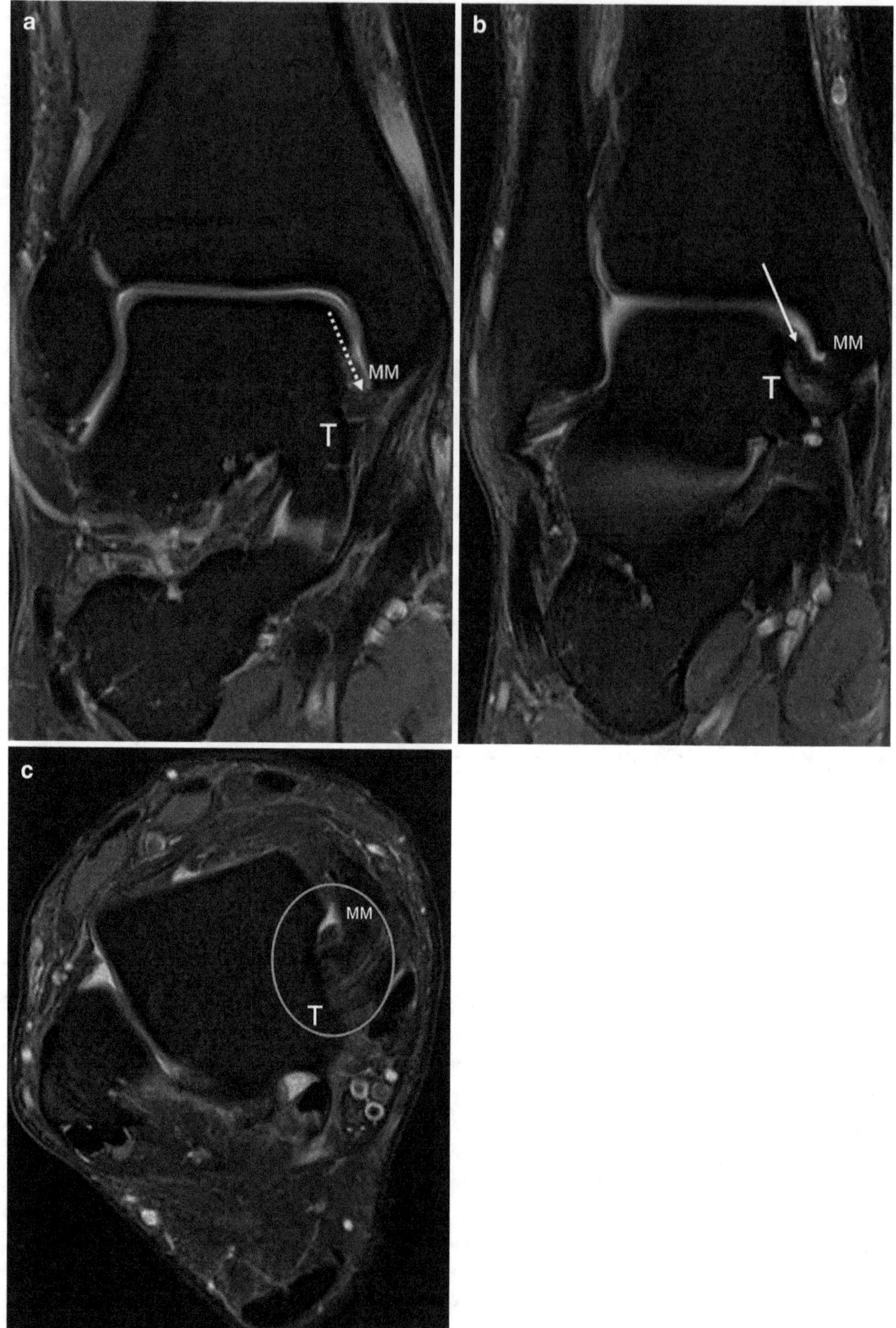

Fig. 2 The normal deep tibiotalar ligament on PD FS MRI. (**a**) On an anterior coronal MRI, the intact aTTL (dotted arrow) is a thin, striated small fascicle that originates from the medial malleolus (*MM*) and inserts on the anterior aspect of body and neck of talus bone (*T*), (**b**) More posteriorly, the pTTL (block arrow) has a striated appearance. It originates from the intercollicular groove of the medial malleolus (*MM*) and inserts on the fovea at the medial aspect of the body of the talus (*T*), (**c**) Axial MRI; the pTTL (circle) is intra-articular and surrounded by synovium

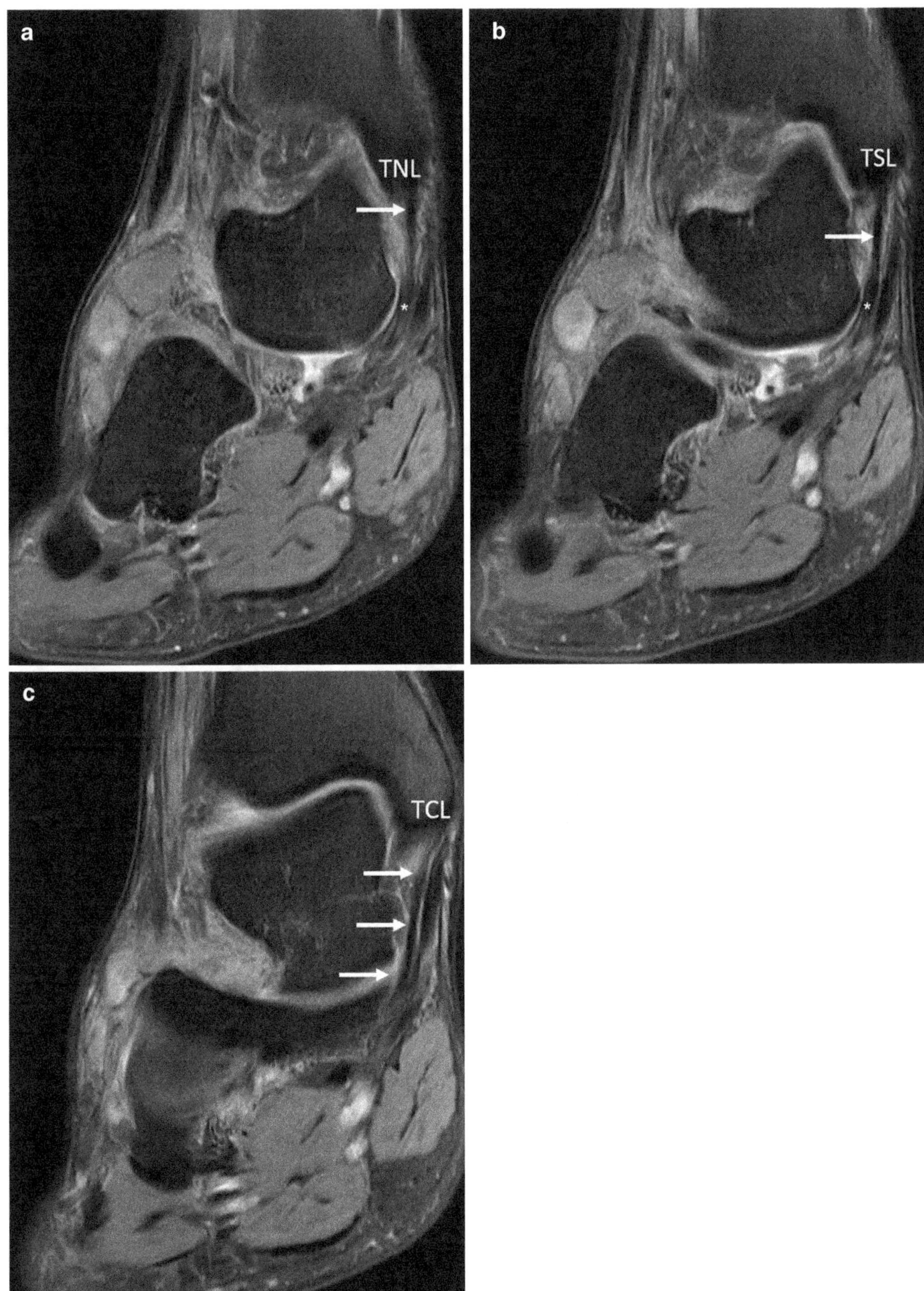

Fig. 3 The normal superficial deltoid ligament origins on MRI. Coronal PD FS images from anterior to posterior (**a**) origin of the intact TNL (arrow). Due to an oblique course, the entire ligament is not visible on a single coronal image. Also seen in the same image is the smCNL (asterisk), (**b**) TSL (arrow) is seen to merge with the smCNL (asterisk), (**c**) TCL (arrows)

the superficial deltoid ligament complex called the superficial posterior tibiotalar ligament (spTTL) has been inconsistently and variably described in literature (Chhabra et al. 2010; Yammine 2017) and has doubtful clinical significance.

The deltoid ligament complex delivers medial stability to the tibiotalar joint by firmly fixing the medial malleolus to the talus and preventing valgus drift of the talus.

3.2 Medial Malleolar Fascial Sleeve

The medial malleolar fascial sleeve at the outer surface of the MM is formed by the blending of three structures (Fig. 4). From anterior to posterior, these three structures are the common origin of the superficial deltoid ligaments, the periosteum of the medial malleolus, and the flexor retinaculum (Fig. 5). The flexor retinaculum maintains the flexor tendons in position posterior to the medial malleolus and also provides a roof to the tarsal tunnel.

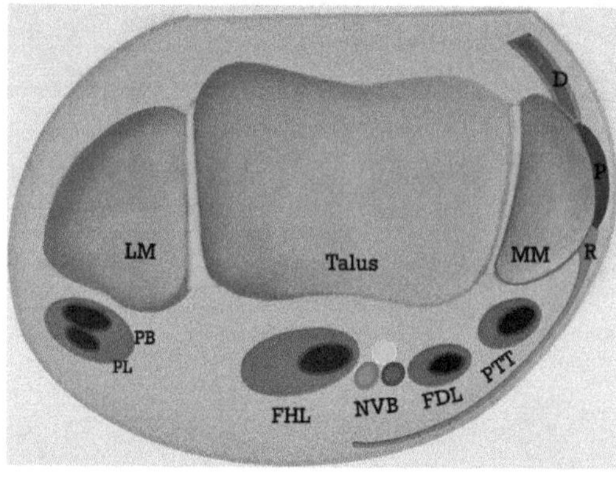

Fig. 4 Normal anatomy of the medial malleolar sleeve formed from anterior to posterior by the common origin of the superficial deltoid ligament (*D*) in green, the outer periosteum (*P*) of the MM in brown, and the flexor retinaculum (*R*) in blue

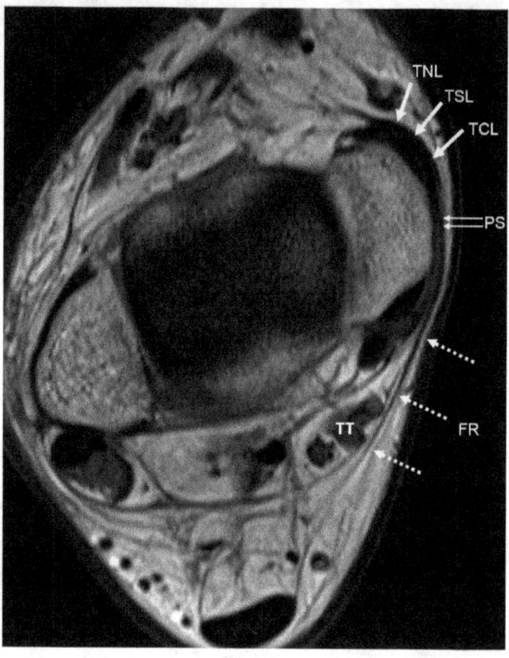

Fig. 5 Medial malleolar sleeve. Axial T1 weighted MRI. The common origin of the three components of the superficial deltoid ligament (solid arrows) includes the origins of the tibionavicular ligament (*TNL*), tibiospring ligament (*TSL*), and tibiocalcaneal ligament (*TCL*). More posteriorly, the superficial deltoid ligament origin fuses with the medial malleolar periosteal sleeve (*PS*, double arrows) and the flexor retinaculum (*FR*, dotted arrows) to form the medial malleolar sleeve. Note the neurovascular bundle in the tarsal tunnel (*TT*) between the FR and the bony structures

3.3 Spring Ligament (Calcaneonavicular Ligament) Complex

The spring ligament (SL) or calcaneonavicular complex consists of three components (Fig. 6). From superomedial to inferolateral; these components are the larger superomedial calcaneonavicular ligament (smCNL) and two smaller successive plantar ligaments which are the medioplantar oblique calcaneonavicular ligament (mpoCNL) and the inferoplantar longitudinal calcaneonavicular ligament (iplCNL) (Fig. 7). The bulk of the sagittal oriented smCNL occupies the space between the talus and the PTT as its stretches from the sustentaculum tali to the naviculum. The inner margin of the curved smCNL parallels and articulates with the talar head. The outer margin of the smCNL is separated from the PTT by a gliding layer of loose connective tissue. The gliding layer between the smCNL and PTT is not clearly discerned on MRI. The upper margin of the smCNL merges with TSL (Fig. 8). Inferolateral to the robust smCNL, the two smaller plantar calcaneonavicular ligaments have a shorter course, extending from the anterior calcaneum to the adjacent navicular bone in the plantar mid foot (Fig. 9). The mpoCNL originates from the coronoid fossa in anterior calcaneum, courses anteromedially and inserts just below the insertion of the PTT on the navicular tuberosity. The mpoCNL is separated from the iplCNL by the fluid containing spring ligament recess (SLR). The iplCNL has the shortest course, originating from the calcaneum anterior and lateral to the origin of the mpoCNL and inserting into the navicular beak.

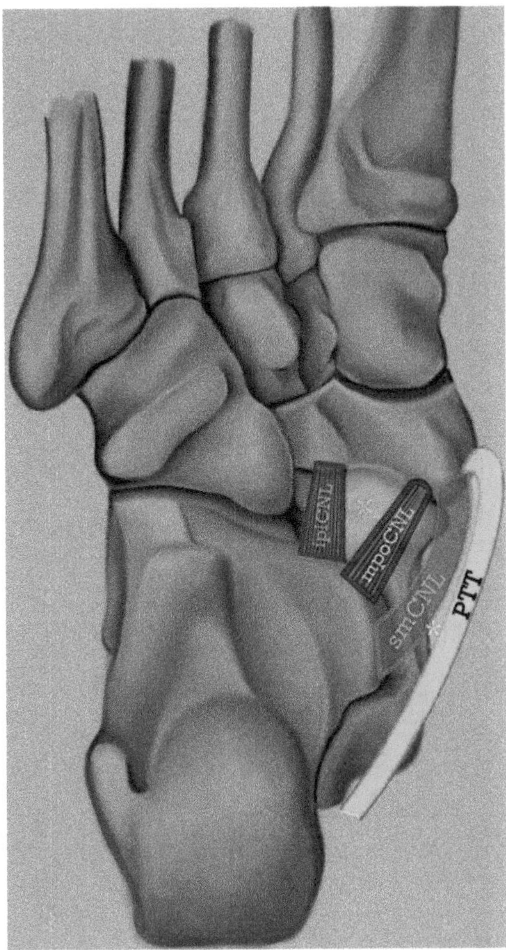

Fig. 6 Normal anatomy of the spring ligament or calcaneonavicular ligament complex. The superomedial calcaneonavicular ligament (*smCNL*) is separated from the posterior tibial tendon (*PTT*) by the gliding zone (asterisk) and is the strongest component. The smaller medioplantar oblique calcaneonavicular ligament (*mpoCNL*) and inferoplantar longitudinal calcaneonavicular ligament (*iplCNL*) are separated by the spring ligament recess (x)

On MRI, the intact smCNL has homogeneous low signal whereas the intact plantar CNLs have more heterogeneous signal intensities due to interposed fat.

The smCNL is the primary static stabilizer of the longitudinal arch and functions synergistically with the PTT which is the chief dynamic stabilizer. The spring and deltoid ligament complex form an anatomic and functional entity for load bearing functions. The iplCNL and mpoCNL have greater tensile load functions as compared to the smCNL (Szaro et al. 2022).

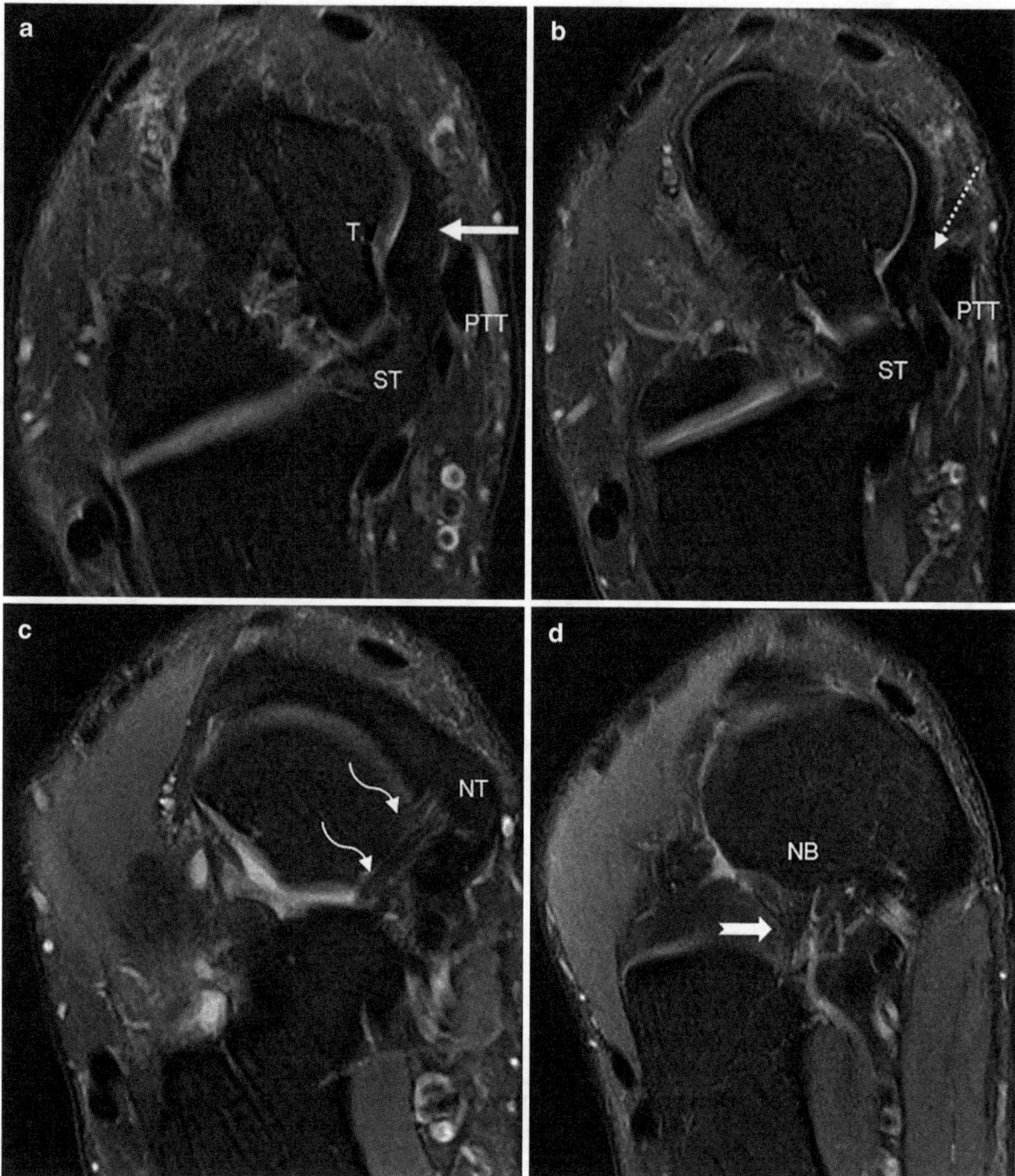

Fig. 7 The normal Spring Ligament (SL) or Calcaneonavicular Ligament (CNL) complex on sequential axial PD FS MRI. (**a**) The smCNL (straight arrow) is the largest component of the SL complex and occupies the sagittal oriented space between the posterior tibial tendon (*PTT*) and Talus (*T*). The smCNL articulates with the talar head as it extends from the sustentaculum tali (*ST*) to the navicular tuberosity, (**b**) a gliding layer (dotted arrow) of loose connective tissue is faintly discerned between the PTT and the smCNL, (**c**) the mpoCNL (curved arrows) originates from the anterior calcaneum and inserts into the navicular tuberosity (*NT*) below the insertion of the smCNL, (**d**) the iplCNL (block arrow) normally has a striated appearance and the shortest course from the anterior calcaneum to the navicular beak (*NB*)

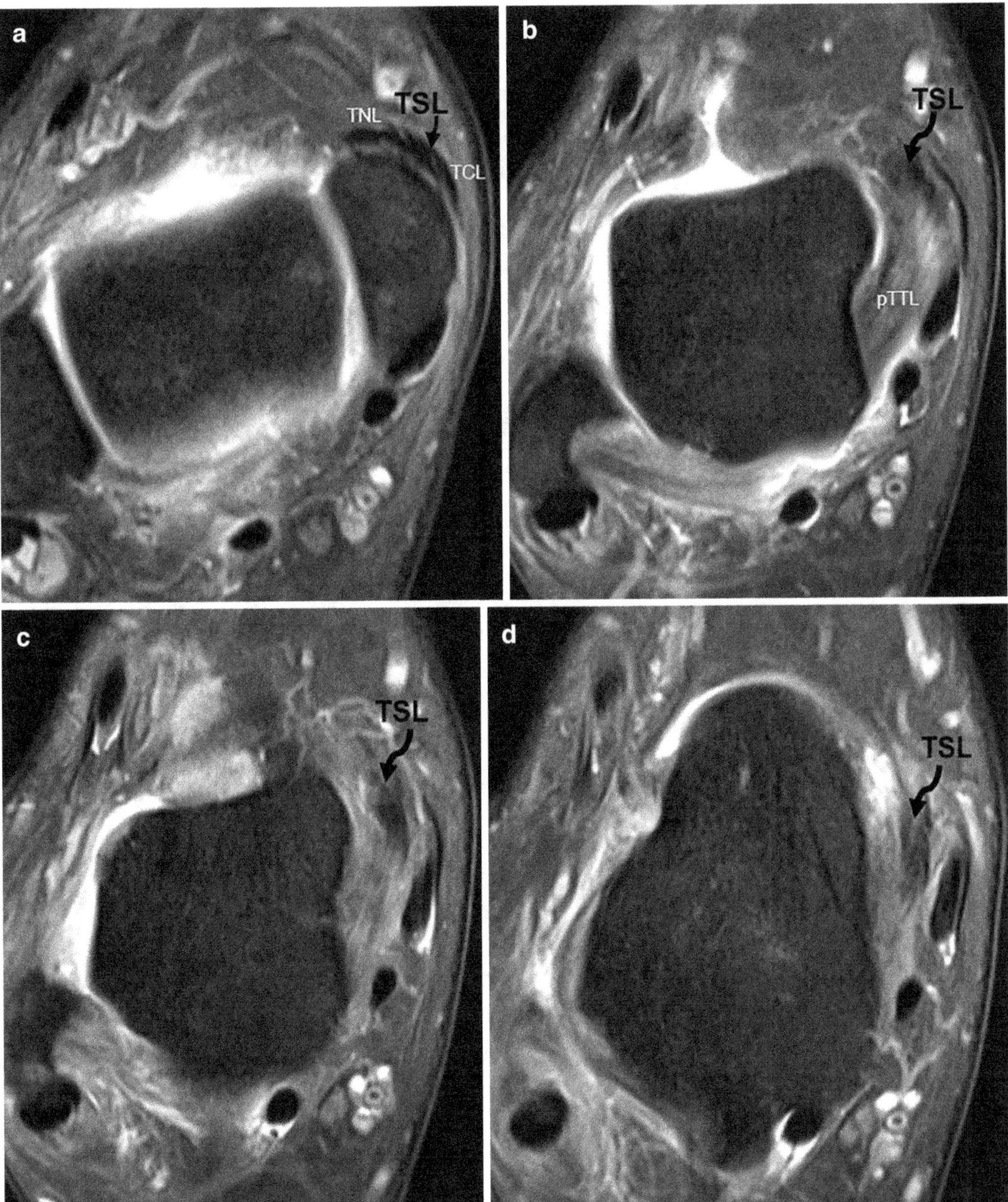

Fig. 8 TSL and smCNL on sequential PD FS MRI; intact ligaments except for mild sprains (**a**–**f**). The middle segment of the common origin of the superficial deltoid ligament forms the *TSL* (arrows) which extends inferiorly to merge with the cranial border of the smCNL (asterisk). Other structures seen are the *pTTL*, origins of the *TNL*, *TCL*, and the *PTT* which is superficial to the smCNL (asterisk)

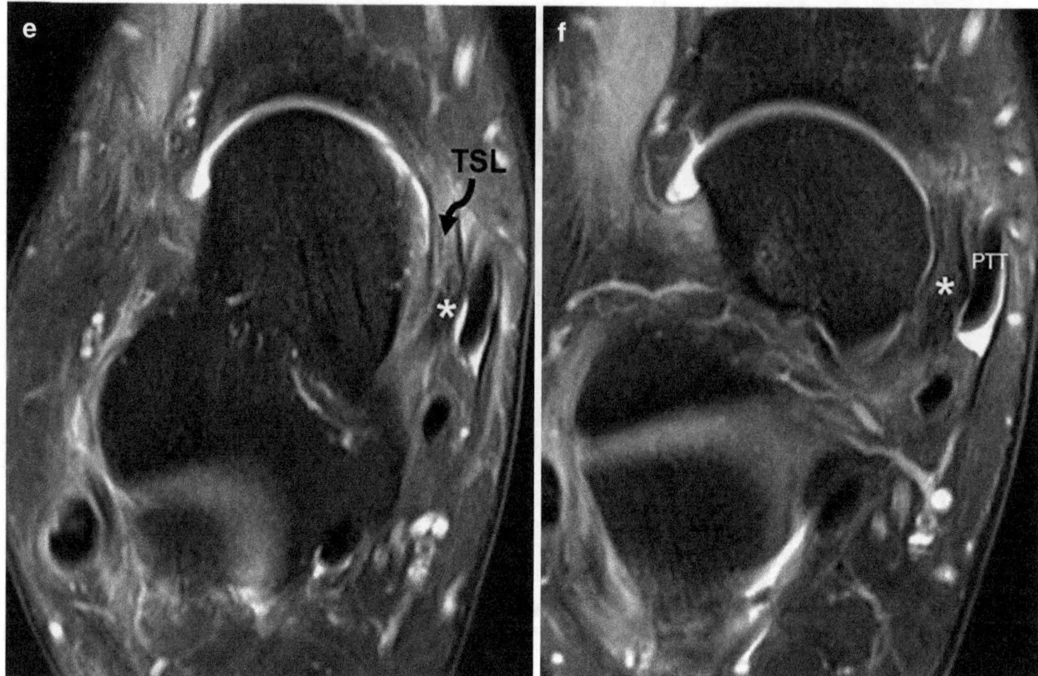

Fig. 8 (continued)

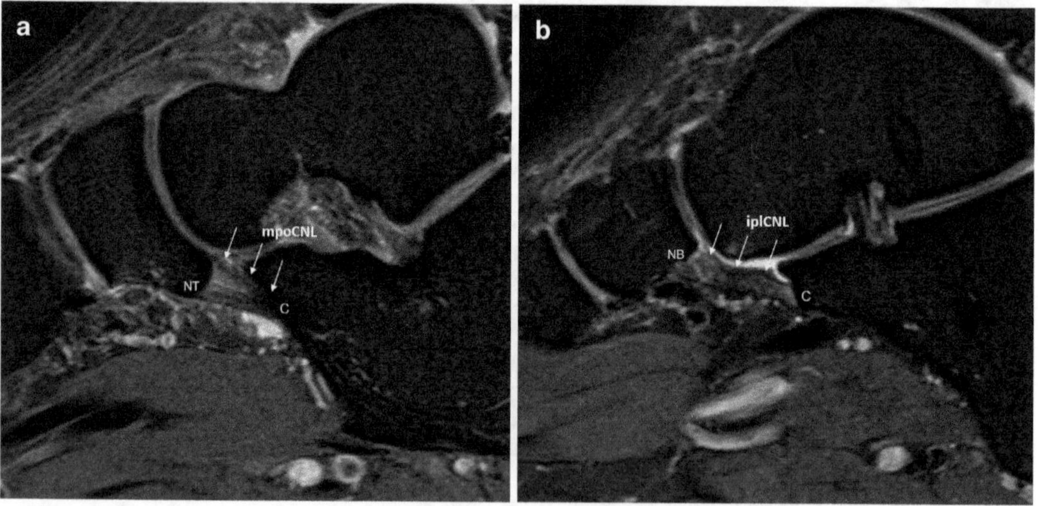

Fig. 9 The normal plantar calcaneonavicular ligaments on sequential oblique sagittal PD FS MRI (**a**) The *mpoCNL* (arrows) originates from the anterior calcaneum (*C*) and inserts into the navicular tuberosity (*NT*), (**b**) The *iplCNL* (arrows) extends from the anterior calcaneum (*C*) to the navicular beak (*NB*)

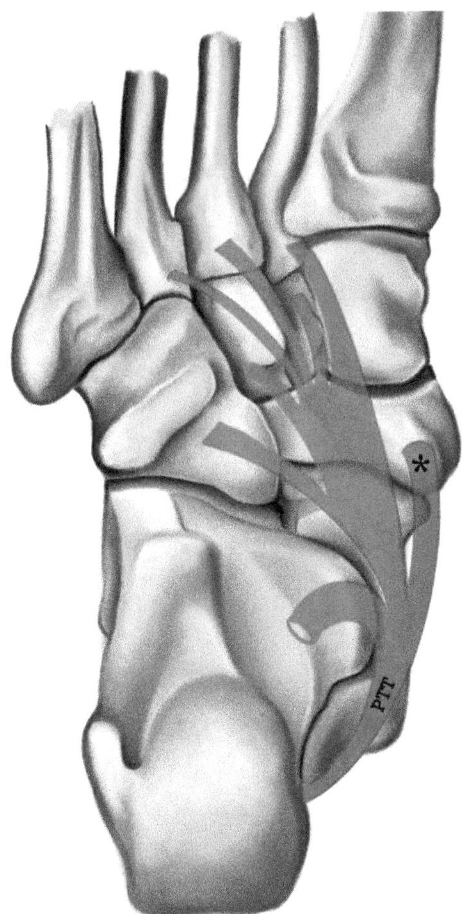

Fig. 10 The normal PTT and its insertions. The main insertion of the *PTT* is on the navicular tuberosity (asterisk). Multiple other insertions are seen in the plantar midfoot into the metatarsals and tarsals including a recurrent calcaneal slip

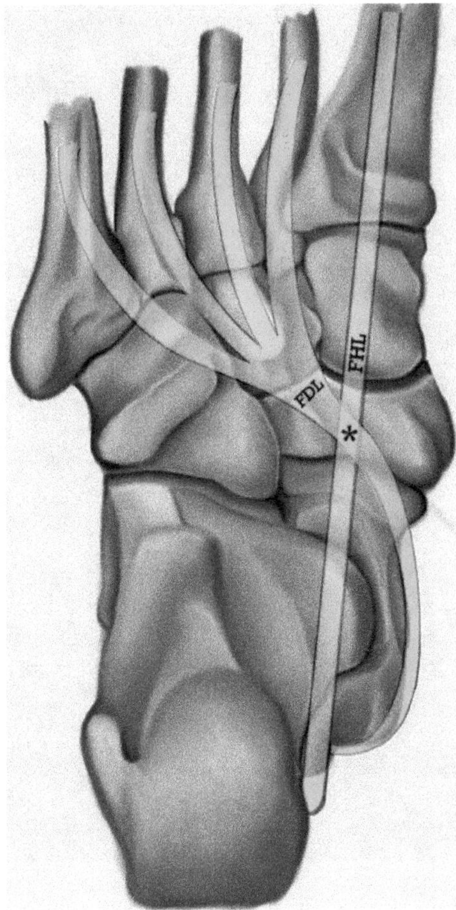

Fig. 11 The knot of Henry (asterisk) is the crossing of the flexor digitorum longus (*FDL*) and flexor hallucis longus (*FHL*) in the plantomedial midfoot

3.4 Flexor Tendons

From anterior to posterior, three tendons occupy the posteromedial compartment of the ankle. The most anterior and medial tendon is the posterior tibial tendon. The PTT has a larger diameter as compared to the other two tendons in the posteromedial compartment of the ankle. The PTT originates in the calf and the tendon is formed in the distal third of the leg. It changes direction from vertical to horizontal as it occupies a shallow groove on the posterior aspect of the medial malleolus. It enters the foot via the tarsal tunnel and terminates in the midfoot. The main insertion of the PTT is medial and into the navicular tuberosity. Additional smaller plantar and lateral insertions are into various tarsal bones in the sole (Fig. 10).

Posterior to the PTT are the tendons of the flexor digitorum longus (FDL) and flexor hallucis longus (FHL) separated from one another by the neurovascular structures of the tarsal tunnel. The distal myotendinous junction of the flexor hallucis longus is relatively low in the ankle, its tendon occupies the tunnel between the medial and lateral tubercles of the posterior talar process. The knot of Henry (Fig. 11) at the level of the naviculum is the plantar and medial crossing of the FDL tendon over the FHL tendon.

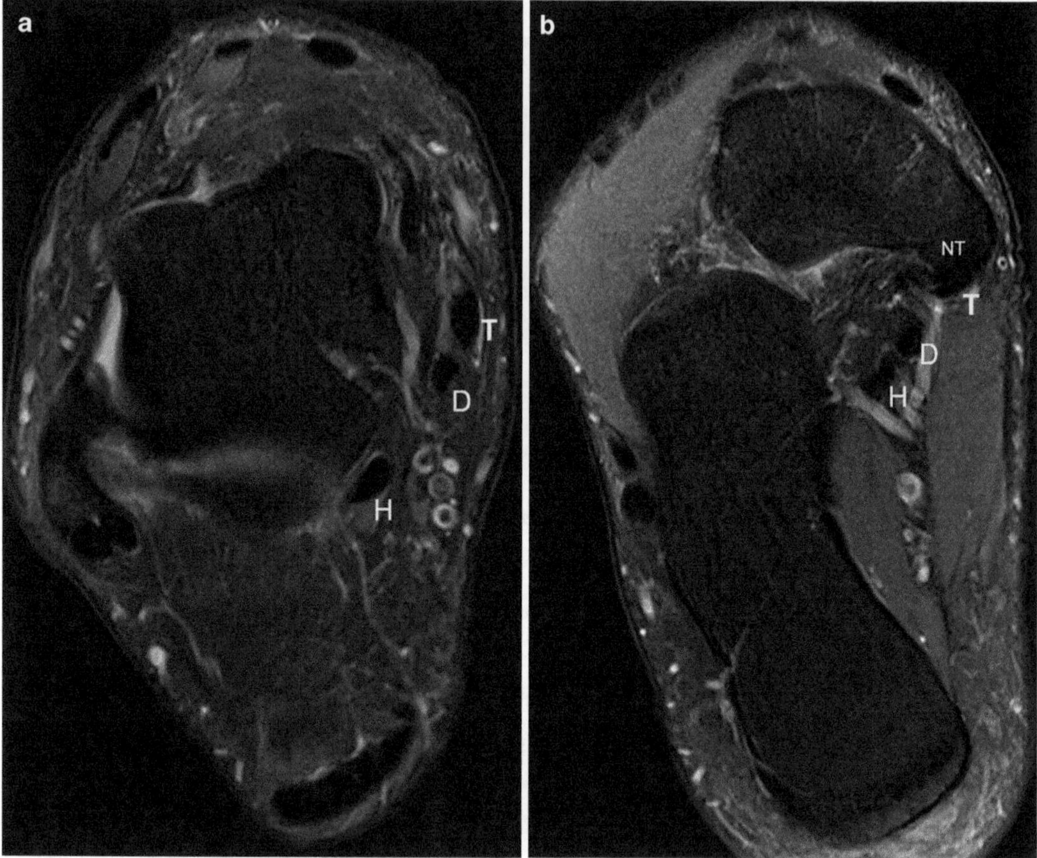

Fig. 12 The normal flexor tendons on sequential axial PD FS MRI (**a**) From anterior to posterior the three tendons in the posteromedial ankle compartment are the PPT (*T*), FDL (*D*), and FHL (*H*). (**b**) On a more caudal section, the FDL (*D*) and FHL (*H*) are seen just prior to their intersection at the knot of Henry. The main insertion of the PTT (*T*) is on the navicular tuberosity (*NT*)

On MRI, the normal flexor tendons (Fig. 12) show expected low signal on all pulse sequences due to poor water content. A small volume of fluid in the tendon sheaths of the PTT and FHL is a normal finding that should not be misinterpreted as tenosynovitis. USG depicts the PTT clearly due to its superficial location.

The PTT is the primary stabilizer of the medial ankle and maintains the longitudinal arch.

3.5 Accessory Navicular Bone

The accessory navicular bone or os naviculare is a commonly encountered ossicle in the foot and ankle, though it is symptomatic only in a fraction of the population (Al-Khudairi et al. 2019). Female predominance has been recorded (Al-Khudairi et al. 2019). Three types of the os naviculare have been described (Fig. 13). Type 1 accessory navicu-

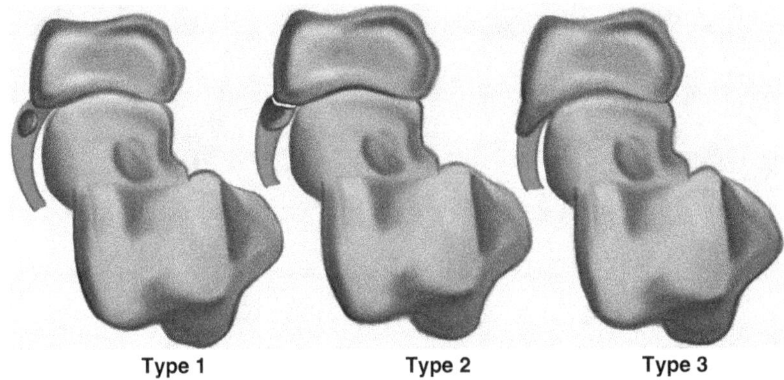

Fig. 13 Types of accessory navicular bones and their relation to the PTT. Type 1 is a sesamoid bone in the PTT tendon. Type 2 forms a synchondrosis with the main navicular body. Type 3 is a prominent or hooked navicular tuberosity

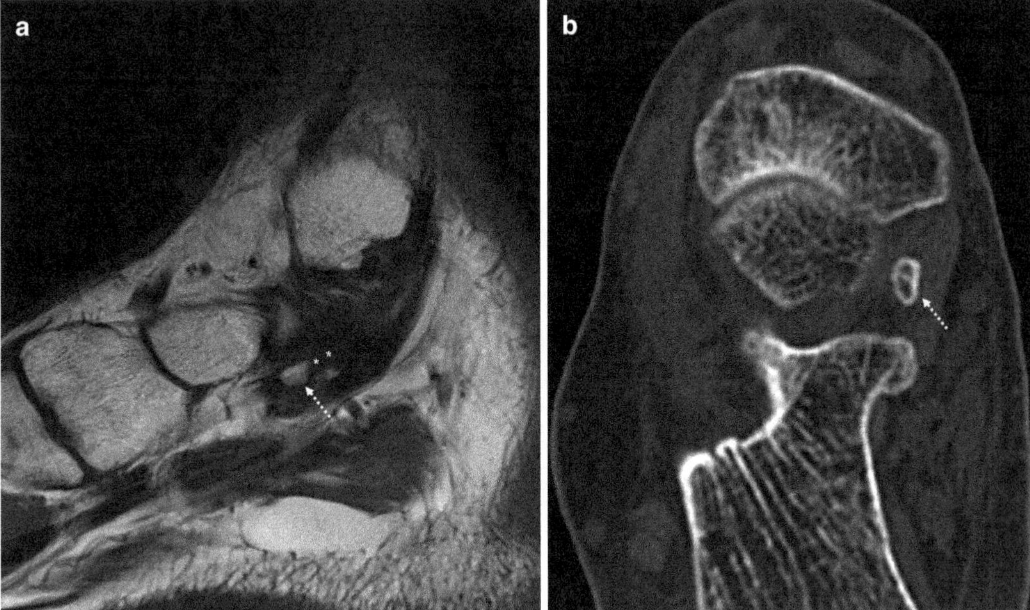

Fig. 14 Type 1 accessory navicular bone. (**a**) On sagittal T1 MRI, a sesamoid bone (dotted arrow) is seen in the PTT tendon (double asterisk) close to the navicular insertion. (**b**) Axial CT confirms a type I accessory navicular bone (dotted arrow)

lar bone is a sesamoid bone in the distal tendon of the tibialis posterior close to its insertion (Fig. 14). Type 2 accessory navicular bone forms a synchondrosis with the main part of the navicular bone (Fig. 15). Type 3 accessory navicular bone is likely a fused type 2 os naviculare, forming a conspicuous and protuberant navicular tuberosity (cornuate navicular) (Fig. 16).

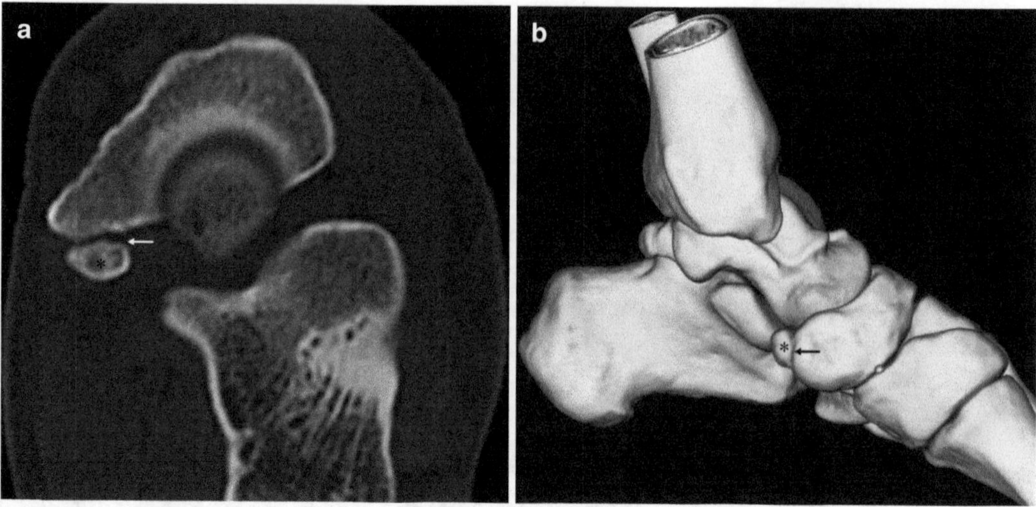

Fig. 15 Type 2 accessory navicular bone. (**a**) Axial CT and (**b**) 3D reconstruction CT show a synchondrosis (arrows) between the accessory navicular (asterisk) and the parent bone

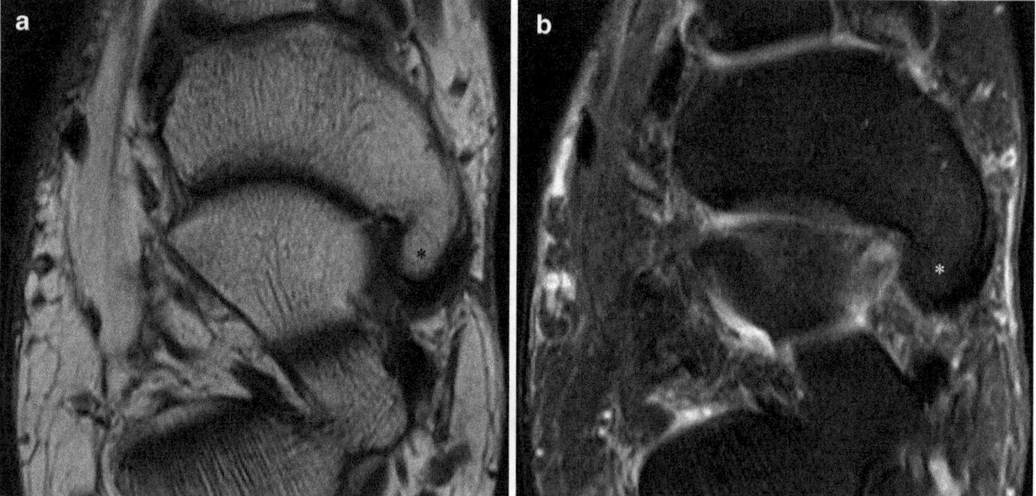

Fig. 16 Type 3 accessory navicular bone (**a**) Axial T1 and (**b**) axial STIR MRI show a hooked (asterisk) type 3 acromion

3.6 Tarsal Tunnel

The tarsal tunnel in the medial ankle is a fibro-osseous canal with a connective tissue roof and a bony floor. The roof of the tarsal tunnel is created by the flexor retinaculum and its floor is formed by the medial surfaces of the distal tibia, talus, and calcaneum (Fig. 17). It contains the posterior tibial artery, veins, and nerve (Fig. 18). Inside the tunnel, the tibial nerve divides into the medial and lateral plantar nerves. The neurovascular bundle of the tarsal tunnel is located between the tendons of the FDL and FHL.

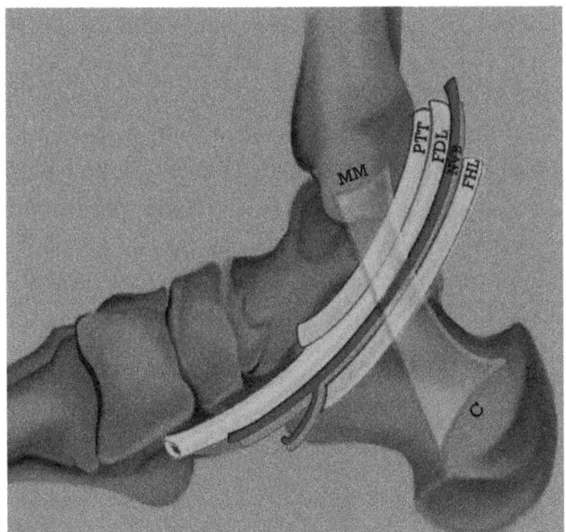

Fig. 17 Normal tarsal tunnel. The flexor retinaculum extending from the medial malleolus (*MM*) to the calcaneus (*C*) forms a fibro-osseous tunnel for the flexor tendons (*PTT, FDL, FHL*) and the neurovascular bundle (*NVB*)

4 Pathology

4.1 Deltoid Ligament Injuries

Tear of the deltoid ligament accounts for approximately 15% of ligamentous ankle injury (Mengiardi et al. 2016). Deltoid ligament tears rarely occur in isolation and are often a part of multiligamentous injury that also involves the lateral, syndesmotic, and/or spring ligament complexes. Associated malleolar fractures are similarly a common occurrence. The pTTL is the strongest ligament of the ankle, and tears of this ligament are often accompanied by disruption of the superficial deltoid complex. In contrast, only half of superficial deltoid ligament injuries have concomitant tears of the pTTL (Mengiardi et al. 2016).

MRI is the modality of choice for assessment of complex ligamentous ankle injuries and in particular for delineation of tears of the deep deltoid ligament. MRI accurately predicts prognosis in deltoid ligament disruptions, assists in planning of physical therapy and surgery when indicated. The intact and normal deep deltoid ligament has a striated appearance; the hyperintensity on MRI between the dark striations must not be interpreted as edema. The intact and normal common origin of the superficial deltoid ligament appears as a band of profoundly low signal intimately attached to the anterior periosteum of the medial malleolus. USG can only depict injuries of the superficial deltoid ligament. Although widening of the medial lucency on a weight-bearing mortise X-rays is historically employed as indirect evidence of deep del-

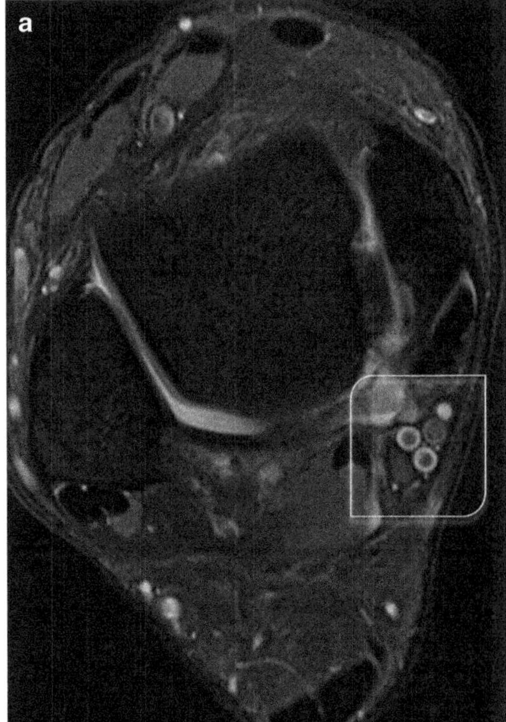

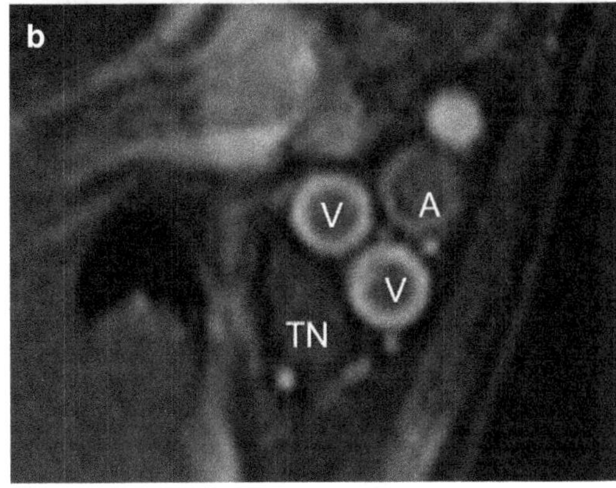

Fig. 18 Normal tarsal tunnel on PD FS axial MRI. (**a**) The neurovascular bundle lies within the fibro-osseous tunnel. (**b**) Inset shows the posterior tibial nerve (*TN*), posterior tibial artery (*A*), and veins (*V*)

toid ligament tear, it has low overall sensitivity (Schuberth et al. 2004). Stable fractures demonstrated on X-rays are known to actually have radiographically occult disruptions of the pTTL (Schuberth et al. 2004).

Acute tears of the deep deltoid ligament most often involve the mid-substance (Crim and Longenecker 2015) with a resulting loss of the normal striated appearance and visualization of intra and periligamentous edema on fluid sensitive MR sequences (Fig. 19). *Acute tears of the superficial deltoid ligament* usually involve the tibial origin (Jeong et al. 2014) often with associated stripping of the medial malleolar periosteum and may extend posteriorly as disruption of the flexor retinaculum. The acutely avulsed common

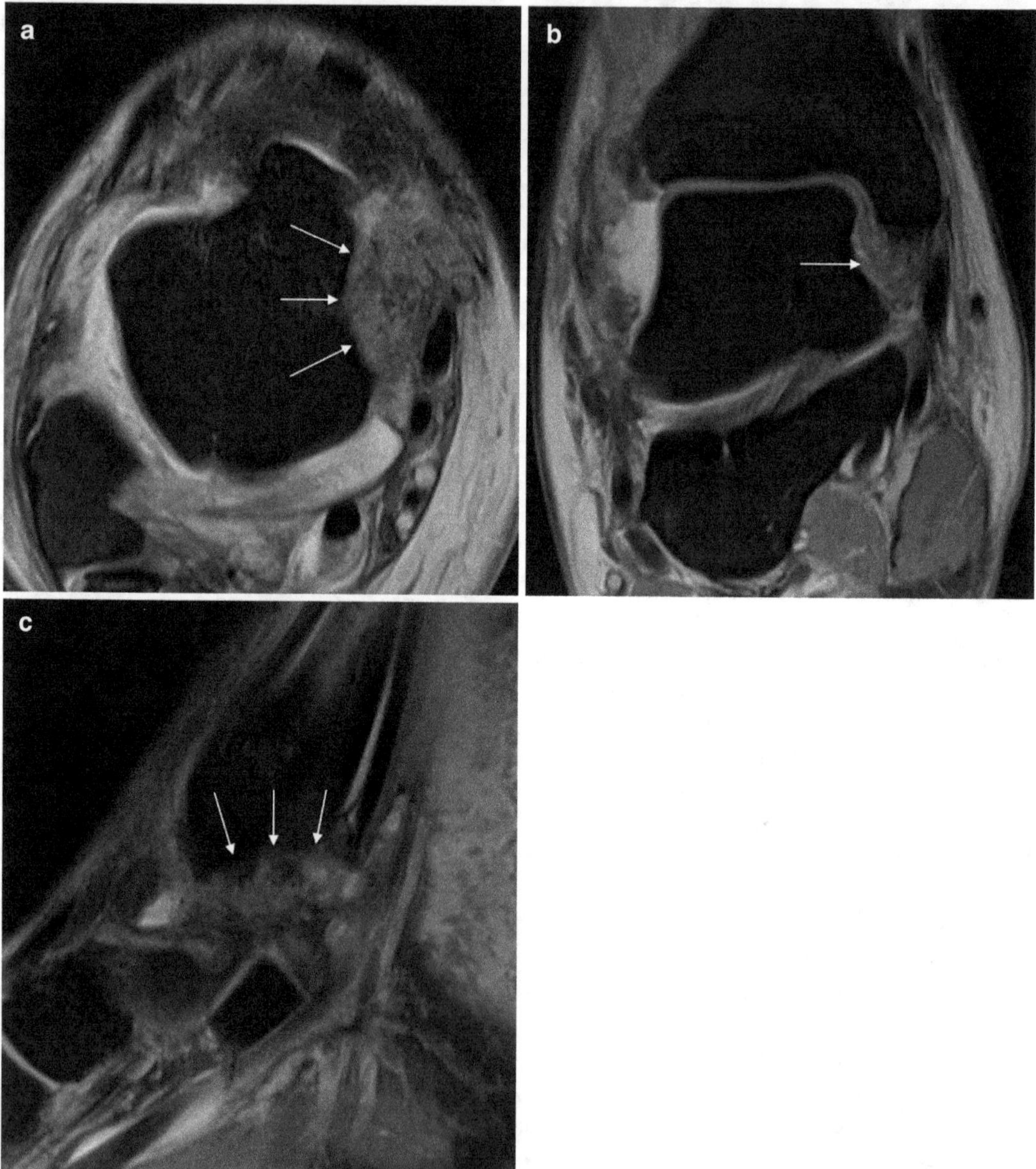

Fig. 19 Acute tear of the pTTL in a case of multiligamentous ankle injury. (**a**) Axial, (**b**) coronal, and (**c**) sagittal PD FS MRI shows edema in the pTTL with loss of the normal striated pattern (arrows)

origin of the superficial deltoid ligaments (Fig. 20) is diagnosed by the presence of a rim of fluid between the medial malleolus and the ligament on MRI or USG. On MRI, the stripped anterior colliculus appears characteristically bare.

Chronic tears of the deep deltoid ligament appear on MRI as ill-defined medial gutter soft tissue lacking striations but with no intra or periligamentous edema. *Chronic tears of the superficial deltoid ligament* have subtle imaging findings. With a high index of suspicion, the chronically torn origin of the superficial deltoid ligament is seen on MRI as well as USG as soft tissue thickening paralleling the anteromedial cortex of the medial malleolus often accompanied by periosteal thickening and periosteal spurs. The bony avulsion fractures (Fig. 21) or bony periosteal appositions of chronic superficial deltoid ligament origin injury are well appreciated on CT.

Most cases of deltoid ligament injuries are treated conservatively with surgical reconstruction reserved for elite athletes, in cases with significant medial ankle instability or while addressing concomitant fractures (Hintermann et al. 2006).

4.2 Medial Impingement Syndromes

Medial impingement syndromes present clinically with painful limitation of movement. The two recognized entities related to medial ankle impingement are anteromedial impingement and posteromedial impingement. The diagnosis of impingement is primarily a clinical verdict validated by certain imaging features. *Posteromedial impingement* correlative findings on MRI are poorly defined scar in the deep medial gutter between the medial talus and medial malleolus (Fig. 22). The scar tissue represents sequalae of remote deep deltoid ligament tears with synovitis and hemarthrosis that heal with fibrosis. The chronically torn pTTL may appear attenuated with reduced volume or enlarged due to hypertrophic scar and synovium. Intraligamentous ossicles are often seen on MRI and CT within the scar tissue showing bone signal intensity/density, respectively. Historically, these ossicles are thought to represent osseous avulsions. However, discordance in the size of the bony fragment relative to the supposed parent bone gives credence to an alternative hypothesis sug-

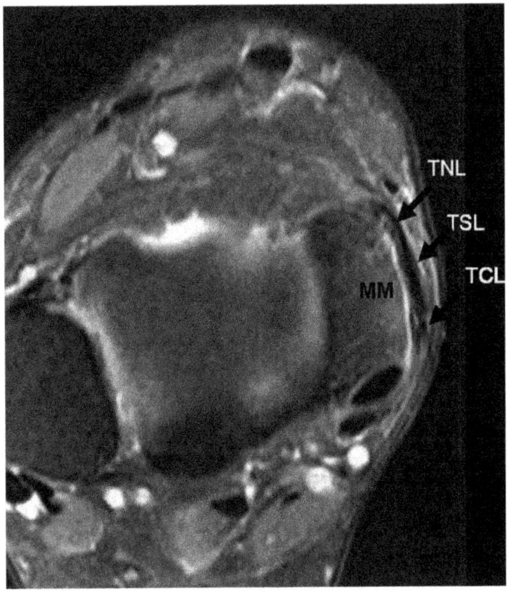

Fig. 20 Acute tear of the common origin of the superficial deltoid ligaments. Axial PD FS MRI shows a rim of fluid between the medial malleolus (*MM*) and the common origins of the *TNL*, *TSL*, and *TCL* (arrows)

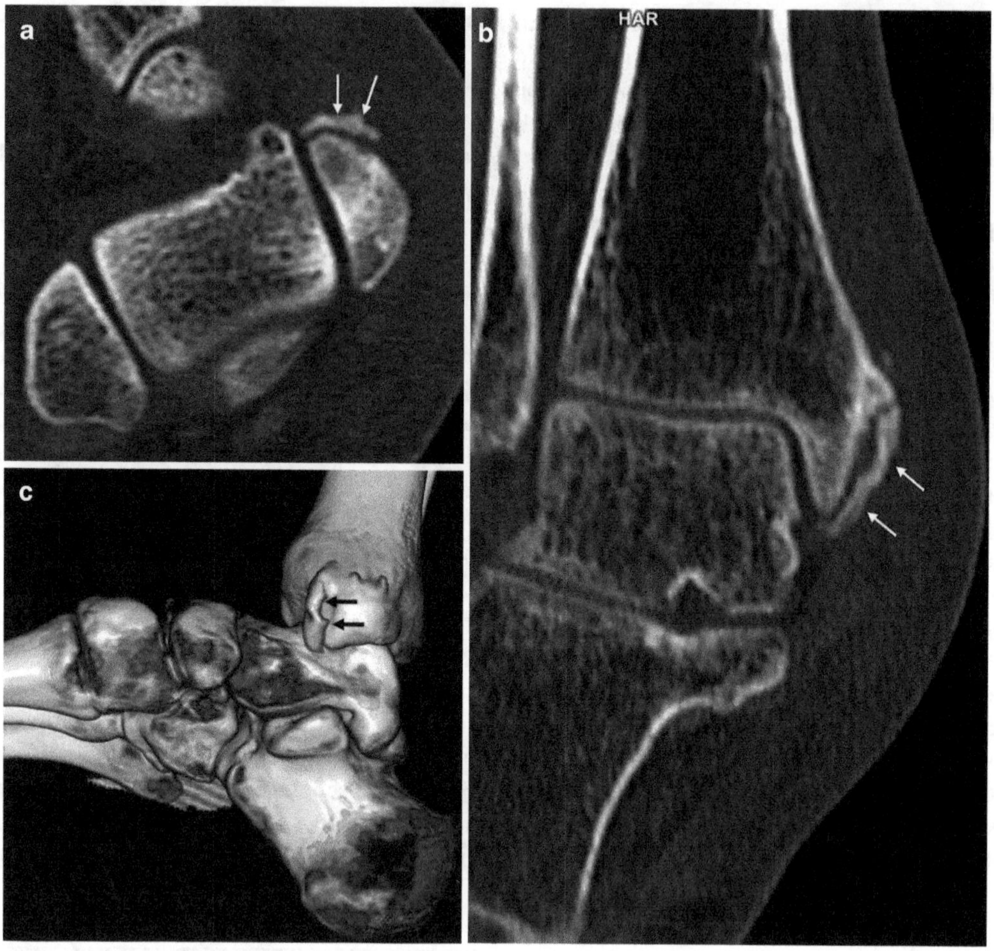

Fig. 21 Chronic avulsion fracture of the common superficial deltoid ligament origin. (**a**) Axial, (**b**) coronal, and (**c**) 3D reconstructed CT shows a well corticated avulsion fracture at the anterior aspect of the MM (arrows)

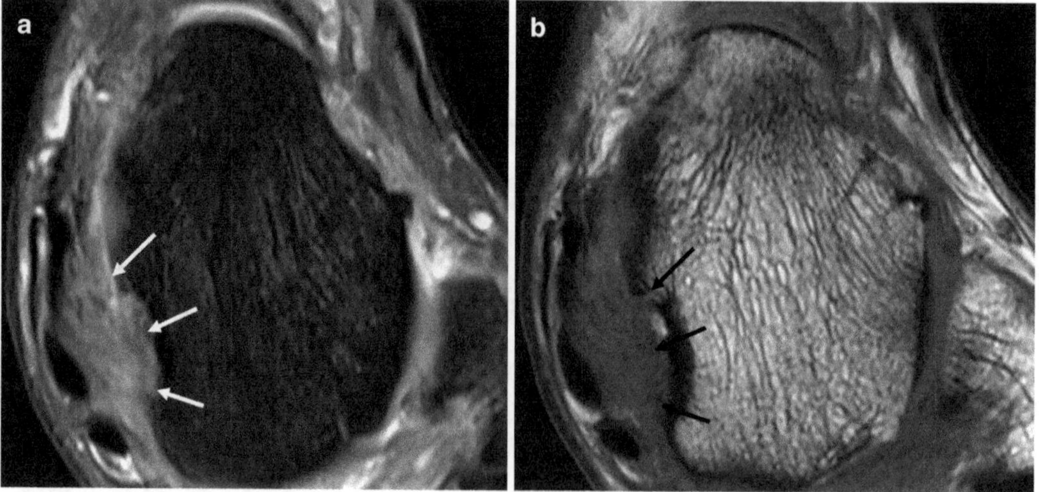

Fig. 22 Posteromedial impingement. (**a**) Axial PD FS and (**b**) axial T1 MRI shows abnormal soft tissue (arrows) in the posteromedial gutter representing fibrous scar from a remote pTTL injury

gested by few authors (Mengiardi et al. 2016) that the ossicles represent heterotopic new bone formation in disrupted collagen fibers. The alternate hypothesis is further validated by observed increase in size of the ossicles over time on imaging. *Anteromedial impingement* occurs due to local capsular injury that subsequently heals with scar and presents on MRI with localized thickening of the capsule and aTTL, focal chronic synovitis, and bony spur formation at the anterior talar process.

4.3 Medial Malleolar Fascial Sleeve Injuries

Detachment of the entire sleeve can be seen in twisting injuries and is appreciated on fluid sensitive MRI sequences as well as USG. The acute injury pattern is an avulsion and delamination of the contiguous common superficial deltoid ligament origin, medial malleolar periosteal sleeve, and flexor retinaculum from anterior to posterior. The chronic pattern of stress injury appears as bony periosteal appositions at the outer surface of the medial malleolus (Fig. 23). MRI has reported sensitivity of 83.3% and specificity of 93.9% in the diagnosis of disruptions of the medial malleolar fascial sleeve (Crim and Longenecker 2015).

4.4 Spring Ligament Injuries

Acute, isolated tears of the SL without associated PTT injury are rare (Kimura et al. 2020). The more commonly encountered concomitant chronic insufficiency of the SL and PTT results in pes planovalgus/acquired flatfoot deformity (AFFD) from loss of the medial longitudinal arch. Due to its relative deep location, MRI is superior to USG in demonstration of SL tears. MRI findings include attenuation of the normal caliber of the ligament or abnormal thickening of the ligament, increased signal on fluid sensitive sequences, waviness, and visible gap/discontinuity (Fig. 24). The presence of associated PTT tendinopathy on imaging improves confidence for diagnosis of SL tear.

Three anatomical peculiarities of the intact SL seen on MRI merit particular attention by the radiologist to avoid false positive interpretation as tears (Fig. 25). Firstly, the normal gliding zone

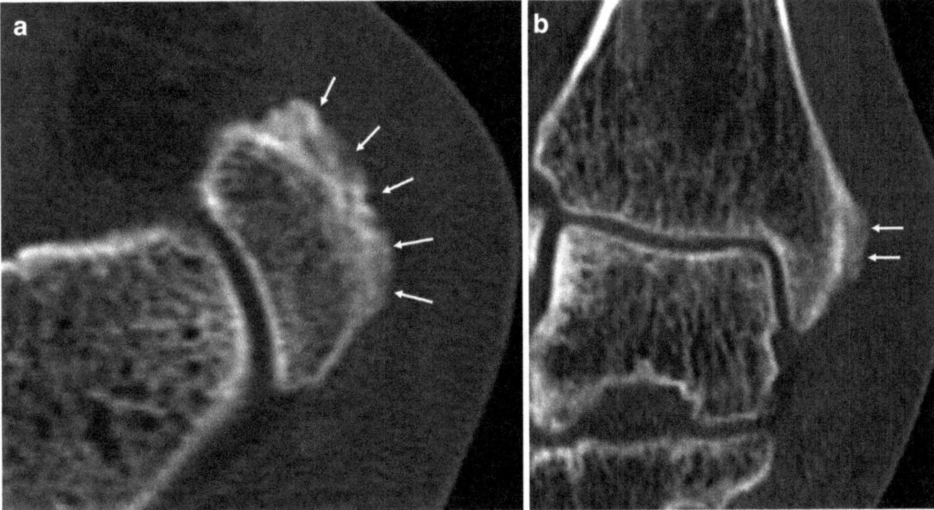

Fig. 23 Chronic stress injury of the medial malleolar sleeve. (**a**) Axial and (**b**) coronal CT shows bony periosteal thickening and appositions (arrows) at the entire outer margin of the medial malleolus involving the attachment of the medial malleolar sleeve from anterior to posterior

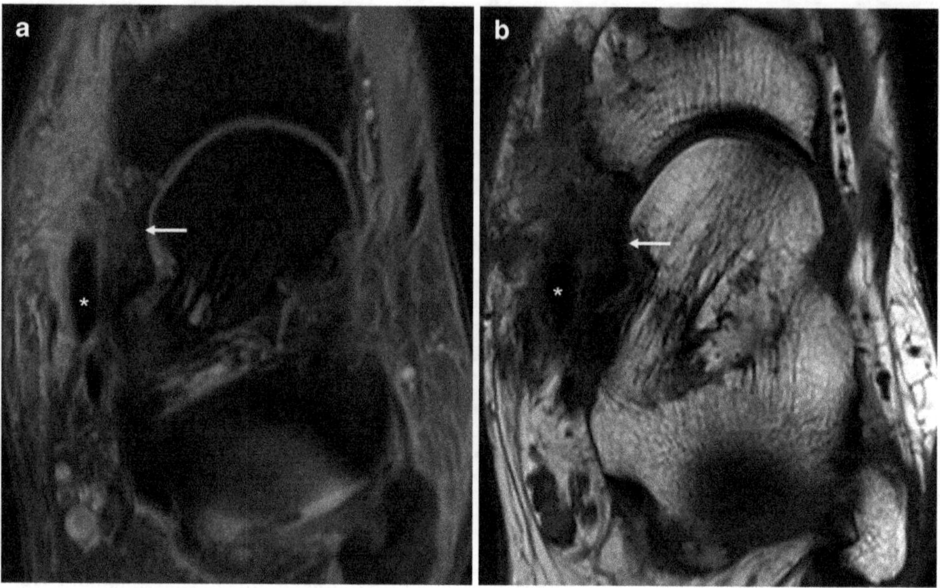

Fig. 24 Spring ligament tear. (**a**) Axial PD FS and (**b**) axial T1 MRI shows swelling and altered signal in the smCNL (arrows). Mild PTT tendinosis is seen (asterisk)

between the SL and PTT may falsely simulate pathological waviness/thickening of the SL. Secondly, the spring ligament recess (SLR) normally contains a small quantity of fluid as it is contiguous with the talocalcaneonavicular joint space. Fluid in the SLR occupies the gap between the two plantar CNLs and must not be misinterpreted as tear. Finally, the intact iplCNL has a striated appearance which must not be incorrectly diagnosed as an injury.

Departing from historical narratives, recent studies (Williams et al. 2014) have indicated that SL disruptions seen on MRI may be more significantly associated with radiographic pes planus foot position as compared to PTT abnormalities seen on MRI. Recognizing the role of the SL as the primary static stabilizer of the medial midfoot, studies from recent literature (Fogleman et al. 2021; Lui 2017) have advocated additional surgical repair of spring ligament tears during PTT repair in pes planovalgus reconstruction.

4.5 Flexor Tendon Injuries

Of the three flexor tendons in the posteromedial ankle compartment, biomechanically, the PTT is more important as compared to the FDL and FHL. The PTT is functionally synergistic with the deltoid ligament complex, spring ligament, and flexor retinaculum. Hence injuries of these structures are usually seen in conjunction.

Due to its superficial location, the PTT is amenable to assessment by USG (Fig. 26) in addition to MRI. The spectrum of PTT abnormalities depicted on imaging includes tendinosis, tenosynovitis, tendon elongation, partial and complete tears. On MRI, altered signal at the PTT navicular insertion may be due to magic angle and must be reported with caution. Early tendinosis is also seen as increased signal on short TE sequences rendering differentiation from magic angle artifact challenging. A method prescribed in literature, albeit less practical is to reimage in prone position with plantar flexion thus eliminating the

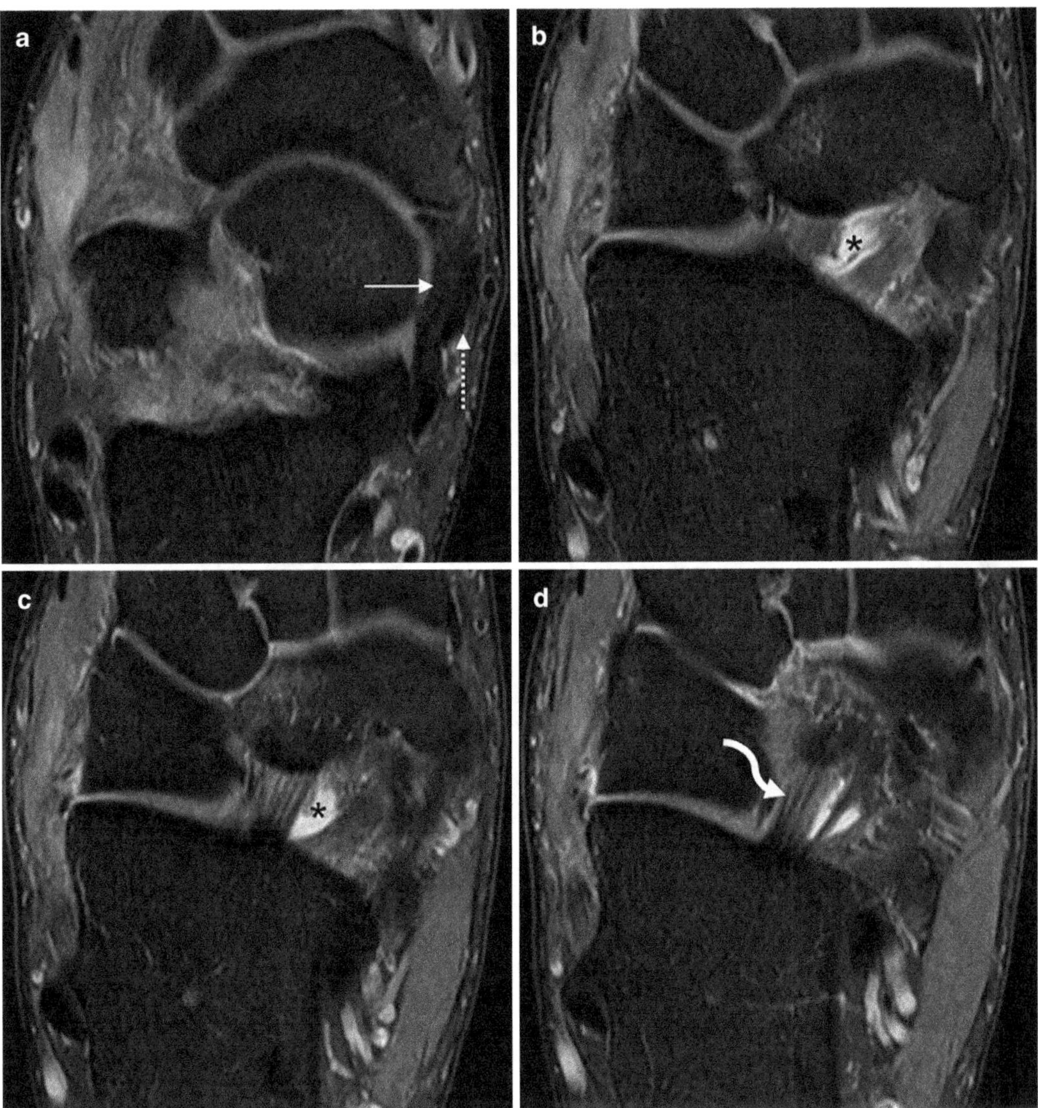

Fig. 25 Potential pitfalls in MRI assessment of the spring ligament complex. Sequential axial PD FD images (**a**) the poorly visualized gliding zone between the smCNL (arrow) and PTT (dotted arrow) should not lead to an incorrect impression of ligament thickening, (**b**, **c**) the fluid filled spring ligament recess (asterisk) between the two plantar CNLs should not be mistaken for a tear, (**d**) the normal striations of the iplCNL (curved arrow) should not be labeled as a tear

possibility of magic angle. Tenosynovitis must also be reported with caution as a small quantity of fluid in the PTT tendon sheath is considered a normal finding. Tenosynovitis of the PTT with significant fluid is easily recognized on imaging and when isolated may be secondary to overuse. PTT tenosynovitis is seen in conjunction with tenosynovitis of other tendons in systemic inflammatory conditions. Tendon elongation is difficult to diagnose on imaging but can cause PTT insufficiency even in the absence of tendon discontinuity. Partial split tears present with the appearance of two subtendons (Fig. 27) which may reunite prior to the navicular insertion.

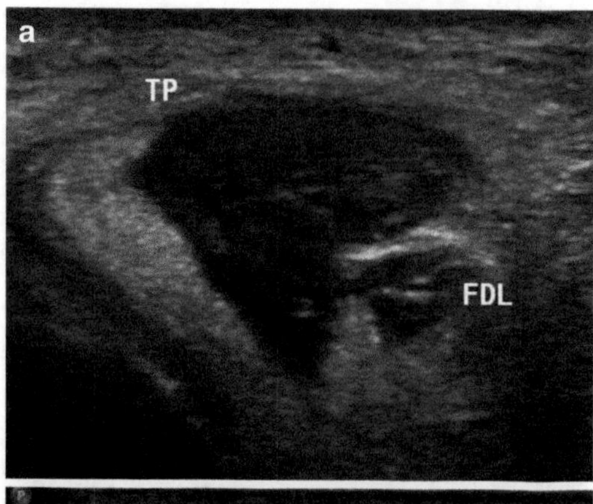

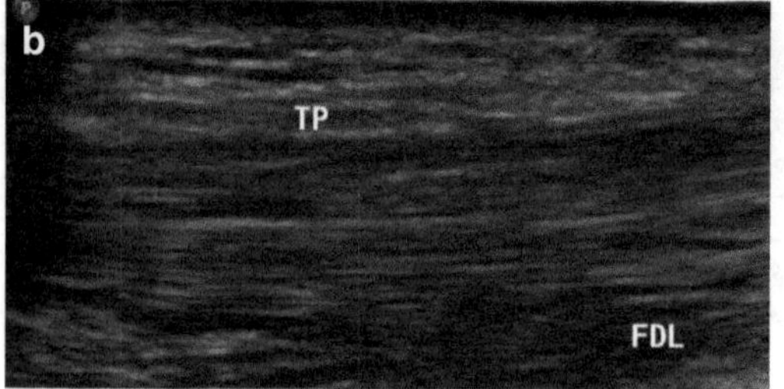

Fig. 26 Posterior tibial tendon tendinosis. (**a**) Transverse and (**b**) longitudinal USG images show a thickened posterior tibial tendon (*TP*) with heterogeneous architecture. The flexor digitorum longus (*FDL*) tendon is also mildly thickened. Image courtesy Dr Rolly Chowdhri

Finally, complete tears are diagnosed by the discontinuity of the tendon with a fluid filled gap and varying degrees of proximal retraction.

Chronic PTT insufficiency leads radiographic and clinical flatfoot due to loss of the longitudinal arch. Imaging shows inferior subluxation of the "keystone" talonavicular joint and forefoot abduction. Further progression of the deformity is associated with increase in heel valgus. On MRI, the normal hindfoot valgus angle has been described as equal to or less than 6° (Donovan and Rosenberg 2009). The angle is measured on coronal images posterior to the plane of the sustentaculum tali where the long axis of the distal tibia subtends the medial calcaneal wall. The degree of heel valgus is likely underestimated on MRI and more accurately determined on erect radiographs reflecting the altered biomechanics on weight bearing. Heel valgus eventually leads to hindfoot impingement syndrome consisting of talocalcaneal impingement and subsequent subfibular impingement. On radiographs and MRI, talocalcaneal impingement is seen at subcortical cystic change and marrow edema at the opposing lateral talar facet and calcaneum at the angle of Gissane due to bony opposition. Subfibular impingement represents soft tissue entrapment between the fibular tip and calcaneum and is seen on imaging as subfibular tissue thickening. Rarely subfibular impingement occurs in isolation without preceding talocalcaneal impingement. Hence pathology of the medial ankle and midfoot eventually leads to lateral ankle abnormalities as a result of transfer of weight-bearing and altered biomechanics (Sanghvi 2021). When conservative treatment of advanced AAFD and hindfoot impingement fails; triple arthrodesis may be performed for pain amelioration.

4.6 Accessory Navicular Bone Pathology

Type 2 accessory navicular is often symptomatic with medial ankle and foot pain (Leonard and Fortin 2010). The likely cause of pain is repeated tension and shear forces from the pull of the powerful PTT stressing the synchondrosis. Although X-rays demonstrate the os (Huang et al. 2014), they may not be helpful in directing clinical management. Bone scans and MRI provide more pertinent clinical information (Takahashi et al. 2014). The MRI features of a painful os naviculare are marrow edema which corresponds to chronic stress and later osteonecrosis. Edema in the synchondrosis is seen on fluid sensitive sequences and indicates inflammation and destruction of the cartilage cap. Soft tissue thickening, edema, and synovitis are seen adjacent to the painful accessory bone and appears as periosseous obliteration of high T1 fat signal with corresponding intermediate T2 signal (Fig. 28). All symptomatic patients have concurrent PTT pathology. The PTT appears enlarged with vari-

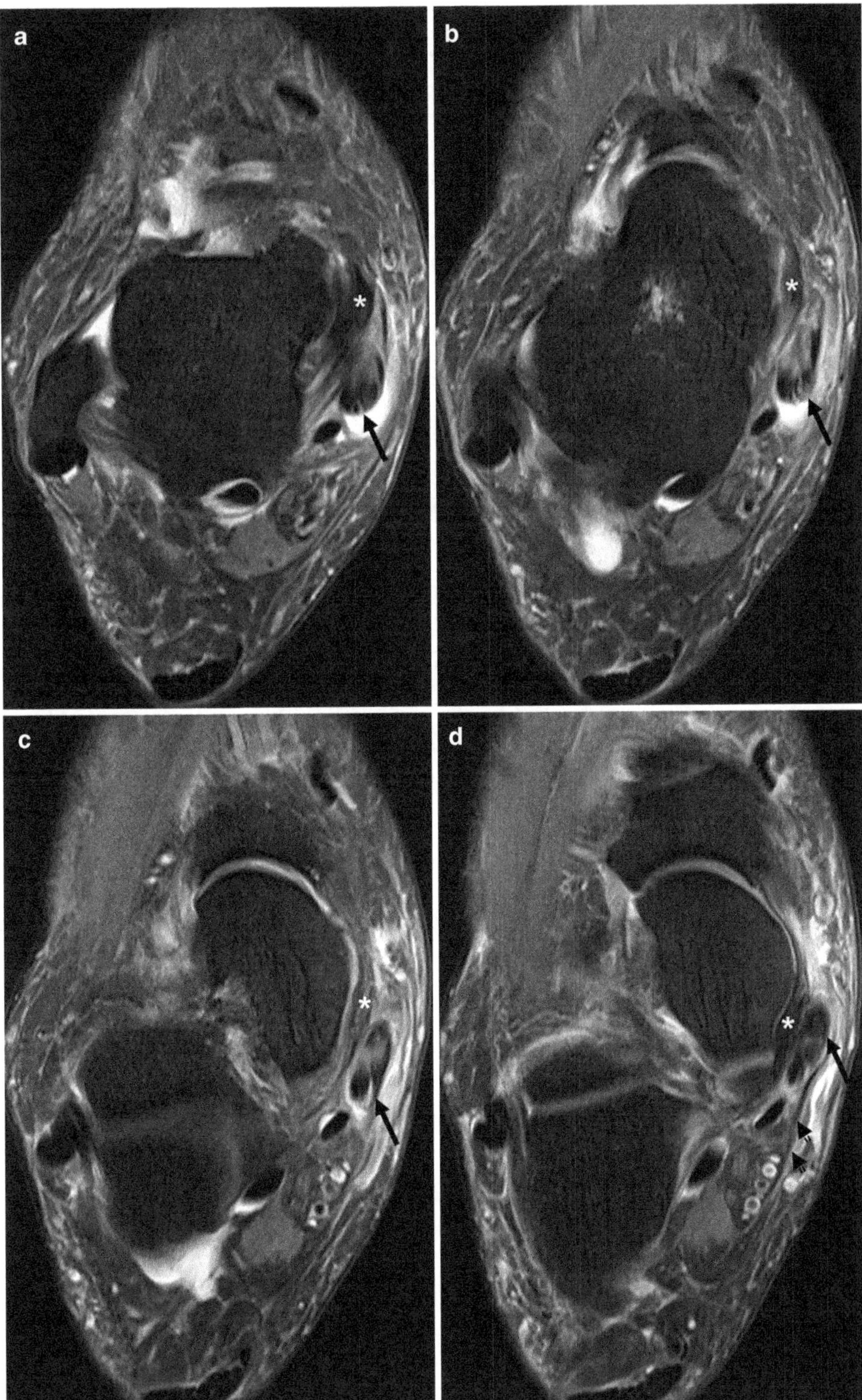

Fig. 27 PTT split tear. Sequential axial PD FS images. (**a**–**d**) Fragmentation and altered signal are seen in the PTT (arrows). Related structures seen include a degenerated tibiospring ligament merging with the superomedial calcaneonavicular ligament (asterisk) and the slightly thickened flexor retinaculum (arrowheads)

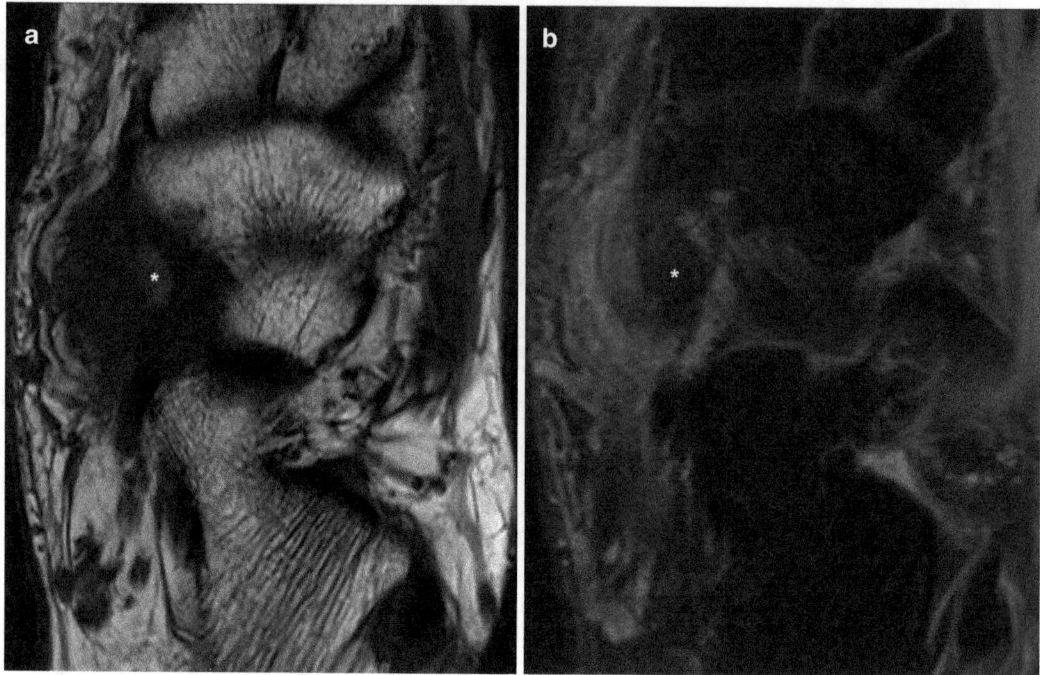

Fig. 28 Accessory navicular bone syndrome. (**a**) Axial T1 and (**b**) PDFS MRI shows extensive soft tissue thickening around an os naviculare (asterisk)

able tendinosis, tenosynovitis, partial or even complete tears.

Surgical treatment involves excision of the accessory navicular bone (Park et al. 2022). The synchondrosis and adjacent margin of the naviculum may also be excised. Additionally, the PTT may be repositioned or FDL transfer may be performed.

4.7 Tarsal Tunnel Syndrome

Tarsal tunnel syndrome occurs from posterior tibial nerve entrapment in the fibro-osseous tunnel that houses the posteromedial tendons and neurovascular bundle. The syndrome presents as paresthesia and pain along the distribution of the nerve in the medial and plantar foot (Nelson 2021). In advanced cases, gait disturbances may occur. Repetitive stress may cause fibrosis and scar in the fibro-osseous canal. The syndrome is also often seen in inflammatory arthritis and diabetes. USG may be used to guide the injection of local anesthetics and steroids into the canal, which is also a useful diagnostic test.

The role of imaging is in demonstration of mass lesions that compress the nerve. USG (de Souza Reis Soares et al. 2022) and MRI effectively demonstrate entrapment of the nerve by a spectrum of pathologies than includes ganglion cyst, lipomas, accessory flexor tendons, osseous excrescences, neurogenic tumors, varicosities, and significant tenosynovitis (Fig. 29). In advanced cases, denervation atrophy of the intrinsic foot muscles is seen.

When trial of conservative treatment fails or in instances when imaging demonstrates space occupative lesions compressing the nerve, surgery is offered. The mainstay of surgical treatment is release of the flexor retinaculum to decompress the entrapped posterior tibial nerve (Gültaç et al. 2020).

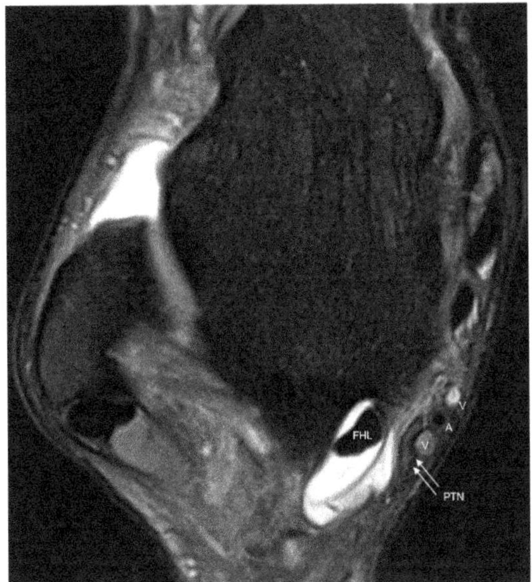

Fig. 29 Tarsal tunnel syndrome. Axial PD FS MRI shows tenosynovitis of the *FHL* compressing and flattening the posterior tibial nerve (arrows, *PTN*). Also seen in the neurovascular bundle are the posterior tibial artery (*A*) and veins (*V*)

4.8 Tarsal Coalition

Vague medial ankle pain can be caused by the two common types of tarsal coalition (Golshteyn and Schneider 2022) which are calcaneonavicular coalition and talocalcaneal (or subtalar coalition). Many coalitions are bilateral and may be fibrous (syndesmosis), cartilaginous (synchondrosis), or osseous (synostosis). Radiographs clearly demonstrate osseous coalition. However, the diagnosis of fibrous and cartilaginous coalitions is subtle and incomplete on X-rays. MRI is the modality of choice for the assessment of biomechanical alterations secondary to tarsal coalition. Overall, MRI is better suited to assess all types of coalitions as it is sensitive to marrow edema. Fluid sensitive sequences are useful to demonstrate stress induced bone marrow edema and soft tissue edema adjacent to the coalition. CT is performed prior to elective surgery in a fraction of cases.

Calcaneonavicular coalition is the commonest type of tarsal coalition. The calcaneum and navicular bones do not normally form a joint. Radiographically, on oblique view, calcaneonavicular coalitions are recognized by the "anteater sign." The osseous bar formed by the elongated anterior process of the calcaneum extending toward the adjacent navicular resembles the snout of an anteater (Ridley et al. 2018). The "reverse anteater sign" refers to a posterolateral elongation of the naviculum to approximate with the anterior process of the calcaneum (Fig. 30).

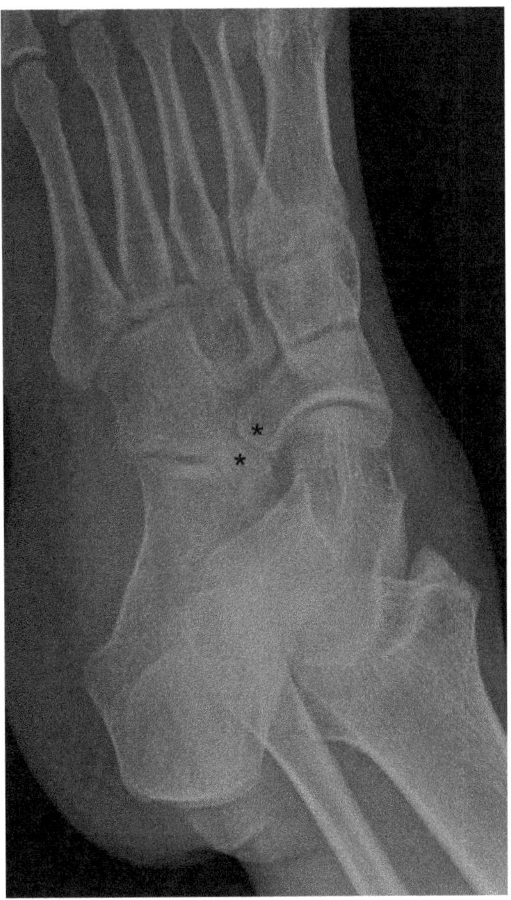

Fig. 30 Calcaneonavicular coalition (non-osseous). Oblique radiograph of the foot shows that the calcaneal and navicular bones (asterisk) are approximated with narrowing and irregularity of the bony interfaces. Normally, the calcaneum and navicular bones do not articulate

Talocalcaneal coalitions usually involve the middle calcaneal facet. On lateral radiographs, talocalcaneal coalitions are recognized by the "C sign" and "talar beak sign." The "C sign" is the continuous column of bone from the posterior talus to the sustentaculum tali. The "talar beak sign" alludes to a prominent osseous spur at the anterior and dorsal talus near the talonavicular joint. It is seen in both the common types of coalition (Phyo et al. 2020). The anterior talar osseous spur seen in talar coalitions is a traction osteophyte developing due to ligamentous laxity and increased stress on the neighboring talonavicular joint.

5 Summary

Injuries to the medial soft tissue structures of the ankle are often eclipsed by lateral compartment abnormalities. Medial ankle injuries may occur simultaneously or in sequence with lateral compartment injury. To guide therapy and for prediction of eventual clinical outcome, imaging assessment must comprehensively cover all compartments of the ankle.

Injuries of the medial soft tissue structures include possible disruptions of four major structures which are the deltoid ligament complex, PTT, flexor retinaculum, and spring ligament complex. These injuries are usually seen in conjunction due to the synergistic nature of their function. Additionally, medial ankle pain may emanate from tarsal tunnel syndrome, type 2 accessory navicular bone, or subtalar coalitions.

References

Al-Khudairi N, Welck MJ, Brandao B, Saifuddin A (2019) The relationship of MRI findings and clinical features in symptomatic and asymptomatic os naviculare. Clin Radiol 74(1):80.e1–80.e6

Chhabra A, Subhawong TK, Carrino JA (2010) MR imaging of deltoid ligament pathologic findings and associated impingement syndromes. Radiographics 30(3):751–761

Crim J (2017) Medial-sided ankle pain: deltoid ligament and beyond. Magn Reson Imaging Clin N Am 25(1):63–77

Crim J, Longenecker LG (2015) MRI and surgical findings in deltoid ligament tears. AJR Am J Roentgenol 204(1):W63–W69

de Souza Reis Soares O, Duarte ML, Brasseur JL (2022) Tarsal tunnel syndrome: an ultrasound pictorial review. J Ultrasound Med 41(5):1247–1272

Donovan A, Rosenberg ZS (2009) Extraarticular lateral hindfoot impingement with posterior tibial tendon tear: MRI correlation. AJR Am J Roentgenol 193(3):672–678

Fogleman JA, Kreulen CD, Sarcon AK, Michelier PV, Giza E, Doty JF (2021) Augmented spring ligament repair in pes planovalgus reconstruction. J Foot Ankle Surg 60(6):1212–1216

Golshteyn G, Schneider HP (2022) Tarsal coalitions. Clin Podiatr Med Surg 39(1):129–142

Gültaç E, Kılınç B, Kılınç CY, Yücens M, Aydogan NH, Öznur A (2020) Comparison of tunnel ligament release instrument assisted minimally open surgery and conventional open surgery in the treatment of tarsal tunnel syndrome. J Orthop Surg (Hong Kong) 28(3):2309499020971868

Hintermann B, Knupp M, Pagenstert GI (2006) Deltoid ligament injuries: diagnosis and management. Foot Ankle Clin 11(3):625–637

Huang J, Zhang Y, Ma X, Wang X, Zhang C, Chen L (2014) Accessory navicular bone incidence in Chinese patients: a retrospective analysis of X-rays following trauma or progressive pain onset. Surg Radiol Anat 36(2):167–172

Jeong MS, Choi YS, Kim YJ, Kim JS, Young KW, Jung YY (2014) Deltoid ligament in acute ankle injury: MR imaging analysis. Skeletal Radiol 43(5):655–663

Kimura Y, Yamashiro T, Saito Y, Kitsukawa K, Niki H, Mimura H (2020) MRI findings of spring ligament injury: association with surgical findings and flatfoot deformity. Acta Radiol Open 9(12):2058460120980145

Leonard ZC, Fortin PT (2010) Adolescent accessory navicular. Foot Ankle Clin 15(2):337–347

Lui TH (2017) Arthroscopic repair of superomedial spring ligament by talonavicular arthroscopy. Arthrosc Tech 6(1):e31–e35

Mengiardi B, Pfirrmann CWA, Vienne P, Hodler J, Zanetti M (2007) Medial collateral ligament complex of the ankle: MR appearance in asymptomatic subjects. Radiology 242(3):817–824

Mengiardi B, Pinto C, Zanetti M (2016) Medial collateral ligament complex of the ankle: MR imaging anatomy and findings in medial instability. Semin Musculoskelet Radiol 20(1):91–103

Nelson SC (2021) Tarsal tunnel syndrome. Clin Podiatr Med Surg 38(2):131–141

Park YH, Kim W, Choi JW, Kim HJ (2022) Risk factors for persistent pain requiring surgical treatment in adult symptomatic accessory navicular. Clin J Sport Med 32(3):e308–e312

Phyo N, Pressney I, Khoo M, Welck M, Saifuddin A (2020) The radiological diagnosis of extra-articular posteromedial talocalcaneal coalition. Skeletal Radiol 49(9):1413–1422

Ridley LJ, Han J, Ridley WE, Xiang H (2018) Anteater nose and reverse anteater signs: calcaneo-navicular coalition. J Med Imaging Radiat Oncol 62(Suppl 1):118–119

Sanghvi D (2021) MRI of lateral hindfoot impingement. Diagn Interv Radiol 27(3):432–439

Schuberth JM, Collman DR, Rush SM, Ford LA (2004) Deltoid ligament integrity in lateral malleolar fractures: a comparative analysis of arthroscopic and radiographic assessments. J Foot Ankle Surg 43(1): 20–29

Szaro P, Ghali Gataa K, Ciszek B (2022) Anatomical variants of the medioplantar oblique ligament and inferoplantar longitudinal ligament: an MRI study. Surg Radiol Anat 44(2):279–288

Takahashi M, Sakai T, Sairyo K, Takao S, Mima S, Yasui N (2014) Magnetic resonance imaging in adolescent symptomatic navicular tuberosity. J Med Investig 61(1–2):22–27

Williams G, Widnall J, Evans P, Platt S (2014) Could failure of the spring ligament complex be the driving force behind the development of the adult flatfoot deformity? J Foot Ankle Surg 53(2):152–155

Yammine K (2017) The morphology and prevalence of the deltoid complex ligament of the ankle. Foot Ankle Spec 10(1):55–62

Lateral Ankle Pain

Ali Shah, Christine Azzopardi,
and Karthikeyan P. Iyengar

Contents

A. Shah
Department of Musculoskeletal Radiology, Nottingham University Hospital NHS Trust, Nottingham, UK

C. Azzopardi (✉)
Department of Musculoskeletal Radiology, The Royal Orthopaedic Hospital, Birmingham, UK
e-mail: christine.azzopardi1@nhs.net

K. P. Iyengar
Department of Orthopedics, Southport and Ormskirk Hospital NHS Trust, Southport, UK

1 Introduction

Lateral ankle pain is a complex entity with a variety of etiologies ranging from trauma, inflammatory conditions, impingement, mass lesions, and other miscellaneous causes, both in acute and chronic presentations. An understanding of the anatomical relations is essential for assessment and work up in order to reach a correct diagnosis. It is equally important to have a sound knowledge of the pathologies, their etiology, imaging appearances, and differential diagnosis to assist the clinicians with the appropriate management plan.

The chapter focuses on the relevant anatomy, available imaging modalities and how to optimize review of structures including preferred sequences, and then finally an overview of various pathologies related to lateral ankle pain.

2 Anatomy

The ankle joint, also referred to as the talocrural joint, is a hinged type of a synovial joint comprising articulation between tibia, fibula, and talus. It can be likened to a mortice formed by the medial malleolus (tibia), distal part of tibia, and the lateral malleolus (fibula), which articulates with the body of talus. Some authors include the subtalar joint as part of the ankle, with the talocrural joint being the true ankle joint (Sawant and Sanghvi 2018).

Med Radiol Diagn Imaging (2023)
https://doi.org/10.1007/174_2023_390,
Published Online: 28 May 2023

The joint capsule is attached around the articulating surfaces and is weak anteriorly and posteriorly but reinforced from ligaments laterally (Table 1) and medially (Ellis and Mahadevan 2010).

Focusing on the lateral side of the joint, the main ligament complex is referred to as the collateral ligament complex including the syndesmosis, posterior talofibular ligament (PTFL—strongest, thick, intracapsular, extrasynovial) (Sawant and Sanghvi 2018) (Figs. 1 and 2), calcaneofibular ligament (CFL—cord-like, extracapsular), and the anterior talofibular (ATFL—flat and weak, intracapsular) ligament. The ATFL (Figs. 1 and 2) is best viewed on axial MRI images where the fibula appears crescent shaped and dome of talus is oblong on the same slice and elongates more during plantar flexion and supination. The CFL conversely elongates on dorsiflexion and pronation. There are different length proposed for the two ligaments ranging from 15.8 mm ± 2.9 mm for the ATFL and 27.7 mm ± 2.7 mm in neutral position (de Asla et al. 2009). The average width of the ATFL is approximately 7.8 mm and that of CFL between 6 and 8 mm (Hertel 2002; Le and Tiu

Table 1 Summary of lateral ankle ligaments

Ligament	Proximal	Distal	Function
Posterior talofibular	Posterior aspect of lateral malleolar fossa	Lateral tubercle of talus	Resists posterior displacement of talus
Calcaneofibular	Depression anterior to apex of lateral malleolus	Lateral tubercle of calcaneum	Resists talar tilt into inversion. Restrains inversion of calcaneum with respect to fibula. Stabilizes talus and fibula during dorsiflexion
Anterior talofibular	Anterior margin of fibula	Inferior to lateral articular facet and lateral aspect of neck of talus	Resists anterior displacement of talus and inversion during plantar flexion
Syndesmosis • Posterior inferior tibiofibular • Transverse tibiofibular • Anterior inferior tibiofibular	• Posterolateral tubercle of tibia • Posterior distal margin of plafond • Distal tibia	• Posterior tubercle of fibula • Proximal edge of malleolar fossa • Anterior aspect of lateral malleolus	• Strong ligament of syndesmosis • Reinforces syndesmosis • Reinforces syndesmosis

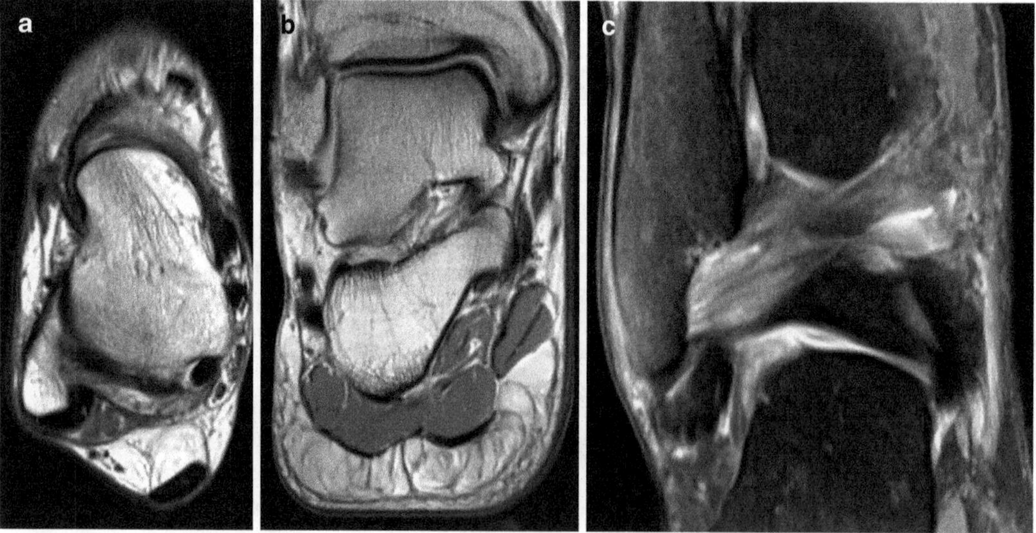

Fig. 1 Ankle ligaments. (**a**) Axial T1W image, (**b**) Coronal T2W image, (**c**) Coronal STIR image

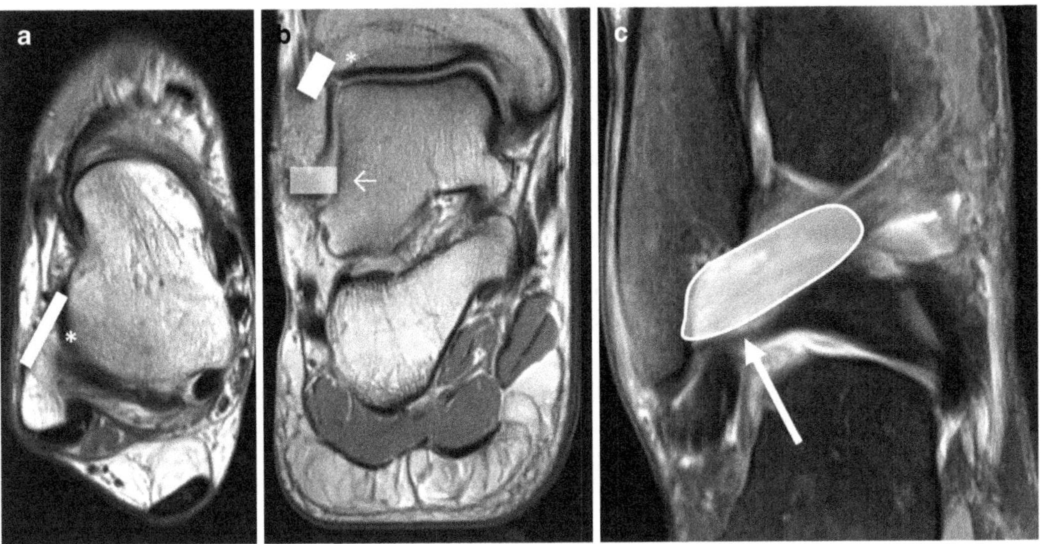

Fig. 2 Ankle ligaments annotated. (**a**) Asterisk = ATFL, (**b**) Asterisk = AITFL, Arrow = ATFL, (**c**) Arrow = PITFL

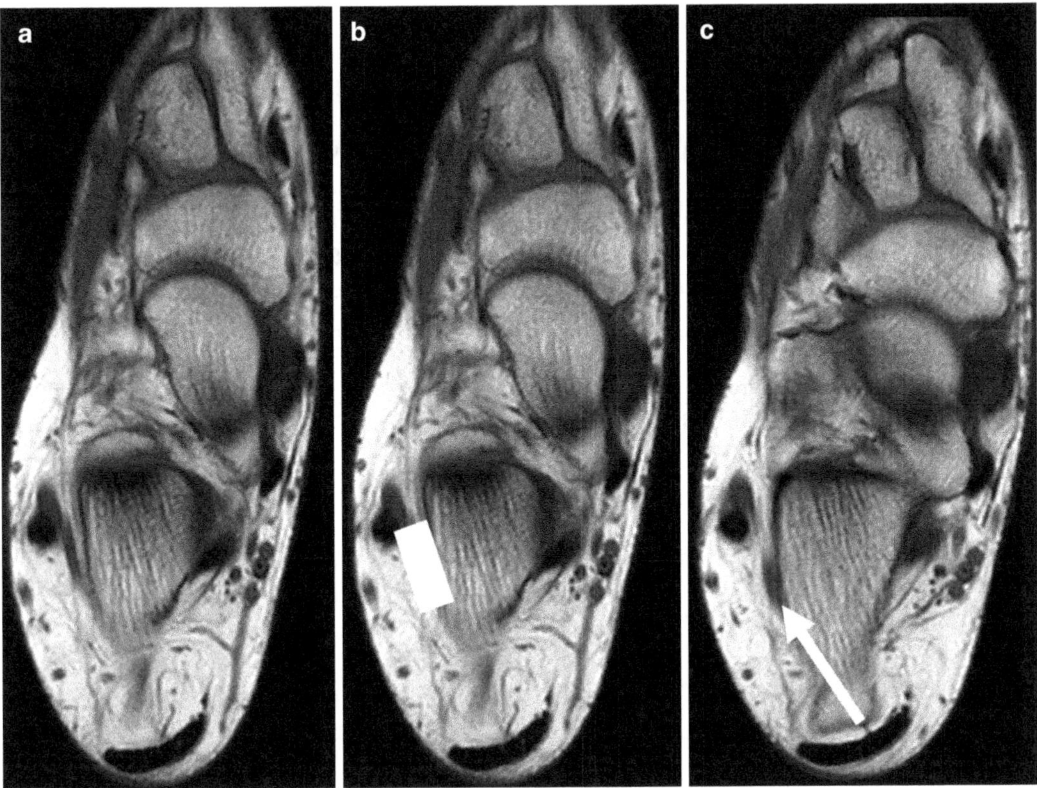

Fig. 3 Ankle ligaments axial T1W images. (**a**) CFL, (**b**) Annotated CFL, (**c**) Arrow = CFL

2022). The CFL (Fig. 3) courses from lateral malleolus posteroinferiorly to lateral aspect of calcaneum posterior to the peroneal tubercle, at mean angle of 133° from long axis of fibula. It can have morphological variation as a V or Y shaped CFL where proximal component has attachment to both tibia and fibula (Hegde et al. 2021). Additionally an accessory ligament has been described coursing posteromedially toward peroneus brevis from fibular origin of PITFL to the lateral part of calcaneum posterior to the peroneal tubercle but deep and separate from CFL. This is referred to as the "Botchu Beale" ligament (Hegde et al. 2021).

The syndesmosis includes three components: posterior inferior tibiofibular (PITFL) (Figs. 2, 4, 5, and 6), inferior transverse tibiofibular (TTFL or ITL), and anterior inferior tibiofibular ligament (AITFL) (Figs. 2 and 5). There is an anatomical variant called the accessory anterior inferior tibiofibular ligament (accessory AITFL or Bassett's ligament) (Fig. 5) which is a distal and separate bundle located parallel to the AITFL and attaching between tibia and fibula. This can vary in width, obliquity, and length, and pathological thickening may be seen in inversion injury which can cause pain due to impingement and minor anterior instability (Nikolopoulos et al. 2004).

In addition to the collateral ligament complexes, it is useful to understand and appreciate the retinaculae around the ankle, which reinforce the deep fascia and also prevent bowstringing of tendons. These are essentially regions of localized thickening of deep fascia and are grouped into the flexor retinaculum, the extensor retinaculum, and the peroneal retinaculum. Knowledge of the extensor retinaculum is important to appreciate the anatomy of the peroneal retinaculum.

At the dorsal aspect of the ankle and foot is the extensor retinaculum which is divided into a superior and inferior component. The superior extensor retinaculum as the name suggests is proximal, transverse, and band like, attaching across the anterior tibial crest and medial malleolus (medially) and the anterior border of fibula and anterior aspect of lateral malleolus (laterally). It contains the dorsal tendons and neurovascular structures as (from medial to lateral) tibialis anterior, extensor hallucis longus, extensor digitorum longus, the dorsalis pedis vessels, the deep peroneal nerve, and peroneus tertius (Win et al. 2022; Geppert et al. 1993).

The inferior extensor retinaculum is X or Y shaped located distally and originates as two limbs, a proximal limb from medial malleolus and a distal limb from planter aponeurosis. They run medial to lateral to converge and form a single band which attaches to the lateral aspect of the calcaneum. This also forms the anterior tarsal tunnel with the roof via the inferior extensor retinaculum and the floor from talonavicular joint and its fascia. Similar to the superior extensor retinaculum, it contains the dorsal tendons and neurovascular structures as (from medial to lateral) tibialis anterior, the dorsalis pedis vessels, the deep peroneal nerve, extensor hallucis longus, extensor digitorum longus, and peroneus tertius (Win et al. 2022).

The traversing lateral tendons (Fig. 7) include the peroneus longus and brevis which pass through the peroneal retinaculum, posterior to the

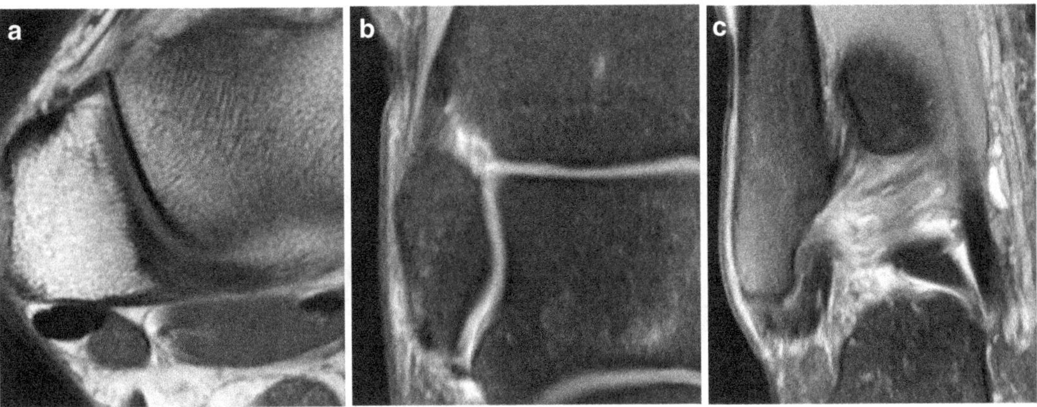

Fig. 4 Ankle syndesmosis complex. (**a**) Axial T2W image, (**b**) Coronal STIR, (**c**) Coronal STIR

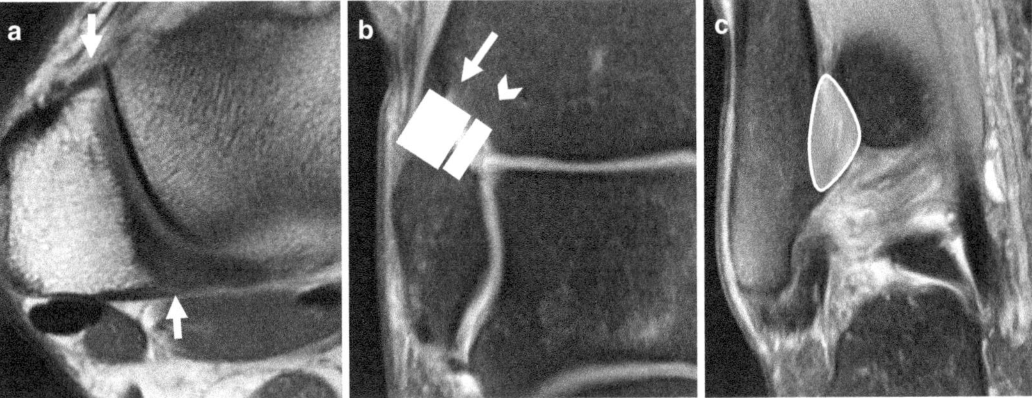

Fig. 5 Ankle syndesmosis complex. (**a**) Arrow = AITFL, Arrowhead = PITFL, (**b**) Arrow = AITFL, Arrowhead = Basset's, (**c**) Annotated = Interosseous

lateral malleolus. The peroneal retinaculum (Fig. 8) is also divided into a superior and inferior component. The superior peroneal retinaculum attaches across the lateral malleolus and lateral aspect of calcaneum and deep fascia of leg. The inferior peroneal retinaculum is essentially a continuation of the inferior extensor retinaculum (see above) which extends posteriorly and laterally to attach to the lateral aspect of the calcaneum. In a cadaveric study, a superior band inserting onto anterior aspect of Achilles tendon and an inferior band inserting into peroneal tubercle of calcaneal has been described (Geppert et al. 1993).

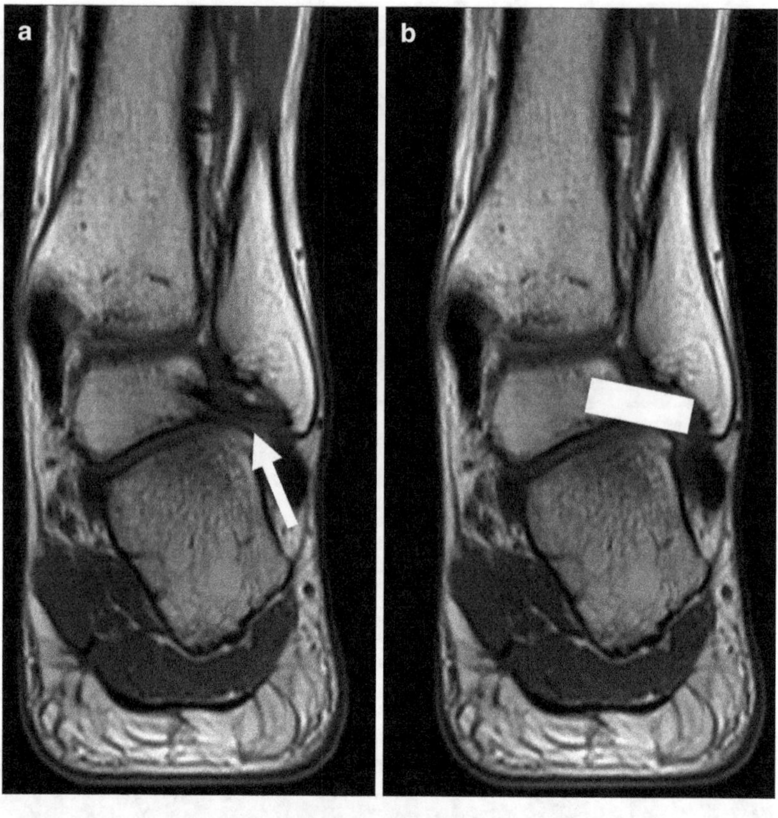

Fig. 6 (**a**, **b**) Axial T1W images demonstrating PITFL

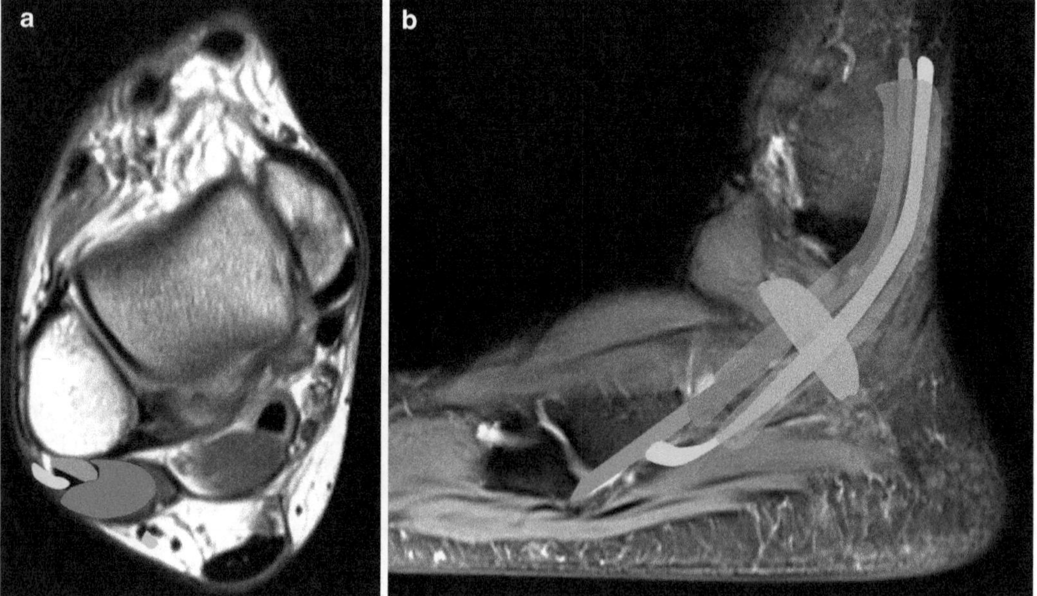

Fig. 7 Peroneal tendons. (**a**) Axial T1W image demonstrating peroneus longus tendon (green), peroneus brevis tendon (blue) and peroneus brevis muscle belly (red). (**b**) Superior peroneal retinaculum (light green), peroneal tendon sheath (orange), peroneus longus (green), peroneus brevis (blue)

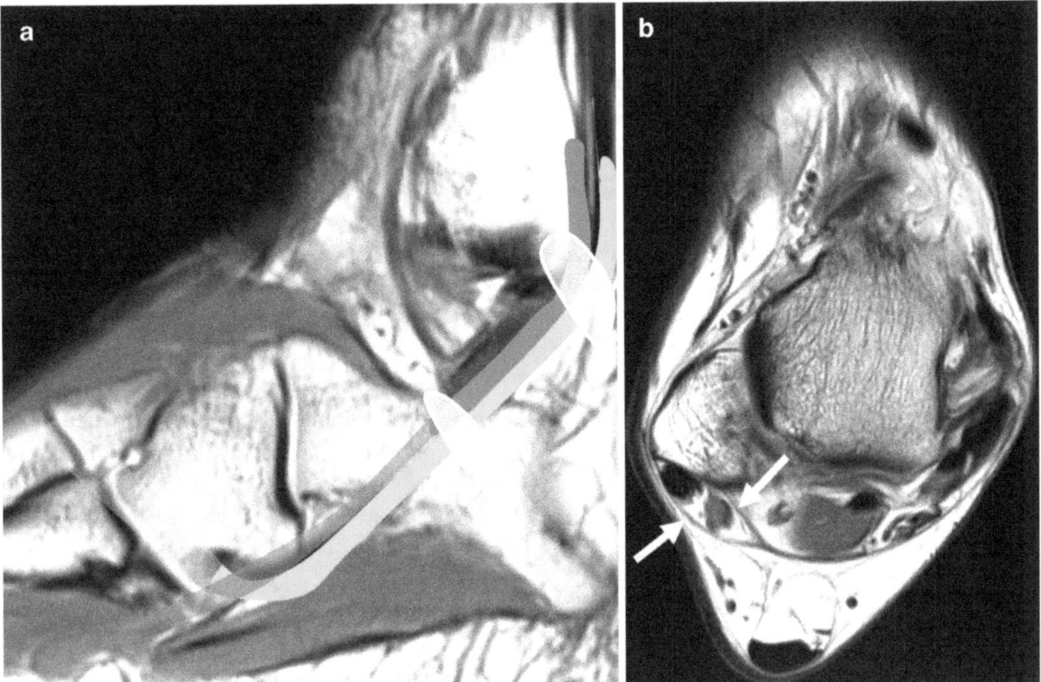

Fig. 8 Peroneal retinaculae. (**a**) Axial T1W image demonstrating peroneus longus tendon (green), peroneus brevis tendon (blue) and the superior and inferior peroneal retinacula (white). (**b**) Layers of the superior peroneal retinaculum (arrowed)

3 Imaging Tools

Assessment of the bone and soft tissue structures on imaging is the cornerstone of diagnosis of pathology, which include plain radiographs, ultrasound (USS), magnetic resonance imaging (MRI), and computer tomography (CT). Plain radiographs usually include an anteroposterior (AP) and lateral (LAT) view with a mortise view to assess the tibiotalar and tibiofibular spaces. Weight-bearing or stress radiographs may be useful for ankle sprains and suspected ligament injuries. CT imaging should include imaging reformats in axial, coronal, and sagittal planes along the axis of talus. Specifically weight-bearing CTs are being used for preoperative planning and diagnostic assessment of deformities which are not easily identified on radiographs for, e.g., valgus subtalar joint alignment in flatfoot deformity or lateral ankle instability by recreating physiological movement with weight-bearing stress (Conti and Ellis 2020).

USS is more of a dynamic study, and the position of the foot and ankle is often dependent on individual patient and operator. Linear high-frequency probes are used for assessments of ligaments and soft tissues.

It is also important to appreciate that there need to be dedicated protocols with MRI where imaging should be aligned with the axis of talus, the axial plane being parallel to long axis of talus and the coronal plane being perpendicular to it. Ideally T1 axial and coronal sequences along with three plane fluid sensitive sequences should be obtained with a 12–14 cm field of view and a dedicated ankle coil. In addition to the bone anatomy described, there are a number of soft tissue structures which include the joint capsule, ligaments, tendons, and neurovascular bundle. Table 2 summarizes the best sequences for assessment of individual lateral ankle ligaments on MRI.

When reviewing the anatomy on MRI, the magic angle artifact needs to be taken into account. This is an artifact which occurs on sequences with short time to echo (TE) for, e.g., T1W, PD, and gradient-echo sequences because of areas of tightly bound collagen, such as peroneal tendons, at 55° from main magnetic field. The result is hyperintense appearance of the structures which can be mistaken for tendon pathology and therefore its awareness can help differentiate physiological appearances from pathology. Some studies have suggested using prone body position with planter flexion of the foot instead of supine body position with neutral foot position to avoid this artifact (Mengiardi et al. 2006).

Table 2 Ligament MRI sequences

Ligament	MRI sequence
Posterior talofibular	Axial or coronal
Calcaneofibular	Axial (partially imaged) or coronal
Anterior talofibular	Axial (6–10 mm long and 2 mm thick)
Syndesmosis • Posterior inferior tibiofibular • Transverse tibiofibular • Anterior inferior tibiofibular	Axial

4 Traumatic Injuries

4.1 Ankle Fracture

Ankle fracture may include an isolated bone injury of the tibia or fibula, or injuries comprising both bones with associated ligament injuries.

Classically the Lauge-Hansen classification is a good method to predict the mechanism of injury and also to predict any associated structural damage. It also incorporates the other commonly used classification for ankle fractures which is based on whether the injury has occurred below (Weber A), at (Weber B), or above the syndesmosis (Weber C).

There are four described mechanisms (Table 3) which result in 13 injury patterns, most of which affect the lateral aspect of the ankle (Lauge-Hansen 1954; Okanobo et al. 2012; Gardner et al. 2006).

Table 3 Ankle injury patterns

Injury pattern	Stage	Injury
Supination—Adduction (SA)	1	Lateral ligament complex with or without fracture of fibula below syndesmosis
	2	Stage 1 + oblique/vertical medial malleolar fracture
Supination—External Rotation (SER)	1	Rupture of AITFL
	2	Stage 1 + oblique/spiral fracture of fibular at syndesmosis
	3	Stage 1 + 2 + Rupture of PITFL
	4	Stage 1 + 2 + 3 + Rupture of deltoid ± medial malleolus fracture
Pronation—Abduction (PAbd)	1	Deltoid rupture or medial malleolus fracture
	2	Posterior malleolus fracture
	3	Fracture of fibula above level of syndesmosis
Pronation—External Rotation (PER)	1	Deltoid rupture or medial malleolus fracture
	2	AITFL + interosseous membrane injury
	3	Fracture of fibula above level of syndesmosis
	4	Posterior malleolus or PITFL injury
	Maisonneuve	Deltoid + distal tibiofibular syndesmosis + proximal fibula

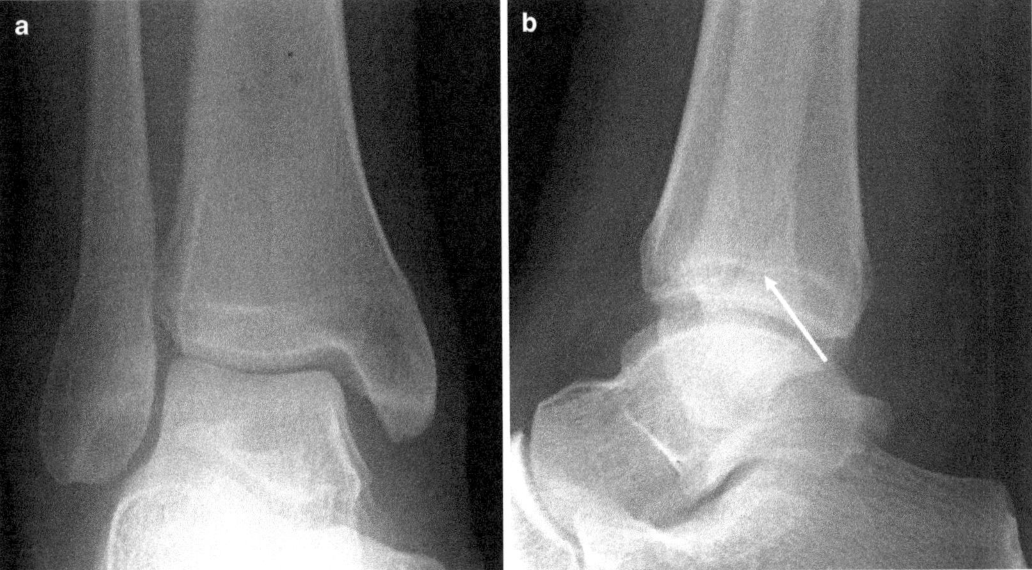

Fig. 9 Weber B ankle fracture. (**a**) Anteroposterior mortise view radiograph demonstrating subtle cortical step at the lateral border of fibula. (**b**) Lateral view radiograph confirming an oblique fracture of fibula at level of syndesmosis

- Supination-adduction
  - Stage 1: rupture of the lateral collateral ligament complex with or without avulsion fracture of lateral malleolus below syndesmosis (without medial malleolar fracture—Weber A)
  - Stage2: with oblique or vertical medial malleolar fracture
- Supination-external rotation (40–70%)
  - Stage 1: rupture/avulsion of anterior inferior tibiofibular ligament
  - Stage 2: true Weber B fracture—the talus displaces and fractures the fibula in an oblique or spiral fracture, starting at the level of syndesmosis (Fig. 9)
  - Stage 3: rupture of the posterior inferior tibiofibular ligament or fracture posterior malleolus
  - Stage 4: rupture of the deltoid ligament or transverse avulsion fracture medial malleolus
- Pronation-abduction
  - Stage 1: deltoid ligament disruption or transverse medial malleolus fracture
  - Stage 2: posterior malleolus fracture
  - Stage 3: oblique fibular fracture above level of syndesmosis (Weber C)
- Pronation-external rotation
  - Stage 1: deltoid ligament rupture or transverse avulsion fracture of the medial malleolus
  - Stage 2: involvement of the anterior inferior tibiofibular ligament with extension into the interosseous membrane results in widening of the distal tibiofibular distance
  - Stage 3: a spiral or oblique fibular fracture above level of syndesmosis (Weber C)
  - Stage 4: involvement of the posterior inferior tibiofibular ligament (PITFL) or posterior malleolus fracture
  - Maisonneuve fracture is a special type of pronation-external rotation injury with lig-

amentous component including the deltoid ligament, distal tibiofibular syndesmosis as well as the proximal fibula.

It is important to appreciate each of these stages to evaluate the described potentially injured structures and request further imaging, for, e.g., on a plain radiograph of the ankle, the only abnormality maybe a widening of the medial tibiotalar space which would miss a proximal fibula fracture in case of a Maisonneuve fracture. Therefore, a radiologist suspecting the same based on clinical information and radiographic appearance may suggest a knee radiograph to assess the proximal tibiofibular joint. Supination-adduction stage 2, supination-external rotation stages 3 and 4, and pronation-external rotation stage 3 and 4 are generally considered to be unstable injuries requiring stabilization and fixation.

CT is very useful for assessment and involvement of articular surfaces and also for identifying intra-articular bone fragments in comminuted fractures. Nowadays with readily available radiology software, surgeons prefer 3D reconstruction models to help with preoperative planning. Furthermore careful assessment with a good understanding of anatomy may also predict ligament injuries from avulsion osseus flakes at or in vicinity of ligament attachment sites.

USS and MRI are both excellent modalities for assessment of soft tissues and ligaments, although in the acute setting USS maybe limited with caveats of swelling and cast.

MRI is highly sensitive for detecting occult fractures and osteochondral defects. One such fracture is the lateral talus process fracture also known as the "Snowboarder's talus fracture" which if missed can result in adverse consequences such as non-union and chronic pain. Posterior process of talus fracture is rare but also easily missed as it is confused with an os trigonum. MRI is the definitive test for differentiation between the two.

4.2 Lateral Ligament Complex Injury

Classically occurs with supination-adduction in a planter flexed foot. One of the commonest injury in sports is an inversion sprain with ATFL being the most commonly injured ligament (up to 95%) and in ~20% the CFL is also injured. The PTFL is only ever injured in a dislocation of the ankle joint being the least commonly sprained (Hertel 2002).

On plain radiographs, lateral ligament complex injury can be predicted with an avulsion flake of bone adjacent to the tip of the lateral malleolus. Similarly on CT scan undertaken for ankle fractures ligament, injuries can be predicted from avulsion osseous fragments at ligament attachment sites. Soft tissue windows (Width: 400 Center:40) can be used to evaluate ligaments, traversing tendons and the neurovascular bundle, and any osseous fragments in close proximity of vital structures.

USS can comfortably and effectively diagnose ligament discontinuity, laxity, or thickening. Stress USS can further improve diagnosis over regular USS especially in chronic cases.

MRI (Figs. 10, 11, and 12) is very accurate particularly in the diagnosis of ATFL and CFL, although the appearances of PTFL (Fig. 10) can be confusing due to its inhomogeneous signal from its thickness and fat tissue located between ligament fibers. A useful finding with MRI is the appearances of a previously ruptured but now healed ligament demonstrating thickening and continuity while incompetent ligaments demonstrate elongation, thinning, waviness, or complete discontinuity.

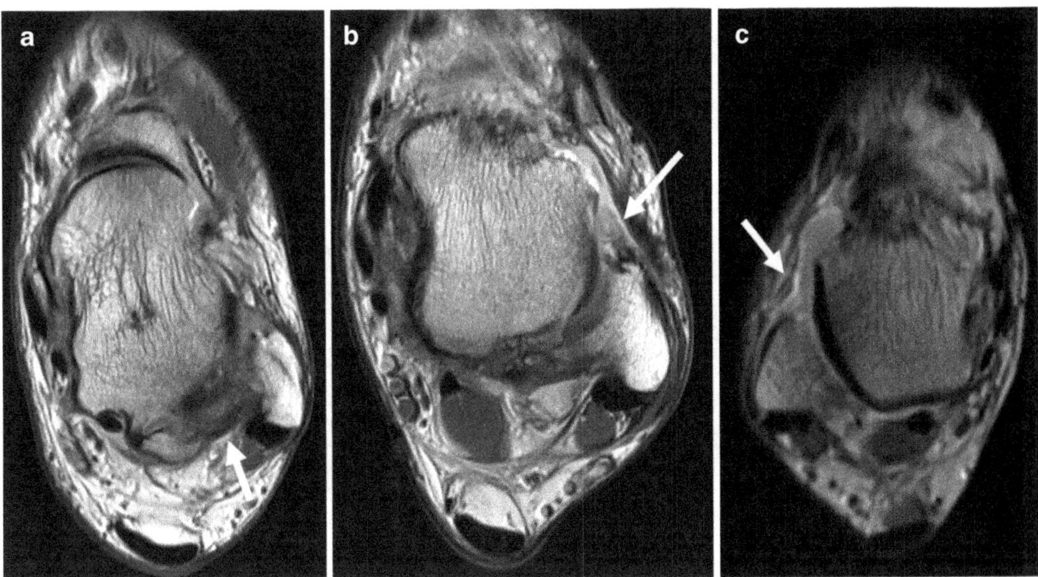

Fig. 10 Axial MRI sequences. (**a**) Arrow = PTFL tear, torn ATFL visible anteriorly, (**b**) ATFL tear from talar attachment with scarring, (**c**) ATFL tear

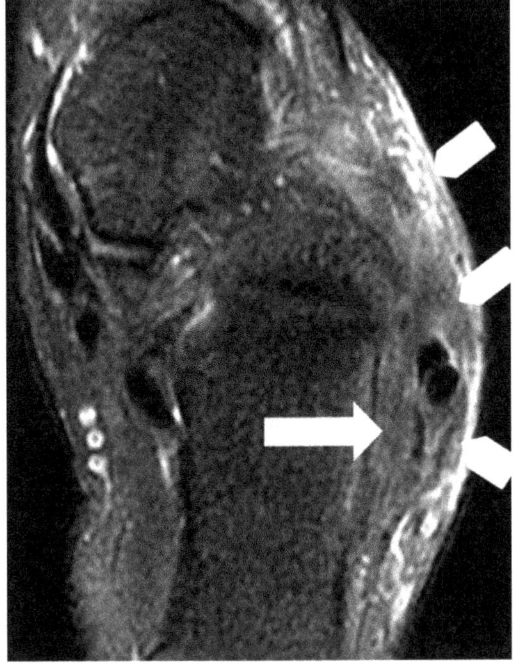

Fig. 11 High-grade CFL injury (arrows and arrowhead delineate edematous and indistinct CFL)

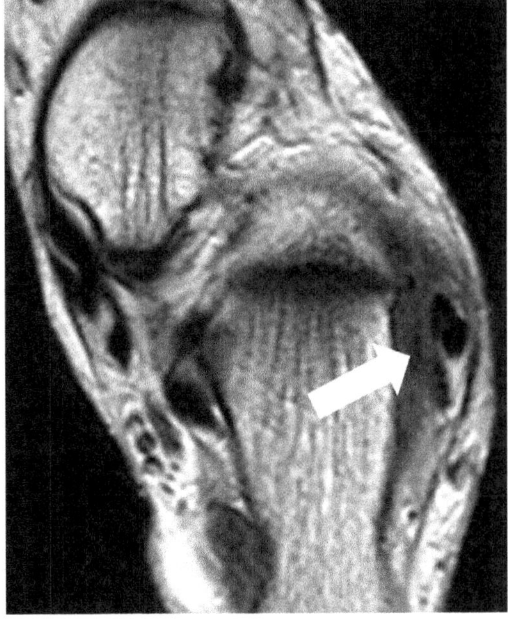

Fig. 12 Axial T1W sequence demonstrating high-grade CFL injury

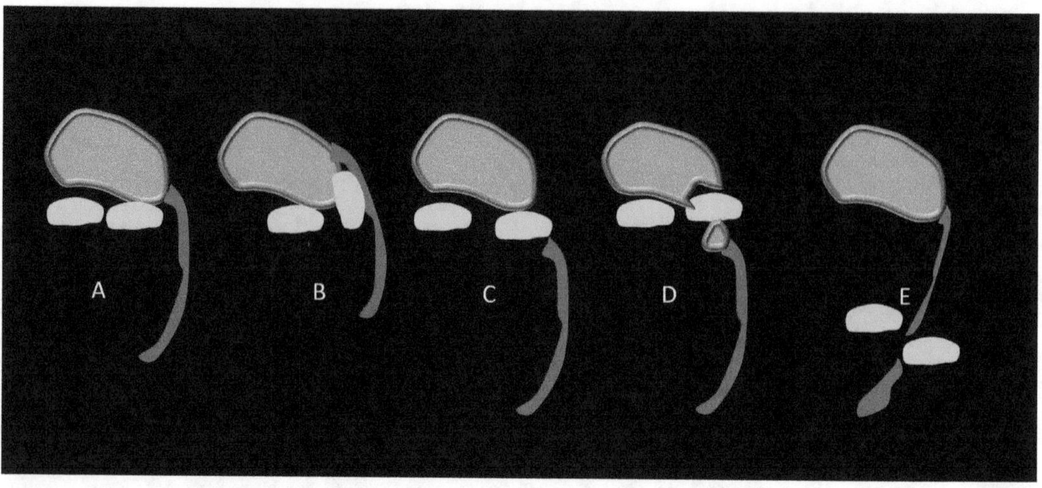

Fig. 13 Oden's classification of superior peroneal retinaculum injuries. Normal (A), Type 1 (B), Type 2 (C), Type 3 (D), Type 4 (E). Peroneus longus (PL), peroneus brevis (PB), fibula (F), superior peroneal retinaculum (red)

4.3 Peroneal Retinaculum Injury

This can be acute or chronic. Oden's classification grades the injuries into four types (Fig. 13): elevation of the periosteal attachment at level of fibular groove of lateral malleolus (type 1), tear of the distal fibular attachment (type 2), avulsion fracture at its attachment on lateral malleolus (type 3), and tear of posterior attachment (type 4).

Plain radiographs may demonstrate an avulsed osseous fragment in type 3 injuries (lateral to lateral malleolus).

Dynamic USS in resisted eversion and dorsiflexion may demonstrate subluxation of peroneal tendons in complete rupture of the retinaculum. MRI is sensitive and can diagnose injury in cases where the tendons do not explicitly sublux and remain within the retrofibular groove. What happens in these cases is that the peroneal tendon's relationship changes with respect to each other and the peroneus longus comes posterior (deep) to peroneus brevis (type A), or the peroneus brevis splits longitudinally with the peroneus longus subluxes anteriorly through the split giving the pseudo appearance of three tendons (Choudhary and McNally 2011).

5 Impingement

5.1 Anterolateral Impingement

This usually refers to pain from a synovial mass in the anterolateral gutter (Figs. 14 and 15), which is a potential space demarcated by tibia (medially), fibula (laterally), ATFL and AITFL (anteriorly), distal tibiofibular syndesmosis (superiorly), and CFL (inferiorly). Normally physiological joint fluid is present in this space, however injury to ATFL (±AITFL), capsule, usually in young athletic patient results in enthesopathy, thickening or thinning of the ligament/s with resultant synovial hyperplasia, scarring and formation of an inflammatory synovial mass which causes pain and impingement. The mass has been referred to as a "meniscoid lesion" (Donovan and Rosenberg 2010).

On MRI, a soft tissue mass with abnormal synovium can be seen as low T1 and low or intermediate T2 signal. USS may demonstrate the ligament abnormality and bone spurs (Choudhary and McNally 2011).

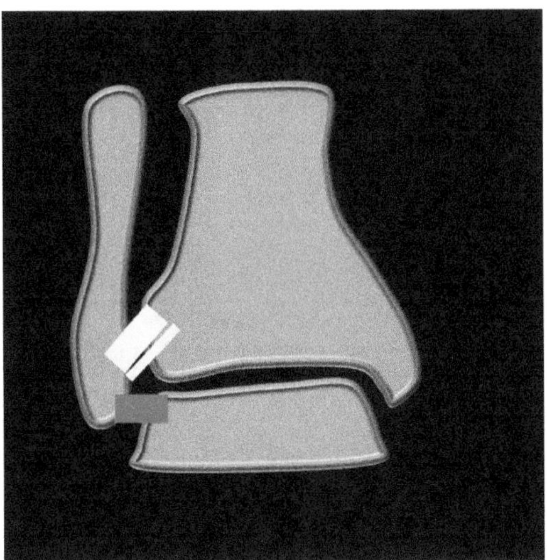

Fig. 14 Schematic diagram demonstrating the anterolateral gutter with marked AITFL (yellow) and ATFL (red)

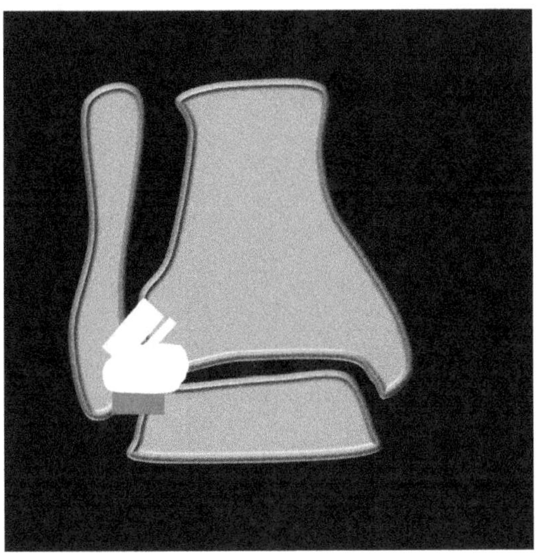

Fig. 15 Anterolateral gutter with synovial mass (meniscoid lesion)

5.2 Posterolateral Impingement

Occurs with plantar flexion activities for, e.g., ballet dancers and gymnasts, the cause being hypertrophy or tear of the PITFL or TTFL. Synovitis, capsulitis, and fibrosis of the ligaments may also result in posterolateral impingement.

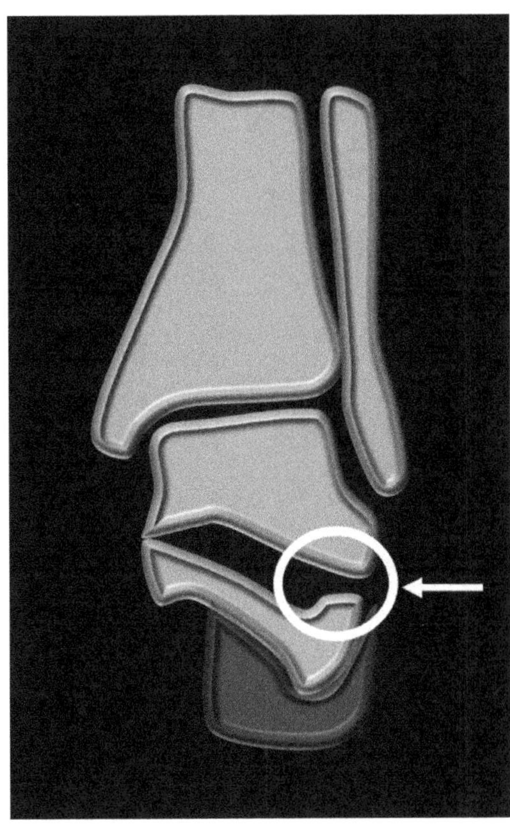

Fig. 16 Lateral impingement involves the osseous structures at the junction of the posterior STJ and the sinus tarsi. In the normal hindfoot, there is no osseous contact between the lateral talar process and calcaneum

USS examination can demonstrate fluid and synovitis with thickening of the ligaments, as well as ganglion cysts. MRI findings are similar (Choudhary and McNally 2011).

5.3 Lateral Impingement

Two types have been commonly described as subfibular impingement and talocalcaneal impingement (Figs. 16, 17, 18, 19, 20, 21, and 22). These present with flatfoot and hind foot valgus deformity and resultant extra-articular impingement from shifting of weight-bearing load frit lar dome to lateral talus and fibula, which can also result in talocalcaneal joint subluxation (Donovan and Rosenberg 2010).

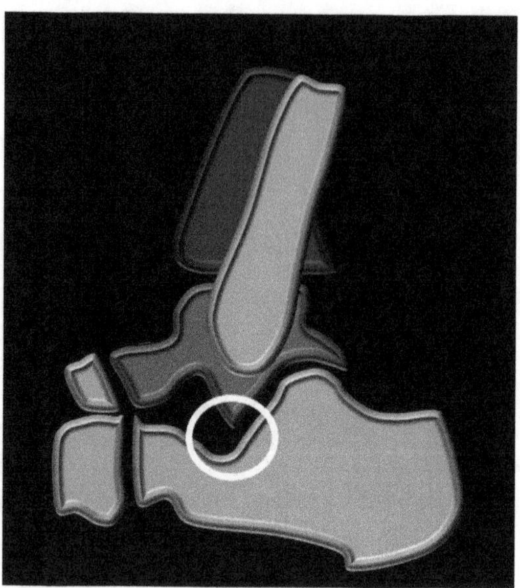

Fig. 17 Lateral impingement involves the osseous structures at the junction of the posterior STJ and the sinus tarsi. In the normal hindfoot, there is no osseous contact between the lateral talar process and calcaneum

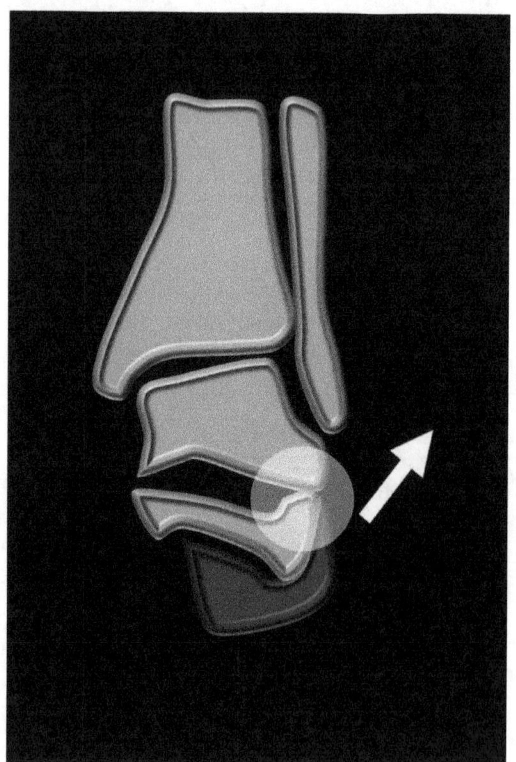

Fig. 18 Mild hindfoot valgus

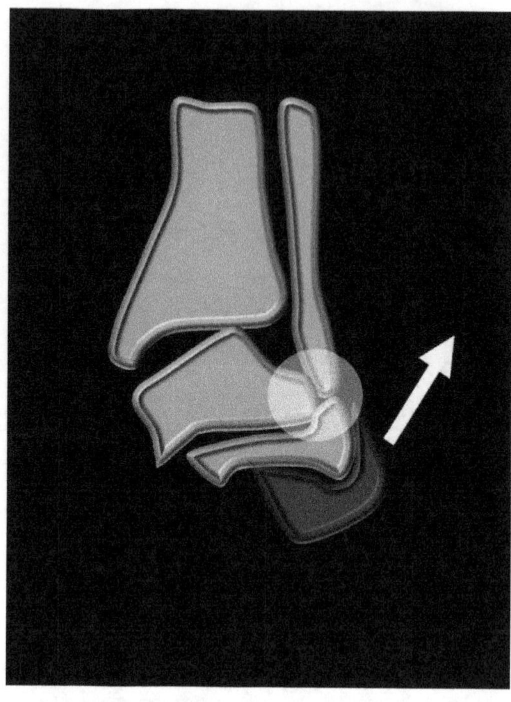

Fig. 19 Severe hindfoot valgus

Plain radiograph may help with assessment of medial arch and valgus deformity; however, CT is more sensitive for detecting sclerosis and/or cystic changes. MRI is very helpful in detecting early impingement with bone edema, as well as other causes for pain for, e.g., lateral malleolar bursitis or distal fibula stress fracture.

5.4 Sinus Tarsi Syndrome

Seen in athletes such as volleyball and basketball players or overweight patients, it results from inflammation within the synovial layers of sinus tarsi, which is a tunnel on the lateral side formed by the talus and calcaneum. It contains interosseous talocalcaneal ligaments, fat, and medial origin of the inferior extensor retinaculum.

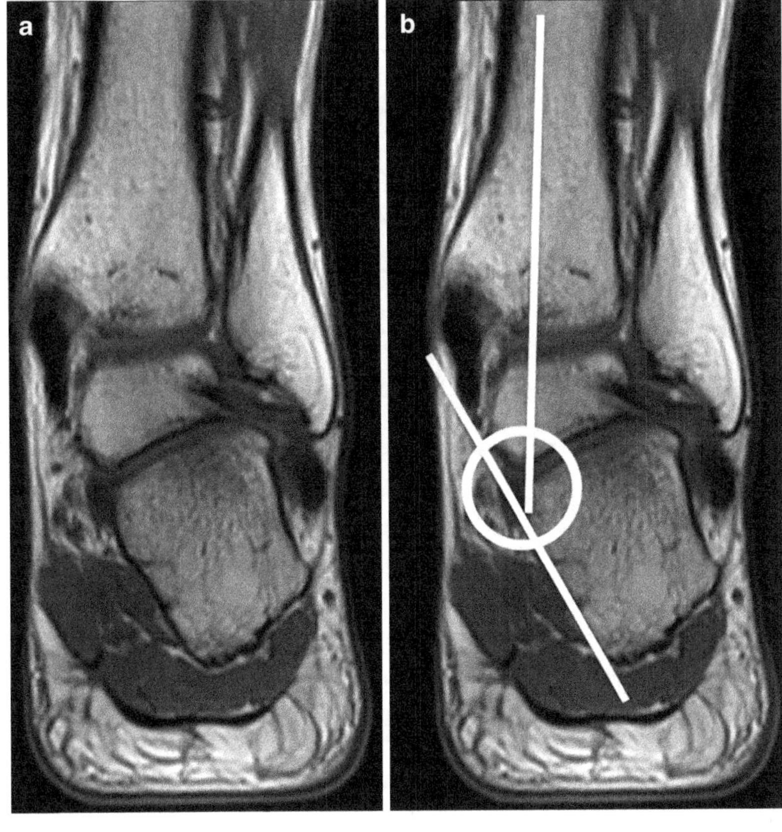

Fig. 20 Coronal T1W images. (**a**) With increased hindfoot valgus angle, (**b**) ankle marked

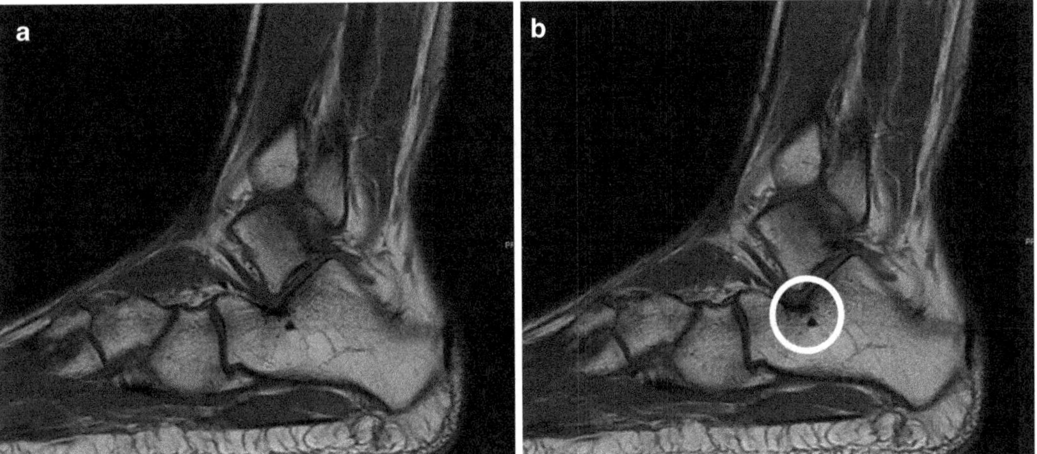

Fig. 21 Sagittal T1W images. (**a**) Demonstrating impingement with sclerosis at angle of Gissane, (**b**) area of sclerosis circled

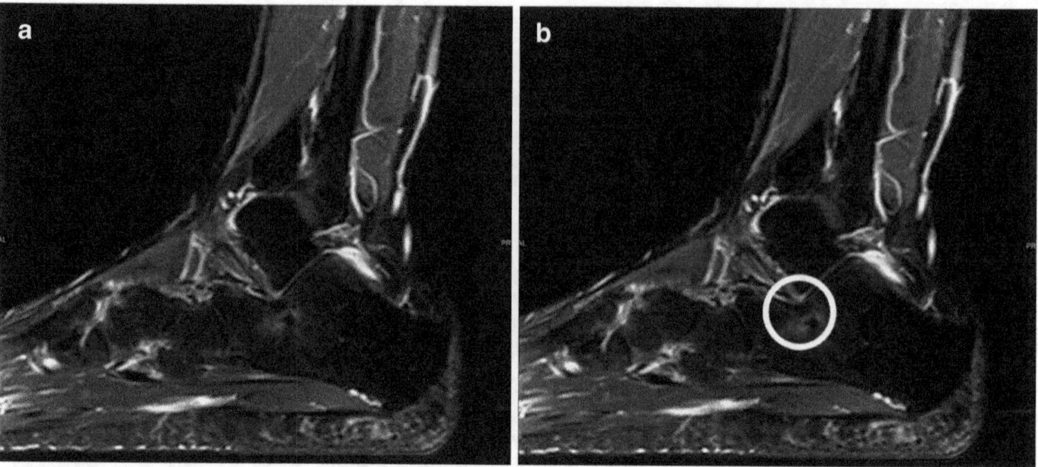

Fig. 22 Sagittal STIR images. (**a**) Demonstrating impingement with oedema at angle of Gissane, (**b**) area of oedema circled

Cause of pain is mainly secondary to trauma secondary to ankle sprains, with other causes being inflammatory arthritis or ganglion cysts. Additional causes include lateral or posterolateral ankle impingement.

CT may demonstrate early bone changes for, e.g., arthritis of the subtalar joint and intraosseous cysts.

On MRI, the fat demonstrates decreased intensity on T1- and T2-weighted sequences, which is a sequelae of fibrosis. Ruptured ligaments can also be seen (Choudhary and McNally 2011).

6 Miscellaneous Syndromes and Other Causes

6.1 Peroneal Tendon Syndrome

Three entities have been described in this syndrome as peroneal tendon subluxation (Fig. 23), peroneal tendonitis (Fig. 24), and peroneal tendon tears. With high impact activities, sudden contraction can result in acute tear of the peroneal tendons. These can be associated with peroneal retinaculum injuries. Attrition longitudinal tears can happen from friction over posterolateral fibula or from chronic subluxation (Fig. 23). The latter can result in tendinitis. Other causes of chronic subluxation include lateral ankle instability, anatomical deformities of the retro-malleolar groove, or abnormal hind foot alignment. Peroneal tendon tenosynovitis can happen at the lateral aspect of the calcaneum where the tendons share a common synovial sheath with individual sheaths further distally at level of peroneal tubercle of calcaneum. Enlarged peroneal tubercle (Figs. 25 and 26), trauma with resultant injury to os peroneum with callous formation can all cause stenosing tenosynovitis of the peroneus longus tendon (Palmanovich et al. 2020).

On USS and MRI, the findings would include fluid around the tendons, thickening, discontinuity, as well as subluxation on dynamic studies.

6.2 Peroneus Quartus Syndrome

Peroneus quartus (Figs. 27, 28, 29, 30, and 31) is an accessory muscle that often originates from peroneus brevis muscle and can be seen posteromedial to it with a fat plane separating the two distally. It attaches at the retro-trochlear eminence at the lateral surface of calcaneum (Walt and Massey 2022; Cheung 2017). It is the commonest tendon variant of the ankle and foot and associated hypertrophied peroneal tubercle (Choudhary and McNally 2011). It can cause peroneus brevis tears and subluxation by narrowing the retro-malleolar groove. Knowledge of this

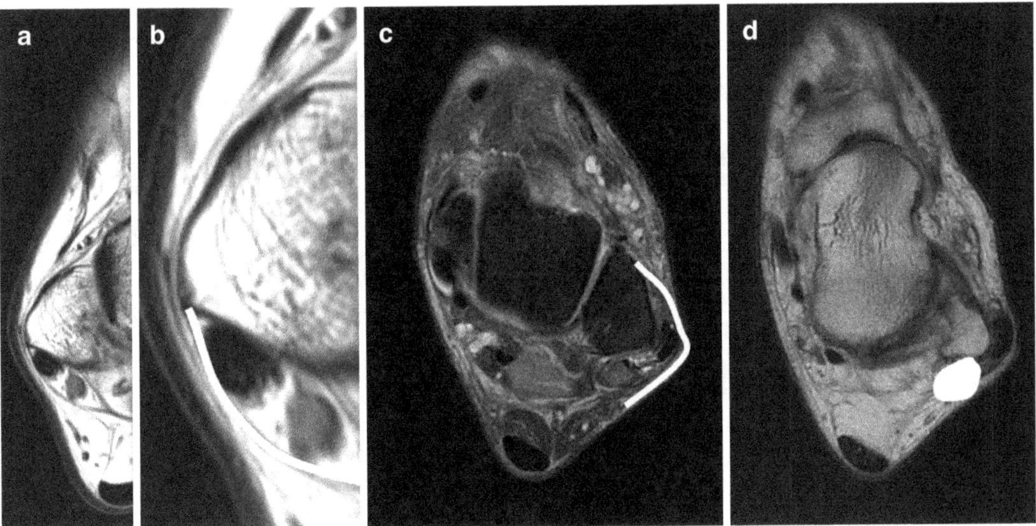

Fig. 23 Axial MRI images demonstrating peroneal tendon subluxation. (**a**) and (**b**) Peroneal retinaculum marked with normal position of the peroneal tendons, (**c**) peroneal retinaculum marked with subluxed peroneal tendons, (**d**) subluxed peroneal tendons with their expected normal position annotated (white)

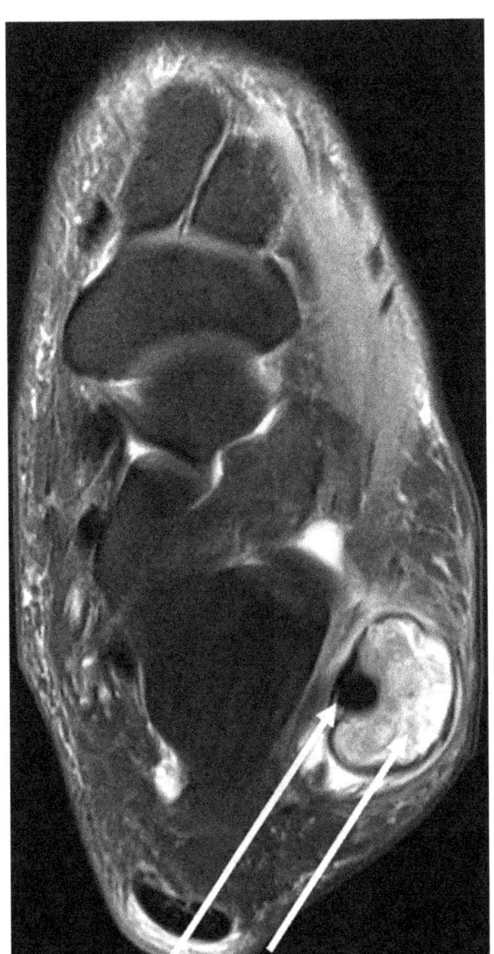

Fig. 24 Peroneal tendonitis

variant is also useful as it can be used in reconstructive surgery.

6.3 Os Peroneum Syndrome

Os peroneum is an accessory bone and common anatomical variant located within the tendon of the peroneus longus in vicinity of the cuboid bone. Its symptomatic presentation, also known as the painful os peroneum syndrome (POPS), can be secondary to acute fracture, diastases of a multipartite os peroneum or old fracture with callous causing irritation, inflammation, and resultant tenosynovitis (Choudhary and McNally 2011). Other complications include partial or complete rupture of the peroneus longus tendon, or entrapment of the peroneus longus muscle ± os peroneum in cases of a large peroneal tubercle at calcaneum.

6.4 Cubital Tunnel Syndrome

The peroneus longus tendon after its course at the lateral aspect of the ankle travels into the planter aspect of the foot to insert at medial cuneiform and base of first metatarsal. During its course, it is intimately related to the cuboid bone within a fibro-osseous tunnel.

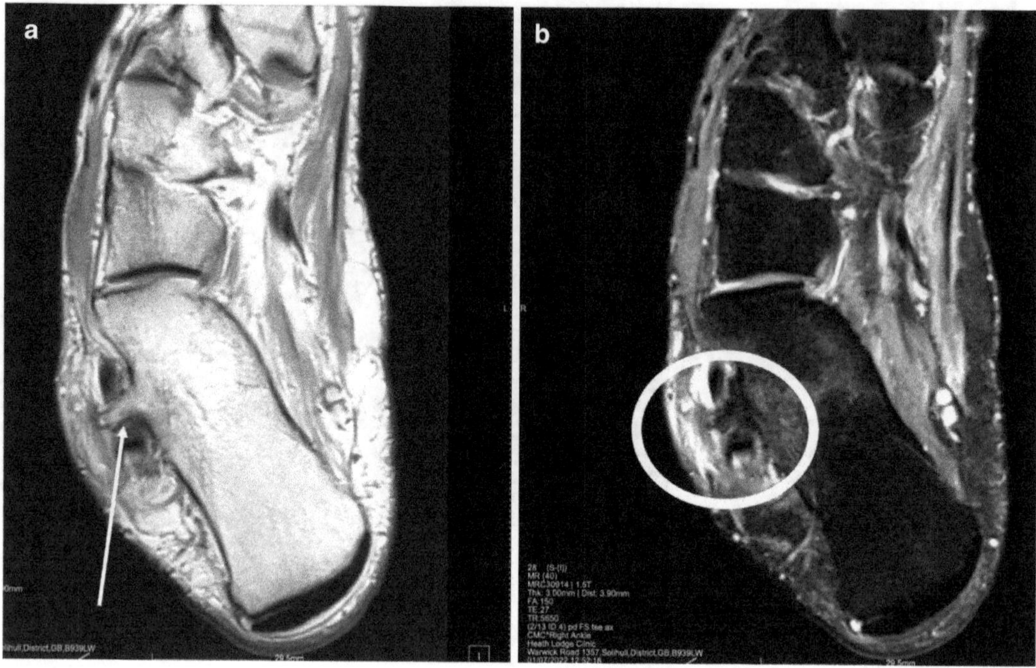

Fig. 25 Enlarged peroneal tubercle. (**a**) Axial proton density (PD) image demonstrating peroneal tubercle (arrowed). (**b**) Axial STIR images demonstrating enlarged peroneal tubercle (circled)

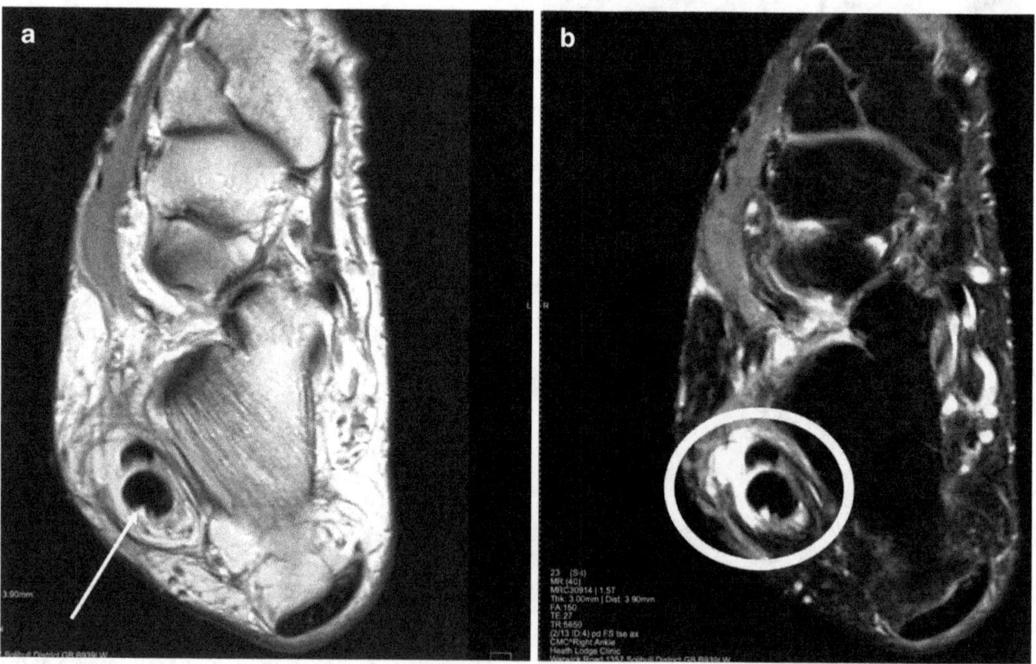

Fig. 26 Same patient as in figure 25 with enlarged peroneal tubercle. (**a**) Axial PD image with thickened peroneus longus (arrowed) and peroneus brevis tendons and peritendinous fluid. (**b**) Axial STIR image with peritendinous fluid (circled)

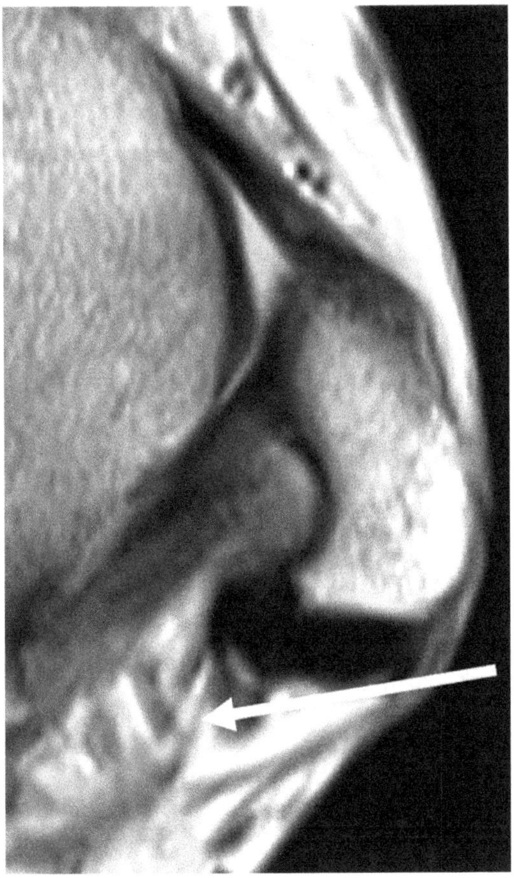

Fig. 27 Accessory peroneus muscle expected location

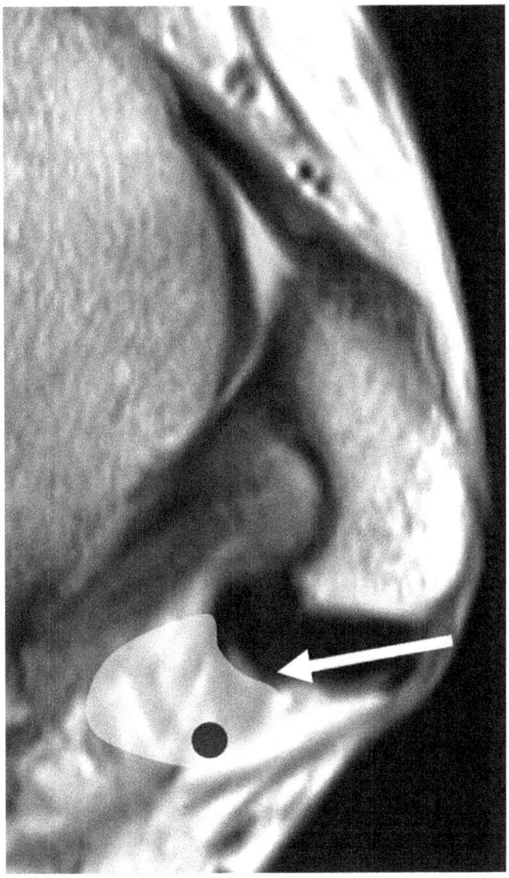

Fig. 28 Accessory peroneus muscle expected location (annotated)

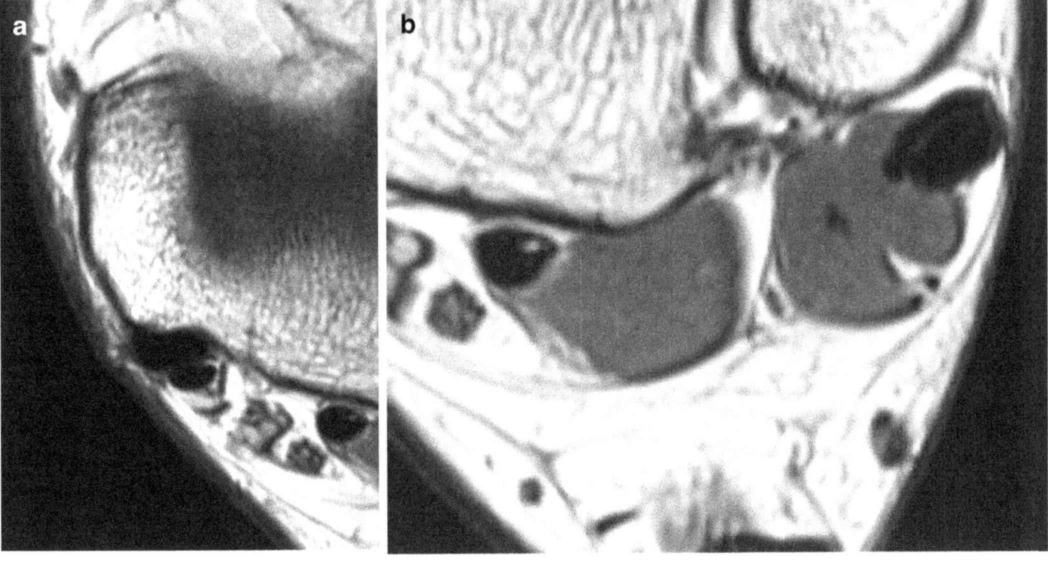

Fig. 29 Peroneus quartus. Accessory muscle seen posteromedial to peroneus brevis

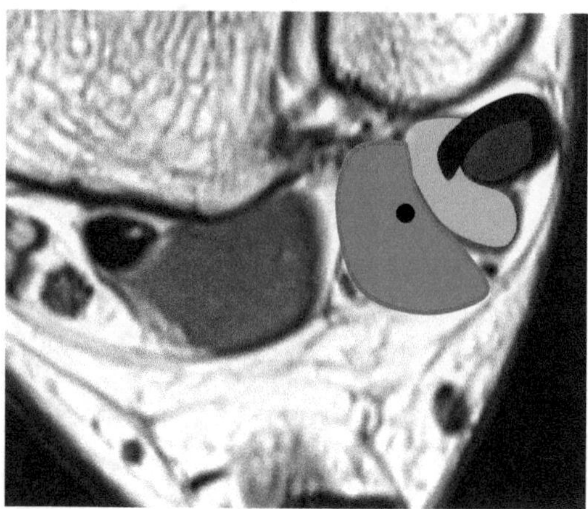

Fig. 30 Peroneus quartus annotated (red)

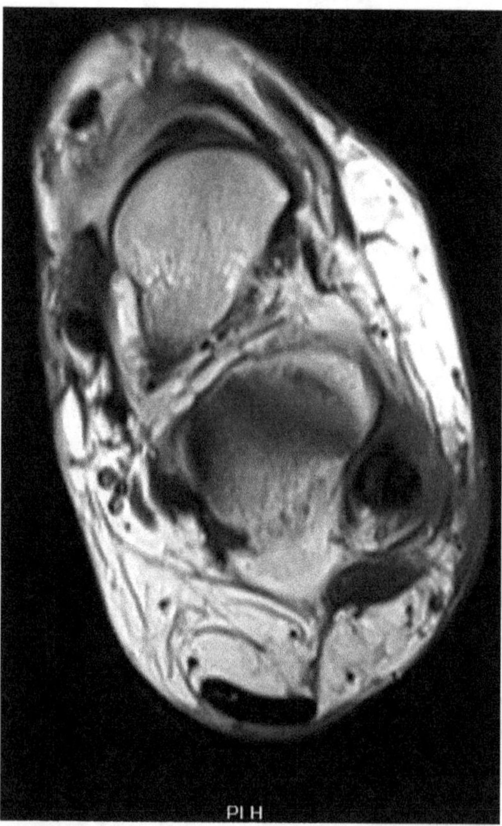

Fig. 31 Accessory peroneus muscle

Given the mechanics and the oblique course of the tendon, this is a potential site for isolated injury of this tendon, as well tendinopathy and tenosynovitis. Additionally there maybe edema of the cuboid, with erosions and/or periosteal reaction. MRI is the best modality for assessment (Figs. 32 and 33).

Furthermore, there is a spectrum of local and systemic pathologies which can result in symptomatic ankle presentations clinically. These are not entirely specific to the ankle and share similar imaging features when found elsewhere (Table 4). They can be summarized as:

Soft Tissue Masses

- Ganglion cysts
- Giant cell tumors of tendon sheath
- Pigmented villonodular synovitis (Fig. 34)
- Nerve sheath tumors
- Neuromas for, e.g., sural nerve neuroma
- Hemangiomas
- Lipomas

Bone Lesions

- Primary lesions for, e.g., ABC, osteoid osteoma, Ewings (Figs. 35 and 36)
- Metastases
- Osteomyelitis (Fig. 37)

Joint Pathologies

- Degenerative arthritis
- Inflammatory arthritis
- Septic arthritis

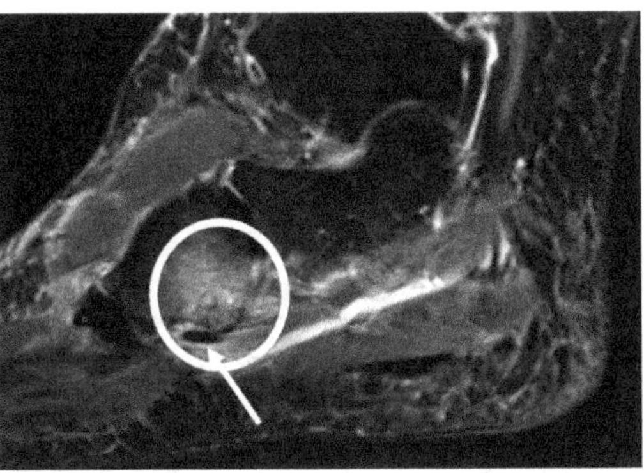

Fig. 32 Cubital tunnel syndrome. Sagittal image demonstrating bone oedema at cuboid (circled) with adjacent coursing peroneus longus tendon (arrowed)

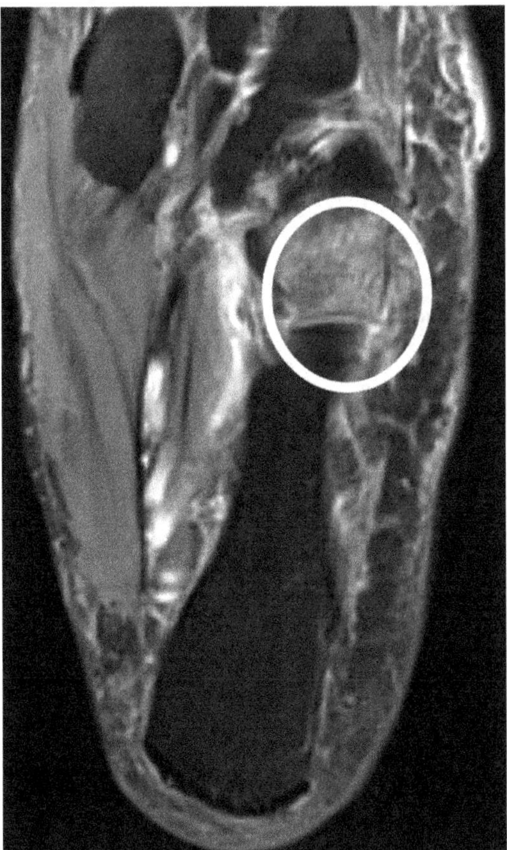

Fig. 33 Cubital tunnel syndrome. Axial image demonstrating bone oedema at cuboid (circled)

Table 4 Summary of causes of lateral ankle pain

Trauma
• Fracture
• Lateral ligament complex injury
• Peroneal retinaculum injury
Impingement
• Anterolateral
• Posterolateral
• Lateral
• Sinus tarsi syndrome
Miscellaneous syndromes
• Peroneal tendon syndrome
• Peroneus quartus syndrome
• Os peroneum syndrome
• Cubital tunnel syndrome
Soft tissue masses
• Ganglion cysts
• Giant cell tumors of tendon sheath
• Pigmented villonodular synovitis
• Nerve sheath tumors
• Neuromas for, e.g., sural nerve neuroma
• Hemangiomas
• Lipomas
Bone lesions
• Primary lesions for, e.g., ABC, osteoid osteoma, Ewings
• Metastases
• Osteomyelitis
Joint pathologies
• Degenerative arthritis
• Inflammatory arthritis
• Septic arthritis

Identification of the causative pathology is naturally dependent on good clinical history, examination, and imaging findings, some of which are unique to each pathology. Understanding of these conditions would help assist in a safe and effective patient management.

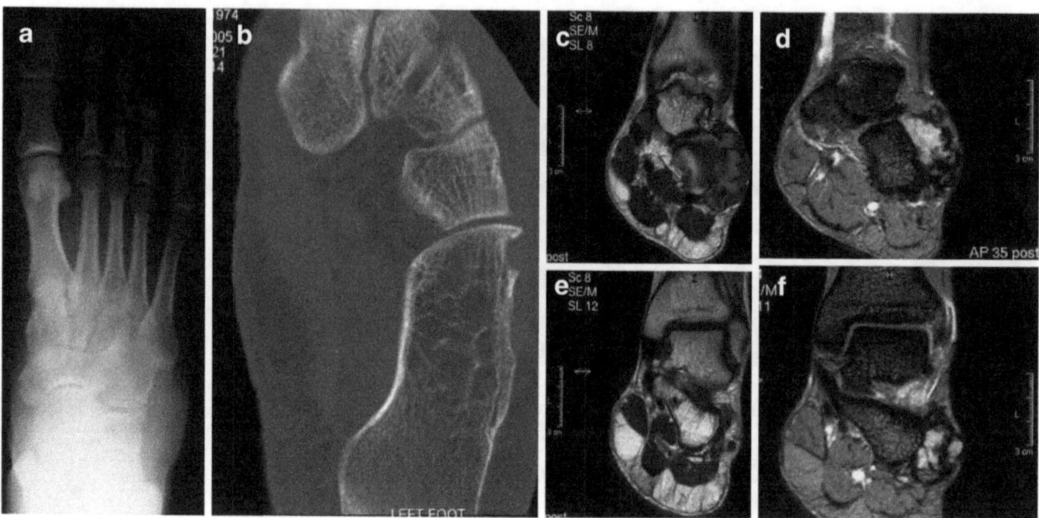

Fig. 34 PVNS. (**a**) Plain radiograph demonstrating lateral ankle soft tissue swelling. (**b**) CT scan demonstrating osseous change and soft tissue. (**c–f**) Coronal MRI images demonstrating PVNS

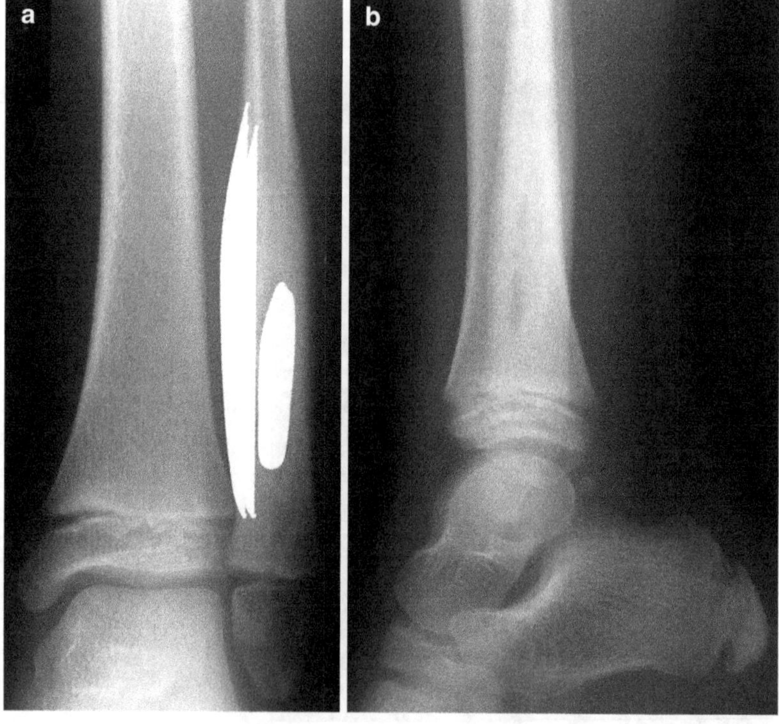

Fig. 35 Plain radiographs **a** and **b** demonstrating onion peel periosteal reaction with cortical lysis in a case of Ewings Sarcoma

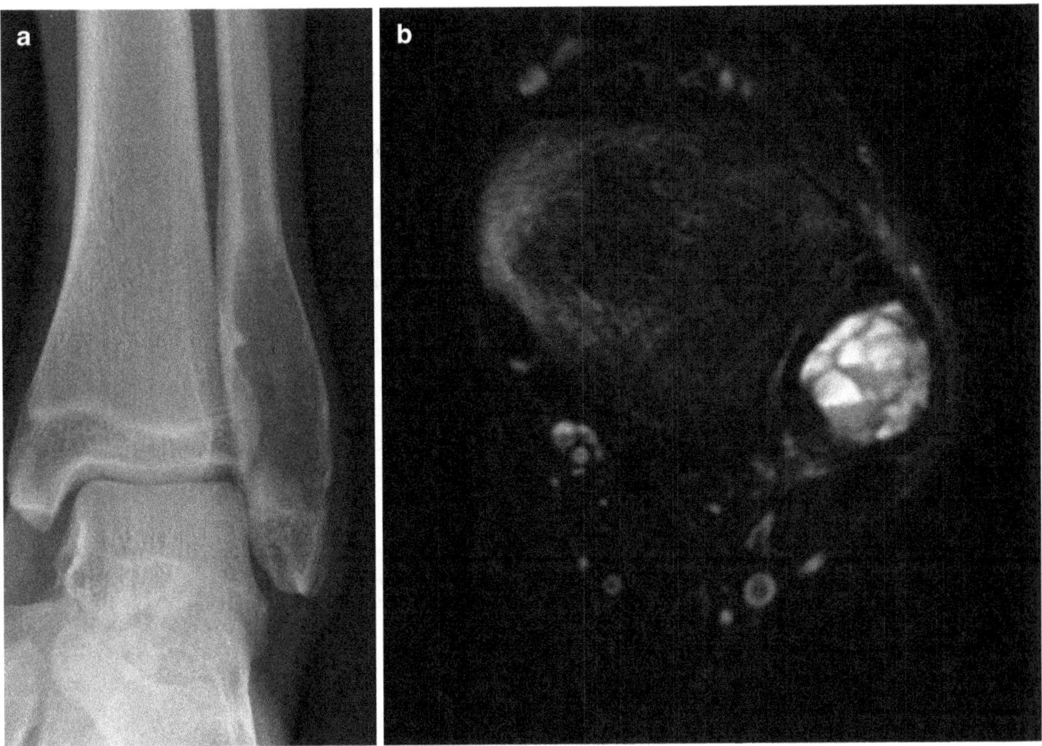

Fig. 36 (**a**) Plain radiograph demonstrating expansile lucent bone lesion. (**b**) MRI demonstrating fluid-fluid levels (ABC)

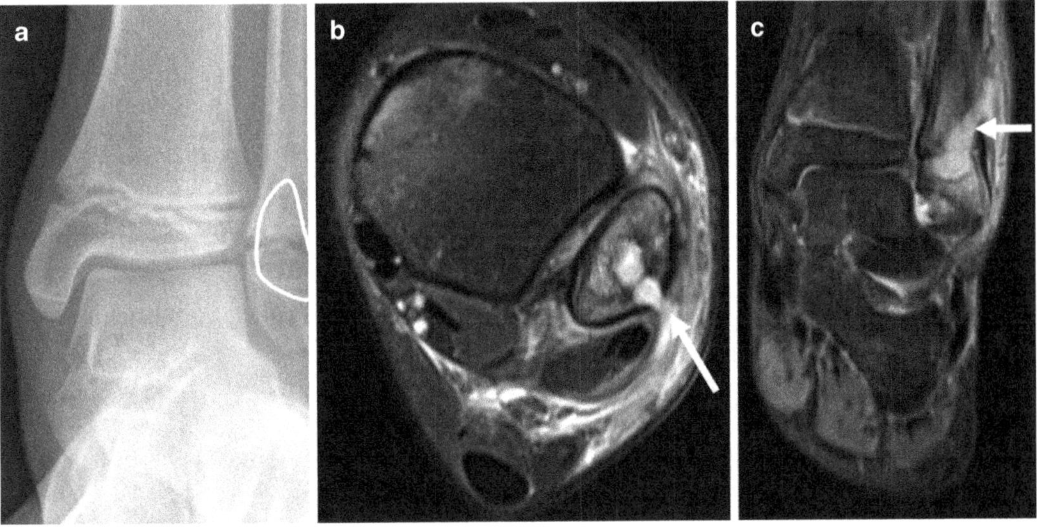

Fig. 37 Osteomyelitis. (**a**) Plain radiograph demonstrating epiphyseal lucency. (**b**) Axial MRI image demonstrating intramedullary abscess and sinus formation. (**c**) Coronal MRI image demonstrating intramedullary abscess

Key: *ATFL* anterior talofibular ligament, *AITFL* anterior inferior tibiofibular ligament, *PITFL* posterior inferior tibiofibular ligament, *CFL* calcaneofibular ligament, *AP* anteroposterior, *LAT* lateral, *PTFL* posterior talofibular ligament, *STJ* subtalar joint, *PVNS* pigmented villonodular synovitis.

References

Cheung Y (2017) Normal variants: accessory muscles about the ankle. Magn Reson Imaging Clin N Am 25(1):11–26. https://doi.org/10.1016/j.mric.2016.08.002. PMID: 27888843

Choudhary S, McNally E (2011) Review of common and unusual causes of lateral ankle pain. Skelet Radiol 40(11):1399–1413. https://doi.org/10.1007/s00256-010-1040-z. Epub 2010 Oct 24. PMID: 20972871

Conti MS, Ellis SJ (2020) Weight-bearing CT Scans in foot and ankle surgery. J Am Acad Orthop Surg 28(14):e595–e603. https://doi.org/10.5435/JAAOS-D-19-00700. PMID: 32692095

de Asla RJ, Kozánek M, Wan L, Rubash HE, Li G (2009) Function of anterior talofibular and calcaneofibular ligaments during in-vivo motion of the ankle joint complex. J Orthop Surg Res 4:7. https://doi.org/10.1186/1749-799X-4-7. PMID: 19291289; PMCID: PMC2666648

Donovan A, Rosenberg ZS (2010) MRI of ankle and lateral hindfoot impingement syndromes. AJR Am J Roentgenol 195(3):595–604. https://doi.org/10.2214/AJR.09.4199. PMID: 20729435

Ellis H, Mahadevan V (2010) Clinical anatomy: applied anatomy for students and junior doctors, 14th edn. Wiley-Blackwell, Hoboken, NJ

Gardner MJ, Demetrakopoulos D, Briggs SM et al (2006) The ability of the Lauge-Hansen classification to predict ligament injury and mechanism in ankle fractures: an MRI study. J Orthop Trauma 20(4):267–272

Geppert MJ, Sobel M, Bohne WH (1993) Lateral ankle instability as a cause of superior peroneal retinacular laxity: an anatomic and biomechanical study of cadaveric feet. Foot Ankle 14(6):330–334. https://doi.org/10.1177/107110079301400604. PMID: 8406248

Hegde G, Penakacherla N, Beale D, Botchu R (2021) Botchu-Beale accessory ligament of lateral ankle. Semin Musculoskelet Radiol. https://doi.org/10.25259/IJMSR_42_2021

Hertel J (2002) Functional anatomy, pathomechanics, and pathophysiology of lateral ankle instability. J Athl Train 37(4):364–375. PMID: 12937557; PMCID: PMC164367

Lauge-Hansen N (1954) Fractures of the ankle. III. Genetic roentgenologic diagnosis of fractures of the ankle. Am J Roentgenol Radium Ther Nucl Med 71(3):456–471

Le MQT, Tiu TK (2022) Calcaneofibular ligament injury. StatPearls Publishing, Treasure Island, FL. https://www.ncbi.nlm.nih.gov/books/NBK557378/

Mengiardi B, Pfirrmann CW, Schöttle PB, Bode B, Hodler J, Vienne P, Zanetti M (2006) Magic angle effect in MR imaging of ankle tendons: influence of foot positioning on prevalence and site in asymptomatic subjects and cadaveric tendons. Eur Radiol 16(10):2197–2206. https://doi.org/10.1007/s00330-006-0164-y. Epub 2006 Mar 28. PMID: 16568266

Nikolopoulos CE, Tsirikos AI, Sourmelis S, Papachristou G (2004) The accessory anteroinferior tibiofibular ligament as a cause of talar impingement: a cadaveric study. Am J Sports Med 32(2):389–395. https://doi.org/10.1177/0095399703258697

Okanobo H, Khurana B, Sheehan S, Duran-Mendicuti A, Arianjam A, Ledbetter S (2012) Simplified diagnostic algorithm for Lauge-Hansen classification of ankle injuries. Radiographics 32(2):E71–E84. https://doi.org/10.1148/rg.322115017

Palmanovich E, Nyska M, Ohana N, Vidra M, Atzmon R (2020) Stenosing tenosynovitis of the peroneal tendons along the lateral wall of the calcaneus. In: Sobel M (ed) The peroneal tendons. Springer, Cham. https://doi.org/10.1007/978-3-030-46646-6_16

Sawant YN, Sanghvi D (2018) Magnetic resonance imaging of ankle ligaments: a pictorial essay. Indian J Radiol Imaging 28(4):419–426. https://doi.org/10.4103/ijri.IJRI_77_16

Walt J, Massey P (2022) Peroneal tendon syndromes. StatPearls Publishing, Treasure Island, FL. https://www.ncbi.nlm.nih.gov/books/NBK544354/

Win K, Gillett M, Botchu R, Suokas A, Seth A, James S (2022) Asymptomatic professional footballers: prevalence of ankle retinacula injury with associated lateral ligament and tendon abnormalities. Muscles Ligaments Tendon J. https://doi.org/10.32098/mltj.03.2020.22

Compressive Neuropathies and Plantar Fascia

Violeta Vasilevska Nikodinovska
and Slavcho Ivanoski

Contents

V. Vasilevska Nikodinovska (✉)
Medical Faculty, University "Ss. Cyril and Methodius", Skopje, Macedonia

Radiology Department, University Surgical Clinic "St. Naum Ohridski", Skopje, Macedonia
e-mail: v_vasilevska@yahoo.com

S. Ivanoski
St. Erasmo Hospital for Orthopaedic Surgery and Traumatology, Ohrid, Macedonia

1 Introduction

Nerve compression neuropathies are a group of several nerve disorders associated with sensory and/or motor loss resulting from nerve compression. Peripheral neuropathies are relatively common clinical disorders, which according to the cause are classified into compressive and non-compressive neuropathies. The nerve compression/entrapment occurs at specific locations, where a nerve courses through fibromuscular or fibro-osseous tunnels or at the areas where it penetrates within the muscles. Variable anatomy of the nerves and adjacent structures may produce a spectrum of symptoms and diagnostic findings. It is critical for the radiologists to be familiar with the appearance of normal nerves on imaging modalities, the anatomy of nerve passages, the muscular innervations of the affected nerve, and imaging features of various compressive neuropathies.

Compressive neuropathy about the foot and ankle may involve any of the five major nerves: tibial, deep peroneal, superficial peroneal, sural, and saphenous nerve. Their branches may also be entrapped at various locations.

Med Radiol Diagn Imaging (2023)
https://doi.org/10.1007/174_2023_437,
Published Online: 15 July 2023

The diagnosis can be based on clinical history, and symptoms, in combination with comprehensive physical examination, and electrodiagnostic studies. Sufficient information in making an accurate diagnosis can be provided by further imaging, being used often to localize the area of nerve compression and to confirm the diagnosis. A focused clinical history and physical examination supplemented with appropriate imaging studies can guide clinicians in the diagnosis and management of compressive neuropathies (Mohile et al. 2020).

1.1 Imaging of Compressive Neuropathies

Imaging modalities should be used to identify the nerve and any bony or soft-tissue etiologies responsible for its compression. Radiologic evaluation should be performed to rule out bony and structural abnormalities, including stress fractures, bone lesions, or arthritis, which may assist in diagnosing foot deformities, whereas electrodiagnostic studies may assist in determining the exact location of the nerve compression (Patel et al. 2005). These modalities should be used in conjunction with a careful history and physical examination. High-resolution ultrasonography, using a high-frequency transducer with more than 12 MHz is a tool for the diagnosis of nerve entrapments in complex anatomical ankle and foot regions (Iborra et al. 2018; Martinoli et al. 2000; Presley et al. 2013). It allows the detection of any space-occupying lesions (Iborra et al. 2018; Martinoli et al. 2000), but also helps in performing a dynamic study or stress assessment. A problem-based approach is recommended for a more accurate diagnosis, consistent with the radiologist's awareness of the patient's symptoms, pain location, and knowledge of the common etiologies of pain sources and imaging findings (Kim et al. 2022a). Knowing the anatomic location of the pain may help to narrow the differential diagnosis. Ultrasonography allows direct visualization of the nerve, presence of focal swelling, changes in shape, and echotexture, with the symptoms correlation that is helpful in identifying the sites of abnormality (Lopez-Ben 2011). However, visualization with ultrasound can sometimes be limited in the plantar aspect of the foot because the nerves dive deep into the plantar foot muscles, or in cases with marked plantar keratosis (Martinoli et al. 2010). Extrinsic causes of entrapment, such as tenosynovitis, ganglia, soft-tissue tumors, bone and joint abnormalities, and accessory muscles, can also be diagnosed with ultrasound (Martinoli et al. 2000).

Magnetic resonance imaging (MRI) provides valuable spatial information by direct visualization of a particular nerve, capable of identifying the cause of the nerve compression, detecting space-occupying lesions, localizing pathologies within the fibro-osseous tunnels around the ankle joint, depicting the lesion extent, and relationship to the nerve and its branches (Donovan et al. 2010). MRI has the ability to demonstrate signal abnormalities within the nerve and is considered superior in delineating the associated indirect signs related to muscle denervation such as consecutive denervation edema of the affected muscles (Donovan et al. 2010). On MRI neurography, the entire pathway of the complex nerve structures can be visualized by distinguishing the nerves from adjacent structures (Ku et al. 2021).

The normal peripheral nerve on MRI is of intermediate to low signal intensity on T1-weighted MR imaging (T1WI) with its fascicular pattern on axial imaging demonstrating clustered low (relative to normal muscle) signal intensity spots of fascicles surrounded by high signal intensity connective tissue containing perineurial and epineural fat components. It is better seen in bigger-sized nerves such as sciatic and common peroneal nerves (Maravilla and Bowen 1998). Its visualization on MR imaging is limited in the small distal nerves, when small nerve fascicles are rarely visualized, due to limited spatial resolution with a large FOV and a small number of matrices (Kim et al. 2007a). On T2-weighted MR imaging (T2WI), the nerve is isointense to mildly hyperintense relative to normal muscle. Prominent nerve fascicles can have slightly higher signal intensity than surrounding perineurial and epineurial tissue, due to the endoneurial fluid (Kuntz et al. 1996). On fast spin-echo (FSE)

T2WI, epineural or perineurial fat remains bright and bright fat from the surrounding tissue can obscure pathological changes within the nerve, which usually appear bright in this sequence. Thus fat suppression (STIR or chemical fat saturation) should be used. On axial fat-saturated T2WI, T2* fat suppression 3D sequence (Kim et al. 2022b) of the nerve, the fascicles demonstrate high signal intensity spots that are embedded within low signal intensity fatty tissue.

1.2 Direct Signs for Nerve Compressive Neuropathy

Nerve size enlargement presented with focal enlargement relative to the unaffected normal segment is considered an abnormal MRI appearance (Martinoli et al. 2010). Hyperintensity of the nerve signal on T2WI is also considered abnormal, but it can be affected by variations in window levels, thus the assessment of signal intensity itself may be subjective (Spratt et al. 2002). This can be minimized in focal neuropathy, by comparison with the signal of the nearby normal segments of the nerve (Britz et al. 1996). The high signal intensity of the affected nerve can be due to changes in the blood–nerve barrier and axoplasmic flow in degeneration of the axon and nerve sheath and endoneurial/perineurial edema, but still, it is with uncertain pathogenesis (Martinoli et al. 2010; Ku et al. 2021; Kim et al. 2007a; Kuntz et al. 1996). Another finding that suggests a nerve abnormality is an altered, non-uniform fascicular patterns, such as clumping of the fascicles or an irregular size of visualized fascicles (Maravilla and Bowen 1998; Kim et al. 2022b) (Fig. 1). This is difficult to be differentiated in small nerves of the foot and ankle.

1.3 Indirect Signs for Nerve Compressive Neuropathy

Compression of nerves produces characteristic MRI findings due to muscle denervation with the muscle signal change. It suggests neurogenic edema in the subacute phase and atrophy with fatty degeneration in the chronic phase (Bendszus et al. 2002; Rodrigues et al. 2015). Even when a small nerve shows no definite abnormalities itself due to spatial resolution, and there is no evidence of a space-occupying lesion compressing the nerve, the signal and configuration changes in the muscle may suggest peripheral nerve abnormality. The muscle through which the nerve passes is never affected at the level of entrapment. Thus when the muscle is affected, the site of entrapment should be looked at more proximally.

MRI is the most sensitive method to detect the involvement of muscle tissues as compared with ultrasonography and computed tomography, and it has some advantages over electromyography (Kim et al. 2011; Farooki et al. 2001). In an acute episode of nerve entrapment on MRI, a hyperintense signal of the denervated muscle usually is seen, due to increased extracellular water content and decreased muscle fiber volume (Polak et al. 1988a, b). In acute and subacute muscle denervation at fluid-sensitive MRI sequences such as PD/T2-weighted sequences with fat suppression or STIR sequences, neurogenic muscle edema is presented with increased signal intensity (Sallomi et al. 1998) of the muscle belly innervated by a particular nerve, as compared with the normal muscle (Kim et al. 2011) (Fig. 2). Contrast enhancement of the muscle by gadolinium occurs either in the acute or subacute phase of denervation (Kim et al. 2011). The MR signal change of denervated muscle occurs as early as 4 days after a traumatic nerve injury, whereas the change in electromyography requires a longer period of 2–3 weeks for detection of denervation change. The signal intensity changes in the denervated muscles are reversible and can be normalized with re-innervation, especially in the subacute phase (West et al. 1994).

Chronic denervation, lasting for more than 1 year, leads to chronic changes in muscle manifested as muscle atrophy and subsequent irreversible fatty infiltration (Sallomi et al. 1998). MRI findings can be clearly depicted in T1-weighted images without fat suppression (Kim et al. 2022b; Brzezinski and Meyn 1977), where atrophy and fat infiltration have a homogeneous appearance in the muscle belly, with high signal intensity in the irreversible chronic phase of muscle denervation (Sallomi et al. 1998). However, when there is double or redun-

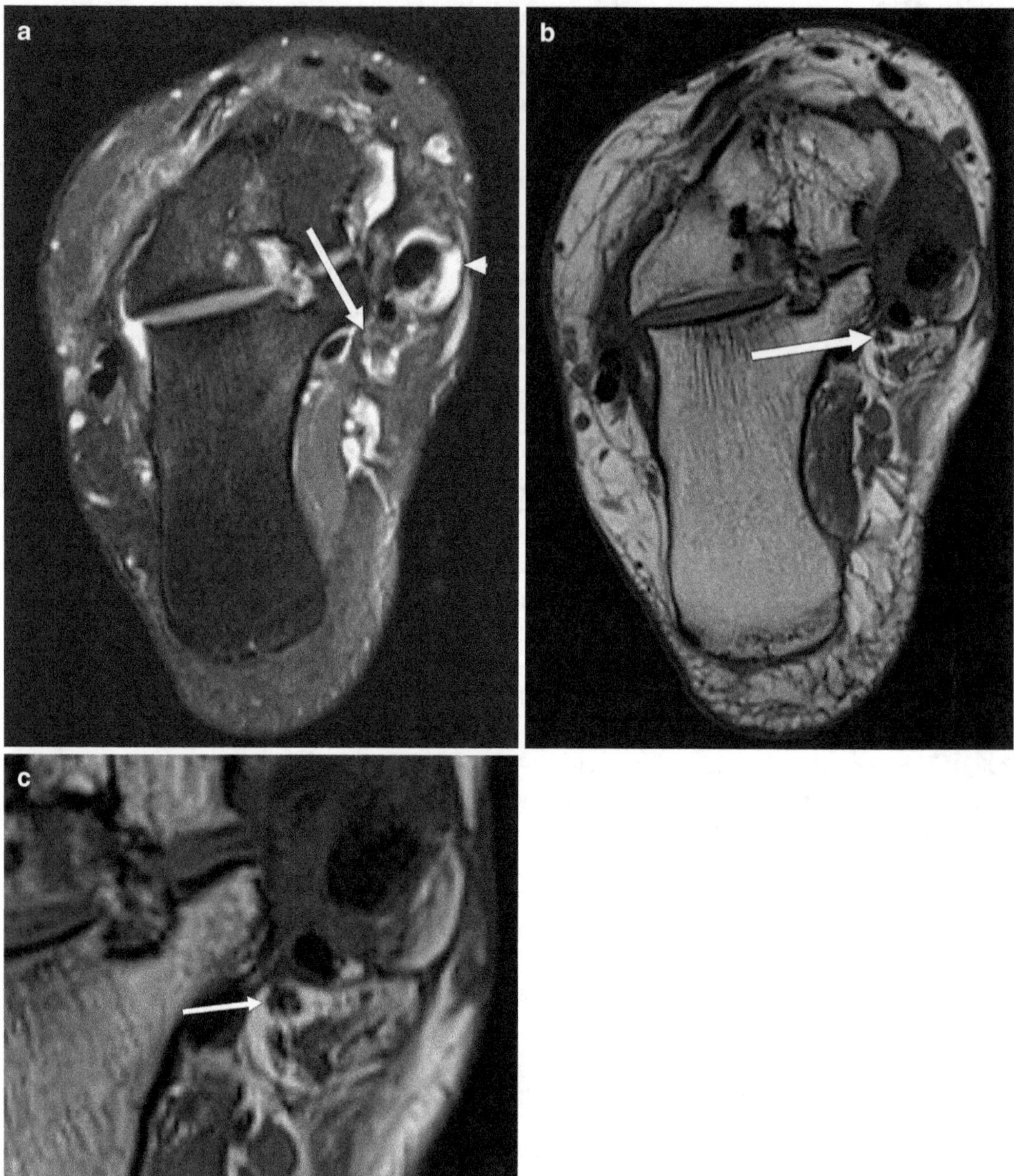

Fig. 1 Tarsal tunnel syndrome due to tenosynovitis and varices. A 37-year-old male patient with symptoms of tarsal tunnel syndrome. On axial PD, fat-suppressed (**a**), fluid is seen in the posterior tibial tendon sheath (arrowhead) with mild reactive changes posteriorly. The posterior tibial nerve is enlarged with high signal intensity (arrow) and surrounded by dilated veins from the medial-posterior aspect. There is little fluid in the flexor hallucis longus tendon sheath laterally to the nerve indicative of tenosynovitis. On T1 axial image within the enlarged nerve, the thickened fascicles can be seen (**b**, **c** arrow)

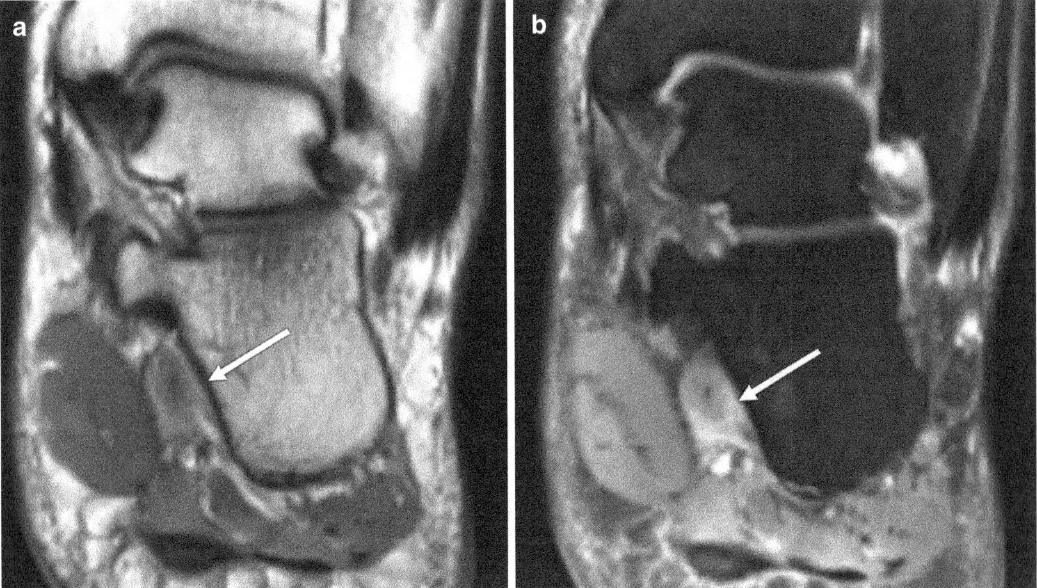

Fig. 2 Baxter's neuropathy. Coronal PD (**a**) and PDFS (**b**) showing denervation edema of quadratus plantae (arrow). (Courtesy of Rajesh Botchu)

dant innervation, then those changes may occur with heterogeneous patterns or not occur at all (Kim et al. 2011).

2 Posterior Tibial Nerve Compressive Neuropathy: Tarsal Tunnel Syndrome

Tarsal tunnel syndrome is a well-known compression neuropathy that refers to pain resulting from compression of the posterior tibial nerve and its branches as they pass through the tarsal tunnel, posterior to the medial malleolus, and medial to the talus and calcaneus. Sometimes the term tarsal tunnel syndrome implies compression of any of the major terminal branches after they leave the tarsal tunnel.

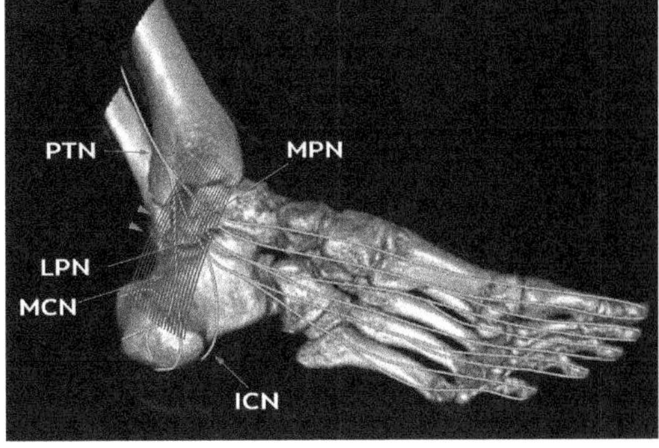

Fig. 3 Posterior tibial nerve and its branches, with their course along the ankle and foot. The posterior tibial nerve (PTN) and its branches travel within the tarsal tunnel, deep to the flexor retinaculum (arrowheads). The medial calcaneal nerve (MCN) is the first branch of the posterior tibial nerve, and then it bifurcates into medial (MPN) and lateral (LPN) plantar nerves. The first branch of the lateral plantar nerve is the inferior calcaneal nerve (ICN). At the level of metatarsal bases, the medial and lateral plantar nerves divide into interdigital nerves

The tibial nerve is a branch of the sciatic nerve. It starts near the popliteal fossa and descends into the posterior compartment of the lower leg deep to the soleus, plantaris, and gastrocnemius muscles. Posteriorly to the medial malleolus, it crosses the ankle and is named the posterior tibial nerve. Deep to the flexor retinaculum, it enters the proximal tarsal tunnel where it divides into its terminal branches: medial plantar nerve, lateral plantar nerve, and medial calcaneal nerve (Fig. 3). The bifurcation of the posterior tibial nerve can be at a very variable level, ranging from 9.6 cm proximal to 1.6 cm distal to the ankle (Brzezinski and Meyn 1977). In most cases

(95%), bifurcation of the posterior tibial nerve occurs within the tarsal tunnel, only in a small percentage of cases (5%), bifurcation occurs proximally to the tarsal tunnel (Lau and Daniels 1999; Inthasan et al. 2020).

The tarsal tunnel is a continuation of the deep posterior compartment of the lower leg into the posteromedial aspect of the ankle and medial plantar aspect of the foot. It is referred to as a fibro-osseous tunnel in the medial aspect of the ankle located posteriorly and inferiorly to the medial malleolus with a roof formed by the flexor retinaculum, which joins the medial malleolus to the calcaneus (Donovan et al. 2010), tibia as an anterior wall, and the lateral wall formed by talus and calcaneus. The wall and floor of the tarsal tunnel are formed by their own flexor sheaths, and without exposed synovium of the tibialis posterior, flexor digitorum longus, and flexor hallucis longus tendons.

The tarsal tunnel is divided into an upper compartment (tibiotalar) at the level of the ankle joint and a lower compartment, the talocalcaneal tunnel in the hindfoot, the latter considered a true anatomic tarsal tunnel (Donovan et al. 2010).

The upper tarsal tunnel is covered by deep aponeurosis. The posterior aspect of the tibia and the talus forms the osseous floor. The tendon of the tibialis posterior and flexor digitorum longus, the tendon and muscle of the flexor hallucis longus, and the posterior tibial neurovascular bundle pass through this space (Donovan et al. 2010; Hansen 2014).

The lower tarsal tunnel is covered by the flexor retinaculum (created by the fusion of the superficial and deep aponeurosis of the leg) and the abductor hallucis muscle with its fascia. The posteromedial aspect of talus, the inferomedial aspect of the navicular bone, and the medial aspects of the sustentaculum tali and calcaneus form the osseous floor (Delfaut et al. 2003) (Fig. 3). On the other hand, the distal part of the tarsal tunnel is separated into independent medial and lateral plantar tunnels by a connective tissue septum, known as medial septum (Singh and Kumar 2012), which is a dorsal extension of the medial border of the plantar aponeurosis. This septum lies between the medial calcaneus which forms the tunnel floor and the deep fascia of the abductor hallucis muscle which forms the tunnel roof. Through these tunnels, the tendons, vessels, and nerves transit their path further into the foot (Hochman and Zilberfarb 2004; Dellon 2008). The close relationship of the tibial nerve branches with the medial intermuscular septum is of greater clinical relevance since might be a possible point of nerve compression if pathological anomalies occur (Moroni et al. 2019; Ling and Kumar 2008). The vessels run superficially to the nerves inside the osteofibrous tubes (Heimkes et al. 1987), within the very limited space, with a high danger of nerve entrapment as blood vessels and the osteofibrous structures could compress the nerves (Moroni et al. 2019) (Fig. 4). Compressive neuropathy can be caused by a change in the girth of any structure that crosses these confined areas.

Tarsal tunnel syndrome (TTS) is a common entrapment syndrome whose diagnosis can be difficult and is often based on clinical history and examination. Nerve conduction and electromyographic studies may be used to assess for nerve compression, although negative studies do not exclude the diagnosis of compression neuropathy (Bowley and Doughty 2019). Consequently,

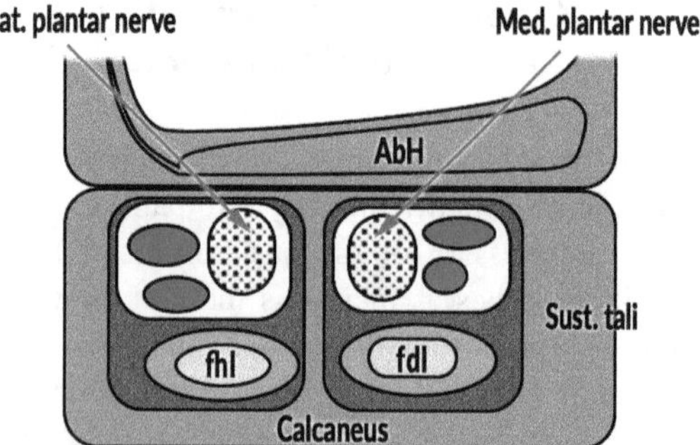

Fig. 4 Drawing of the area immediately distal to the upper tarsal tunnel. It demonstrates medial and lateral plantar tunnels, separated by a septum known as the medial septum. The medial septum extends between the tunnel fibrous roof consisting of the deep abductor hallucis fascia, and the calcaneus as the floor. The abductor hallucis overlies the roof. The lateral plantar nerve lies within the lateral plantar tunnel near the septum, with vessels peripherally and the flexor hallucis longus tendon (fhl). The medial plantar nerve lies in the medial plantar tunnel, near the septum, with vessels peripherally and the flexor digitorum longus (fdl)

there is no gold standard examination, and the diagnosis and treatment of TTS tend to be based on clinical findings (McSweeney and Cichero 2015; Doneddu et al. 2017; Vega-Zelaya et al. 2021).

Tarsal tunnel compressive neuropathy is divided into proximal and distal syndromes. Proximal tarsal tunnel syndrome is compression of the tibial nerve in the retromalleolar region, within the tunnel, whereas a distal syndrome involves the divisions of the tibial nerve, implies compression of one or more of the terminal branches of the tibial nerve. Since in most cases, the tibial nerve branching is within the tunnel (Kim et al. 2014), the distal compressions may be within the tarsal tunnel. However, the compression may happen distal to the tunnel when terminal branches traverse the fascial planes of the foot. Compression of the terminal branches, distally and outside of the tarsal tunnel includes compression of the medial plantar nerve (i.e., jogger's foot) and compression of the first branch of the lateral plantar nerve (i.e., Baxter's nerve). The medial calcaneal nerve demonstrates several anatomic variations in its origin: within the tunnel (34%), proximal to the tarsal tunnel (35–45%), origin from the lateral plantar nerve (16%), or from multiple branches (21%) (Doneddu et al. 2017; Vega-Zelaya et al. 2021; Kim et al. 2014; Radin 1983). It provides sensory innervation to the medial portion of the heel and part of the calcaneus. When this branch arises proximal to the tarsal tunnel, the symptoms of tarsal tunnel syndrome do not involve the heel. The medial plantar nerve originates in the cutaneous branches innervating the medial two-thirds of the plantar aspect of the foot, whereas the lateral one-third of the plantar aspect of the foot is innervated by the lateral plantar nerve (Fig. 5).

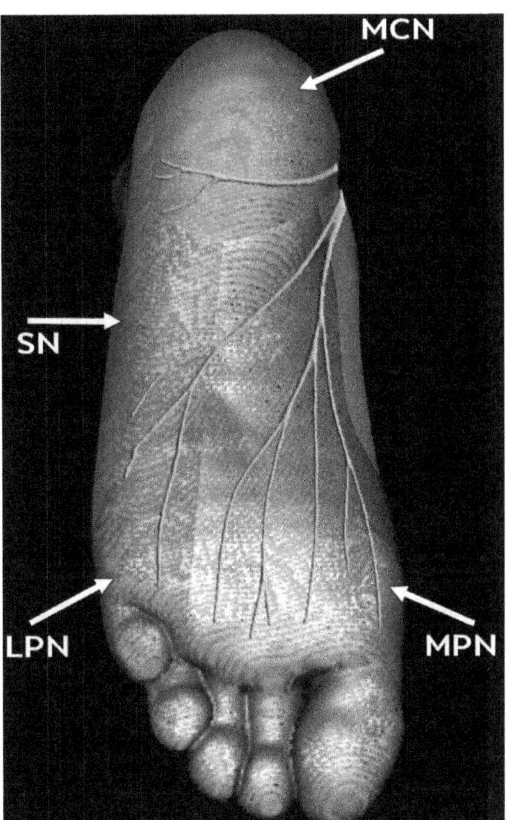

Fig. 5 Sensory map of the plantar aspect of the foot. The medial calcaneal nerve (MCN) gives sensory branches to the heel and medial plantar nerve (MPN), innervating the medial two-thirds of the plantar aspect of the foot. The lateral plantar nerve (LPN) innervates the lateral one-third of the foot's plantar aspect. The inferior calcaneal nerve (ICN) has no cutaneous branches for the heel. The sural nerve gives sensory branches for the mid-third of the lateral border of the foot (SN)

Most patients with tarsal tunnel syndrome report pain at the posteromedial ankle and plantar aspect of the foot manifested as burning pain and paraesthesia along the plantar foot and toes described as shooting, or electric pain, with a plantar foot intermittent numbness, or tingling in the toes or the sole of the foot. Typically, it is described as diffuse pain along the medial ankle and plantar foot with worsening of symptoms as the day goes on, exacerbated by activity and alleviated by rest, symptoms worsened at night as well, with nocturnal awakening and foot tingling. The symptoms may radiate distally along tibial nerve terminal branches or may radiate proximally into the calf (i.e., Valleix phenomenon) (Kalçık Ünan et al. 2021). Approximately half of the patients with tarsal tunnel syndrome report cold sensation, where neuropathic rather than vascular factors are involved (Radin 1983; Del Toro and Nelson 2018). All symptoms are included in the symptom complex termed tarsal tunnel syndrome (Kinoshita et al. 2001; Rydevik et al. 1981). Percussion over the tarsal tunnel may elicit pain along with the distribution of the medial and lateral plantar nerves, known as Tinel's test, but also during the dorsiflexion-eversion test, the symptoms may appear as well (Dahlin et al. 1986). Misdiagnosing TTS can lead to sensory loss, muscle weakness, and difficulty running, walking, and even standing as the condition progresses (Kinoshita et al. 2001; Rydevik et al. 1981).

A mechanism of compression of the distal tibial nerve in the presence of space-occupying lesions within the narrow canals is explained by increased pressure that influences compressed nerve physiology. Pressure on a peripheral nerve greater than 20 mmHg leads to blood flow reduction within the veins, whereas the blood flow within the arteries of the nerve can be reduced when pressure is greater than 40 mmHg (Manske et al. 2016). At pressures greater than 80 mmHg, structural changes with irreversible nerve damage appear (Spinner et al. 2007). Peripheral nerve ischemia results in the symptoms of numbness and tingling referred to as paresthesias, due to an ischemic conduction block of electrical activity in that nerve with longer decreased oxygen content (Tladi et al. 2017).

The presence of space-occupying lesions within the tarsal tunnel causes compression of the tibial nerve which is most commonly compressed in this area of its course, resulting in tarsal tunnel syndrome. It can be caused by tenosynovitis (Fig. 1), ganglion cyst (Ettehadi et al. 2022) (Fig. 6), lipoma, neurilemmoma,

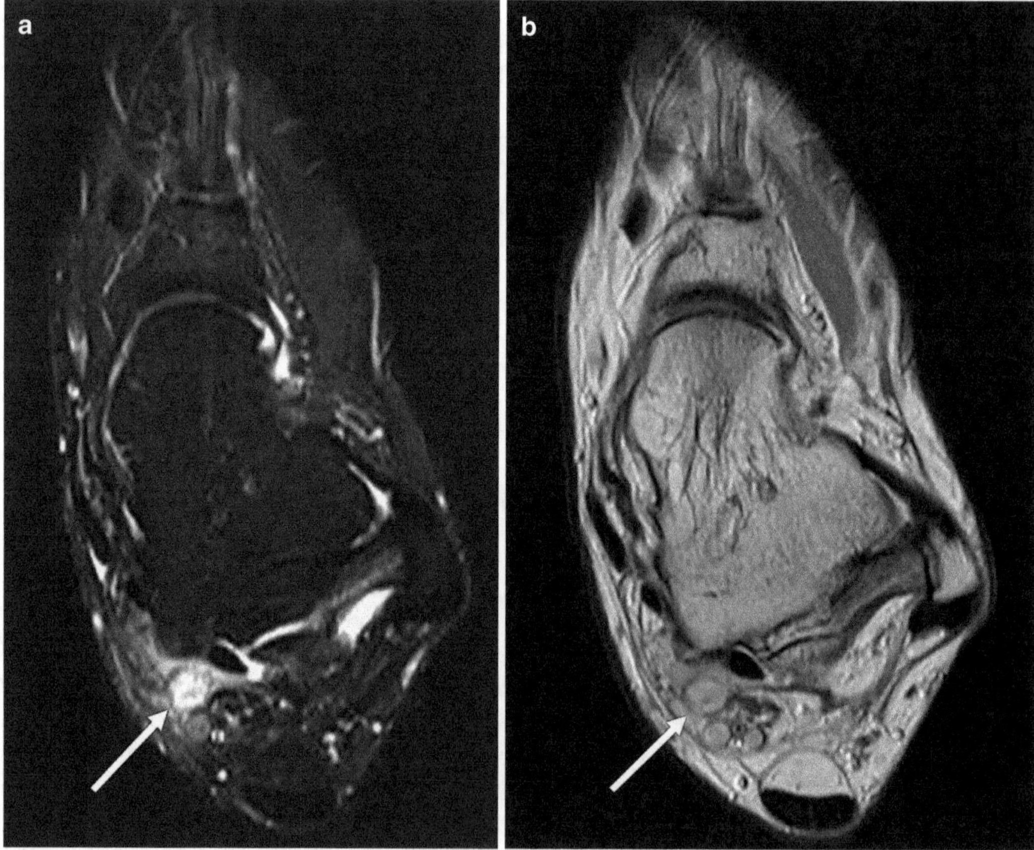

Fig. 6 MR imaging of tarsal tunnel syndrome. A patient presented with typical symptoms of tarsal tunnel syndrome. On MRI with axial T2 fat-suppressed (**a**) and PD (**b**) sequences in the midtarsal tunnel cystic lesion were found, suggestive of ganglion cyst. Edema noted adjoining cyst related to fluid decompression from cyst, was found to compress the posterior tibial nerve and vessels

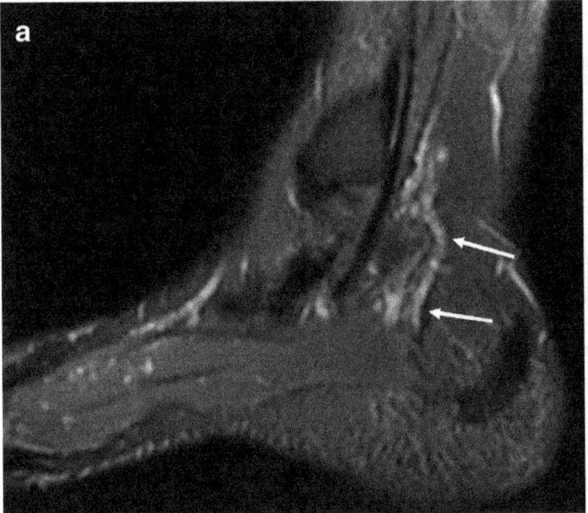

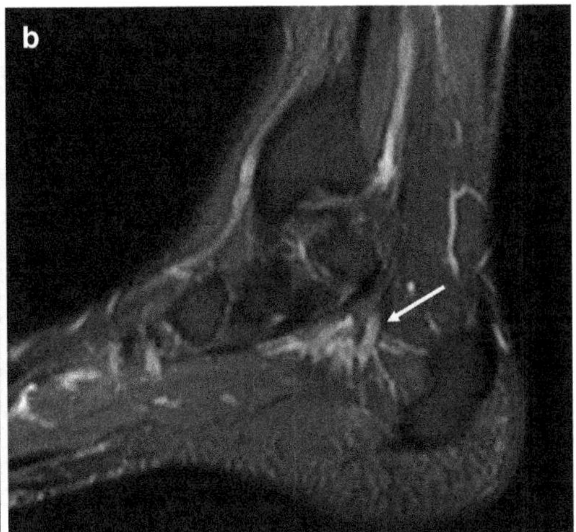

Fig. 7 Tarsal tunnel syndrome due to varicosities. A 42-year-old male presented with tarsal tunnel syndrome. A sagittal PD fat-saturated MR images (**a**, **b**) dilated posterior tibial veins in a tarsal tunnel (arrows) can be seen demonstrating as tubular intermediate signal intensity structures that extend from the posterior ankle, through the tarsal tunnel, and into the plantar soft tissue of the forefoot

exostosis, dilated or tortuous veins (Baba et al. 1997) (Figs. 7 and 8), accessory muscle within the canal (Badr et al. 2020; Bhat et al. 2017; Tassler et al. 2000), fibrous tarsal coalition and sustentaculum tali hypertrophy (Baba et al. 1997). Neuropathy is predisposed due to metabolic problems within the peripheral nerve such as in diabetes (Oh 2007) and in inflammatory changes reported in rheumatoid arthritis (Del Toro and Nelson 2018). Longstanding inflammation (Fig. 9), even posttraumatic fibrosis due to fracture, bony or cartilaginous prominences within the canal, and flexor retinaculum fibrosis or thickening may narrow the tarsal tunnel and compress the nerve (Trepman et al. 1999; Berachilovic et al. 2006). Excessive nerve tension in affected biomechanics while positioning the ankle joint may increase pressure on the tibial nerve in the tarsal tunnel (Barker et al. 2007; Mackinnon et al. 1984; Nagaoka and Matsuzaki 2005). The pressure increases in the medial plantar tunnel with ankle pronation and flexion with similar pressure changes within the lateral plantar tunnel. Surgical excision of the septum between the two tunnels will prevent increasing the pressures with ankle pronation and flexion (Hoffman and Bianchi 2013).

If even minimal pressure persists about a peripheral nerve for 2 months, there is a loss of endoneurial microvessel integrity, resulting in endoneurial edema. After 6 months perineurial fibrosis and demyelination occur, whereas persistence of the pressure for 12 months, the further loss of demyelination and loss of large myelinated fibers will follow, resulting in incomplete remyelination after nerve decompression (Tawfik et al. 2016).

Radiographs should be used to identify any bony or soft-tissue etiologies. Weight-bearing X-rays should be done to exclude bony causes and foot and ankle malalignment such as hyper pronation, and valgus and varus foot deformities with a comparative study of the contralateral joint. On MRI, axial view on the heel, the hypertrophy of the sustentaculum tali and corresponding beaking of the talus can be seen if present. A CT scan may reveal a presence of talar coalition as well, but a fibrous coalition of the middle (medial) talocalcaneal facet and hypertrophic sustentaculum tali can be presented on MRI without other compressive pathology within the tarsal tunnel nor changes of the nerve. A diagnostic blockade (2% Lidocain) in the tarsal tunnel with transient symptoms relief points toward the diagnosis of tarsal tunnel syndrome.

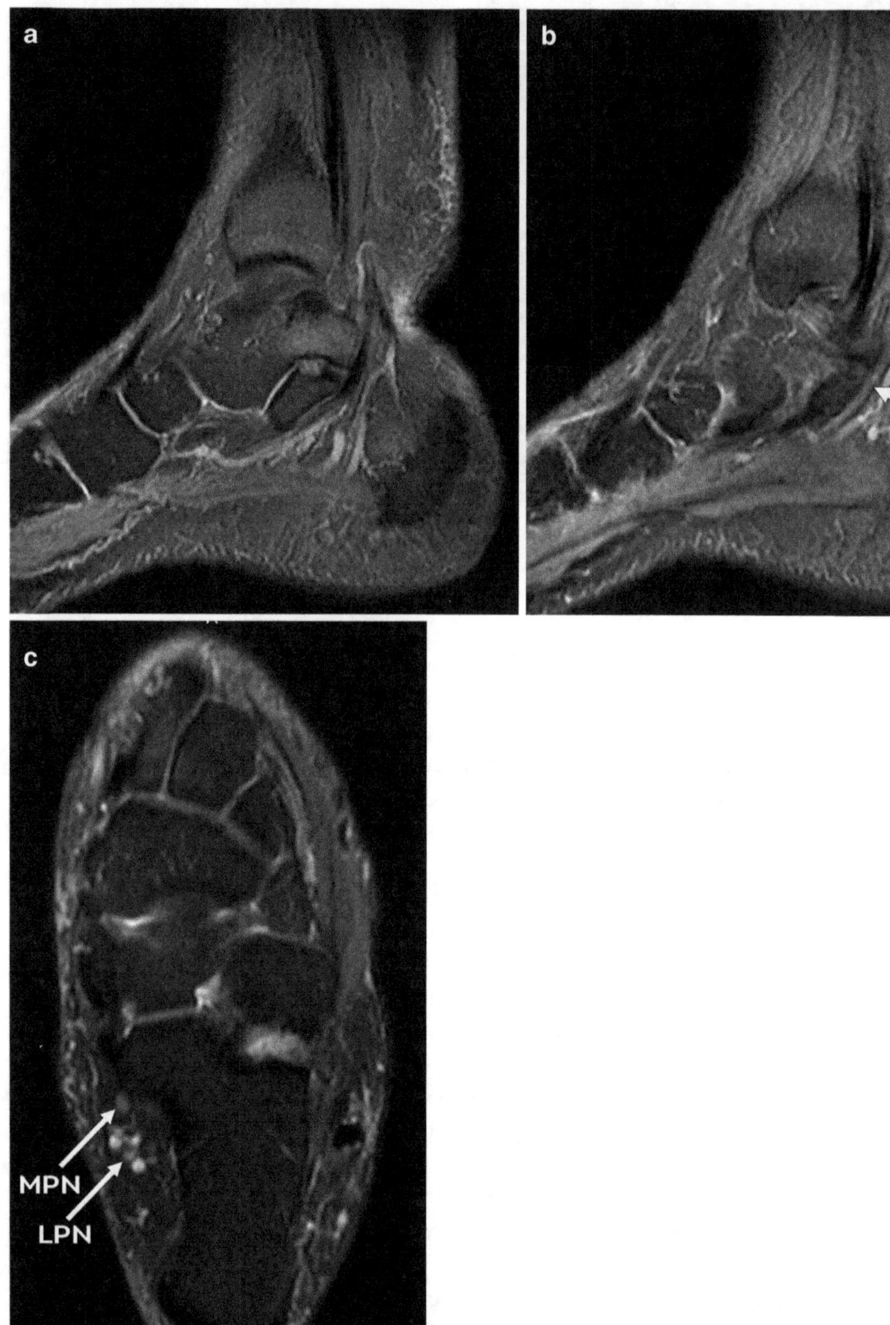

Fig. 8 MRI evidence of compressive neuropathy of medial and lateral plantar nerves in a 37-year-old male with tarsal tunnel syndrome. On sagittal PD fat-suppressed MR images (**a**, **b**), mildly dilated veins can be seen, with an enlarged and high signal intensity on the medial plantar nerve (**b**, arrow). Axial PD fat-suppressed image demonstrates an increase in the caliber of medial and lateral plantar nerves with increased signal intensity (**c**, arrows). The signal intensity of the nerves (arrows) is less than the signal intensity of the adjacent vessels (**c**)

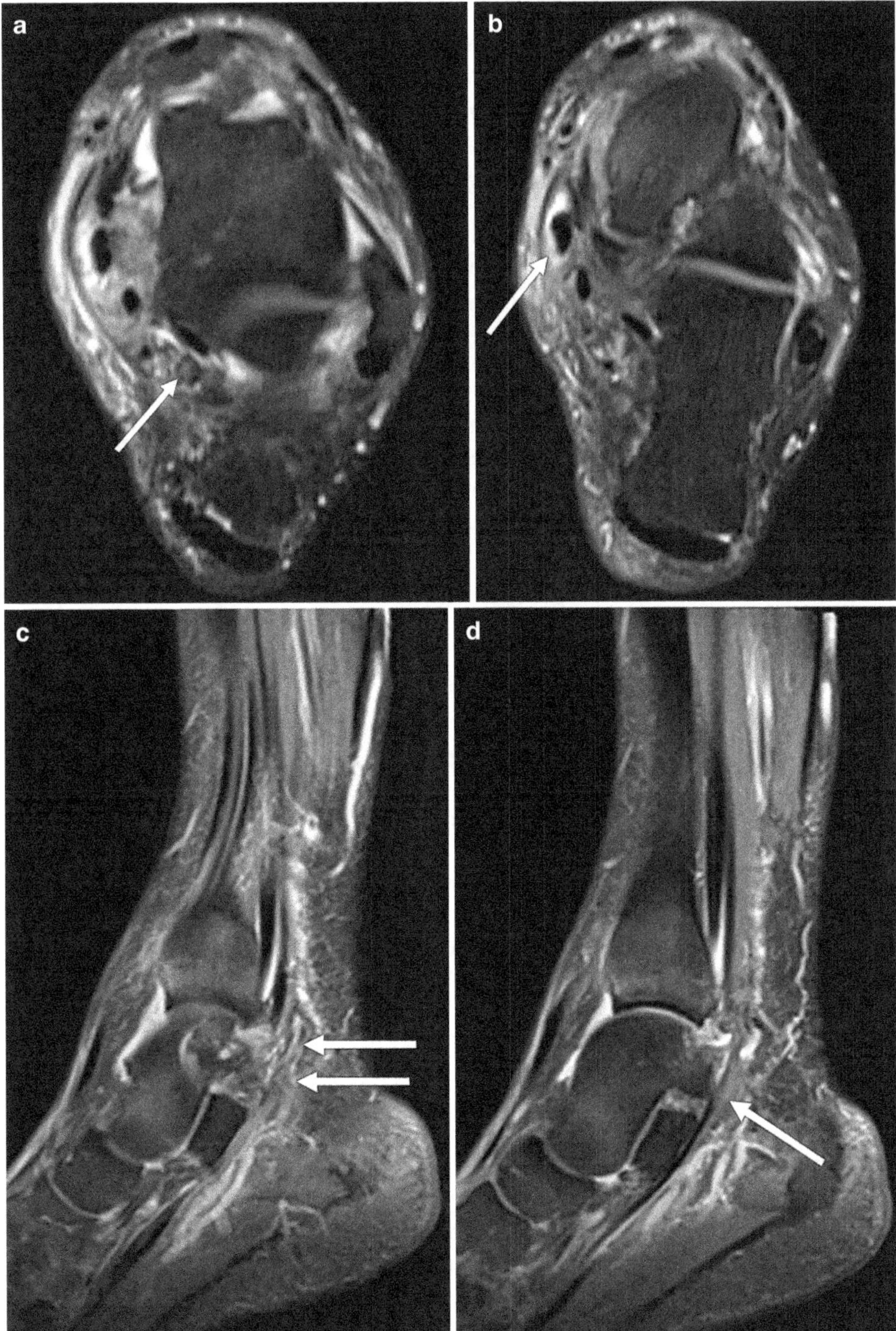

Fig. 9 Tarsal tunnel syndrome. On axial PD fat-saturated, chronic inflammation and edema within the tarsal tunnel (**a**, **c**) are seen. There is a consecutive posterior tibial nerve increase in the caliper and in signal intensity (**a**, arrow). Fluid is seen in the posterior tibial tendon indicative of tenosynovitis (**b**, arrow). On sagittal PD fat-saturated posterior to flexor hallucis longus tendon, the posterior tibial nerve and its branches are visible with an increased caliper and high signal intensity (**d**, arrow). (Courtesy of Gjorgji Damjanovski)

On ultrasound, the tibial nerve can be visualized as it passes deep to the flexor retinaculum and between the medial malleolus and the medial wall of the calcaneus. With high-resolution transducers, US is able to demonstrate the complex anatomy of the tarsal tunnel, where under the hypoechoic retinaculum three tendons can be evaluated (tibialis posterior, flexor digitorum longus, flexor hallucis longus), the posterior tibial vessels (artery and veins) and the tibial nerve division into its branches (medial and lateral plantar nerves and calcaneal sensory branch) posteroinferior to the medial malleolus (Iborra et al. 2018; Martinoli et al. 2000; Lopez-Ben 2011; Therimadasamy et al. 2011). The tibial nerve lies posteriorly to the flexor digitorum longus tendon and superficially to the flexor hallucis longus tendon, close to the posterior tibial vessels that can be visualized with color Doppler imaging as a useful landmark for visualizing the nerve. US can provide exact information on the nature and extent of the space-occupying lesions within the tunnel and help assume the pathologic condition that exists in both proximal and distal tarsal tunnels (Martinoli et al. 2000).

Ganglion cysts appear as well-demarcated anechoic to hypoechoic masses with multiple internal septations without vascularity (Hoffman and Bianchi 2013), that displace adjacent arteries, veins, and the enlarged nerve. A varicose vein is a frequently underdiagnosed, but common cause of tarsal tunnel syndrome, which may appear as bulbous enlargements of the venous structure on US, being tortuous with signs of venous stasis in standing position (Tladi et al. 2017). Comparison with the contralateral side is important. A dynamic examination during the movements of the ankle and local compression by the US transducer can help to confirm the diagnosis by reproducing the patient's symptoms (US Tinel test) (Ghosh et al. 2013). Other causes for tarsal tunnel syndrome such as hypertrophic retinaculum, tendinopathies, inflammatory arthritis, tumors, or supernumerary muscles can be evaluated on US, but especially the flexor digitorum accessorius longus muscle (Tladi et al. 2017) and accessory abductor hallucis muscle (Kim et al. 2022a). Tunnel-to-inlet CSA ratio and the tunnel CSA are accurate sonographic parameters and can be helpful in the assessment of idiopathic tarsal tunnel syndrome which represents about 20–40% of the cases (Hochman and Zilberfarb 2004). Transducer should be orthogonal to the nerve, with minimal pressure with the transducer by using Doppler to delineate the nerve's outer rim from the adjacent vascular structures (Tawfik et al. 2016; Therimadasamy et al. 2011).

On MRI, space-occupying lesions within the tarsal tunnel are readily identified with the assessment of hindfoot alignment, such as scar tissue within the tarsal tunnel presenting with low signal intensity, but also the presence of small ganglia arising from the subtalar joint or medial compartment tendon sheaths, adjacent osteophytes, and talocalcaneal coalition. Direct tibial nerve evaluation for caliber change, signal intensity, and fascicular pattern and uniformity is limited due to the small nerve size at this distal level. In idiopathic cases, patients have clinical signs of tarsal tunnel syndrome, but no imaging abnormalities are observed. In the absence of focal mass lesions, and normal nerve appearance, the MRI can be partially useful for diagnosing idiopathic tarsal tunnel syndrome (Kim et al. 2022b; McSweeney and Cichero 2015) by not providing details required for surgical planning. It is suggested that clinicians should always correlate MRI findings with clinical symptoms, caution is required for a diagnosis based on MRI studies alone (Kim et al. 2022b).

MRI reveals the presence of accessory muscle on the posterior medial aspect of the ankle with a signal consistent with the surrounding normal musculature in all sequences performed. The key features that differentiate these muscles include their position with respect to the flexor hallucis longus muscle, to the neurovascular bundle, and to the flexor retinaculum and deep aponeurosis of the lower leg (Ettehadi et al. 2022; Canter and Siesel 1997). The flexor digitorum accessorius longus tendon may travel with the posterior tibial neurovascular bundle in the tarsal tunnel and inserts on the quadratus plantae muscle which can be associated with tarsal tunnel syndrome (Donovan et al. 2010) (Figs. 10 and 11).

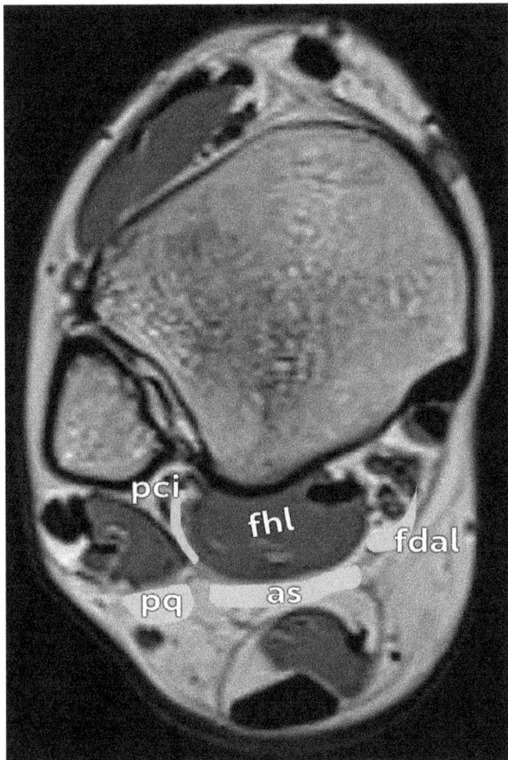

Fig. 10 Accessory muscles of the ankle. Axial T1 WI drawing shows the location of common accessory muscles relative to the flexor hallucis longus (fhl) muscle, deep aponeurosis, and neurovascular bundle. The accessory soleus muscle (as) is located superficially to the deep aponeurosis. Peroneal calcaneus internus (pci) muscle is situated laterally to FHL. Both flexor digitorum accessories longus (fdal) and tibiocalcaneus internus (tci) muscles are located deep to the aponeurosis and posteromedial to the fhl; they can be differentiated by tracing their insertions distally. Peroneus quartus (pq) travels posteromedial to the peroneal tendons encircled by the superior peroneal retinaculum

Treatment of tarsal tunnel syndrome starts with a conservative approach such as wearing a brace, neuropathic pain medication, and activity modification (Rydevik et al. 1981). When non-surgical measures fail, surgical release of the tibial nerve and its terminal branches is recommended, which includes releasing of entire flexor retinaculum. An incomplete release can cause continued pain after surgery. Resection of space-occupying lesions will improve the outcomes compared with those of patients who have no identifiable lesion to be resected (Gould 2014; Ferkel et al. 2015). In idiopathic entrapment, without identified etiology of nerve compression on MRI, nerve involvement of varices, small vessel branches, and connective tissue (Kim et al. 2022b) with entrapment due to adhesions due to trauma, or distortion of an artery can be found during surgery (Doneddu et al. 2017). Potential postsurgical complications include the persistence of the symptoms due to scar formation, incomplete nerve release, and iatrogenic neurovascular injury (Ghosh et al. 2013).

2.1 Compressive Neuropathy of Medial Plantar Nerve: Jogger's Foot

Medial plantar nerve neuropathy is characterized by medial foot and arch pain, which is common in clinical practice, present in 24% of older adults, ≥45 years, and is more common in women, causing moderate disability in most of the patients (Thomas et al. 2011).

The medial plantar nerve is important for the balance of the body, walking, and many sports activities (Unlü et al. 2008; McKeon et al. 2015).

It is a larger branch of the posterior tibial nerve, which runs anterior to the lateral plantar nerve into the medial plantar tunnel known as an abductor tunnel, through an opening in the deep fascia of the abductor hallucis muscle. By remaining deep and close to the abductor hallucis muscle, it runs to its terminal branches division. It moves more lateral to a narrow space under the flexor digitorum brevis, between the abductor halluces muscle and the crossing of the flexor hallucis longus tendon and flexor digitorum longus tendons, known as the Master knot of Henry or the chiasma tendineum plantare, located under the junction of the talus and navicular bones (Amlang et al. 2012; Ghosh et al. 2013). The medial plantar nerve has four terminal branches: the medial plantar cutaneous nerve of the hallux and three medial common digital nerves that divide into the proper digital nerve (Beltran et al. 2010) (Fig. 12). With the motor branches, the medial plantar nerve innervates the flexor digitorum brevis muscle, abductor hallucis muscle,

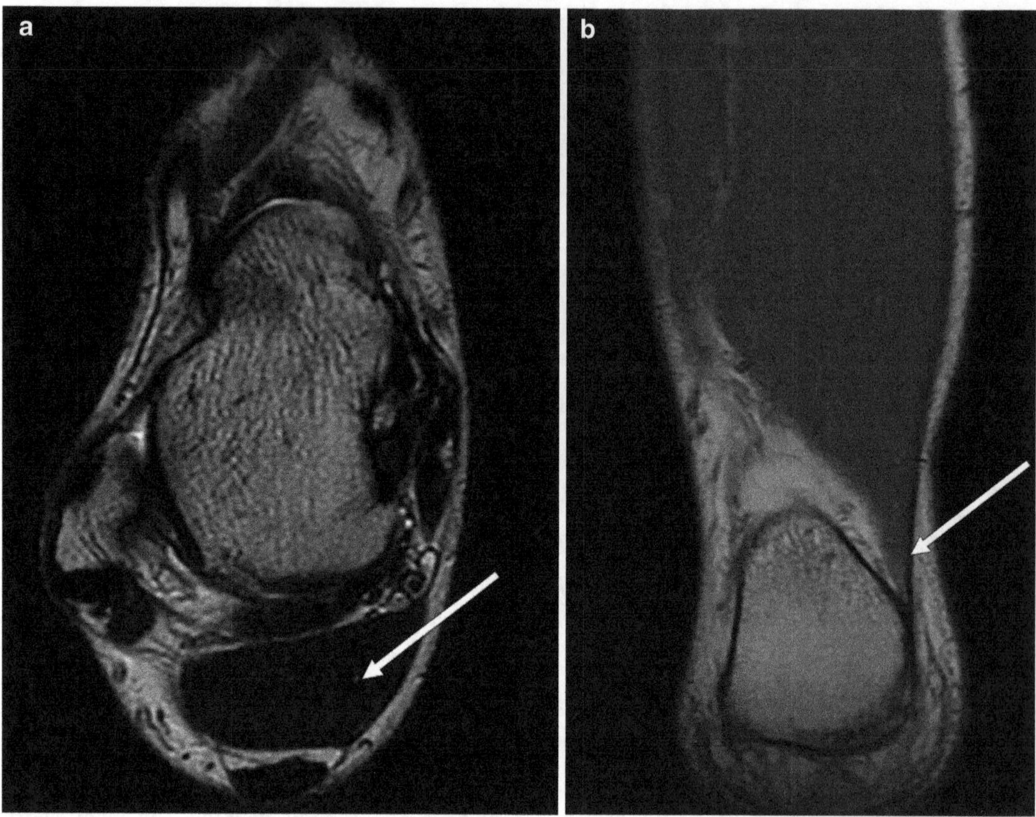

Fig. 11 Accessory soleus muscle. Axial (**a**) and Coronal (**b**) T1 MRI images of the hindfoot show mass-like accessory soleus muscle which extends low, inserted on the medial aspect of the calcaneus. (Courtesy of Harun Gupta)

flexor hallucis brevis, and the first lumbrical muscles. These are the plantar muscles that flex the toes, especially at the metatarsophalangeal joint of the great toe (Kopell and Thompson 1976). The sensory branches of the medial plantar nerve provide sensation from the medial two-thirds of the plantar surface of the foot, from the plantar sides of the first to third toes, and the medial half of the fourth toe as the proper digital nerves. The sensation of the lateral aspect of the fourth toe, of the whole fifth toe, and the lateral third of the plantar surface of the foot is provided from the lateral plantar nerve through the proper digital nerves (Kopell and Thompson 1976) (Fig. 5). Persistence of the connecting branch between the deep branch of the lateral plantar nerve and the medial plantar nerve, which are in the space between the flexor hallucis brevis muscle and flexor hallucis longus tendon, was found to be important since can be subject to friction during walking or running. Those are reported to be present in 86% of the patients (Arakawa et al. 2011). Superficial connections have been described as well (Govsa et al. 2005).

Isolated entrapment of the medial plantar nerve is relatively rare, appearing only in 5% of patients with foot and ankle pain (Murphy and Baxter 1985), but it can be seen in 40% of patients with foot pain due to tarsal tunnel syndrome. The medial plantar nerve, by crossing midfoot deep to the talonavicular joint is vulnerable to compression and irritation in patients with a high medial arch or with hyperpronation.

Entrapment of the medial plantar nerve may happen at different levels. Proximal entrapment of the medial plantar nerve can be at the proximal tarsal tunnel, close to its origin, and deep to the flexor retinaculum. It may also be part of a tarsal tunnel syndrome that includes other branches of the tibial nerve. Nevertheless, the medial plantar

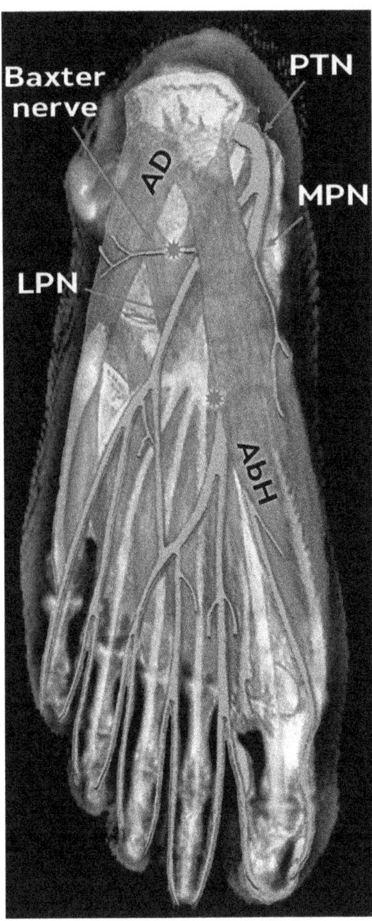

Fig. 12 Normal anatomy of the plantar nerves. The posterior tibial nerve (PTN) divides into the lateral plantar nerve (LPN) and medial plantar nerve (MPN), and both nerve branches course under the abductor hallucis muscle (AbH). The first branch of the lateral plantar nerve is the inferior calcaneal nerve or Baxter's nerve, which innervates the abductor digiti minimi muscle (AD). The potential site of compression of the medial plantar nerve at the knot of Henry and of the Baxter nerve is marked with star

nerve can be entrapped at the distal tarsal tunnel as it passes through the fascial leash in the deep fascia of the abductor hallucis muscle when entering the medial plantar tunnel. The openings of the fascia of the abductor hallucis muscle can be constricted by a high arch (pes cavus) if present, or excessive pronation may lead to medial plantar nerve stretching against the tunnel (Kopell and Thompson 1976).

Medial plantar nerve neuropathy can be caused by a fascial sling at the knot of Henry, when the nerve can be trapped between the plantar prominence of the navicular bone tuberosity and the talar bone, between the abductor hallucis muscle belly and the knot of Henry (Donovan et al. 2010). A repetitive motion of the talonavicular joint accompanied by eversion of the foot with the collapse of the arch can injure the medial plantar nerve at this particular location, presenting a condition known as "jogger's foot" (Murphy and Baxter 1985) (Fig. 12). In 16% of the cases, medial plantar nerve crosses through the medial intermuscular septum which could be an additional area where the nerve can be entrapped (Singh and Kumar 2012) (Fig. 4). In pronation of the ankle with or without plantar flexion, the pressure within the medial and lateral plantar tunnels and in the tarsal tunnel can be significantly elevated, during walking on a pronated foot that causes compressive neuropathy (Hoffman and Bianchi 2013).

Patients with medial plantar nerve entrapment complain of burning pain, dysesthesias along the heel, medial arch, and first to third toes, pain at the medial arch, and medial plantar surface of the foot. Pain increase with activity with radiation distally toward the plantar aspect of the first through third toes or may radiate proximally into the heel and ankle. On clinical examination, there is tenderness over the medial arch, just posterior to the navicular tuberosity, with a positive Tinel sign at the plantar border of the navicular tuberosity, with decreased sensation on the foot behind the great toe (Oh and Lee 1987; Schon and Baxter 1990). The nerve can be compressed in acute settings due to the presence of posttraumatic hematoma and edema locally in fracture of the navicular tuberosity causing the symptoms (Figs. 13 and 14). More complex is the clinical presentation and diagnosis of medial plantar nerve entrapment if it coexists with compression of the tibial nerve (double crush syndrome), or with simultaneous entrapment of other branches of the posterior tibial nerve, most commonly the medial calcaneal nerve (Rose et al. 2003). Even more challenging is the evaluation of medial plantar nerve dysfunction in coexisting small fiber neuropathy as seen in diabetes mellitus. However, the medial plantar nerve has consistent

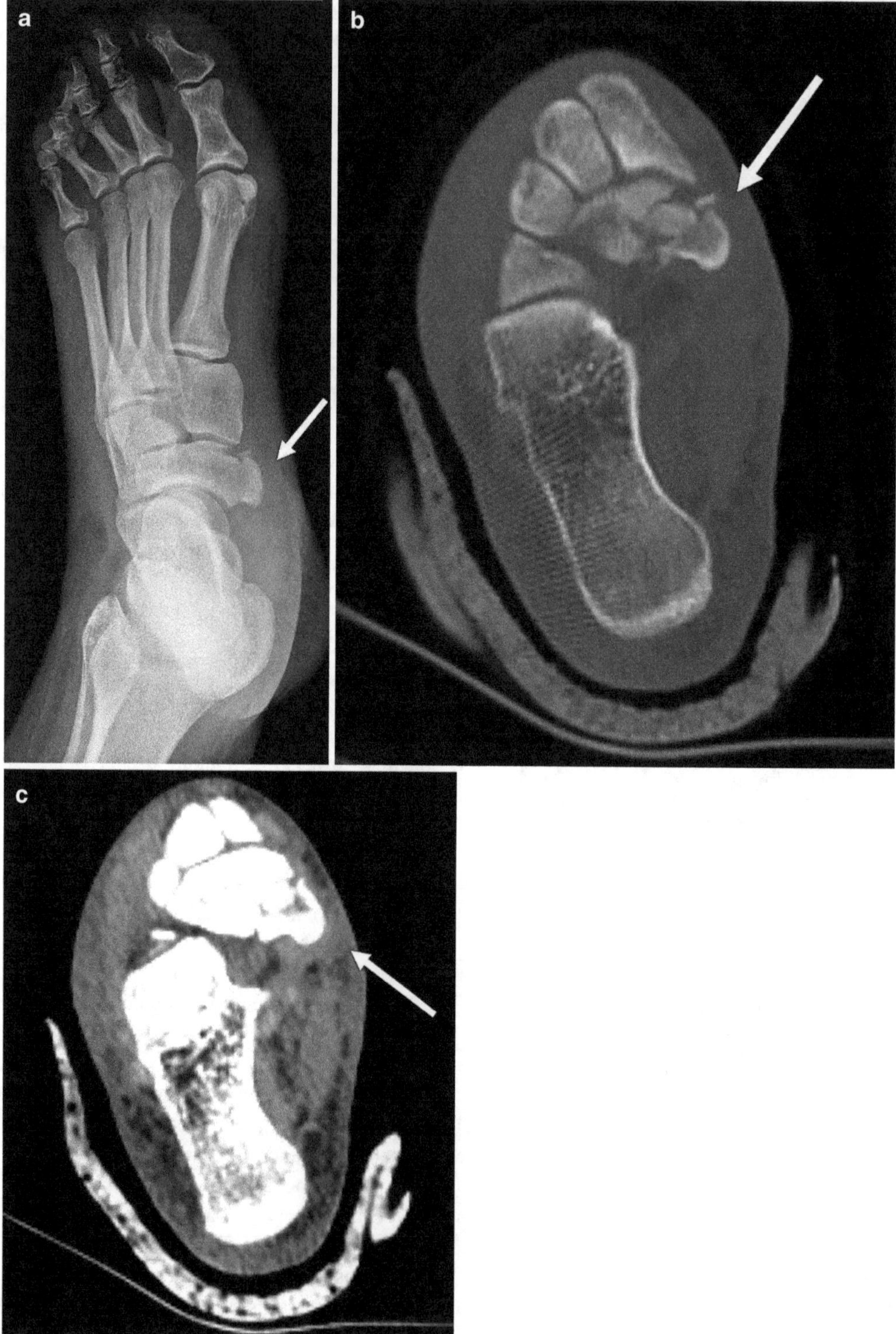

Fig. 13 Medial plantar nerve neuropathy. A 48-year-old female 14 days after fracture of the medial aspect of the navicular bone, presented with burning pain, dysesthesias along the medial arch, and first to third toes, symptoms suggestive of medial plantar nerve neuropathy. The plain film shows the fragment with small dislocation (**a**, arrow), which is better presented on CT (**b**, **c**, arrow). There are signs of posttraumatic hematoma and edema locally near fractured navicular tuberosity causing the symptoms due to nerve compression

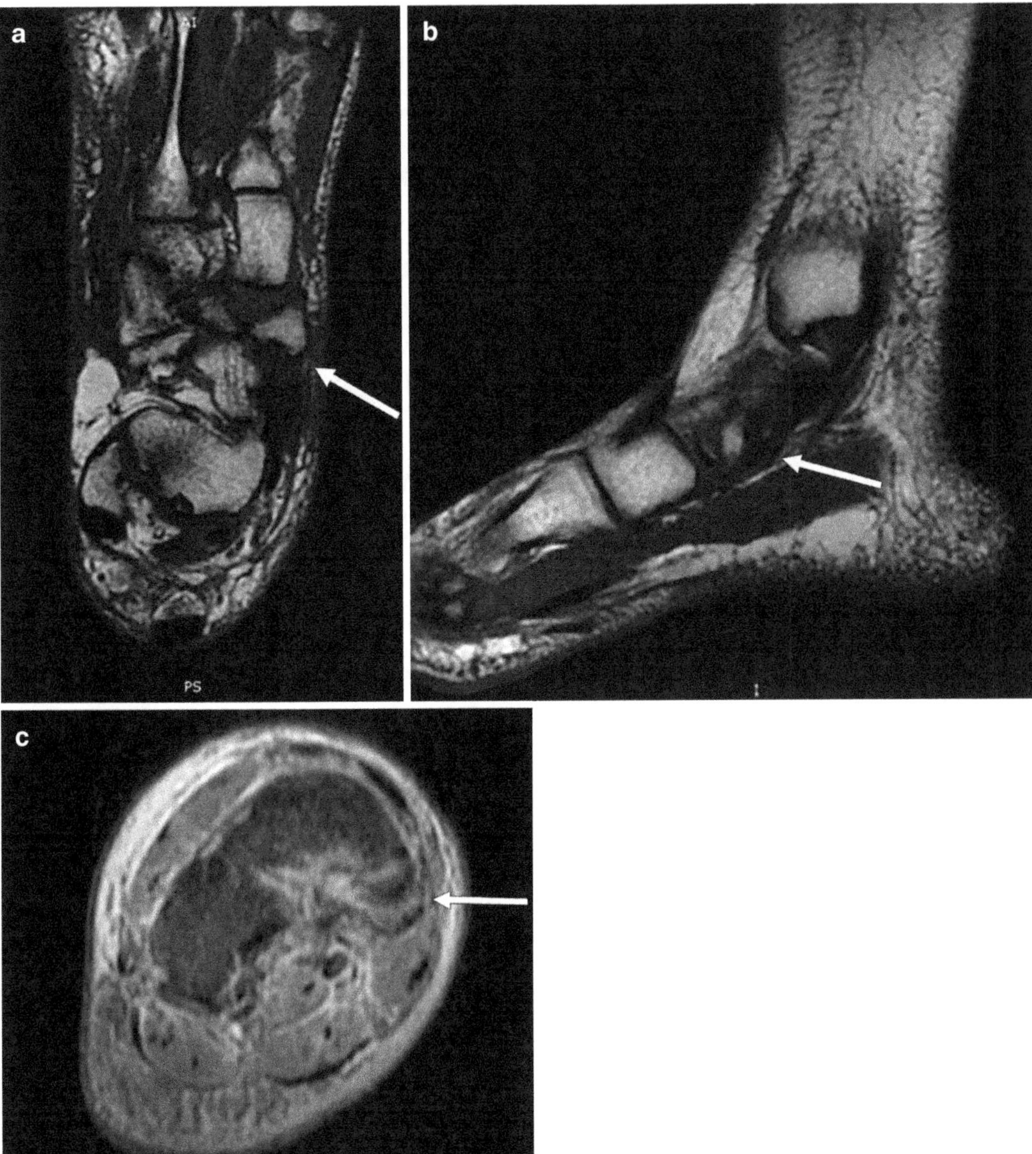

Fig. 14 Medial plantar nerve neuropathy, MR imaging. The same case from Fig. 13. On coronal PD (**a**), sagittal PD (**b**) and axial PD fat-saturated (**c**) displacement of navicular tuberosity (**a**, **c**, arrow) can be seen with infiltration of the adjacent soft tissue due to hematoma and edema with medial plantar nerve compression (**b**, arrow)

cutaneous sensory distribution, and the clinical diagnosis of its dysfunction may be established by performing sensory nerve testing (Oh et al. 1985). More susceptible to jogger's foot are long-distance runners with valgus hindfeet or when running on a slanted track or road that increases pronation, and in patients with hindfoot valgus and pes planus, when the shoe with excessive or rigid arch support wear can be a source of external nerve compression (Rose et al. 2003).

In differential diagnosis, a compressive neuropathy of the medial plantar nerve can mimic plantar fasciitis, although patients with medial plantar nerve dysfunction usually will not experience the "first-step" foot pain which is characteristic of plantar fasciitis and have tenderness more distally. In some cases, medial plantar nerve entrapment can be confused with the presence of intermetatarsal (Morton's) "neuroma" (D'Orazi et al. 2014).

Radiographs may be used for the assessment of any bony abnormalities and eventually diagnosing foot deformities.

Neurological deficits in the setting of the subtalar coalition have been reported, tarsal tunnel syndrome, with sensory loss involving the distribution of branches of the posterior tibial nerve, most commonly along the distribution of the medial plantar nerve (Takakura et al. 1991). The talocalcaneal coalition can be shown with MRI or CT, lying in close proximity to or impinging on neurovascular structures within the tunnel.

On MRI compressed medial plantar nerve can demonstrate high nerve signal on fat-suppressed, fluid-sensitive images, suggestive of underlying neuritis, with less intense signal intensity than the adjacent vessels which can reflect the magic angle effect. The mild increase in the T2 signal can be seen in the medial plantar nerve at the inferior aspect of the tarsal tunnel, where the nerve transit from more vertical to a relatively horizontal course (Alaia et al. 2016). Indirect signs of compressive neuropathy include denervation changes within innervated muscles.

Initial nonsurgical management is similar to the care provided for proximal tarsal tunnel syndrome. When conservative treatment fails in providing relief of the symptoms, surgical release of the deep fascia of the abductor hallucis from its origin on the calcaneus to the knot of Henry could be done, with the release of the flexor retinaculum and the tibial nerve proximally (Lopez-Ben 2011; Kim et al. 2014).

2.2 Compressive Neuropathy of the First Branch of the Lateral Plantar Nerve: Baxter's Neuropathy

Compressive neuropathy of the first branch of the lateral plantar nerve, a compression of the inferior calcaneal nerve is a condition known as Baxter's neuropathy (Baxter and Thigpen 1984; Recht et al. 2007a). It is compressive neuropathy presented clinically with a mixed sensory-motor pattern and typical recalcitrant heel pain, with maximal tenderness over the medial border of the calcaneus on the place of the entrapment. Clinical features overlap with those of plantar fasciitis, which is often concurrently present. The inferior calcaneal nerve entrapment is estimated to involve 20% of the patients with chronic heel pain (Shon and Easly 2000). Referred to as distal tarsal tunnel syndrome or Baxter's neuropathy, this condition often presents in athletes such as runners, ballet dancers, and gymnasts (Ferkel et al. 2015). In athletes with chronic heel pain, it may occur from minor trauma, mimicking an overuse injury (Mohile et al. 2020).

The inferior calcaneal nerve arises either as the first branch of the lateral plantar nerve or directly from the posterior tibial nerve (11.7%) (Govsa et al. 2006; Chundru et al. 2008), within the tarsal tunnel in 82%, at the level of the medial malleolus, with an anatomical variation to originate from a common branch with the posterior branch to the lateral plantar nerve and with the medial calcaneal branch (4.1%) (Chundru et al. 2008).

At the level of the medial malleolus, the nerve courses plantar from its origin deep in relation to the abductor halluces muscle, courses between the abductor hallucis muscle and the quadratus plantae, and runs along the medial border of the long plantar ligament (Fig. 15) The nerve transfers from a vertical to a horizontal direction at the inferior margin of the abductor hallucis muscle, turns laterally between the abductor hallucis muscle and anteriorly to the medial calcaneal tuberosity between the quadratus plantae dorsally and the plantar fascia and flexor digitorum brevis muscle on its plantar aspect. The nerve continues laterally to insert into the proximal aspect of the muscle abductor digiti quinti to give motor branches to the muscle. It is a small (<2 mm) mixed nerve that sends out motor branches beside abductor digiti quinti muscles, to the flexor digitorum brevis, and quadratus plantae and gives sensory fibers to the long plantar ligament, and calcaneal periosteum (medial tuberosity or medial process of the calcaneus) (Fig. 5). The

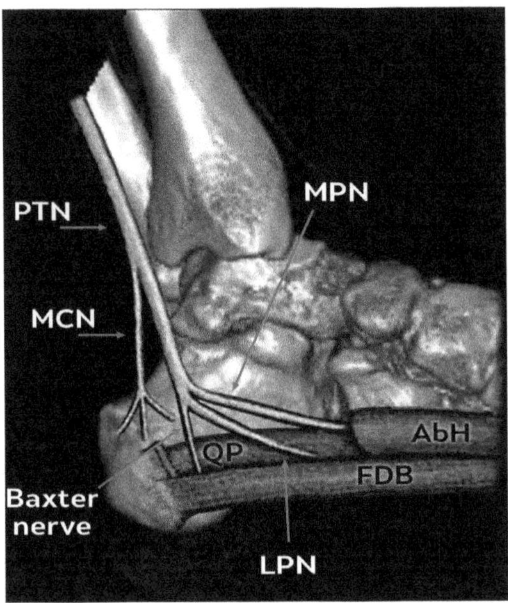

Fig. 15 Drawing of the posterior tibial nerve (PTN) and its branches at the upper tarsal tunnel (tibiotalar) and lower tarsal tunnel (talocalcaneal) showing the relationship of medial (MPN) and lateral plantar nerve (LPN) with adjacent muscles: quadratus plantae (QP), flexor digitorum brevis (FDB), abductor halluces (AbH)

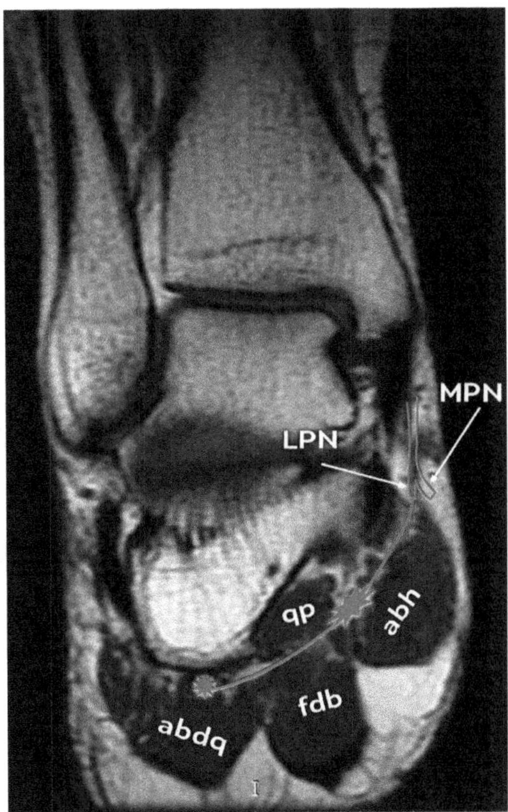

Fig. 16 Coronal T1 MR image of the hindfoot with a schematic presentation of two areas (stars) of possible compression of the first branch of the lateral plantar nerve (Baxter's nerve): one in the nerve pathway between the deep fascia of the abductor muscle of the hallux and the medial plantar margin of the quadratus plantae muscle (qp). Distally, possible compression is in the nerve pathway along the medial calcaneal tuberosity. *Abdq* abductor digiti quinti, *fdb* flexor digitorum brevis, *abh* abductor halluces muscle

nerve is located on average 5.5 mm anteriorly to the medial process of the calcaneal tuberosity (Arenson et al. 1990). Any pathology causing increased volume in the region of the nerve might cause a focal compressive effect with consequential neuropathy.

The first branch of the lateral plantar nerve may be entrapped at two regions: proximally, at the point where the nerve changes direction from vertical to horizontal as it travels toward the lateral foot, at the inferior margin of the abductor hallucis muscle where it is compressed between the fascia of the abductor hallucis muscle and the medio-caudal margin of the medial aspect of the quadratus plantae muscle, between the medial intermuscular septum and the quadratus plantae muscle, more precisely at the hiatus, where the nerve enters within the tarsal tunnel as it travels to innervate the abductor digiti quinti muscle which is the most often site for nerve compression in athletes (Delfaut et al. 2003; Chundru et al. 2008). The second point of compression is slightly more distally, as the nerve may be entrapped at the anterior aspect of the medial calcaneal tuberosity passing laterally, with compression between the flexor digitorum brevis muscle plantarly and the quadratus plantae dorsally (Baxter and Thigpen 1984) (Fig. 16).

Contributory factors include soft-tissue inflammatory changes of plantar fasciitis (Figs. 17 and 18) or can interfere mechanically due to microtrauma of the nerve by plantar calcaneal spur formation or the nerve can be stretched in the pronated foot as it courses anteriorly to the medial calcaneal tuberosity (Delfaut et al. 2003; Baxter and Thigpen 1984; Chundru et al. 2008).

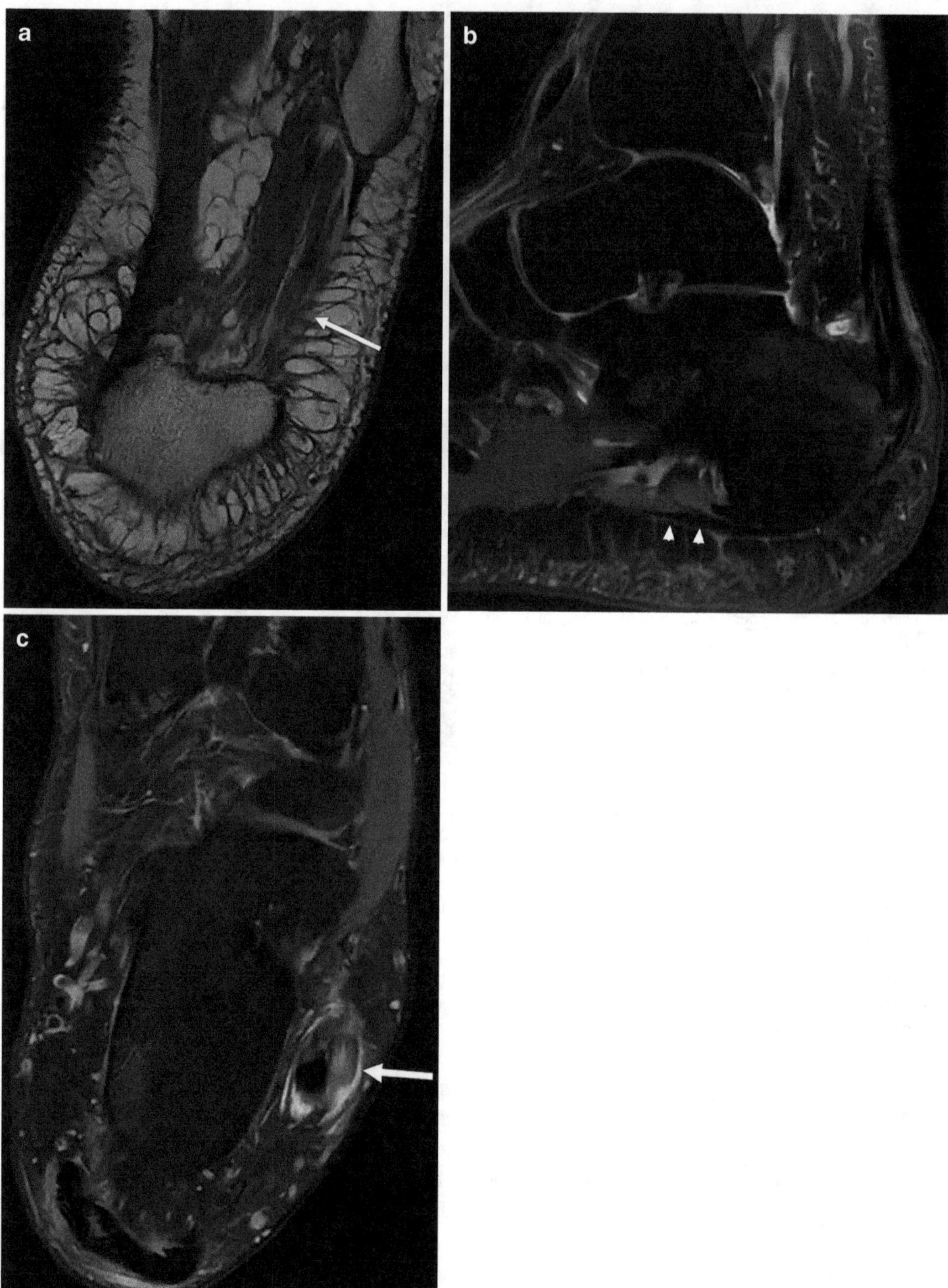

Fig. 17 Baxter's neuropathy in a 69-year-old male patient with plantar fasciitis and Achilles tendinopathy. Axial T1 image demonstrates a fatty replacement of the abductor digiti minimi (**a**, arrow) indicating atrophy. Intrafascial and perifascial focal high signal indicating plantar fasciitis (**b**, arrowheads), and insertional Achilles tendinopathy are visible. Also, note the tear of the peroneus brevis tendon with surrounding edema (**c**, arrow). (Courtesy of MP Aparisi Gomez)

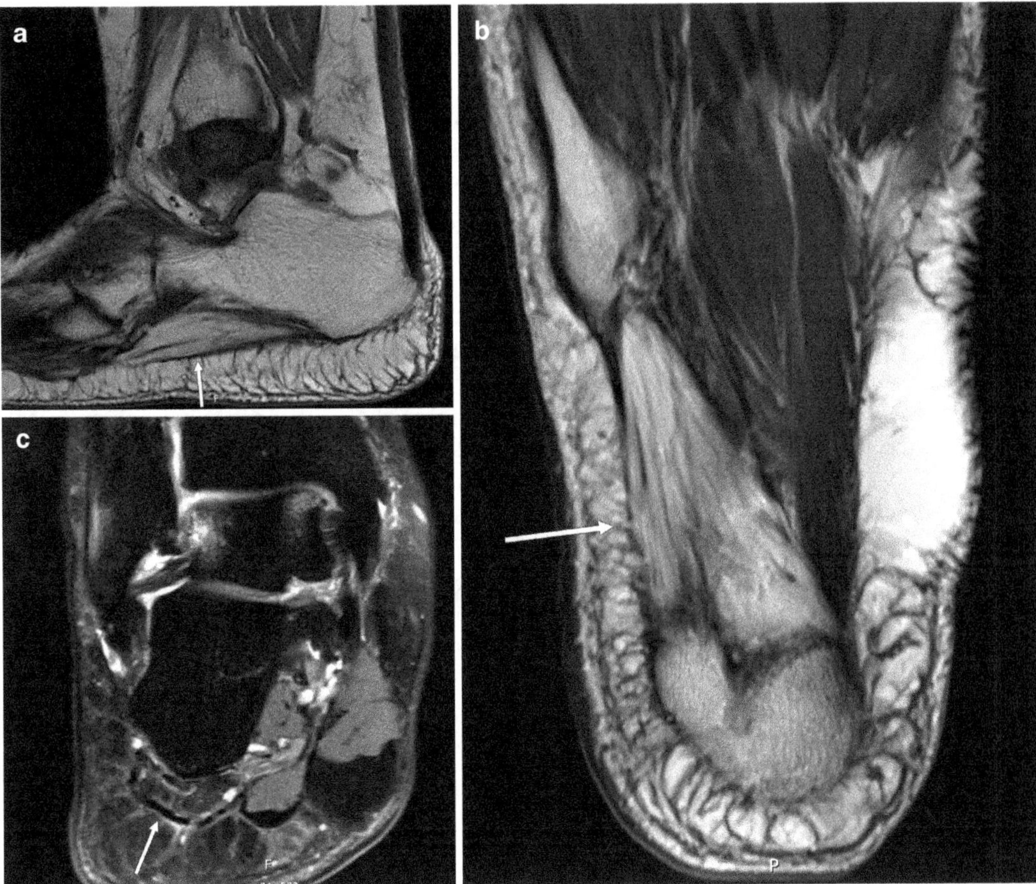

Fig. 18 Sagittal (**a**) and axial T1 (**b**) demonstrating fatty replacement of the abductor digiti minimi (arrow) indicating atrophy, with decreased muscle volume (**c**, arrow), in keeping with a chronic first branch of lateral plantar nerve entrapment—Baxter's neuropathy. Coronal T2 FS shows mild edema in the lateral plantar fascia (**c**). (Courtesy of Harun Gupta)

In runners, the nerve can be stretched and compressed by hypertrophied abductor hallucis muscle. The isolated nerve entrapment presents as neuropathic pain after prolonged activity, likely due to ischemia of the nerve from engorgement of the accompanying branches of the lateral plantar artery (Lui 2016). Another possible site of nerve entrapment is in cases with altered biomechanics, such as excessive pronation, with compression in the movement of lateral rotation between the plantar square and abductor hallucis muscle.

Clinically the compression of the inferior calcaneal nerve is presented with chronic medial plantar heel pain, which is difficult to differentiate from pain secondary to plantar fasciitis, most often with symptoms overlapping (Offutt and DeHeer 2004). However, in contrast to plantar fasciitis, symptoms are located medial and more proximal, worsening with activity, with pain exacerbation in foot eversion and abduction. The patient may report pain radiation proximally into the medial aspect of the ankle or distally and laterally along the plantar foot. Pain radiates to the medial inferior aspect of the heel and proximally into the medial aspect of the ankle region and even may radiate across the plantar aspect of the heel to the lateral aspect of the foot. In chronic cases, the adductor digiti quinti muscle weakness is present, with decreased fifth toe abduction strength, determined by muscle degeneration. Unless there is more proximal entrapment of the nerve (tarsal tunnel syndrome), patients usually do not complain of heel or foot numbness. Palpation provokes maximal tenderness over the course of the nerve in the area of entrapment, typically located on the plantar medial aspect of the foot, anterior to the medial aspect of the calcaneus, and deep to the abductor hallucis muscle. The local symptoms are provoked, like paraesthesia with nerve compression and motor weakness of the adductor digiti minimi muscle. Palpation may even cause radiation of the pain proximally or distally (Baxter and Thigpen 1984).

Plain radiography can identify the presence of plantar calcaneal spurs which may give additional information in symptomatic patients. However, in many patients, calcaneal spurs are asymptomatic (Fuller 2000). On ultrasonography, direct visualization of an enlarged inferior calcaneal nerve can be traced with a dedicated technique and high-resolution US (Martinoli et al. 2010). Muscle atrophy and fatty changes of the adductor digiti minimi muscle caused by chronic denervation are readily recognized on US. A comparison with the adjacent muscles or with the adductor digiti minimi muscle on the contralateral side may aid in the determination of atrophic changes (Hoffman and Bianchi 2013). However, visualization of early denervation changes of the adductor digiti minimi muscle or soft tissue edema around the nerve in neuropathy is better demonstrated by MRI (Donovan et al. 2010; Alshami et al. 2008; Recht et al. 2007b). On MRI no muscle signal changes appear immediately after denervation, but within 4–15 days, with prolongation of both T1 and T2 relaxation times. STIR may be helpful in questionable nerve entrapment cases, presenting as an increased signal. However, in some cases, the MRI may not show evidence of an increased signal in the two muscles innervated by the lateral plantar nerve, the abductor digiti quinti, and flexor digitorum brevis (Fredericson et al. 2001). In later phases, signs of muscle atrophy may be seen in patients with compressive neuropathies, graded as grade 0 no fat or minimal fatty streaks within the muscle, grade 1, increased fat within the muscle but a greater amount of muscle, grade 2, is when there are equal amounts of fat and muscle (Fig. 19); and grade 3, is when there is a greater amount of fat within the muscle compared to muscle tissue (Draghi et al. 2017). Chronic changes of muscle denervation (>1 year) are manifested as atrophy and irreversible fatty replacement which is best evaluated with T1WI. An isolated fatty atrophy of the abductor digiti quinti muscle is a typical MR imaging sign secondary to this neuropathy (Donovan et al. 2010), reflecting a chronic compression of the inferior calcaneal nerve and contributing to the clinical diagnosis of Baxter's neuropathy (Donovan et al. 2010; Recht et al. 2007b). However, few authors reported that selective fatty atrophy of the adductor digiti minimi is also prevalent in patients without entrapment (Recht et al. 2007b), seen in 6.3–7.5% of all MR examinations of the foot and ankle (Recht et al. 2007b). There is a strong correlation between muscle atrophy of adductor digiti minimi and plantar fasciitis and calcaneal spur (Chundru et al. 2008). Plantar enthesophytes, prominent plantar calcaneal spur, and inflammatory changes around even smaller plantar spur may be symptomatic. Chronic plantar fasciitis and local varicosities represent the findings most frequently associated with entrapment of the abductor digiti quinti nerve (Sinnaeve and Vandeputte 2008).

Initially, heel pain should be treated with conservative measures (use of a nocturnal orthosis, therapeutic footwear, physical therapy, anti-inflammatory drugs, and corticoid infiltration) (Thomas et al. 2010; Draghi et al. 2017). In chronic cases, with a lack of improvement after 6 months of conservative treatment (Thomas et al. 2010; Latt et al. 2020), surgical nerve release can be performed. A small portion of bone spur that impinges the nerve in this area can be removed by performing a partial resection (Baxter and Thigpen 1984).

The enthesopathy of the plantar fascia, or plantar fasciitis, is the most important differential diagnosis of the Baxter's neuropathy.

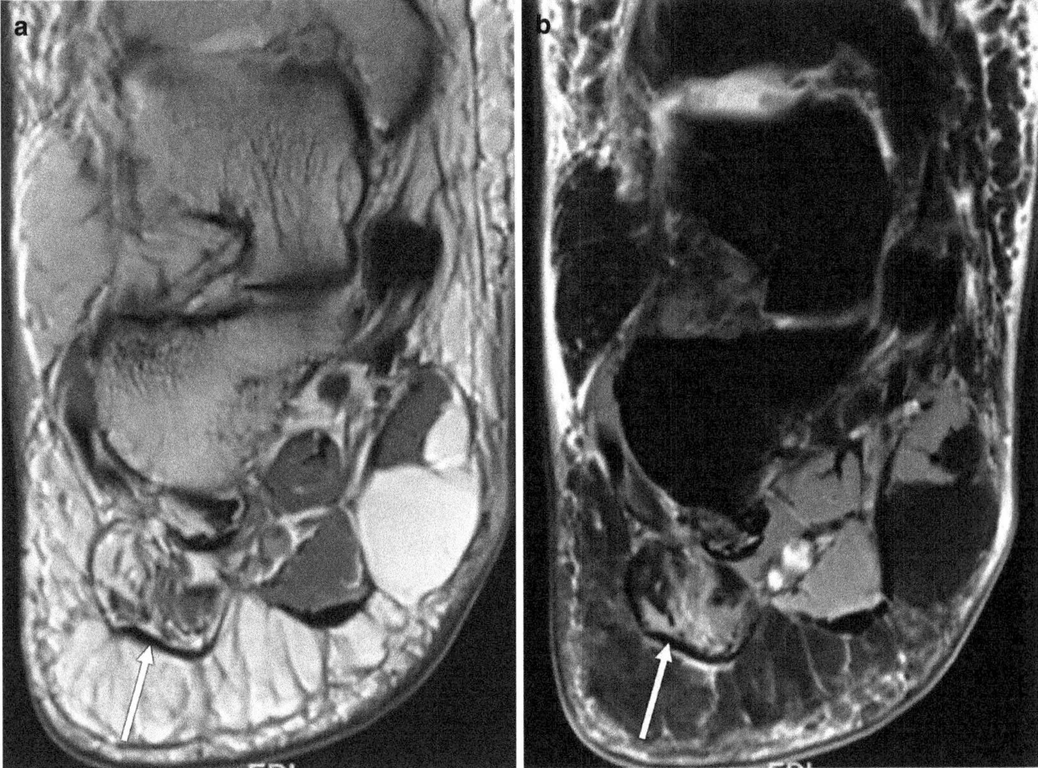

Fig. 19 Coronal PD (**a**) and PDFS (**b**) show grade 2 fatty atrophy of abductor digiti minimi (arrow) with preserved muscle volume in keeping with the first branch of lateral plantar nerve entrapment—Baxter's neuropathy

2.3 Plantar Fascia

The plantar fascia, a thick fibrous connective tissue structure, originates from the calcaneal tuberosity and attaches to the proximal phalanges, the deep soft-tissue forefoot structures, and the skin. It is a band of longitudinally oriented fibers made of three different components: the central band, which is the thickest, and sometimes referred to as plantar aponeurosis; the thinner medial band which inserts at the m. abductor hallucis; lateral band, which inserts at the m. abductor digiti minimi (Draghi et al. 2017; Latt et al. 2020). The central band or the aponeurosis, from its calcaneal attachment extends anteriorly to the forefoot, divides into five separate bundles at the midtarsal level, reaches all proximal phalanxes, and attaches at their plantar plates (Draghi et al. 2017; Chen et al. 2014). It is the part of the plantar fascia that is most commonly involved in plantar fasciitis (Latt et al. 2020). The thickness of the plantar fascia can be clearly depicted and measured by ultrasound or MRI. The primary function of the plantar fascia is supporting the foot during the weight-bearing and maintaining the medial longitudinal arch. It opposes the vertical forces and prevents flattening of the medial longitudinal arch and foot collapse with its longitudinal orientation and stretch tension (Bolgla and Malone 2004).

Normal plantar fascia in the longitudinal plane is a thick, fibrillary structure. Its maximum thickness should not exceed 4 mm in any segment of the fascia (McMillan et al. 2009). The most common pathological condition affecting the plantar fascia is the plantar fasciitis.

Plantar fasciitis is a pain (acute or chronic) appearing at the anteromedial calcaneal prominence, on the attachment of the medial bend of plantar fascia to the calcaneal medial tubercle. It is the most common cause of heel pain in adults (Trojian and Tucker 2019), and a common orthopedic diagnosis, although its name is a misnomer. Plantar fasciitis is an enthesopathy, most probably of a degenerative than inflammatory origin. The histopathological changes consist of fiber disorganization, collagen degeneration, and ground substance increase, which are more similar to fasciosis or fasciopathy than fasciitis (Latt et al. 2020; Trojian and Tucker 2019; Tahririan et al. 2012). The proposed mechanism of the condition is chronic overload due to extensive exercise in young athletes or sedentariness in mature individuals (Trojian and Tucker 2019). The primary symptom is heel pain, appearing during the initial steps usually in the morning or after a prolonged rest period. The pain might reduce or even diminish during the day but deteriorates in the evening (Tahririan et al. 2012).

Ultrasound is usually a first-line diagnostic modality for evaluation of plantar fasciitis. A longitudinal view of the plantar fascia is a preferred plane for the examination. Although the prone position is a preferred method for the examination of plantar fascia, some authors disagree and favor the supine position, because of the theoretically decreased time needed for the exam and increased patient comfortability if lying supine (Ahn et al. 2016).

Ultrasound signs of plantar fasciitis include focal thickening of the plantar fascia, hypoechoic part of the fascia, edema, increased vascularity, and elasticity changes of the fascia (Draghi et al. 2017) (Fig. 20).

A focal fusiform thickening of the plantar fascia, measuring more than 4 mm, in proximity to the fascial attachment at the calcaneal tuberosity is the most common and most reliable sonographic sign for plantar fasciitis diagnosis, which is frequently used by clinicians (McMillan et al. 2009). Focal areas of decreased echogenicity in the proximal plantar fascia also suggest the presence of the condition (McMillan et al. 2009; Cardinal et al. 1996). The changes most possibly are a result of a reparatory process (McMillan et al. 2009). Moderate or strong vascularity in the area near the fascial thickening on Power Doppler ultrasound can be a useful additional sign of plantar fasciitis (Walther et al. 2004). Shear wave elastography of the plantar fascia is a beneficial additional evaluation method (Wu et al. 2022). The plantar fascia is less stiff in patients with plantar fasciitis. The elasticity changes are independent of the thickness and echogenicity of the plantar fascia, adding a new value of SWE in plantar fasciitis diagnosis.

The normal plantar fascia on sagittal MRI images presents as a thin, homogenous band of low signal in T1 and T2 sequences, which is thickest at its origin and becomes thinner distally. Sagittal images are preferred for MR evaluation of the plantar fascia, allowing a longitudinal view of the fascia's total length. Coronal images can be useful in the evaluation of all three bands of the plantar fascia (Theodorou et al. 2002; McNally and Shetty 2010).

MRI signs of plantar fasciitis include thickening of the plantar fascia at its calcaneal attachment similar to US exam, intrafascial high signal in the fluid sensitive sequences and intermediate signal in T1 sequence, high signal in perifascial soft tissue in fluid sensitive sequences representing edema, and osseous edema at the calcaneal attachment (Draghi et al. 2017; Theodorou et al. 2002; McNally and Shetty 2010; Lawrence et al. 2013) (Figs. 17 and 20).

Plantar fasciitis is a self-limiting condition in the majority of cases, which response to conservative treatment, and imaging is required and necessary primarily for refractory cases, or more invasive therapy strategies are considered (Tahririan et al. 2012).

2.4 Plantar Interdigital Nerve Compressive Neuropathy: Morton Neuroma

At the level of metatarsal bases, the medial and lateral plantar nerves divide into interdigital nerves, which pass deep to the transverse intermetatarsal ligament into a relatively small space between the metatarsal heads, where with the plantar skin the tunnel is formed. The interdigital nerve can be entrapped near the distal edge of the intermetatarsal ligament, most commonly in the third web space (Fig. 21). Occasionally it may appear in the second web space. The primary

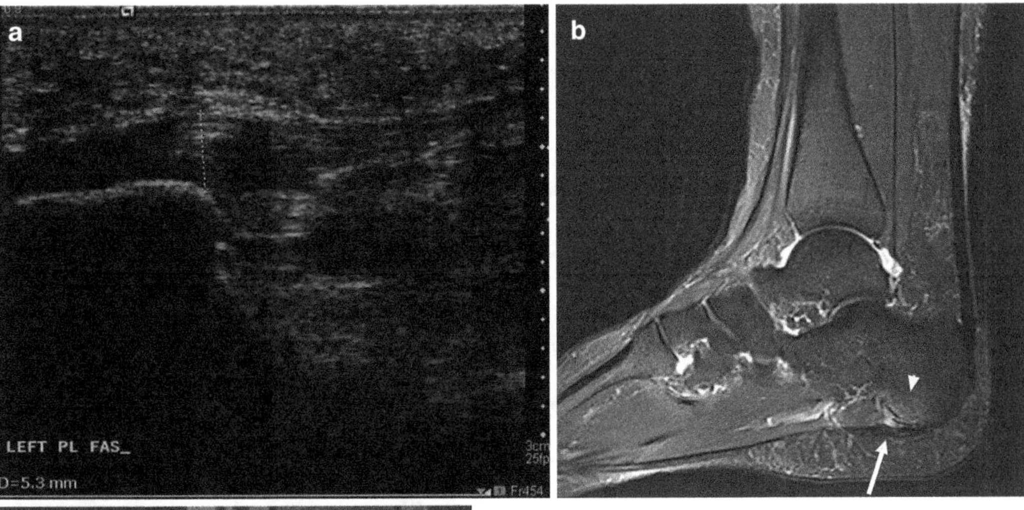

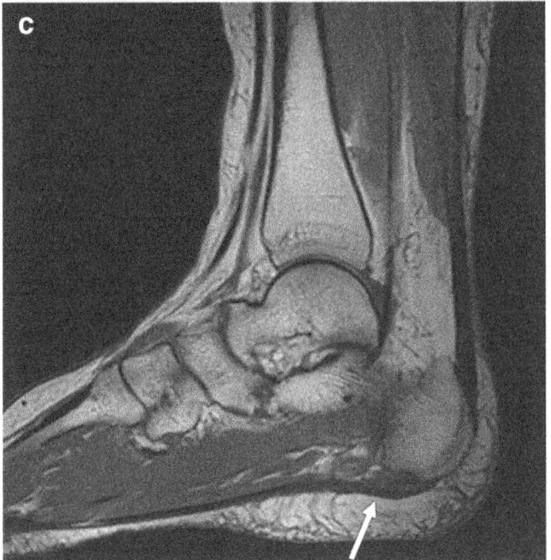

Fig. 20 US and MRI of plantar fasciitis. A longitudinal US image of the plantar fascia reveals an area of focal thickening measuring 5.3 mm and hypoechoic changes in the same area (**a**). A focal thickening, perifascial edema (**b**, **c**, arrow), and osseous edema of the calcaneal tuberosity at the fascial attachment are noted (**b**, arrowhead)

cause of the entrapment is not clear yet. Possibly the nerve is compressed by the metatarsal heads and the surrounding soft tissue of metatarsophalangeal joints due to repetitive microtraumas, or the compression appears by the intermetatarsal ligament (Giannini et al. 2004; Kim et al. 2007b; Peters et al. 2011). However, it demonstrates a soft-tissue lesion, mass-like enlargement called a "Morton neuroma" with consequent loss of normal fat in the intermetatarsal space. Repetitive mechanical stress with subsequent perineural fibrosis results in the development of Morton neuroma, often associated with the presence of inflamed and enlarged intermetatarsal bursa that may cause compression and ischemia of the nerve. The term "neuroma" is a misnomer, because it is not a true neoplasm. It is formed from nerve degeneration, endoneurial edema, epineurial and endoneurial vascular hyalinization, and perineural fibrosis along common plantar digital nerve suggesting nonneoplastic lesion (Bencardino et al. 2000). Women are more often affected as the result of wearing narrow-toe box shoes that cause forefoot compression during walking, associated with metatarsophalangeal joint injury. Excessive pronation and dorsiflexion

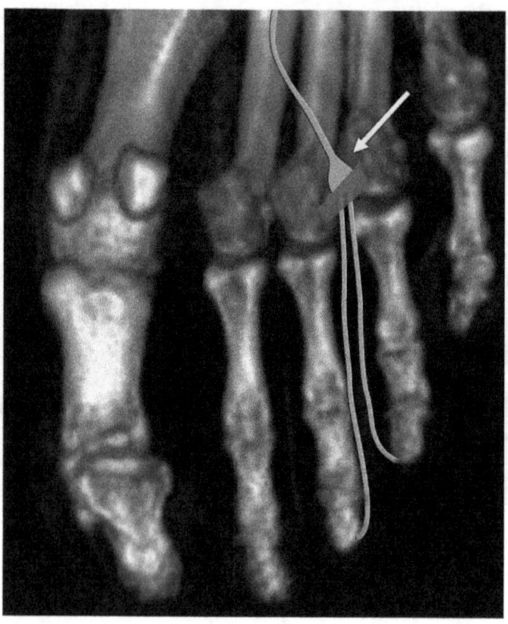

Fig. 21 Illustration of interdigital nerve compressive neuropathy—Morton neuroma. Medial and lateral plantar nerves, at the level of metatarsal bases, divide into interdigital nerves, which pass deep to the transverse intermetatarsal ligament (gray thick line) into a relatively small space between the metatarsal heads. The interdigital nerve is entrapped near the distal edge of the intermetatarsal ligament, forming a mass Morton's neuroma (arrow)

of the metatarsal bones, arthritis, ganglion cysts, Freiberg's infarction, and repetitive traumas due to sports activities such as running and ballet dancing are included in the etiology.

Symptoms are burning or electric pain and paresthesias in the typical location of affected web space with a sensation of walking on a lump, with symptoms of Morton's metatarsalgia that arise from mechanical stress and compression of the transverse forefoot arch. Direct pressure placed plantarly between the metatarsal heads that can reproduce the symptoms or findings indicates a positive Mulder sign. The Morton neurinoma in most patients can be diagnosed clinically, and clinician may ask for imaging only in atypical presentations to help confirm the diagnosis.

Radiographs can be used to exclude differential diagnoses such as osteonecrosis, stress fracture, or arthritis at the metatarsophalangeal joint. Direct reliable identification of neuroma can be done on ultrasonography and MRI (Lopez-Ben 2011; Donovan et al. 2010; Musson et al. 2012) which are recommended to confirm as well as rule out other soft-tissue masses. Nevertheless, asymptomatic patients may also have positive MRI or ultrasonography findings of neuroma (Bencardino et al. 2000; Symeonidis et al. 2012; Sharp et al. 2003).

US evaluation can be performed with a dorsal approach. The toes are in plantar flexion, and manual pressure in the affected web space is applied on the plantar side. Due to the thinner skin and the absence of keratosis, the quality of sonograms is better in the dorsal probe approach to the lesion. For the plantar approach, the toes are dorsiflexed and finger pressure is exerted in the web spaces on the dorsal side. Doppler imaging demonstrates adjacent intermetatarsal arteries and veins which serve as a valuable landmark for the localization of the nerve (Fessell and van Holsbeeck 1999). An ultrasound dynamic study with the probe pressed on the plantar area in both axis, by the spread of the metatarsal heads, shows the deep tarsometatarsal ligament between them as a hyperechoic band that pushes the tissues and/area to the plantar area of the foot allowing further exploration of the region (Petscavage-Thomas 2014; Del Mar Ruiz-Herrera et al. 2022; Del Mar et al. 2022). On US, neuromas are identified as fusiform, non-compressible, hypoechoic masses displacing the expected hyperechoic fat within the intermetatarsal spaces (Lopez-Ben 2011) that may not have intralesional Doppler signal (Fig. 22a, b). Performing a sonographic Mulder test, by squeezing the metatarsal bones together and visualizing the neuroma popping up plantarly, can improve the sensitivity (Torriani and Kattapuram 2003). Intense tenderness elicited by pressure with the transducer over the suspected neuroma supports the diagnosis. Identification of small lesions, less than 5 mm in diameter, can be difficult with US.

On MRI, Morton's neuroma is best seen in the true coronal view (perpendicular axis to the long axis of the foot), best visualized with an extremity coil while the patient is in the prone body position with the foot in plantar flexion (Zanetti et al. 1997; Weishaupt et al. 2003). The MRI

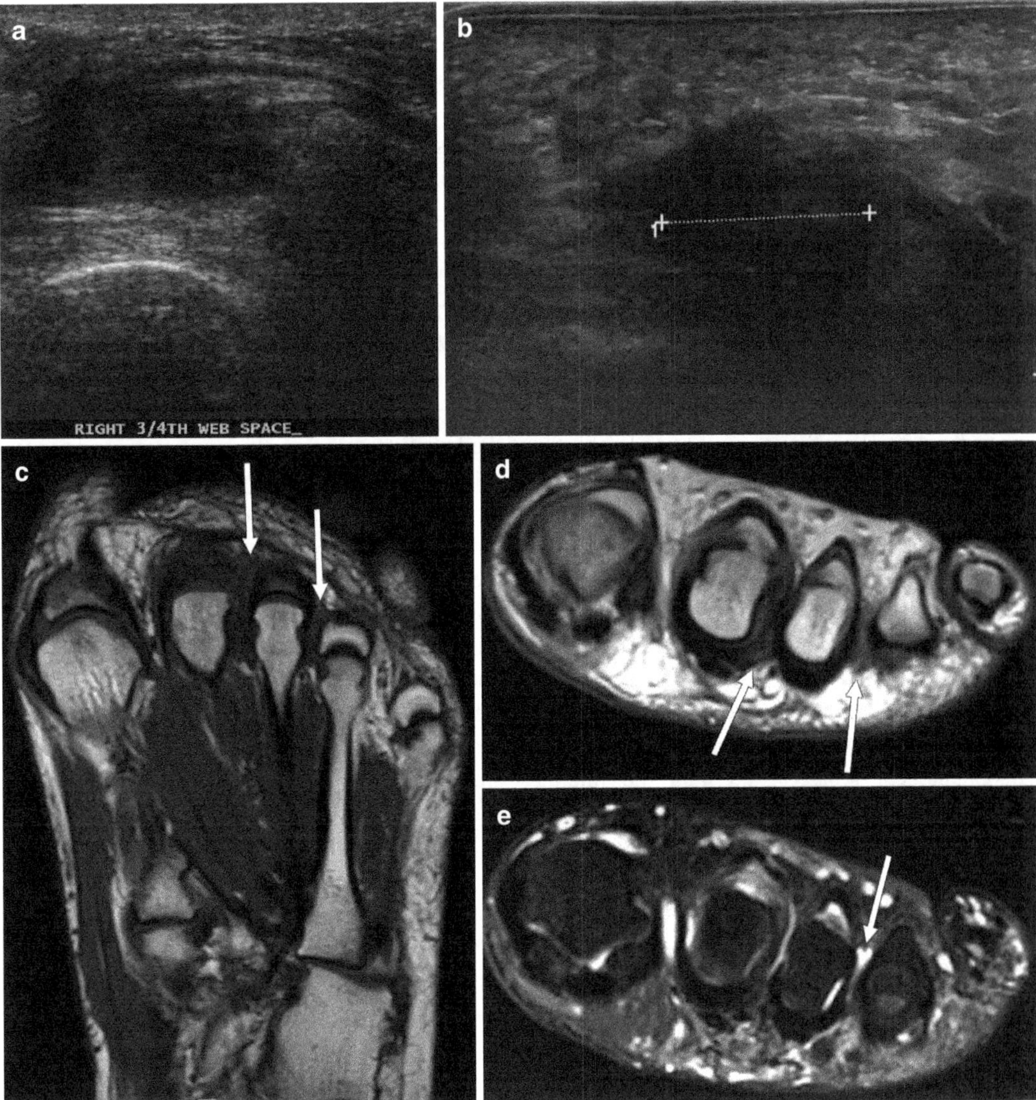

Fig. 22 Intermetatarsal neuropathy (Morton's neuroma). A 43-year-old female with paresthesias and electric pain in the second and third web space with a sensation of walking on a lump. Longitudinal (**a**) and transverse (**b**) US image, long-axis T1WI (**c**), short-axis T2WI (**d**), PD fat-suppressed (**e**) MRI. US scans of the third intermetatarsal space show a hypoechoic and fusiform mass (between the caliper markings) consistent with a Morton neuroma. Thickening of the digital nerve was also noted. On MRI note the hypointense plantar mass located in the second and third metatarsal space (**c**, **d**, arrows). On the T2WI the masses are with intermediate signal intensity (**d**, arrow). An intermetatarsal bursa in the third web space is present (**e**, arrow)

appearance of the Morton's neuroma is characteristic, seen as an enhancing tear-drop-shaped or a dumbbell soft-tissue mass with intermediate to low signal intensity signal on both T1WI and T2WI sequences, and with a highly variable appearance on STIR and contrast-enhanced T1WI with fat suppression because of variable composition of the inflammatory and fibrotic tissue (Bencardino et al. 2000). The T1-weighted sequence allows more reliable identification of this lesion, showing neuroma as a mass isointense to the muscle replacing normal fat at the plantar aspect of the intermetatarsal space with a variable degree of dorsal intermetatarsal extension. Its typical localization is centered between the metatarsal heads (Fig. 22c, d). The diagnosis of a Morton neuroma on MR imaging should be considered when the diameter of the lesion is 5 mm or greater but with a correlation with clinical symptoms. An intermetatarsal bursa may contain a small amount of fluid, seen between the metatarsal heads located dorsal to the neuroma. The normal transverse diameter of the bursa is 3 mm or less (Zanetti et al. 1997) (Fig. 22e). Pericapsular fibrosis associated with plantar plate and capsular tears can mimic Morton's neuroma but it has an eccentric location of the mass, adherent to the capsule rather than centered over the interdigital space (Umans et al. 2014; Gorbachova 2020).

Nonsurgical management includes orthoses, metatarsal pads, accommodative footwear, NSAIDs, and injections. Corticosteroid injections provide good short-term pain relief but little long-term improvement (Markovic et al. 2008), with possible complications after repeated corticosteroid injections such as damage to the metatarsophalangeal joint capsule and the plantar plate. Serial injections of alcohol sclerosing agents should be performed with adequate precautions as it may damage the surrounding tissues (Espinosa et al. 2011; Gurdezi et al. 2013).

Surgical treatment is typically through a dorsal approach with removal of the primary lesions, (Title and Schon 2008) with excellent results and good outcomes (Peters et al. 2011; Title and Schon 2008; Womack et al. 2008). If symptoms are left untreated, there may be persistent foot pain, motor deficits, and severe numbness, potentially leading to plantar ulcerations and complex regional pain syndrome (Greene 2001).

3 Deep Peroneal Nerve Compressive Neuropathy: Anterior Tarsal Tunnel Syndrome

Deep peroneal nerve compression neuropathy might occur within the anterior tarsal tunnel beneath the inferior extensor retinaculum which is known as anterior tarsal tunnel syndrome. The deep peroneal nerve is one of two terminal branches of the common peroneal nerve which runs between the tibialis anterior and the extensor hallucis longus five centimeters above the ankle mortise. At the ankle, it courses under the superior extensor retinaculum to enter the anterior tarsal tunnel, approximately 1 cm proximal to the ankle joint. The nerve divides into medial and lateral branches (Donovan et al. 2010; Flanigan and DiGiovanni 2011; Aktan Ikiz et al. 2007). Both branches cross under the inferior extensor retinaculum. The lateral branch provides sensation to the ankle joint (critical for ankle stability), the lateral tarsal joint, the sinus tarsi, and the tarsal and metatarsophalangeal joints of the middle three digits (Kennedy et al. 2007), whereas the motor innervation is for the extensor digitorum brevis. The medial branch path is parallel to the dorsalis pedis artery, dorsally to the talonavicular joint, and between the bases of the first and second metatarsals to provide sensation to the first web space and occasional motor supply to the first web space (Donovan et al. 2010; Flanigan and DiGiovanni 2011; Aktan Ikiz et al. 2007) (Fig. 23).

Neuropathy may result from the compression of the deep peroneal nerve and either of its branches, as the nerve passes through the anterior tarsal tunnel. The anterior tarsal tunnel is a fibro-osseous tunnel along the dorsal midfoot, superficially defined by the inferior extensor retinaculum (roof), laterally by the fibula, medially by the medial malleolar process of the distal tibia, and the talonavicular joint capsule deeply, forming the floor (Aktan Ikiz et al. 2007). It is a flat space between the medial and lateral malleoli. Contents include the extensor musculature of the foot (tibialis anterior, extensor halluces longus, extensor digitorum longus, and peroneus tertius tendon as anatomical variant (Derrick et al. 2016), the dorsalis pedis artery and vein, and the deep peroneal nerve) (Ferkel et al. 2015; Manoharan et al. 2021).

The symptom resulting from the compression of the lateral branch of the deep peroneal nerve is dorsal foot pain that radiates to the region of the lateral tarsometatarsal joints, whereas in medial branch compression patients often complain of

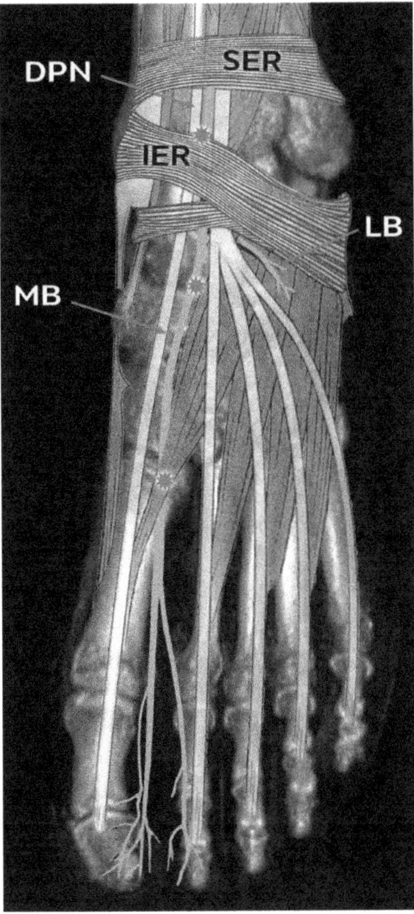

Fig. 23 Deep peroneal nerve anatomy and sites of entrapment. The deep peroneal nerve (DPN) courses under the superior extensor retinaculum (SER) and under and below inferior extensor retinaculum (IER) bifurcates to its medial (MB) and lateral branches (LB). The three most common sites for DPN entrapment (stars) are: one deep to the inferior extensor retinaculum, along the superior border as the nerve dives under the retinaculum, second deep to the extensor hallucis longus tendon at the level of the talonavicular joint, and the third location is deep to the extensor hallucis brevis muscle (at the level of the first and second tarsal-metatarsal joints)

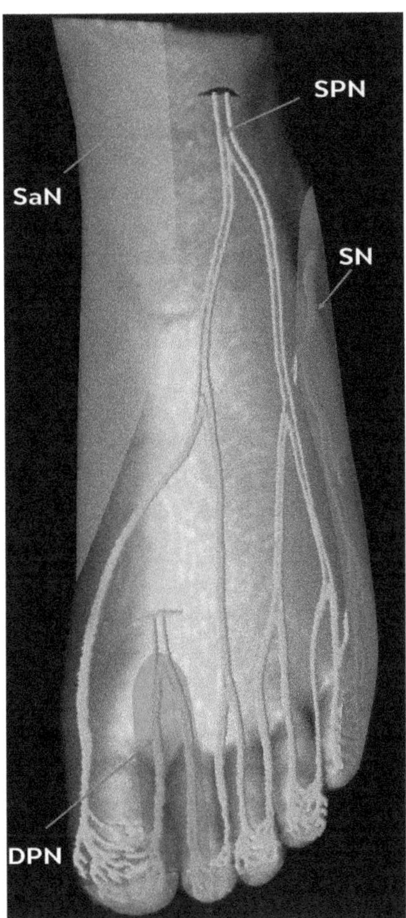

Fig. 24 Sensory innervation of the dorsum of the foot. *DPN* deep peroneal nerve, *SPN* superficial peroneal nerve, *SN* sural nerve, *SaN* saphenous nerve

the presence of pain and/or numbness to the first web space. Patients with a lesion of the deep peroneal nerve experience sensory changes along the dorsal/medial aspect of the foot (Fig. 24). Extensor digitorum weakness may be present. The entire deep peroneal nerve from behind the neck of the fibula to the first web space should be examined clinically. The precise site of the compression may often be confirmed with a local nerve block.

The deep peroneal nerve may become entrapped at three anatomic locations (Fig. 23). The first one is deep to the inferior extensor retinaculum along the superior border as the nerve dives under the retinaculum, at the inferior extensor retinaculum where the extensor hallucis longus tendon crosses over it (Lopez-Ben 2011). The second location is deep to the extensor hallucis longus tendon at the level of the talonavicular joint. The third one is deep to the extensor hallucis brevis muscle at the level of the first and second tarsal-metatarsal articulations, caused by dorsal osteophytes in the tarsometatarsal joints,

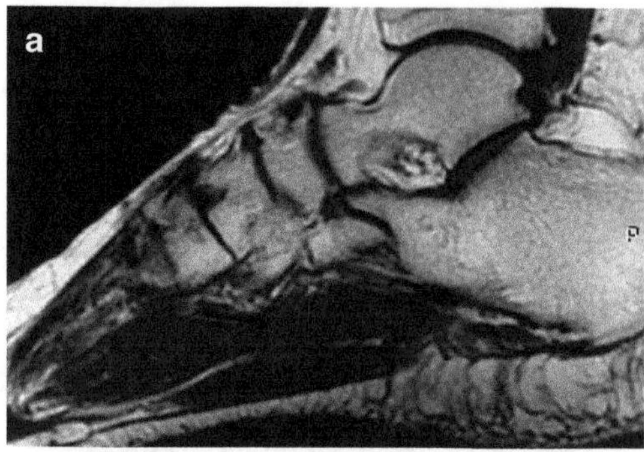

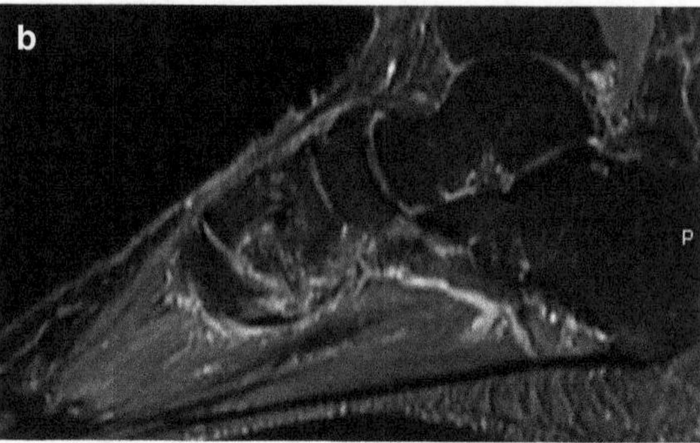

Fig. 25 Anterior tarsal syndrome due to osteoarthritis of the talonavicular joint and navicular/cuneiform joint. Sagittal T1WI and PD fat-saturated image shows dorsally directed osteophytes around the talonavicular joint and navicular/cuneiform joints (**a**) causing reactive changes of the soft tissue compressing the deep peroneal nerve (**b**)

secondary to underlying degenerative joint disease (Beltran et al. 2010; Parker 2005). Dorsally directed osteophytosis (Fig. 25) and reactive changes caused by repetitive external compression at tight shoe wear (Fig. 26) may compressed the nerve. The reactive changes at the talonavicular and/or navicular-cuneiform joints dorsally directed ganglia (Fig. 27), and intraneural ganglion formation has been described as a cause of the nerve compression (Aktan Ikiz et al. 2007). The sensory branch of the deep peroneal nerve courses over the dorsum of the foot, so trauma in this area from tight shoe wear, or repetitive blows as is seen with soccer players, can cause chronic injury (Martinoli et al. 2010).

In anterior tarsal tunnel syndrome, a radiographic evaluation is critical in the workup since the most common causes are trauma and impingement of the nerve by dorsally directed osteophytes around the talonavicular joint and navicular/cuneiform joints. They can be identified on CT and MRI. MRI is relatively poor in nerve identification at the foot and ankle level, because of its small size and its close apposition to the dorsal surfaces of the foot bones. Using US, the nerve can be seen as it becomes more superficial under the extensor retinaculum between the extensor hallucis longus and extensor digitorum longus, just lateral to the dorsalis pedis artery which may serve as a landmark for nerve identification. MRI may be used if a space-occupying lesion is suspected (Donovan et al. 2010). Denervation changes within a deep peroneal nerve distribution include the anterior tibial, extensor hallucis longus, extensor digitorum longus, and peroneus tertius musculature.

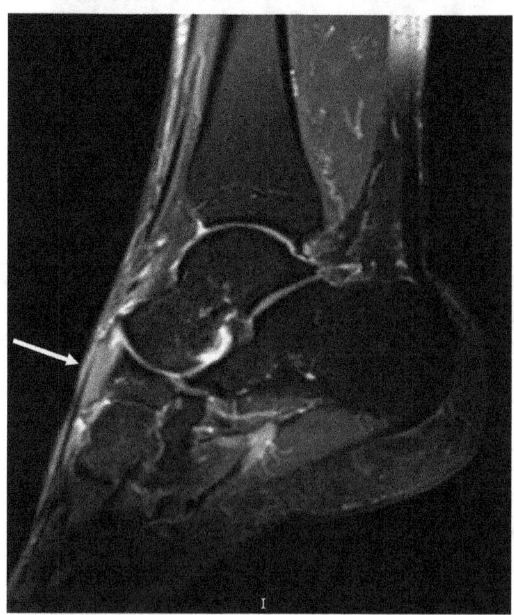

Fig. 26 MRI of deep peroneal neuropathy—anterior tarsal tunnel syndrome. The patient presented with disturbance of the sensation of the first web space which appear after wearing a tight shoe wear. On the sagittal PD fat-saturated image, an area of increased signal intensity can be seen at the level of the dorsal aspect of the navicular/cuneiform joint (arrow), indicating chronic reactive changes that involve the medial branch of the deep peroneal nerve

Nonsurgical management consists of physical therapy, reducing external compression, and sta-

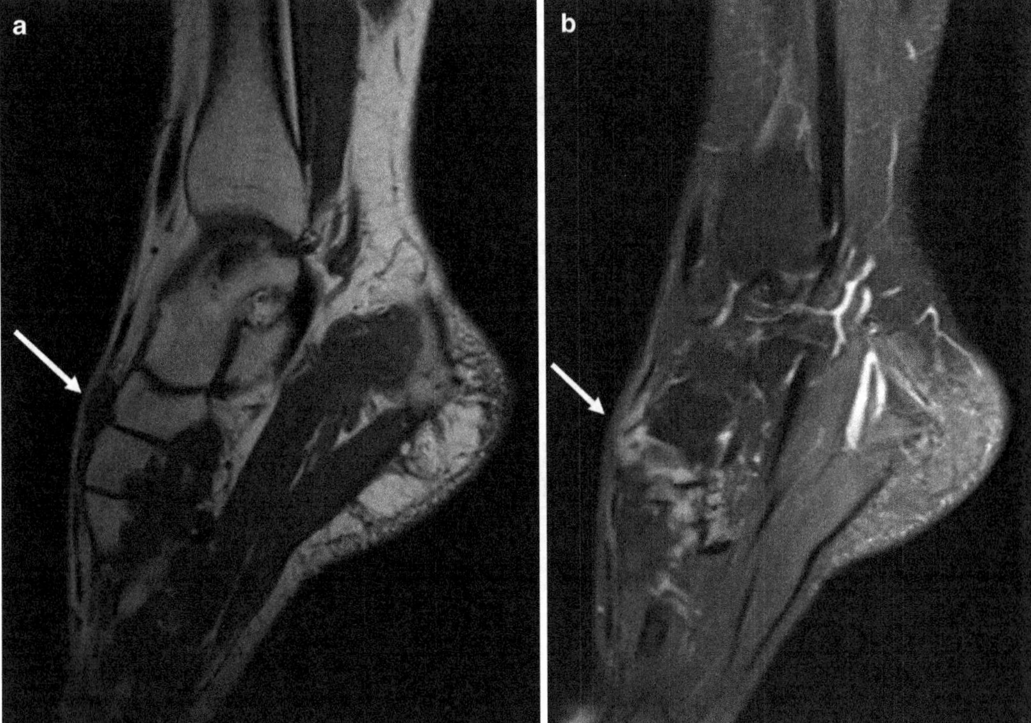

Fig. 27 Deep peroneal neuropathy. A 46-year-old male patient presented with a sensory deficit at the first web space after operative treatment of a dorsally directed ganglion cyst at the level of the navicular-cuneiform joint. On T1 WI sagittal image, a small residual ganglion is presented locally with low signal intensity (**a**, arrow). The medial branch of the deep peroneal nerve is entrapped in a postoperative scar and adjacent reactive changes are seen on sagittal PD fat-saturated images (**b**, arrow)

bilizing any ankle laxity. Surgical release is performed with releasing of the extensor retinaculum, and scarring reduction from extensive nerve dissection. Removal of the osteophytes over the ankle joint or over the dorsal edge of the talonavicular joint can be beneficial. If the extensor halluces brevis tendon is compressing the nerve, partial resection and transfer to the extensor halluces longus can be recommended (Flanigan and DiGiovanni 2011).

4 Superficial Peroneal Nerve Compressive Neuropathy

The superficial peroneal nerve is the superficial terminal branch of the common peroneal nerve. It courses through the lateral leg compartment, between the peroneal muscles and m. extensor digitorum longus, near to the anterior intermuscular septum. The nerve pierces the crural fascia at the distal part of the leg and divides into its terminal sensory branches, the medial and intermediate dorsal cutaneous nerves, in the subcutaneous fat tissue (Tzika et al. 2015; Canella et al. 2009). The terminal branches innervate the skin of the dorsum of the foot and toes, with the exception of the lateral side of the little toe and the medial foot part (Fig. 24). Proximally to its bifurcation, the nerve gives motor branches for m. peroneus longus and brevis (Tzika et al. 2015).

Compressive neuropathy of the superficial peroneal nerve is a rare entrapment syndrome and seldom an isolated nerve abnormality. The symptoms can overlap with common peroneal nerve entrapment or L5 radiculopathy (Fortier et al. 2021). There are two common sites of nerve entrapment. At the level of the ankle, or at the

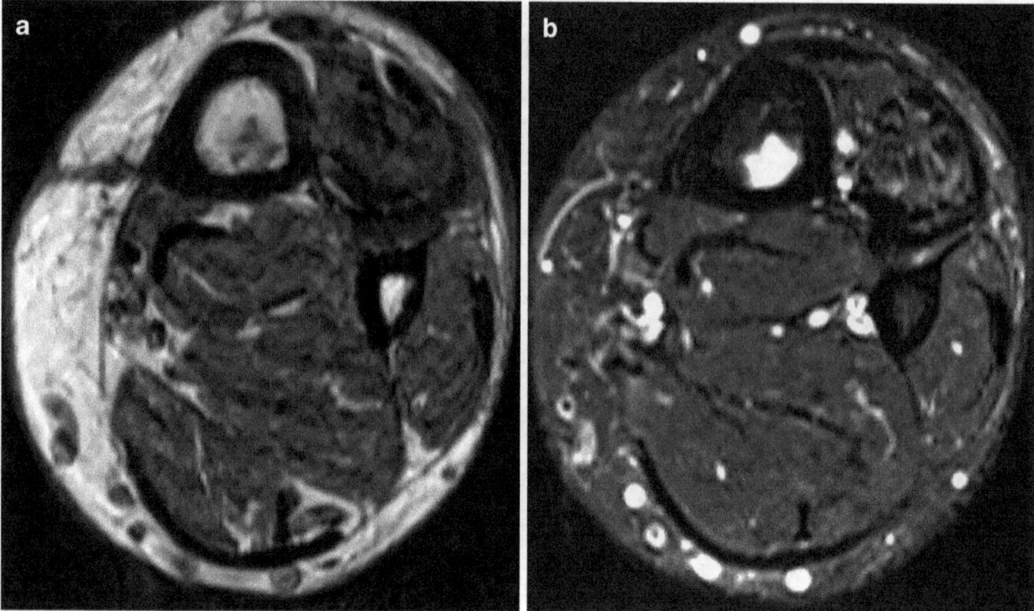

Fig. 28 Superficial peroneal nerve compressive neuropathy. Previous Ilizarov fixation of the tibia for knee distraction—problematic anterolateral pin-site scarring changes. Developed pain on the dorsum of the foot suspected for superficial peroneal nerve involvement. On axial MRI T1WI (**a**) and PD fat-saturated (**b**) images present scarring changes in the anterior extensor compartment encroaching on the superficial peroneal nerve. (Courtesy of Harun Gupta)

point where it passes through the crural fascia, which is the most usual site of the nerve entrapment. The entrapment can be a result of recurrent microtrauma—stretch injury, peroneal hypertrophy like in ballet dancers, soft-tissue masses (ganglion cyst), muscle or fat herniation through the fascia, direct trauma (fibular fracture or ankle sprain), surgery, etc. (Canella et al. 2009; Fortier et al. 2021; Luz et al. 2014) (Fig. 28).

The diagnosis is usually clinical, based on the patient's symptoms. Common entrapment clinical sign is a sensory disorder of the foot dorsum and/or lateral lower leg, without associated weakness of the peroneal muscles (Tzika et al. 2015).

Radiography can exclude osseous changes such as fractures and bone tumors near the nerve course. MRI can be useful for identifying the exact compression spot, focal edema, nerve diameter, and the possible muscle herniation with muscle edema (Donovan et al. 2010). The total length of the nerve can be visualized adequately with high-resolution ultrasound (Canella et al. 2009), which can be a primary imaging method for the evaluation of superficial peroneal nerve entrapment (Luz et al. 2014). Perineural corticosteroid injections with ultrasound guidance can be a useful therapeutic technique (Luz et al. 2014).

5 Sural Nerve Compressive Neuropathy

The sural nerve is a purely sensory nerve located in the subcutaneous fat along the lateral Achilles tendon that continues inferiorly below the lateral malleolus and the peroneal tendons and bifurcates into terminal branches at the level of the fifth metatarsal base.

Although rare, the most common sites of entrapment of the sural nerve are along the lateral border of the ankle, lateral malleolus, the area of the calcaneus, and the fifth metatarsal. It is often due to bony overgrowth secondary to trauma, and/or surgery, or in a sequel of prior fractures involving the lateral malleolus the cuboid, or base of the fifth metatarsal base (Lopez-Ben 2011) due to soft-tissue scarring (Seror 2002; Yuebing and Lederman 2014). However, atraumatic entrapment of the nerve can occur along the lateral border of the proximal Achilles tendon which is the area where the nerve passes through a fibrous arcade when it moves from a deep to a superficial position (Fabre et al. 2000). Sural neuropathy may be secondary to tendinopathy of the adjacent Achilles and peroneal tendons or in the setting of prior trauma (Fig. 29).

Symptoms are burning pain, numbness, or aching in the posterolateral aspect of the leg, lateral ankle, or lateral aspect of the foot. In young athletes, the pain is often exclusive to the posterolateral leg adjacent to the musculotendinous junction of the Achilles tendon (Fabre et al. 2000).

Bony abnormalities may be identified on radiography and confirmed with CT or MRI. They may tense the nerve due to impingement or structural abnormalities. The lesser saphenous vein lies adjacent to the sural nerve which serves as an accurate landmark for sonographic localization of this small nerve on its course down the calf near the Achilles tendon (Martinoli et al. 2010). The sonographic findings of entrapment include focal nerve enlargement proximal to the site of entrapment and focal narrowing at the site of entrapment from adjacent scarring or other extrinsic causes. MRI is less useful in direct visualization of the nerve entrapment, given the small size of this nerve. However, MRI may be helpful in assessing the degree of tendinopathy, and other underlying causes, which can be ruled out, like soft-tissue masses or other space-occupying lesions that may compress the nerve (Fig. 30). The treatment of sural nerve entrapment is dependent on the accurate identification of the causative factors and the location of the entrapment (Fabre et al. 2000). Surgical intervention should address any bony abnormalities, deformities, or

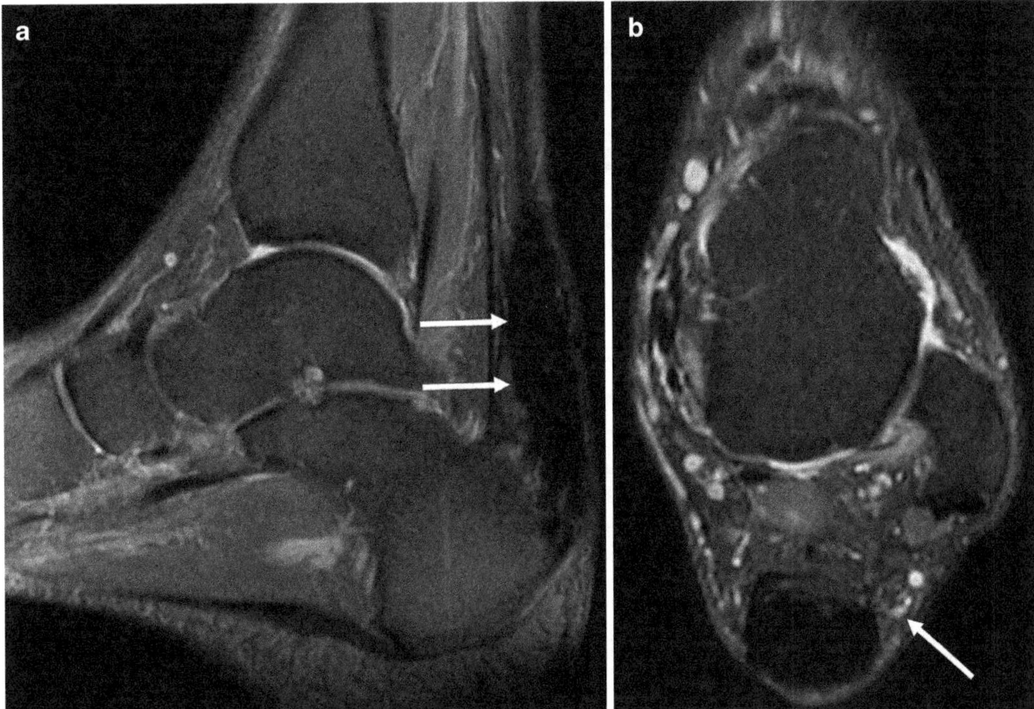

Fig. 29 Sural nerve neuropathy. Status post Achilles tendon rupture with operative treatment. Due to foreign body reactions on the surgical material, chronic reactive changes on the tendon appear with subsequent bacterial inflammation. Chronic inflammation was healed with more extensive scaring tissue (**a**, arrows) with involvement of the sural nerve, retracted by the scaring tissue (**b**, arrow), when a sensory deficit appeared

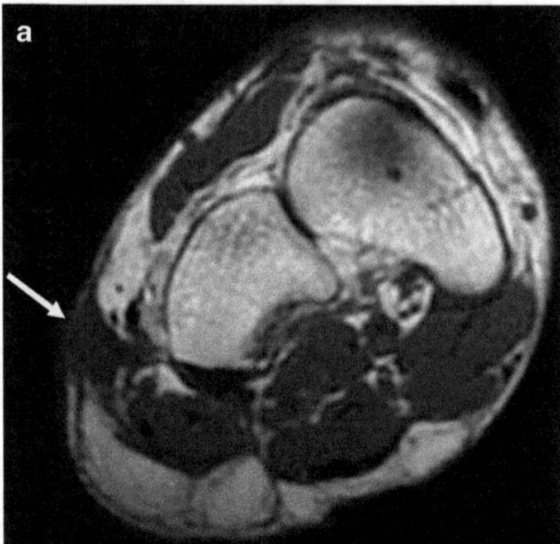

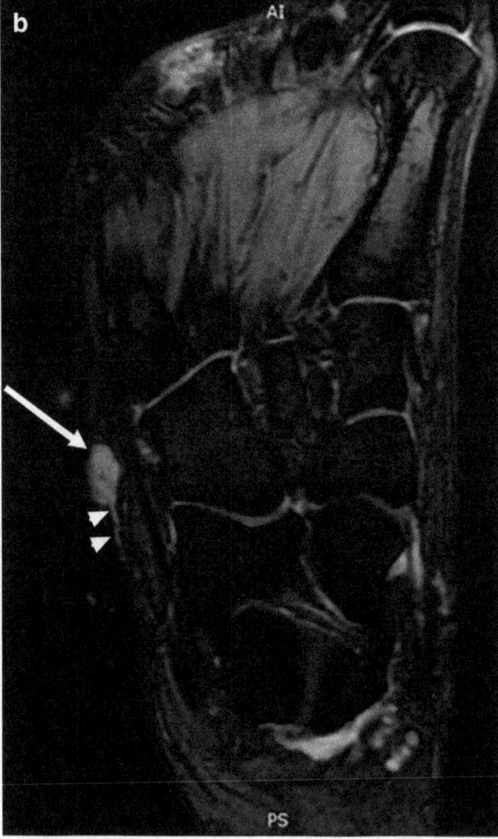

Fig. 30 Sural nerve neuropathy due to ganglion cyst. A 27-year-old female presented with a lump of the lateral aspect of the midfoot with a sensory deficit. A polylobulated high signal intensity lesion is presented on axial T2WI and PD FS images (**a**, **b**, arrow) with enlarged and with high signal intensity presented sural nerve (arrowheads)

joint instability. If no causative factor is identified, efforts should be directed at establishing the exact location of the entrapment and the nerve released from the constrictive tissue. A nerve resection may also be performed, with satisfactory results (Fabre et al. 2000).

6 Saphenous Nerve Compressive Neuropathy

The saphenous nerve is the longest, purely sensory terminal branch of the femoral nerve (Flanigan and DiGiovanni 2011). The nerve at the level of the foot and ankle is called the superficial or distal saphenous nerve. It gives innervation to the medial part of the distal foot (Brown et al. 2016). Entrapment of the distal saphenous nerve is a very rare condition, the rarest of all entrapment neuropathies of the foot and ankle.

Patients with saphenous entrapment can present with pain and paresthesias at the anteromedial side of the foot and ankle, proximally to the metacarpophalangeal joints (Kalenak 1996). Typically, entrapment occurs more proximally. Distal entrapment of this nerve is most often secondary to trauma, including ankle fractures or distortion, but can be iatrogenic trauma, soft tissue or bone tumors, ganglion cyst, varices, and muscle or tendon abnormalities (Flanigan and DiGiovanni 2011). Radiography can exclude fracture and a subsequent osseous impingement, CT exam can be helpful to rule out bony or soft-tissue obstructions, or for preoperative planning. MRI and ultrasound are complementary methods, which can identify the compression cause (Flanigan and DiGiovanni 2011; Brown et al. 2016). In addition, ultrasound-guided local anesthetic infiltration for pain relief can be performed, or preoperative nerve block, which can be useful as a part of ankle block (Brown et al. 2016). Surgical intervention (decompression, neurolysis, or neurectomy) should be delayed until it is determined that nonsurgical management options have failed to provide relief. Decompression and neurolysis may be the preferred options because neurectomy inevitably leads to permanent sensory deficits (Flanigan and DiGiovanni 2011; Kalenak 1996).

References

Ahn JH, Lee CW, Park C, Kim YC (2016) Ultrasonographic examination of plantar fasciitis: a comparison of patient positions during examination. J Foot Ankle Res 9:38

Aktan Ikiz ZA, Ucerler H, Uygur M (2007) Dimensions of the anterior tarsal tunnel and features of the deep peroneal nerve in relation to clinical application. Surg Radiol Anat 29(7):527–530

Alaia EF, Rosenberg ZS, Bencardino JT, Ciavarra GA, Rossi I, Petchprapa CN (2016) Tarsal tunnel disease and talocalcaneal coalition: MRI features. Skeletal Radiol 45(11):1507–1514

Alshami AM, Souvlis T, Coppieters MW (2008) A review of plantar heel pain of neural origin: differential diagnosis and management. Man Ther 13:103–111

Amlang M, Rosenow MC, Friedrich A, Zwipp H, Rammelt S (2012) Direct plantar approach to Henry's knot for flexor hallucis longus transfer. Foot Ankle Int 33(1):7–13

Arakawa T, Sekiya S, Terashima T, Miki A (2011) Pseudoganglion on the connecting branch between the deep branch of the lateral plantar nerve and medial plantar nerve. Clin Anat 24(5):646–651

Arenson DJ, Cosentino GL, Suran SM (1990) The inferior calcaneal nerve: an anatomic study. J Am Podiatry Assoc 70:552–560

Baba H, Wada M, Annen S, Azuchi M, Imura S, Tomita K (1997) The tarsal tunnel syndrome: evaluation of surgical results using multivariate analysis. Int Orthop 21(2):67–71

Badr IT, Hassan S, Fotoh DS, Moawad MM (2020) Extrinsic compression neuropathy of the tibial nerve secondary to accessory soleus muscle in a young teenager. J Clin Orthop Trauma 11(2):302–306

Barker AR, Rosson GD, Dellon AL (2007) Pressure changes in the medial and lateral plantar, and tarsal tunnels related to ankle position: a cadaver study. Foot Ankle Int 28:250–254

Baxter DE, Thigpen CM (1984) Heel pain: operative results. Foot Ankle 5(1):16–25. le Surg. 2010;49(3 Suppl):S1–S19

Beltran LS, Bencardino J, Ghazikhanian V, Beltran J (2010) Entrapment neuropathies III: lower limb. Semin Musculoskelet Radiol 14(5):501–511

Bencardino J, Rosenberg ZS, Beltran J, Liu X, Marty-Delfaut E (2000) Morton's neuroma: is it always symptomatic? AJR Am J Roentgenol 175(3):649–653

Bendszus M, Koltzenburg M, Wessig C, Solymosi L (2002) Sequential MR imaging of denervated muscle: experimental study. AJNR Am J Neuroradiol 23:1427–1431

Berachilovic A, Nihal A, Houston VL et al (2006) Effect of foot and ankle position on tarsal tunnel compartment volume. Foot Ankle Int 27:431–437

Bhat AK, Madi S, Mane PP, Acharya A (2017) Bilateral tarsal tunnel syndrome attributed to bilateral fibrous tarsal coalition and symmetrical hypertrophy of the sustentaculum tali. BMJ Case Rep 2017:bcr2017220087

Bolgla LA, Malone TR (2004) Plantar fasciitis and the windlass mechanism: a biomechanical link to clinical practice. J Athl Train 39(1):77–82

Bowley MP, Doughty CT (2019) Entrapment neuropathies of the lower extremity. Med Clin North Am 103(2):371–382

Britz GW, Haynor DR, Kuntz C et al (1996) Ulnar nerve entrapment at the elbow: correlation of magnetic resonance imaging, clinical, electrodiagnostic, and intraoperative findings. Neurosurgery 38:458–465; discussion 465

Brown MN, Pearce BS, Karl HW, Trescot AM (2016) Distal saphenous nerve entrapment. In: Peripheral nerve entrapments, vol 1. Springer, Cham, pp 645–654

Brzezinski PF, Meyn NP (1977) The level of bifurcation of the tibial nerve into the medial and lateral plantar nerves. J Am Podiatry Assoc 67(8):553–555

Canella C, Demondion X, Guillin R, Boutry N, Peltier J, Cotten A (2009) Anatomic study of the superficial peroneal nerve using sonography. AJR Am J Roentgenol 193(1):174–179

Canter DE, Siesel KJ (1997) Flexor digitorum accessories longus muscle: an etiology of tarsal tunnel syndrome. J Foot Ankle Surg 36:226–229

Cardinal E, Chhem RK, Beauregard CG, Aubin B, Pelletier M (1996) Plantar fasciitis: sonographic evaluation. Radiology 201(1):257–259

Chen DW, Li B, Aubeeluck A, Yang YF, Huang YG, Zhou JQ, Yu GR (2014) Anatomy and biomechanical properties of the plantar aponeurosis: a cadaveric study. PloS One 9(1):e84347

Chundru U, Liebeskind A, Seidelmann F, Fogel J, Franklin P, Beltran J (2008) Plantar fasciitis and calcaneal spur formation are associated with abductor digiti minimi atrophy on MRI of the foot. Skeletal Radiol 37(6):505–510

D'Orazi V, Venditto T, Panunzi A et al (2014) Misdiagnosis of plexiform neurofibroma of the medial plantar nerve: case report. Foot (Edinb) 24(3):143–145

Dahlin LB, Danielsen N, Ehira T et al (1986) Mechanical effects of compression of peripheral nerves. J Biomech Eng 108:120–122

Del Mar Ruiz-Herrera M, Marcos-Tejedor F, Aldana-Caballero A et al (2022) Novel ultrasound anatomical measurement of the deep transverse metatarsal ligament: an intra-rater reliability and inter-rater concordance study. J Clin Med 11(9):2553

Del Mar Ruiz-Herrera M, Criado-Álvarez JJ, Suarez-Ortiz M, Konschake M, Moroni S, Marcos-Tejedor F (2022) Study of the anatomical association between Morton's neuroma and the space inferior to the deep transverse metatarsal ligament using ultrasound. Diagnostics (Basel) 12(6):1367

Del Toro D, Nelson PA (2018) Guiding treatment for foot pain. Phys Med Rehabil Clin N Am 29(4):783–792

Delfaut EM, Demondion X, Bieganski A, Thiron MC, Mestdagh H, Cotten A (2003) Imaging of foot and ankle nerve entrapment syndromes: from well demonstrated to unfamiliar sites. Radiographics 23:613–623

Dellon AL (2008) The four medial ankle tunnels: a critical review of perceptions of tarsal tunnel syndrome and neuropathy. Neurosurg Clin N Am 19(4):629–648, vii

Derrick E, Flores M, Scherer K, Bancroft L (2016) Peroneus tertius tendon tear: a rare cause of lateral ankle pain. Cureus 8(4):e577

Doneddu PE, Coraci D, Loreti C, Piccinini G, Padua L (2017) Tarsal tunnel syndrome: still more opinions than evidence. Status of the art. Neurol Sci 38:1735–1739

Donovan A, Rosenberg ZS, Cavalcanti CF (2010) MR imaging of entrapment neuropathies of the lower extremity: Part 2. The knee, leg, ankle, and foot. Radiographics 30(4):1001–1019

Draghi F, Gitto S, Bortolotto C, Draghi AG, Ori Belometti G (2017) Imaging of plantar fascia disorders: findings on plain radiography, ultrasound and magnetic resonance imaging. Insights Imaging 8(1):69–78

Espinosa N, Seybold JD, Jankauskas L, Erschbamer M (2011) Alcohol sclerosing therapy is not an effective treatment for interdigital neuroma. Foot Ankle Int 32(6):576–580

Ettehadi H, Saragas NP, Ferrao P (2022) A rare case of flexor digitorum accessorius longus muscle presenting as tarsal tunnel syndrome. Arch Bone Jt Surg 10(1):112–116

Fabre T, Montero C, Gaujard E, Gervais-Dellion F, Durandeau A (2000) Chronic calf pain in athletes due to sural nerve entrapment: a report of 18 cases. Am J Sports Med 28(5):679–682

Farooki S, Theodorou DJ, Sokoloff RM, Theodorou SJ, Trudell DJ, Resnick D (2001) MRI of the medial and lateral plantar nerves. J Comput Assist Tomogr 25(3):412–416

Ferkel E, Davis WH, Ellington JK (2015) Entrapment neuropathies of the foot and ankle. Clin Sports Med 34(4):791–801

Fessell DP, van Holsbeeck MT (1999) Foot and ankle sonography. Radiol Clin North Am 37:831–858

Flanigan RM, DiGiovanni BF (2011) Peripheral nerve entrapments of the lower leg, ankle, and foot. Foot Ankle Clin 16(2):255–274

Fortier LM, Markel M, Thomas BG, Sherman WF, Thomas BH, Kaye AD (2021) An update on peroneal nerve entrapment and neuropathy. Orthop Rev (Pavia) 13(2):24937

Fredericson M, Standage S, Chou L, Matheson G (2001) Lateral plantar nerve entrapment in a competitive gymnast. Clin J Sport Med 11(2):111–114

Fuller EA (2000) The windlass mechanism of the foot: a mechanical model to explain pathology. J Am Podiatr Med Assoc 90:35–46

Ghosh SK, Raheja S, Tuli A (2013) Potential sites of compression of tibial nerve branches in foot: a cadaveric and imaging study. Clin Anat 26(6):768–779

Giannini S, Bacchini P, Ceccarelli F, Vannini F (2004) Interdigital neuroma: clinical examination and histopathologic results in 63 cases treated with excision. Foot Ankle Int 25(2):79–84

Gorbachova T (2020) Magnetic resonance imaging of the ankle and foot. Pol J Radiol 85:e532–e549

Gould JS (2014) Recurrent tarsal tunnel syndrome. Foot Ankle Clin 19(3):451–467

Govsa F, Bilge O, Ozer MA (2005) Anatomical study of the communicating branches between the medial and lateral plantar nerves. Surg Radiol Anat 27(5):377–381

Govsa F, Bilge O, Ozer A (2006) Variations in the origin of the medial and inferior calcaneal nerves. Arch Orthop Trauma Surg 126:6–14

Greene B (2001) Essentials of musculoskeletal care, 2nd edn. Illinois, American Academy of Orthopedic Surgeons

Gurdezi S, White T, Ramesh P (2013) Alcohol injection for Morton's neuroma: a five year follow-up. Foot Ankle Int 34(8):1064–1067

Hansen JT (2014) Netter's clinical anatomy, 3rd edn. Elsevier

Heimkes B, Posel P, Stotz S, Wolf K (1987) The proximal and distal tarsal tunnel syndromes. An anatomical study. Int Orthop 11(3):193–196

Hochman MG, Zilberfarb JL (2004) Nerves in a pinch: imaging of nerve compression syndromes. Radiol Clin North Am 42:221–245

Hoffman D, Bianchi S (2013) Sonographic evaluation of plantar hindfoot and midfoot pain. J Ultrasound Med 32:1271–1284

Iborra A, Villanueva M, Barrett SL, Rodriguez-Collazo E, Sanz P (2018) Anatomic delineation of tarsal tunnel innervation via ultrasonography. J Ultrasound Med 37(6):1325–1334

Inthasan C, Vaseenon T, Mahakkanukrauh P (2020) Anatomical study and branching point of neurovascular structures at the medial side of the ankle. Anat Cell Biol 53(4):422–434

Kalçık Ünan M, Ardıçoğlu Ö, Pıhtılı Taş N, Aydoğan Baykara R, Kamanlı A (2021) Assessment of the frequency of tarsal tunnel syndrome in rheumatoid arthritis. Turk J Phys Med Rehabil 67(4):421–427

Kalenak A (1996) Saphenous nerve entrapment. Arthroscopy 4:40–45

Kennedy JG, Brunner JB, Bohne WH, Hodgkins CW, Baxter DB (2007) Clinical importance of the lateral branch of the deep peroneal nerve. Clin Orthop Relat Res 459:222–228

Kim S, Choi J-Y, Huh Y-M et al (2007a) Role of magnetic resonance imaging in entrapment and compressive neuropathy—what, where, and how to see the peripheral nerves on the musculoskeletal magnetic resonance image: Part 1. Overview and lower extremity. Eur Radiol 17:139–149

Kim JY, Choi JH, Park J, Wang J, Lee I (2007b) An anatomical study of Morton's interdigital neuroma: the

relationship between the occurring site and the deep transverse metatarsal ligament (DTML). Foot Ankle Int 28(9):1007–1010
Kim SJ, Hong SH, Jun WS et al (2011) MR imaging mapping of skeletal muscle denervation in entrapment and compressive neuropathies. Radiographics 31:319–332
Kim K, Isu T, Morimoto D et al (2014) Neurovascular bundle decompression without excessive dissection for tarsal tunnel syndrome. Neurol Med Chir (Tokyo) 54:901–906
Kim YH, Chai JW, Kim DH, Kim HJ, Seo J (2022a) A problem-based approach in musculoskeletal ultrasonography: heel pain in adults. Ultrasonography 41(1):34–52
Kim K, Kokubo R, Isu T et al (2022b) Magnetic resonance imaging findings in patients with tarsal tunnel syndrome. Neurol Med Chir (Tokyo) 62(12):552–558
Kinoshita M, Okuda R, Morikawa J, Jotoku T, Abe M (2001) The dorsiflexion-eversion test for diagnosis of tarsal tunnel syndrome. J Bone Joint Surg Am 83(12):1835–1839
Kopell HP, Thompson WAL (1976) Peripheral entrapment neuropathies, 2nd edn. R. E. Krieger Pub. Co, New York
Ku V, Cox C, Mikeska A, MacKay B (2021) Magnetic resonance neurography for evaluation of peripheral nerves. J Brachial Plex Peripher Nerve Inj 16(1):e17–e23
Kuntz CT, Blake L, Britz G et al (1996) Magnetic resonance neurography of peripheral nerve lesions in the lower extremity. Neurosurgery 39:750–756; discussion 756–757
Latt LD, Jaffe DE, Tang Y, Taljanovic MS (2020) Evaluation and treatment of chronic plantar fasciitis. Foot Ankle Orthop 5(1):2473011419896763
Lau JT, Daniels TR (1999) Tarsal tunnel syndrome: a review of the literature. Foot Ankle Int 20:201–209
Lawrence DA, Rolen MF, Morshed KA, Moukaddam H (2013) MRI of heel pain. AJR Am J Roentgenol 200(4):845–855
Ling ZX, Kumar VP (2008) The myofascial compartments of the foot: a cadaver study. J Bone Joint Surg Br 90(8):1114–1118
Lopez-Ben R (2011) Imaging of nerve entrapment in the foot and ankle. Foot Ankle Clin 16(2):213–224
Lui TH (2016) Endoscopic decompression of the first branch of the lateral plantar nerve and release of the plantar aponeurosis for chronic heel pain. Arthrosc Tech 5(3):e589–e594
Luz J, Johnson AH, Kohler MJ (2014) Point-of-care ultrasonography in the diagnosis and management of superficial peroneal nerve entrapment: case series. Foot Ankle Int 35(12):1362–1366
Mackinnon SE, Dellon AL, Hudson AR et al (1984) Chronic nerve compression—an experimental model in the rat. Ann Plast Surg 13:112–120
Manoharan D, Sudhakaran D, Goyal A, Srivastava D, Ansari M (2021) Clinico-radiological review of peripheral entrapment neuropathies – Part 2 Lower limb. Eur J Radiol 135:109482
Manske MC, McKeon KE, McCormick JJ, Johnson JE, Klein SE (2016) Arterial anatomy of the posterior tibial nerve in the tarsal tunnel. J Bone Jt Surg 98(6):499–504
Maravilla KR, Bowen BC (1998) Imaging of the peripheral nervous system: evaluation of peripheral neuropathy and plexopathy. AJNR Am J Neuroradiol 19:1011–1023
Markovic M, Crichton K, Read JW, Lam P, Slater HK (2008) Effectiveness of ultrasound-guided corticosteroid injection in the treatment of Morton's neuroma. Foot Ankle Int 29(5):483–487
Martinoli C, Bianchi S, Gandolfo N, Valle M, Simonetti S, Derchi LE (2000) US of nerve entrapments in osteofibrous tunnels of the upper and lower limbs. Radiographics 20 Spec No:S199–S213; discussion S213–S217
Martinoli C, Court-Payen M, Michaud J et al (2010) Imaging of neuropathies about the ankle and foot. Semin Musculoskelet Radiol 14(3):344–356
McKeon PO, Hertel J, Bramble D, Davis I (2015) The foot core system: a new paradigm for understanding intrinsic foot muscle function. Br J Sports Med 49(5):290
McMillan AM, Landorf KB, Barrett JT, Menz HB, Bird AR (2009) Diagnostic imaging for chronic plantar heel pain: a systematic review and meta-analysis. J Foot Ankle Res 13(2):32
McNally EG, Shetty S (2010) Plantar fascia: imaging diagnosis and guided treatment. Semin Musculoskelet Radiol 14(3):334–343
McSweeney SC, Cichero M (2015) Tarsal tunnel syndrome - a narrative literature review. Foot 25:244–250
Mohile N, Perez J, Rizzo M et al (2020) Chronic lower leg pain in athletes: overview of presentation and management. HSS J 16(1):86–100
Moroni S, Zwierzina M, Starke V, Moriggl B, Montesi F, Konschake M (2019) Clinical-anatomic mapping of the tarsal tunnel with regard to Baxter's neuropathy in recalcitrant heel pain syndrome: Part I. Surg Radiol Anat 41(1):29–41
Murphy PC, Baxter DE (1985) Nerve entrapment of the foot and ankle in runners. Clin Sports Med 4(4):753–763
Musson RE, Sawhney JS, Lamb L, Wilkinson A, Obaid H (2012) Ultrasound guided alcohol ablation of Morton's neuroma. Foot Ankle Int 33(3):196–201
Nagaoka M, Matsuzaki H (2005) Ultrasonography in tarsal tunnel syndrome. J Ultrasound Med 24(8):1035–1040
Offutt S, DeHeer P (2004) How to address Baxter's nerve entrapment. Podiatry Today 17:52–58
Oh SJ (2007) Neuropathies of the foot. Clin Neurophysiol 118:954–980
Oh SJ, Lee KW (1987) Medial plantar neuropathy. Neurology 37(8):1408–1410
Oh SJ, Kim HS, Ahmad BK (1985) The near-nerve sensory nerve conduction in tarsal tunnel syndrome. J Neurol Neurosurg Psychiatry 48(10):999–1003
Parker RG (2005) Dorsal foot pain due to compression of the deep peroneal nerve by exostosis of the

metatarsocuneiform joint. J Am Podiatr Med Assoc 95(5):455–458
Patel AT, Gaines K, Malamut R, Park TA, Toro DR, Holland N (2005) American Association of Neuromuscular and Electrodiagnostic Medicine: usefulness of electrodiagnostic techniques in the evaluation of suspected tarsal tunnel syndrome: an evidence-based review. Muscle Nerve 32(2):236–240
Peters PG, Adams SB Jr, Schon LC (2011) Interdigital neuralgia. Foot Ankle Clin 16(2):305–315
Petscavage-Thomas J (2014) Clinical applications of dynamic functional musculoskeletal ultrasound. Rep Med Imaging 7:27–39
Polak JF, Joresz FA, Adama DF (1988a) MRI of skeletal muscle: prolongation of T1 and T2 subsequent to denervation. Invest Radiol 23:365–369
Polak JF, Joresz FA, Adama DF (1988b) NMR of skeletal muscle differences in relaxation parameters related to extracellular/intracellular fluid spaces. Invest Radiol 23:107–112
Presley JC, Maida E, Pawlina W, Murthy N, Ryssman DB, Smith J (2013) Sonographic visualization of the first branch of the lateral plantar nerve (Baxter's nerve): technique and validation using perineural injections in a cadaveric model. J Ultrasound Med 32(9):1643–1652
Radin EL (1983) Tarsal tunnel syndrome. Clin Orthop Relat Res 181:167–170
Recht MP, Grooff P, Ilaslan H et al (2007a) Selective atrophy of the abductor digiti quinti: an MRI study. AJR Am J Roentgenol 189:W123–W127
Recht MP, Grooff P, Ilaslan H, Recht HS, Sferra J, Donley BG (2007b) Selective atrophy of the abductor digiti quinti: an MRI study. AJR Am J Roentgenol 189(3):W123–W127
Rodrigues RN, Lopes AA, Torres JM, Mundim MF, Silva LL, Silva BR (2015) Compressive neuropathy of the first branch of the lateral plantar nerve: a study by magnetic resonance imaging. Radiol Bras 48(6):368–372
Rose JD, Malay DS, Sorrento DL (2003) Neurosensory testing of the medial calcaneal and medial plantar nerves in patients with plantar heel pain. J Foot Ankle Surg 42(4):173–177
Rydevik B, Lundborg G, Bagge U (1981) Effects of graded compression on intraneural blood blow. An in vivo study on rabbit tibial nerve. J Hand Surg (Am) 6A:3–12
Sallomi D, Janzen DL, Munk PL, Connell DG, Tirman PFJ (1998) Muscle denervation patterns in upper limb nerve injuries: MR imaging findings and anatomic basis. AJR Am J Roentgenol 171:779–784
Schon LC, Baxter DE (1990) Neuropathies of the foot and ankle in athletes. Clin Sports Med 9(2):489–509
Seror P (2002) Sural nerve lesions: a report of 20 cases. Am J Phys Med Rehabil 81(11):876–880
Sharp RJ, Wade CM, Hennessy MS, Saxby TS (2003) The role of MRI and ultrasound imaging in Morton's neuroma and the effect of size of lesion on symptoms. J Bone Joint Surg Br 85(7):999–1005
Shon LC, Easly ME (2000) Chronic pain. In: Myerson M (ed) Foot and ankle disorders. WB Saunders, Philadelphia, PA, pp 815–881
Singh G, Kumar VP (2012) Neuroanatomical basis for the tarsal tunnel syndrome. Foot Ankle Int 33(6):513–518
Sinnaeve F, Vandeputte G (2008) Clinical outcome of surgical intervention for recalcitrant infero-medial heel pain. Acta Orthop Belg 74(4):483–488
Spinner RJ, Dellon AL, Rosson GD et al (2007) Tibial intraneural ganglia in the tarsal tunnel: is there a joint connection? J Foot Ankle Surg 46:27–31
Spratt JD, Stanley AJ, Grainger AJ, Hide IG, Campbell RS (2002) The role of diagnostic radiology in compressive and entrapment neuropathies. Eur Radiol 12:2352–2364
Symeonidis PD, Iselin LD, Simmons N, Fowler S, Dracopoulos G, Stavrou P (2012) Prevalence of interdigital nerve enlargements in an asymptomatic population. Foot Ankle Int 33(7):543–547
Tahririan MA, Motififard M, Tahmasebi MN, Siavashi B (2012) Plantar fasciitis. J Res Med Sci 17(8):799–804
Takakura Y, Sugimoto K, Tanaka Y, Tamai S (1991) Symptomatic talocalcaneal coalition. Its clinical significance and treatment. Clin Orthop Relat Res 269:249–256
Tassler PL, Dellon AL, Lesser G et al (2000) Utility of decompressive surgery in the prophylaxis and treatment of cisplatin neuropathy in adult rats. J Reconstr Surg 16:457–463
Tawfik EA, El Zohiery AK, Abouelela AA (2016) Proposed sonographic criteria for the diagnosis of idiopathic tarsal tunnel syndrome. Arch Phys Med Rehabil 97(7):1093–1099
Theodorou DJ, Theodorou SJ, Resnick D (2002) MR imaging of abnormalities of the plantar fascia. Semin Musculoskelet Radiol 6(2):105–118
Therimadasamy AK, Seet RC, Kagda YH, Wilder-Smith EP (2011) Combination of ultrasound and nerve conduction studies in the diagnosis of tarsal tunnel syndrome. Neurol India 59(2):296–297
Thomas JL, Christensen JC, Kravitz SR et al (2010) The diagnosis and treatment of heel pain: a clinical practice guideline-revision 2010. J Foot Ankle Surg 49(3 Suppl):S1–S19
Thomas MJ, Roddy E, Zhang W, Menz HB, Hannan MT, Peat GM (2011) The population prevalence of foot and ankle pain in middle and old age: a systematic review. Pain 152(12):2870–2880
Title CI, Schon LC (2008) Morton neuroma: primary and secondary neurectomy. J Am Acad Orthop Surg 16(9):550–557
Tladi MJ, Saragas NP, Ferrao PN, Strydom A (2017) Schwannoma and neurofibroma of the posterior tibial nerve presenting as tarsal tunnel syndrome: review of the literature with two case reports. Foot 32:22–26

Torriani M, Kattapuram SV (2003) Technical innovation: dynamic sonography of the forefoot. The sonographic Mulder sign. AJR Am J Roentgenol 180:1121–1123

Trepman E, Kadel NJ, Chisholm K et al (1999) Effect of foot and ankle position on tarsal tunnel compartment pressure. Foot Ankle Int 20:721–726

Trojian T, Tucker AK (2019) Plantar fasciitis. Am Fam Physician 99(12):744–750

Tzika M, Paraskevas G, Natsis K (2015) Entrapment of the superficial peroneal nerve: an anatomical insight. J Am Podiatr Med Assoc 105(2):150–159

Umans H, Srinivasan R, Elsinger E et al (2014) MRI of lesser metatarsophalangeal joint plantar plate tears and associated adjacent interspace lesions. Skeletal Radiol 43:1361–1368

Unlü RE, Orbay H, Kerem M, Esmer AF, Tüccar E, Sensöz O (2008) Innervation of three weight-bearing areas of the foot: an anatomic study and clinical implications. J Plast Reconstr Aesthet Surg 61(5):557–561

Vega-Zelaya L, Iborra Á, Villanueva M, Pastor J, Noriega C (2021) Ultrasound-guided near-nerve needle sensory technique for the diagnosis of tarsal tunnel syndrome. J Clin Med 10:3065

Walther M, Radke S, Kirschner S, Ettl V, Gohlke F (2004) Power Doppler findings in plantar fasciitis. Ultrasound Med Biol 30(4):435–440

Weishaupt D, Treiber K, Kundert HP et al (2003) Morton neuroma: MR imaging in prone, supine, and upright weightbearing body positions. Radiology 226:849–856

West GA, Haynor DR, Goodkin R et al (1994) Magnetic resonance imaging signal changes in denervated muscles after peripheral nerve injury. Neurosurgery 35:1077–1085; discussion 1085–1076

Womack JW, Richardson DR, Murphy GA, Richardson EG, Ishikawa SN (2008) Long-term evaluation of interdigital neuroma treated by surgical excision. Foot Ankle Int 29(6):574–577

Wu CH, Chiu YH, Chang KV, Wu WT, Özçakar L (2022) Ultrasound elastography for the evaluation of plantar fasciitis: a systematic review and meta-analysis. Eur J Radiol 155:110495

Yuebing L, Lederman RJ (2014) Sural mononeuropathy: a report of 36 cases. Muscle Nerve 49(3):443–445

Zanetti M, Strehle JK, Zollinger H, Hodler J (1997) Morton neuroma and fluid in the intermetatarsal bursae on MR images of 70 asymptomatic volunteers. Radiology 203:516–520

Infection

Aanand Vibhakar, Ian Reilly, and Amit Shah

Contents

A. Vibhakar
Department of Radiology, Royal National Orthopaedic Hospital, Stanmore, UK
e-mail: aanand.vibhakar@nhs.net

I. Reilly
Department of Podiatric Surgery, Northamptonshire Healthcare NHS Foundation Trust, Northampton, UK
e-mail: ianreilly@nhs.net

A. Shah (✉)
Department of Radiology, University Hospitals of Leicester, Leicester, UK
e-mail: amit.shah2@nhs.net

1 Introduction

Infection involving the foot and ankle can occur in any age group and is classically described as occurring via one of the three routes: (1) contiguous spread, (2) direct implantation, or (3) hematogenous spread. The infective process can be acute, subacute, or chronic in onset and is associated with complications and high morbidity and mortality if not accurately or promptly diagnosed. The clinical presentation can vary based on the infective organism type, location within the foot and ankle, and clinical status of the patient: poor host resistance (e.g., immunocompromised or diabetic), poor blood supply (e.g., peripheral vascular disease), or reduced sensation (e.g., leprosy). In children and adolescents, hematogenous osteomyelitis is the most frequently encountered diagnosis, while in adults,

Med Radiol Diagn Imaging (2023)

https://doi.org/10.1007/174_2023_406,
Published Online: 19 April 2023

the majority of ankle and foot infections result from an ulcer with contiguous spread of infection, from surgery or direct implantation, or from a puncture wound. An infective organism within a bone gives rise to a pathogenic cascade causing alteration in pH, increased capillary permeability causing edema, cytokine release, leukocyte recruitment, tissue breakdown, increased localized pressure, and subsequent bone deterioration. Once the infective process tracks to the medullary cavity, there is subsequent extension into the cortex via the Haversian and Volkmann canals. Further progression involves spread to the subperiosteal and periosteal space and finally into the soft tissues.

Despite there being considerable debate regarding the precise anatomic configuration of the compartments of the foot, there is a general consensus that the muscles of the plantar aspect of the foot are separated into three compartments by fascial planes that extend the length of the plantar aspect of the foot. These three compartments are the lateral, medial, and central compartments and are defined by the medial and lateral intermuscular septa that arise from the plantar aponeurosis. The lateral compartment contains the muscles of the fifth toe. The medial compartment contains the muscles of the great toe, which include abductor hallucis, flexor hallucis brevis, and flexor hallucis longus tendon. The central compartment contains the remaining plantar muscles, which include flexor digitorum brevis, lumbrical muscles, quadratus plantae muscle, adductor hallucis muscle, and flexor digitorum longus tendon. Some authors also acknowledge the existence of interosseous and dorsal compartments. A study by Lederman et al. in 2002 analyzing compartmental involvement of 115 feet found that soft tissue inflammation in the forefoot had a propensity to spread into neighboring compartments with little respect for fascial planes, whereas inflammation in the hindfoot usually stayed confined. In addition, it found that spread from the foot to the lower leg was rare.

Diabetic pedal infection, covered in the chapter "Diabetic Foot", accounts for the majority of cases of pedal infection. The most common infective organisms responsible for pedal infection are bacterial; however, viral, fungal, and parasitic infections do also occur. Pedal infections are subcategorized and include cellulitis of the subcutaneous tissues, abscesses, osteomyelitis and osteitis, necrotizing fasciitis, infection secondary to a retained foreign body, infected hardware, and septic arthritis. The following sections consider each of these entities in turn. It is crucial that early diagnosis of acute osteomyelitis is made as prompt antibiotic therapy may prevent bone necrosis. An initial in-depth clinical examination, demarcation of the affected area, and an appropriate biochemical and microbiological workup (C-reactive protein, erythrocyte sedimentation rate, full blood count, liver function tests, and blood cultures) are recommended prior to starting treatment. In some cases, these laboratory tests have no yield and ultimately biopsy may be required. Imaging has a key role in diagnosing infection, assessing disease extent and associated complications, planning and performing biopsies, and monitoring treatment response. Imaging modalities performed depend on the type of infection, age of patient, and extent of involvement of infection suspected. Radiographs are the initial imaging modality in most scenarios, with MRI usually being the gold standard. Ultrasound (US), CT, and radionuclide studies can play an important role depending on the clinical context. It is important that the appropriate imaging modality is performed to evaluate pedal infection in a timely manner, which will enable and help expedite the correct medical and surgical treatment options.

2 Glossary of Terms

Term	Definition	Relevant images
Cellulitis	Superficial, non-necrotizing infection involving the skin and subcutaneous tissues. Does not extend to the deep fascia or musculature	Figures 2, 3, 4
Infectious myositis	Infection of skeletal muscle. Pyomyositis refers to suppuration and abscess formation secondary to bacterial myositis	
Soft tissue abscess	Organized collection of pus secondary to invasion by an infectious organism. Macrophages, fibrin, and granulation tissue form a peripheral capsule	Figures 5, 6
Phlegmon	Poorly defined, nonencapsulated mass-like inflammatory soft tissue. Not yet organized enough to be described as an abscess	
Retained foreign body		Figures 5, 7
Devitalized tissue	Ischaemic or necrotic tissue, usually near or overlying ulcer margin	
Necrotizing fasciitis	Aggressive soft tissue infection of the subcutaneous tissues and deep fascia by toxin producing organisms. The infection spreads rapidly and causes liquefaction or necrosis of fat and muscle	
Superficial fascia	Fascia that is located within the subcutaneous tissues, in between the muscle and the skin	Figure 8
Deep peripheral fascia	The deep peripheral fascia envelopes the surface of muscles. *[The deep intermuscular fascia lies between muscles]*	Figure 8
Septic tenosynovitis	Infection of a synovial tendon sheath	Figures 6, 8
Skin ulceration	Break in the skin resulting in discontinuity of the skin surface	Figures 2, 3, 9
Sinus tract	Abnormal connection between the site of inflammation and the skin surface. Often overlying an ulcer	Figure 3
Infectious periostitis	Infection that invades only the periosteum and does not involve the cortex and bone marrow	Figures 10, 14
Infectious osteitis	Infection that penetrates the cortex but does not invade medullary bone	
Osteomyelitis	Infection involving both cortex and bone marrow	Figures 3, 6, 10, 11, 12, 13
Brodie abscess	Subacute or chronic intramedullary abscess	Figures 6, 13
Sequestrum	Segment of devascularized bone that becomes separated ("sequestered") from its host bone due to surrounding necrosis	
Involucrum	Reactive bone sclerosis surrounding the sequestrum. It isolates the sequestrum from the bloodstream in a similar fashion to a walled-off abscess	
Cloaca	Opening or rupture of the involucrum that allows granulation tissue to be discharged, and which can give rise to a subperiosteal abscess	Figure 13
Confluent intramedullary pattern of T1 signal alteration	Geographic area of T1 hypointensity involving medullary canal. Very high association with osteomyelitis	
Hazy reticular pattern of T1 signal alteration	Interspersed areas of low T1 signal within regions of normal marrow. Rarely associated with hematogenous osteomyelitis. Not associated with contiguous-focus osteomyelitis	
Subcortical pattern of T1 signal alteration	T1 hypointensity limited to thin linear region subjacent to the cortex. Not associated with osteomyelitis	
Chronic osteomyelitis	Continuation of osseous infection for greater than 30 days. May manifest as indolent low-grade infection with possible episodes of superimposed active inflammation	Figures 10, 11
Sclerosing osteomyelitis of Garré	Distinctive type of chronic osteomyelitis that leads to extensive periosteal new bone formation with minimal suppuration	
Septic arthritis	Infection of a joint	Figures 1, 6, 10, 11, 14, 15, 16, 17, 18, 19
Periprosthetic infection	Infection involving a prosthesis and the adjacent tissue	Figures 11, 14, 15, 17, 18, 19

3 Imaging Modalities in Infection

Multiple imaging modalities can be used in the evaluation of suspected foot and ankle infection. Plain radiographs traditionally were and still currently are considered first-line imaging, mainly to provide bony anatomy and overview of pathology. Computed tomography (CT) and magnetic resonance imaging (MRI) are considered standard in the imaging for osteomyelitis; however, it must be appreciated that no one specific imaging modality can definitively diagnose or rule out infection. More recently, nuclear medicine techniques are being used to assess for infection, which, although is highly sensitive and useful in multifocal infective involvement, can sometimes be nonspecific and in certain cases contribute to incorrect interpretation. A combination of imaging modalities is usually required to confer a diagnosis.

3.1 Conventional Radiography

A two-projection plain radiograph is the initial imaging of choice for suspicion of foot or ankle infection, as it is readily available, inexpensive, and reproducible and provides high-resolution characterization of the bones.

Radiographs provide a useful overview and an anatomical baseline for diagnostic interpretation. They are insensitive and usually normal during the early stages of infection. Prior to any osseous infective changes becoming apparent on plain radiography, soft tissue changes are usually first apparent, which manifest as blurring of the soft tissue planes and muscle swelling. These signs are however nonspecific and can be seen in both soft tissue infection and following trauma to the bone. The bony changes that can be visualized range across subtle osteopenia, periosteal thickening, lytic destruction or erosion, endosteal scalloping, new bone apposition, and loss of the normal trabecular architecture. Radiographic osseous changes of osteomyelitis do not appear for at least 10–14 days or until 30–50% of the bone has been destroyed. For pyogenic infections, osseous change suggests that the infective process has been present for at least 2–3 weeks. Radiolucent intra-osseous abscess formation is usually circumscribed in appearance and suggests a subacute or chronic phase. Osseous mineralization and alignment, soft tissues, joint spaces, and radiopaque implants and retained foreign bodies are routinely assessed. Given that plain radiographs are not sensitive for infection, further characterization with cross-sectional imaging such as MRI is often the next imaging step (Fig. 1).

3.2 Ultrasound

Ultrasound (US) is a readily accessible, cheap, and nonionizing radiation imaging modality. It is frequently used in the assessment of musculoskeletal infection and particularly helpful in distinguishing acute and chronic infections from tumorous and noninfective complications. It reliably distinguishes soft tissue and fluid collections. The ability for real-time dynamic imaging, power Doppler vascularity, and characterizing of hyperemia is valuable in more complex presentations. In addition to diagnosis, US can be used for image-guided diagnostic and therapeutic procedures such as aspiration and biopsy.

During US assessment, an approximation of the size and involvement of the soft tissues affected by the infection and any evidence of collections and abscess formation should be assessed. US also provides high image resolution with good soft tissue contrast and spatial resolution in a relatively small field of view and in this context can be deemed superior to MRI and CT. US imaging is a good first-line imaging modality for the assessment of radiolucent soft tissue retained foreign bodies.

Hypoechoic layering of purulent material corresponding with elevation of the periosteal layer of bone can be recognized in acute osteomyelitis. In children, acute osteomyelitis can be detected on US several days earlier than its presentation on conventional radiographs. In adults, US has limited to no value in the assessment of deep-seated infections or osseous pathology due to the inherent inability of sound waves to penetrate through bone. The lack of ionizing radiation and

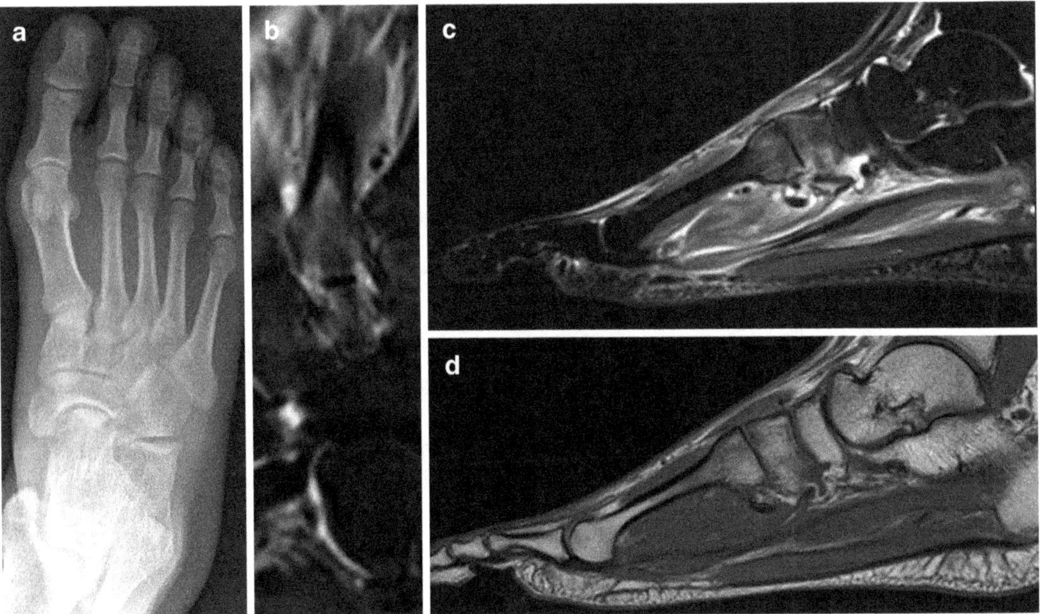

Fig. 1 Septic arthritis. Normal appearances of a frontal radiograph of the right foot (**a**). Axial and sagittal STIR images of a contemporaneous MRI demonstrate contiguous edema in the second metatarsal base and the intermediate cuneiform (**b** and **c**) with inflammation in the adjacent soft tissues in keeping with septic arthritis. A sagittal T1 image (**d**) reveals subtle corresponding T1 hypointensity. These images highlight the importance of MRI in the setting of radiographically occult septic arthritis. Radiographic manifestations of septic arthritis are a late finding, and MRI must not be delayed in such cases

the ability to scan a distressed patient without the use of sedation make US an important tool, particularly in the pediatric population.

In chronic osteomyelitis, US is extremely powerful for assessing the surrounding soft tissues and providing information on abscesses, which are typically hypoechoic fluid collections extending around the bony contours. US is also useful in the assessment of joint effusions, turbid fluid material, and septic arthritis. Often, these findings will be present before becoming apparent on plain radiographs.

3.3 Computed Tomography

Cross-sectional imaging evaluation of pedal infection is better appreciated on MRI; however, computed tomography (CT) provides excellent multiplanar reconstructions of axial imaging to allow delineation of subtle osseous changes. In chronic osteomyelitis, the presence of a sequestrum, draining sinus, and/or involucrum is better seen on CT than MRI. CT offers excellent detail on bony architecture, cortical destruction, periosteal changes, and also presence of intraosseous gas, which is less conspicuous on MRI and not likely to be seen on plain radiography. In addition, CT imaging can also be used in the guidance of intervention for joint aspiration, biopsy, or abscess drainage. CT imaging does involve exposure to ionizing radiation and has inferior soft tissue contrast resolution to MRI and hence is less desirable than MRI for soft tissue characterization. CT is excellent in being able to rapidly image a large anatomic region and is thus an important test in the emergency department in the assessment of infection.

3.4 Magnetic Resonance Imaging

Magnetic resonance imaging (MRI) is the modality of choice for most musculoskeletal infections. It is a nonionizing modality that gives excellent soft tissue contrast, anatomical detail, and spatial resolution and can be acquired and formatted in multiple planes. Most pathologic processes including infection exhibit edema, and MRI is excellent in its detection. Certain MRI sequences also enable the detection of tumors, fluid collections, and blood products. Gadolinium-enhanced postcontrast sequences enable accurate detection of devitalized tissue, abscesses, and sinus tracts. MRI can also help determine whether infection or necrosis has spread to critical contiguous structures such as the physes and joint spaces. If these regions are involved, specialist management is likely to be needed to minimize morbidity and complications.

In pedal infection, MRI is very sensitive in detecting osteomyelitis within the first 3–5 days. It also provides excellent information regarding the extent of bone involvement when a diagnosis of osteomyelitis has already been established.

Whole-body MRI (WBMRI) combines good anatomical resolution, and diffusion-weighted MRI sequences can add functional molecular qualitative and quantitative information. WBMRI can help identify targets for collection of microbiological samples in multifocal disease. WBMRI is also useful in detecting chronic recurrent multifocal osteomyelitis especially in indeterminate clinical cases where subclinical edema may be detected. It may also be used to identify a focus of infection in children with fever of unknown origin.

Limitations of MRI include cost, long scanning times, available scan slots, presence of cardiac pacemakers or certain metallic implants, claustrophobia, and patient size.

3.5 Nuclear Medicine

Nuclear medicine complements conventional radiological modalities and plays a key role in the evaluation of musculoskeletal infections. In patients with equivocal findings for infection using conventional imaging modalities, nuclear medicine studies can be used for further evaluation. There are several studies that use single photon-emitting radiotracers that can be used for the assessment of musculoskeletal infections. These include leukocyte scintigraphy, bone marrow scintigraphy, IgG scintigraphy, bone scans, and gallium scans. PET has also been used in the evaluation of osteomyelitis, with the most common tracer being FDG. Pedal infection in the diabetic foot is difficult to differentiate from neuropathic arthropathy (Charcot joint) on conventional imaging such as radiography and MRI, and FDG PET/CT has been shown to be able to help with this. In neuropathic osteoarthropathy, the SUV_{max} ranges from 0.7 to 2.4, and in osteomyelitis, the SUV_{max} is usually above 2.5. FDG/PET is also a valuable diagnostic modality in the monitoring of treatment response to musculoskeletal infections, in the workup of patients with pyrexia of unknown origin, in helping differentiate insufficiency fractures from pathological fractures, in patients with metallic hardware where metal-induced artifacts interfere with MRI and CT characterization, and in excluding superimposed infection when assessing fracture nonunion. Research efforts are focusing on the development of specific probes for imaging infections such as 18F-fluorodeoxysorbitol (a radiolabeled sugar) and ^{68}Ga-DOTA-TBIA[101] (a gallium-68-labeled antimicrobial peptide).

4 Soft Tissue

4.1 Cellulitis

Cellulitis is defined as localized or diffuse soft tissue inflammation of skin and subcutaneous tissues. It is most commonly observed close to areas of puncture wounds, cuts, and skin ulceration. It is an acute inflammatory reaction, which produces an acute inflammatory infiltrate and capillary dilatation secondary to contiguous spread of organisms into the subcutaneous fat. The most common causative organisms are *Streptococcus pyogenes* and *Staphylococcus aureus*. Cellulitis is usually diagnosed clinically and treated conservatively. Imaging is useful for the detection of associated complications such as abscess formation, osteomyelitis, and necrotizing fasciitis.

Plain radiography is not a useful test and may only demonstrate soft tissue swelling with displacement or loss of the intermuscular fat planes. US is a good test for the assessment of cellulitis, and particularly in distinguishing it from superficial venous thrombosis; however, both these conditions can coexist. Cellulitis manifests as edema and hyperemia of the subcutaneous fat together with skin thickening. Edematous fat is hyperechoic. In addition, thickened interlobular septa manifesting as a cobblestoned morphology can be seen. Periseptal fluid and fluid around the surrounding fascia can sometimes be seen. The sonographic diagnosis of cellulitis requires both hyperemia and edema, as hyperemia is not seen in noninflammatory edematous states such as congestive cardiac failure or venous insufficiency. Cellulitis can also give rise to secondary tenosynovitis with tendon thickening and synovial proliferation. With increasing severity of cellulitis, the morphology of the subcutaneous dermal-hypodermal layers changes from generalized swelling with indistinct lobules to a cobblestoned appearance with well-defined lobules due to the accumulation of anechoic exudate along the interlobular septations. US-guided intervention can be used to aspirate fluid for microscopy, culture, and sensitivity, and it can be used to drain associated abscesses. CT demonstrates fat stranding of the affected area with associated skin thickening. On MRI, cellulitis manifests as variable patterns of T2 hyperintense and T1 hypointense signal in the subcutaneous tissues and along the outer layer of the deep muscular fascia, often with a linear pattern. Contrast enhancement of the infected subcutaneous tissue is variable. MRI can also help differentiate cellulitis from pedal edema and necrotic tissue: pedal edema has minimal to no enhancement, and the fat signal in the subcutaneous tissues is not replaced (Figs. 2, 3, and 4).

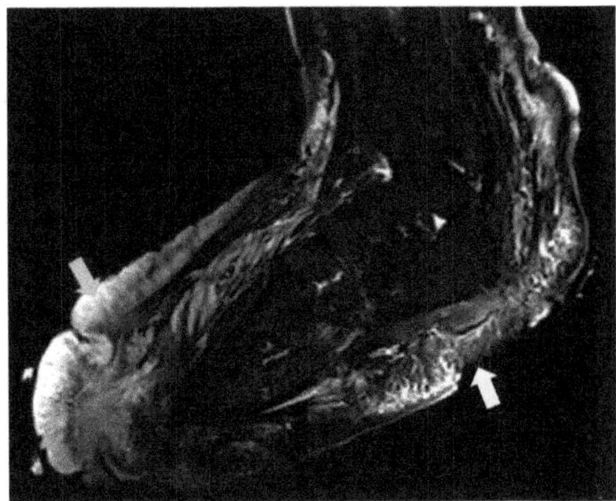

Fig. 2 Cellulitis and heel ulceration. A sagittal STIR image of the foot and ankle demonstrates extensive subcutaneous edema along the dorsal surface of the forefoot in keeping with known cellulitis (blue arrow). A disruption in the cutaneous signal line at the posterior aspect of the plantar surface of the foot represents a skin ulcer (yellow arrow)

4.2 Abscess Formation

An abscess is a localized collection of pus. It is a common complication of cellulitis. In the acute setting, before liquefaction, an abscess is termed phlegmon. In the muscle, infectious myositis can lead to suppurative bacterial infection, and this is termed pyomyositis. Pyomyositis frequently gives rise to intramuscular abscess formation as the enclosed nature of muscle and fascial compartments lends to the accumulation of pus and consequent abscess formation. On plain radiography, an abscess may be seen as a mass-like opacity with air-fluid levels and/or gas within it. If the abscess is chronic, it may demonstrate peripheral calcification. On US, posterior acoustic enhancement is a key feature. However, depending on the maturity and contents, the echogenicity varies from hypoechoic to hyperechoic. An abscess may mimic a solid mass if thick fluid or debris is present. Internal septations, peripheral hyperemia, and gas locules manifesting as comet tail or shadowing artifact may be present. The more chronic the abscess, the thicker the wall. On CT, abscesses are typically hypodense fluid collections with peripheral rim enhancement. Internal hemorrhagic or proteinaceous content can result in variable internal attenuation. If the internal contents approach the density of soft tissue, abscesses can be difficult to detect on CT. In the absence of penetrating injury, internal gas locules are strongly suggestive of an abscess with gas-forming organisms. On MRI,

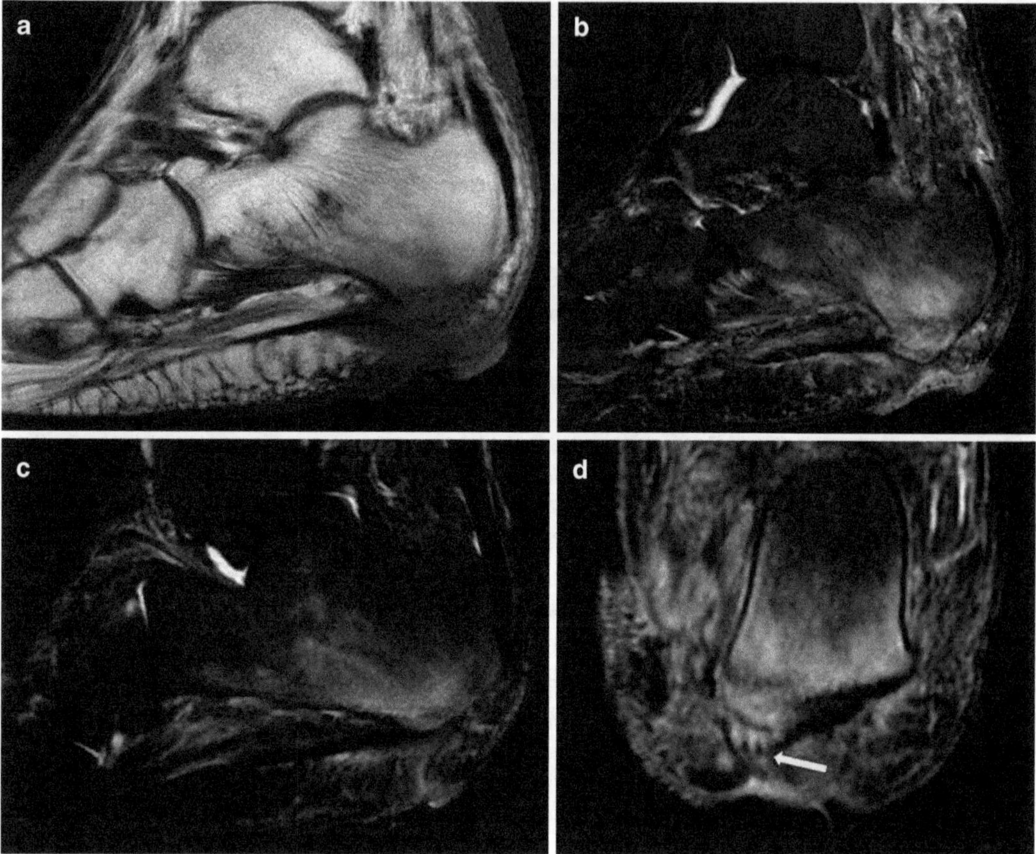

Fig. 3 Heel ulceration with sinus tract formation and osteomyelitis. Sagittal T1 (**a**) and STIR images (**b** and **c**) demonstrate focal loss of the cutaneous signal line overlying the heel with cellulitis, and a coronal STIR image demonstrates a sinus tract (yellow arrow, **d**) to the posterior surface of the calcaneus which has STIR hyperintensity (and T1 hypointensity in **a**) in keeping with osteomyelitis

abscesses are T1 hypointense and T2 hyperintense collections with peripheral enhancement. Gas locules are seen as foci of signal dropout. As with other imaging modalities, variable internal contents can give rise to varied T1/T2 signal intensities, particularly T1 as its signal increases with hemorrhagic or proteinaceous content. Abscesses demonstrate diffusion restriction (Figs. 5 and 6).

4.3 Retained Foreign Bodies

The vast majority of retained foreign bodies (RFBs) in the foot and ankle are due to penetrating injury. Patients may present acutely, or they may present several weeks after removing an RFB with persistent pain, discharge, or a non-healing wound. Wood, glass, and metal account for the majority of penetrating RFB injuries. Radiographs are the best (and first) imaging tool. US is the usual next step if the radiograph is negative. US can also be used to guide intervention to remove the RFB. Radiographs will detect 80% of all retained foreign bodies. Glass (including non-leaded glass) and metal are radiopaque compared to soft tissues. More than 90% of glass RFBs are visible on radiographs. Plastic and wood are often of similar density to muscle and are not easily identified on radiographs. Large pieces of aerated wood may contain enough air to create a lucency in soft tissues.

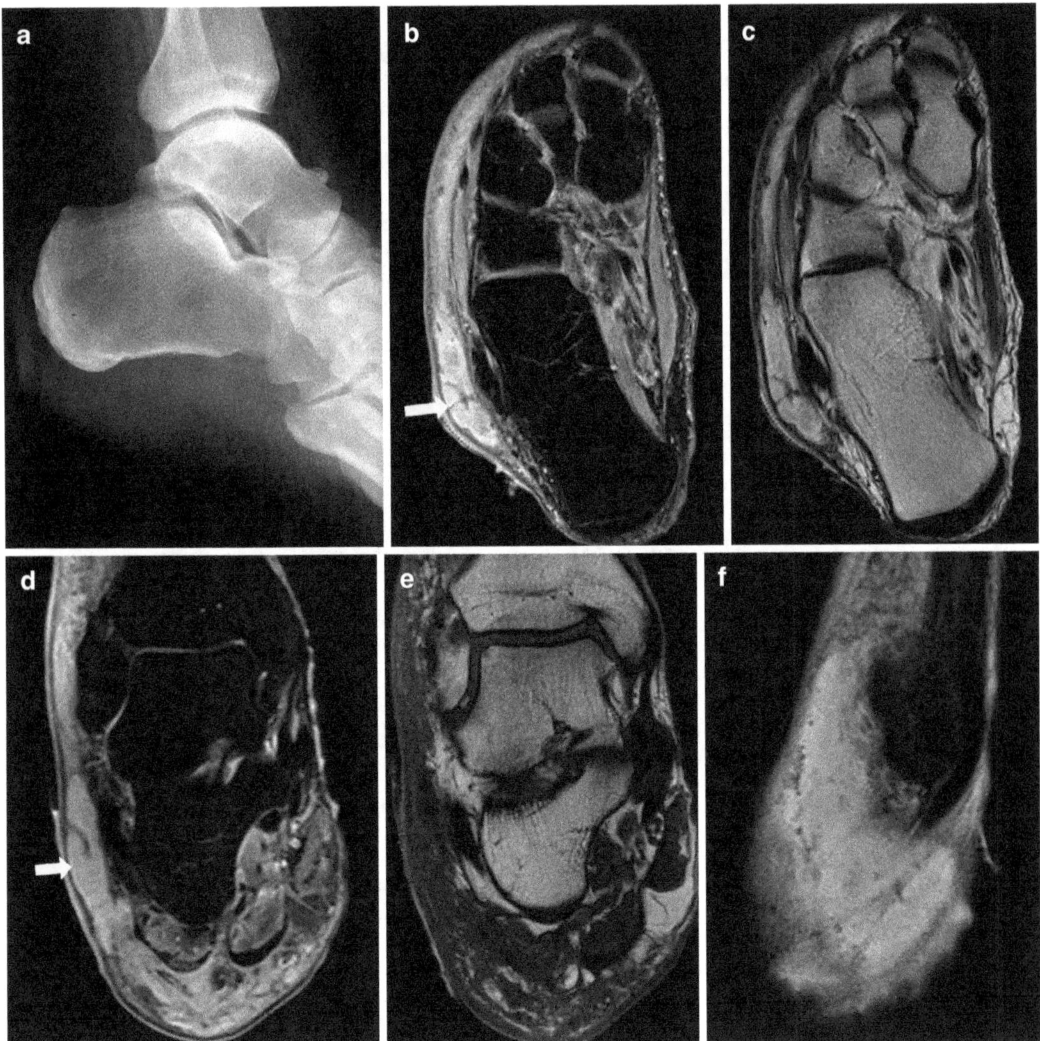

Fig. 4 Soft tissue collection with cellulitis. Lateral radiograph (**a**) of the ankle reveals nonspecific soft tissue swelling at the plantar aspect of the hindfoot. Axial PD (**b**) and T2 (**c**), coronal STIR (**d**) and T1 (**e**), and sagittal STIR (**f**) images reveal a subcutaneous collection with surrounding cellulitis lateral to the calcaneus (yellow arrows). Note that there is no evidence of osteomyelitis

For small, nonmetallic RFBs, decreasing the X-ray tube voltage (kV) and increasing the tube current (mA) may help enhance detection. It is important when reviewing radiographs to triangulate the location of the RFB on at least two views. On CT, metal and glass have a high attenuation and are easily identified. Acutely, wood is of low density on CT due to its air content; however, over time, its density increases due to absorption of exudate and blood products. MRI is not usually performed nor is it useful in the acute setting. In the subacute setting, postcontrast T1 fat-saturated sequences can be useful in identifying an RFB as a central defect within surrounding inflamed and enhancing tissue. MRI can also help assess for complications of RFBs including osteomyelitis, abscesses, scar formation, and granulomas. Glass and wood

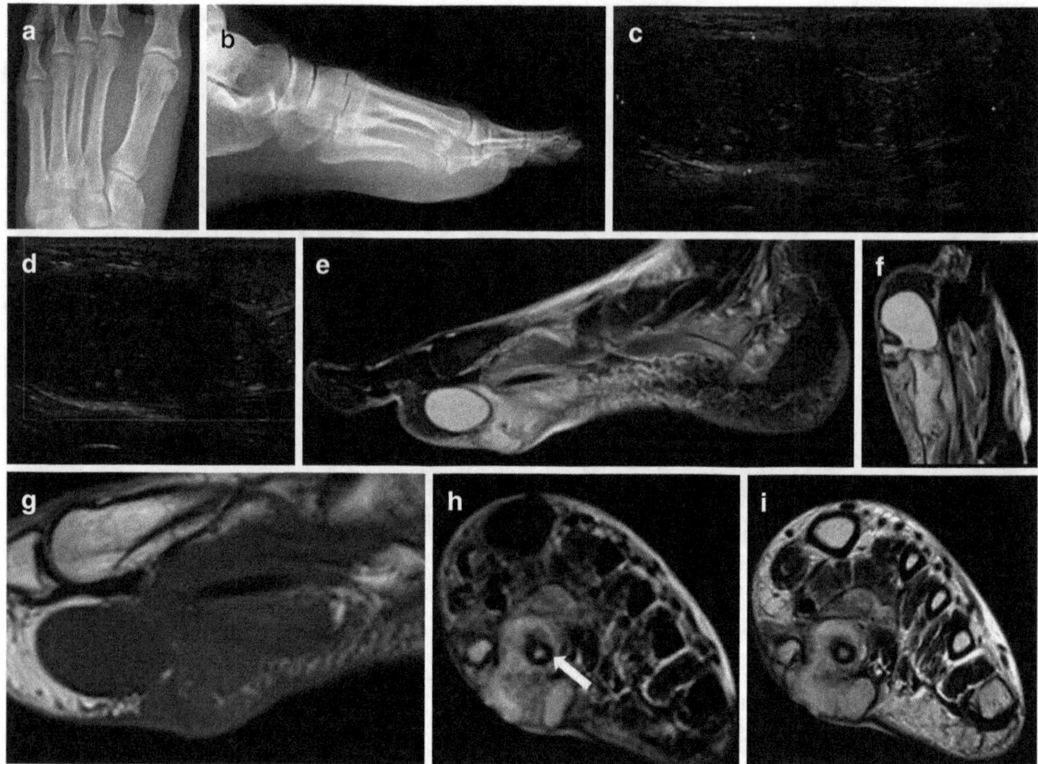

Fig. 5 Abscess and retained foreign body. Frontal (**a**) and lateral (**b**) radiographs demonstrate soft tissue swelling surrounding the first left metatarsal. Ultrasonography (**c** and **d**) reveals an avascular, hypoechoic lesion with innumerable internal echogenic foci. Sagittal STIR (**e**), axial STIR (**f**), and sagittal T1 (**g**) weighted images reveal a multilocular collection at the plantar surface of the foot extending to the skin surface in keeping with an abscess. Coronal STIR (**h**) and (**i**) T2-weighted images reveal a geometric, circular hypointense structure (yellow arrow) within the collection in keeping with a foreign body. This case demonstrates the utility of a multimodality diagnostic approach, with both radiography and ultrasonography unable to visualize the retained foreign body

will create well-defined areas of signal void but will demonstrate no susceptibility artifact. Wood is usually T1 and T2 hypointense to skeletal muscle.

Metallic RFBs will generate susceptibility artifact. US is a useful tool for identifying RFBs; however, in the acute setting, an open wound may preclude the application of a probe to the skin. High-frequency transducers with high resolution and low penetration enable optimal visualization. All RFBs are initially hyperechoic. Over time, wooden RFBs become less echogenic. RFBs usually become more conspicuous with time as a hypoechoic halo of hemorrhage, edema, or granulation tissue begins to develop after about 24 h. Different types of RFBs can exhibit different artifacts on US, which can help in their identification. RFBs with a smooth surface such as metal or glass will exhibit reverberation artifact and dirty shadowing. RFBs with rough surfaces such as wood will exhibit clean posterior acoustic shadowing. Plastic RFBs are less echogenic but will exhibit significant posterior acoustic shadowing (Figs. 5 and 7).

4.4 Devitalized Tissue

Devitalized tissue is almost exclusively a sequela of the diabetic foot or peripheral vascular dis-

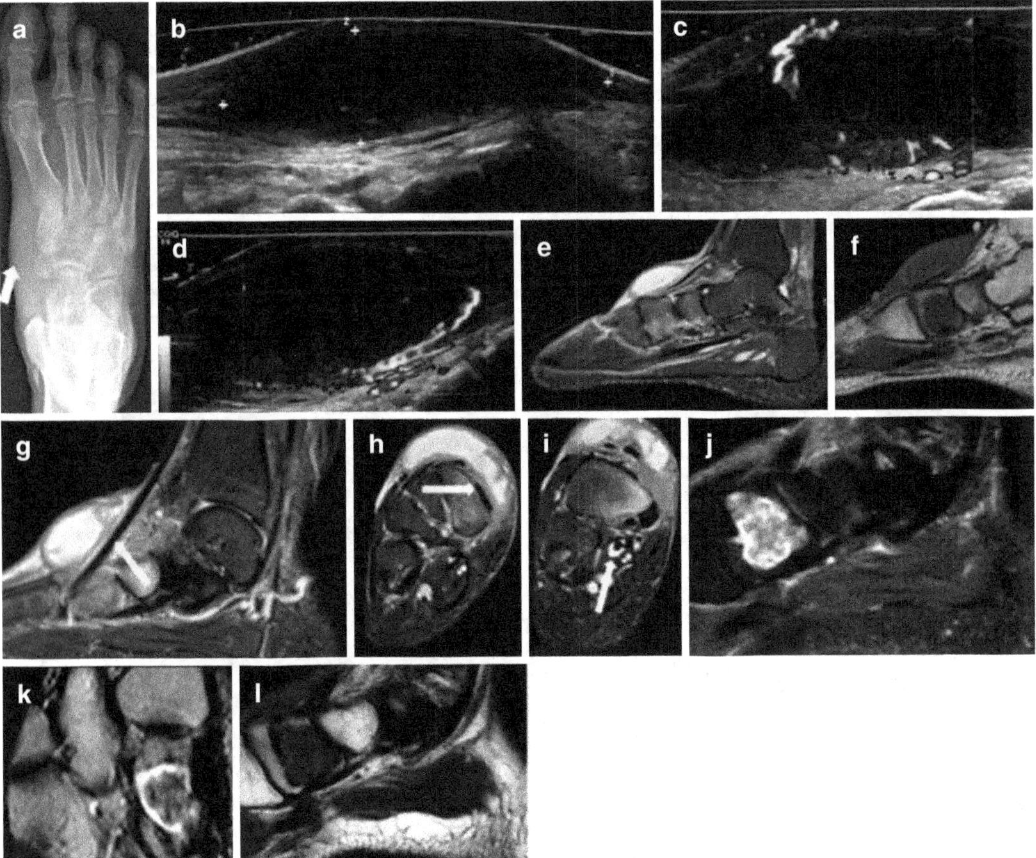

Fig. 6 Osteomyelitis with subcutaneous and intra-osseous (Brodie's) abscess. A frontal radiograph of the right foot (**a**) demonstrates soft tissue swelling medially at the level of the tarsus. Ultrasonography (**b–d**) reveals a subcutaneous lesion overlying the extensor tendons of the midfoot. No internal vascularity. Sagittal STIR (**e**) and (**f**) T1-weighted images confirm the lesion identified on ultrasound to be a well-defined fluid-filled collection. Furthermore, STIR hyperintensity and T1 hypointensity are noted in the medial cuneiform and navicular in keeping with osteomyelitis and septic arthritis. Sagittal (**g**) and coronal (**h**) STIR images demonstrate the tibialis anterior tendon (yellow arrows) to be intimately related to the infective change at its insertion at the medial aspect of the medial cuneiform. The infection has been tracked along the extensor tendons (not depicted) and to the subcutaneous collection. A coronal STIR image (**i**) reveals fluid surrounding the flexor hallucis longus tendon in keeping with infective tenosynovitis (yellow arrow). The collection was proven to be *Mycobacterium tuberculosis* on histopathological analysis. An interval MRI 9 months later (**j–l**) revealed some resolution in the inflammatory changes previously seen, with the persistence of an intra-osseous abscess in the medial cuneiform (Brodie's abscess)

ease. Devitalized tissue includes necrotic and ischemic soft tissue. Necrosis occurs in the critically ischemic extremity because the metabolic requirements to heal an injury are far greater than those required to maintain normal tissue viability. It is important to evaluate the extent of soft tissue and osseous infection on MRI as this can significantly alter plans for medical or surgical management. Foot-preserving surgery in pedal infection is of great importance. Here, only the infected and/or necrotic tissue is optimally removed because extensive amputation of the foot leads to more rapid progression of disease in the contralateral foot due to shifting of weight-bearing stresses. Here, MRI can provide a "surgical map" of the infected, necrotic, and viable tissue. The radiologist should thoroughly interrogate the soft tissues proximal from the source of infection as

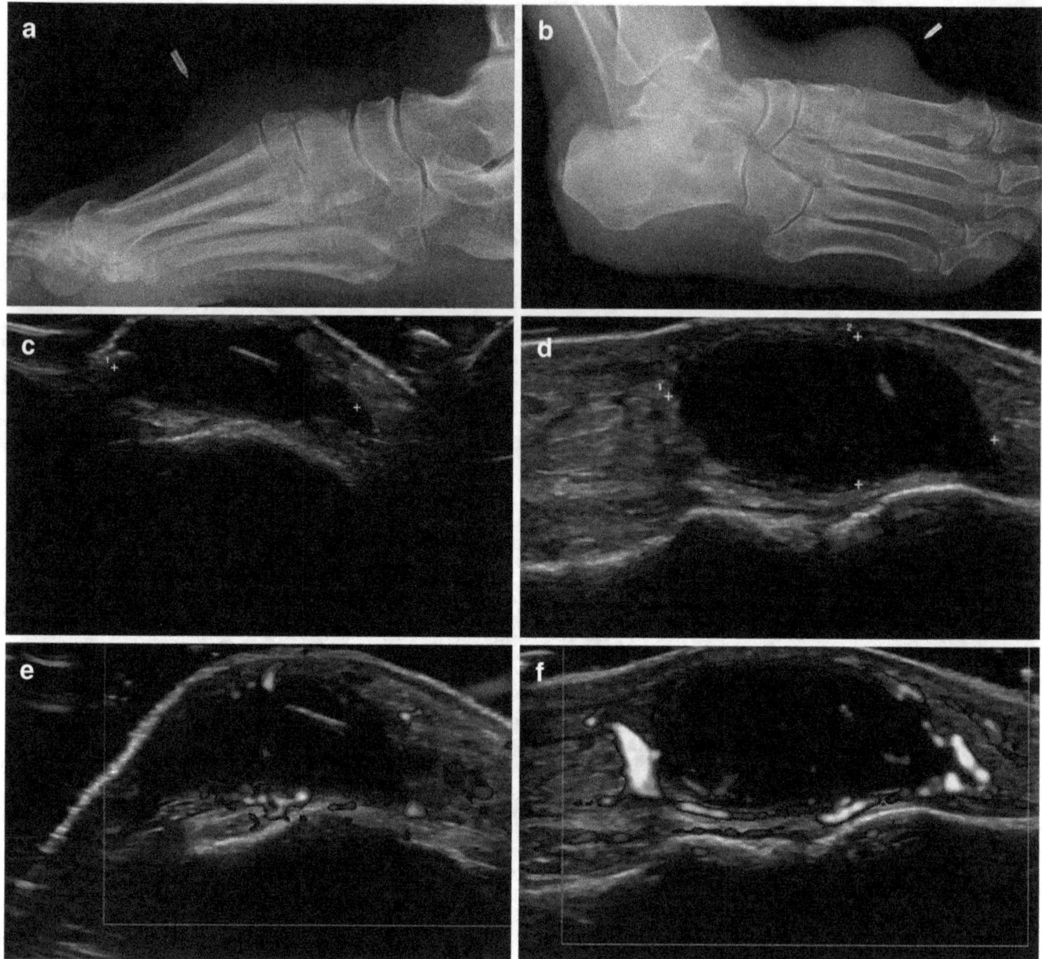

Fig. 7 Retained foreign body granuloma. Frontal (**a**) and oblique (**b**) radiographs of the foot demonstrate focal soft tissue swelling overlying the dorsal aspect of the midfoot. Longitudinal (**c**) and transverse (**d**) ultrasound demonstrates a hypoechoic fluid collection with an internal echogenic linear structure in keeping with a retained foreign body. Peripheral hypervascularity on color Doppler (**e** and **f**) is in keeping with a surrounding granulomatous reaction

pedal infection readily spreads into and across joints, through tendons and across fascial planes. If all the infected tissue is not debrided, then the patient may fail their foot-sparing procedure and need more extensive amputation.

4.5 Necrotizing Fasciitis

Necrotizing fasciitis is an aggressive soft tissue infection of the subcutis and deep fascia by toxin-producing organisms that spread rapidly and cause liquefaction/necrosis of muscle and fat. This condition warrants urgent and aggressive combinations of medical and surgical management.

Necrotizing fasciitis has a high mortality rate of up to 29% in recent years. The high mortality rate is thought to be related to sepsis secondary to the release of endotoxins from liquefactive tissue necrosis and widespread and rapid bacterial dissemination. Group A beta-hemolytic streptococci is the main causative organism. Predisposing conditions in the lower leg or ankle include soft tissue ischemia or diabetes mellitus. Once bacteria infiltrate the subcutis, exotoxins and enzymes are thought to cause local tissue destruction. Necrotic or poorly perfused tissue serves as a nidus for bacterial proliferation, enabling further toxin production and tissue destruction. Tissue destruction initially spreads horizontally within the subcutaneous tissues and superficial fascia. Rapid bacterial proliferation leads to disease progression of the underlying muscle and overlying skin due to ischemic necrosis from toxin-induced thrombosis or vasoconstriction of the feeding vasculature. Clinically, progressive necrosis of the skin and subcutaneous tissues is seen. Blisters and bullae are common with Group A beta-hemolytic streptococcal infections. Severe infection and subcutaneous necrosis extend well beyond the borders of the superficially apparent wound necrosis.

Plain radiographs contribute little to the diagnosis. There may be increased soft tissue opacification and gas within the soft tissues. CT is a good modality in the acute setting due to its speed and availability. In deep fascial planes, fat infiltration, fascial thickening and focal fluid collections may be seen. Gas in the deep soft tissues is almost diagnostic of necrotizing fasciitis; however, it is seen in less than half of cases. On MRI, the subcutis, fascia, and muscle can be characterized in detail. Subcutaneous edema is less prominent in necrotizing fasciitis than in cellulitis. Deep fascial thickening ($\geq$3 mm) with enhancement is observed. The thickening is generally smooth, usually extending the length of the muscle/compartment. Enhancement may be heterogeneous or uniform. Necrotic regions will be nonenhancing. Both the superficial and the deep fascia are usually involved in necrotizing fasciitis. If only the peripheral deep fascia is involved, then the differential also includes cellulitis. However, long segment involvement, fascial thickening, necrosis, and fascial gas confined to the superficial fascia should raise concern for necrotizing fasciitis. Fluid pockets can also be seen within the fascia. Gas within the fascia is seen as foci of T2 hypointensity or "blooming" artifact on gradient-echo sequences. Rim-enhancing fascial abscesses may be present. Muscle is generally not enhancing or swollen in necrotizing fasciitis. There may be peripheral reactive edema in muscles due to adjacent fascial inflammation. Intramuscular fluid is uncommon. There may be reactive inflammation of the intermuscular layer of deep fascia. Necrotizing fasciitis is a clinical diagnosis, and imaging can be used for problem-solving. MRI should not be undertaken in an unstable patient. Imaging in necrotizing fasciitis can be useful to aid surgical planning.

4.6 Septic Tenosynovitis

Septic tenosynovitis is typically the result of contiguous spread from an underlying ulcer, or septic arthritis or direct inoculation through trauma. It rarely occurs due to hematogenous seeding. The tendons of the toes course below commonly ulcerated areas such as the interphalangeal and metatarsophalangeal joints and are frequently involved in deep infection. Infection of the flexor hallucis longus sheath can also result from septic arthritis of the subtalar or ankle joint with which it communicates. Radiography is of limited value and may demonstrate soft tissue swelling and/or gas. Ultrasonography may show synovial hyperemia and fluid distension of the tendon sheath. CT may demonstrate fluid and/or gas within the tendon sheath, synovial thickening, and enhancement. MRI is the gold standard for assessment of tenosynovitis and may reveal complex heterogenous signal within the tendon sheath, synovial thickening and contrast enhancement, thickened tendons with variable signal alterations and/or enhancement, and soft tissue edema like signal surrounding the tendon sheath. Occasionally, there may also be subjacent osteomyelitis. Septic tenosynovitis of the flexor tendons of the toes can result in proximal spread of infection into the central plantar compartment with abscess formation. In the hindfoot, infection spreading proximally along the flexor tendons from the central plantar compartment into the lower leg has been reported. Notwithstanding this, most cases of tenosynovitis tend to remain confined to the local area of infection (Figs. 6 and 8).

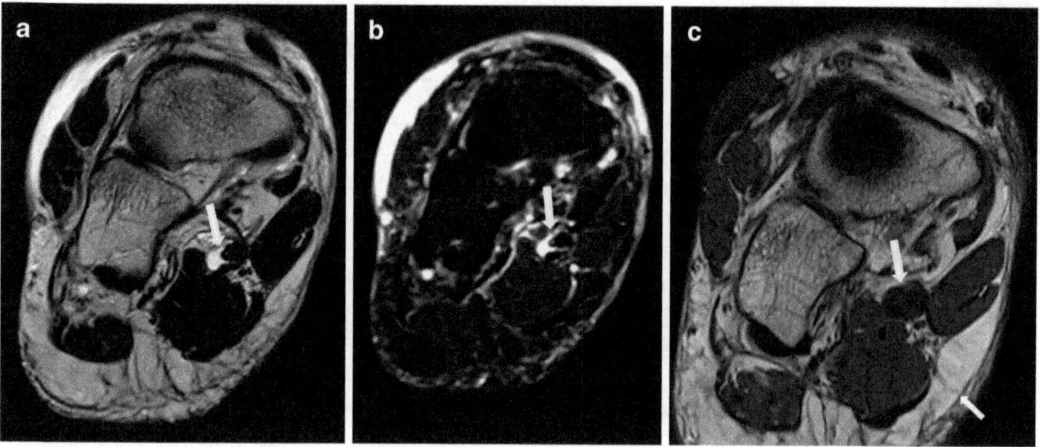

Fig. 8 Septic tenosynovitis. T2 (**a**), STIR (**b**), and (**c**) T1-weighted coronal MRI images at the level of the navicular demonstrate fluid within the tendon sheaths surrounding the flexor digitorum longus and flexor hallucis longus tendons at the knot of Henry, where the tendons cross over each other. This is a known site of tendon intersection syndrome. The blue arrow depicts the deep peripheral fascia, and the white arrow depicts the superficial fascia

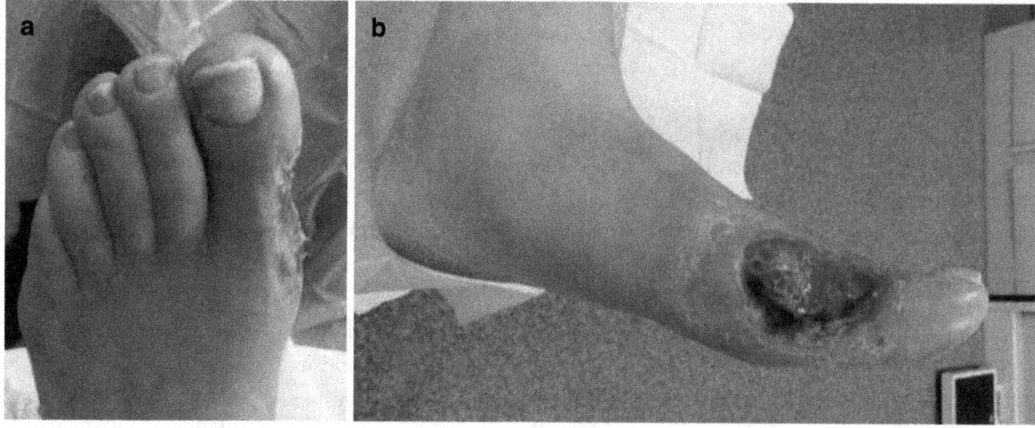

Fig. 9 Hallux ulceration. Frontal (**a**) and lateral (**b**) clinical photographs of a patient's left foot show a large ulcer centered overlying the left hallux with full-thickness skin loss in keeping with a neuro-ischemic ulcer. The green and yellow material within the ulcer represents slough from underlying infection

4.7 Skin Ulceration

Skin ulcers can be seen as an interruption of the cutaneous signal line on MR. Superficial erosions can be subtle. Ulcers in the plantar-posterior heel, and in the plantar aspect of the toes and at the metatarsophalangeal joints, are readily detected on MRI. However, ulcers at the medial and lateral aspect of the toes and dorsum may be more difficult to recognize. Contrast-enhanced sequences can help delineate the break in the cutaneous line more clearly, and ulcers typically display peripheral rim enhancement. Deep ulceration is frequently associated with underlying osteomyelitis and/or septic arthritis (Figs. 2, 3, and 9).

4.8 Sinus Tracts

Sinus tracts are commonly found in case of osteomyelitis and adjacent skin ulceration. On imaging, a thin line of near-fluid signal is seen on MRI in most cases. The best sequence for assessing sinus tracts is a post-contrast and fat suppressed T1 weighted sequence. Here, a sinus tract will be seen as parallel lines of enhancement in a tram-track pattern. However, if the tract is not actively draining, fluid signal may not be apparent and thus the tract may not be detected (Fig. 3).

5 Osteomyelitis

Osteomyelitis (OM) is defined as inflammation of the bone caused by an infectious organism. It is a difficult clinical problem to diagnose, classify, and manage; often requiring a multidisciplinary approach. OM is particularly a challenging diagnosis when there are coexisting pathologies such as Charcot neuropathic osteoarthropathy, osteoarthritis, or prior surgery. Patients usually present to the emergency department with clinical concern for possible OM, or with signs and symptoms relating to underlying OM. Over the last few decades, OM has nearly tripled in incidence largely due to an increase in diabetes-related pedal OM. Improved survival following traumatic injury with open fractures has contributed to an increased incidence of post-traumatic OM.

Staphylococcus aureus is the most common organism that causes OM; however, other common organisms such as *Escherichia coli* or *Streptococcus* spp. may also be responsible in some cases. OM secondary to contiguous soft tissue infection depends on the mechanism of infection. For instance, an animal bite from a cat or dog can cause infection from *Pasteurella multocida*, whereas a puncture wound is commonly complicated by *Staphylococcus* or *Pseudomonas aeruginosa*. Patients with diabetes usually have polymicrobial wound infections, which then track to the underlying bone. Maduromycosis is a rare granulomatous infection endemic to the tropics that affects the plantar surface of the foot. The common route of infection is contaminated soil coming into contact with breaks in the skin, and infection subsequently tracking to the deep tissues and underlying bone. *Actinomycoses bacteria* (60%) and *Madurella fungus* (40%) are the causative organisms.

Osteomyelitis can be acute, subacute, or chronic in presentation, and the definitions of these are variably described. The acute phase is generally defined as being either less than 10 days or 2 weeks in duration. The subacute phase constitutes disease lasting less than 3 months but lacking acute symptoms. The chronicity of osteomyelitis can also be divided into acute and non-acute, and non-acute includes both the subacute and chronic phases. Chronic osteomyelitis is generally regarded as infection lasting longer than 6 weeks. The development of bone necrosis is the key feature in the development of chronic osteomyelitis. The necrotic bone is usually surrounded by sclerotic hypovascular bone, a thickened periosteum, and inflamed surrounding soft tissues. The Cierny-Mader classification describes anatomic involvement, host, treatment, and prognosis.

Osteomyelitis can spread via either hematogenous dissemination or contiguous spread. Contiguous spread involves direct extension of infection into bone from adjacent soft tissue infection or from direct inoculation secondary to trauma. Non-spinal hematogenous osteomyelitis is predominantly a disease of childhood due to its predilection to involve the highly vascularized metaphyseal region of growing bone. Understanding age-related vascular anatomy will help to unpack this concept. In infants up to 12 months of age, some of the metaphyseal vessels penetrate the physis and anastomose with epiphyseal vessels. Hence, infections in infants under 12 months of age often involve the metaphysis, epiphysis, and joint and may result in osteonecrosis, slipped epiphysis, and growth deformity. In children older than 12 months, blood vessels do not cross the physis and metaphyseal vessels terminate in loops which have sluggish blood flow. The combination of a relative lack of phagocytes in the metaphysis together with this vascular anatomy results in the metaphyses of long bones being the most common site of infection in a child. In adults, the epiphyseal vessels anastomose with the terminal metaphyseal vessels across the physis. Therefore, joint involvement secondary to osteomyelitis is more common in adults. However, hematogenous pedal osteomyelitis in adults is rare and pedal osteomyelitis secondary to contiguous spread is by far the most common route of spread.

In non-acute osteomyelitis, there are four entities that need to be understood: Brodie's abscess, sequestrum, involucrum, and cloaca. Brodie's abscess, first described by Sir Benjamin Brodie in 1832, is an intra-osseous abscess. It is considered a form of subacute osteomyelitis, although a variable time course from 1 week to 1 year after symptom onset has been reported. The signs and symptoms of acute osteomyelitis such as recent-onset pain and fever are typically absent. Robert's classification of Brodie's abscesses defines six types depending on the anatomic location: with the most classic case of a metaphyseal lucent lesion with sclerotic borders. It should be highlighted that Brodie's abscess has a protean radiographic appearance and can occur at any location and in a patient of any age. It may or may not be expansile, has a sclerotic or nonsclerotic border, etc. On MRI, the typical appearance of a Brodie's abscess is a fluid intensity signal lesion, sometimes with a peripheral penumbra sign. The penumbra sign represents a thin rim of vascularized granulation tissue and is reflected as hyperintense signal on T1-weighted imaging at the periphery of the intra-osseous abscess. The penumbra sign has been reported to have a specificity of 96% for the presence of infection (and a sensitivity of 27%) and has been suggested as being a reliable way to differentiate subacute osteomyelitis (penumbra sign) from neoplasm. It can be challenging distinguishing a cyst from a Brodie's abscess. Cloaca, involucrum, and sequestrum are interrelated entities of chronic osteomyelitis. A sequestrum is a segment of devascularized bone that becomes separated ("sequestered") from host bone due to surrounding necrosis, which can therefore act as a harbor for bacteria, which is inaccessible to antibiotics. The definitive treatment is surgical resection. A sequestrum is best imaged with CT and appears as a mineralized segment of bone with circumferential surrounding lucency. Several primary bone tumors may produce a mineralized matrix that can simulate a sequestrum such as an osteoid osteoma or osteoblastoma. The margins of a sequestrum are irregular, in contrast with the smooth and round center of an osteoid osteoma nidus. An involucrum is a reactive bone sclerosis that surrounds the sequestrum. It isolates the sequestrum from the bloodstream similar to a walled-off abscess. A cloaca is an opening or rupture of the involucrum that allows granulation tissue to be discharged, and which can give rise to a subperiosteal abscess. A sinus tract may eventually form if the cloaca communicates with the skin surface through the soft tissues. Over time, sinus tracts may undergo malignant transformation most frequently to squamous cell carcinoma.

5.1 Imaging of Osteomyelitis

5.1.1 Radiography

Radiographs are the common first-line investigations for suspected osteomyelitis, which are often negative. They can help exclude alternative differential diagnoses such as a fracture. Radiographic findings of osteomyelitis may differ depending on the route of spread. The imaging findings mirror the pathophysiology in both contiguous focal and hematogenous osteomyelitis. The earliest radiographic changes of hematogenous osteomyelitis occur in the soft tissues, with soft tissue swelling evident within 2–3 days of symptom onset. Bony changes of hematogenous osteomyelitis are not typically seen until at least 10–12 days, and they begin in the medullary cavity and extend outward. Approximately 30% of the bone matrix must be destroyed for changes to be evident on radiography. The earliest osseous changes include focal osteopenia and periosteal reaction. It usually takes 2–3 weeks for cortical erosion to develop, and bone destruction may be apparent in only the late stage of the disease. In contiguous-focus osteomyelitis, an ulcer tract should be sought, which can be seen on radiographs as a lucent soft tissue defect extending from the skin surface often with foci of gas to the underlying bone. Other radiographic findings include focal osteopenia corresponding to trabecular lysis and ill-defined cortical erosion that is contiguous with the ulcer tract. Bony destruction and soft tissue or intra-osseous gas can be present in advanced cases (Fig. 10).

5.1.2 CT

Although CT is less sensitive than MRI or nuclear medicine studies for detecting early intramedullary changes of osteomyelitis, it is an excellent modality to evaluate soft tissue infection in the acute setting as it can reliably detect soft tissue abscesses and soft tissue gas. In addition, the ability to rapidly image a large anatomic region on CT makes it an excellent modality in the emergency department for assessment of osteomyelitis. CT also provides superior contrast resolution and detail for detecting retained foreign bodies that may be acting as a nidus for infection. CT findings of osteomyelitis also depend on the route of spread, though they generally include soft tissue swelling, decreased attenuation of the medullary space, and periosteal reaction. CT is also excellent at characterizing the bony changes of chronic osteomyelitis, including sequestrum, involucrum, and cloaca.

5.1.3 US

US is not the first-line modality for the assessment of suspected OM. It can be useful in visualizing subperiosteal abscesses, joint effusions, or superficial fluid collections in pediatric patients.

5.1.4 Radionuclide Imaging

Radionuclide imaging can play a role in problem-solving in pedal infection. In particular, it has an important role in the setting of extensive orthopedic hardware, and in helping to differentiate osteomyelitis from neuropathic arthropathy. Both osteomyelitis and neuropathic arthropathy cannot be differentiated from one another on a three-phase bone scan as they both demonstrate uptake (i.e., it is sensitive but not specific), and a three-phase bone scan is rarely a helpful test in isolation. In contrast, a radiolabeled leukocyte scan is both sensitive and specific and is considered the radionuclide test of choice for the evaluation of osteomyelitis. It has an accuracy of approximately 90% when combined with sulfur colloid imaging. In the evaluation of diabetic pedal infection, a systematic review found that a radiolabeled leukocyte HMPAO study had a specificity of 92% and sensitivity of 91% compared to a specificity of 75% and sensitivity of 93% using MRI. Nevertheless, MRI is still the preferred modality for assessment of pedal infection (Fig. 11).

5.1.5 MRI

MRI is the most accurate imaging test for the evaluation of suspected osteomyelitis, with a meta-analysis demonstrating a sensitivity of 90% and a specificity of 79%. Intravenous contrast is useful but not essential for the assessment of suspected osteomyelitis. Soft tissue abscesses may not be apparent without contrast to delineate the typical peripheral enhancement pattern. Contrast also assists in identification and demarcation of areas of necrotic, nonenhancing soft tissue or bone. Fluid-sensitive sequences are the most sensitive for detecting osteomyelitis. Fluid-sensitive sequences include T2, PD with fat suppression, or STIR sequences.

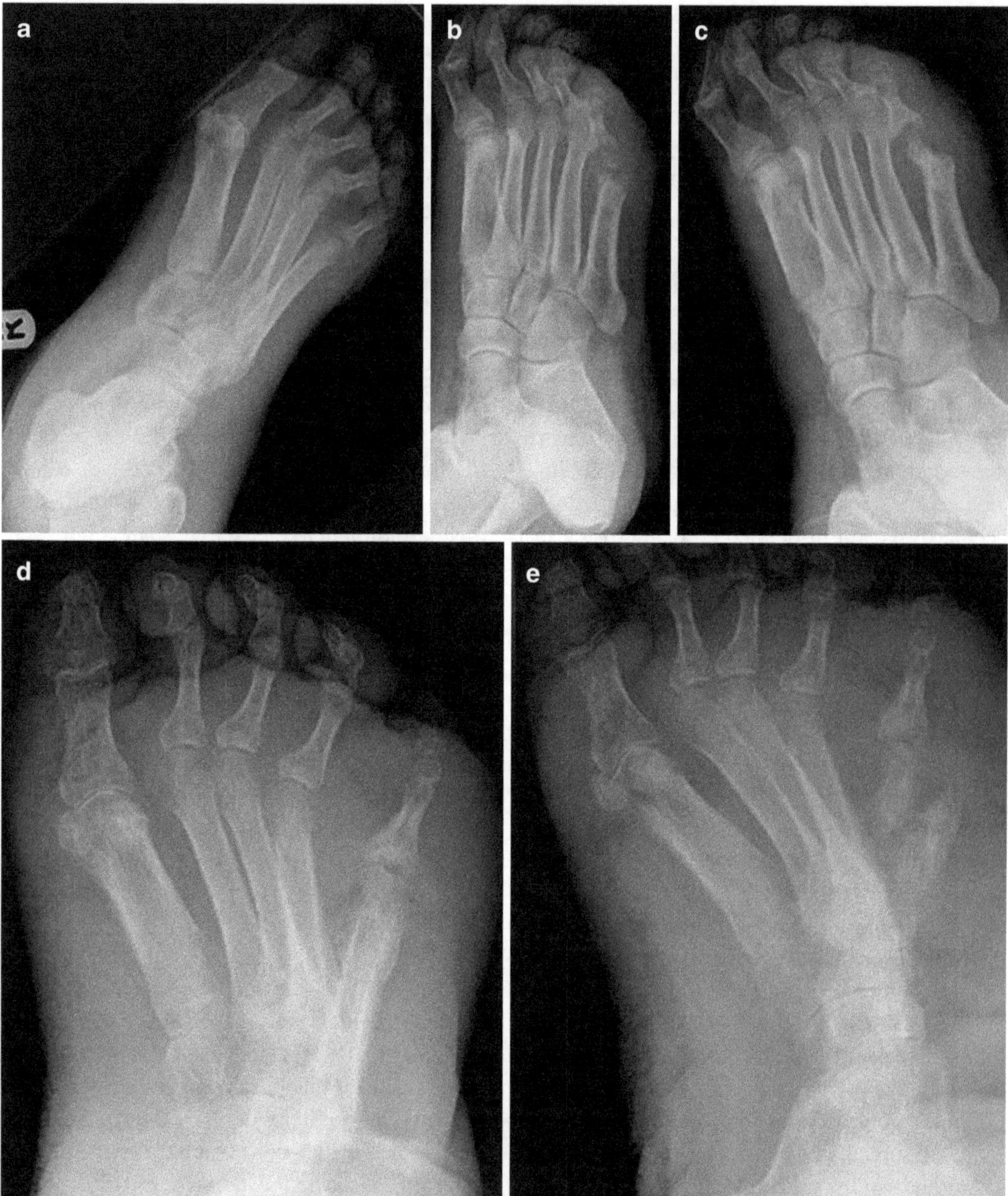

Fig. 10 Evolution of septic arthritis and chronic osteomyelitis. An oblique radiograph of the foot (**a**) demonstrates osteolysis and destruction at the head of the right fifth metatarsal and base of the right fifth proximal phalanx in keeping with septic arthritis. A dressing overlying an ulcer at the lateral aspect of the fifth proximal phalanx is demonstrated and is the likely source of infection. An interval oblique radiograph performed 4 weeks later (**b**) demonstrates marked destruction at the fifth metatarsophalangeal joint. An oblique radiograph (**c**) approximately 10 weeks after the initial onset of infection demonstrates inhomogeneous sclerotic and deformed bone at the distal aspect of the fifth metatarsal with surrounding soft tissue swelling in keeping with chronic osteomyelitis. A frontal radiograph 12 months later (**d**) demonstrates proximal dislocation of the fifth metatarsal and progression of the infective change to involve the entire fifth metatarsal, which is diffusely sclerotic and has surrounding periosteal reaction. A subsequent oblique radiograph 1 month later (**e**) demonstrates near-total destruction of the fifth metatarsal with a pathological fracture through its shaft in keeping with ongoing infection

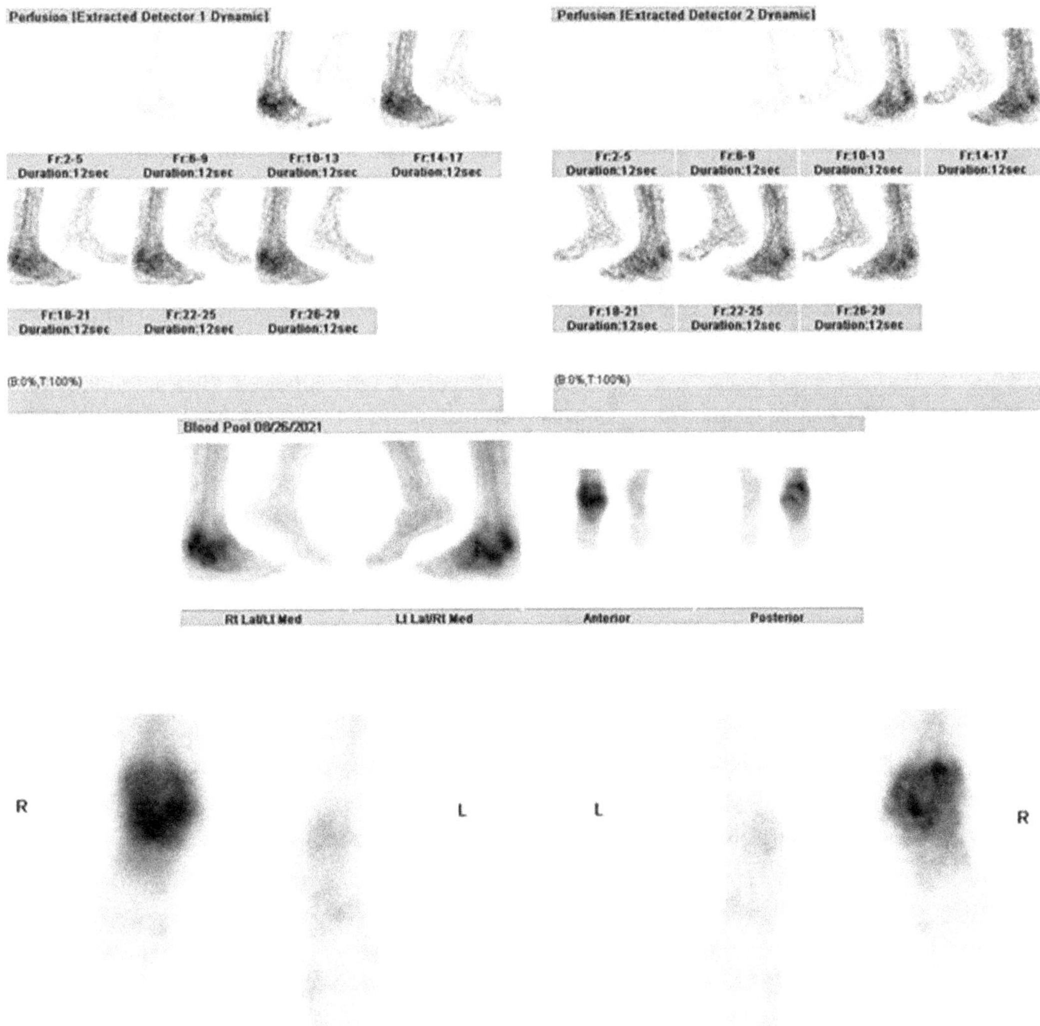

Fig. 11 Infected hardware and septic arthritis. Triple-phase bone scan demonstrates increased uptake on arterial, blood pool, and delayed (bottom row) images in the right ankle joint. Linear photopenic defects within the regions of high uptake best seen on the perfusion images represent the fixation screws. Overall findings are suggestive of chronic osteomyelitis and septic arthritis of the ankle joint. Infection involving the fixation screws cannot be objectively assessed on this examination

If the fluid-sensitive sequence is normal, osteomyelitis is extremely unlikely. However, the presence of bone marrow edema-like signal is nonspecific and only indicates possible osteomyelitis. Corresponding decreased T1 signal is key in diagnosing osteomyelitis. If there is bone marrow edema on T2-weighted imaging but the T1-weighted images are normal, this is considered to represent "osteitis" rather than osteomyelitis, suggesting that infection is not thought to be present. Three patterns of altered T1 signal have been described: confluent intramedullary, hazy reticular, and subcortical. The confluent intramedullary pattern describes a geographic

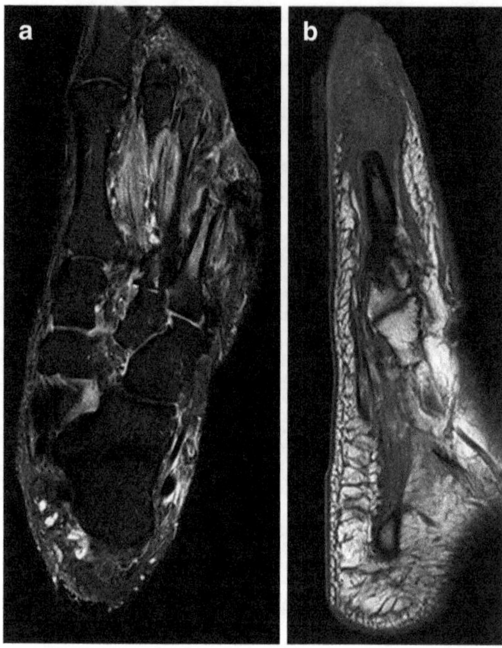

Fig. 12 Osteomyelitis. Axial STIR (**a**) and sagittal T1 (**b**) MRI images of the left foot demonstrate STIR hyperintensity in the shaft of the fourth metatarsal with corresponding T1 hypointensity in keeping with osteomyelitis

area of decreased T1 signal intensity involving the medullary canal. It is associated with osteomyelitis with a sensitivity of 95% and a specificity of 91%. The hazy reticular pattern describes interspersed areas of low T1 signal within regions of normal marrow. This is not associated with contiguous-focus osteomyelitis. It is rarely associated with hematogenous osteomyelitis. The subcortical pattern describes a thin linear region of T1 hypointensity subjacent to the cortex. This is not associated with osteomyelitis. Although decreased T1 signal intensity is almost always present in osteomyelitis, there have been rare reports of culture or pathologically proven osteomyelitis corresponding to regions of normal T1 signal. These regions possibly reflect necrotic bone with fatty marrow signal. In addition, if there is high T2 but normal T1 signal in an area subjacent to an ulcer; this should be interpreted with caution as a study demonstrated that 61% of patients with these findings ultimately developed osteomyelitis (Figs. 3, 6, 12, and 13).

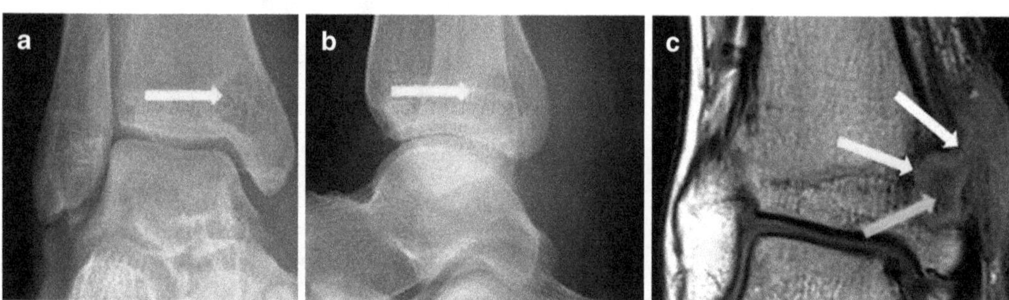

Fig. 13 Osteomyelitis with intra-osseous abscess (Brodie's abscess) and sinus tract formation. Frontal (**a**) and lateral (**b**) radiographs of the right ankle demonstrate a well-defined lucent lesion with a faint sclerotic border at the posteromedial aspect of the tibia (yellow arrows). Coronal T1 (**c**) and STIR (**d**) images reveal the penumbra sign of an intra-osseous abscess with the peripheral ring of higher T1 signal intensity (yellow arrow in **c**) than its cavity (blue arrow in **c**) and a peripheral halo of bone marrow edema (**d**). A cloaca (white arrow in **c**) is demonstrated draining pus into the subcutaneous tissues (yellow arrow in **d**). Interval frontal (**e**) and lateral (**f**) radiographs 2 months later demonstrate a more well-defined lucency (yellow arrows). Coronal T1 (**g**), axial STIR (**h**), and sagittal STIR (**i**) images of an MRI performed 7 months post-treatment reveal complete resolution of the soft tissue collection and a more homogenous fluid signal within the abscess cavity also in keeping with resolution of the infective change (yellow arrows). A thin rim of fluid in the posterior tibial tendon sheath (blue arrow) is likely reactive

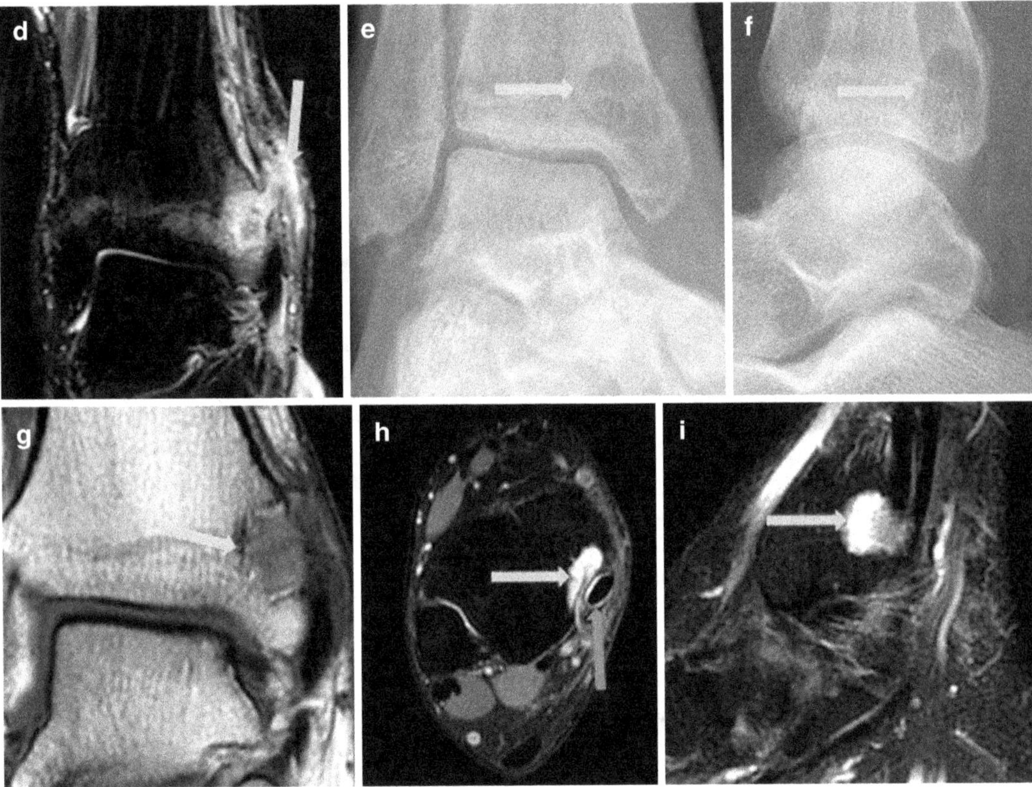

Fig. 13 (continued)

6 Septic Arthritis

Septic arthritis is a clinical diagnosis which does not usually require imaging. Joint aspiration is the test of choice. Nevertheless, imaging studies are sometimes requested. The first radiological sign of septic arthritis is usually a joint effusion. As it progresses, hyperemia-induced bone turnover and net increased bone resorption result in periarticular osteopenia. Cartilage destruction occurs and is evidenced by joint space narrowing. Cortical bone becomes indistinct. The margins of the joint lose cartilage and become "bare"; this results in marginal erosions. Bone destruction ensues, and osteomyelitis may develop by means of contiguous spread. There may be a sclerotic host reaction if the septic arthritis is bacterial in origin. Ankylosis may eventually result. Fungal and tuberculous septic arthritides are more chronic processes and may elicit little or no host bone reaction; cartilage destruction is much slower, joint space width is largely unaffected, and erosions are slow to progress and may appear well delineated.

In the foot and ankle, septic arthritis may arise via hematogenous spread; however, it is more commonly seen as a complication of adjacent soft tissue infection. At the metatarsophalangeal joints, septic arthritis usually occurs due to communication with plantar ulcers or medial ulceration at the first metatarsophalangeal joint. Septic arthritis at the midfoot may be seen in patients with foot deformity related to neuropathic disease; in these cases, the loss of the arch can lead to ulcer formation directly under the Chopart (midtarsal) or Lisfranc (tarsometatarsal) joints.

Septic arthritis involving the subtalar or ankle joint is often related to infection arising over the posterior calcaneal tubercle or malleoli. The ankle and subtalar joints communicate in approximately 20% of feet, and thus in these patients, infection can spread to both joints simultaneously. Septic arthritis in the phalanges is often due to breakdown of callus at the dorsal aspect of the toes.

6.1 Radiography

Early in the course of septic arthritis, radiographs are likely to be normal. The earliest sign is a joint effusion. In the ankle, this manifests as a rounded or irregular density extending from the anterior tibiotalar joint. Effusions in the smaller joints of the foot are more difficult to appreciate. Marginal juxta-articular bone erosion and joint space loss are seen with progression of the infection. Moth-eaten bone destruction and periosteal reaction result from involvement of adjacent osseous involvement. Infected joint prostheses usually have no early abnormality visible. As the infection progresses, periprosthetic loosening and rarely osteolysis and/or periosteal reaction may be visible (Figs. 1, 10, and 14).

6.2 CT

CT is less sensitive and specific than MRI. Findings are similar to radiography with joint effusion, bone erosion (if there is concurrent osteomyelitis), and surrounding soft tissue swelling. CT is better than radiography for evaluation of erosions or sclerosis, and to guide aspiration of joints difficult to visualize on fluoroscopy or US (Fig. 15).

6.3 MRI

MRI is sensitive (100%) and more specific (77%) than other imaging; abnormalities are detected

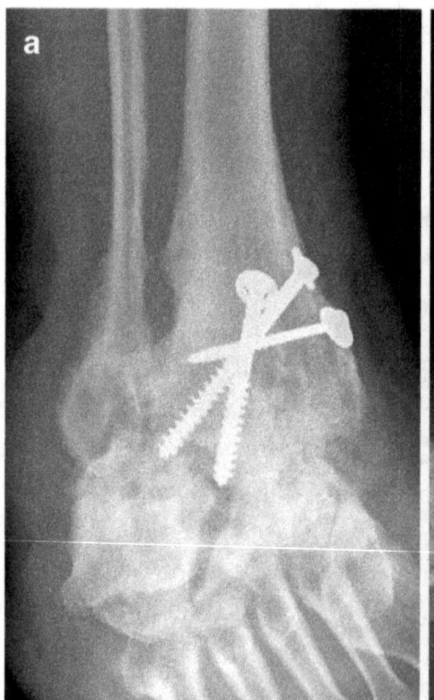

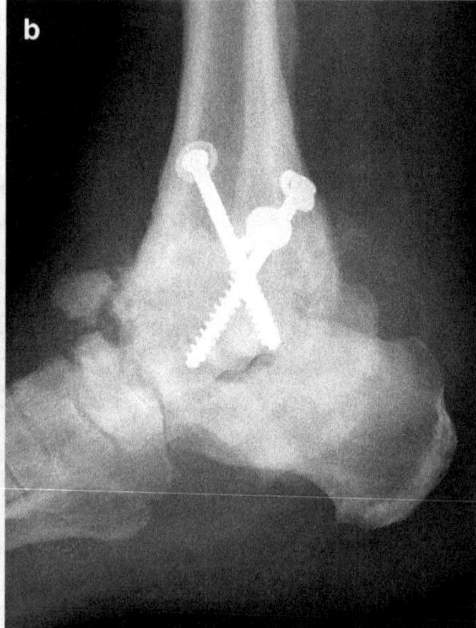

Fig. 14 Infected hardware and septic arthritis. Frontal (**a**) and lateral (**b**) radiographs demonstrate cortical destruction, disorganization, sclerosis, and periosteal reaction in the ankle and hindfoot in a patient with suspected septic arthritis. Radiographic appearances are long-standing and in keeping with a Charcot joint. Radiographic features are not specific for infected hardware or septic arthritis

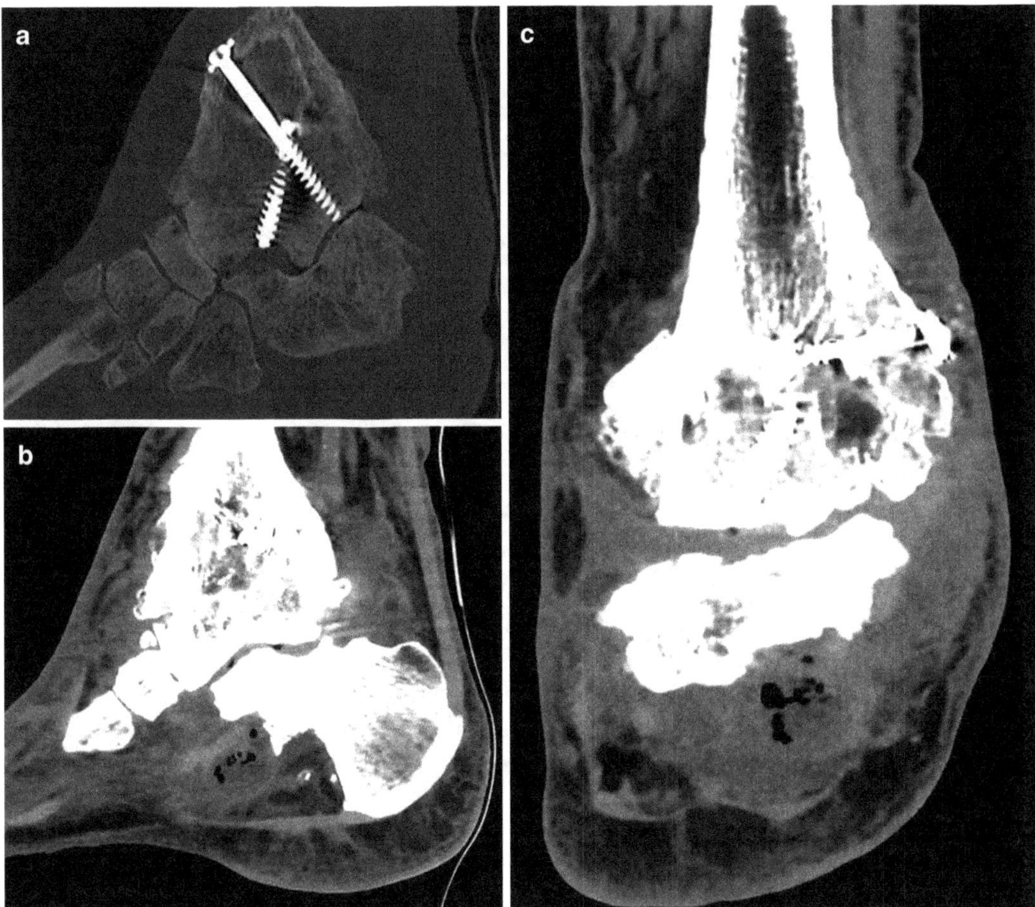

Fig. 15 Infected hardware and septic arthritis. A sagittal CT image in a bone window (**a**) demonstrates the internal fixation screws in situ with no evidence of surrounding lucency or osteolysis. There are background changes of known Charcot arthropathy. Sagittal (**b**) and coronal (**c**) soft tissue windows reveal soft tissue swelling surrounding the ankle joint and a well-defined collection containing internal gas locules in the plantar aspect of the foot abutting the calcaneus. CT features are not specific for infected hardware or septic arthritis

within 24 hours of onset. In the early stages, joint effusion, synovial enhancement, and perisynovial edema and enhancement are seen. As the infection progresses, there is subchondral bone involvement on both sides of the joint with increased T2 signal, decreased T1 signal, and increased contrast enhancement. There may also be an adjacent soft tissue abscess.

Synovial thickening and enhancement may be subtle in the small joints of the digits. MRI diagnosis of a septic joint in pedal infection may be more specific than in other parts of the body as there will likely be adjacent skin ulceration in the vast majority of cases. In addition, sinus tracts can sometimes be seen extending to the infected joint. Following treatment, abscesses and joint effusions decrease in size. However, marrow edema, synovial thickening, cellulitis, and enhancement can persist even after resolution of infection (Figs. 1, 6, 16, and 17).

6.4 US

US is sensitive for joint fluid if the joint is superficial enough to evaluate. Debris within the syno-

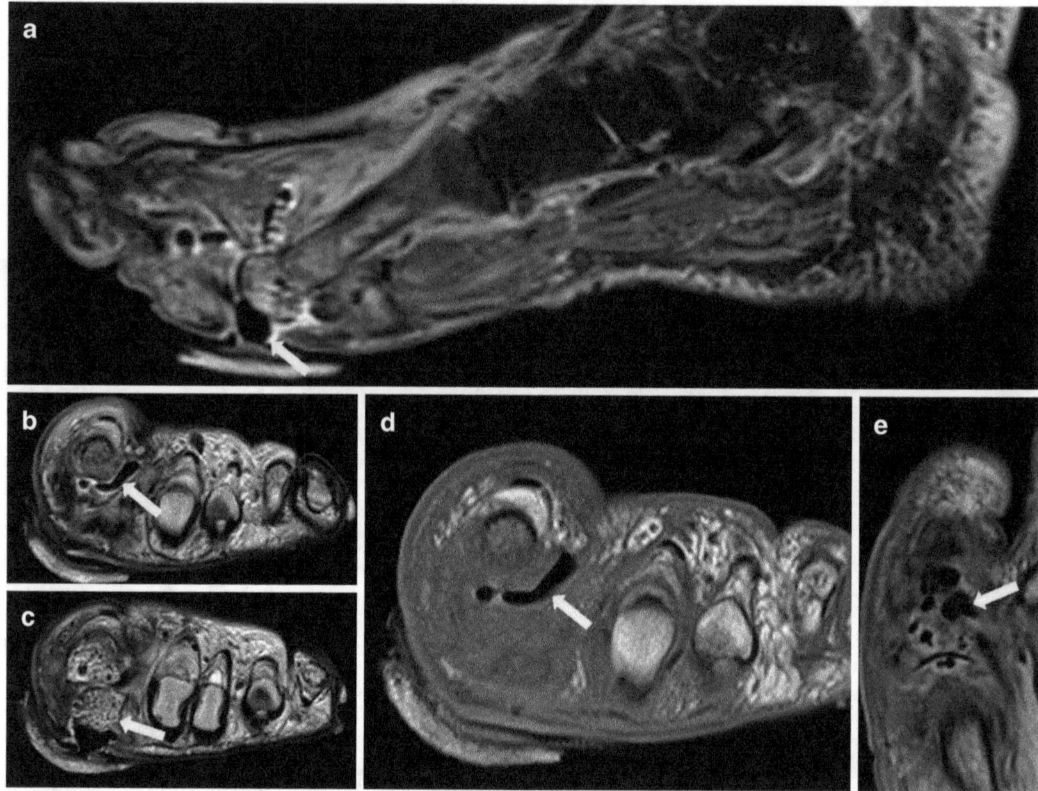

Fig. 16 Septic arthritis with an infected collection and gas-forming organisms. Sagittal STIR MRI image (**a**) demonstrates hyperintensity in the distal first metatarsal and contiguously with the proximal phalanx of the first left toe in keeping with septic arthritis. Markedly hypointense locule abutting the inferior border of the left first metatarsophalangeal joint (yellow arrow) represents a gas locule. This is likely secondary to infection with gas-forming organisms. The yellow arrows in **b** (T2-weighted images), **d** (T1-weighted images), and **e** (PD-weighted images) all depict gas locules, which are uniformly hypointense on all sequences. The yellow arrow in **c** points to a collection immediately plantar to the first metatarsophalangeal joint and contains multiple punctate hypointense gas locules

vial fluid is indicative of increased cellularity or blood within the joint. Synovial thickening and increased vascularity on color Doppler are sometimes seen. US can also help guide aspiration.

6.5 Radionuclide Studies

Bone scans are sensitive (90–100%) but not specific (75%) for a septic joint. Blood flow and blood pool images show increased activity on both sides of the joint. Delayed phase shows continued increase in activity if septic arthritis has resulted in contiguous osteomyelitis. PET/CT is highly specific in the setting of a prosthetic joint infection. Ga-67 scintigraphy has a high specificity but a significant false-positive rate. Similarly, labeled leukocyte scintigraphy has a high specificity but significant false-positive rate (Figs. 18 and 19).

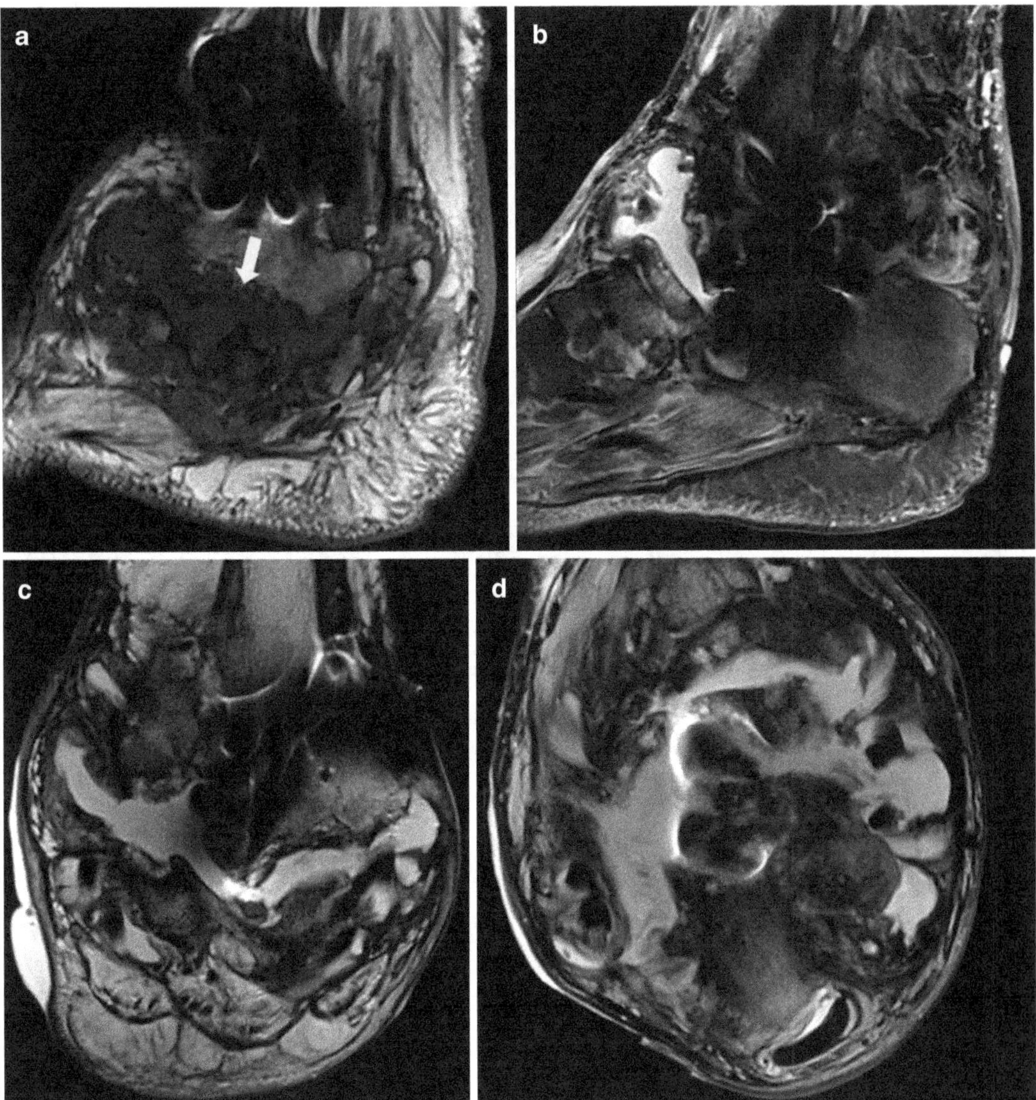

Fig. 17 Sagittal T1 weighted (**a**) and STIR (**b**) with corresponding axial T1 weighted (**c**) and STIR (**d**) of the ankle infected hardware and septic arthritis. These images demonstrate osseous destruction with fluid collections in the ankle joint. The yellow arrow (**a**) depicts destruction at the subtalar joint. Findings are in keeping with septic arthritis

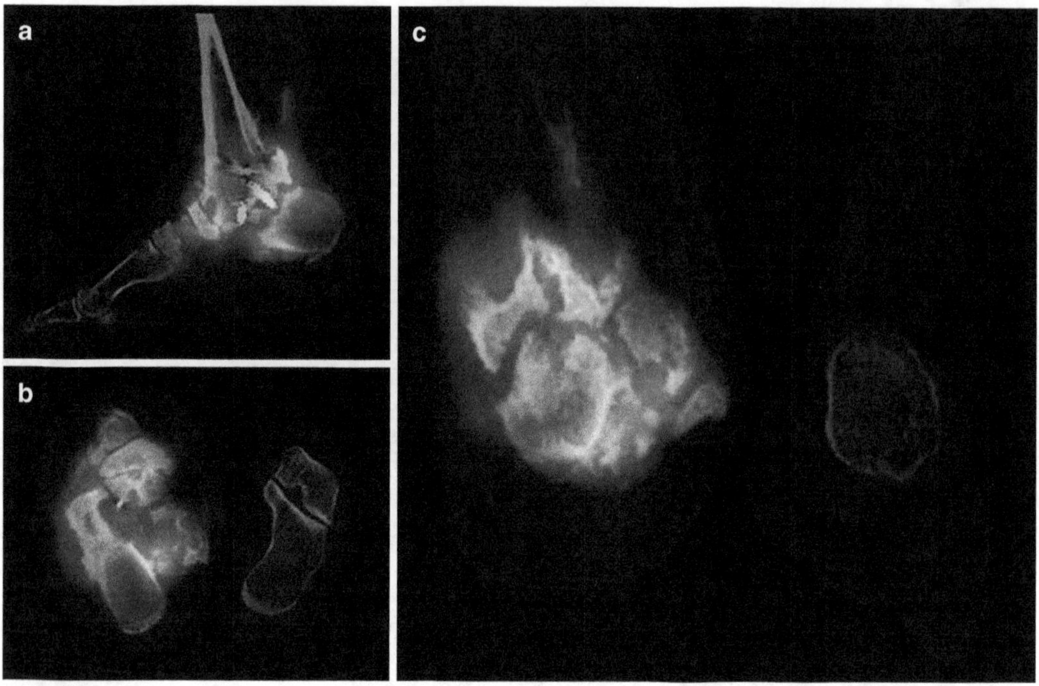

Fig. 18 Infected hardware and septic arthritis. Sagittal (**a**), axial (**b**), and coronal (**c**) delayed SPECT-CT images reveal intense uptake within the ankle joint and fragmentation of the subtalar joint. Findings are in keeping with septic arthritis and infection of the fixation screws

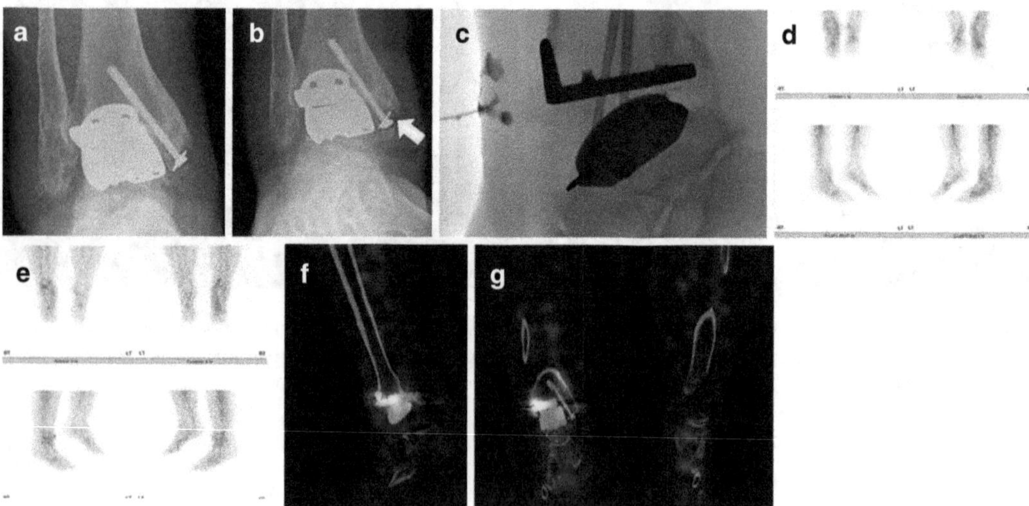

Fig. 19 Infected hardware and septic arthritis. Initial frontal radiograph of the right ankle (**a**) demonstrates a total ankle prosthesis. A subsequent frontal radiograph (**b**) a year later demonstrates osteolysis at the tip of the medial malleolus (yellow arrow). A sinogram (**c**) was performed to assess the extent of an ulcer anterior to the right talocrural joint. Contrast filled the ulcer crater, and no sinus tract was demonstrated. A white cell HMPAO scan demonstrated focal uptake in the right tibial component of the prosthesis on the planar images at 1 h (**d**), which revealed more focal intense uptake on the 4-h planar images (**e**). On SPECT-CT (**f–h**), the focal intense uptake localizes to the lateral aspect of the tibial component of the prosthesis. This proves leukocyte migration to the site of infection in the tibial prosthesis. This is a more specific test than the triple-phase bone scan in Figs. 7 and 8. Consequently, the ankle prosthesis was explanted (**i**)

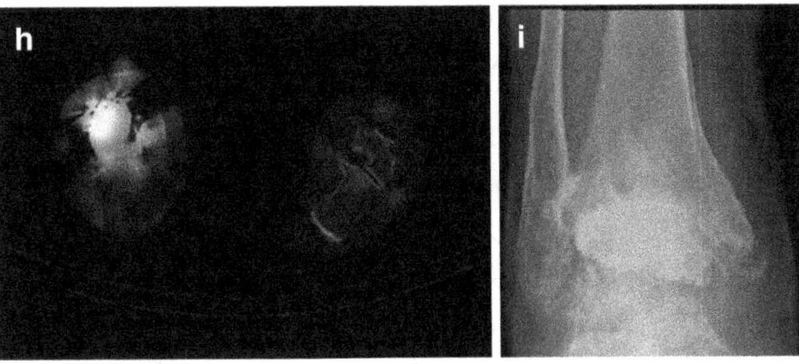

Fig. 19 (continued)

7 Infected Hardware

Periprosthetic infection is an important complication which can lead to joint and/or bone failure, including loss of osteosynthesis in the early post-procedure stage. Diagnosis can be extremely challenging as infective and noninfective causes for hardware/surgical failure overlap clinically and radiographically. Radiographs are the initial imaging modality despite their low specificity and sensitivity in assessing a prosthetic joint: peri-implant osteolysis, transcortical sinus tracts, osteopenia, and periosteal reaction may be identified. Radiographs add significant value in being able to compare serial appearances over time. CT will provide more detail about the above osseous changes; however, beam-hardening artifact from metallic implants obscures detailed characterization and assessment of pathology. US cannot penetrate bone or metal, and thus its utility is limited to detecting peri-implant inflammation and fluid collections. MRI with metal artifact reduction sequences (MARS) improves the assessment of pathologies such as peri-osseous fluid and collections, bone marrow edema, and pathological enhancement. A common difficult scenario for the orthopedic or podiatric surgeon is to try and assess whether their patient with a painful prosthetic joint is presenting with a loosening prosthesis or an infected joint replacement. Nuclear medicine imaging studies such as ^{99m}Tc MDP and combined ^{111}indium/marrow imaging play an important role in helping answer this question. Although a ^{99m}Tc MDP three-phase bone scan is positive in all three phases in infection (sensitivity 90–100%), on its own, it is not specific for infection (18–35% specificity) as aseptic loosening can also be positive in all three phases, and in addition their respective patterns of uptake have been described as indistinguishable. Bone scans can also demonstrate uptake for a year following surgery. Radiolabeled white blood cell (WBC) scintigraphy can help differentiate between aseptic loosening and an infected joint prosthesis; however, combined ^{111}In-oxine WBC and ^{99m}Tc-sulfur colloid scintigraphy is the gold standard nuclear medicine study to evaluate this. If there is uptake of radiolabeled WBCs surrounding the prosthesis different in distribution to the uptake on the sulfur colloid scan, then this is considered to be positive for an infected joint prosthesis (Figs. 11, 14, 15, 17, 18, and 19).

8 MR Imaging Protocols in Pedal Infection

Although MR imaging protocols vary widely, observation of some general principles can help optimize the examination. The MR protocol should be tailored to the patient and specific clinical scenario. It is recommended that surface markers are placed over shallow ulcers that may not easily be detected on imaging. The practical difficulty with this is that ulcers are often covered in dressings. The field of view should include the region of interest with the foot normally divided into the hindfoot, midfoot, or forefoot regions. A large field of view should ideally be avoided, as it sacrifices detail. A small field of view and thin slices optimize spatial resolution. Notwithstanding this, the whole foot may need to be imaged to include the entire extent of infection. Coil selection and imaging planes are also important. Extremity coils are excellent for imaging the ankle and foot; however, they result in suboptimal examination of the toes. Three-inch or five-inch surface coils are preferred for imaging the toes; however, if there is concern for proximal spread of infection then the surface coils may not suffice. Imaging should be performed in at least two planes for optimum visualization. The different planes can also provide specific benefits. For instance, the coronal and axial planes are good for visualizing medial and lateral hindfoot ulcers, and the sagittal plane is useful for visualizing posterior calcaneal ulcers and midfoot neuroarthropathic changes. For imaging the toes, a plane perpendicular to the toes in short-axis view is recommended as the small bones in the toes easily acquire average volume in sagittal and axial planes. T1-weighted sequences are excellent for depicting anatomy. In addition, they are sensitive to marrow changes and are very specific in detecting osteomyelitis. T2-weighted sequences detect bone marrow and soft tissue edema and soft tissue collections with exquisite sensitivity. However, with fast-spin echo, the bright signal of fatty bone marrow can mask the bright signal of marrow edema. Thus, T2-weighted sequences with chemical fat suppression eliminate this problem. To achieve homogenous fat suppression however, the foot has to be positioned in the center of the magnet. The natural curvature of the foot can cause some inhomogeneity in the fat suppression using this technique, and alternately short tau inversion recovery (STIR) sequences can be used to offset this problem. The trade-off with STIR sequences is poorer image resolution. The acquisition of contrast-enhanced sequences is still a subject of debate. In patients with renal failure, there is a risk of gadolinium-induced nephrogenic systemic fibrosis, and it should be used judiciously in this setting. There is no conclusive evidence that intravenous contrast increases the accuracy in detection of osteomyelitis. It does however improve the assessment of soft tissue complications such as necrosis, abscesses, and sinus tracts. It also provides crucial information in preoperative planning of limb resection.

Further Reading

Beaman FD, von Herrmann PF, Kransdorf MJ et al (2017) ACR appropriateness criteria® suspected osteomyelitis, septic arthritis, or soft tissue infection (excluding spine and diabetic foot). J Am Coll Radiol 14:S326–S337. https://doi.org/10.1016/j.jacr.2017.02.008

Berquist T (2014) Imaging of the foot and ankle. Wolters Kluwer, Philadelphia

Cardinal E, Bureau NJ, Aubin B, Chhem RK (2001) Role of ultrasound in musculoskeletal infections. Radiol Clin North Am 39(2):191–201. https://doi.org/10.1016/s0033-8389(05)70272-4

Chin TY, Peh WC (2021) Imaging update on musculoskeletal infections. J Clin Orthop Trauma 22:101600. https://doi.org/10.1016/j.jcot.2021.101600

Christman R (2014) Foot and ankle radiology, 2nd edn. LWW

Donovan A, Schweitzer ME (2010) Use of MR imaging in diagnosing diabetes-related pedal osteomyelitis. Radiographics 30(3):723–736. https://doi.org/10.1148/rg.303095111

Goodwin DW, Salonen DC, Yu JS, Brossmann J, Trudell DJ, Resnick DL (1995) Plantar compartments of the foot: MR appearance in cadavers and diabetic patients. Radiology 196(3):623–630. https://doi.org/10.1148/radiology.196.3.7644621

Hayeri MR, Ziai P, Shehata ML, Teytelboym OM, Huang BK (2016) Soft-tissue infections and their imaging mimics: from cellulitis to necrotizing fasciitis. Radiographics 36(6):1888–1910. https://doi.org/10.1148/rg.2016160068

Ingraham CR, Mannelli L, Robinson JD, Linnau KF (2015) Radiology of foreign bodies: how do we image them? Emerg Radiol 22(4):425–430. https://doi.org/10.1007/s10140-015-1294-9

Ledermann HP, Schweitzer ME, Morrison WB (2002a) Nonenhancing tissue on MR imaging of pedal infection: characterization of necrotic tissue and associated limitations for diagnosis of osteomyelitis and abscess. AJR Am J Roentgenol 178(1):215–222. https://doi.org/10.2214/ajr.178.1.1780215

Ledermann HP, Morrison WB, Schweitzer ME (2002b) MR image analysis of pedal osteomyelitis: distribution, patterns of spread, and frequency of associated ulceration and septic arthritis. Radiology 223(3):747–755. https://doi.org/10.1148/radiol.2233011279

Ledermann HP, Morrison WB, Schweitzer ME (2002c) Pedal abscesses in patients suspected of having pedal osteomyelitis: analysis with MR imaging. Radiology 224(3):649–655. https://doi.org/10.1148/radiol.2243011231

Ledermann HP, Morrison WB, Schweitzer ME, Raikin SM (2002d) Tendon involvement in pedal infection: MR analysis of frequency, distribution, and spread of infection. AJR Am J Roentgenol 179(4):939–947. https://doi.org/10.2214/ajr.179.4.1790939

Ledermann HP, Morrison WB, Schweitzer ME (2002) Is soft-tissue inflammation in pedal infection contained by fascial planes? MR analysis of compartmental involvement in 115 feet. AJR Am J Roentgenol 178(3):605–612. https://doi.org/10.2214/ajr.178.3.1780605

Lim W, Barras CD, Zadow S (2021) Radiologic mimics of osteomyelitis and septic arthritis: a pictorial essay. Radiol Res Pract 2021:9912257. https://doi.org/10.1155/2021/9912257

Llewellyn A, Jones-Diette J, Kraft J, Holton C, Harden M, Simmonds M (2019) Imaging tests for the detection of osteomyelitis: a systematic review. Health Technol Assess 23(61):1–128. https://doi.org/10.3310/hta23610

Mandell JC, Khurana B, Smith JT, Czuczman GJ, Ghazikhanian V, Smith SE (2018) Osteomyelitis of the lower extremity: pathophysiology, imaging, and classification, with an emphasis on diabetic foot infection. Emerg Radiol 25(2):175–188. https://doi.org/10.1007/s10140-017-1564-9

Naidoo SL, Campbell DL, Miller LM, Nicastro A (2005) Necrotizing fasciitis: a review. J Am Anim Hosp Assoc 41(2):104–109. https://doi.org/10.5326/0410104

Palestro CJ (2020) Molecular imaging of infection: the first 50 years. Semin Nucl Med 50(1):23–34. https://doi.org/10.1053/j.semnuclmed.2019.10.002

Parisi MT, Otjen JP, Stanescu AL, Shulkin BL (2018) Radionuclide imaging of infection and inflammation in children: a review. Semin Nucl Med 48(2):148–165. https://doi.org/10.1053/j.semnuclmed.2017.11.002

Pineda C, Espinosa R, Pena A (2009) Radiographic imaging in osteomyelitis: the role of plain radiography, computed tomography, ultrasonography, magnetic resonance imaging, and scintigraphy. Semin Plast Surg 23(2):80–89. https://doi.org/10.1055/s-0029-1214160

Salmanoglu E, Kim S, Thakur ML (2018) Currently available radiopharmaceuticals for imaging infection and the holy grail. Semin Nucl Med 48(2):86–99. https://doi.org/10.1053/j.semnuclmed.2017.10.003

Sambri A, Spinnato P, Tedeschi S et al (2021) Bone and joint infections: the role of imaging in tailoring diagnosis to improve patients' care. J Pers Med 11(12):1317. https://doi.org/10.3390/jpm11121317

Sconfienza LM, Signore A, Cassar-Pullicino V et al (2019) Diagnosis of peripheral bone and prosthetic joint infections: overview on the consensus documents by the EANM, EBJIS, and ESR (with ESCMID endorsement). Eur Radiol 29(12):6425–6438. https://doi.org/10.1007/s00330-019-06326-1

Seltzer A, Xiao R, Fernandez M, Hasija R (2019) Role of nuclear medicine imaging in evaluation of orthopedic infections, current concepts. J Clin Orthop Trauma 10(4):721–732. https://doi.org/10.1016/j.jcot.2019.04.024

Simpfendorfer CS (2017) Radiologic approach to musculoskeletal infections. Infect Dis Clin North Am 31(2):299–324. https://doi.org/10.1016/j.idc.2017.01.004

Thakolkaran N, Shetty AK (2019) Acute hematogenous osteomyelitis in children. Ochsner J 19(2):116–122. https://doi.org/10.31486/toj.18.0138

Turecki MB, Taljanovic MS, Stubbs AY et al (2010) Imaging of musculoskeletal soft tissue infections. Skeletal Radiol 39(10):957–971. https://doi.org/10.1007/s00256-009-0780-0

Stress Injuries of Ankle and Foot

Ganesh Hegde, K. P. Iyengar, and R. Botchu

Contents

G. Hegde (✉)
Department of Radiology, University Hospitals of Morecambe Bay NHS Foundation, Lancaster, UK
e-mail: ganesh.hegde@nhs.net

K. P. Iyengar
Department of Orthopaedics, Southport and Ormskirk Hospital NHS Trust, Southport, UK

R. Botchu
Department of Musculoskeletal Radiology, Royal Orthopaedic Hospital, Birmingham, UK

Abstract

Stress injuries of foot and ankle are common, especially in military recruits and athletically active individuals. Their treatment and outcome depend on the location and the bone involved. Imaging is essential for their diagnosis, treatment planning, and follow-up and also in assessing the response. In this chapter, we describe the pathophysiology and imaging features of stress injuries involving the bones of the ankle and foot.

1 Introduction

Stress injuries of the foot and ankle are not uncommon and are frequently encountered in clinical practice. They are overuse injuries, more frequently encountered in individuals who indulge in strenuous activities such as military recruits and athletes. Their incidence is rising due to ever-increasing competitiveness in sports, the intensity of fitness regimens in athletes, and the number of people engaging in activities such as running and cycling due to increasing emphasis

Med Radiol Diagn Imaging (2023)
https://doi.org/10.1007/174_2023_393,
Published Online: 18 April 2023

on weight loss and an active lifestyle (Berger et al. 2007; Patel et al. 2020). They can be seen in any bones of the ankle and foot, and their clinical management and outcome depend on the type of bone involved and the location of the fracture. Their initial diagnosis may be delayed as they present with nonspecific symptoms, which may overlap with other conditions and are often undetectable on initial radiographs resulting in increased morbidity (Liong and Whitehouse 2012).

2 Terminologies

Stress fractures occur due to the summation of repetitive submaximal stress on the bone, which on their own are inefficient in causing a fracture. They can be of two types, fatigue fracture and insufficiency fracture (Marshall et al. 2018).

Fatigue fractures occur due to repetitive stress on a normal bone and are commonly seen in athletically active individuals. Insufficiency fractures are secondary to normal stress acting on a weakened bone, which could be due to various causes such as metabolic disorders, medication, inflammatory disorders, or neurological conditions (Hedge et al. 2021).

3 Pathophysiology

Unlike post-traumatic fractures which occur due to a single maximum load that exceeds the failure load of the bones, stress fractures occur due to cumulative damage by repetitive submaximal force. Bones are constantly subjected to stress by various forces, mainly originating from the direct action of the muscles and indirectly from transmitted ground contact forces. These stress/forces are of different types, such as compressive, tensile, shearing, bending, and torsion forces. Bone responds to the applied submaximal stress through remodeling, which increases the strength of the bones. Stress fractures develop when the remodeling response cannot keep up to the progressive, repetitive overload of stress on the bone (Mandell et al. 2017a).

The remodeling process is initiated when a complex combination of the above mentioned forces act on the bone, resulting in a microfracture. These microfractures stimulate osteoclasts, which resorb the trabeculae at the microfracture site. This is followed by an osteoblastic response, which results in stronger new bone formation at the microfracture site, thus strengthening the bone. This osteoblastic response begins approximately 10–14 after the onset of remodeling process, and during this time, the bone is relatively weak (Berger et al. 2007; Mandell et al. 2017a).

Stress fractures develop when the remodeling response fails to heal the microfractures resulting in the accumulation and propagation of these microfractures (Miller and Best 2016). The factors responsible for this propagation are poorly understood. Although the number and density of microfractures increase with each stress and loading cycle, this has not been shown to be responsible for the microfracture propagation; however, the length of the microfracture seems to have a role. Longer microfractures take more time to heal and are more likely to propagate (Berger et al. 2007; O'Brien et al. 2005). Another cause proposed to explain the propagation is repetitive stress on the bone during the remodeling process. The bone is relatively weak during the remodeling process till the osteoblastic reaction is complete. Although periosteal inflammatory responses try to counterbalance this, bone is susceptible to breaking down if there is persistent continued repetitive stress during this healing period.

The remodeling process is seen in both cortical and cancellous bones. In cortical bone, it is seen in periosteal, endosteal, and intracortical surfaces, whereas in the cancellous bone, it is along the trabecular surface.

The action of the muscles plays a vital role in the dissipation of the forces (particularly tensile) on the bone and joint during athletic activity. This protective action reduces as the muscles get fatigued during the activity, resulting in an increased force on the bone, which can result in stress injuries. Most of the stress injuries in the foot and ankle are fatigue injuries. In addition, when there is excessive repetitive stress on a muscle group, they respond to it by hypertrophy and strengthening. Muscular hypertrophy and strengthening happen earlier than the bone, resulting in an increased force on the bone at the muscle attachments due to the action of the muscle group, which can contribute to mechanical failure of the bone, microfractures, and, finally, stress fracture. Relative imbalance of the muscle and reduced bulk are also associated with the stress injuries (Berger et al. 2007; Mandell et al. 2017a; Miller and Best 2016).

4 Predisposing Factors

Multiple risk factors are known to predispose the occurrence of stress fractures in an individual. These risk factors can be broadly categorized into intrinsic and extrinsic. Intrinsic factors are related to an individual's internal characteristics such as structure and variations of the bony anatomy; metabolic, hormonal status; and muscle strength. Extrinsic factors such as type of activity, intense excessive training, abrupt changes in the frequency and intensity of the training regimen, ill-fitting equipment and footwear, and type of training surface also increase the likelihood of developing stress injuries.

Certain anatomical variations such as cavus feet, tarsal coalition, forefoot varus, limb-length discrepancies, and knee alignment are known to predispose the bones of ankle and foot for stress injuries. Preexisting metabolic disorders such as osteoporosis, hypophosphatasia, and vitamin D deficiency are associated with a higher incidence of stress injuries. Hormonal factors such as delayed menarche and contraceptive use may also influence.

Female athletes and military recruits have a higher incidence of stress injuries than their male counterparts. Relatively wider pelvis, more frequent genu valgum which can result in a compensatory increase in Q angle and foot pronation, and relatively less muscle mass are some of the factors thought to be responsible for this. Apart from this, a triad of eating disorders, amenorrhea, and osteoporosis, also called the "female athlete triad," can also increase the risk of stress fracture by 15–50% (Mandell et al. 2017a; Miller and Best 2016; Mayer et al. 2014).

5 Epidemiology

Stress injuries of the foot and ankle are uncommon in the general population; however, they are frequently seen in sports medicine clinics accounting for up to 20% of the clinic visits (Abbott et al. 2020). Their incidence is rising due to the popularity of the sports, increased intensity of the sporting activities and training regimens, increased awareness and use of imaging modalities in evaluating the clinical symptoms. They are more frequent in athletes, military recruits, and athletically active population, with a reported prevalence of as high as 49% in athletes. Their incidence varies with age, and they are more common between 19 and 30 years. Higher incidences are noted in women than men. Although stress fractures of many bones have been described, their incidence is highest in the bones of the lower limbs. The distal tibia (24–73%) is the commonest site for stress fractures, followed by metatarsals (17–35%) and calcaneus (21–28%) (Mayer et al. 2014).

6 Clinical Presentation

Stress injuries present with insidious onset of pain. Initially, the pain is experienced typically with activity or weight-bearing, which relieves on rest. However, on continuing activity, the intensity of pain increases and may be felt even after the cessation of the activity. In later stages, pain may be felt even at rest. A history of a recent change in the activity level, start of a new training program, change in the intensity of an existing training regimen, or change in the training surface should raise the suspicion of a stress injury.

On clinical examination, if the involved bone is superficial, a tender point may be identified with or without mild swelling and warmth of the affected site. There may be a limitation in the range of movement due to pain (Berger et al. 2007; Mandell et al. 2017a; Mayer et al. 2014).

7 Imaging

Imaging is central in diagnosing stress injuries and their follow-up and prognosis. As these injuries are frequently seen in athletes, early diagnosis and treatment are vital for early recovery/return to play and also to prevent further progression of the injury.

Radiographs are commonly used as an initial modality for imaging. Radiographs are often negative, and identification of early stress injuries on radiographs may be difficult. Initial radiographs have sensitivity as low as 15%, which improves to 30–70% in the follow-up radiographs. Stress injuries are occult on initial radiographs. They become evident once the reparative response has begun, and the average time taken from the onset of symptom to radiographic evidence is approximately 2–6 weeks (Nussbaum et al. 2022). Hence, follow-up radiographs are often useful if the initial radiographs are negative. Their radiographic appearance depends on the site of involvement, chronicity, and grade of the injury (Mandell et al. 2017a).

In cancellous bones such as tarsal bones or metaphysis of the long bones, initially, they manifest as subtle sclerosis or blurring of trabeculae, which progress to more diffuse sclerosis in a later stage due to healing response, which results in microcallus formation. In the cortical bone, their initial appearance is described as "gray cortex sign," which is characterized by the presence of a cortical lucency at the site of microfracture. With the progression of injury and onset of healing response, they demonstrate cortical thickening, periosteal reaction, and endosteal callus formation. A clear fracture line may be visible in high-grade injuries (Marshall et al. 2018; Hedge et al. 2021; Mandell et al. 2017a).

Although radiographs have low sensitivity in identifying stress injuries, they should be used as an initial imaging modality as they can help evaluate the symptoms by ruling out other causes with a similar presentation, such as tumors or infection.

MRI is highly sensitive in identifying changes of a stress injury in bone and is the preferred modality in evaluating stress injuries. In a suspected stress injury, if the radiographs are negative, MRI is the next investigation of choice, and MRI can demonstrate changes weeks before they can be seen on radiographs. T1 and fluid-sensitive sequences such as STIR or proton density fat-saturated sequences play an essential role in the evaluation of changes in stress injuries seen in bone and surrounding soft tissues. While the marrow and soft tissue edema related to the stress injuries are best visualized on fluid-sensitive images, bony anatomy, cortical changes, and fracture lines are better seen on T1 images.

Stress injuries can manifest in the bone in the form of stress reactions or stress fractures. Stress reaction precedes stress fracture. The stress reaction is considered an early stress injury due to the accumulation of microfractures with edema and hyperemia. On MRI, it is seen as a focus of marrow edema without any identifiable fracture line. If the stress on the bone continues, a frank fracture may develop called a stress fracture. This is seen on MRI as a serpiginous or linear low signal intensity line. MRI is also helpful in depicting subtle related abnormalities such as periosteal edema and surrounding soft tissue edema.

Although not used as a routine imaging modality, ultrasound is sensitive in identifying stress fractures of superficial bones such as the anterior tibia or, more commonly, metatarsals. Occasionally, metatarsal fractures are incidentally detected on ultrasound performed for the evaluation of forefoot pain or metatarsalgia. Stress fractures appear as a focal cortical irregularity, buckling, or discontinuity with adjacent echogenic callus.

CT scan is used as a problem-solving tool in the evaluation of suspected stress injuries. They are mainly used to identify a subtle fracture line to differentiate a stress fracture from a stress reaction, to assess if the fracture is complete or incomplete, and to rule out other causes such as osteoid osteoma or infection, which can present with a similar clinical picture.

Radionuclide bone scan has high sensitivity in identifying the stress fractures, and changes can be visible within 48–72 h of injury. However, it is nonspecific and, with the availability of MRI, rarely used as a primary imaging modality in stress injuries (Datir et al. 2007; Kaiser et al. 2018).

8 Classification of Stress Injuries of Foot and Ankle

Stress fractures of the ankle and foot can be broadly classified into low-risk and high-risk fractures (Table 1). Low-risk fractures show a high propensity to heal with conservative management. High-risk fractures occur along the tensile side of the bone, which receives relatively poor blood supply. They show a higher propensity for delayed union and nonunion, requiring more proactive management with restricted weight-bearing, immobilization, or even early surgical intervention for optimal outcomes (Mandell et al. 2017b).

8.1 Low Risk Fractures

8.1.1 Posteromedial Distal Tibia

The tibia is the commonest bone involved in stress injuries accounting for approximately one-third to half of the reported stress fractures. The posteromedial aspect of the tibia is the most frequently affected site (Liong and Whitehouse 2012; Nussbaum et al. 2022; Zadpoor and Nikooyan 2011). This injury is predominantly due to compressive forces; however, tensile forces resulting from the pull of gastrocnemius-soleus complex and deep plantar flexors also contribute. On occasions, these injuries can be bilateral.

Table 1 Classification of stress injuries of foot and ankle

Low-risk fractures	High-risk fractures
Posteromedial distal tibia	Anterior cortex of tibia
Calcaneum	Medial malleolus
Metatarsals	Navicular
Distal fibula	Talus
Cuboid	Base of the fifth metatarsal
Cuneiforms	Hallux sesamoid

Most of these fractures are oriented transversely, and a longitudinal fracture is rare, and they are likely to result from the action of rotational forces. When encountered, they are frequently seen in the superomedial aspect of nutrient foramen (Craig et al. 2003).

Radiographs may be negative initially; however, if positive, their appearance depends on the site of involvement. When the stress fracture is located in the metaphysis, where trabecular bone predominates, they appear as a subtle sclerotic line interrupting the trabeculae. In the diaphysis where cortical bone predominates, they appear as faint lucency in the cortex with adjacent periosteal reaction.

MRI is the most sensitive and specific imaging modality for stress fractures and also the earliest imaging modality to demonstrate the abnormality. MRI is often recommended for evaluating stress fracture even when initial radiographs are negative and in cases of high clinical suspicion. Fluid-sensitive sequences demonstrate edema, which is a key feature of stress injury. T1- and T2-weighted sequences may show a hypointense fracture line (Fig. 1). Although cortical changes are sometimes difficult to appreciate on MRI, T1 sequences are preferred for assessing them. Fredericson classification (Fredericson et al. 1995) is based on MRI findings and is widely used to grade the stress injuries of the tibia and also to estimate the return to playtime. Kijowski et al. further classified Fredericson grade 4 fracture into 4a and 4b (Table 2) (Kijowski et al. 2012).

CT scan is not the preferred imaging modality in stress fractures owing to its low sensitivity. However, it is helpful as a problem-solving tool in selected cases. It demonstrates cortical changes well and helps differentiate stress reaction from a fracture by identifying a subtle fracture line. CT has been found helpful in identifying longitudinal fractures, which can be sometimes challenging to diagnose on MRI.

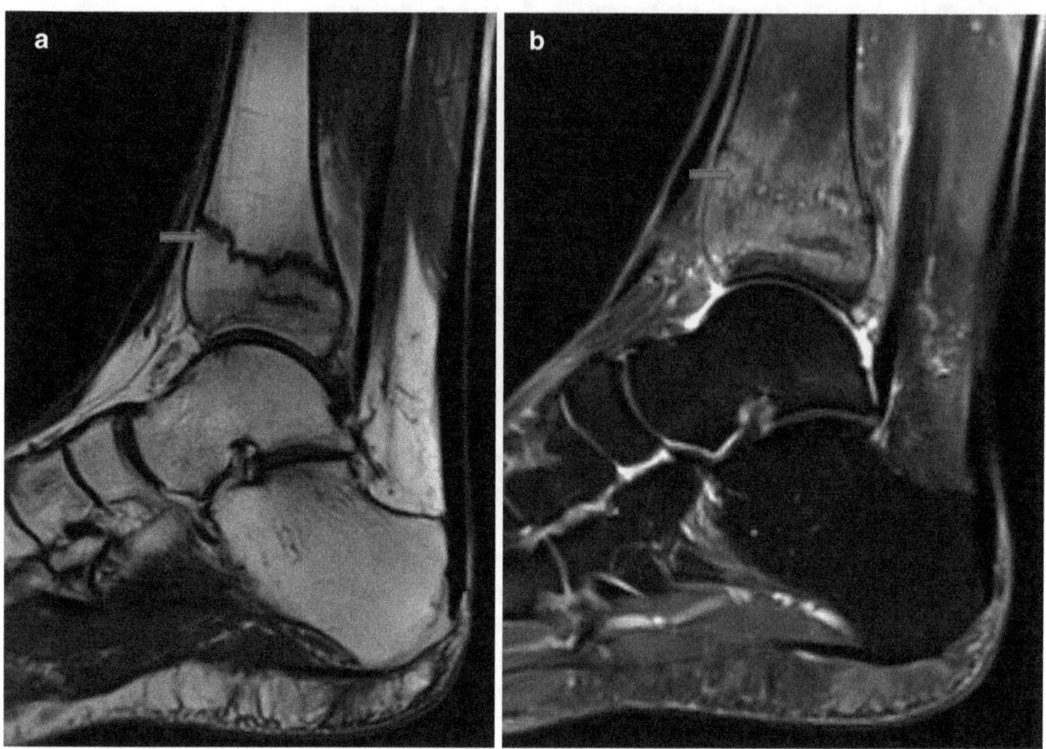

Fig. 1 Stress fracture of the distal tibia—T1 and proton density fat-saturated sagittal MRI images of the distal tibia demonstrating a T1 hypointense fracture line with extensive surrounding marrow edema

Table 2 Fredericson classification

Grade	MRI appearances	Mean return to playtime
0	No abnormality	
1	Periosteal edema with no associated marrow edema	16
2	Periosteal edema with marrow edema visible on only T2-weighted images	39
3	Periosteal edema with marrow edema visible on both T1- and T2-weighted images	48
4a	Grade 3 changes with multiple focal areas of intracortical signal abnormality	43
4b	Grade 3 changes with linear areas of intracortical signal abnormality (fracture line)	71

8.2 Calcaneal Fracture

The calcaneum is the second most common site for stress fractures in the foot and ankle, and it is more frequently seen in military recruits and long-distance runners and slightly more common in females. Repetitive striking force to the heel, particularly on a non-cushioned surface, and opposing pull of the Achilles tendon are thought to be responsible for calcaneal stress fractures. Pain on weight-bearing is a common presenting symptom. On clinical examination, conditions such as plantar fasciitis, Baxter neuropathy, Achilles tendinopathy, retrocalcaneal bursitis, and Sever's disease can mimic the symptoms of stress fracture and can delay the diagnosis (Kaiser et al. 2018; Sormaala 2006).

These stress fractures may be located in the posterior, middle, or anterior portion of the calcaneus. Posterior fractures are more common. Fractures of the anterior process are less frequent and may be associated with the coalition and prominent anterior process (Sormaala 2006). The calcaneum is made up of cancellous bone with arc-like trabeculae running perpendicular to the posterior cortex (Figs. 2 and 3). Early

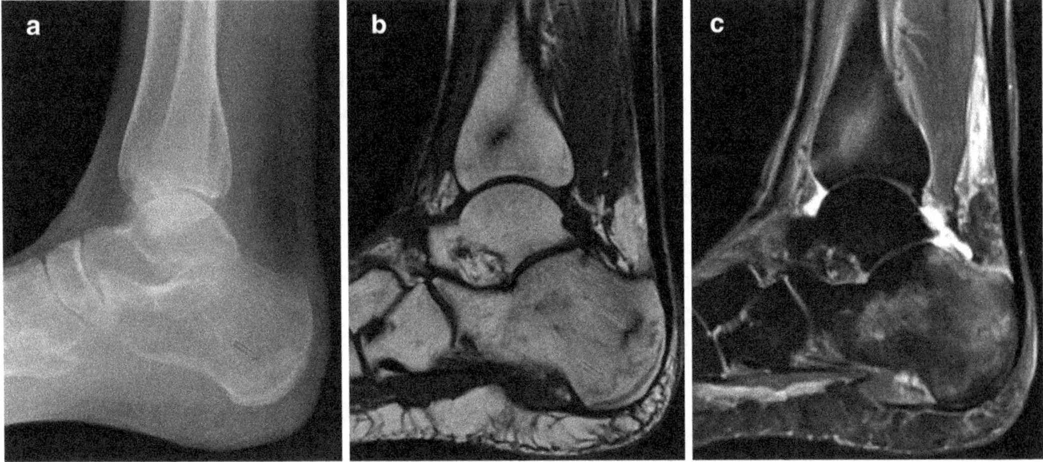

Fig. 2 Stress fracture calcaneum—lateral radiograph of the ankle (**a**) demonstrating a sclerotic focus in the posterior aspect of the calcaneus with obliteration of the trabeculae. Sagittal T1 (**b**) MRI image demonstrates a fracture line corresponding to the sclerotic focus on radiograph. (**c**) Proton density fat-saturated sagittal MRI image of the ankle demonstrating extensive marrow edema in the calcaneum

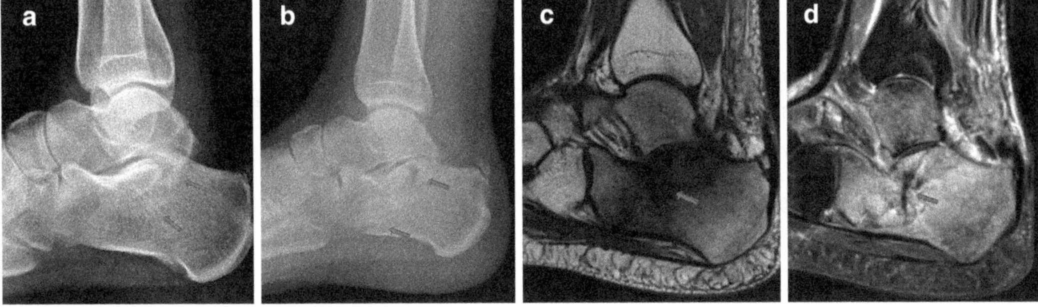

Fig. 3 Stress fracture of the mid-calcaneum—42-year-old runner presenting with pain in the foot. Initial radiograph (**a**) demonstrating a subtle sclerotic line in the mid-calcaneum with obliteration of the trabeculae. A follow-up radiograph (**b**) done after 1 month shows a facture at the same location. Sagittal T1 (**c**) and PDFS (**d**) MRI images demonstrating a hypointense fracture line (arrows) with extensive edema

radiographic manifestation of this fracture is in the form of a faint sclerotic line, which is frequently seen in the posterior aspect of the calcaneum, oriented parallel to the posterior cortex, interrupting the trabeculae. The changes can be seen as early as 10 days of the onset of the symptoms. MRI demonstrates a T1 hypointense fracture line with extensive marrow edema. MRI is particularly useful in identifying the fracture located in the mid- and anterior calcaneum (Fig. 3). Calcaneal stress injuries, particularly located in the anterior aspect, could be associated with calcaneonavicular coalition and elongated anterior process.

Undisplaced non-comminuted fractures of the calcaneum are treated conservatively with non-weight-bearing, immobilization, and limitation of training (Oji 2021).

8.3 First to Fourth Metatarsal Fractures

Metatarsals are the commonest site for stress fractures in the foot. These fractures are also called as march fractures, as they were first described in military recruits subjected to long marches. They are also commonly seen in ballet dancers and athletes who engage in jumping and running. Due to the fixed base and proximal hinged metatarsophalangeal joints, second and third metatarsals are subjected to maximum bending strain and shear force during the stance phase of the gate compared to the rest of the metatarsals. Hence, most stress fractures are seen in second (52%) and third (35%) metatarsals. As the second metatarsal is relatively long and the first ray of the foot is relatively more mobile, there is an increase in the forces acting on the distal second metatarsals, making it the most common location.

These fractures are commonly diaphyseal. Fractures involving the first metatarsals tend to be metaphyseal and located predominantly on the medial aspect. Distal diaphyseal fractures tend to heal early with treatment, whereas fractures involving the proximal second metatarsals take longer to heal. The patient presents with pain, which is aggravated by activity. Clinical examination elicits tenderness at the site of the fracture, and sometimes callus may be palpable.

Radiographs demonstrate cortical thickening, periosteal reaction, and sometimes a thin lucent fracture line, which is generally oriented transversely. On occasions, cortical thickening and irregularities can also be seen on ultrasound. MRI is more sensitive and specific than radiographs and demonstrates marrow edema, cortical thickening, and sometimes a fracture line (Fig. 4). There may be associated surrounding soft tissue edema.

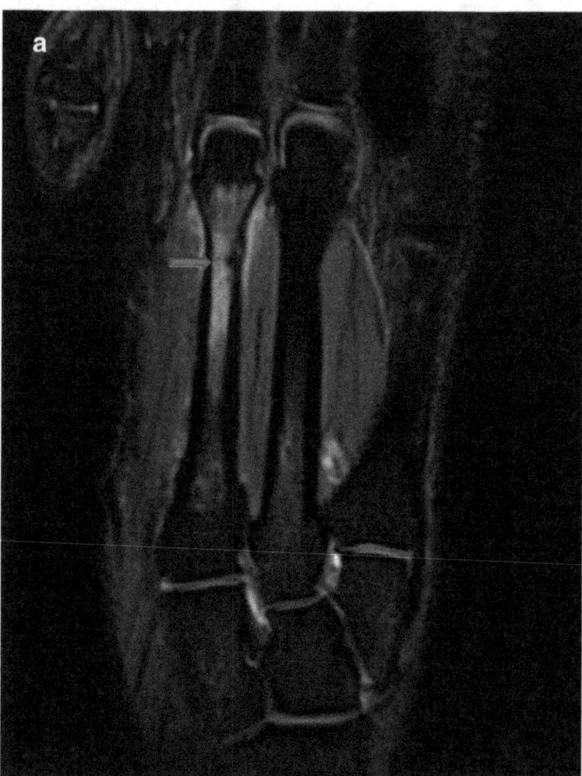

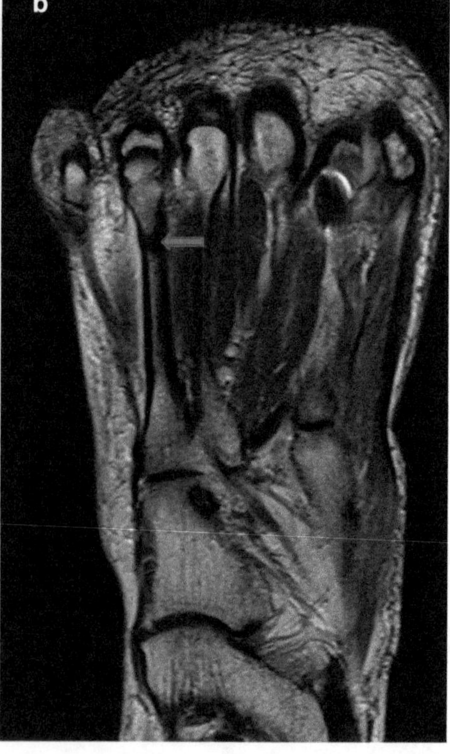

Fig. 4 (**a**) Metatarsal stress fractures—proton density fat-saturated MRI image of the foot demonstrating a stress fracture of the third metatarsal, which is seen as a hypointense line (arrow) with surrounding marrow edema and periosteal reaction. Image (**b**) demonstrating another example of metatarsal fracture involving the fourth metatarsal, which is seen as a hypointense line with cortical thickening (arrow) in the T1 image

Fractures of the first metatarsal present as linear sclerosis perpendicular to the direction of the stress, and periosteal reaction is uncommon in this location (Mandell et al. 2017b; Anderson and Cohen 2014).

8.4 Distal Fibula

Fibular stress fractures are usually encountered in the distal end, commonly involving the lateral cortex, frequently located just proximal to the incisura. This location acts as a physiological weak point, juxtaposed between the strong ligamentous attachments. Contraction of the plantar flexors, which causes to-and-fro movement of the fibula in coronal plain; compressive forces during the activity; and subfibular impingement, which can occur in repetitive eversion, especially in patients with pes planus, can contribute to the occurrence of the stress fracture at this location.

Radiographic findings become evident 2–3 weeks following the onset of clinical symptoms. Radiographic findings include a periosteal reaction, cortical thickening, and occasionally a frank fracture line. Less frequently, the injury can manifest in the form of a sclerotic line or callus formation. MRI shows marrow edema, cortical thickening, periosteal edema, and periosteal reaction (Fig. 5). Peroneal tendon abnormalities and subfibular impingement are common differentials, and MRI helps exclude these differentials.

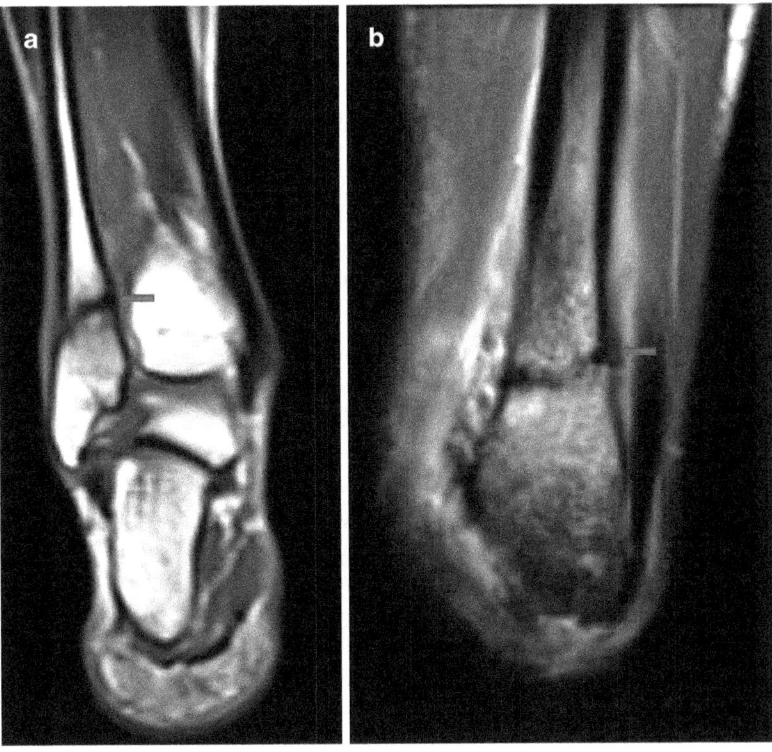

Fig. 5 Stress fracture lateral malleolus—coronal T1 (**a**) and sagittal PDFS (**b**) images demonstrating a stress fracture in the lateral malleolus (arrow) with surrounding edema

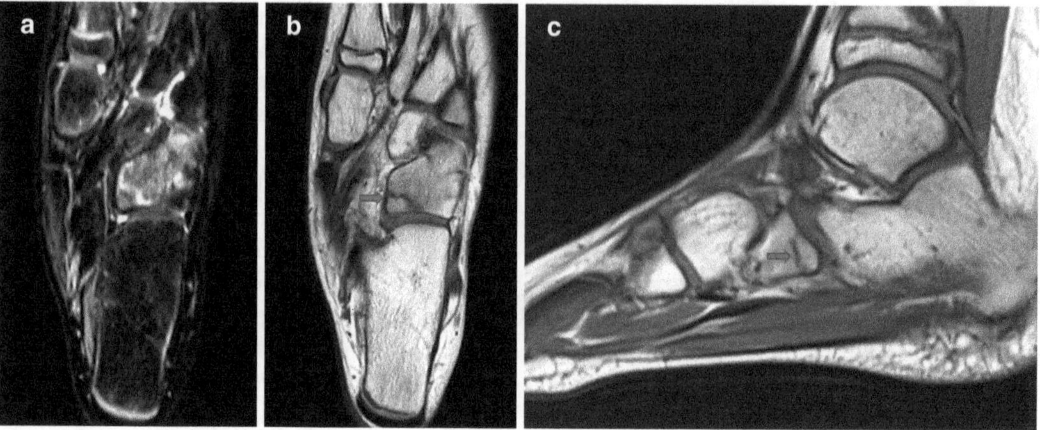

Fig. 6 Stress fracture of cuboid—axial PDFS images of the foot demonstrating extensive marrow edema involving the cuboid. Axial and coronal T1 images demonstrating a hypointense fracture line

These fractures are treated conservatively with cessation of the activity with the patient being allowed to weight bear (Woods et al. 2008).

8.5 Cuboid

The cuboid is a constituent of the lateral column of the foot. Since it is not a critical weight-bearing bone, stress fractures of the cuboid are uncommon. Stress injuries of the cuboid are associated with a tear of the plantar fascia or plantar fasciotomy, which is thought to cause destabilization of the lateral column resulting in excessive force along the peroneus tendon, which may play a role in cuboid stress fracture. Clinical findings are nonspecific and may mimic sinus tarsi syndrome and fractures of other tarsal bones or the base of the metatarsals. These fractures are often occult on the radiographs requiring MRI for confirmation. MRI demonstrates edema in the cuboid with a hypointense fracture line (Fig. 6). These fractures are more common on the lateral aspect than medial. A CT scan may be helpful in some cases by demonstrating a sclerotic fracture line. Cuboid fractures are managed conservatively with activity modification (Franco et al. 2005).

8.6 Cuneiform

Stress fractures of the cuneiform are extremely rare. They are secondary to compression and bending/torsion forces due to their location between the planted forefoot and hindfoot. Relatively rich blood supply of the cuneiforms compared to the rest of the tarsal bones makes them less prone for structural failure when subjected to stress and protects them from stress injuries. As the medial cuneiform lies between the navicular and first metatarsal, it is subjected to relatively more stress and hence prone to injury compared to intermediate and lateral cuneiform.

Cuneiform fractures, like cuboid stress fractures, are challenging to visualize in radiographs and often require MRI for diagnosis. MRI demonstrates marrow edema in the cuneiform with or without a hypointense fracture line (Fig. 7). These fractures are managed conservatively (Krebs and Borchers 2019).

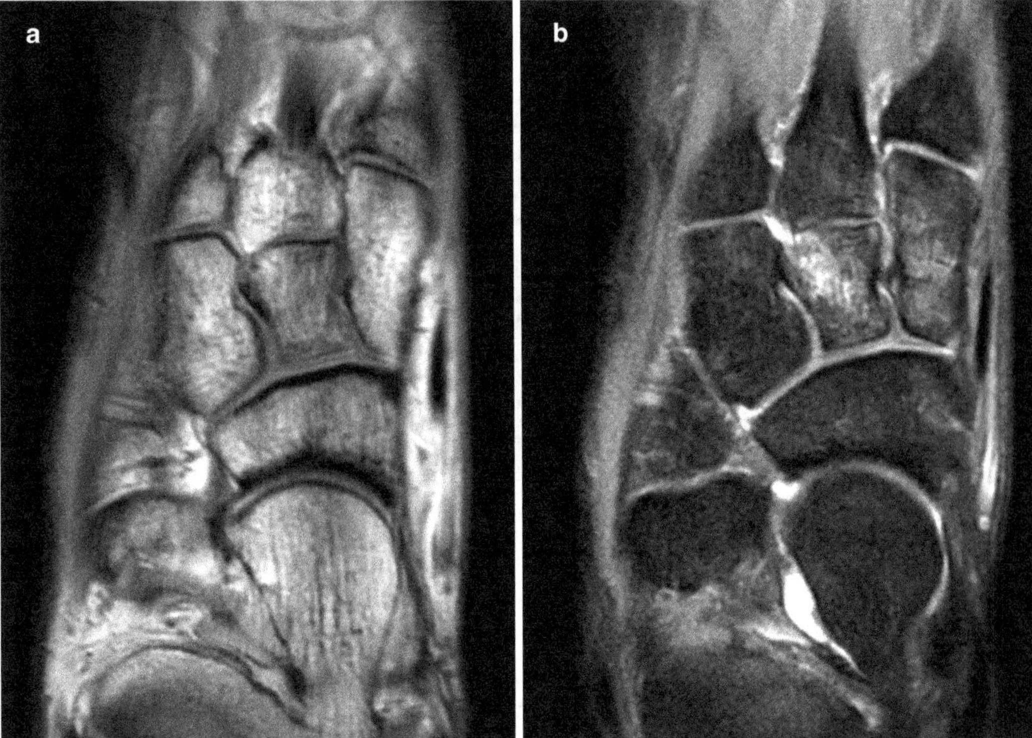

Fig. 7 Stress injury cuneiform—axial T1 (**a**) and PDFS (**b**) MRI images showing marrow edema in the medial and intermediate cuneiform suggesting a stress injury

9 High-Risk Stress Fractures

9.1 Anterior Tibial Cortex

They are relatively uncommon, constituting only 4–5% of all the stress fractures involving the tibia. They are usually seen in people who engage in repetitive jumping activities. The anterior cortex of the tibia is relatively hypo-vascular and is subjected to tensile forces. In addition, lack of supporting musculotendinous attachment may result in the propagation of fracture, delayed or nonunion, making them difficult to treat. Anterior leg pain and tenderness are common presenting symptoms.

A thin lucent line representing a cortical fracture, also called the "dreaded black line," is often visible on radiographs. MRI helps in early diagnosis before the radiographic changes become visible (Fig. 8). Their treatment is controversial; while some prefer early operative management, others advise a trial of conservative management. In complications such as delayed union or nonunion, operative management such as intramedullary nailing or compression plating helps to reduce the healing time (Orava and Hulkko 1984; Orava et al. 1991).

9.2 Medial Malleolus

Stress fracture of the medial malleolus is uncommon, and it is almost exclusively seen in athletes who play sports which involve running and jumping. Shear and tensile forces acting on medial malleolus typically due to repetitive dorsiflexion and rotatory movements and in conditions where medial malleolus impinges on talus as seen in anterior ankle impingement are thought to be responsible for this injury. They present with pain in the

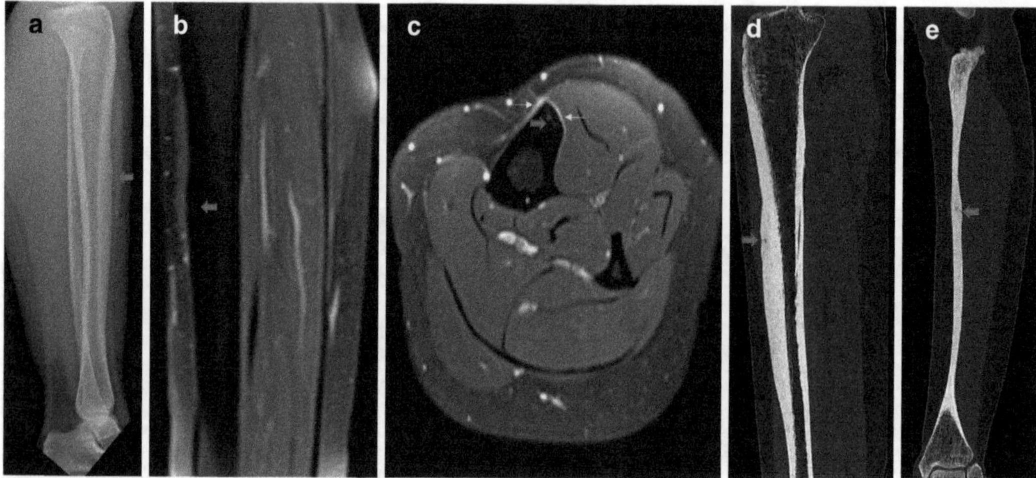

Fig. 8 Anterior tibial fracture—lateral radiograph of the leg (**a**) demonstrating a lucent focus (arrow) in the anterior cortex with surrounding cortical sclerosis. Sagittal and axial PDFS MRI sequences (**b**, **c**) demonstrating cortical thickening and a subtle fracture line (arrow) with minimal periosteal edema (yellow arrows). Sagittal and coronal reformatted CT images of the tibia clearly demonstrating a cortical fracture line with surrounding extensive sclerosis (**d**, **e**)

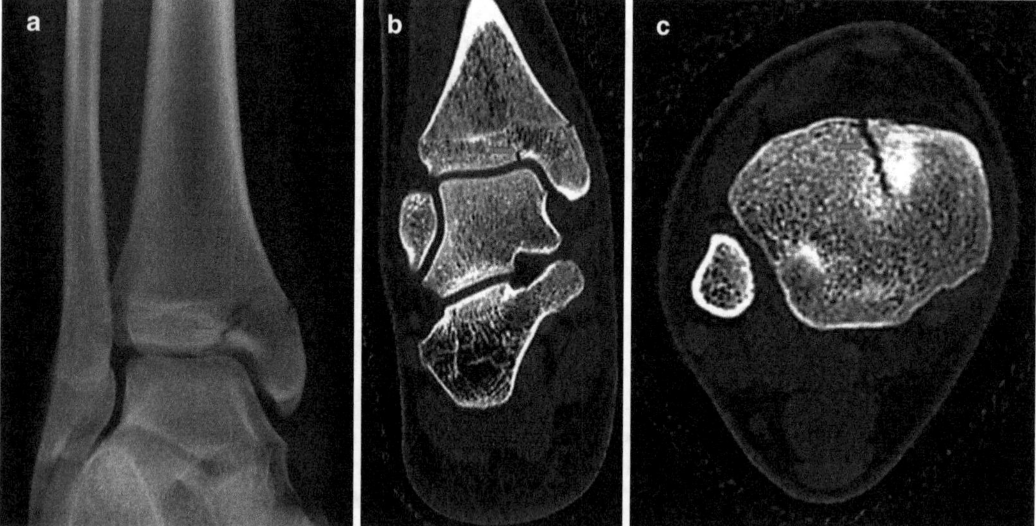

Fig. 9 Stress fracture medial malleolus—AP radiograph (**a**), coronal and axial CT images (**b**, **c**) demonstrating a fracture of the medial malleolus in a footballer extending from medial aspect of the tibial plafond

anterior or anteromedial aspect of the ankle and can be mistaken for anterior ankle impingement.

This can be occult on initial radiographs. When visible, they appear as thin lucencies extending from the shoulder of the tibial plafond toward the medial malleolus or vertically upwards. CT is often helpful in identifying subtle fracture line and fracture pattern, which are sometimes difficult to appreciate on radiographs (Fig. 9). MRI is often required to identify the fracture early.

Treatment of this fracture is often challenging. Conservative treatment is attempted initially if the fracture line is not well visible in the radiograph. However, if the fracture is visualized and refractory to conservative management, surgery may be required (Jowett et al. 2008; Shelbourne et al. 1988; Irion et al. 2014).

9.3 Navicular Bone

Navicular stress fractures are relatively uncommon; however, their incidence is increasing with more frequent use of cross-sectional imaging in evaluating foot pain. They are predominantly seen in high-performance athletes. Compressive forces acting along the medial column of the foot in combination with tensile forces produced by the action of the spring ligament and tibialis posterior tendon are likely to be responsible for this injury. The action of these forces is maximum in the central part of the navicular bone. In addition, the central third of the navicular is relatively more avascular than the rest of the bone as the medial navicular receives blood supply from posterior tibial vessels and lateral navicular from the dorsalis pedis, making the central part a watershed zone. As a result, the central third is the most common location for stress injuries.

Clinically, it presents as vague pain over the dorsum of the midfoot and sometimes over the navicular region, which is aggravated by activity. On examination, a point tenderness may be present in the navicular region. Radiographs are poor in diagnosing these fractures and can miss up to two-thirds of incomplete and one-fifth of complete fractures. MRI usually demonstrates marrow edema indicating a stress reaction, and a fracture line may or may not be visible (Fig. 10). CT scan is helpful to identify the fracture line and to characterize it as complete or incomplete based on the involvement of the distal articular surfaces. Based on the extent of the fracture, Saxena et al. classified them into three types (Table 3). These fractures are seen in the sagittal plane, beginning from the proximal aspect involving the dorsal cortex and propagating distally over time. There may be associated surrounding sclerosis.

Management of these fractures is challenging as they have a high chance of complications such as delayed union and nonunion. In general, con-

Table 3 Saxena et al classification of navicular fractures

Type	Imaging	Treatment
1	Fracture involving only the dorsal cortex	Conservative or ORIF in athletes
II	Fracture extending to the navicular body	Conservative, ORIF in athletically active individuals
III	Fracture involving another cortex (plantar, medial, or lateral)	Often ORIF

ORIF—open reduction and internal fixation

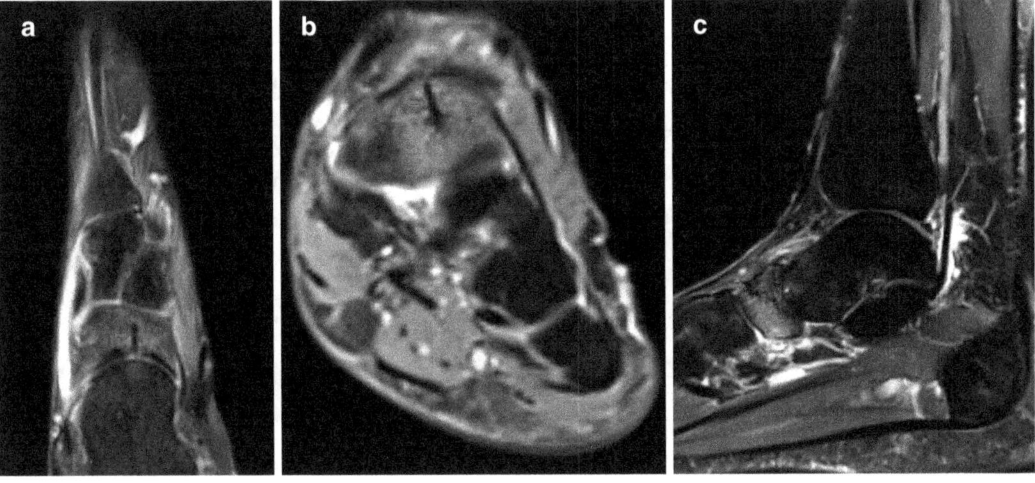

Fig. 10 Stress fracture of the navicular—axial (**a**), coronal (**b**), and sagittal PDFS MRI images (**c**) demonstrating a linear hypointense fracture line in the central third of the navicular with surrounding marrow edema

servative management is used initially for nondisplaced or incomplete fractures. Surgical treatment is preferred for complete fractures, displaced fractures, or fractures with delayed or nonunion (Mandell et al. 2017b; Gross and Nunley 2015; Saxena et al. 2000).

9.4 Proximal Fifth Metatarsal

Stress fractures of the proximal fifth metatarsal are rare, accounting for approximately 2% of the metatarsal stress fractures. The proximal aspect of the fifth metatarsal has been divided into three different zones. Zone 1 contains the tuberosity to which peroneus brevis tendon inserts. Zone 2 corresponds to the metaphysis, extending up to the meta-diaphyseal junction, which articulates with the base of the fourth metatarsal. Zone 3 corresponds to the proximal diaphysis and distal to the meta-diaphyseal junction. Avulsion fractures of the base of the fifth metatarsal involve zone 1, Jones fracture is seen in zone 2, and stress fractures of proximal fifth metatarsals are located in zone 3. These fractures are at risk for delayed or nonunion due to relatively avascular proximal diaphysis.

As these fractures occur at the meta-diaphyseal junction, their radiographic features are a combination of the findings seen in the fractures involving the cortical and cancellous bones. They often present with cortical thickening and periosteal reaction with intramedullary sclerosis. Fracture line may be visible in some with a cortical break (Fig. 11). The gap between the fracture lines in the plantar aspect is called a plantar gap, and a larger gap (>1 mm) is associated with delayed or poor fracture healing. MRI demonstrates marrow edema with cortical thickening and periosteal reaction. Fracture line may be seen in high-grade injuries (Lee et al. 2011a, b; Lawrence and Botte 1993).

Acute, nondisplaced fractures can be treated conservatively. However, displaced fractures and fractures with delayed or nonunion require surgery. Early operative management may benefit athletes as it reduces the healing time and, thus, the return to playtime (Kerkhoffs et al. 2012).

9.5 Sesamoids

Stress injuries of sesamoid are less frequently encountered, accounting for approximately 4% of stress injuries seen in the foot. Among the two sesamoid bones, the medial one is larger than the lateral and is more commonly involved in stress injuries as more weight-bearing forces act on it.

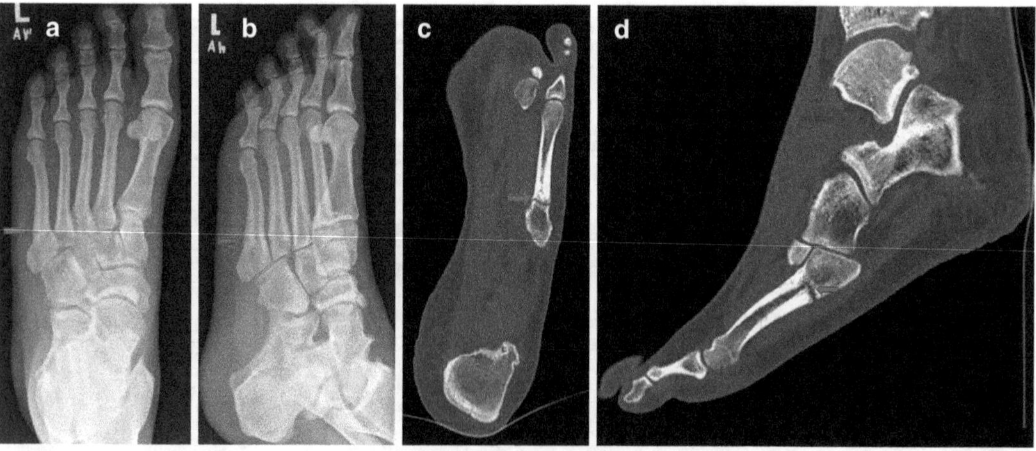

Fig. 11 Stress fracture base of the fifth metatarsal—AP (**a**) and oblique (**b**) radiograph of the foot demonstrating a fracture line at the base of the fifth metatarsal (arrow). A follow-up CT images (**c**, **d**) done after 6 months showing nonunion of the fracture

These injuries are more common in sports persons participating in sports requiring forced dorsiflexion. Excessive compressive forces acting on the sesamoid bones and tensile forces mainly through the flexor hallucis brevis are thought to be responsible for stress injuries of sesamoid bones.

Clinically, these injuries present with insidious onset of vague pain. Sesamoid fractures are difficult to diagnose on standard foot radiographs, and special views such as axial, oblique, and tangential views may be required. Fractures appear as transversely oriented lucencies. Unlike bipartite sesamoids, which show corticated margins, stress fracture lines have sharp linear margins. MRI is helpful in doubtful cases and demonstrates edema and may also demonstrate the fracture line (Fig. 12).

These fractures are treated conservatively with anti-inflammatory medication, activity reduction, and non-weight-bearing by using casts or boots. Operative procedures such as partial or complete sesamoidectomy and screw fixation with or without bone grafting are reserved for patients with failed conservative management with persistent symptoms even after 6 months or with function loss (Robertson et al. 2017; Biedert and Hintermann 2003).

9.6 Talus

Stress fractures of the talus are rare and often seen in athletes or individuals who indulge in excessive physical activity, such as military recruits. They present with vague pain in the ankle joint, sometimes mimicking ankle impingement.

These injuries may be occult on the radiograph, and MRI is frequently required. MRI demonstrates marrow edema, and a fracture line may or may not be visible (Fig. 13). The important thing to note here is that ill-defined marrow edema-like signal is frequently seen in athletes and should not be mistaken for a stress fracture. They are managed conservatively by non-weight-bearing (McInnis and Ramey 2016).

10 Differential Diagnosis

Important differential diagnosis of stress fracture includes osteoid osteoma, osteomyelitis, and neoplasms with osteoid matrix.

Osteoid osteoma is relatively uncommon in the bones of the foot and ankle. They typically present with pain, which is relieved by nonsteroidal anti-inflammatory drugs, whereas stress frac-

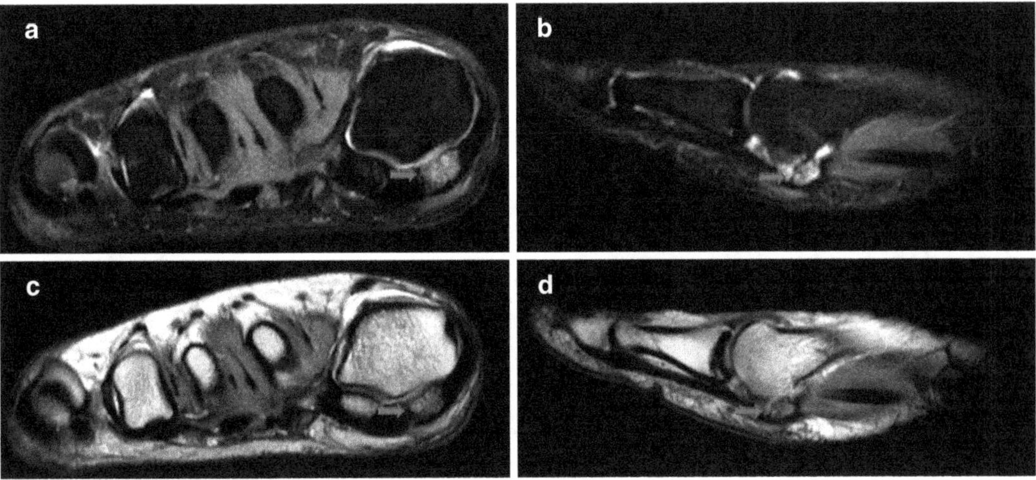

Fig. 12 Stress fracture of the medial sesamoid—axial and sagittal PDFS (**a**, **b**) and axial and sagittal PD (**c**, **d**) images demonstrating a fracture of the medial sesamoid with marrow edema

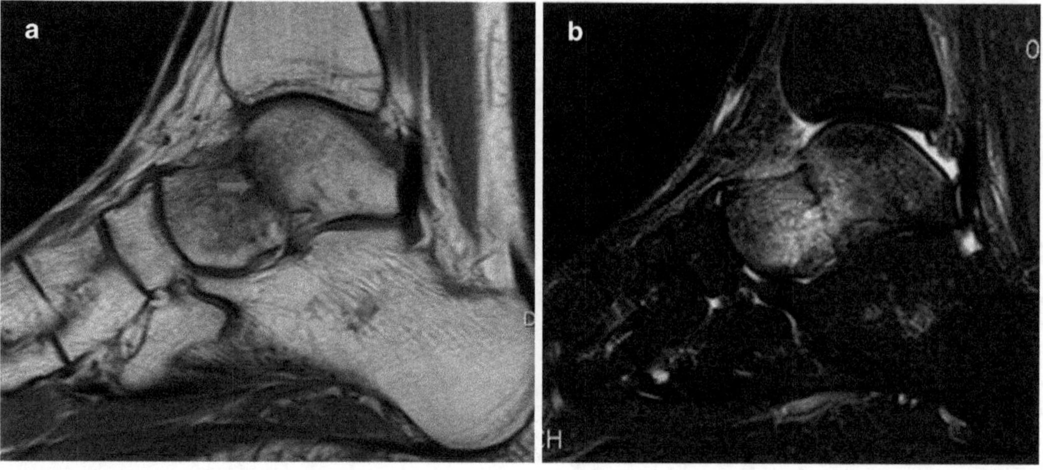

Fig. 13 Stress fracture talus—sagittal T1 (**a**) and PDFS (**b**) MRI images of the ankle demonstrating a stress fracture of the talus (arrow)

tures are more symptomatic during an activity. On radiographs, osteoid osteoma may appear as a sclerotic lesion with cortical thickening and periosteal reaction mimicking a stress fracture. Central nidus may not be detectable on radiographs. MRI may demonstrate cortical thickening and marrow edema. CT is the modality of choice and helps to differentiate osteoid osteoma from stress fracture by identifying a nidus.

Changes in chronic osteomyelitis are usually more diffuse, involve a wider area of the bone, and demonstrate relatively more inflammatory changes in the surrounding soft tissues. In addition, there may be intracortical or intraosseous abscess formation. On serial follow-up imaging, stress fracture shows rapid evolution, whereas chronic osteomyelitis remains stable.

Some of the highly aggressive malignant lesions such as Ewing sarcoma and osteosarcoma may present with pathological fractures mimicking stress injuries. Malignant lesions with pathological fracture tend to demonstrate aggressive periosteal reaction, and on MRI, a distinct mass lesion is often visible (Mandell et al. 2017b).

11 Conclusion

Stress injuries of the ankle and foot are common and are more prevalent in athletically active individuals. They present with nonspecific symptoms, and a high level of clinical suspicion is required for their early diagnosis. Radiographs, although less sensitive, are the preferred initial imaging modality. The radiographic appearance of the stress injuries depends on the location and grade. MRI has high sensitivity and specificity in detecting these injuries and is the modality of choice in evaluating stress injuries. CT scan is used selectively to identify the fracture line and to rule out other differentials. Management and outcome of these injuries depend on the location, and imaging is central for their early diagnosis and appropriate management.

References

Abbott A, Bird ML, Wild E, Brown SM, Stewart G, Mulcahey MK (2020) Part I: epidemiology and risk factors for stress fractures in female athletes. Phys Sportsmed 48:17–24 [cited 2022 Jul 18]. Available from: https://www.tandfonline.com/doi/full/10.1080/00913847.2019.1632158

Anderson RB, Cohen BE (2014) Chapter 31—Stress fractures of the foot and ankle. In: Mann's surgery of the foot ankle, 9th edn. Elsevier Inc.

Berger FH, de Jonge MC, Maas M (2007) Stress fractures in the lower extremity. Eur J Radiol 62:16–26 [cited 2022 Jul 17]. Available from: https://linkinghub.elsevier.com/retrieve/pii/S0720048X07000393

Biedert R, Hintermann B (2003) Stress fractures of the medial great toe sesamoids in athletes. Foot Ankle Int 24:137–41 [cited 2022 Jul 19]. Available from: http://journals.sagepub.com/doi/10.1177/107110070302400207

Craig JG, Widman D, van Holsbeeck M (2003) Longitudinal stress fracture: patterns of edema and the importance of the nutrient foramen. Skeletal Radiol 32:22–7 [cited 2022 Jul 18]. Available from: http://link.springer.com/10.1007/s00256-002-0597-6

Datir AP, Saini A, Connell D, Saifuddin A (2007) Stress-related bone injuries with emphasis on MRI. Clin Radiol 62:828–36 [cited 2022 Jul 18]. Available from: https://linkinghub.elsevier.com/retrieve/pii/S0009926007001481

Franco M, Albano L, Kacso I, Gaïd H, Jaeger P (2005) An uncommon cause of foot pain: the cuboid insufficiency stress fracture. Joint Bone Spine 72:76–8 [cited 2022 Jul 18]. Available from: https://linkinghub.elsevier.com/retrieve/pii/S1297319X04000466

Fredericson M, Bergman AG, Hoffman KL, Dillingham MS (1995) Tibial stress reaction in runners: correlation of clinical symptoms and scintigraphy with a new magnetic resonance imaging grading system. Am J Sports Med 23:472–81 [cited 2022 Jul 18]. Available from: http://journals.sagepub.com/doi/10.1177/036354659502300418

Gross CE, Nunley JA (2015) Navicular stress fractures. Foot Ankle Int 36:1117–22 [cited 2022 Jul 19]. Available from: http://journals.sagepub.com/doi/10.1177/1071100715600495

Hedge G, Thaker S, Botchu R, Fawcett R, Gupta H (2021) Atraumatic fractures of the femur. BJR 94:20201457 [cited 2022 Jul 17]. Available from: https://www.birpublications.org/doi/10.1259/bjr.20201457

Irion V, Miller TL, Kaeding CC (2014) The treatment and outcomes of medial malleolar stress fractures: a systematic review of the literature. Sports Health 6:527–30 [cited 2022 Jul 19]. Available from: http://journals.sagepub.com/doi/10.1177/1941738114546089

Jowett AJL, Birks CL, Blackney MC (2008) Medial malleolar stress fracture secondary to chronic ankle impingement. Foot Ankle Int 29:716–21 [cited 2022 Jul 19]. Available from: http://journals.sagepub.com/doi/10.3113/FAI.2008.0716

Kaiser PB, Guss D, DiGiovanni CW (2018) Stress fractures of the foot and ankle in athletes. Foot Ankle Orthop 3:247301141879007 [cited 2022 Jul 18]. Available from: http://journals.sagepub.com/doi/10.1177/2473011418790078

Kerkhoffs GM, Versteegh VE, Sierevelt IN, Kloen P, van Dijk CN (2012) Treatment of proximal metatarsal V fractures in athletes and non-athletes. Br J Sports Med 46:644–8 [cited 2022 Jul 19]. Available from: https://bjsm.bmj.com/lookup/doi/10.1136/bjsports-2011-090389

Kijowski R, Choi J, Shinki K, Del Rio AM, De Smet A (2012) Validation of MRI classification system for tibial stress injuries. Am J Roentgenol 198:878–84 [cited 2022 Jul 18]. Available from: http://www.ajronline.org/doi/abs/10.2214/AJR.11.6826

Krebs P, Borchers J (2019) A middle cuneiform stress fracture in an adolescent athlete: a case report and literature review. Clin Med Insights Arthritis Musculoskelet Disord 12:117954411987871 [cited 2022 Jul 18]. Available from: http://journals.sagepub.com/doi/10.1177/1179544119878712

Lawrence SJ, Botte MJ (1993) Jones' fractures and related fractures of the proximal fifth metatarsal. Foot Ankle 14:358–65 [cited 2022 Jul 19]. Available from: http://journals.sagepub.com/doi/10.1177/107110079301400610

Lee KT, Kim KC, Park YU, Kim TW, Lee YK (2011a) Radiographic evaluation of foot structure following fifth metatarsal stress fracture. Foot Ankle Int 32:796–801 [cited 2022 Jul 19]. Available from: http://journals.sagepub.com/doi/10.3113/FAI.2011.0796

Lee KT, Park YU, Young KW, Kim JS, Kim JB (2011b) The plantar gap: another prognostic factor for fifth metatarsal stress fracture. Am J Sports Med 39:2206–11 [cited 2022 Jul 19]. Available from: http://journals.sagepub.com/doi/10.1177/0363546511414856

Liong SY, Whitehouse RW (2012) Lower extremity and pelvic stress fractures in athletes. BJR 85:1148–56 [cited 2022 Jul 17]. Available from: http://www.birpublications.org/doi/10.1259/bjr/78510315

Mandell JC, Khurana B, Smith SE (2017a) Stress fractures of the foot and ankle, part 1: biomechanics of bone and principles of imaging and treatment. Skeletal Radiol 46:1021–9 [cited 2022 Jul 17]. Available from: http://link.springer.com/10.1007/s00256-017-2640-7

Mandell JC, Khurana B, Smith SE (2017b) Stress fractures of the foot and ankle, part 2: site-specific etiology, imaging, and treatment, and differential diagnosis. Skeletal Radiol 46:1165–86 [cited 2022 Jul 18]. Available from: http://link.springer.com/10.1007/s00256-017-2632-7

Marshall RA, Mandell JC, Weaver MJ, Ferrone M, Sodickson A, Khurana B (2018) Imaging features and management of stress, atypical, and pathologic fractures. Radiographics 38:2173–92 [cited 2022 Jul 17]. Available from: http://pubs.rsna.org/doi/10.1148/rg.2018180073

Mayer SW, Joyner PW, Almekinders LC, Parekh SG (2014) Stress fractures of the foot and ankle in athletes. Sports Health 6:481–91 [cited 2022 Jul 17]. Available from: http://journals.sagepub.com/doi/10.1177/1941738113486588

McInnis KC, Ramey LN (2016) High-risk stress fractures: diagnosis and management. PM&R 8:S113–24 [cited 2022 Jul 19]. Available from: https://onlinelibrary.wiley.com/doi/abs/10.1016/j.pmrj.2015.09.019

Miller TL, Best TM (2016) Taking a holistic approach to managing difficult stress fractures. J Orthop Surg Res 11:98 [cited 2022 Jul 17]. Available from: http://josr-online.biomedcentral.com/articles/10.1186/s13018-016-0431-9

Nussbaum ED, Holtzman B, Rizzone KH, Tenforde AS et al (2022) Evaluation and diagnosis of tibial bone stress injuries in adolescents: imaging and nomenclature. J Pediatr Orthop Soc N Am 4:1–13 [cited 2022 Jul 18]. Available from: https://www.jposna.org/ojs/index.php/jposna/article/view/386

O'Brien F, Hardiman D, Hazenberg J, Mercy M, Mohsin S, Taylor D et al (2005) The behaviour of microcracks in compact bone. Eur J Morphol 42:71–9 [cited 2022 Jul 17]. Available from: http://access.portico.org/stable?au=pggtrn2fjx

Oji DE. Foot and ankle high-risk injuries. In: Tenforde AS, Fredericson M, editors. Bone stress injuries. 1st ed. New York: Springer Publishing Company; 2021. [cited 2022 Jul 18]. Available from: http://connect.springerpub.com/lookup/doi/10.1891/9780826144249.0010

Orava S, Hulkko A (1984) Stress fracture of the mid-tibial shaft. Acta Orthop Scand 55:35–7 [cited 2022 Jul 19]. Available from: http://www.tandfonline.com/doi/full/10.3109/17453678408992308

Orava S, Karpakka J, Hulkko A, Väänänen K, Takala T, Kallinen M et al (1991) Diagnosis and treatment of stress fractures located at the mid-tibial shaft in athletes. Int J Sports Med 12:419–22 [cited 2022 Jul 19]. Available from: http://www.thieme-connect.de/DOI/DOI?10.1055/s-2007-1024705

Patel NM, Mai DH, Ramme AJ, Karamitopoulos MS, Castañeda P, Chu A (2020) Is the incidence of paediatric stress fractures on the rise? Trends in New York State from 2000 to 2015. J Pediatr Orthop B 29:499–504 [cited 2022 Jul 17]. Available from: https://journals.lww.com/10.1097/BPB.0000000000000650

Robertson GAJ, Goffin JS, Wood AM (2017) Return to sport following stress fractures of the great toe sesamoids: a systematic review. Br Med Bull 122:135–49 [cited 2022 Jul 19]. Available from: https://academic.oup.com/bmb/article-lookup/doi/10.1093/bmb/ldx010

Saxena A, Fullem B, Hannaford D (2000) Results of treatment of 22 navicular stress fractures and a new proposed radiographic classification system. J Foot Ankle Surg 39:96–103 [cited 2022 Jul 19]. Available from: https://linkinghub.elsevier.com/retrieve/pii/S1067251600800332

Shelbourne KD, Fisher DA, Rettig AC, McCarroll JR (1988) Stress fractures of the medial malleolus. Am J Sports Med 16:60–3 [cited 2022 Jul 19]. Available from: http://journals.sagepub.com/doi/10.1177/036354658801600111

Sormaala MJ (2006) Stress injuries of the calcaneus detected with magnetic resonance imaging in military recruits. J Bone Joint Surg Am 88:2237 [cited 2022 Jul 18]. Available from: http://jbjs.org/cgi/doi/10.2106/JBJS.E.01447

Woods M, Kijowski R, Sanford M, Choi J, De Smet A (2008) Magnetic resonance imaging findings in patients with fibular stress injuries. Skeletal Radiol 37:835–41 [cited 2022 Jul 18]. Available from: http://link.springer.com/10.1007/s00256-008-0488-6

Zadpoor AA, Nikooyan AA (2011) The relationship between lower-extremity stress fractures and the ground reaction force: a systematic review. Clin Biomech 26:23–8 [cited 2022 Jul 18]. Available from: https://linkinghub.elsevier.com/retrieve/pii/S0268003310002251

Diabetic Foot

Rahul Shetty and Amit Shah

Contents

R. Shetty
Bristol Royal Infirmary, Bristol, UK
e-mail: rahul.shetty@nhs.net

A. Shah (✉)
Department of Radiology, University Hospitals of Leicester, Leicester, UK
e-mail: amit.shah2@nhs.net

1 Background and Epidemiology

Diabetes mellitus (DM) is a major public health concern throughout the world. Type 2 DM accounts for approximately 90% of cases. According to the World Health Organization, the number of people with DM rose from 108 million in 1980 to 422 million in 2014. In the UK, 4.1 million people have been diagnosed with DM, and there are approximately 850,000 who are yet to be diagnosed. This means that the number of DM diagnoses have more than doubled in the last 15 years and by 2030 the total number of cases will exceed 5.5 million (González et al. 2009).

Diabetes cost the UK approximately £23.7bn in 2010/2011 and is projected to reach £39.8bn by 2035/2036. This currently accounts for approximately 10% of the total health resource expenditure and is estimated to reach around 17% in 2035/2036 (Hex et al. 2012). The economic impact of ulceration and amputation due to diabetes in the UK in 2014–2015 was estimated to be between £837 million and £962 million (Kerr et al. 2019).

Diabetic foot is a chronic complication of diabetes that is associated with peripheral vascular disease and neuropathy of the lower limb. Its incidence has been rising due to the increase in incidence of diabetes coupled with the increase in the life expectancy of diabetic patients (Zhang et al. 2017). Worldwide, diabetic foot has an

Med Radiol Diagn Imaging (2023)
https://doi.org/10.1007/174_2023_401,

Published Online: 03 May 2023

annual incidence of between 9.1 and 26.1 million (Armstrong et al. 2017). Roughly 15–25% of patients with DM will have a diabetic foot ulcer during their lifetime (Mutluoglu et al. 2012).

Diabetes is the leading cause of non-traumatic amputations worldwide. Approximately 40–60% of non-traumatic lower limb amputations throughout the world are caused by complications due to diabetes and 80% of them follow a foot ulcer (Hingorani et al. 2016). It is estimated that in the UK, diabetes leads to a foot amputation every 1 h (Hex et al. 2012). A diabetic foot leading to a major amputation has a high mortality rate with a 5-year survival rate of 41–48% (Tseng et al. 2008) and in minor amputations, the 5-year survival rate is only 59% (Hambleton et al. 2009).

2 Pathophysiology of Diabetic Foot

Diabetes is a chronic, complex disease which has various complications acting in conjunction. They include peripheral neuropathy, neuropathic osteoarthropathy, foot deformity, peripheral vascular disease, and immunopathy.

2.1 Peripheral Neuropathy

Peripheral neuropathy is one of the most common complications of diabetes. Neuropathic complications can be acute or chronic and can affect the peripheral nerve from the root to the distal axon. It is the most common diabetic complication and has a prevalence of 50% (Singh et al. 2014; Tesfaye and Selvarajah 2012). The neuropathy commonly starts with the toes and over time starts affecting the hands in a characteristic "stocking and glove" presentation. More than 40% of patients with diabetes develop neuropathy despite good glycemic control (Callaghan et al. 2015). Patients with peripheral neuropathy have a higher risk of falls due to muscle imbalance and atrophy; in addition to this, neuropathy causes a 15% increased risk of developing ulcers and an estimated 6–43% of those with ulcers will go on to have an amputation (Callaghan et al. 2012).

Early MRI studies attempted the use of a proton density-weighted Dixon sequence at 1.5 T to measure the water content of the sural nerve. Higher nerve water content was demonstrated in patients with peripheral neuropathy which coincided with nerve conduction deficits (Griffey et al. 1988; Koechner et al. 1995; Eaton et al. 1996). More recent studies (Felisaz et al. 2017) used a 3-point Dixon sequence and a T1-weighted TSE and demonstrated an increase in tibial nerve and fascicle volume, along with a decreased nerve-fascicle ratio in patients with diabetic neuropathy, which was suggestive of expansion of the epineurial connective tissue and fascicular enlargement.

2.2 Neuropathic Osteoarthropathy (Charcot Arthropathy)

Neuropathic osteoarthropathy also known as Charcot arthropathy or Charcot joint is a degenerative joint disorder in chronic and advanced diabetic patients who have altered pain sensation, proprioception, and muscular reflexes that regulate joint movement (Rajbhandari et al. 2002). The loss of the above three mechanisms causes chronic repeated trauma leading to progressive bone and cartilage damage. Charcot joint almost exclusively affects the foot. Clinical symptoms include a swollen and tender ankle, progressing to multiple dislocations and fractures leading to severe deformities. Charcot arthropathy can produce significant deformities in the midfoot or hindfoot, resulting in plantar and medial prominences causing eventual ulceration.

The incidence of Charcot arthropathy ranges from 0.1% to 0.4% in diabetic patients and increases to 35% in patients with peripheral neuropathy (Schoots et al. 2010). Charcot joint is most commonly seen in diabetics over the age of

50 and those with symptoms of diabetes for over 10 years (Ergen et al. 2013).

Jeffcoate in 2005 defined Charcot arthropathy as an inflammatory response to a lesion that induces increased bone lysis. Multiple studies support this theory and have looked at inflammatory factors such as CRP, TNF-a, and IL6 and bone modeling in people with Charcot joint (Schara et al. 2017; Petrova et al. 2015; Uccioli et al. 2010).

The most commonly used classification of staging for Charcot arthropathy is that by Eichenholtz in his monograph "Charcot Joint" in 1966, which was based on clinical and radiological signs. Stage 0 is characterized by mild inflammation, soft tissue edema, and normal radiographs, but MRI demonstrates signs of microfracture, bone marrow edema, and contusion (Chantelau and Richter 2013). Early recognition of stage 0 is highly imperative to halt the disease activity and prevent formation of any foot deformities. Stage 1 is characterized by severe inflammation, soft tissue edema, abnormal radiographs with macro-fractures. On MRI, macro-fractures, bone marrow edema, resorption of the bone, and signs of articular dislocation can be seen. Stage 2 is also known as the coalescence stage, which is the end of bone resorption and start of remodeling with healing of fractures and debris resorption. Finally, stage 3 is characterized by reconstruction of the bone, followed by the chronic phase of Charcot arthropathy, which is characteristic for the appearance of ulcers following significant changes to the arch of the foot.

Sanders and Frykberg used an anatomical classification system which divided the site of involvement into five patterns (Frykberg 1991) The phalanges, interphalangeal and the metatarsophalangeal joints include pattern 1; pattern 2 involves the tarsometatarsal joint; pattern 3 the talonavicular, cuneonavicular, and calcaneocuboid joints (Chopart joint); the talocrural joint is pattern 4 and the posterior calcaneus involves pattern 5 (Fig. 1). Patterns 2 and 3 were found to be the most commonly affected with an incidence of 45% and 35%, respectively (Sella and Barrette 1999). Trepman classified Charcot arthropathy anatomically with respect to the articulation of the foot which helped elaborate its multisite presence (Trepman et al. 2005) (Table 1). The tarsometatarsal joint, commonly known as the Lisfranc joint, is the most common site of neuropathic osteoarthropathy in diabetic foot (Chisholm and Gilchrist 2011). If the TMTJ is affected, the metatarsal bases get displaced superiorly, causing the tarsal bones to become weight-bearing, resulting in abnormal plantar pressures; this eventually leads to the collapse of the longitudinal arch and results in the characteristic "rocker bottom" deformity.

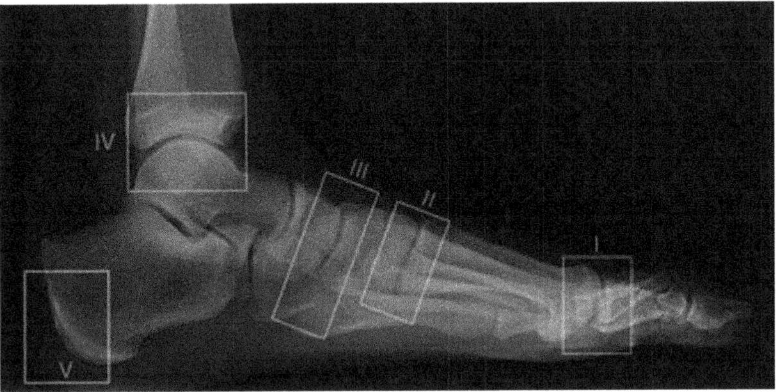

Fig. 1 Frykberg classification. Pattern I: phalanges, interphalangeal and the metatarsophalangeal joints; pattern II: the tarsometatarsal joints; pattern III: the cuneonavicular, talonavicular, and calcaneocuboid articulations; pattern IV: the talocrural joint; pattern V: the posterior calcaneal involvement

Table 1 Trepman classification

Type	Localization	Joint
1	Plantar	Tarsometatarsal, naviculocuneiform
2	Medio plantar	Subtalar, talonavicular
3A	Bassi ankle	Calcaneocuboid tibiotalar
3B	Calcaneus	Tuberosity fracture
4	Multiregions	Sequential, simultaneous
5	Forefoot	Metatarsophalangeal

Charcot joints are typically unilateral but are bilateral in ~20% (range 5.9–39.3%) of cases (Mautone and Naidoo 2015). There are two patterns of Charcot joint: atrophic and hypertrophic.

Atrophic form is the most common form which occurs earlier than the hypertrophic form. It has an acute progression characterized by reabsorption of the ends of the affected bone, joint destruction, resorption of fragments, an absence of osteosclerosis, and osteophytes. It mainly occurs in non-weight-bearing joints of the upper limb.

In contrast, in hypertrophic form, only sensory nerves affected and therefore has a slow progression, joint destruction with periarticular debris/bone fragmentation. Joint space is initially widened and subsequently narrows. There is osteosclerosis and osteophytes with absence of osteoporosis (unless joint is infected).

The radiographic features of a Charcot joint are often remembered using the following mnemonics of the 5 Ds: *D*ensity change (subchondral osteopenia or sclerosis), *D*estruction (osseous fragmentation and resorption), *D*ebris (intra-articular loose bodies), *D*istension (joint effusion), *D*isorganization/*D*islocation (joint malalignment due to ligamentous laxity).

2.3 Foot Deformities

Foot deformities are an integral component in the formation of diabetic foot ulcers. Atrophy of the intrinsic foot muscles due to motor neuropathy leads to loss of muscle balance, subluxations, and dislocations. This leads to various types of deformities such as hammer and claw toe deformities, prominent metatarsal heads, plantar fat pad atrophy, pes cavus and equinus, hallux valgus, and Charcot foot deformity (Bus Sicco et al. 2009; Heitzman 2010). Claw toes are a deformity in diabetic patients that arises as a result of hyperextension of the metatarsophalangeal joints with distal displacement of the submetatarsal fat pads. This leaves the metatarsal head prominences without the protective fat pads and causes an increase of plantar foot pressures.

Hallux valgus is the most common forefoot deformity with a prevalence of 23–35% (Wülker and Mittag 2012). Hallux valgus may also occur as a result of amputation of the second toe. There is medial deviation of the MTP joint, causing an increase in pressure by footwear over the eminence. This leaves the feet of diabetic patients extremely prone to ulceration. Loss of joint mobility was a common finding with about 30–40% of the diabetic population being affected (Formosa et al. 2013). Studies showed that joint mobility reduced progressively with the duration of diabetes (García-Álvarez et al. 2013). This loss of joint mobility will lead to a loss of shock absorption, pronation of the foot and ultimately lead to various foot deformities (Formosa et al. 2013).

2.4 Peripheral Vascular Disease

Peripheral arterial disease (PAD) is one of the major macrovascular complications of DM. PAD involves a complete or partial blockage of peripheral arteries due to atherosclerosis of the vessel wall, embolism, thrombosis, or vasculitis, resulting in reduced blood flow and tissue loss (Kullo and Rooke 2016). In diabetic patients, studies show that the distal arteries of the lower limbs are mostly commonly involved; the dorsalis pedis artery being the most commonly involved artery (Fig. 2) (Forbang et al. 2014; Marso and Hiatt 2006).

There is uncertainty regarding the prevalence of PAD in DM as a large number of PAD patients are asymptomatic due to the altered pain perception in peripheral neuropathy. However, one study found that 20.1% of ≥40-year-old diabetics had symptomatic PAD (Belch et al. 2008). Other studies have found the prevalence to be

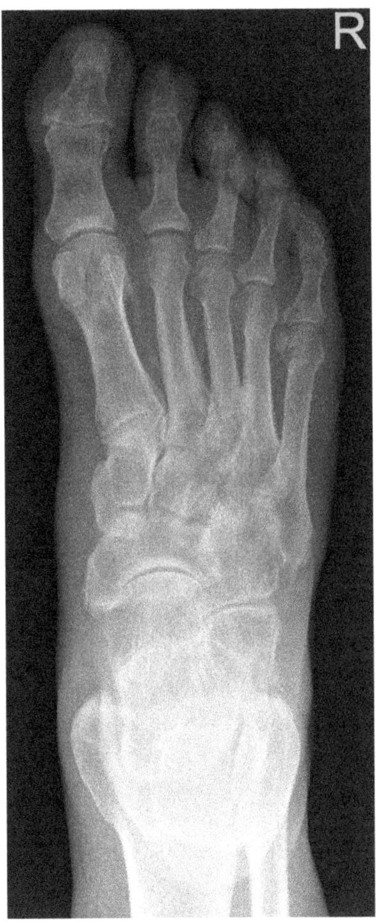

Fig. 2 DP radiograph of a patient newly diagnosed with diabetes demonstrating calcification of dorsalis pedis artery

much higher in diabetics, ranging from 20% to 50%, in comparison to 10–26% in nondiabetics (Stoberock et al. 2021; Mostaza et al. 2008; Marso and Hiatt 2006). DM increases the likelihood of developing PAD by two folds. Just a 1% increase in HbA1c leads to a 28% increase in the risk of developing PAD (Jude et al. 2010; Selvin et al. 2004). The PAD in diabetic patients progresses much more rapidly with poorer outcomes in comparison to nondiabetics; the frequency of amputation was much higher, with a significant increase in mortality (Rhee et al. 2007; Forbang et al. 2014).

Studies have shown impaired fibrinolytic activity, with an increase in the circulating levels of procoagulants like tissue factor, factor VII, and decreased levels of anticoagulants like antithrombin-III and protein C. This results in a tendency to coagulate and leads to an environment favoring thrombosis (Marso and Hiatt 2006). PAD has a major contribution to the development of diabetic foot ulcers. Diabetic foot ulcers in the presence of PAD can ultimately result in lower limb amputation, due to significant tissue loss, infection, and gangrene (Klein 2021).

Mönckeberg's sclerosis, a particular type of atherosclerosis with radiological significance, can be observed in diabetic patients (Fishbein and Fishbein 2009). It affects the medium-large arteries of the body through calcification of the medial wall, resulting in a characteristic image of a network of calcified arteries on radiograph (Fig. 3). It is a variant of atherosclerosis consisting of calcification combined with an inflamma-

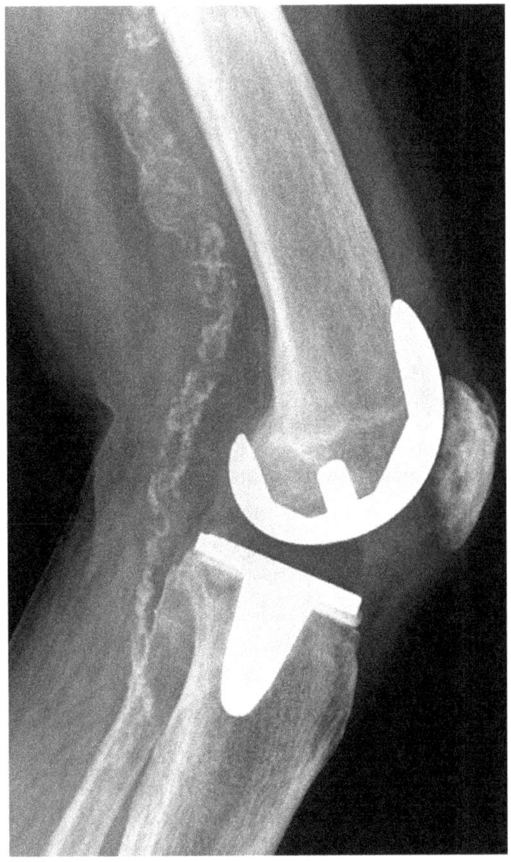

Fig. 3 Lateral radiograph of the knee with total knee replacement demonstrating Mönckeberg's sclerosis of the popliteal artery

tory component (McCullough et al. 2008). If seen on a radiograph, it can be used as an indication for diabetes screening in individuals or as an indicator for surgical intervention in a known diabetic (David Smith et al. 2008).

2.5 Immunopathy

Type 2 DM has been recognized to alter the functioning of immune cells including B cells, and this plays an important role in diabetic foot infections (Hammad et al. 2018). Studies have shown a significant decrease in interferon-γ (IFN-γ) in diabetic patients, making them more susceptible to infections (Kartika et al. 2020; Jayakumar Sunandhakumari et al. 2018). In one study examining wound swabs from patients with diabetic ulcers, IFN-γ was undetectable in the wound fluid, however 100% IFN-γ recovery was found during the period of healing (Schmohl et al. 2012). IFN-γ plays a vital role initiating the inflammatory responses and cellular immunity and is pivotal in the activation of macrophages.

3 Radiologic Findings

3.1 Ulceration and Callus

Diabetic patients with peripheral neuropathy develop calluses along areas of excess friction or abnormal pressures, such as underneath the metatarsal heads, the tips of the toes, over eminences arising due to digital foot deformities, over the heel, and over the malleoli. This can eventually lead to hemorrhagic keratosis and eventual ulceration from skin erosion and breakdown of the callus from friction (Klein 2021). Doppler ultrasound (US) examination can provide valuable insight on the vascular changes in patients with diabetic foot (Gupta and Singh 2012).

Callus formation occurs commonly under the first and fifth metatarsal head and over the tip of the great toe in the forefoot. In DF patients with neuropathy and rocker-bottom deformity, callus formation in the midfoot occurs under the cuboid bone, and in the hindfoot, they develop over the heel (Ledermann et al. 2002). Skin calluses on MRI are seen as focal subcutaneous lesions showing low T1-W signal intensity along with low to intermediate T2-W signal intensity. An infection may be mimicked if there is enhancement of the callus, however, its location and lack of surrounding soft tissue signal change help in differentiating it. Adventitial bursa may be visualized as minimal fluid collection over bony prominences, without subcutaneous inflammatory fat stranding. They may occur over the same sites as the calluses as they both arise due to chronic friction (Low and Peh 2015). Long-standing friction will eventually lead to breakdown of the callus, preceding the formation of an ulcer.

A skin ulcer on MRI is visualized as a local discontinuity of the cutaneous line associated with surrounding soft tissue defects and raised margins, if succeeding a callus. High T2-W signal intensity with peripheral enhancement is seen in acute ulcers, indicative of granulation tissue at the base of the ulcer. Whereas chronic ulcers are seen as an induration of intermediate to low T2-W signal intensity in the subcutaneous layer, which demonstrates healing by fibrosis (Low and Peh 2015).

3.2 Diabetic Edema and Cellulitis

Soft tissue edema and cellulitis are common findings of diabetic neuropathy and are demonstration of soft tissue infection. DM complicated by PVD causes decreases in venous drainage, which leads to soft tissue edema and thus compounds the ischemic process (Hill et al. 1999). Plain radiographs can be utilized to detect soft tissue swelling, which can be seen as increased opacity within the infected tissue. CT can visualize skin edema and subcutaneous fat stranding in diabetic patients with cellulitis. CT imaging in cellulitis shows a homogeneous enhancement within the edematous soft tissue planes (Loredo et al. 2010). Cellulitis appears on MRI as loss of the normal subcutaneous fat signal intensity on T1-weighted images along with an associated increase in

T2-weighted signal intensity. Diffuse enhancement with gadolinium is a characteristic feature of cellulitis and differentiates it from edema of neuropathic disease (Ledermann et al. 2002).

3.3 Vascular Disease

The use of imaging of the arterial circulation in vascular disease associated with diabetes is fundamental in the planning of revascularization procedures. Due to vascular disease commonly being multisegmental in diabetes, arterial imaging can be challenging. Arteriography remains the gold standard in imaging PVD due to its diagnostic as well as therapeutic functions. Imaging modalities that are commonly used include magnetic resonance angiography with contrast (MRA), computerized tomographic angiography (CTA), and intra-arterial digital subtraction angiography (DSA) (Pomposelli 2010). There are more recent modalities which include 3D intravascular ultrasound, MR spectroscopy, and optical coherence tomography that assist in the study of intricate details of metabolic function and coronary anatomy that routine imaging cannot visualize (Levitt et al. 2014).

The Doppler ultrasound signal characterizes arterial waveforms into triphasic, biphasic, or monophasic. With the progression in PVD, the Doppler signal changes from triphasic to biphasic, and finally to monophasic in severe forms of PVD. A Duplex ultrasound scan is a reliable imaging method which is noninvasive and helps in hemodynamic vascular assessments. It has been shown to be a more reliable indicator than Ankle Brachial Index (ABI) to screen for PVD (Santoro et al. 2018). US visualizes the vascular structure directly and helps identify the anatomic site of obstruction. Furthermore, it assists in the measurement of the velocity of blood flow and demonstrates the hemodynamic information while screening for PVD without the need for invasive arteriography (Andersen 2010).

Magnetic resonance angiography (MRA) and computerized tomography angiography (CTA) are newer modalities that are commonly being used as noninvasive alternatives for imaging in PVD. Administration of contrast dye such as gadolinium helps in differentiating blood and soft tissue structures (Fleischmann et al. 2006). The images can be visualized with 3D data reconstruction showing sagittal and coronal views in extensive detail.

PVD causes microvasculopathy in diabetic patients, leading to ischemia, which may in turn lead to gangrene. Contrast-enhanced MRI is particularly useful in gangrene as they help to delineate areas of soft tissue necrosis and assist with further surgical planning. Gangrene is visualized as a region of non-enhanced devascularized soft tissue with a well-demarcated border from adjacent normal soft tissue. A paradoxical reactive hyperemia and enhancement are seen in the surrounding soft tissue (Ledermann et al. 2002). Gas seen in wet gangrene is found within the fascial layers, which normally show low MR imaging signal intensity similar to gas, thus making it difficult to visualize on MRI. Thus, the radiologist needs to be aware and differentiate the gas in the soft tissue secondary to wet gangrene from the gas seen with a skin ulcer. Characteristic findings to differentiate the two is the visualization of an unenhanced devitalized soft tissue with greater extent of soft tissue gas in comparison to a surrounding a skin ulcer (Panchbhavi and Hecox 2006).

3.4 Tendon, Muscle, and Joint Dysfunction

Tendon inflammation and degeneration can occur due to extension of adjacent ulcer or sinus. The most commonly affected sites in the hindfoot include the peroneal and Achilles' tendon due to the adjacent spread of calcaneal skin and malleolus skin ulcers; forefoot involvement is seen commonly in flexor tendons due to ulceration in the plantar skin (Donovan and Schweitzer 2010). Tenosynovitis on MRI can be visualized as an enhanced area surrounding the tendon associated with a skin ulcer, tendon thickening, and hyperintense T2-weighted signals.

Septic arthritis of the ankle occurs as a direct consequence of neighboring soft tissue infection, commonly affecting the lateral IP and MTP joints. MRI shows joint effusion, perisynovial edema, marked enhancement, and thickening of the synovium with notable fluid outpouching (Ledermann et al. 2002; Karchevsky et al. 2004). Extension of joint fluid to a neighboring sinus tract may be seen, with perisynovial edema of the adjacent soft tissue, as well as reactive subchondral marrow edema with marginal erosion.

Peripheral neuropathy in diabetes can eventually lead to denervation of muscles, which is divided into an acute, subacute, and chronic phase. Acute phase shows no changes on MR images, while subacute phase shows diffuse edema within the affected muscle, presenting as a hyperintense signal on T2 and STIR. If muscle innervation does not occur within the subacute phase, chronic atrophy develops which is irreversible. The involved muscle will show a larger amount of fat associated with a high T1-weighted signal and decreased overall muscle bulk.

3.5 Osteomyelitis

Osteomyelitis is often present when there is a deep ulceration in diabetic foot and shows characteristic soft tissue defects on MRI (Ledermann et al. 2002). Between 20% and 50% of diabetic foot infections were accompanied with osteomyelitis (Lavery et al. 2009; Richard et al. 2011), however, OM can also occur in the absence of an overlying evidence of inflammation (Newman et al. 1991).

Diagnosing OM with the help of plain radiographs of the foot has shown variable accuracy and depends on the chronicity of the infection. A bone loss of approximately 40% is required to visualize OM changes on X-ray (Game 2013). The radiographic findings of OM include osteopenia, periosteal reaction or elevation, loss of cortex, new bone formation, sequestrum, involucrum, and cloacae (Mettler 2005; Pineda et al. 2009). Ultrasound can be used to visualize soft tissue abscesses and joint effusion and is a useful tool in their aspiration. US can detect a hypoechoic layer of purulent material elevating the periosteum in acute OM and hypoechoic or anechoic surrounding soft tissue abscesses in chronic OM (Simpfendorfer 2017). CT imaging in OM has a sensitivity of roughly 70% and is superior to MRI in detecting sequestra, involucra, cloacae, and intraosseous gas in chronic OM. A sequestrum appears as a mineralized segment of bone with a surrounding lucency enclosing it, and the involucrum consists of reactive bone sclerosis surrounding the sequestrum. Furthermore, CT can be used for needle biopsies and joint aspirations. However, due to their poor soft tissue contrast, it is difficult to identify marrow edema and diagnose early OM. Thus, they are reserved for when MRI is unavailable or contraindicated (Mandell et al. 2018).

MRI is the imaging of choice in OM due to a high sensitivity of approximately 90% (Pineda et al. 2009) and its ability to visualize alterations in the water content of bone marrow with very good spatial resolution and structural definition (Meyers and Wiener 1991). MRI can detect OM changes within 5 days of the onset of the infection and is an extremely useful tool in planning surgical management (Flemming et al. 2005). The MRI findings are dependent on the pulse sequences used as well as the disease stage. Early findings of acute OM consist of a poorly defined low-signal intensity on the T1-weighted images and a high signal intensity on the T2-weighted images and STIR sequences due to exudates and edema within the medullary space.

Sequestrum is visualized by low signal intensity on T1-weighted and STIR sequences. The bordering granulation tissue shows an intermediate to low signal intensity on T1-weighted sequences and high signal intensity with STIR or T2-weighted images. A contrast medium such as gadolinium can be utilized to enhance the granulation tissue. The involucrum, which consists of an ossified periosteal shell and dead tubular cortical bone, has low signal intensity on all pulse sequences. The cloaca is visualized by a periosteum with low signal intensity, interspersed by high signal intensity gaps on T2-weighted images. A sinus tract or abscess may be noted by seeing the high signal intensity extend from the cloaca into the soft tissues (Pineda et al. 2009; Lipsky et al. 2012; Low and Peh 2015).

Osteitis, which consists of reactive marrow changes secondary to a neighboring soft tissue infection, should not be confused with OM. Both osteitis and OM appear as hyperintense signals in T2-weighted images, however, on T1-weighted images, OM demonstrates a characteristic low signal, whereas osteitis does not (Donovan and Schweitzer 2010).

Technique	Findings
Plain radiograph	Periosteal thickening or elevation
	Loss of cortex with bony erosion
	Focal loss of trabecular architecture or marrow radiolucency
	New bone formation
	Bone sclerosis with or without erosion
Ultrasound	Periosteal elevation
	Joint effusion
	Soft tissue abscess
Computed tomography	Periosteal elevation
	Cortical erosion or destruction
	Sequestra and involucra
	Intraosseous gas
Magnetic resonance imaging	T1-weighted images—Low signal intensity
	T2-weighted images—High signal intensity
	High bone marrow signal in STIR sequences
	Adjacent cutaneous ulcer
	Sinus tract formation
	Adjacent soft tissue inflammation or edema
	Gadolinium-enhanced area of necrosis

3.6 Neuropathic Osteoarthropathy

Long-standing peripheral neuropathy leads to decreased trauma perception, which coupled with PVD and ischemia, leads to poor healing, deformities, joint instability, and progressive arthropathy. Neuropathic osteoarthropathy is typically seen at the Lisfranc joint (tarsometatarsal joints) and leads to a collapse of the normal longitudinal arch of the foot, causing various foot deformities such as rocker bottom deformity. Other common sites of fractures include the distal tibia and fibula, as well as adulation fractures of the calcaneus (Wukich et al. 2011; Sagray et al. 2013).

Plain radiography and CT does not play a considerable role in the acute stages of neuroarthropathy. This is because the early stages of Charcot's arthropathy is characterized by soft tissue inflammation and bone marrow edema and poorly seen. With long-term progression of the disease, foot deformity due to bone destruction and debris is visualized well on CT imaging. Fractures of all ages, dislocations, calcifications, and callus formation are visualized well on CT. The initial most finding in PR includes focal demineralization and flattening of the metatarsal heads, most commonly the second metatarsal bone (Loredo et al. 2010; Yeoh et al. 2008).

MRI is the gold standard imaging modality for the detection and assessment of changes in all the stages of Charcot neuroarthropathy. MRI plays a significant role right from stage 0 of Charcot neuroarthropathy, which is characterized by extensive inflammation and diffuse edema. Due to its fluid sensitivity, MRI sequences can report the anatomical location as well as the degree of edema in bones and soft tissues (Morrison and Ledermann 2002). MR imaging can also reveal early joint dislocation, especially in the Lisfranc joint, ligamentous disruptions, and occult fractures that cannot be visualized on X-ray or CT (Figs. 4 and 6).

MR diffusion-weighted imaging is important for the early detection of osteomyelitis and can help differentiate it from noninfectious neuroarthropathy (Starr et al. 2008; Roug and Pierre-Jerome 2012). A significant factor responsible for spontaneous onset of neuropathic fractures is inflammatory osteolysis. This inflammatory osteolysis eventually causes one or many bones of the

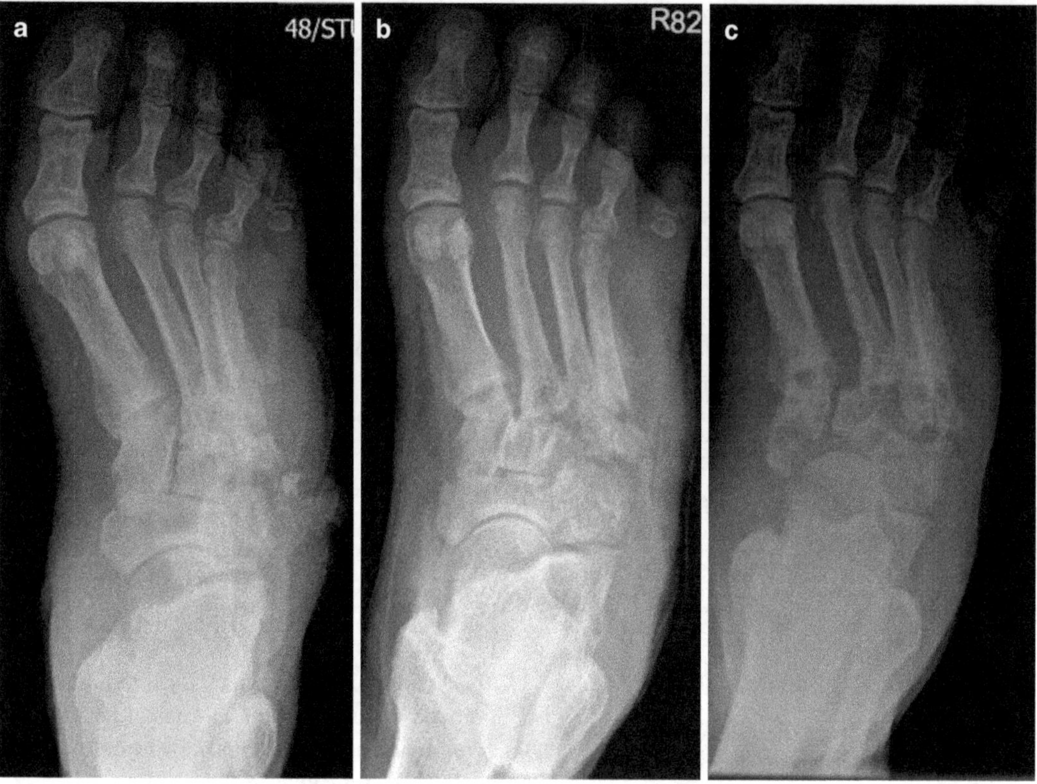

Fig. 4 (**a**) T1 coronal, (**b**) PDFS coronal, and (**c**) STIR sagittal of a known diabetic patient. There is florid marrow edema centered at the midfoot (Charcot) with disorganization and marked soft tissue swelling. There is osteolysis of the fifth metatarsal. It is difficult to distinguish neuropathic arthropathy from osteomyelitis. This case had both pathologies with a small soft tissue abscess (not shown)

foot to progressively disappear or "vanish" and can be mistaken for osteomyelitis (Figs. 5 and 6) (Lipsky et al. 2004; Sinacore et al. 2017).

3.7 Differentiating Osteomyelitis from Neuroarthropathy

It is important to differentiate OM from noninfectious neuroarthropathy, however, this has been a long-standing challenge for clinicians in evaluating diabetic foot complications. There are certain radiological and clinical findings that can help differentiate the two, and have been summarized in Table 2.

Neuroarthropathy is primarily articular, whereas osteomyelitis always arises by direct extension of infection to the bone from skin ulcers at adjacent sites. The presence of periarticular marrow edema with no adjacent ulcer is highly indicative of noninfective neuroarthropathy. Location of bone marrow signal changes is one of the most helpful features in differentiating between OM and neuroarthropathy. Neuroarthropathy commonly involves the Lisfranc joints (Fig. 4), whereas OM tends to involve the talus, calcaneum, malleoli and can occur anywhere distal to the TMT joint. The midfoot causes the biggest diagnostic problem, especially when neuroarthropathy is pre-existent. In such an instance, secondary signs of infection such as a direct spread from an ulcer or a sinus tract present over a rocker bottom foot indicates the presence of osteomyelitis, which can be confirmed by bone biopsy or diffusion-weighted imaging (Ledermann et al. 2002; Morrison and Ledermann 2002).

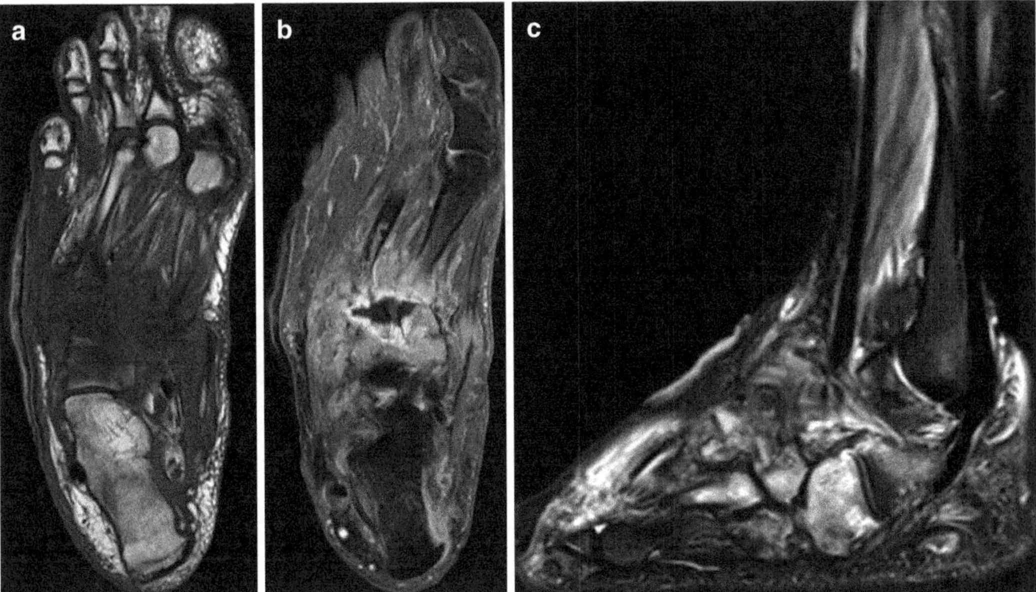

Fig. 5 (**a**–**c**) Three DP radiograph of the right foot of a diabetic patient taken at monthly intervals. There is gradual subluxation and disorganization of the Lisfranc joint from **a** to **c**. There is destruction and fragmentation at the midfoot best in image (**b**). There is increased soft tissue swelling. There is patchy mixed sclerotic lucency of the metatarsal bases in keeping with concurrent chronic osteomyelitis. There is osteolysis of the fifth metatarsal which has "vanished"

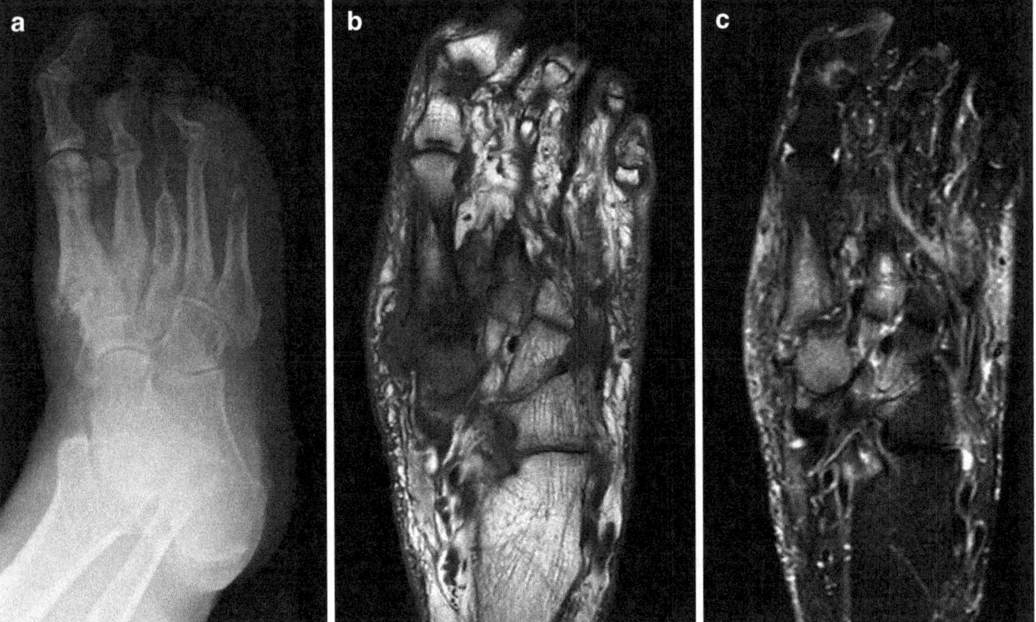

Fig. 6 (**a**) Oblique radiograph of the right of a diabetic patient demonstrating multiple metatarsal osteolysis. (**b**) T1 coronal and corresponding STIR (**c**) MRI of the same patient demonstrating soft tissue and marrow edema, disorganization at the Lisfranc joint and joint destruction in keeping with Charcot arthropathy

Table 2 Differentiation of osteomyelitis from neuropathic osteoarthropathy

	Osteomyelitis	Neuroarthropathy
Common location	• Toes (dorsum and tips) • Metatarsal heads (esp. 1st, 5th) • Calcaneus • Malleoli	• Lisfranc joint • Chopart joint
Distribution	Focal, local, centripetal spread	Multiple joints in a region
Pattern of edema/ enhancement	Predominant involvement of one bone	Epicenter in joint and subchondral bone
Deformity	Uncommon (unless there is underlying neuropathic disease)	Common
Soft tissues	Adjacent ulcer, cellulitis, sinus tract Enhancement limited to periarticular soft tissues; skin, subcutaneous tissues intact	Diffuse subcutaneous edema is typical in diabetic feet

References

Andersen CA (2010) Noninvasive assessment of lower-extremity hemodynamics in individuals with diabetes mellitus. J Am Podiatr Med Assoc 100(5):406–411. https://doi.org/10.7547/1000406. PMID: 20847355

Armstrong DG, Boulton AJM, Bus SA (2017) Diabetic foot ulcers and their recurrence. N Engl J Med 376(24):2367–2375. https://doi.org/10.1056/NEJMra1615439

Belch J, MacCuish A, Campbell I, Cobbe S, Taylor R, Prescott R, Lee R, Bancroft J, MacEwan S, Shepherd J, Macfarlane P, Morris A, Jung R, Kelly C, Connacher A, Peden N, Jamieson A, Matthews D, Leese G, McKnight J, O'Brien I, Semple C, Petrie J, Gordon D, Pringle S, MacWalter R, Prevention of Progression of Arterial Disease and Diabetes Study Group; Diabetes Registry Group; Royal College of Physicians Edinburgh (2008) The prevention of progression of arterial disease and diabetes (POPADAD) trial: factorial randomised placebo controlled trial of aspirin and antioxidants in patients with diabetes and asymptomatic peripheral arterial disease. BMJ 337:a1840. https://doi.org/10.1136/bmj.a1840. PMID: 18927173; PMCID: PMC2658865

Bus Sicco A, Maas M, Michels RP, Levi M (2009) Role of intrinsic muscle atrophy in the etiology of claw toe deformity in diabetic neuropathy may not be as straightforward as widely believed. Diabetes Care 32(6):1063–1067. https://doi.org/10.2337/dc08-2174. Epub 2009 Mar 11. PMID: 19279305; PMCID: PMC2681028

Callaghan BC, Cheng HT, Stables CL, Smith AL, Feldman EL (2012) Diabetic neuropathy: clinical manifestations and current treatments. Lancet Neurol 11(6):521–534. https://doi.org/10.1016/S1474-4422(12)70065-0. Epub 2012 May 16. PMID: 22608666; PMCID: PMC4254767

Callaghan B, Kerber K, Langa KM et al (2015) Longitudinal patient-oriented outcomes in neuropathy: importance of early detection and falls. Neurology 85(1):71–79. https://doi.org/10.1212/WNL.0000000000001714

Chantelau EA, Richter A (2013) The acute diabetic Charcot foot managed on the basis of magnetic resonance imaging—a review of 71 cases. Swiss Med Wkly 143:w13831. https://doi.org/10.4414/smw.2013.13831

Chisholm KA, Gilchrist JM (2011) The Charcot joint: a modern neurologic perspective. J Clin Neuromuscul Dis 13(1):1–13. https://doi.org/10.1097/CND.0b013e3181c6f55b. PMID: 22361621

David Smith C, Gavin Bilmen J, Iqbal S, Robey S, Pereira M (2008) Medial artery calcification as an indicator of diabetic peripheral vascular disease. Foot Ankle Int 29(2):185–190. https://doi.org/10.3113/FAI.2008.0185. PMID: 18315974

Donovan A, Schweitzer ME (2010) Use of MR imaging in diagnosing diabetes-related pedal osteomyelitis. Radiographics 30(3):723–736. https://doi.org/10.1148/rg.303095111. PMID: 20462990

Eaton RP, Qualls C, Bicknell J, Sibbitt WL Jr, King MK, Griffey RH (1996) Structure-function relationships within peripheral nerves in diabetic neuropathy: the hydration hypothesis. Diabetologia 39(4):439–446. https://doi.org/10.1007/BF00400675. PMID: 8777993

Ergen FB, Sanverdi SE, Oznur A (2013) Charcot foot in diabetes and an update on imaging. Diabet Foot Ankle 4:1. https://doi.org/10.3402/dfa.v4i0.21884

Felisaz PF, Maugeri G, Busi V, Vitale R, Balducci F, Gitto S, Leporati P, Pichiecchio A, Baldi M, Calliada F, Chiovato L, Bastianello S (2017) MR microneurography and a segmentation protocol applied to diabetic neuropathy. Radiol Res Pract 2017:2761818. https://doi.org/10.1155/2017/2761818. Epub 2017 Apr 16. PMID: 28567306; PMCID: PMC5439248

Fishbein GA, Fishbein MC (2009) Arteriosclerosis: rethinking the current classification. Arch Pathol Lab Med 133(8):1309–1316. https://doi.org/10.5858/133.8.1309. PMID: 19653731

Fleischmann D, Hallett RL, Rubin GD (2006) CT angiography of peripheral arterial disease. J Vasc Interv

Radiol 17(1):3–26. https://doi.org/10.1097/01.RVI.0000191361.02857.DE. PMID: 16415129

Flemming DJ, Murphey MD, McCarthy K (2005) Imaging of the foot and ankle: summary and update. Curr Opin Orthop 16(2):54–59. https://doi.org/10.1097/01.bco.0000154176.29585.8b

Forbang NI, McDermott MM, Liao Y, Ix JH, Allison MA, Liu K, Tian L, Evans N, Criqui MH (2014) Associations of diabetes mellitus and other cardiovascular disease risk factors with decline in the ankle-brachial index. Vasc Med 19(6):465–472. https://doi.org/10.1177/1358863X14554033. Epub 2014 Oct 30. PMID: 25358555; PMCID: PMC4515111

Formosa C, Gatt A, Chockalingam N (2013) The importance of clinical biomechanical assessment of foot deformity and joint mobility in people living with type-2 diabetes within a primary care setting. Prim Care Diabetes 7(1):45–50. https://doi.org/10.1016/j.pcd.2012.12.003. Epub 2013 Jan 16. PMID: 23332418

Frykberg RG (ed) (1991) The high risk foot in diabetes mellitus. Churchill Livingstone

Game FL (2013) Osteomyelitis in the diabetic foot: diagnosis and management. Med Clin North Am 97(5):947–956. https://doi.org/10.1016/j.mcna.2013.03.010. Epub 2013 May 4. PMID: 23992902

García-Álvarez Y, Lázaro-Martínez JL, García-Morales E, Cecilia-Matilla A, Aragón-Sánchez J, Carabantes-Alarcón D (2013) Morphofunctional characteristics of the foot in patients with diabetes mellitus and diabetic neuropathy. Diabetes Metab Syndr 7(2):78–82. https://doi.org/10.1016/j.dsx.2013.02.029. Epub 2013 Mar 15. PMID: 23680245

González EL, Johansson S, Wallander MA, Rodríguez LA (2009) Trends in the prevalence and incidence of diabetes in the UK: 1996–2005. J Epidemiol Commun Health 63(4):332–336. https://doi.org/10.1136/jech.2008.080382. Epub 2009 Feb 24. Erratum in: J Epidemiol Community Health. 2009 Oct;63(10):864. PMID: 19240084

Griffey RH, Eaton RP, Sibbitt RR, Sibbitt WL Jr, Bicknell JM (1988) Diabetic neuropathy. Structural analysis of nerve hydration by magnetic resonance spectroscopy. JAMA 260(19):2872–2878. https://doi.org/10.1001/jama.260.19.2872. PMID: 3141635

Gupta SK, Singh SK (2012) Diabetic foot: a continuing challenge. Adv Exp Med Biol 771:123–138. PMID: 23393676

Hambleton IR, Jonnalagadda R, Davis CR, Fraser HS, Chaturvedi N, Hennis AJ (2009) All-cause mortality after diabetes-related amputation in Barbados: a prospective case-control study. Diabetes Care 32(2):306–307. https://doi.org/10.2337/dc08-1504. Epub 2008 Nov 4. PMID: 18984775; PMCID: PMC2628698

Hammad RH, El-Madbouly AA, Kotb HG, Zarad MS (2018) Frequency of circulating B1a and B2 B-cell subsets in Egyptian patients with type 2 diabetes mellitus. Egypt J Immunol 25(1):71–80. PMID: 30242999

Heitzman J (2010) Foot care for patients with diabetes. Top Geriatr Rehabil 26(3):250–263. https://doi.org/10.1097/TGR.0b013e3181ef31c9

Hex N, Bartlett C, Wright D, Taylor M, Varley D (2012) Estimating the current and future costs of Type 1 and Type 2 diabetes in the UK, including direct health costs and indirect societal and productivity costs. Diabet Med 29(7):855–862. https://doi.org/10.1111/j.1464-5491.2012.03698.x. PMID: 22537247

Hill SL, Holtzman GI, Buse R (1999) The effects of peripheral vascular disease with osteomyelitis in the diabetic foot. Am J Surg 177(4):282–286. https://doi.org/10.1016/s0002-9610(99)00050-1

Hingorani A, LaMuraglia GM, Henke P, Meissner MH, Loretz L, Zinszer KM, Driver VR, Frykberg R, Carman TL, Marston W, Mills JL Sr, Murad MH (2016) The management of diabetic foot: a clinical practice guideline by the Society for Vascular Surgery in collaboration with the American Podiatric Medical Association and the Society for Vascular Medicine. J Vasc Surg 63(2 Suppl):3S–21S. https://doi.org/10.1016/j.jvs.2015.10.003. PMID: 26804367

Jayakumar Sunandhakumari V, Sadasivan A, Koshi E, Krishna A, Alim A, Sebastian A (2018) Effect of nonsurgical periodontal therapy on plasma levels of IL-17 in chronic periodontitis patients with well controlled type-II diabetes mellitus-a clinical study. Dent J (Basel) 6(2):19. https://doi.org/10.3390/dj6020019. PMID: 29899268; PMCID: PMC6023374

Jeffcoate WJ (2005) Theories concerning the pathogenesis of the acute Charcot foot suggest future therapy. Curr Diab Rep 5(6):430–435. https://doi.org/10.1007/s11892-005-0050-z

Jude EB, Eleftheriadou I, Tentolouris N (2010) Peripheral arterial disease in diabetes—a review. Diabet Med 27(1):4–14. https://doi.org/10.1111/j.1464-5491.2009.02866.x

Karchevsky M, Schweitzer ME, Morrison WB, Parellada JA (2004) MRI findings of septic arthritis and associated osteomyelitis in adults. AJR Am J Roentgenol 182(1):119–122. https://doi.org/10.2214/ajr.182.1.1820119. PMID: 14684523

Kartika R, Purnamasari D, Pradipta S, Larasati RA, Wibowo H (2020) Impact of low interferon-γ and IL-10 levels on TNF-α and IL-6 production by PHA-induced PBMCs in type 2 diabetes mellitus. J Inflamm Res 22(13):187–193. https://doi.org/10.2147/JIR.S245064. PMID: 32425577; PMCID: PMC7190380

Kerr M, Barron E, Chadwick P et al (2019) The cost of diabetic foot ulcers and amputations to the National Health Service in England. Diabet Med 36(8):995–1002. https://doi.org/10.1111/dme.13973

Klein RJ (2021) Etiology of diabetic foot wounds. https://dialoguesinwoundmanagement.com/etiology-of-diabetic-foot-wounds/

Koechner D, Petropoulos H, Eaton RP, Hart BL, Brooks WM (1995) Segmentation of small structures in MR images: semiautomated tissue hydration measurement. J Magn Reson Imaging 5(3):347–351. https://doi.org/10.1002/jmri.1880050320. PMID: 7633113

Kullo IJ, Rooke TW (2016) Clinical practice. Peripheral artery disease. N Engl J Med 374(9):861–871.

https://doi.org/10.1056/NEJMcp1507631. PMID: 26962905

Lavery LA, Peters EJ, Armstrong DG, Wendel CS, Murdoch DP, Lipsky BA (2009) Risk factors for developing osteomyelitis in patients with diabetic foot wounds. Diabetes Res Clin Pract 83(3):347–352. https://doi.org/10.1016/j.diabres.2008.11.030. Epub 2008 Dec 30. PMID: 19117631

Ledermann HP, Morrison WB, Schweitzer ME (2002) MR image analysis of pedal osteomyelitis: distribution, patterns of spread, and frequency of associated ulceration and septic arthritis. Radiology 223(3):747–755. https://doi.org/10.1148/radiol.2233011279. PMID: 12034944

Levitt K, Vivas L, Courtney B, Connelly KA (2014) Vascular imaging in diabetes. Curr Atheroscler Rep 16(4):399. https://doi.org/10.1007/s11883-014-0399-z. PMID: 24493479

Lipsky BA, Berendt AR, Deery HG, Embil JM, Joseph WS, Karchmer AW, LeFrock JL, Lew DP, Mader JT, Norden C, Tan JS, Infectious Diseases Society of America (2004) Diagnosis and treatment of diabetic foot infections. Clin Infect Dis 39(7):885–910. https://doi.org/10.1086/424846. Epub 2004 Sep 10. PMID: 15472838

Lipsky BA, Peters EJ, Senneville E, Berendt AR, Embil JM, Lavery LA, Urbančič-Rovan V, Jeffcoate WJ (2012) Expert opinion on the management of infections in the diabetic foot. Diabetes Metab Res Rev 28(Suppl 1):163–178. https://doi.org/10.1002/dmrr.2248. PMID: 22271739

Loredo R, Rahal A, Garcia G, Metter D (2010) Imaging of the diabetic foot diagnostic dilemmas. Foot Ankle Spec 3(5):249–264. https://doi.org/10.1177/1938640010383154

Low KT, Peh WC (2015) Magnetic resonance imaging of diabetic foot complications. Singapore Med J 56(1):23–33; quiz 34. https://doi.org/10.11622/smedj.2015006. PMID: 25640096; PMCID: PMC4325563

Mandell JC, Khurana B, Smith JT, Czuczman GJ, Ghazikhanian V, Smith SE (2018) Osteomyelitis of the lower extremity: pathophysiology, imaging, and classification, with an emphasis on diabetic foot infection. Emerg Radiol 25(2):175–188. https://doi.org/10.1007/s10140-017-1564-9. Epub 2017 Oct 20. PMID: 29058098

Marso SP, Hiatt WR (2006) Peripheral arterial disease in patients with diabetes. J Am Coll Cardiol 47(5):921–929. https://doi.org/10.1016/j.jacc.2005.09.065. Epub 2006 Feb 9. PMID: 16516072

Mautone M, Naidoo P (2015) What the radiologist needs to know about Charcot foot. J Med Imaging Radiat Oncol 59(4):395–402. https://doi.org/10.1111/1754-9485.12325

McCullough PA, Agrawal V, Danielewicz E, Abela GS (2008) Accelerated atherosclerotic calcification and Monckeberg's sclerosis: a continuum of advanced vascular pathology in chronic kidney disease. Clin J Am Soc Nephrol 3(6):1585–1598. https://doi.org/10.2215/CJN.01930408. Epub 2008 Jul 30. PMID: 18667741

Mettler MA (2005) Essentials of radiology. Elsevier Saunders, Philadelphia, PA

Meyers SP, Wiener SN (1991) Magnetic resonance imaging features of fractures using the short tau inversion recovery (STIR) sequence: correlation with radiographic findings. Skeletal Radiol 20(7):499–507. https://doi.org/10.1007/BF00194246. PMID: 1754911

Morrison WB, Ledermann HP (2002) Work-up of the diabetic foot. Radiol Clin North Am 40(5):1171–1192. https://doi.org/10.1016/s0033-8389(02)00036-2. PMID: 12462475

Mostaza JM, Suarez C, Manzano L, Cairols M, López-Fernández F, Aguilar I, Diz Lois F, Sampedro JL, Sánchez-Huelva H, Sanchez-Zamorano MA, Merito Study Group (2008) Sub-clinical vascular disease in type 2 diabetic subjects: relationship with chronic complications of diabetes and the presence of cardiovascular disease risk factors. Eur J Intern Med 19(4):255–260. https://doi.org/10.1016/j.ejim.2007.06.018. Epub 2008 Feb 21. PMID: 18471673

Mutluoglu M, Uzun G, Turhan V, Gorenek L, Ay H, Lipsky BA (2012) How reliable are cultures of specimens from superficial swabs compared with those of deep tissue in patients with diabetic foot ulcers? J Diabetes Complications 26(3):225–229. https://doi.org/10.1016/j.jdiacomp.2012.03.015

Newman LG, Waller J, Palestro CJ, Schwartz M, Klein MJ, Hermann G, Harrington E, Harrington M, Roman SH, Stagnaro-Green A (1991) Unsuspected osteomyelitis in diabetic foot ulcers. Diagnosis and monitoring by leukocyte scanning with indium in 111 oxyquinoline. JAMA 266(9):1246–1251. https://doi.org/10.1001/jama.266.9.1246. PMID: 1908030

Panchbhavi VK, Hecox SE (2006) All that is gas is not gas gangrene: mechanical spread of gas in the soft tissues. A case report. J Bone Joint Surg Am 88(6):1345–1348. https://doi.org/10.2106/JBJS.E.01172. PMID: 16757770

Petrova NL, Dew TK, Musto RL et al (2015) Inflammatory and bone turnover markers in a cross-sectional and prospective study of acute Charcot osteoarthropathy. Diabet Med 32(2):267–273. https://doi.org/10.1111/dme.12590

Pineda C, Espinosa R, Pena A (2009) Radiographic imaging in osteomyelitis: the role of plain radiography, computed tomography, ultrasonography, magnetic resonance imaging, and scintigraphy. Semin Plast Surg 23(2):80–89. https://doi.org/10.1055/s-0029-1214160. PMID: 20567730; PMCID: PMC2884903

Pomposelli F (2010) Arterial imaging in patients with lower extremity ischemia and diabetes mellitus. J Vasc Surg 52(3 Suppl):81S–91S. https://doi.org/10.1016/j.jvs.2010.06.013. PMID: 20804938

Rajbhandari SM, Jenkins RC, Davies C, Tesfaye S (2002) Charcot neuroarthropathy in diabetes mellitus. Diabetologia 45(8):1085–1096. https://doi.

org/10.1007/s00125-002-0885-7. Epub 2002 Jul 11. PMID: 12189438

Rhee SY, Guan H, Liu ZM, Cheng SW, Waspadji S, Palmes P, Tai TY, Suwanwalaikorn S, Kim YS, PAD-SEARCH Study Group (2007) Multi-country study on the prevalence and clinical features of peripheral arterial disease in Asian type 2 diabetes patients at high risk of atherosclerosis. Diabetes Res Clin Pract 76(1):82–92. https://doi.org/10.1016/j.diabres.2006.07.029. Epub 2006 Sep 6. PMID: 16950543

Richard JL, Lavigne JP, Got I, Hartemann A, Malgrange D, Tsirtsikolou D, Baleydier A, Senneville E (2011) Management of patients hospitalized for diabetic foot infection: results of the French OPIDIA study. Diabetes Metab 37(3):208–215. https://doi.org/10.1016/j.diabet.2010.10.003. Epub 2010 Dec 18. PMID: 21169044

Roug IK, Pierre-Jerome C (2012) MRI spectrum of bone changes in the diabetic foot. Eur J Radiol 81(7):1625–1629. https://doi.org/10.1016/j.ejrad.2011.04.048. Epub 2011 May 28. PMID: 21620598

Sagray BA, Stapleton JJ, Zgonis T (2013) Diabetic calcaneal fractures. Clin Podiatr Med Surg 30(1):111–118. https://doi.org/10.1016/j.cpm.2012.09.001. Epub 2012 Oct 11. PMID: 23164444

Santoro L, Flex A, Nesci A, Ferraro PM, De Matteis G, Di Giorgio A, Giupponi B, Saviano L, Gambaro G, Franceschi F, Gasbarrini A, Landolfi R, Santoliquido A (2018) Association between peripheral arterial disease and cardiovascular risk factors: role of ultrasonography versus ankle-brachial index. Eur Rev Med Pharmacol Sci 22(10):3160–3165. https://doi.org/10.26355/eurrev_201805_15076. PMID: 29863271

Schara K, Štukelj R, Krek JL et al (2017) A study of extracellular vesicle concentration in active diabetic Charcot neuroarthropathy. Eur J Pharm Sci 98:58–63. https://doi.org/10.1016/j.ejps.2016.09.009

Schmohl M, Beckert S, Joos TO, Königsrainer A, Schneiderhan-Marra N, Löffler MW (2012) Superficial wound swabbing: a novel method of sampling and processing wound fluid for subsequent immunoassay analysis in diabetic foot ulcerations. Diabetes Care 35(11):2113–2120. https://doi.org/10.2337/dc11-2547. Epub 2012 Jul 26. PMID: 22837363; PMCID: PMC3476897

Schoots IG, Slim FJ, Busch-Westbroek TE, Maas M (2010) Neuro-osteoarthropathy of the foot—radiologist: friend or foe? In: Seminars in musculoskeletal radiology, vol 14(03). Thieme Medical Publishers, pp 365–376

Sella EJ, Barrette C (1999) Staging of Charcot neuroarthropathy along the medial column of the foot in the diabetic patient. J Foot Ankle Surg 38(1):34–40. https://doi.org/10.1016/s1067-2516(99)80086-6

Selvin E, Marinopoulos S, Berkenblit G, Rami T, Brancati FL, Powe NR, Golden SH (2004) Meta-analysis: glycosylated hemoglobin and cardiovascular disease in diabetes mellitus. Ann Intern Med 141(6):421–431. https://doi.org/10.7326/0003-4819-141-6-200409210-00007. PMID: 15381515

Simpfendorfer CS (2017) Radiologic approach to musculoskeletal infections. Infect Dis Clin North Am 31(2):299–324. https://doi.org/10.1016/j.idc.2017.01.004. Epub 2017 Mar 30. PMID: 28366223

Sinacore DR, Hastings MK, Bohnert KL, Strube MJ, Gutekunst DJ, Johnson JE (2017) Immobilization-induced osteolysis and recovery in neuropathic foot impairments. Bone 105:237–244. https://doi.org/10.1016/j.bone.2017.09.009. Epub 2017 Sep 20. PMID: 28942120; PMCID: PMC5650927

Singh R, Kishore L, Kaur N (2014) Diabetic peripheral neuropathy: current perspective and future directions. Pharmacol Res 80:21–35. https://doi.org/10.1016/j.phrs.2013.12.005. Epub 2013 Dec 25. PMID: 24373831

Starr AM, Wessely MA, Albastaki U, Pierre-Jerome C, Kettner NW (2008) Bone marrow oedema: pathophysiology, differential diagnosis, and imaging. Acta Radiol 49(7):771–786. https://doi.org/10.1080/02841850802161023. PMID: 18608031

Stoberock K, Kaschwich M, Nicolay SS, Mahmoud N, Heidemann F, Rieß HC, Debus ES, Behrendt CA (2021) The interrelationship between diabetes mellitus and peripheral arterial disease. Vasa 50(5):323–330. https://doi.org/10.1024/0301-1526/a000925. Epub 2020 Nov 11. PMID: 33175668

Tesfaye S, Selvarajah D (2012) Advances in the epidemiology, pathogenesis and management of diabetic peripheral neuropathy. Diabetes Metab Res Rev 28(Suppl 1):8–14. https://doi.org/10.1002/dmrr.2239. PMID: 22271716

Trepman E, Nihal A, Pinzur MS (2005) Current topics review: Charcot neuroarthropathy of the foot and ankle. Foot Ankle Int 26(1):46–63. https://doi.org/10.1177/107110070502600109

Tseng CH, Chong CK, Tseng CP, Cheng JC, Wong MK, Tai TY (2008) Mortality, causes of death and associated risk factors in a cohort of diabetic patients after lower-extremity amputation: a 6.5-year follow-up study in Taiwan. Atherosclerosis 197(1):111–117. https://doi.org/10.1016/j.atherosclerosis.2007.02.011. Epub 2007 Mar 28. PMID: 17395186

Uccioli L, Gandini R, Giurato L et al (2010) Long-term outcomes of diabetic patients with critical limb ischemia followed in a tertiary referral diabetic foot clinic. Diabetes Care 33(5):977–982. https://doi.org/10.2337/dc09-0831

Wukich DK, McMillen RL, Lowery NJ, Frykberg RG (2011) Surgical site infections after foot and ankle surgery: a comparison of patients with and without diabetes. Diabetes Care 34(10):2211–2213. https://doi.org/10.2337/dc11-0846. Epub 2011 Aug 4. PMID: 21816974; PMCID: PMC3177737

Wülker N, Mittag F (2012) The treatment of hallux valgus. Dtsch Arztebl Int 109(49):857–67; quiz 868. https://doi.org/10.3238/arztebl.2012.0857.

Epub 2012 Dec 7. PMID: 23267411; PMCID: PMC3528062

Yeoh J, Muir KR, Dissanayake AM, Tzu-Chieh WY (2008) Lisfranc fracture-dislocation precipitating acute Charcot arthopathy in a neuropathic diabetic foot: a case report. Cases J 1(1):290. https://doi.org/10.1186/1757-1626-1-290. PMID: 18973700; PMCID: PMC2584082

Zhang P, Lu J, Jing Y, Tang S, Zhu D, Bi Y (2017) Global epidemiology of diabetic foot ulceration: a systematic review and meta-analysis. Ann Med 49(2):106–116. https://doi.org/10.1080/07853890.2016.1231932

Foot and Ankle Inflammatory Arthritis

Iwona Sudoł-Szopińska, Anne Cotten, and James Teh

Contents

I. Sudoł-Szopińska (✉)
Department of Radiology, National Institute of Geriatrics, Rheumatology and Rehabilitation, Warsaw, Poland
e-mail: sudolszopinska@gmail.com

A. Cotten
Service de Radiologie et Imagerie Musculosquelettique, CHU de Lille, Lille University, Lille Cedex, France

J. Teh
Department of Radiology, Nuffield Orthopaedic Centre, Oxford University Hospitals NHS Foundation Trust, Oxford, UK

Abstract

This chapter discusses imaging findings in the most common inflammatory arthropathies affecting the foot and ankle, belonging to the two main subgroups: connective tissue diseases and spondyloarthritis. The connective tissue subgroup is comprised of rheumatoid

Med Radiol Diagn Imaging (2023)
https://doi.org/10.1007/174_2023_398,
Published Online: 11 April 2023

arthritis, juvenile idiopathic arthritis, adult-onset Still's disease, systemic lupus erythematosus, systemic sclerosis, polymyositis, and dermatomyositis. The spondyloarthritis subgroup is comprised of ankylosing spondylitis, reactive arthritis, arthritis associated with inflammatory bowel diseases, psoriatic arthritis, and undifferentiated spondyloarthritis.

Radiography, ultrasonography and magnetic resonance imaging features are listed for each of the aforementioned entities in adults and juveniles. Pathological findings and imaging features for a wide spectrum of diseases are presented. The main roles of imaging in achieving an early diagnosis, monitoring disease progression, and assessing remission are illustrated.

Abbreviations

AOSD	Adult-onset Still's disease
AP	Anteroposterior
AS	Ankylosing spondylitis
CD	Crohn's disease
CMC	Carpometacarpal
DIP	Distal interphalangeal
DM	Dermatomyositis
DP	Dorsoplantar
IP	Interphalangeal
JAS	Juvenile ankylosing spondylitis
JIA	Juvenile idiopathic arthritis
JPsA	Juvenile psoriatic arthritis
JSN	Joint space narrowing
MCTD	Mixed connective tissue disease
MTP	Metatarsophalangeal
OA	Osteoarthritis
PA	Posteroanterior
PDUS	Power Doppler ultrasound
PIP	Proximal interphalangeal
PM	Polymyositis
PsA	Psoriatic arthritis
RA	Rheumatoid arthritis
ReA	Reactive arthritis
SAPHO	Synovitis, acne, pustulosis, hyperostosis, and osteitis syndrome
SLE	Systemic lupus erythematosus
SpA	Spondyloarthritis/spondyloarthropathy
SSc	Systemic sclerosis/scleroderma
UA	Undifferentiated arthritis
UC	Ulcerative colitis
USpA	Undifferentiated arthritis

1 Introduction

The most common arthropathies affecting the foot and ankle are osteoarthritis (OA), rheumatoid arthritis (RA), and gout. This chapter focuses on inflammatory rheumatic diseases, which form a heterogeneous group of predominantly chronic autoimmune disorders that can be divided into two main subgroups: connective tissue diseases and spondyloarthritis (SpA). The former includes rheumatoid arthritis (RA), juvenile idiopathic arthritis (JIA), adult-onset Still's disease (AOSD), systemic lupus erythematosus (SLE), systemic sclerosis (SSc), polymyositis (PM), and dermatomyositis (DM), less frequent diseases. The latter includes ankylosing spondylitis (AS), reactive arthritis (ReA), arthritis associated with inflammatory bowel diseases (IBD-related arthritis), psoriatic arthritis (PsA), and undifferentiated spondyloarthritis (USpA).

The foot and ankle are most often affected by RA, PsA, SSc, SLE, and JIA. Other rarer conditions are DM, PM, other than PsA forms of SpA, and other than JIA rare diseases of the developmental age, such as juvenile scleroderma. Overlapping syndromes may also be encountered. These are conditions where patients present with a clinical picture of at least two rheumatic diseases along with the presence of a specific serological marker (Znajdek et al. 2019). Mixed connective tissue disease (MCTD) is an example of an overlapping syndrome, as it may give a clinical picture of SLE, SS, PM or DM, and RA or PsA (Thibaut et al. 2018) (Fig. 1).

The main roles of imaging in inflammatory arthritis are to achieve an early diagnosis, establish the extent of abnormality, and assess for disease progression or remission. US and MRI are the primary methods utilized for the early diagnosis of disease, as they allow visualization of

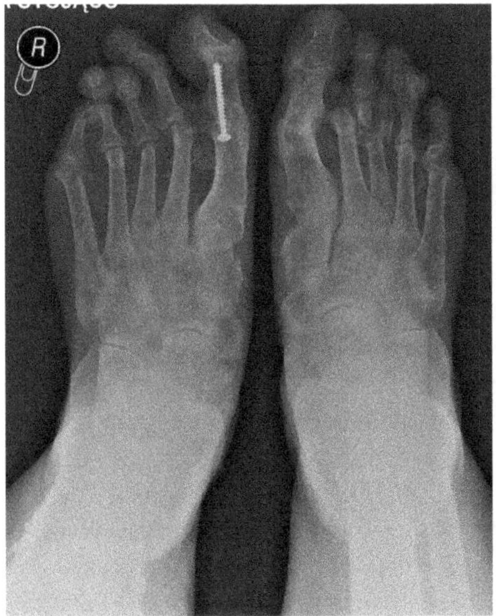

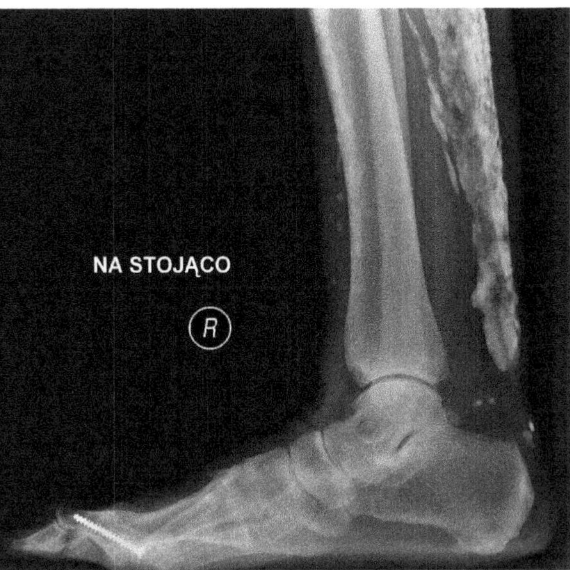

Fig. 1 A 64-year-old female with an overlapping syndrome: RA and DM, following surgery for hallux valgus deformity and osteotomies. X-ray of feet demonstrates osteoporosis and diffuse calcifications in the soft tissues of the right calf

pre-radiographic inflammatory changes such as synovitis, tenosynovitis, and bursitis. MRI may demonstrate bone marrow changes, which may predict future joint damage such as erosions, and may be useful for monitoring the course of the disease. In the early stages of disease, radiography may show no abnormality but remains a useful technique as a baseline for future follow-up and for determining the pattern of disease involvement, which may be useful in establishing a specific diagnosis.

2 Differential Diagnosis

2.1 Monoarthritis, Oligoarthritis, or Polyarthritis

In patients presenting with ankle monoarthritis (defined as arthritis affecting one joint), the diagnostic considerations are different from patients with oligoarthritis (defined as arthritis affecting two to four joints) and with polyarthritis (five and more joints are affected), in whom the ankle is involved.

Mjaavatten et al. (2009) evaluated the pattern of joint involvement in 634 patients with arthritis. At initial presentation, around a third of inflammatory arthritis patients were found to have ankle synovitis. Involvement of the ankle was more frequent in those presenting with oligoarthritis (43.5%) than in those presenting with monoarthritis (18.9%) or polyarthritis (33.7%) (Mjaavatten et al. 2009). In those presenting with oligoarthritis, the ankle was the most common involved joint followed by the knee. In patients with polyarthritis, the small joints were most commonly involved (Mjaavatten et al. 2009).

Norli et al. (2020) found that in a group of 347 patients with acute monoarthritis of less than 16 weeks' duration, the ankle was involved in 16.7%, which was the second most commonly affected joint after the knee (49.3%). They followed the patients over 2 years, and in nearly 90% of cases, the eventual outcome of ankle monoarthritis was resolution, degenerative disease, or gout, with around 10% progressing to a chronic inflammatory arthritis, classified as either SpA or undifferentiated arthritis (Norli et al. 2020). In their cohort however, they had no cases of RA or psoriatic arthritis (PsA). The ankle was found to have an odds ratio of 0.5 (0.2–1.2) on multivariate analysis for developing any chronic inflammatory arthritis compared to 2.0 (1.0–4.2) for the wrist (Norli et al. 2020).

Jeong et al. (2013) found in a group of 171 arthritis patients that the ankle was the third most affected joint in 18.7%, after the knee (24%) and wrist (22.8%). In 32 patients with ankle monoarthritis, progression occurred in 20 cases (62.5%) and multivariate analysis showed that ankle monoarthritis was predictive of a final diagnosis of peripheral SpA with an odds ratio of 3.04 (Jeong et al. 2013).

2.2 Non-autoimmune arthropathies

Many of the imaging features of inflammatory arthritis in the foot and ankle are nonspecific. The imaging findings need to be taken in conjunction with the clinical history, examination, and further investigations, including blood tests to establish a specific diagnosis. In patients who present with an acutely inflamed ankle or foot, in the absence of trauma, it is important to determine if it is a monoarthritis, oligoarthritis, or polyarthritis. With any acute inflammatory monoarthritis, infection should always be excluded. When infection has been excluded, the findings are more likely to represent undifferentiated arthritis or peripheral SpA than RA. If the cause is crystal arthritis, gout is more common than calcium pyrophosphate dihydrate deposition disease (CPPD). If the presentation is of a polyarthritis with involvement of the ankle, the findings are likely to represent peripheral SpA or RA.

In patients who present with a chronic history or established arthropathy of the ankle, it is again crucial to ascertain if it is a monoarthritis or polyarthritis. Another important feature to determine is if the findings are predominantly of osteoarthritis or synovitis. If osteoarthritis is the main feature, then previous trauma should be considered. If there is no history of trauma, hemochromatosis and hemophilia should be excluded. If the patient is diabetic, a Charcot joint is the primary consideration. If synovitis is the predominant feature, then RA and peripheral spondyloarthritis are the main considerations, particularly if other joints are involved. In established inflammatory arthropathy of the ankle and foot, there may be patterns of involvement that can suggest a specific disease process, and radiographs assume a key role in the diagnostic process.

3 Imaging Modalities

3.1 Radiography (X-rays)

Plain radiography remains an important imaging technique for the diagnosis of foot and ankle arthropathy although early pathological changes such as synovitis are poorly demonstrated. In established disease, radiography has a key role in delineating the pattern of disease involvement, which may indicate a specific diagnosis. For instance, RA typically involves joints bilaterally, while SpA or gout often affects only one foot or ankle. Furthermore, radiography has an important role in determining the degree of progression and surgical planning. Typically, for the evaluation of suspected arthritis of the foot and ankle, bilateral X-rays are taken in two standard projections to avoid bone superimposition. For the feet, these are the dorsoplantar (DP) and oblique views, and for the ankle joint, these are the anteroposterior (AP) and lateral views. The oblique and lateral projections of the foot and ankle increase the detectability of lesions (e.g., cysts, erosions, joint space narrowing) and joints (e.g., inferior ankle joint). Additional views can be useful when static deformities have developed.

3.2 Ultrasonography (US)

Foot and ankle ultrasound is frequently performed for the evaluation of inflammatory lesions in peripheral joints, tendon sheaths, bursae, as well as entheses. In contrast to radiography, US allows assessment of soft tissues for synovitis, tenosynovitis, bursitis, and enthesitis and is also able to detect erosions and cartilage lesions.

US is performed for (Plagou et al. 2016; Miller et al. 2017):

- Early diagnosis—important as early treatment before joint damage prevents progression

- Disease activity assessment
- Follow-up/therapy monitoring
- Interventions—for both diagnosis and treatment

Foot and ankle US should be performed using a high-frequency linear transducer (Plagou et al. 2016; Miller et al. 2017; Taljanovic et al. 2015). Tissue harmonic imaging, spatial compound imaging, and extended field-of-view (panoramic) imaging are some of the software capabilities that may be useful (Miller et al. 2017). Matrix array probes, sensitive Doppler techniques including even more sensitive than power and color Doppler that evaluate microcirculation, elastography including strain and shear wave elastography, and microcalcification imaging increase the diagnostic capacity of US. The ESSR (*European Society of Musculoskeletal Radiology*) arthritis subcommittee has produced Musculoskeletal Ultrasound Technical Guidelines (Plagou et al. 2016; Miller et al. 2017; Martinoli 2010). A dynamic scanning technique by means of slight movements of translation (side-to-side, back-to-front), angulation, and rotation of the probe should be carried out in order to allow the best visualization of the structure of interest (Miller et al. 2017). To avoid anisotropy (the anisotropic artifact refers to a darkening and loss of resolution of the image, which occurs when the approach of the ultrasound waves is less than perpendicular) and the common pitfalls that accompany it, the probe should be continuously adjusted to maintain the beam perpendicular to the fibers especially at insertions (Miller et al. 2017).

Familiarity with the normal US features of joints, tendons, ligaments, and surrounding tissues is a prerequisite for performing US (Plagou et al. 2016). The Outcome Measures in Rheumatology (OMERACT) group has published a consensus of US definitions of pathologic findings seen in inflammatory arthropathies that are widely used (Plagou et al. 2016; Taljanovic et al. 2015; Bruyn et al. 2019).

The ankle joint is evaluated with the patient in the supine position with flexed knees and the foot resting on the bed and extended anteriorly to enable exact contact of the probe with the anterior tibiotalar joint surface. As for the foot, the dorsal and plantar aspects are evaluated with the latter being scanned with the patient in the prone position or with the foot crossed over the contralateral knee. Apart from the static assessment, the scanning also involves the evaluation of the pronation and supination movements in order to assess joint movement, anterior drawer test, or examination of the intermetatarsal bursae while squeezing the forefoot.

The tibiotalar joint should be assessed in the sagittal plane from side to side. The subtalar joint should be evaluated from both the lateral and medial aspects in the coronal plane. The talonavicular and the calcaneocuboid joints are best assessed in the sagittal plane, as are the joints of the foot.

The flexor tendons (tibialis posterior tendon, flexor digitorum longus, hallucis longus), extensor tendons (tibialis anterior tendon, extensor hallucis longus, and digitorum longus), and peroneal tendons (longus and brevis) should be evaluated in both the longitudinal and axial planes. The Achilles tendon and plantar fascia entheses should specifically be interrogated as this is frequently affected by inflammatory arthritis. The so-called enthesis organ also includes the bursa and the Kager's fat pad and is often affected in SpA, as well as RA (Benjamin and McGonagle 2009).

3.3 Magnetic Resonance Imaging (MRI)

MRI with its multiplanar capability, excellent soft tissue contrast resolution, and ability to visualize the bone marrow has an important role in the early diagnosis of inflammation, monitoring response to therapy and identification of disease complications (Sudoł-Szopińska et al. 2015a, b, c).

Foot and ankle MRI should be performed using a dedicated coil. In certain situations, such as a large patient, or the presence of a plaster cast, a head and neck coil or a flex coil can be used.

MRI protocols should be adjusted taking into consideration the scanner specifications, available coils, and image quality in particular sequences (Sudoł-Szopińska et al. 2015a, b, c).

Short-tau inversion recovery (STIR) or turbo inversion recovery magnitude (TIRM), T2-weighted sequences with fat suppression (T2FS), T2-weighted Dixon, proton density (PD) FS, T1-weighted sequences with or without FS, and pre- and/or postcontrast imaging may be used (Sudoł-Szopińska et al. 2015a, b, c). Isotropic 3D sequences can also be very useful in the feet, mainly for detection of erosions. Diffusion tensor imaging (DTI) is potentially relevant for the diagnosis of muscle diseases (e.g., dermatomyositis) and for the assessment of cartilage structure. MR spectroscopy allows assessment of tissue metabolism and biochemical composition, e.g., in juvenile dermatomyositis (attempts to use 31P-MRS phosphorus).

The size of the field of view and the matrix as well as the slice thickness should be appropriately adjusted; the recommended maximal slice thickness for ankle is 3 mm, with interslice gap of 0.3 mm; the slice thickness for foot is 2 mm with interslice gap of 0.3 mm.

The sequences recommended by the ESSR Arthritis Subcommittee for ankle and foot scanning are listed in the Recommendation paper (Sudoł-Szopińska et al. 2015a, b, c). The images should be obtained in at least two (usually three) perpendicular planes. MRI with intravenous contrast injection is performed mainly to determine the degree of inflammation of thickened synovium. In JIA, there are ongoing discussions about the standard use of contrast in MRI due to accumulation of contrast in the central nervous system and kidneys (Damasio et al. 2013; Nusman et al. 2016; Gulani et al. 2017; Ranga et al. 2017).

3.4 Computed Tomography (CT)

CT with its multiplanar capability and excellent depiction of bone is the best method for the assessment of erosions. Dual-energy CT has an important role for the diagnosis of gout (Teh et al. 2018).

3.5 Nuclear Medicine Imaging

Scintigraphy is a functional imaging modality that entails the administration of a radioisotope and mapping of its distribution in a given tissue. It is possible both to perform dynamic and static acquisitions and to combine the images with CT (SPECT-CT) to provide improved anatomical depiction. The lesions detected on bone scintigraphy can significantly precede the signs shown on X-rays.

3.6 Positron Emission Tomography (PET)

PET scans using 18-fluorodeoxyglucose (FDG) enable semiquantitative evaluation of the uptake and metabolism of glucose in inflammatory cells and can play a useful role in the assessment of inflammatory arthritides.

4 Pathological Findings in Inflammatory Arthritis of the Foot and Ankle

4.1 Periarticular Soft Tissues and Synovium

Juxta-articular soft tissue thickening seen on X-rays results from intra-articular or periarticular tissue inflammation (synovitis, tenosynovitis, bursitis, periarticular fat tissue inflammation). In RA, the thickening is usually bilateral, whereas in SpA it is more often unilateral or may just affect one toe (dactylitis/"sausage toe").

Synovitis is the hallmark feature of rheumatic diseases. It manifests as an effusion with synovial thickening of joint capsules, tendon sheaths, or bursae.

On US, the echogenicity of the inflamed synovium is low, similar to that of an effusion, which usually accompanies synovial pathologies. In chronic conditions, the echogenicity of thickened synovium increases. Probe compression can be helpful in distinguishing a compressible fluid collection from a non-compressible synovium (Miller et al. 2017). Minimal compression is important when performing Doppler examination to avoid blocking blood flow in small vessels within the synovium (Miller et al. 2017). As the disease develops, increased vascularity is visible on Doppler interrogation. Following treatment, reduced vascularity of the synovium or tenosynovium indicates a good response, while the lack of vascularity is one of the features indicative of remission.

On MRI, joint effusions are hyperintense on T2- and PD-weighted images and hypointense on T1-weighted images and do not enhance immediately after intravenous gadolinium (Sudoł-Szopińska et al. 2015a, b, c). Normal synovium is very thin and only enhances slightly following intravenous contrast administration. Thickened synovium has intermediate to high signal on T2-weighted images. Synovitis should be assessed in postcontrast T1 FS sequences, especially in small joints of feet (and hands). The enhancement within the synovial membrane should be examined optimally within 10 min after contrast administration (Ostergaard and Klarlund 2001). After this time, the contrast agent permeates into the synovial fluid. In chronic inflammation, synovial enhancement is lower due to the presence of fibrosis. Fibrotic synovium does not enhance and is isointense in relation to muscle. Dynamic contrast-enhanced MRI (DCE-MRI) allows the quantitative assessment of the degree of enhancement of inflamed synovium and has a role in diagnosing and evaluating inflammatory arthritis (Axelsen et al. 2012; Boesen et al. 2018).

In chronic conditions, thickened, hypertrophied synovium may undergo fragmentation, which may result in loose intra-articular bodies, which can resemble "rice bodies." Joint destruction may result in intra-articular mineralized bodies, and osteochondral lesions may become apparent. Lipoma arborescens is another finding that may coexist with the thickened synovium, and RA may cause secondary lipoma arborescens (Coll et al. 2011).

4.2 Tendons and Tendon Sheaths

Inflammation of the tendon sheath is described as tenosynovitis. It is manifest by a thickened tenosynovium and increased vascularity, frequently with an accompanying effusion. With chronicity, the tenosynovium may exhibit increased echogenicity without hyperemia. In the foot and ankle, the long flexors and peroneal tendons are most frequently affected. In inflammatory arthropathies, a combination of intrinsic tendon inflammation (tendinitis), usually secondary to tenosynovitis, and microtears with collagen degeneration (tendinosis) may result in macroscopic tendon tears or complete tendon rupture.

US has a useful role in assessing tendon tears. It can help determine the presence of injury, the exact site, and the distance between tendon stumps. Dynamic examination may be used to determine tendon excursion and reveal adhesions or scarring in the tendon sheath. A dynamic examination may also demonstrate subluxation of the peroneal tendons resulting from a tear of the peroneal retinaculum.

On MRI, fluid in the tendon sheath is seen as high T2 signal. Following intravenous contrast, there may be variable enhancement depending on the degree of synovial thickening. Features of tendinopathy include tendon thickening and loss of normal, low signal on T1- and T2-weighted images. Partial tendon tears are seen as hyperintense areas on T2-weighted images with loss of continuity of fibers or as longitudinal splits along the length of the tendon. Full-thickness tears result in complete loss of continuity of fibers with retraction of tendon ends.

4.3 Bursae

The pre-Achilles and retro-calcaneal bursae are frequently inflamed in rheumatic diseases, particularly in RA. Bursitis is manifest by thickening and increased blood flow in the synovium as well as effusion and internal septations in chronic stages. Pre-Achilles bursitis can lead to inflammation of the Kager's fat pad and to erosions in the adjacent bone/bony wall of the bursa. The Achilles tendon itself may become secondarily inflamed and tendinopathic.

Intermetatarsal and adventitial submetatarsal bursal inflammation may also occur in inflammatory arthropathies. These bursae are often missed by clinical examination (US vs. clinical examination: 92.6% vs. 23.5% in RA) (Fodor et al. 2022). In patients with metatarsalgia, US-detected intermetatarsal bursa distension was the most common underlying pathology (Fodor et al. 2022).

4.4 Entheses

The "enthesis organ" is comprised of the tendon, its bony insertion, and the adjacent bursa and fat tissue (Benjamin and McGonagle 2009; Sudoł-Szopińska et al. 2015a, b, c). Enthesitis is the hallmark feature of SpA. The calcaneal entheses of the Achilles tendon, plantar fascia and flexor digitorum brevis tendon are most frequently affected. Enthesopathic lesions on US include enthesis thickening, low echogenicity, delamination, and enthesophytes. Cysts and erosions may be seen at the bony attachment. Hyperemia of the enthesis in patients with inflammatory arthritis indicates active inflammation. However, in the context of trauma, it prognosticates a favorable reparative outcome (Sudoł-Szopińska et al. 2015a, b, c). In the lower limb, degenerative enthesopathic findings are common. The criteria for differentiation between inflammation-related enthesitis from metabolic, age, and overload-driven enthesopathy are yet to be firmly established (Pracoń et al. 2021; Dubash et al. 2020). Therefore, it is important to avoid overdiagnosis of inflammatory arthritis based on US findings alone (Plagou et al. 2016). Correlation with clinical and laboratory data is essential. Lack of correlation between US features of enthesitis and clinical, laboratory data has been shown by several researchers (Mandl et al. 2015). However, an enthesitis score developed in a recent GRAPPA study has reported the ability to differentiate between PsA and healthy controls (Tom 2019).

MRI is an excellent modality for visualizing active enthesitis as it is able to depict abnormal signal in the fibrous and bony parts of an enthesis, as well as peri-entheseal soft tissue involvement. On MRI, an abnormal enthesis demonstrates hyperintense signal on fluid-sensitive sequences and hypointense signal on T1-weighted images (Sudoł-Szopińska et al. 2015a, b, c). Bone marrow edema (BME) may be present. Both fibrous and bony parts show enhancement following contrast administration. The inflamed neighboring synovial and adipose tissues may also enhance. Enthesophytes can also be detected.

4.5 Dactylitis

Dactylitis ("sausage toe") is a specific feature of peripheral SpA, mainly PsA and ReA, and may result from a combination of tenosynovitis, synovitis, and subcutaneous inflammation (Sudoł-Szopińska and Pracoń 2016; Coates et al. 2012).

4.6 Nail Involvement

Enthesitis, synovitis, and osteitis are implicated in the pathogenesis of nail involvement in PsA patients. It has been suggested that the entheses, which reach to the nail bed and envelop the DIP joint, transmit the inflammation in this region, or that the inflammation may originate in the bone and subsequently extend to the nail bed (Tan et al. 2006; Scarpa et al. 2006). There might also be a link between DIP joint inflammation and onychopathy (Sudoł-Szopińska et al. 2015a, b, c). Ultrasound and MRI may be used in the evaluation of nail pathologies, namely DIP joint synovitis, distal phalanx osteitis, and enthesopathic lesions at the attachments of collateral ligaments at the DIP joint and at the attachment of the extensor and flexor tendons. Ultrasound with high-frequency probes and sensitive Doppler techniques provides additional information on nail bad, matrix, and nail root vascularity. Performance of nail US has been standardized through a consensus-based methodology by an international expert working group (Fodor et al. 2022).

4.7 Bone

Demineralization/bone loss (osteopenia or osteoporosis) occurs in almost all rheumatic diseases. Initially, increased bone lucency is found on X-rays in the periarticular area, but it may become generalized as the disease progresses. In PsA, bone density tends to be preserved until late stages of the disease.

MRI allows assessment for BME, which indicates bone marrow inflammation believed to represent a pre-erosional stage (Sudoł-Szopińska et al. 2017a, b). Hetland et al. (2010) showed that BME and anti-CCP antibodies predicted radiographic progression in early RA in the CIMESTRA trial. BME may appear within several weeks of the onset of disease and is considered a very early marker of inflammation. In the early stage of disease, BME is a reversible phenomenon and may subside with treatment.

BME is seen as a hyperintense area with ill-defined margins on fluid-sensitive sequences. It is of intermediate/low signal on T1-weighted images, although the underlying bony architecture may still be visible. Following contrast administration, there may be enhancement (Sudoł-Szopińska et al. 2015a, b, c). In PsA, BME in the peripheral joints might be more diffuse than in other forms of SpA (Tom 2019; Narvaez et al. 2012). In DM, PM, and CRMO, bone marrow is the primary site of pathology, and therefore MRI is the basis of early diagnosis (Thibaut et al. 2018; Sudoł-Szopińska et al. 2020; Jurik et al. 2018).

Erosions are the hallmark of many rheumatic diseases. As joint inflammation progresses, ectopic lymphatic tissue that forms in the subintima begins secreting cytokines and enzymes that cause degradation of the connective tissue (Sudoł-Szopińska et al. 2012). The affected synovium hypertrophies and results in pannus, which leads to hyaline cartilage destruction and erosions in a so-called outside-in mechanism. Erosions may occur particularly early in RA. During the first 2 years of the disease, erosions are found in the majority of patients, and in up to 25% during the first 3 months of the disease (van der Heijde et al. 1995). An alternative mechanism by which erosions occur (so-called inside-out mechanism) is by inflammatory infiltration of the subchondral tissue causing inflammatory cysts, which take the form of erosions after cortical damage (Ostrowska et al. 2018).

Joint erosions initially develop in the so-called bare area, i.e., the area not covered by cartilage, between the border of an articular cartilage surface and the site of joint capsule attachment, described as marginal erosions. Subsequently, after the pannus destroys the hyaline cartilage, subchondral erosions develop. Erosions at the bone attachments of entheses are one of the components of enthesopathy, e.g., in the attachment of the Achilles tendon or plantar fascia to calcaneus, and are one of the most typical features of peripheral SpA. Surface erosions may occur beneath inflamed tenosynovium (e.g., erosion of the medial malleolus in the course of tibialis posterior tendon tenosynovitis). Erosions also develop in the bony wall of the bursa, secondary to pre-Achilles bursitis.

An erosion is seen on radiographs as a focal radiolucency reflecting eroded subchondral bone with a discontinuity of the cortical bone layer.

On US, erosions are visible as cortical bone defects of various sizes, in at least two planes. Active erosions may be filled with synovium that demonstrates increased vascularity on Doppler. Inflammatory cysts differ from erosions in that the cortical bone is preserved. Access to the entirety of the joint may be difficult on US, so MRI and CT have been shown to be superior for the detection of erosions (Dohn et al. 2006).

On MRI, a bone erosion is a sharply marginated trabecular bone defect with disrupted cortical bone continuity, seen in at least two planes with low signal intensity on T1-weighted images and T1 FS or in gradient sequences. It may be seen with or without concomitant BME and corresponds to subchondral plate or periostrium disruption and subchondral or subperiosteal tissue infiltrates on biopsy.

An inflammatory cyst/geode is a radiolucent area within the bone, usually round in shape, with a blurred outline and preserved cortical layer. It results from the destruction of the subchondral bone by inflammatory infiltrates. It should be differentiated from a degenerative cyst, which is usually larger and has a sclerotic border.

Osteolysis, progressive bone destruction, most often involves the distal, followed by proximal, phalanges of the feet. Acro-osteolysis refers to resorption of the terminal tuft and is most common in SSc and PsA, and less frequently in DM.

Proliferative changes include enthesophytes and osteophytes. Enthesophytes (bone spurs) mainly develop at the site of the attachment of the Achilles tendon and plantar fascia. They are a hallmark of peripheral SpA. Osteophytes, along with subchondral sclerosis, are a hallmark of OA. In rheumatic diseases, secondary degenerative changes develop.

Periosteal reaction (periostitis) is most often seen along the diaphyses of the metatarsals and phalanges. It develops in the course of JIA, PsA, ReA, juvenile PsA, ReA, or CRMO. Sometimes, it leads to the straightening of the concave diaphyseal outline or even to convex bulging.

Avascular necrosis may be seen in ankle, in patients with SLE.

4.8 Articulations

Joint space narrowing (JSN) on radiography indirectly indicates the destruction of the articular cartilage, which is not visible on radiographs. In inflammatory processes, JSN is uniform, in contrast to OA. The width of the joint space may also increase as a result of joint exudate.

Deformities, including contractures, subluxations, and dislocations, may result from both intra-articular lesions (damage to articular surfaces, like in RA) and extra-articular lesions (inflammation of joint capsule, ligaments, like in SLE).

Ankylosis is a fibrous or bony union of the joint. It is typically observed in patients with PsA, JIA, AS, and RA. The coexistence of ankylosis with destructive lesions (erosions, osteolytic lesions) in the foot is highly specific for PsA (Sudoł-Szopińska et al. 2016a, b).

4.9 The Skin, Subcutaneous Tissue, Fascia, and Muscle

There are several rheumatic diseases that may affect the skin, subcutaneous tissue, fascia, and muscles, including SSc, DM, and PM. For the superficial tissues, high-frequency ultrasound with sensitive Doppler and elastography are a valuable supplementation of the clinical assessment at an early stage of diagnosis, characterization of disease activity, quantifying of soft tissue involvement, and treatment monitoring (Thibaut et al. 2018; Fodor et al. 2022; Sudoł-Szopińska et al. 2020; Idzior et al. 2020). Shear wave elastography is well suited for the diagnostic workup and follow-up of lesions involving the skin, subdermis, fascia, and muscles in the course of scleroderma (Pracoń et al. 2021; Idzior et al. 2020). US can assess tissue thickness, echogenicity, vascularity, possible calcification, and nodules. In the active phase, tissue thickness is increased, echogenicity is reduced, and there is vascularity. As tissue atrophies, the elasticity of the tissues may decrease.

On MRI, fluid-sensitive sequences depict increased "edema-like" signal intensity in affected muscle, fascia, and subcutaneous tissue. Although these findings are nonspecific, MR images are particularly useful in the detection of inflammatory changes within muscles (in DM, PM), superficial and deep fascia, and subcutaneous tissue (DM, scleroderma), which correlate with disease activity (Thibaut et al. 2018; Sudoł-Szopińska et al. 2020; Schanz et al. 2011). Active myositis presents as a high signal on T2-weighted images and in STIR sequence. In the chronic phase, calcification, fibrotic lesions, and muscle fatty degeneration can be observed. The examination can help determine the biopsy site.

4.10 Other Soft Tissue Pathologies

Rheumatoid nodules are firm lumps that appear under the skin in up to 20% of patients with RA.

Soft tissue atrophy is a frequent finding in scleroderma and often coexists with acro-osteolysis (resorption of the distal phalanges) and soft tissue calcification. In certain cases of SLE, periarticular tissue inflammation (ligaments, joint capsule) may lead to contracture and subluxation, referred to as Jaccoud arthropathy. MRI demonstrates characteristic signs of soft tissue pathology, such as capsular swelling, edema and proliferative tenosynovitis, synovial hypertrophy, and occasionally erosions, termed rhupus (Ostendorf et al. 2003).

Soft tissue calcification, in addition to SSc, is also found in adults with DM, PM, and MCTD and in overlap syndromes (Fig. 1).

4.11 Nerve Lesions

US is an excellent modality for assessing for inflammatory, traumatic, and postsurgical causes of nerve compression. In the foot and ankle, particular areas of interest are the tibial nerve which may be compressed at the level of the tarsal tunnel by tenosynovitis and the common digital nerves which may be compressed by the intermetatarsal bursitis.

On MRI, an abnormal nerve is thickened and has a high signal on T2-weighted sequences.

On US, it is typically seen as well-defined, hypoechoic, and swollen (Fodor et al. 2022). A sonographic Mulder's sign may be elicited with the ultrasound probe for a Morton's neuroma.

4.12 Developmental Disorders

JIA may result in bony developmental disorders of the foot and ankle. The ossification may be delayed or accelerated. Accelerated skeletal maturation is secondary to increased vascularization of the bones (e.g., tarsus) or epiphyses and leads to epiphyseal overgrowth/hypertrophy/ballooning (e.g., heads of the metatarsals). Elongation of long bones with deformation of the epiphyses is more common than their shortening. Premature closure of growth plates and bone growth arrest are rarely observed nowadays, but brachydactyly (shortening of the phalanges) of the feet can be found in some children or adults following JIA (Fig. 2) (Sudoł-Szopińska et al. 2016a, b).

Fractures may be associated with disease-related osteoporosis and corticosteroid-induced osteoporosis. In the foot and ankle, posterior talar process, distal metaphysis of tibia, and midfoot are most often involved.

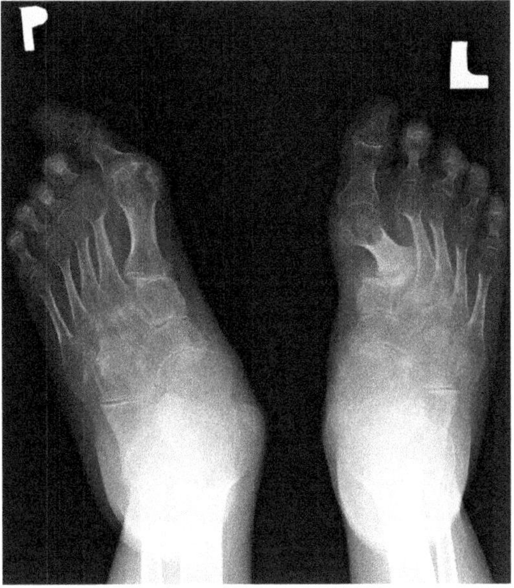

Fig. 2 A 41-year-old female following JIA. X-ray of feet demonstrates demineralization, developmental changes (bone-end hypertrophy, bone hypoplasia, shortening of the first metatarsal of the left foot with sclerotic changes), subchondral cysts, subluxation, JSN, and secondary OA

4.13 Postoperative Complications

Postoperatively, fluid collections related to an endoprosthesis may be due to hematomas, seromas, or abscesses.

5 Imaging Features of Specific Inflammatory Rheumatic Diseases

The most common rheumatic diseases affecting the foot and ankle in adults are RA, SpA, SSc and SLE, DM, PM, and AOSD. In children, the ankle and foot can be the predominant site of JIA, while other forms of arthritis are less common. The toes in particular may be affected by CRMO. The spectrum of radiographic features and their distribution are crucial for the diagnosis of specific rheumatic diseases (Table 1).

5.1 Rheumatoid Arthritis

Rheumatoid arthritis is a chronic, multi-organ autoimmune disease. In the musculoskeletal system, it involves multiple joints, tendon sheaths, and bursae. As a result of synovitis and bone inflammation (osteitis), the disease leads to progressive destruction of hyaline cartilage, bone, and soft tissue (mainly tendons) (Colebatch et al. 2013; Karasick 2009; Resnick et al. 2005a; Brown 2013).

Table 1 Distribution of radiographic lesions in specific rheumatic diseases

Anatomical area or imaging feature	Most frequent disease
Ankle joint	RA, AOSD, SpA (AS, ReA, IBD related), JIA, juvenile SLE, juvenile IBD related, juvenile ReA, SAPHO, DM/PM
Tarsus	JIA, RA
Foot	RA, PsA, SSc, SLE, ReA, AS, JIA, juvenile SSc, CRMO
Hindfoot	RA (Achilles tendon bursitis), PsA, and the remaining SpA (calcaneal enthesopathies)
MTP and PIP joints	RA, PsA, SLE, JIA
DIP joints	PsA, OA
Acro-osteolysis	PsA, SSc
Sausage toe(s)	PsA, ReA
The first toe(s)	RA (IP), PsA (IP), AS, juvenile AS, ReA
Bilateral, often symmetrical joint involvement	RA, OA, SLE

The feet are the second most common anatomical site of RA only preceded by the hands and wrists. The ankles are involved less often, usually after the knees and glenohumeral joints. In up to 20% of the patients, foot involvement may be the first manifestation of the disease. Initially, the lesions can be unilateral, but in advanced RA, both feet and ankles are involved bilaterally, more or less symmetrically. Characteristic anatomical regions involved by RA are presented in Table 2.

Typically, the forefoot is involved first. The midfoot is involved in about 2/3 of patients, whereas the involvement of hindfoot usually occurs at later stages of the disease. Typical locations in the feet and ankles include the metatarsophalangeal (MTP) and proximal interphalangeal (PIP) joints, tarsal joints, ankle joint, Achilles tendon bursa, tendon sheaths of the long flexors (most often the tibialis posterior tendon), and peroneal tendons, rarely the long extensor tendon sheaths (Figs. 3, 4, 5, 6, 7, 8, 9, 10, 11, 12, 13, 14, 15, and 16).

Table 2 Characteristic anatomical regions involved by RA

Most typical locations by RA
• Bilateral involvement
– IP joint of the first toe
– MTP and PIP joints
– Tarsus
• Flexor and peroneal tendon sheaths
• Intermetatarsal, Achilles tendon bursae

Fig. 3 Power Doppler ultrasound (PDUS) shows synovitis at the tarsometatarsal joint

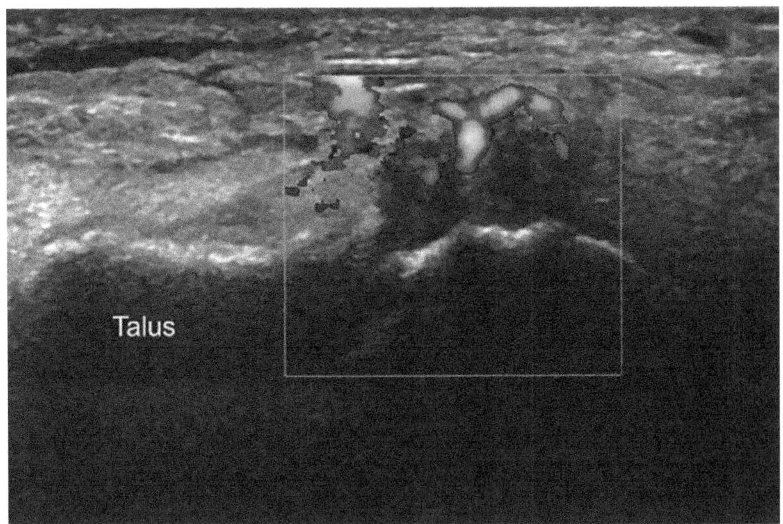

Fig. 4 PDUS with subtalar joint synovitis

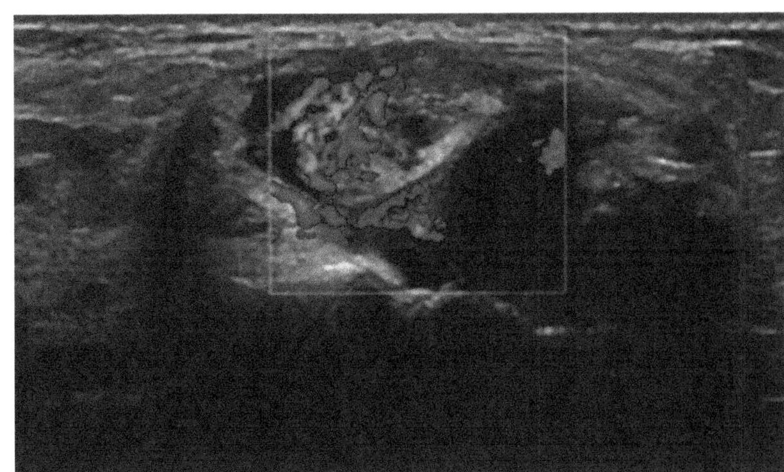

Fig. 5 PDUS shows tibialis posterior tendon tenosynovitis, with secondary tendinitis and partial tears of the tendon

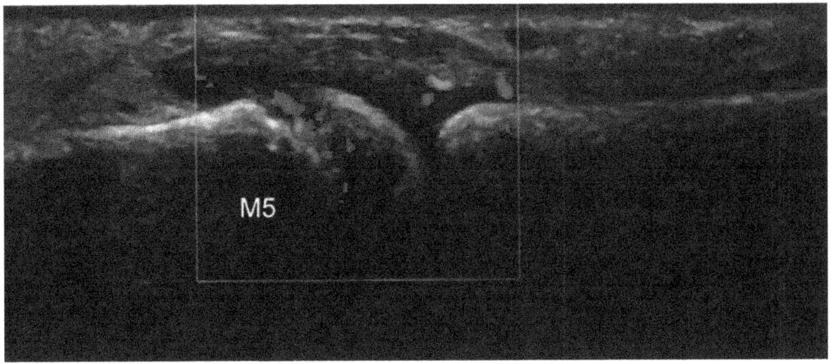

Fig. 6 MTP5 joint synovitis with an active erosion in the metatarsal head (*M5* the fifth metatarsal bone)

Fig. 7 Achilles tendon bursitis with effusions, thickened synovium (arrowheads), erosions in the bony wall of the bursa (arrow), and vascularization of the Kager's fat pad and the tendon; *C* calcaneus

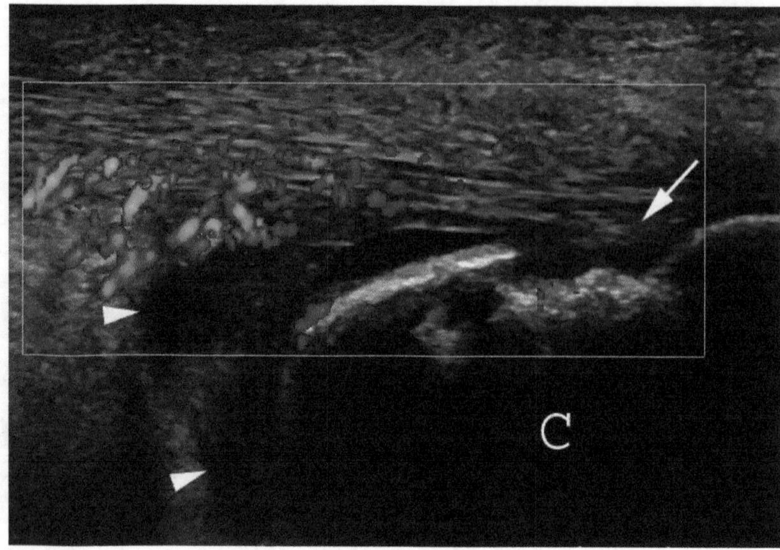

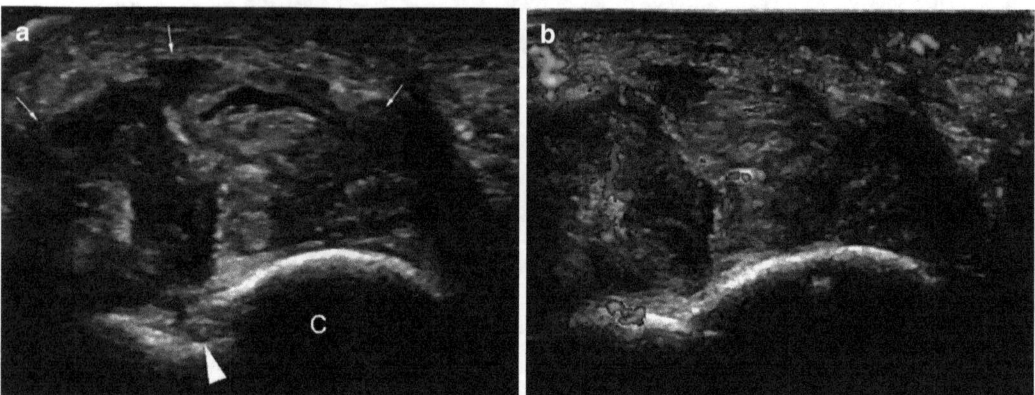

Fig. 8 Nonhomogeneous, large, hypoechoic rheumatoid nodule (arrows) and erosion in the calcaneus (arrowhead) in gray scale (**a**) and PDUS (**b**) demonstrating minor vascularity on Doppler

The typical sequence of involvement is as follows: interphalangeal and MTP joints of first toe, followed by the fourth and fifth MTPJs.

Early inflammatory changes seen on US, MRI, and/or X-rays include:

- Periarticular soft tissue thickening resulting from the presence of joint effusion, synovitis, tenosynovitis, and/or bursitis
- Periarticular demineralization, which may progress to generalized bone loss
- BME

Late changes seen on imaging include the following:

- Inflammatory cysts and erosions in the joints, in the calcaneus adjacent to the pre-Achilles bursa and rarely at the attachment of the Achilles tendon (enthesopathic lesions are more specific for SpA). Erosions may occur at the medial malleolus (secondary to tibialis posterior tendon tenosynovitis).
- A uniform narrowing of the joint space following hyaline cartilage damage.

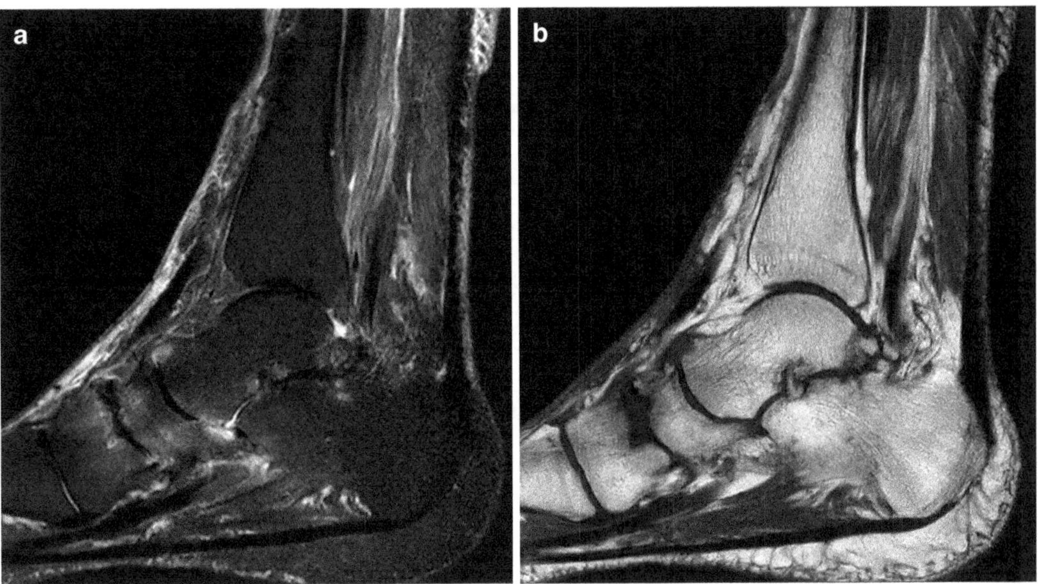

Fig. 9 An 80-year-old female with RA. Sagittal PDFS (**a**) and T1 (**b**) sequences demonstrate BME in midtarsal and subtalar joints, with JSN, erosions, and secondary OA

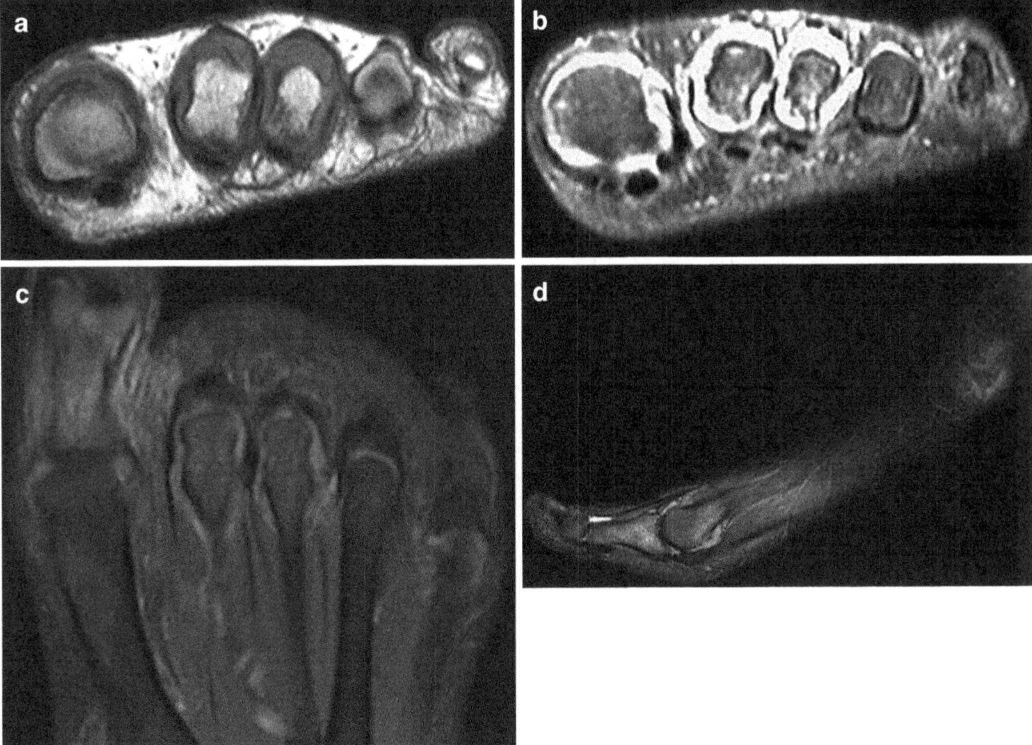

Fig. 10 A 35-year-old female with RA. There is synovitis and osteitis at the MTP1–3 joints seen on coronal T1 (**a**), coronal PDFS (**b**), axial PDFS (**c**), and sagittal PDFS (**d**) sequences

- Ankylosis in the tarsus (the second most common location of ankylosis in RA, the first being the wrist).
- Foot deformities, including hallux valgus, lateral deviations in the second to fifth MTP joints, flat valgus foot, mallet toes arising as a result of joint arthritis leading to the widening of the joint capsule, damage to passive joint stabilizers (collateral ligaments, plantar plate), secondary OA, as well as tenosynovitis, successive secondary tendinitis, and tendon ruptures (most often of the posterior tibial muscle).

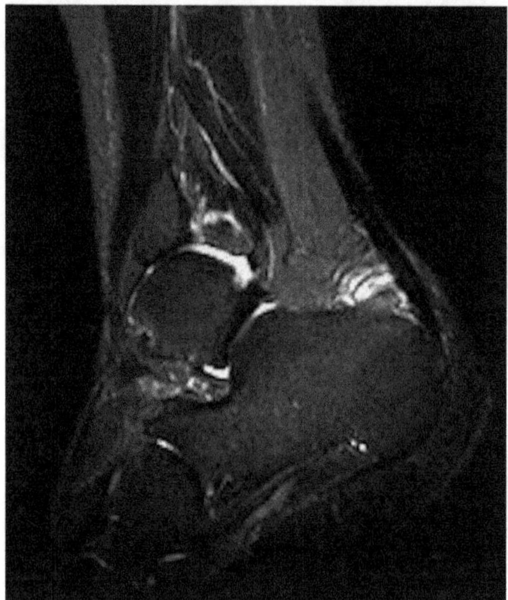

Fig. 11 Sagittal PDFS image demonstrating Pre-Achilles bursitis in a patient with RA

Moreover, in all affected joints, the findings may include:

- Rheumatoid nodules, which occur in about 20–30% of RA patients
- Secondary OA (osteophytes, sclerosis, subchondral cysts)
- Osteoporotic fractures in metatarsals

5.2 Psoriatic Arthritis

PsA is a form of SpA, a group of diseases (Table 3) that typically begin with sacroiliitis (so-called axial SpA), and often with inflammation of a few peripheral joints, mainly of lower limb (oligoarthritis), enthesitis, and dactylitis (so-called peripheral SpA) (Resnick et al. 2005).

The Moll and Wright classification distinguishes five subtypes of PsA (Table 4), of which

Fig. 12 X-ray of feet in a 46-year-old female with RA demonstrates bilateral soft tissue swelling and erosions at the MTP5 joint

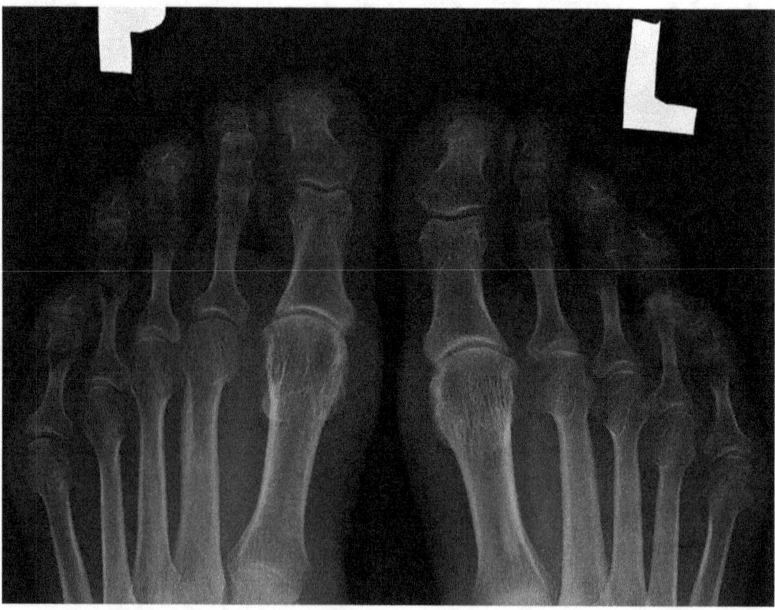

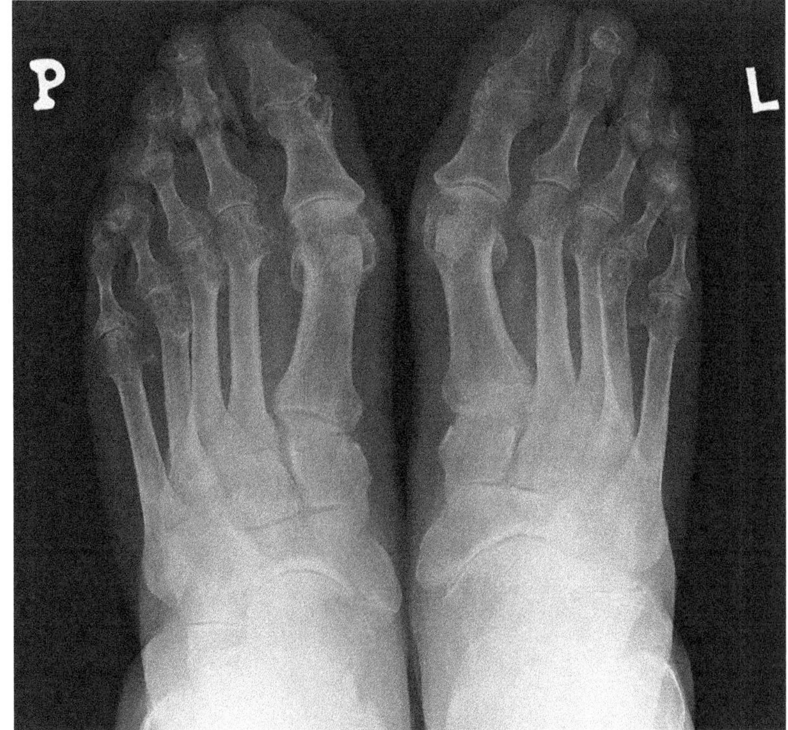

Fig. 13 A 57-year-old male with RA. X-ray of both feet demonstrates cysts, erosions, JSN at the MTP joints bilaterally, IP joints of big toes. There is lateral deviation of the MTP joints, secondary OA at the Chopart joints

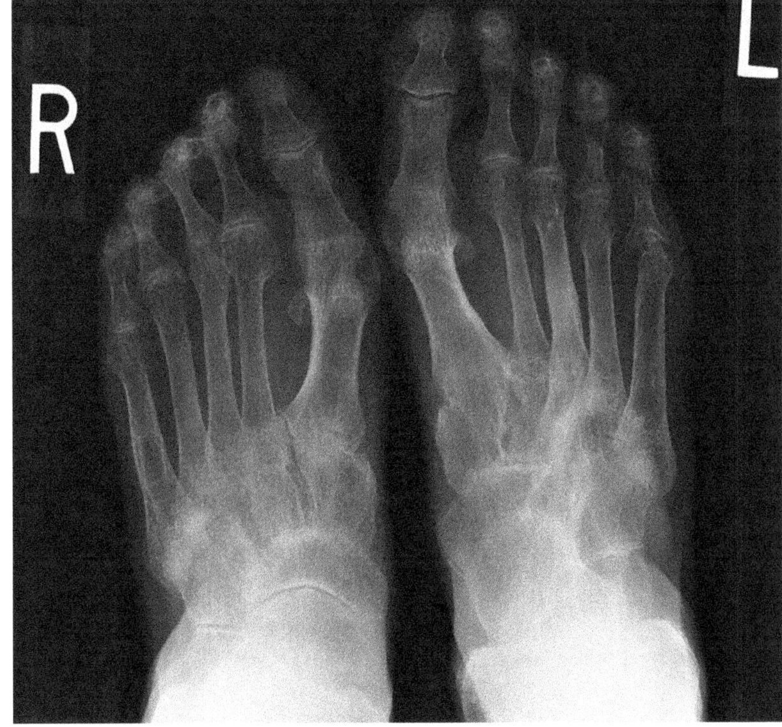

Fig. 14 Feet X-rays in a 61-year-old female show advanced RA with ankylosis of the MTP1 joints bilaterally, and at the tarsometatarsal joints, tarsal and talonavicular joints of the left foot. On the right, there is JSN at several joints. There is a fracture of the third metatarsal of the left foot and of the fifth metatarsal of the right foot

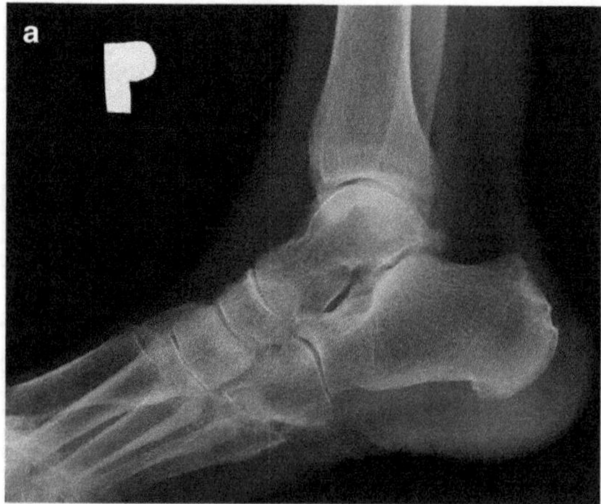

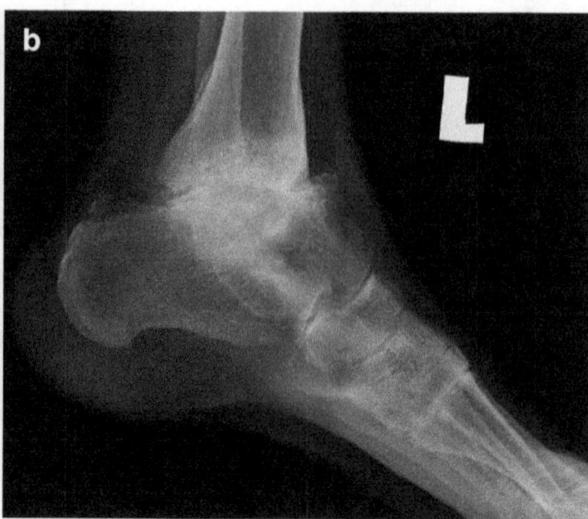

Fig. 15 A 59-year-old female with RA. X-ray demonstrates cysts, erosions in the calcaneus adjacent to the right Achilles tendon bursa (**a**), and unilateral involvement of the left ankle (**b**) with soft tissue thickening, demineralization, cysts, erosions, JSN, and secondary OA in tibiotalar and talocalcaneal joints

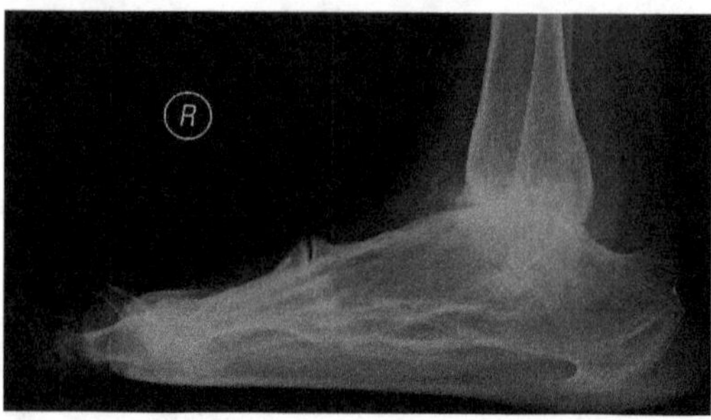

Fig. 16 A 68-year-old female with advanced RA. X-ray demonstrates demineralization, with ankylosis in tarsal, Lisfranc, Chopart, and talocalcaneal joints. Secondary OA. Inferior bone spurs bilaterally. Arthritis in tibiotalar joint

Table 3 Diseases that comprise spondyloarthritis

Spondyloarthritis	
1	Ankylosing spondylitis
2	Enteropathic arthropathies (associated with inflammatory bowel diseases, such as ulcerative colitis and Crohn's disease)
3	Psoriatic arthritis
4	Reactive arthritis
5	Undifferentiated spondyloarthritis
6	Juvenile spondyloarthropathies

Table 4 Five subtypes of PsA as described by Moll and Wright (1973 y.)

1. Symmetrical polyarthritis
2. Asymmetrical oligoarthritis
3. Spondylitis
4. Predominant DIP joint involvement
5. Arthritis mutilans

all but subtype 3 can affect the foot and ankle (Sudoł-Szopińska et al. 2016a, b; Brown 2013).

Subtype 1 is in many cases indistinguishable from RA due to identical radiographic presentation and the fact that the majority of patients are female in both these disease entities. A typical feature of PsA is the lack of demineralization. Subtype 2 may occur in all forms of peripheral SpAs. Subtype 4 is a unique form of PsA that does not occur in other diseases.

In the clinical practice, the CASPAR classification criteria for psoriatic arthritis are used for the diagnosis, with a sensitivity of 91% and specificity of up to 99% (Table 5) (Taylor et al. 2006). Radiographic involvement of the DIP joints, which is the hallmark for PsA, is one of these criteria.

The following features seen on imaging are characteristic of the foot and ankle PsA (Sudoł-Szopińska et al. 2016a, b) (Figs. 17, 18, 19, 20, and 21):

- Asymmetrical joint involvement, from single-joint involvement to polyarthritis in an advanced stage with effusions, synovitis, and BME

- Involvement of one or several toes (sausage toe, dactylitis)
- Involvement of DIP joints with synovitis, concomitant erosions, and juxta-articular bone proliferations
- Destruction of the IP joint of the big toe with synovitis, concomitant cysts, erosions, periostitis, and sclerosis
- No bone loss in most cases
- Fluffy/cloudy or linear periosteal reaction of the metatarsal bones and phalanges
- New bone formation at the terminal tufts
- Acro-osteolysis
- Ankylosis
- Coexistence of osteolysis and ankylosis in the same foot
- Enthesopathic lesions
- Ivory phalanx resulting from extensive periosteal and endosteal reaction (very rare but pathognomonic)
- Arthritis mutilans, which is a destructive, advanced form of PsA with significant toe deformity (subluxations, dislocations), osteolysis with whittling appearance of the toes (pencil-in-cup deformity), or so-called telescopic toes.

Table 5 The 2006 CASPAR criteria for PsA (Taylor et al. 2006)

To meet the CASPAR criteria for PsA, the patient should have inflammatory joint disease (peripheral, axial, or enthesitis) and score 3 or more based on the following categories:	
1	Evidence of psoriasis: Current—2 points Personal history—1 point Family history—1 point
2	Psoriatic nail dystrophy—1 point
3	Negative test result for rheumatoid factor—1 point
4	Dactylitis: Current inflammation—1 point History of dactylitis—1 point
5	Juxta-articular new bone formation in the hands and feet on plain radiography—1 point

5.3 Systemic Sclerosis/Scleroderma

Systemic sclerosis is a multi-organ connective tissue disease that leads to the progressive thickening and fibrosis of the skin and subcutaneous tissue, as well as to the fibrosis of internal organs. In more than a half of the SSc patients, lesions are seen in the joints, with the foot being one of the most frequent locations (Thibaut et al. 2018; Alparslan 2009; Johnson 2015; Resnick and Kransdorf 2005a, b, c).

On imaging, the following features may be present (Figs. 22 and 23):

- Soft tissue atrophy of the distal phalanges of the feet
- Acro-osteolysis of the terminal tufts of the toes

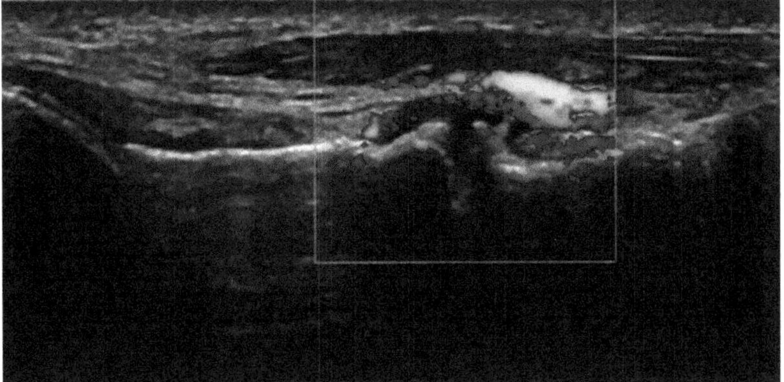

Fig. 17 PDUS demonstrating tarsometatarsal joint synovitis, and enthesophytes

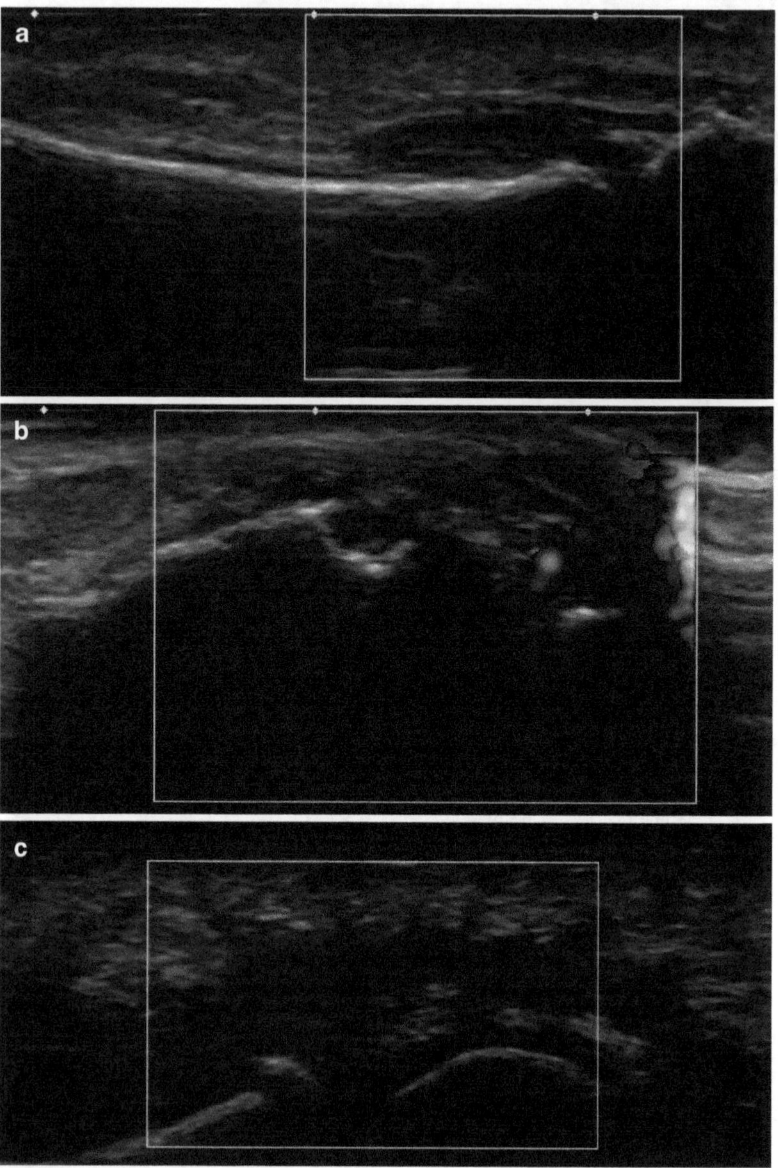

Fig. 18 A 41-year-old female with first toe dactylitis: (**a**) synovitis in MTP1 joint; (**b**) MET1 erosion; (**c**) tenosynovitis of the flexor hallucis longus tendon

- Soft tissue calcifications
- Coexistence of acro-osteolysis with soft tissue calcifications in the tips of toes
- Generalized demineralization
- Soft tissue involvement (skin, subdermis, fascia, muscles)
- Contractures and subluxations, secondary to post-inflammatory lesions (scars and atrophy) of the skin, subcutaneous tissue, ligaments, or tendons

5.4 Systemic Lupus Erythematosus

Systemic lupus erythematosus is an autoimmune inflammatory disease that may affect numerous tissues and organs. Joint inflammation (lupus arthritis) is one of the most common symptoms of SLE. The foot is one of the most frequently affected sites, after the hand, wrist, and knee. The disease leads to nonerosive polyarthritis (Jaccoud arthropathy) with

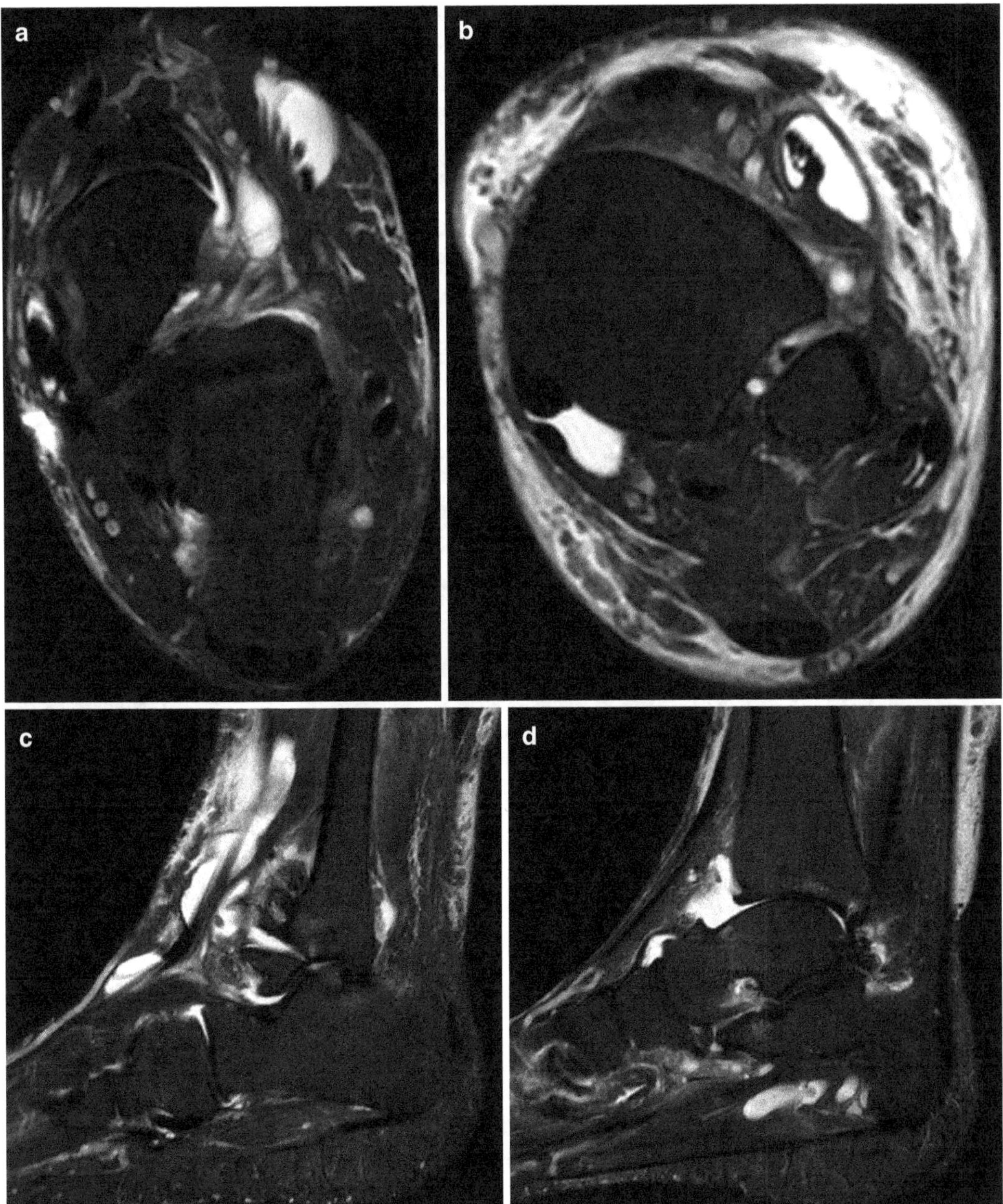

Fig. 19 Psoriatic arthritis. Axial (**a**, **b**) and sagittal (**c**, **d**) PDFS images. Extensor tendon tenosynovitis and tibiotalar and Chopart joint synovitis

characteristic malalignment resulting from post-inflammatory lesions of periarticular tissues (joint capsules, ligaments, tendons) (Thibaut et al. 2018) (Fig. 24). The progressive rheumatoid-like deformities of the hands and feet, occurring in 3–43% of patients with lupus, can be clinically difficult to distinguish from RA (Molina et al. 1995; Sierra-Jimenez et al. 2008), especially since rheumatoid factor may be negative in some RA patients, and anti-citrullinated antibodies may be present in some SLE patients. Rarely, erosive symmetric polyarthritis with deformities similar to those in RA, named

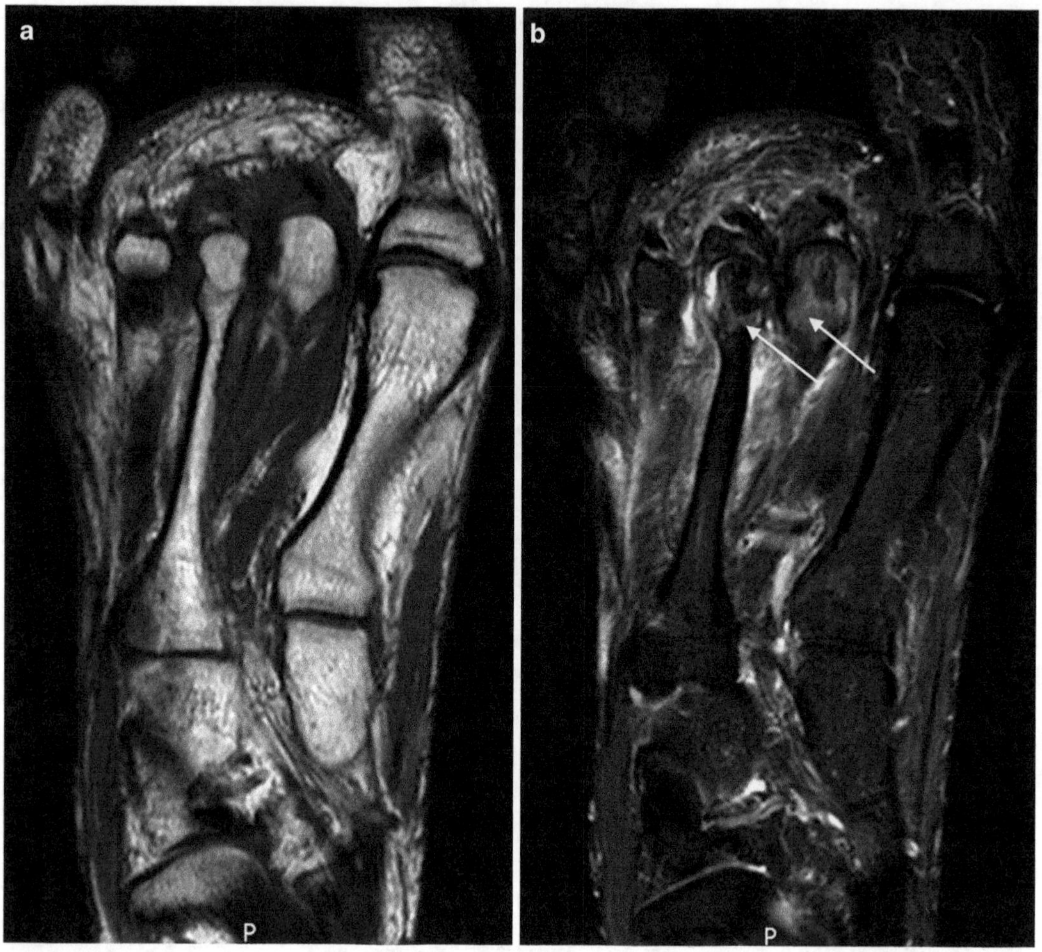

Fig. 20 Psoriatic arthritis of the left foot. BME of the heads of the second and third metatarsals on axial T1 (**a**) and PDFS (**b**) (arrows)

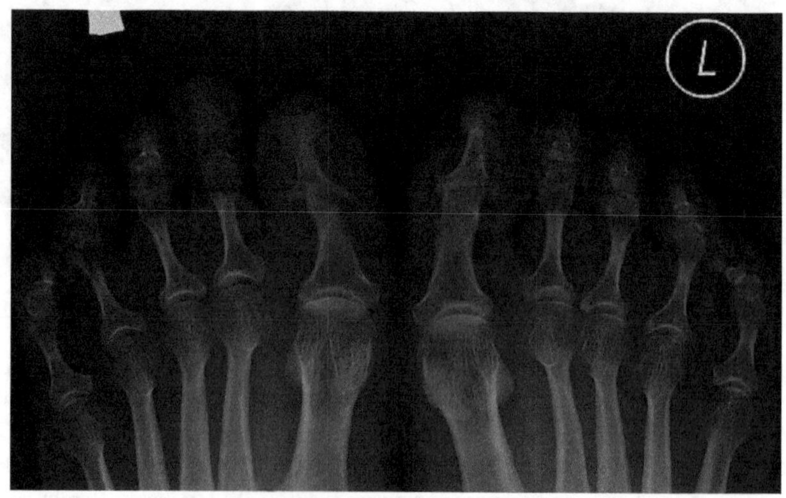

Fig. 21 X-ray of the feet in a 45-year-old female with PsA: soft tissue thickening of first toes bilaterally, osteolysis, new bone formation of the interphalangeal joints of first toes, and acro-osteolysis of the first toes

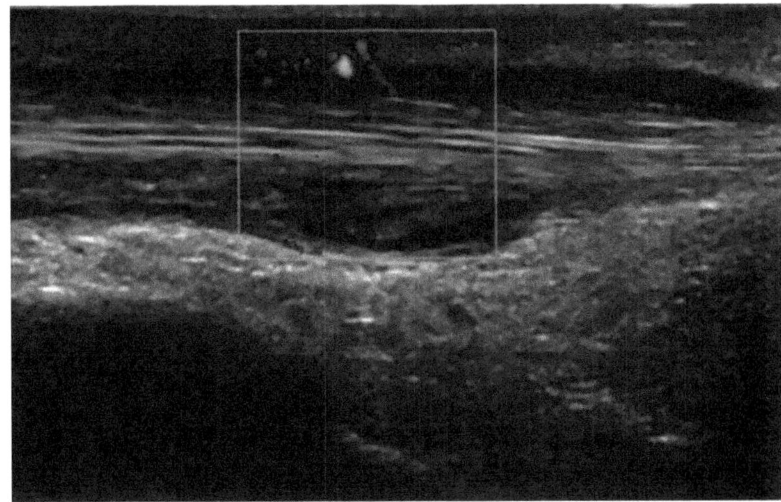

Fig. 22 PDUS demonstrating tenosynovitis of the tibialis anterior tendon

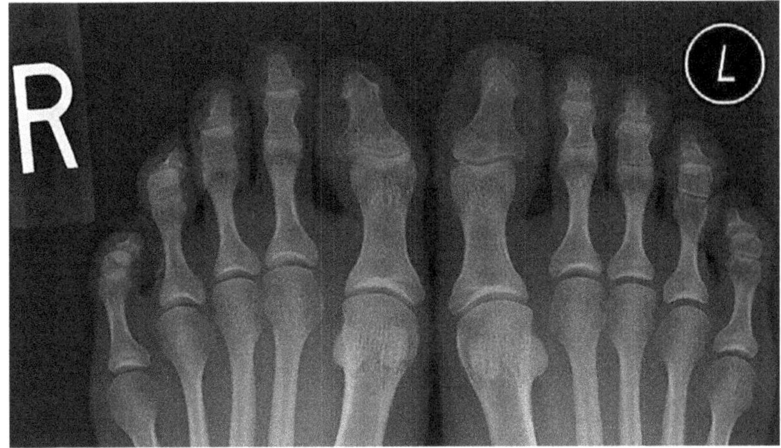

Fig. 23 X-ray of feet in a 19-year-old female with scleroderma demonstrates acro-osteolysis and soft tissue atrophy of the first right toe

rhupus, can occur in SLE and may represent a distinct lupus subset (Fernandez et al. 2004; van Vugt et al. 1998; Weissman et al. 2009), which additionally complicates the differential diagnosis.

The following features seen on imaging are characteristic of the foot and ankle SLE (Thibaut et al. 2018; Resnick and Kransdorf 2005a, b, c; Weissman et al. 2009):

- Symmetrical polyarthritis, and periosteal/periarticular bone loss and BME, as in RA.
- No cysts and erosions in majority of the cases, and preservation of the joint space, unlike RA.
- Reducible deformity, unlike RA. The deformities (Jaccoud arthropathy) are due to tenosynovitis, tendinitis, tendon tears, and capsule and ligament laxity and include contractures, subluxations of the MTP joints with lateral deviations, lateral subluxation of the toes, hallux valgus, or hammer toes.
- Osteonecrosis is reported in 5–30% of patients with SLE (Diaz-Jouanen et al. 1985; Rascu et al. 1996; Cozen and Wallace 1998). Although the epiphysis of the femoral head is particularly vulnerable to ischemic damage, osteonecrosis can develop in other bones, including talus, tibia, and calcaneus, with a tendency to occur at multiple sites among patients with SLE (Fishel et al. 1987). The lesions typically show as bone infarcts characterized by serpiginous well-defined densities with sclerotic borders surrounding areas of bone necrosis.

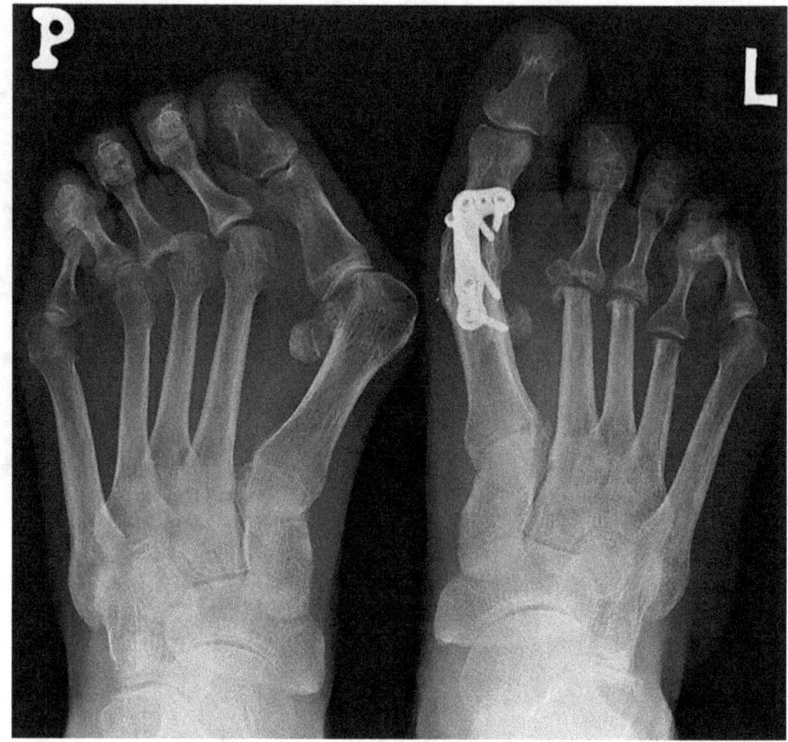

Fig. 24 A 46-year-old female with SLE. X-ray of feet shows postsurgical ankylosis of the first big toe of the left foot, osteotomy of the metatarsal heads 2–4 of the left foot, and soft tissue thickening of the left midfoot. Calcifications in soft tissues of the forefoot right > left. Subluxation at the MTP3 joint; subluxations at the MTP1, -2, -4, and -5 joints on the right; flexion at the PIP2–5 joints of the left foot

5.5 Polymyositis and Dermatomyositis

Polymyositis and dermatomyositis belong to the group of idiopathic inflammatory myopathies affecting the striated muscles, while DM additionally involves the skin.

The following features seen on imaging are characteristic of the foot and ankle PM and DM (Thibaut et al. 2018; Sudoł-Szopińska et al. 2020):

- Soft tissue inflammation
- Soft tissue thickening secondary to the skin, subcutaneous tissue, and muscle inflammation
- Multiform calcifications in the subcutaneous tissue, fascia, and striated muscles
- Bone loss
- Joint malalignment due to muscle weakness, fibrosis, and atrophy of the affected soft tissues

5.6 Adult-Onset Still's Disease

Adult-onset Still's disease is a rare systemic inflammatory disease of the connective tissue that usually affects the knee and wrist (Thibaut et al. 2018; Resnick and Kransdorf 2005a, b, c). Its etiology is unknown. The ankles are less commonly affected, and the imaging features resemble RA.

The following features seen on imaging are characteristic of the foot and ankle AOSD:

- Periarticular soft tissue thickening, effusion, synovitis, or tenosynovitis
- Periarticular demineralization

- Erosions
- Joint space narrowing
- Early formation of bone ankylosis

5.7 Ankylosing Spondylitis

Ankylosing spondylitis is the most common spondyloarthropathy. It is a chronic, progressive inflammatory process that usually begins with sacroiliitis. In up to 20% of patients, the disease begins with asymmetrical involvement of the peripheral joints, mainly in the shoulders and lower limbs. Enthesopathy, mainly of Achilles tendon, is a typical feature. The ankles and feet are among the most frequently affected regions.

The following features seen on imaging are characteristic of the foot and ankle AS (Resnick and Kransdorf 2005a, b, c; Brown 2013; Sudoł-Szopińska et al. 2013, 2014) (Figs. 25, 26, and 27):

- Periarticular soft tissue thickening, effusion, synovitis, tenosynovitis, and bursitis
- BME
- Enthesopathic lesions (most commonly at the calcaneus)
- Demineralization
- Uniform JSN
- Osteophytes
- Single cysts
- Rarely erosions

5.8 Reactive Arthritis and Arthritis Associated with Inflammatory Bowel Disease

Reactive arthritis and IBD-related arthritis are spondyloarthropathies that typically present with asymmetrical inflammation of several peripheral joints (oligoarthritis), but polyarthritis may also be present (Brown 2013). Ankle joint involve-

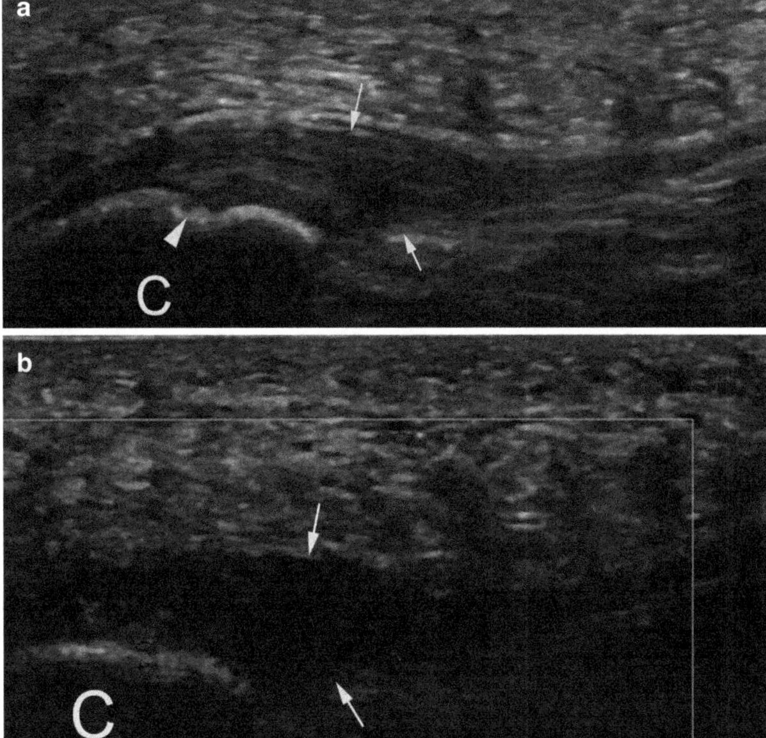

Fig. 25 Plantar fascia enthesopathy (enthesitis) with fascia thickening, loss of fibrillar echostructure, delamination, and erosion at its bony attachment (*C* calcaneus) (**a**) and minor increased vascularity on PDUS (**b**)

ment is common, while the foot is slightly less frequently affected, with the predilection for the first MTP joint. In many cases, the entheses of the calcaneal tuberosity are involved (Resnick and Kransdorf 2005a, b, c; Brown 2013; Sudoł-Szopińska et al. 2013, 2014).

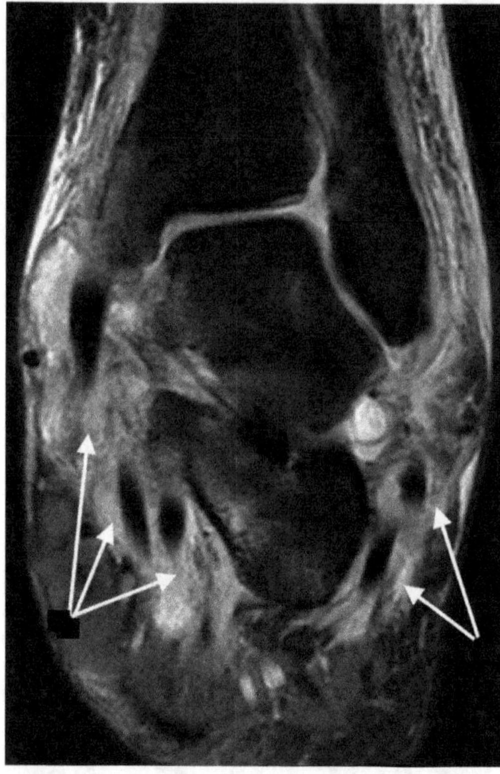

Fig. 26 A 30-year-old male with SpA. Tenosynovitis of the long flexors (triple arrow) and peroneal tendons (double arrow) in coronal T1 FS postcontrast MRI

Imaging features in ReA are similar to PsA and include:

- Periarticular soft tissue thickening, resulting from effusion, synovitis, tenosynovitis, and bursitis
- BME
- Periarticular bone loss
- Periostitis
- Dactylitis
- Enthesopathic lesions
- Single cysts
- Rarely erosions

Imaging findings in enteropathic SpA are similar to AS and include:

- Periarticular soft tissue thickening, effusion, synovitis, tenosynovitis, and bursitis
- BME
- Soft tissue thickening
- Periarticular bone loss
- Enthesopathic lesions (most commonly at the calcaneus)
- Single cysts
- Rarely erosions

5.9 Juvenile Idiopathic Arthritis

Juvenile idiopathic arthritis is the most common, chronic, immune-mediated systemic connective tissue disease affecting children.

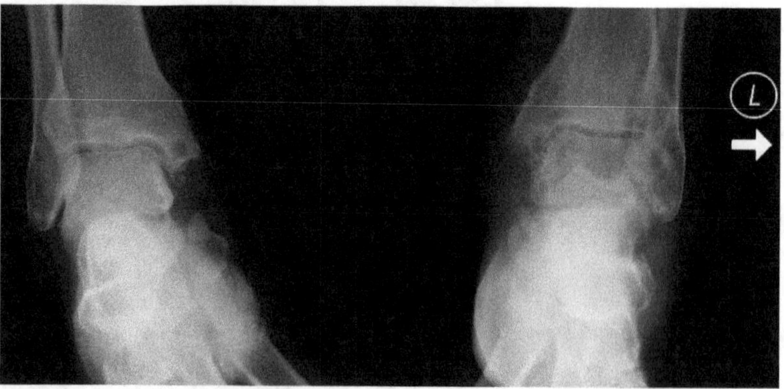

Fig. 27 A 58-year-old man with SpA. X-ray of the ankles demonstrates soft tissue thickening L > R, cysts, and erosions at medial malleolus of the right ankle; demineralization, periostitis of the distal tibia, medial malleolus, and talus of the left ankle

Radiographs show age-specific features of both arthritis-related and bone growth disturbances caused by ongoing inflammation.

The disease involves one or several joints. Lesions may be bilateral and symmetrical or asymmetrical, or unilateral. The ankle is often involved, the foot being a rarer site with a predilection for the tarsal joints.

Conventional radiographs have a lower sensitivity and specificity for detection of disease activity and early destructive change, as compared to MRI or ultrasound (Hemke et al. 2020). Nonetheless, radiography remains important, particularly in narrowing the differential diagnosis and evaluating growth disturbances (Hemke et al. 2020).

The following features seen on imaging are characteristic of the foot and ankle JIA (Pracoń et al. 2021; Sudoł-Szopińska et al. 2016a, b; Resnick and Kransdorf 2005a, b, c; Schwartz Doria and Babyn 2009; Sheybani et al. 2013; Ostrowska et al. 2022) (Figs. 28, 29, 30, and 31):

- Soft tissue thickening, effusions, synovitis, tenosynovitis, and bursitis.
- BME.
- Periarticular bone loss and generalized osteoporosis in chronic cases.
- Periostitis along the shafts of the metatarsals and phalanges.
- Fibrous and bony ankylosis in the interphalangeal and tarsal joints.
- Developmental disorders:
  - Epiphyseal hypertrophy
  - Acceleration or retardation in the appearance and maturation of the ossification centers
  - Bone elongation or shortening, bone modeling disturbances of metatarsals and pha-

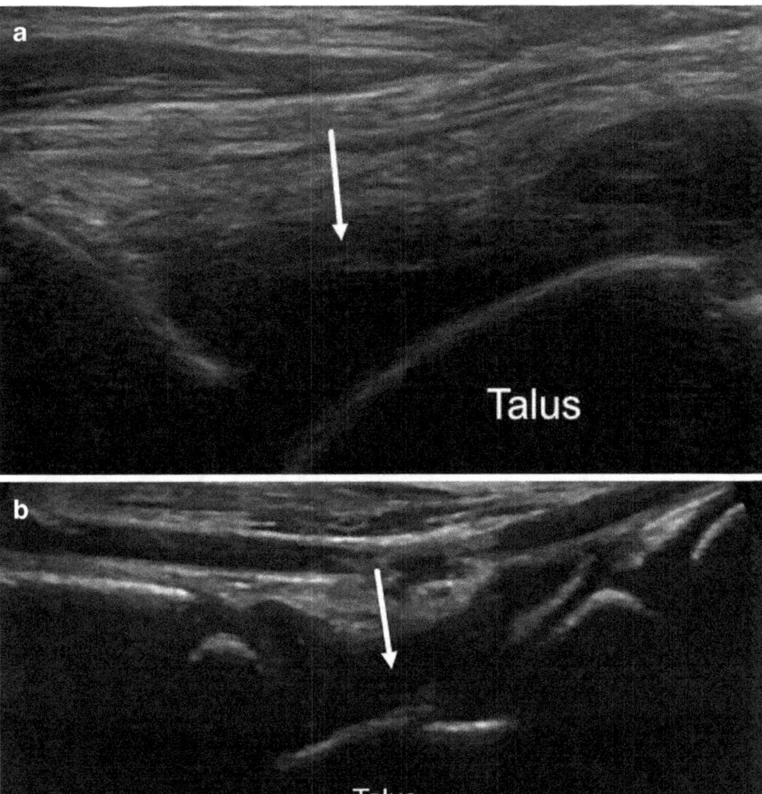

Fig. 28 (**a**, **b**) Tibiotalar joint effusion in two different patients (arrows)

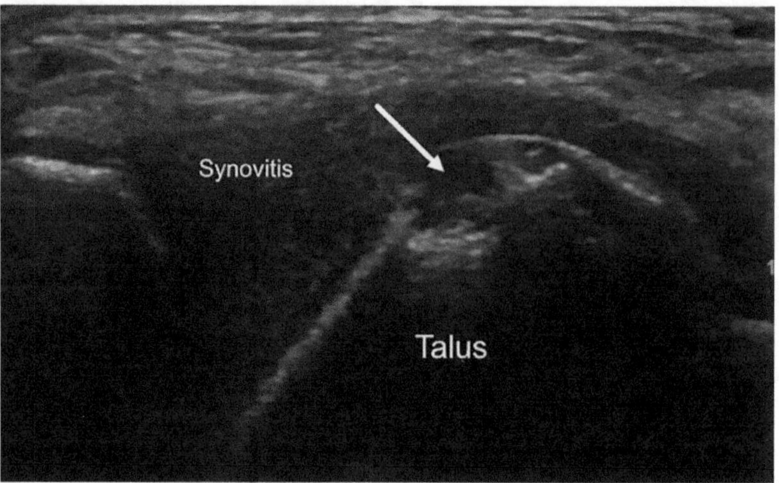

Fig. 29 Chronic synovitis in the tibiotalar joint and erosions of the talar dome (arrow)

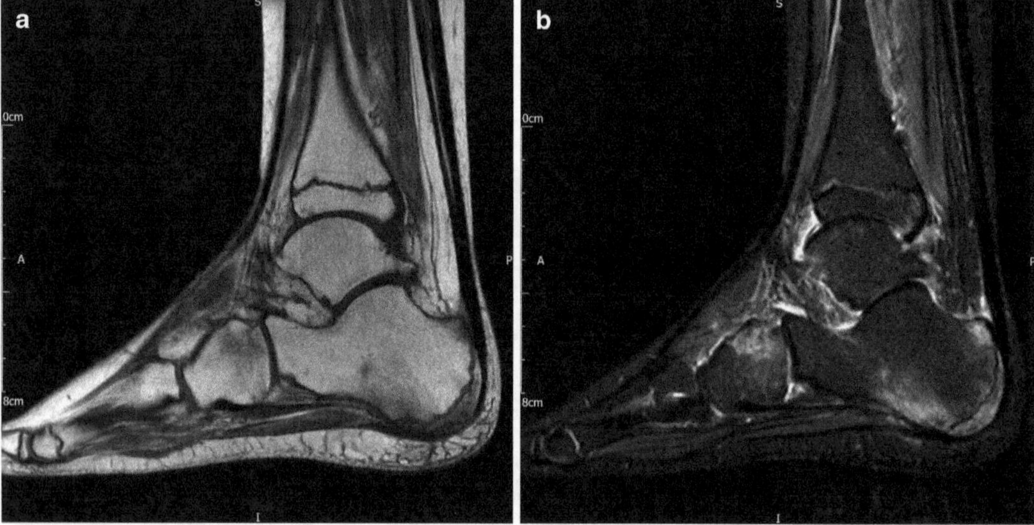

Fig. 30 A 11-year-old male with JIA. Sagittal T1 (**a**) and PDFS (**b**) show pre-Achilles bursitis, plantar fascia enthesitis, and periarticular BME cuboid bone

langes, premature closure of growth plates, and cessation of growth (brachydactyly is currently rarely observed)

- Cysts and erosions and JSN are usually rare and occur late in the course of the disease.

5.10 Juvenile Systemic Lupus Erythematosus

Juvenile form of SLE accounts for up to 15% of SLE cases. The disease may affect the ankle joints.

Imaging features include periarticular soft tissue thickening and US/MRI lesions reflecting transient arthritis (Sudoł-Szopińska et al. 2018a, b). Contractures or subluxations are rare in children.

5.11 Juvenile Dermatomyositis and Polymyositis

Juvenile DM is the most common inflammatory myopathy in children. Inflammatory lesions in the subcutaneous tissue in children are more severe than in adults with DM and PM.

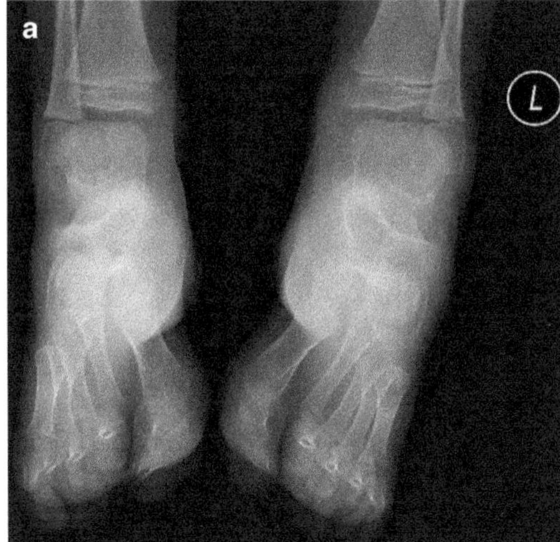

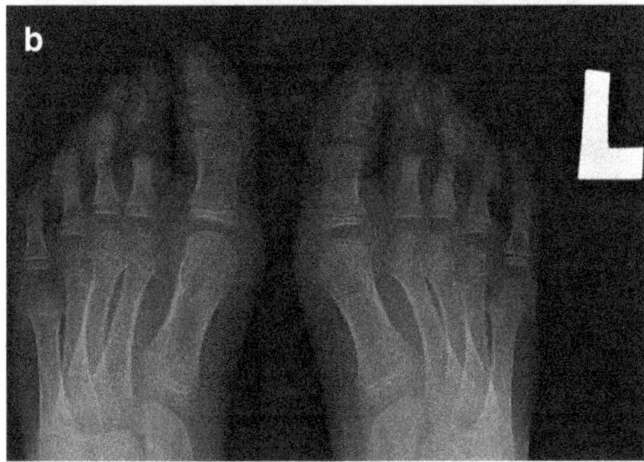

Fig. 31 X-ray of the ankles (**a**) and feet (**b**) in a 6-year-old male. Soft tissue thickening at the left ankle, distal epiphyses hypertrophy of the left tibia and fibula. Soft tissue thickening at the MTP joints bilaterally, hypertrophy of the epiphyses of the MTP1 joint of the right toe

Radiographic features include (Sudoł-Szopińska et al. 2020):

- Soft tissue inflammation
- Soft tissue calcifications that can be very extensive and seen around ankle joints and/or soft tissues within the crura (Fig. 32)
- Bone demineralization due to prolonged use of steroids and disuse

5.12 Juvenile Scleroderma

Localized scleroderma is much more common in children than in adults. The linear type of disease may lead to severe disproportion in bone growth with soft tissue atrophy within the limbs (Idzior et al. 2020). Overlap syndromes of systemic sclerosis, mainly with juvenile DM, may also be evident.

Imaging findings include the following (Sudoł-Szopińska et al. 2018a, b) (Figs. 33 and 34):

- Soft tissue inflammation (skin, subdermis, fascia, muscles).
- Arthritis, tenosynovitis, tendinitis.
- Acro-osteolysis.
- Acro-osteolysis accompanied by soft tissue atrophy.

Fig. 32 A 13-year-old girl with jDM. X-ray of feet demonstrates numerous soft tissue calcifications within the forefeet

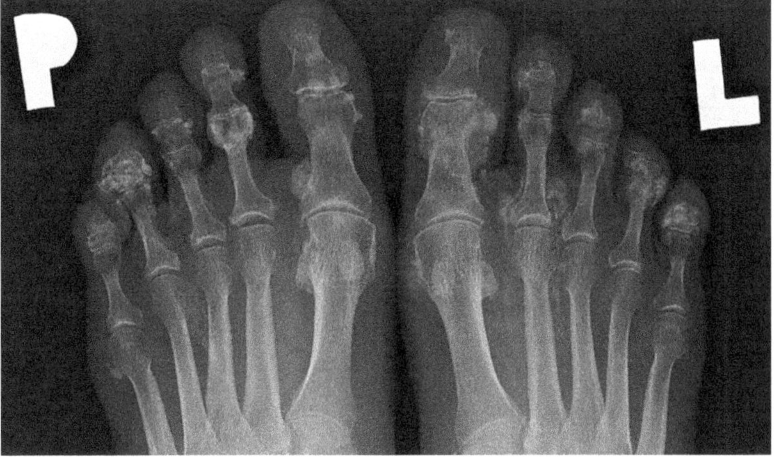

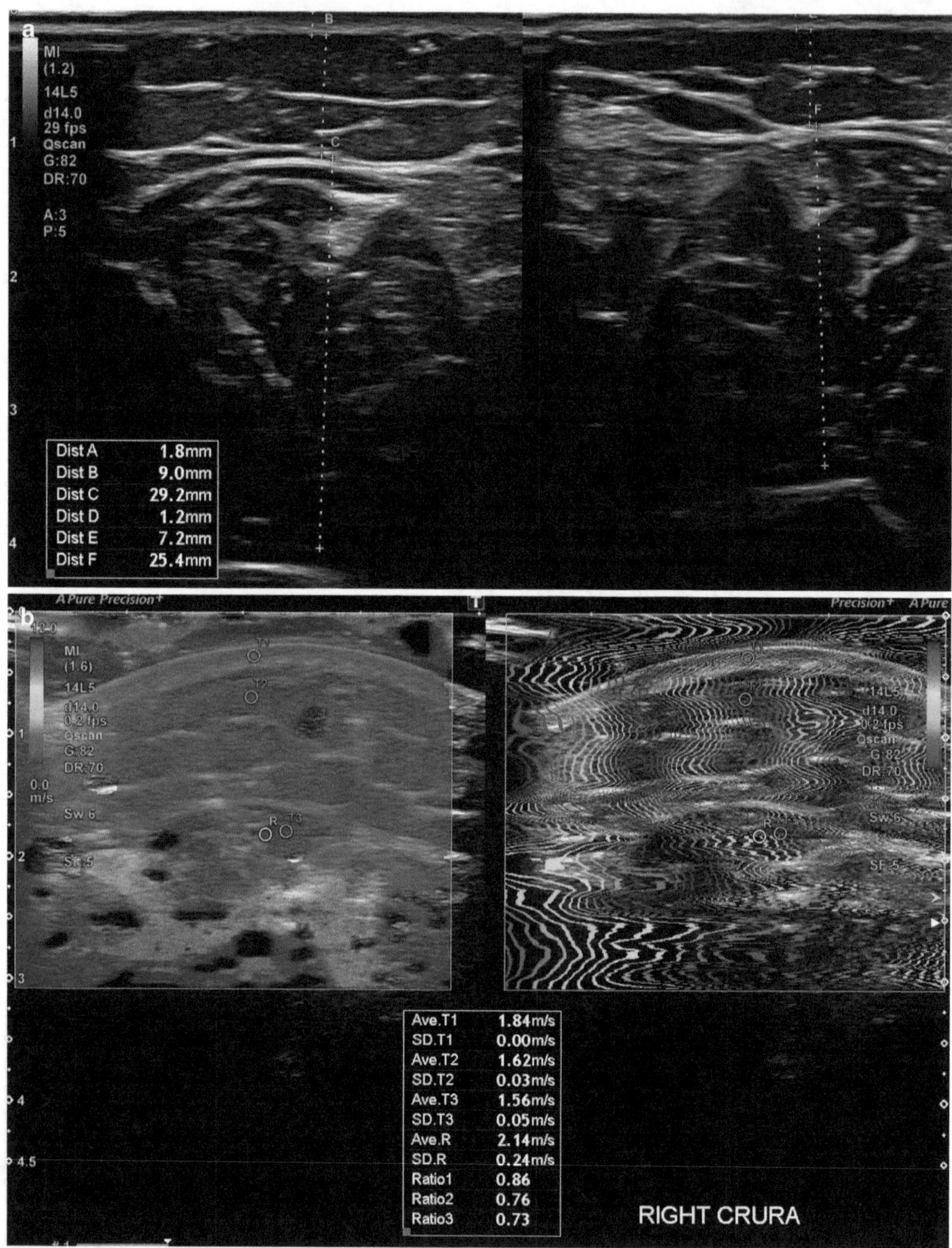

Fig. 33 A 17-year-old girl with linear scleroderma (morphoea) of the left lower limb: (**a**) 24 MHz transducer shows thinning of the skin, subdermis, and muscle on the affected side (right side of the image); shear wave elastography confirms lower elasticity of the skin, subdermis, and muscle on the affected side (**b**) compared to the contralateral crura (**c**)

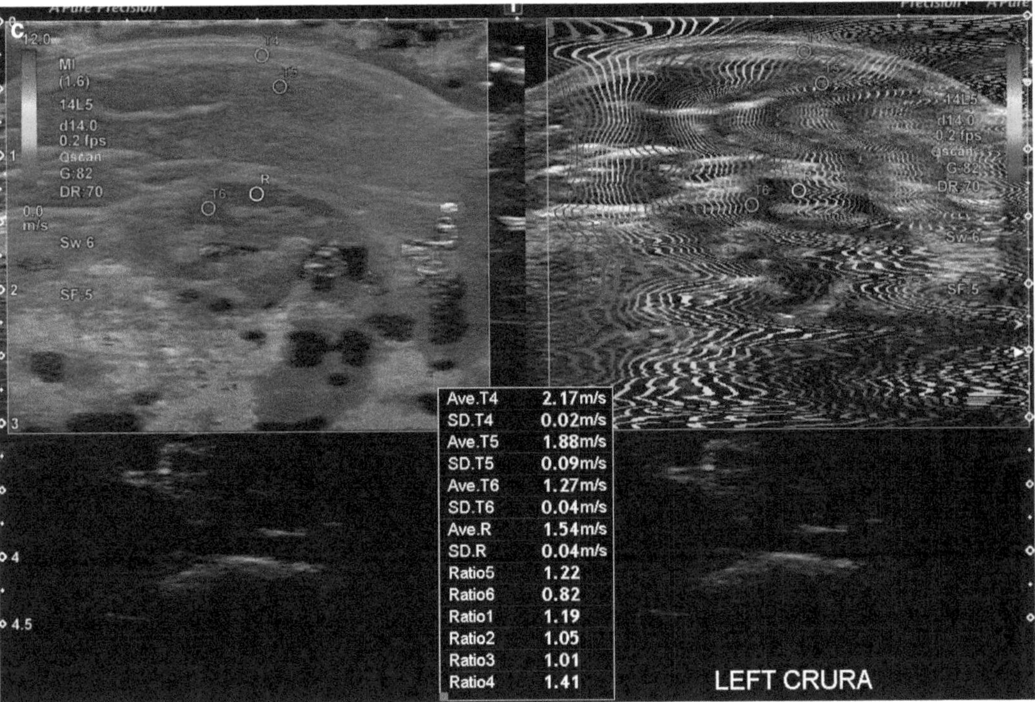

Fig. 33 (continued)

- Calcification/calcinosis in the skin and subcutaneous tissue of a cloud-like or linear appearance, usually in locations exposed to pressure.
- Flexion contractures and subluxations in the MTP and PIP joints are rare.
- Bone demineralization and arthritis are rare.

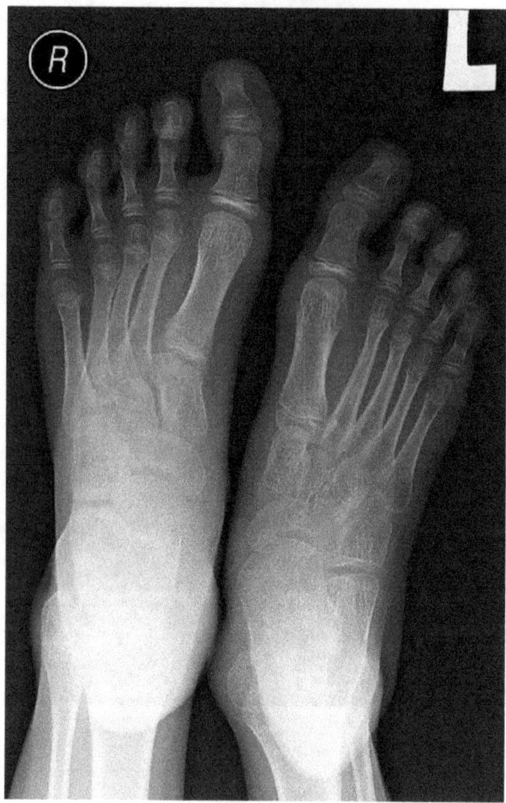

Fig. 34 A 11-year-old female with scleroderma. X-ray of feet shows demineralization, bone hypoplasia of several tarsal bones, and to a lesser extent metatarsals 2–5 in the left foot

5.13 Juvenile Spondyloarthritis

According to the classification of the International League Against Arthritis, juvenile spondyloarthritis (jSpA) is a subtype of JIA. It is characterized by asymmetrical involvement of joints within the lower limb, without erosions, and presence of enthesopathic lesions (Schwartz Doria and Babyn 2009; Sudoł-Szopińska et al. 2017a, b).

Imaging findings include the following:

- The involvement of the MTP and the IP joints of the first toe, which is characteristic at the initial stage of the juvenile AS.
- Ankle joint arthritis.
- Achilles tendon bursitis.
- Acro-osteolysis and DIP joint involvement with erosions and proliferative changes are rare findings in juvenile PsA.

5.14 Chronic Recurrent Multifocal Osteomyelitis (CRMO) and Synovitis, Acne, Pustulosis, Hyperostosis, Osteitis (SAPHO)

The etiology of CRMO and SAPHO remains uncertain, but they are considered autoinflammatory diseases, arising due to dysregulation of the innate immune system (Jurik et al. 2018; Rubenstein 2009; Sudoł-Szopińska et al. 2018a, b).

CRMO occurs in children and adolescents. It is a nonspecific, bilateral, multifocal inflammatory condition of bone. The metaphyses of long bones, anterior chest wall, and clavicle are sites of predilection, but the disease may also involve the spine, pelvis, long bones of the lower limb, and feet (Fig. 35).

Imaging findings include (Jurik et al. 2018; Sudoł-Szopińska et al. 2018a, b):

- Osteolytic lesions (preceded by osteitis which is visible on MRI)
- Mixed sclerotic and lytic lesions
- Bone hypertrophy with secondary narrowing of the bone marrow cavity
- Periostitis as a result of lesions located close to the cortex
- Premature closure of the growth plates

SAPHO affects adults and is characterized by a predilection to the anterior chest wall, spine, and pelvic bones. Of the peripheral joints, the ankle is one of the most frequently involved joints.

Imaging findings include:

- Soft tissue thickening, effusions, and synovitis
- BME

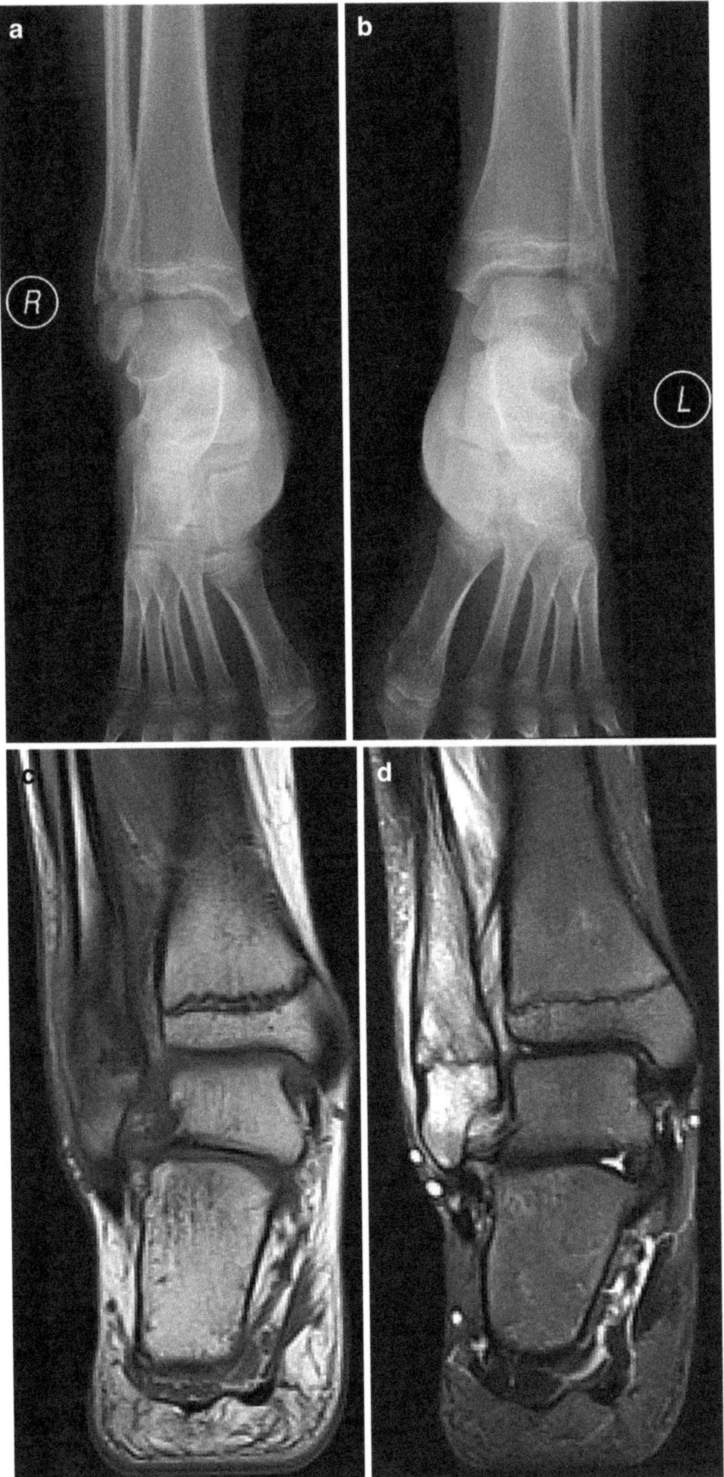

Fig. 35 A 11-year-old female with CRMO. Ankle X-ray (**a**, **b**) demonstrates soft tissue thickening at the lateral part, deformity of the fibula metaphysis, small osteolytic areas, and periosteal thickening; coronal MR in T1 (**c**) and PDFS (**d**) show BME at the distal fibula, with deformity and sclerosis

- Osteolysis, sclerosis, with possible hyperostosis
- Erosions
- Ankylosis

References

Alparslan LH (2009) Scleroderma and related disorders. In: Weissman BN (ed) Imaging of arthritis and metabolic bone disease. Saunders Elsevier, Philadelphia, pp 365–376

Axelsen MB, Stoltenberg M, Poggenborg RP et al (2012) Dynamic gadolinium-enhanced magnetic resonance imaging allows accurate assessment of the synovial inflammatory activity in rheumatoid arthritis knee joints: a comparison with synovial histology. Scand J Rheumatol 41(2):89–94

Benjamin M, McGonagle D (2009) The enthesis organ concept and its relevance to the spondyloarthropathies. Adv Exp Med Biol 649:57–70

Boesen M, Kubassova O, Sudoł-Szopińska I et al (2018) MR imaging of joint infection and inflammation with emphasis on dynamic contrast-enhanced MR imaging. PET Clin 13(4):523–550

Brown AK (2013) How to interpret plain radiographs in clinical practice. Best Pract Res Clin Rheumatol 27:249–269

Bruyn GA, Iagnocco A, Naredo E et al (2019) OMERACT definitions for ultrasonographic pathologies and elementary lesions of rheumatic disorders 15 Years on. J Rheumatol 46:1388–1393

Coates LC, Hodgson R, Conaghan PG et al (2012) MRI and ultrasonography for diagnosis and monitoring of psoriatic arthritis. Best Pract Res Clin Rheumatol 26:805–82230

Colebatch AN, Edwards CJ, Østergaard M et al (2013) EULAR recommendations for the use of imaging of the joints in the clinical management of rheumatoid arthritis. Ann Rheum Dis 72:804–814

Coll JP, Ragsdale BD, Chow B et al (2011) Lipoma arborescens of the knees in a patient with rheumatoid arthritis. Radiographics 31:333–337

Cozen L, Wallace DJ (1998) Avascular necrosis in systemic lupus erythematosus: clinical associations and a 47-year perspective. Am J Orthop (Belle Mead NJ) 27:352–354

Damasio MB, de Horatio LT, Boavida P et al (2013) Imaging in juvenile idiopathic arthritis (JIA): an update with particular emphasis on MRI. Acta Radiol 54(9):1015–1023

Diaz-Jouanen E, Abud-Mendoza C, Inglesias-Gamarra A et al (1985) Ischemic necrosis of bone in systemic lupus erythematosus. Orthop Rev 14:303–309

Dohn UM, Ejbjerg BJ, Court-Payen M et al (2006) Are bone erosions detected by magnetic resonance imaging and ultrasonography true erosions? A comparison with computed tomography in rheumatoid arthritis metacarpophalangeal joints. Arthritis Res Ther 8(4):R110

Dubash SR, De Marco G, Wakefield RJ et al (2020) Ultrasound imaging in psoriatic arthritis: what have we learnt in the last five years? Front Med 7:487

Fernandez A, Quintana G, Matterson E et al (2004) Lupus arthropathy: historical evolution from deforming arthropathy to rhupus. Clin Rheumatol 23:523–526

Fishel B, Caspi D, Eventov I et al (1987) Multiple osteonecrotic lesions in systemic lupus erythematosus. J Rheumatol 14:601–604

Fodor D, Rodriguez-Garcia SC, Cantisani V et al (2022) The EFSUMB guidelines and recommendations for musculoskeletal ultrasound. Part I: Extra-articular pathologies. Ultraschall Med 43(1):34–57

Gulani V, Calamante F, Shellock FG et al (2017) International Society for Magnetic Resonance in Medicine. Gadolinium deposition in the brain: summary of evidence and recommendations. Lancet Neurol 16(7):564–570

Hemke R, Herregods N, Jaremko JL et al (2020) Imaging assessment of children presenting with suspected or known juvenile idiopathic arthritis: ESSR-ESPR points to consider. Eur Radiol 30:5237–5249

Hetland ML, Stengaard-Pedersen K, Junker P et al (2010) Radiographic progression and remission rates in early rheumatoid arthritis - MRI bone oedema and anti-CCP predicted radiographic progression in the 5-year extension of the double-blind randomized CIMESTRA trial. Ann Rheum Dis 69(10):1789–1795

Idzior M, Sotniczuk M, Michalski E et al (2020) Ultrasonography, MRI and classic radiography of skin and MSK involvement in juvenile scleroderma. J Ultrason 20(83):311–317

Jeong H, Kim AY, Yoon HJ et al (2013) Clinical course and predictors of outcomes in patients with monoarthritis: a retrospective study of 171 cases. Int J Rheum Dis 17:502–510

Johnson SR (2015) New ACR EULAR guidelines for systemic sclerosis classification. Curr Rheumatol Rep 17(5):32

Jurik AG, Klicman RF, Simoni P et al (2018) SAPHO and CRMO: the value of imaging. Semin Musculoskelet Radiol 22:207–224

Karasick D (2009) Imaging of rheumatoid arthritis. In: Weissman BN (ed) Imaging of arthritis and metabolic bone disease. Saunders Elsevier, Philadelphia, pp 340–364

Mandl P, Navarro-Compán V, Terslev L et al (2015) EULAR recommendations for the use of imaging in the diagnosis and management of spondyloarthritis in clinical practice. Ann Rheum Dis 74(7):1327–1339

Martinoli C (2010) Musculoskeletal ultrasound: technical guidelines. Insights Imaging 1:99–144

Miller I, Janta J, Backhaus M et al (2017) The 2017 EULAR standardized procedures for ultrasound imaging in rheumatology. Ann Rheum Dis 76(12):1974–1979

Mjaavatten MD, Haugen AJ, Helgetveit K et al (2009) Pattern of joint involvement and other disease characteristics in 634 patients with arthritis of less than 16 weeks' duration. J Rheumatol 36:1401–1406

Molina J, Molina J, Gutierrez S et al (1995) Deforming arthropathy of the hands (Jaccoud's) in systemic lupus erythematosus (SLE): an independent subset of SLE? Arthritis Rheum 38:S347. (abstract)

Narvaez J, Narvaez JA, de Albert M et al (2012) Can magnetic resonance imaging of the hand and wrist differentiate between rheumatoid arthritis and psoriatic arthritis in the early stages of the disease? Semin Arthiritis Rheum 42:234–245

Norli ES, Brinkmann GH, Kvien TK et al (2020) Joint distribution and 2-year outcome in 347 patients with monoarthritis of less than 16 weeks' duration. Arthritis Care Res 72:705–710

Nusman CM, Ording Muller LS, Hemke R et al (2016) Current status of efforts on standardizing magnetic resonance imaging of juvenile idiopathic arthritis: report from the OMERACT MRI in JIA Working Group and Health-e-Child. J Rheumatol 43(1):239–244

Ostendorf B, Scherer A, Specker C et al (2003) Jaccoud's arthropathy in systemic lupus erythematosus: differentiation of deforming and erosive patterns by magnetic resonance imaging. Arthritis Rheum 48:157–165

Ostergaard M, Klarlund M (2001) Importance of timing of post-contrast MRI in rheumatoid arthritis: what happens during the first 60 minutes after IV gadolinium-DTPA? Ann Rheum Dis 60(11):1050–1054

Ostrowska M, Maśliński W, Prochorec-Sobieszek M et al (2018) Cartilage and bone damage in rheumatoid arthritis. Reumatologia 56(2):111–120

Ostrowska M, Michalski E, Gietka P et al (2022) Ankle MRI in JIA versus in non-JIA juveniles with arthralgia. J Clin Med 11(3):760

Plagou A, Teh J, Grainger AJ, Schueller-Weidekamm C, Sudoł-Szopińska I, Rennie W et al (2016) Recommendations of the ESSR Arthritis Subcommittee on ultrasonography in inflammatory joint disease. Semin Musculoskelet Radiol 20(5):496–506

Pracoń G, Simoni OP, Gietka P et al (2021) Conventional radiography and ultrasound imaging of rheumatic diseases affecting the pediatric population. Semin Musculoskelet Radiol 25:68–81

Ranga A, Agarwal Y et al (2017) Gadolinium based contrast agents in current practice: risks of accumulation and toxicity in patients with normal renal function. Indian J Radiol Imaging 27:141–147

Rascu A, Manger K, Kraetsch H et al (1996) Osteonecrosis in systemic lupus erythematosus, steroid-induced or a lupus-dependent manifestation? Lupus 5:323–327

Resnick D, Kransdorf MJ (2005a) Rheumatoid arthritis and related diseases. In: Resnick D, Kransdorf MJ (eds) Bone and joint imaging. Saunders Elsevier, Philadelphia, pp 209–254

Resnick D, Kransdorf MJ (2005b) Connective tissue disease. In: Resnick D, Kransdorf MJ (eds) Bone and joint imaging. Saunders Elsevier, Philadelphia, pp 328–332

Resnick D, Kransdorf MJ (2005c) Juvenile chronic arthritis. In: Resnick D, Kransdorf MJ (eds) Bone and joint imaging. Saunders Elsevier, Philadelphia, pp 255–266

Rubenstein J (2009) Seronegative spondyloarthropathies and SAPHO syndrome. In: Weissman BN (ed) Imaging of arthritis and metabolic bone disease. Saunders Elsevier, Philadelphia, pp 410–427

Scarpa R, Soscia E, Peluso R et al (2006) Nail and distal interphalangeal joint in psoriatic arthritis. J Rheumatol 33:1315–1319

Schanz S, Fierlbeck G, Ulmer A et al (2011) Localized scleroderma: MR findings and clinical features. Radiology 260:817–824

Schwartz Doria A, Babyn P (2009) Imaging investigation of arthritis in children. In: Weissman BN (ed) Imaging of arthritis and metabolic bone disease. Saunders Elsevier, Philadelphia, pp 428–456

Sheybani EF, Khanna G, White AJ et al (2013) Imaging of juvenile idiopathic arthritis: a multimodality approach. Radiographics 33:1253–7324

Sierra-Jimenez G, Sanchez-Ortiz A, Aceves-Avila F et al (2008) Tendinous and ligamentous derangements in systemic lupus erythematosus. J Rheumatol 35:2187–2191

Sudoł-Szopińska I, Pracoń G (2016) Diagnostic imaging of psoriatic arthritis. Part II: Magnetic resonance imaging and ultrasonography. J Ultrason 16:163–174

Sudoł-Szopińska I, Kontny E, Maśliński W et al (2012) The pathogenesis of rheumatoid arthritis in radiological studies. Part I: Formation of inflammatory infiltrates within the synovial membrane. J Ultrason 12(48):202–213

Sudoł-Szopińska I, Kwiatkowska B, Kołodziejczak M (2013) Musculoskeletal extraintestinal manifestations during the course of non-specific bowel diseases. Pol Przegl Chir 85(11):669–675

Sudoł-Szopińska I, Zaniewicz-Kaniewska K, Saied F et al (2014) The role of ultrasonography in the diagnosis of rheumatoid arthritis and peripheral spondyloarthropathies. Pol J Radiol 79:59–63

Sudoł-Szopińska I, Jurik AG, Eshed I et al (2015a) Recommendations of the ESSR Arthritis Subcommittee for the use of magnetic resonance imaging in musculoskeletal rheumatic diseases. Semin Musculoskelet Radiol 19(4):396–411

Sudoł-Szopińska I, Zaniewicz-Kaniewska K, Kwiatkowska B et al (2015b) Enthesopathies and enthesitis. Part II: Imaging studies. J Ultrason 15:196–207

Sudoł-Szopińska I, Kwiatkowska B, Prochorec-Sobieszek M et al (2015c) Enthesopathies and enthesitis. Part 1. Etiopathogenesis. J Ultrason 15:72–84

Sudoł-Szopińska I, Matuszewska G, Kwiatkowska B et al (2016a) Diagnostic imaging of psoriatic arthritis. Part I: Etiopathogenesis, classifications and radiographic features. J Ultrason 16:65–77

Sudoł-Szopińska I, Matuszewska G, Gietka P et al (2016b) Imaging of juvenile idiopathic arthritis. Part I: Clinical classifications and radiographs. J Ultrason 16(66):225–236

Sudoł-Szopińska I, Jans L et al (2017a) Rheumatoid arthritis: what do MRI and ultrasound show. J Ultrason 17(68):5–16

Sudoł-Szopińska I, Gietka P, Znajdek M et al (2017b) Imaging of juvenile spondyloarthritis. Part I: Classifications and radiographs. J Ultrason 17(70):167–175

Sudoł-Szopińska I, Jans L, Jurik AG et al (2018a) Imaging features of the juvenile inflammatory arthropathies. Semin Musculoskelet Radiol 22(2):147–165

Sudoł-Szopińska I, Eshed I, Jans L et al (2018b) Classifications and imaging of juvenile spondyloarthritis. J Ultrason 18:224–233

Sudoł-Szopińska I, Jacques T, Gietka P et al (2020) Imaging in dermatomyositis in adults and children. J Ultrason 20:e36–e42

Taljanovic MS, Melville DMH, Gimber LH et al (2015) High-resolution US of rheumatologic diseases. Radiographics 35(7):2026–2048

Tan AL, Grainger AJ, Tanner SF et al (2006) A high-resolution magnetic resonance imaging study of distal interphalangeal joint arthropathy in psoriatic arthritis and osteoarthritis: are they the same? Arthritis Rheum 54:128–1333

Taylor WJ, Gladman DD, Helliwell P et al (2006) CASPAR Study Group: classification criteria for psoriatic arthritis: development of new criteria from a large international study. Arthritis Rheum 54:2665–2673

Teh J, McQueen F, Eshed I et al (2018) Advanced imaging in the diagnosis of gout and other crystal arthropathies. Semin Musculoskelet Radiol 22(02):225–236

Thibaut J, Sudoł-Szopińska I, Larkman N et al (2018) Musculoskeletal manifestations of non-RA connective tissue diseases: scleroderma, systemic lupus erythematosus, Still's disease, dermatomyositis/polymyositis, Sjögren's syndrome, and mixed connective tissue disease. Semin Musculoskelet Radiol 22: 166–179

Tom S (2019) GRAPPA development of a preliminary ultrasonographic enthesitis score in psoriatic arthritis—GRAPPA ultrasound working group. J Rheumatol 46:384–390

van der Heijde DM, van Leeuwen MA, van Riel PL et al (1995) Radiographic progression on radiographs of hands and feet during the first 3 years of rheumatoid arthritis measured according to Sharp's method (van der Heijde modification). J Rheumatol 22(9):1792–1796

van Vugt R, Derksen R, Kater L et al (1998) Deforming arthropathy or lupus and rhupus hands in systemic lupus erythematosus. Ann Rheum Dis 57:540–544

Weissman BN, Ersoy HE, Hsu L et al (2009) Systemic lupus erythematosus and related conditions and vasculitic syndromes. In: Weissman BN (ed) Imaging of arthritis and metabolic bone disease. Saunders Elsevier, Philadelphia, pp 376–409

Znajdek M, Gazda A, Gietka P et al (2019) Juvenile spondyloarthritis and CRMO overlap syndrome in a 16 y.o. adolescent. A case report and literature review. J Ultrason 19(77):152–157

Metabolic Bone Disease

Niharika Prasad, G. Hegde, K. P. Iyengar, and R. Botchu

Contents

N. Prasad (✉)
Department of Radiology, IOCL, Barauni, Begusarai, India
e-mail: vats.niharika248@gmail.com

G. Hegde
Department of Radiology, University Hospitals of Morecambe Bay NHS Foundation, Lancaster, UK

K. P. Iyengar
Department of Orthopedics, Southport and Ormskirk Hospital NHS Trust, Southport, UK

R. Botchu
Department of Musculoskeletal Radiology, Royal Orthopedic Hospital, Birmingham, UK

1 Introduction

Metabolic bone diseases are frequently encountered in clinical practice, but their presence is often nonspecific (Panwar et al. 2017). Bone is comprised of both extracellular and cellular components. The calcium and phosphate metabolism balance is regulated by complex mechanisms. Metabolic bone diseases result due to disharmony in this very balance (Patel et al. 2015). Thus, on imaging, the picture is of osteosclerosis or osteopenia.

These diverse diseases result in pathology related to (1) bone mass, (2) calcium phosphate homeostasis, (3) bone turnover, and (4) growth (Jadav et al. 2014). The different types of metabolic bone diseases include osteoporosis, osteomalacia, rickets, scurvy, renal osteodystrophy, hyperparathyroidism, Paget's disease, osteogenesis imperfecta, acromegaly, and osteopetrosis.

By their nature, the metabolic bone diseases have their effect throughout the skeleton, and changes observed in the foot and ankle will usually be accompanied by changes elsewhere in the skeleton, which may be more significant. However, since the findings associated with metabolic bone disease may be incidental or unexpected, it is important to be aware of the spectrum of such disease when undertaking a radiological assessment of the foot and ankle. In this chapter, we have emphasized the changes seen in metabolic bone diseases as they apply to the foot and ankle. The reader is referred to the many excellent, more general texts for further discussion of

Med Radiol Diagn Imaging (2023)
https://doi.org/10.1007/174_2023_397,
Published Online: 03 May 2023

changes seen elsewhere in the skeleton and more thorough discussion of the pathophysiology of metabolic bone disease.

2 Pathophysiology of Bone Remodeling

The skeleton changes throughout life, being subject to growth, modeling, and remodeling. In the normal remodeling process, the synthesis of new bone by osteoblasts and the removal of old bone by osteoclasts are closely linked so that a balance is maintained. However, with increasing age, resorption tends to exceed formation. This age-related bone loss occurs irrespective of sex, race, or geographical location (Parfitt 1988). The remodeling process also occurs more rapidly in trabecular bone than in cortical bone, and trabecular bone loss leads to decreased connectivity between trabeculae in the weight-bearing skeleton.

As a result of faster bone loss in trabecular bone and in estrogen-deficient states, fractures may occur, often related to minimal trauma. Cortical bone is lost primarily from the endosteal surface, allowing the marrow space to expand and leading to decreased cortical thickness (Kalender et al. 1989). Higher trabecular bone densities are found in black people than white people, and although white women have more rapid bone loss in the spine and radius at the menopause than black women, the cortical bone loss is similar (Han et al. 1996). The differences between the two groups remain similar with increasing age and would appear to be related to peak adult bone mass rather than rates of bone loss.

Imaging in Metabolic Bone Diseases
Plain Radiographs

Plain radiographs form a key initial element in the workup of metabolic bone diseases. They should be sought, before a magnetic resonance imaging (MRI), so that they add to the diagnosis. They are usually the first line of investigation in osteoporosis (Panwar et al. 2017; Patel et al. 2015; Jadav et al. 2014; Harper 1989; Gerster 2007; Kottamasu et al. 1983). However, conventional radiographs have their limitations:

- Low sensitivity:
  A minimum of 30% bone loss is required to diagnose osteopenia (Panwar et al. 2017).
- Subjective.
- Differences in radiographic technique and quality.
- Overlapping findings as non-metabolic diseases can present with the same features.

Quantitative Ultrasound

It uses wavelengths of less than 1 kHz, unlike conventional diagnostic ultrasound, which uses 2–10 MHz wavelength to detect bone density.

Conventional diagnostic ultrasound is a noninvasive and widely available modality. It is particularly useful for diagnosing infection, inflammation, collections, and tenosynovitis (Lipsky 1997).

Computed Tomography

Quantitative CT (QCT) can help in the estimation of bone mineral density. It gives trabecular and cortical density to assess three-dimensional volumetric CT (Patel et al. 2015). It is mainly used for the spine. Its main limitation is its low spatial resolution.

Conventional diagnostic CT shows characteristic findings in osteoporosis, renal osteodystrophy, and Paget's disease, which will be discussed in the relevant headings later.

MRI

Due to its superior soft tissue resolution and multiplanar imaging capability, MRI is the gold standard investigation and is especially useful in imaging bone marrow (Lipsky 1997). It can aid in differentiating osteomyelitis from a neuropathic joint. It can also help in differentiating sterile joint effusion from septic arthritis.

PET/CT

PET/CT using 18-FDG shows increased uptake of this metabolite at sites of infection. It has high sensitivity and specificity in diabetes-related osteomyelitis and neuropathic joint (sensitivity of 80–95% and specificity of 90–100%) (Lipsky 1997). It has been found superior to a WBC-labeled scan for chronic osteomyelitis.

2.1 Osteoporosis

Osteoporosis may be considered a generalized or a regional abnormality. Regional or localized osteoporosis usually relates to injury, surgery, or infection, and a period of disuse, although it may represent conditions such as transient bone marrow edema of the hip or reflex sympathetic dystrophy.

2.2 Generalized Osteoporosis

In view of the potential for fracture with increasing bone loss, the identification of at-risk groups has been of interest. In defining osteoporosis, attempts have been made to determine the transition from acceptable bone loss to the pathological state in this spectrum of bone physiology.

2.2.1 Definition

As described by the Consensus Development Conference, osteoporosis is "a disease characterised by low bone mass and microarchitectural deterioration of bone tissue, leading to enhanced bone fragility and a consequent increase in fracture risk" (WHO 1994). This definition describes the functional importance of the abnormality but lacks any objective measure. The World Health Organization (WHO) has defined osteoporosis in terms of bone mineral concentration (BMC) or bone mineral density (BMD) values obtained from dual-energy X-ray absorptiometry (DXA) measurements such that a BMC or BMD more than 2.5 standard deviations below peak bone mass represents osteoporosis (referred to as T score < -2.5) (WHO 1994). BMD is normally distributed in the population, and criteria have been proposed to categorize results, although in view of the overlap between normal patients and those with fractures, these should be considered guidelines in the management of osteoporosis (Table 1).

Table 1 WHO definitions of osteoporosis based on bone mineral density (BMD) or bone mineral concentration (BMC)

Normal	BMC/BMD more than I SD below average young adult ($T < -1$)
Osteopenia	BMC/BMD more than I SD below average young adult but not more than 2.5 SD below ($-2.5 < T < -1$)
Osteoporosis	BMC/BMD more than 2.5 SD below young adult ($T < -2.5$)
Established osteoporosis	BMC/BMD more than 2.5 SD below the young adult average and one or more osteoporotic fractures

This has proved a useful definition based on objective measures, although "peak bone mass" cannot be applied consistently for all ages and all bone sites. Application of the female "normal" values to a male population may give spurious results, and application across different racial groups is also questionable. Its use has become established, and the bone mass has been shown to correlate with bone strength (Hodgskinson et al. 1997). The WHO definition is limited by its objectivity and does not consider issues of bone quality and those factors that contribute to it such as the geometric arrangement of trabeculae.

Generalized osteoporosis may be idiopathic or may occur as a result of various risk factors and medical conditions. In addition to genetic and lifestyle factors, chronic diseases of the gastrointestinal or urinary tracts that interfere with calcium and vitamin D metabolism may be responsible. Endocrine disorders such as hyperthyroidism and hyperparathyroidism and prolonged treatment with corticosteroids and anticoagulants have also been implicated.

In the individual patient, it was often the clinical endpoint of a fracture (particularly hip, spine, and forearm) that led to the diagnosis of osteoporosis. The associated morbidity and mortality of such complications remain considerable, and the healthcare costs involved in treatment are escalating as the older population increases. Despite the limitations of the WHO criteria, a greater awareness of the disease and those at risk now means that treatment can be implemented prior to end-stage disease.

2.2.2 Bone Mineral Density and Its Measurement

The radiological changes of osteoporosis reflect the underlying pathology. Radiographs show a reduction in bone density in keeping with osteopenia. The distinction between the different causes of osteopenia, which include osteoporosis, is generally not possible on conventional radiographs.

Accurate quantification of bone loss from conventional radiographs is not possible. In the foot, attempts have been made to quantify bone loss by analysis of the trabecular pattern of the calcaneus (Aggarwal et al. 1986). However, correlation with bone density measurement elsewhere is poor (Cockshott et al. 1984).

Several techniques are available for the noninvasive quantitative assessment of BMD including photon and X-ray absorptiometry (single and dual), quantitative CT (spinal and peripheral), and quantitative ultrasound (Genant 1997). If density is considered to be "mass per unit volume," then the only true volumetric measure of bone density is provided by quantitative CT. In this method, volumetric data are acquired and regions of interest placed selectively around cortical or trabecular bone. Comparison with phantom standards allows BMD to be calculated. Traditionally, however, BMD can also be considered as an "amount per unit area measure" and is given in the form g/cm^2 (mass per unit area) when estimated by X-ray absorptiometry.

2.2.3 Dual-X-Ray Absorptiometry

Dual-X-ray absorptiometry (DXA) is probably the most widely used method of bone density measurement. It is readily available, reproducible, and accurate and delivers a low ionizing radiation dose. Two distinct energy X-ray beams are used with bone and soft tissue standards for calibration. Pencil and fan-beam X-ray sources and single- and multiple-detector arrays are available, and while there is less radiation with the pencil beam types, examination times are shorter with the fan-beam type, and soft tissue and bone composition can be estimated (Mazess et al. 1992). The preferred anatomical sites are the lumbar spine and proximal femur, but peripheral sites can be examined. In fact, dedicated peripheral extremity scanners (pDXA) are available which utilize the high trabecular bone arrangement in the calcaneus for measurement. These have the advantage of being small and hence portable and inexpensive. Generally, examination of the spine is performed in a posteroanterior direction, but in the older population, the presence of aortic calcification, degenerative disk disease, and osteophyte formation may lead to an erroneous increase in the measured bone density. Lateral examination reduces such error, but the method is less reproducible. It is important to note that with DXA methods of BMD assessment, comparison of results is not possible across equipment from different manufacturers without careful cross-calibration. This has implications for serial measurements in the follow-up of patients or in clinical trials.

Such methods allow a measure of bone quantity to be determined, but quality factors like trabecular orientation and connectivity do not influence the result. However, as noted in the earlier definitions of osteoporosis, consideration of the microarchitecture of the bone was deemed important: a factor that cannot be evaluated by standard X-ray or CT methods.

2.2.4 Quantitative Ultrasound

Quantitative ultrasound (QUS) is a more recent innovation that evaluates bone mass and other parameters and hence potentially provides more qualitative information (Jergas and Schmid 1999). The two principal parameters are the speed of sound (SOS) in bone and broadband ultrasound attenuation (BUA). These are altered in osteoporotic bone compared with normal bone. The various manufacturers have further derived other factors to simplify the interpretation such as "stiffness" (Lunar Corp., Madison, WI, USA), "quantitative ultrasound index" (QUI) (Hologic Inc., Bedford, MA, USA), "strength index" (SI) (DMS SA, Montpellier, France), and "soundness" (Norland Inc., Fort Atkinson, WI, USA).

The current devices are used in the calcaneus, patella, tibia, radius, and phalanges, but as with DXA, comparison between manufacturers is difficult.

2.2.5 Fracture Risk

Whichever technique of bone density assessment is chosen, fracture risk prediction for that population is similar. A T score of less than −2.5 is associated with a twofold increase in the risk of fracture. The risk of fracture for the individual cannot be determined, but in conjunction with other lifestyle and medical conditions, a judgement can be made on the appropriateness of instituting therapy. Unless there are exceptional clinical reasons (e.g., corticosteroids or renal transplant), follow-up in osteoporosis is usually not performed more frequently than on a 2-yearly basis. This is felt to be sufficient time to ensure that changes occurring in BMD are greater than the precision error associated with the method.

3 Regional Osteoporosis

3.1 Reflex Sympathetic Dystrophy Syndrome

3.1.1 Etiology and Pathogenesis

The etiology of reflex sympathetic dystrophy or Sudeck's atrophy remains obscure, as suggested by the variety of synonyms that have been applied (Atkins and Duthie 1987). The traditional understanding has been of an alteration in the vasomotor status due to a sympathetic reflex following a local insult. Increased osteoclastic activity occurs as a result of acidic metabolites. The abnormal sympathetic response has also been considered at the spinal cord or even cerebral cortical level. A more recent study found that signs of sympathetic response were infrequent and that early symptoms were more suggestive of an exaggerated inflammatory reaction (Veldman et al. 1993).

A number of diagnostic factors have been described, including pain and tenderness, soft tissue swelling, diminished motor function, trophic skin changes, vasomotor instability, and patchy osteoporosis (Genant et al. 1975; Kozin et al. 1976b).

The vasomotor instability may progress from an early "warm phase" lasting days to weeks in which the skin is warm, red, and swollen to a "cold phase" where the skin is cool, clammy, and cyanosed.

3.1.2 Radiological Appearances

Radiological features include endosteal and intracortical excavation and subperiosteal and patchy trabecular bone resorption (Fig. 1). Juxta-articular and subchondral bone erosions may also be present, and there is increased tracer uptake on bone scintigraphy (Kozin et al. 1976a). More recently, the role of MR imaging has been examined. While one study suggested that it was of little value, a larger study demonstrated that fat-suppressed T2-weighted or STIR images were helpful in identifying those patients with the warm form of the process. Its use in the cold form of the condition was primarily to exclude

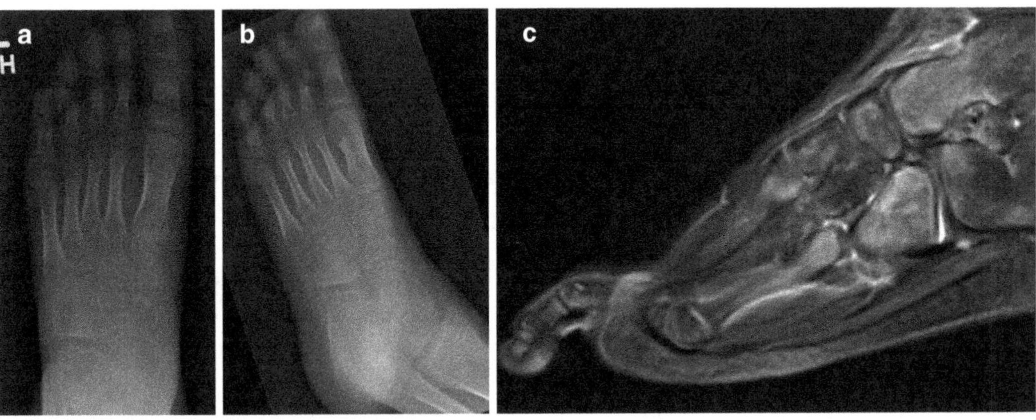

Fig. 1 Radiograph (**a**, **b**) of the foot demonstrating patchy lucency in the tarsal bones. Sagittal proton density fat-saturated MRI (**c**) image of the foot demonstrating edema involving multiple tarsal bones and metatarsals

other causes for the symptoms (Darbois et al. 1999; Koch et al. 1991). Quantitative ultrasound has been evaluated in the diagnosis and monitoring of response to calcitonin in the feet and was found to be a sensitive tool, particularly when BUA and "stiffness" were considered (Cepollaro et al. 1998). The final diagnosis can only be made on the clinical course by regression of findings or the development of aponeurotic and tendinous retractions with bony sclerosis over many months to years.

It should be remembered that the error in judging osteopenia based on conventional radiographic appearances has been estimated at 30–50%. While in most cases osteopenia seen on radiographs of the foot and ankle is likely to be self-limiting and related to the primary pathology and disuse, it may also be the manifestation of an underlying generalized osteoporosis or an indicator of an abnormal response to injury such as RSDS.

3.2 Rickets/Osteomalacia

In contrast to osteoporosis, where there is a reduction in bone mass, osteomalacia and rickets are the result of inadequate mineralization of the osteoid bone matrix. The term rickets is applied to the condition when seen in children, while osteomalacia is the adult form of the disease.

3.2.1 Etiology and Pathogenesis

There are many causes of osteomalacia and rickets, but the underlying etiology usually results in a deficiency of the active (dihydroxy) form of vitamin D, 1,25-$(OH)_2$-cholecalciferol. Vitamin D is synthesized in the skin by the action of sunlight and is obtained from the diet. The initial hydroxylation of the vitamin occurs in the liver, but a second hydroxylation is required to produce the active form of the hormone. This final step occurs in the kidney. As a consequence, deficiency may be the result of dietary insufficiency or inadequate sunlight exposure. However, more common causes relate to malabsorption of the vitamin from the gut or the presence of renal disease resulting in inadequate hydroxylation of the 25-OH-vitamin D molecule to active 1,25-$(OH)_2$-cholecalciferol. Less commonly, osteomalacia and rickets result from liver failure (inadequate primary hydroxylation of vitamin D) or interference in the metabolism of vitamin D by drugs. In some cases, the condition results from phosphate deficiency, usually due to renal tubular disorders.

3.2.2 Radiological Appearances

Although rickets and osteomalacia share a common etiology, they have different radiological manifestations. Rickets affects the immature skeleton and primarily affects the site of bone growth at the cartilaginous growth plate. In contrast, osteomalacia has its effects on the mature bone.

3.2.2.1 Rickets

The generalized, nonspecific skeletal effects of rickets include retarded bone growth and osteopenia. However, more specific findings are growth plate widening (due to the failure of mineralization of the proliferating cartilage) and increasing irregularity at the interface between the growth plate and metaphysis (Pitt 1991). In more advanced cases, the metaphyses become widened and cup shaped. A further feature of rickets is a characteristic bowing seen in the long bones of the arms and legs. These features become more marked as weight-bearing begins to have an effect (Pitt 1981, 1991). The features are most marked at sites where bone growth, and therefore the requirement for mineralization, is most rapid. In the foot, involvement of the metatarsals and phalanges is unusual and only seen in severe cases (Bhargava et al. 1983). However, typical changes may be seen in less severe cases at the distal tibial physis and metaphysis (Fig. 2). Furthermore, bowing deformities commonly involve the tibia and fibula and may be demonstrated on ankle radiographs (Fig. 3). Such a bowing deformity may persist into adulthood (Fig. 4).

3.2.2.2 Osteomalacia

As with rickets, generalized osteopenia is a feature, albeit rather nonspecific. Since osteomalacia affects the mature skeleton, the involvement

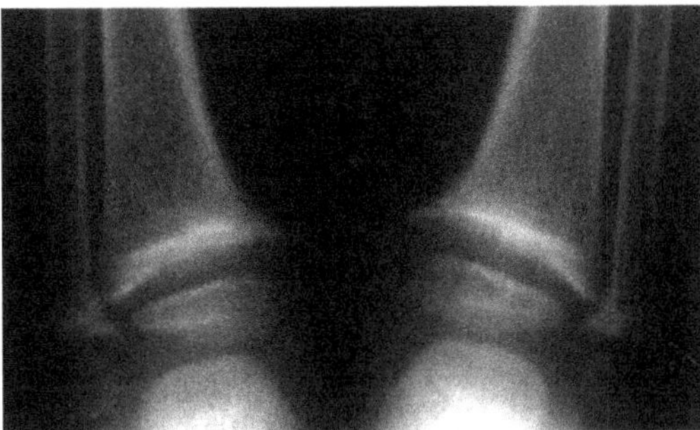

Fig. 2 AP view of both distal tibia and fibular metaphyses. Bilateral metaphyseal changes typical of rickets are apparent in this child who emigrated to the UK from India. There is widening and irregularity of all the metaphyses

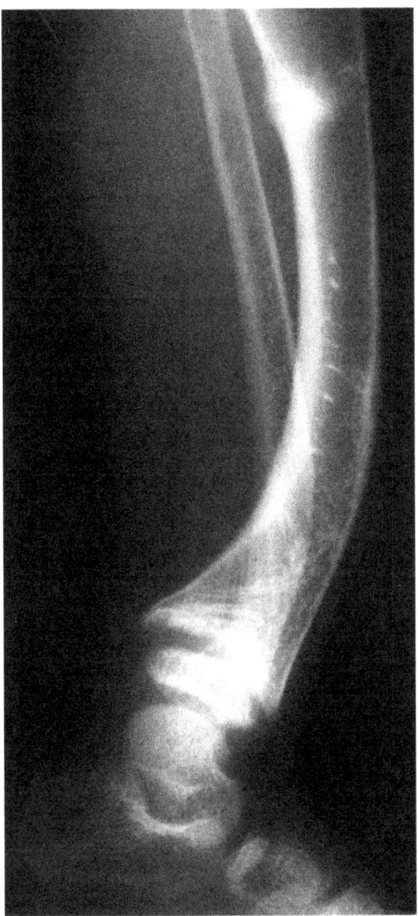

Fig. 3 Lateral view of the tibia and fibula. This child with advanced nutritional rickets shows bowing deformity of both the tibia and fibula. Note also the typical cupped metaphyseal changes of rickets, as well as Looser zone in the tibial shaft

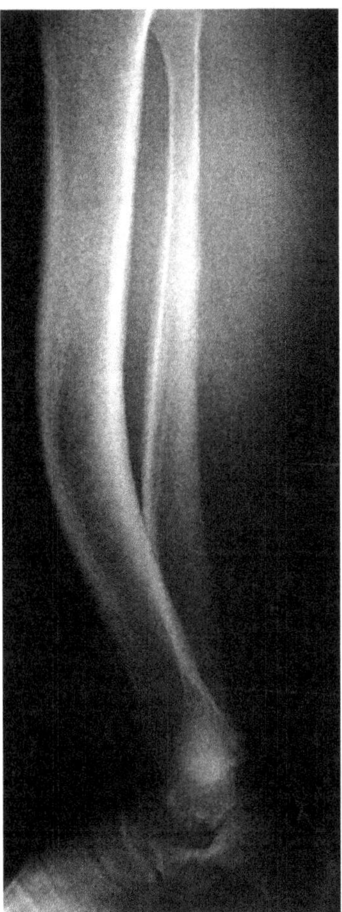

Fig. 4 Lateral view of tibia and fibula. This adult suffered severe rickets as a child and has a persistent bowing deformity of the tibia despite treatment

of the metaphyses is not seen. The most characteristic feature of osteomalacia is the presence of pseudofractures also known as Looser zones. These characteristically occur at sites of stress where there is high bone turnover and histologically consist of unmineralized osteoid. This is deposited during the natural repair processes the bone undergoes at this site (Pitt 1981). They are often symmetrical and appear as linear radiolucencies seen perpendicular to the bone cortex. They extend into the bone, appearing as small fissures, often with sclerotic margins. Pseudofractures are seen at characteristic sites within the skeleton, particularly along the lateral borders of the scapulae and along the pubic rami and medial borders of the femoral neck. They may be

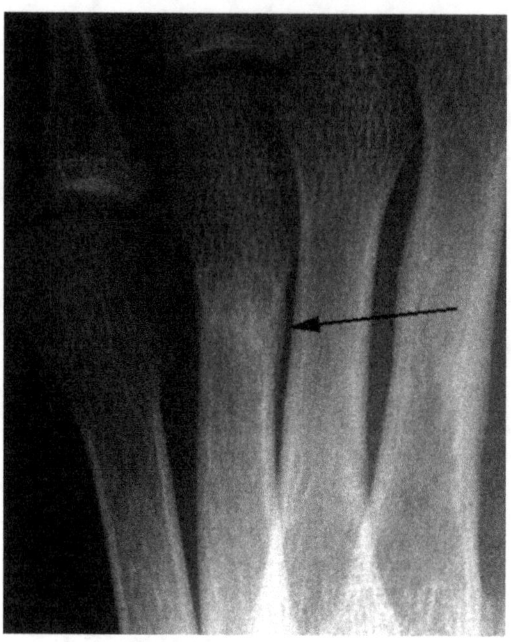

Fig. 5 Dorsoplantar radiograph of the foot. Looser zone (pseudofracture) in the fourth metatarsal in a patient with nutritional osteomalacia (*arrow*)

seen elsewhere in the long bones, including the tibia, where they may be seen during radiological review of the ankle. However, they are only rarely seen in the bones of the foot and ankle themselves (Fig. 5).

Severe hypophosphatemic osteomalacia has been reported as a complication of connective tissue tumors. Crouzet et al. undertook a review of the literature of such cases and found that the underlying tumor was usually located in a limb, generally the lower limb. They themselves described a case in which the underlying tumor was a plantar neurilemmoma. It is thought that the tumor produces substances capable of blocking intracellular phosphate transfer and inhibiting renal vitamin D hydroxylation (Crouzet et al. 1995).

It would be unusual to make a diagnosis of osteomalacia or rickets on the basis of radiographs of the foot and ankle, and if these diagnoses are suspected, then confirmatory evidence from radiographs of other areas along with clinical and biochemical evidence should be sought.

3.3 Hyperparathyroidism

3.3.1 Pathogenesis

The hyperparathyroid disorders result from overactivity of the parathyroid hormone (PTH)-producing parathyroid glands. PTH is of fundamental importance in calcium and phosphate homeostasis. It has two main target organs:

- The bones, where it stimulates osteoclastic activity, thereby releasing calcium and phosphate and bringing about bone resorption
- The kidneys, where it acts to conserve calcium and stimulates phosphate excretion
- The net effect is to increase the serum free-ionized calcium

Hyperparathyroidism is subdivided into three types:

1. Primary hyperparathyroidism: the overproduction of PTH due to parathyroid hyperplasia or adenoma. Rarely, this can also be brought about by a parathyroid carcinoma. Occasionally, the cause lies outside the parathyroids in the form of ectopic production of PTH by non-parathyroid tumors.
2. Secondary hyperparathyroidism: this results from increased PTH production in response to persistent hypocalcemia that fails to correct. The most common cause is chronic renal failure, but the condition is also seen in cases of prolonged vitamin D deficiency such as may be seen with inadequate intestinal absorption following gastrectomy or in cases of malnutrition.
3. Tertiary hyperparathyroidism: this usually occurs in patients receiving renal dialysis when the parathyroid gland has been in a state of prolonged positive feedback due to hypocalcemia (secondary hyperparathyroidism) and becomes autonomous, no longer responding to the normal feedback mechanisms.

3.3.2 Radiological Appearances

The radiological appearances of hyperparathyroidism are the result of the process of bone resorption stimulated by the excess PTH. Typically, bone resorption is first noted radiographically in the form of subperiosteal and cortical bone resorption. Cortical bone resorption may be seen in the form of cortical tunneling (Genant et al. 1973). Typically, these changes are noted first in the bones of the hand, but such changes may be observed in the short bones of the foot (Fig. 6). In severe cases, hyperparathyroidism may bring about resorption of the terminal phalangeal tufts or midportion.

Resorption may also occur at the sites of tendinous and ligamentous insertion. In the foot, resorption may frequently be seen on the inferior aspect of the calcaneum, an appearance that can be confused with inflammatory arthropathies such as Reiter's disease (Hayes and Conway 1991; Resnick et al. 1981).

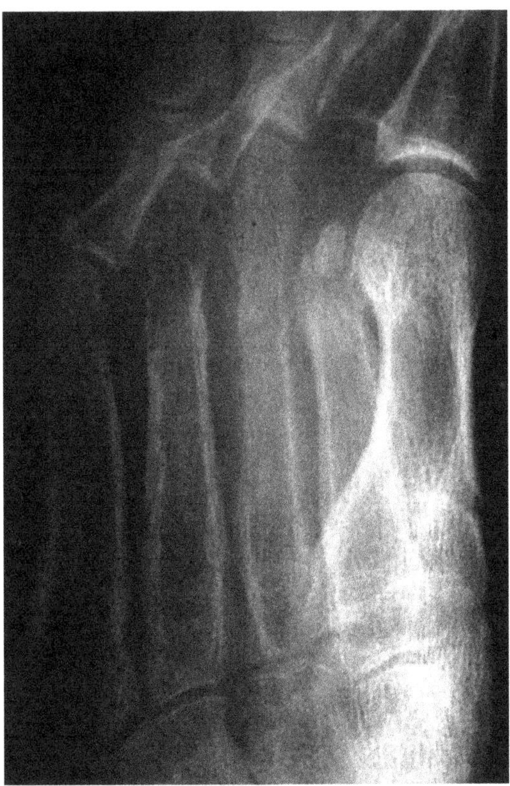

Fig. 6 Dorsoplantar oblique view of the foot. This patient has severe primary hyperparathyroidism. There is marked cortical bone resorption and focal destruction characteristic of brown tumor in the metatarsals. Both subperiosteal resorption and intracortical tunneling can be seen

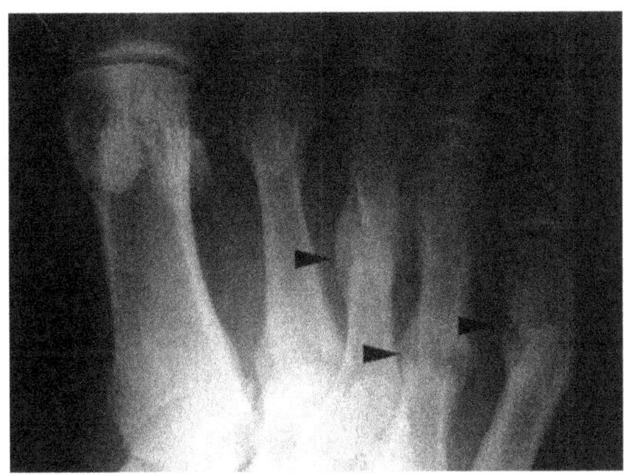

Fig. 7 Dorsoplantar view of foot. There are insufficiency fractures in the third, fourth, and fifth metatarsals in this patient with primary hyperparathyroidism (*arrowheads*). Cortical resorption is also noted

Brown tumors in the form of localized areas of bone lysis may also be observed, although these are not typically found in the feet.

In hyperparathyroidism, the bones will characteristically show generalized osteopenia. The weakened bone may be subject to stress fractures, and this has been described as a complication of hyperparathyroidism in the os calcis (Fishco and Stiles 1999). Fractures of the metatarsals may also be seen (Fig. 7).

In addition to the bone changes seen in hyperparathyroidism, soft tissue changes may be observed. These include vascular and periarticular calcification (Hamilton 1972). Vascular calcification is particularly a feature of secondary hyperparathyroidism.

3.4 Renal Osteodystrophy

3.4.1 Pathogenesis

Renal osteodystrophy has a complex pathogenesis resulting from an interplay between the metabolic pathways involved. Two main processes are involved:

- *Abnormal vitamin D metabolism.* This results from insufficient active 1,25-$(OH)_2$-cholecalciferol as a consequence of inadequate secondary hydroxylation in the damaged kidney.

- *Secondary hyperparathyroidism.* Phosphate retention by the damaged kidney leads to hypocalcemia, which in turn stimulates PTH production by the pituitary gland. PTH secretion attempts to restore the serum calcium. With time, the action of PTH produces characteristic changes in the skeleton with features of both skeletal decalcification and osteosclerosis.

These two processes both play a role in bringing about the radiological appearances seen in renal osteodystrophy. However, the contribution each makes varies, and this results in a spectrum of appearances seen radiologically.

3.4.2 Radiological Appearances

The features of osteomalacia are seen in renal osteodystrophy in the form of reduced bone density and findings of rickets in children. However, Looser zones are rare. The features of secondary hyperparathyroidism usually predominate, with evidence of bone resorption (most usually seen in the hands). Sclerotic changes, or osteosclerosis, may also be seen (Fig. 8). These are most frequently seen in the axial skeleton, most typically in the spine in the form of the "rugger jersey spine." However, these appearances may also be seen in the metaphyses of long bones and in the tarsal bones of the foot (Garver et al. 1981).

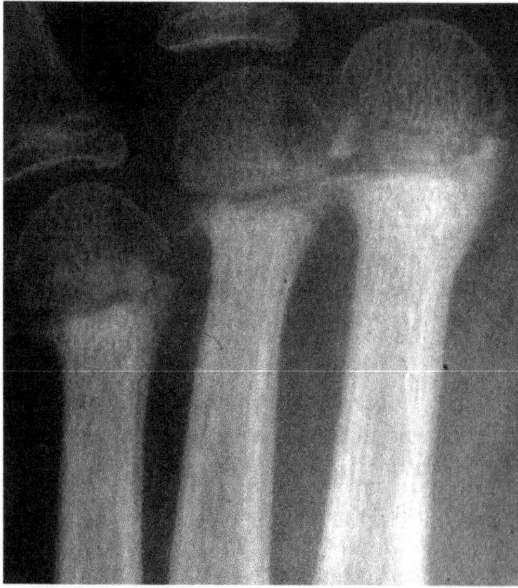

Fig. 8 Dorsoplantar view of the forefoot. Features of renal osteodystrophy with osteosclerosis, intracortical tunneling, and metaphyseal fractures in this child with advanced renal failure

Many patients with renal disease or with renal transplants receive steroid therapy, making them susceptible to developing avascular necrosis (AVN). The talus is a common site for this to occur. Conventional radiographs may show no abnormality in the early stages of AVN, but subsequently an area of subchondral lysis may be seen which later develops into an area of subchondral sclerosis, which may be associated with subchondral collapse. The changes are more sensitively demonstrated on MR imaging, with a characteristic subchondral segmental area of signal abnormality delineated by a sclerotic band of low signal intensity on T1-weighted sequences. On T2 weighting, this marginal zone classically shows an outer low signal band with an inner margin of high signal intensity representing the reactive interface between the normal marrow and the area of ischemia. As with hyperparathyroidism, soft tissue and vascular calcifications may be observed in the feet. Such soft tissue calcification may present as a painful nodule, and ulceration has been described (Chalmers et al. 1998; De Palma et al. 1993; Edwards and Spinner 1994). Calcium deposition in tendons may also occur, and spontaneous tears of tendons have been described in renal osteodystrophy, including avulsion of the tendon at its bony insertion (Meneghello and Bertoli 1983). Such occurrences may be associated with the Achilles tendon (De Palma et al. 1993).

3.5 Hypoparathyroidism

3.5.1 Pathogenesis

Idiopathic hypoparathyroidism is a rare condition in which the parathyroid glands are hypoplastic and produce inadequate PTH. This condition usually presents in childhood.

A more common cause of hypoparathyroidism is the result of surgical damage to the parathyroid glands or their blood supply at the time of thyroid surgery (Sherwood 1993). The effect of reduced PTH levels is to induce hypocalcemia with hyperphosphatemia.

3.5.2 Radiological Appearances

Sclerotic change is the most frequent radiological change in hypoparathyroidism. This may be generalized or focal (Resnick and Niwayama 1995b). Other features include band-like densities in the metaphyses of long bones and premature epiphyseal closure.

3.6 Pseudohypoparathyroidism and Pseudopseudohypoparathyroidism

In addition to primary hypoparathyroidism, a hypoparathyroid state can result from a rare inborn error of metabolism that leads to the impaired response of the end organs (kidneys and bone) to PTH. This condition is known as pseudohypoparathyroidism and is associated with short stature, obesity, mental retardation, and a round face. The condition has several different variants depending on the precise nature of the defect in the metabolism (Levine 1993). However, the radiological features are similar in each. In addition to the changes in the skeleton seen in primary hypoparathyroidism (bone sclerosis and premature epiphyseal closure), the patients characteristically have shortened metatarsals and phalanges affecting the first and fourth digits (Resnick and Niwayama 1995b). Shortening of the metacarpals and phalanges is also seen in the hands.

Pseudopseudohypoparathyroidism is a condition in which the patients have clinical somatypic features similar to pseudohypoparathyroidism (short stature, obesity, etc.) but are normocalcemic. The radiological features are similar to those of pseudohypoparathyroidism.

3.7 Thyroid Disorders

Thyroid hormones play an important part in normal growth and development. They act primarily on cartilage formation. However, they also act to stimulate bone resorption and can be a cause of secondary osteoporosis (Canalis 1993).

3.7.1 Hypothyroidism

Hypothyroidism can either result from a primary deficiency of the thyroid gland or be secondary to the failure of thyroid-stimulating hormone (TSH) secretion by the pituitary gland.

In adults, the effect of hypothyroidism on the skeleton is mild, with a normal or mildly increased bone mass. However, soft tissue calcific deposits and increased radiodensity of the bones have been reported (Chew 1991).

It is in children that the most significant effects of thyroid deficiency are seen radiographically. The changes are most in evidence at the physeal plates and epiphyses. There is delayed skeletal maturation, with late appearance of the secondary ossification centers, which are typically stippled or even fragmented. Delayed or even failure of physeal plate closure is also a feature.

3.7.2 Hyperthyroidism

Thyrotoxicosis most frequently results from Graves' disease, an autoimmune process affecting the thyroid gland and stimulating thyroid hormone production, or from the presence of solitary or multiple thyroid hormone-producing (toxic) nodules. The condition results in increased bone turnover and remodeling and may be associated with hypercalcemia (Chew 1991).

Bone loss results in the progressive development of osteopenia. This is particularly marked in the appendicular skeleton where changes may be prominent in the feet, and there may be associated insufficiency fractures (Chevrot et al. 1978). The appearance in the short tubular bones of the hands and feet is that of "busy bone," namely increased intracortical bone resorption producing striations or tunneling (Fig. 9). This finding is nonspecific and can be seen in disuse osteoporosis, reflex sympathetic dystrophy, hyperparathyroidism, and even radiation-induced osteolysis (Fig. 10).

3.7.2.1 Thyroid Acropachy

This represents a complication of thyrotoxicosis occurring in around 1% of patients (Resnick 1995b). Clubbing of the fingers and toes is

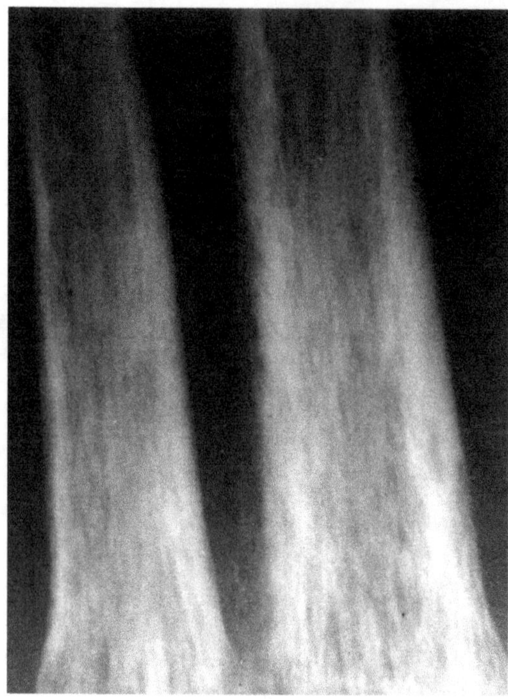

Fig. 9 Close-up view of the metatarsals. Marked intracortical tunneling or "busy bone" in a patient with advanced thyrotoxicosis

seen. Involvement is characteristically limited to the hands and feet where dense periosteal new bone formation is seen along the diaphyses of the metacarpals and metatarsals. There is usually overlying soft tissue swelling, and the bone involvement may be asymmetrical (Chew 1991). This appearance may simulate the periosteal changes of pulmonary hypertrophic osteoarthropathy (Fig. 11).

3.8 Acromegaly

3.8.1 Pathogenesis

Acromegaly results from the inappropriate secretion of growth hormone by the pituitary gland. The action of growth hormone is to promote skeletal growth. Prior to skeletal maturity, such secretion results in gigantism. However, once the growth plates have closed, the action of the growth hormone results in acromegaly. In the majority of cases, the cause is a secreting pituitary adenoma. Other less common causes include ectopic production of growth hormone

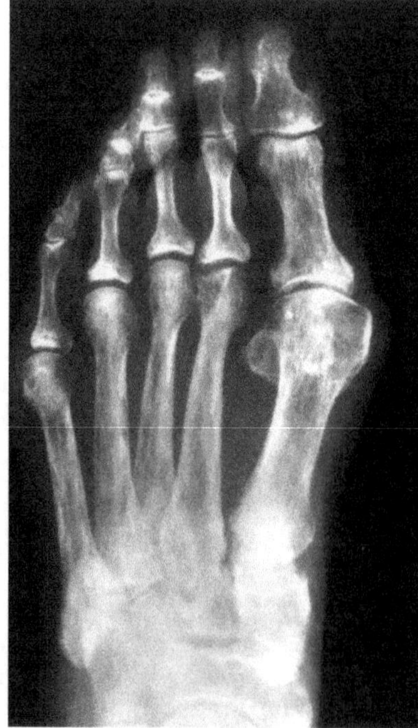

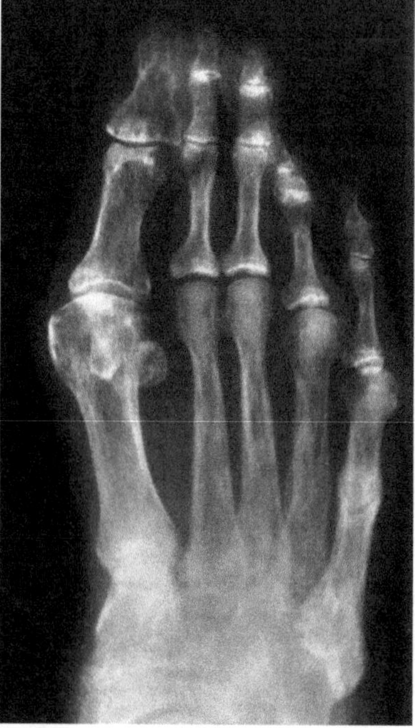

Fig. 10 Dorsoplantar view of the forefeet. Patchy osteolysis and sclerosis of the shafts of the tubular bones with osteonecrosis of the left second metatarsal head and insufficiency fracture of the right fifth metatarsal shaft in a rare patient with radiation necrosis due to radium ingestion

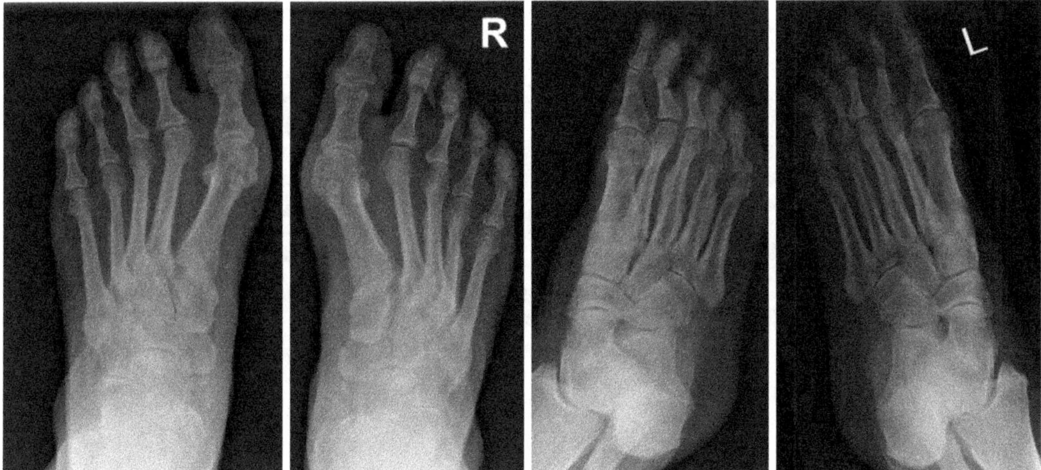

Fig. 11 Thyroid acropachy-prominent smooth periosteal reaction in the bilateral third and fourth metatarsals

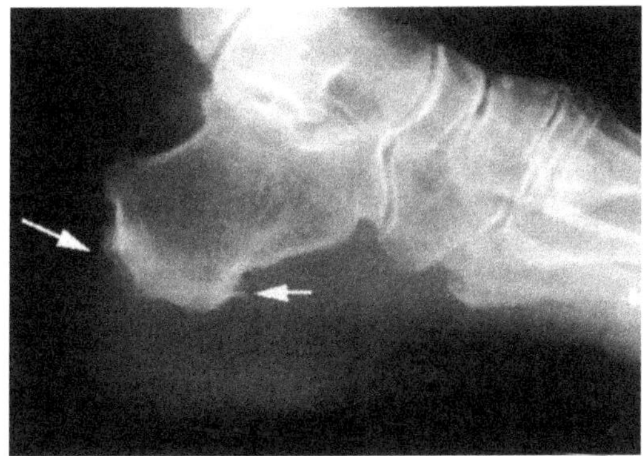

Fig. 12 Lateral radiograph of the calcaneus. There is thickening of the heel pad in this woman with acromegaly. The heel pad was measured at 31 mm. Note also the bone proliferation at the enthesis sites (*arrows*)

by non-pituitary tumors. The condition is seen in both men and women with equal incidence (Chew 1991).

3.8.2 Radiological Appearances

3.8.2.1 Soft Tissue Changes

Acromegaly induces thickening of the soft tissues. Clinically, this is manifest in the coarsened fades characteristic of acromegaly along with thickened oily skin. Radiologically, the soft tissue thickening can be detected, and this is seen characteristically over the calcaneus (Fig. 12). Heel pad thickness has been considered a useful diagnostic tool for acromegaly. However, there has been and still is considerable debate in the literature as to the upper limit of normal heel pad thickness (Gonticas et al. 1969; Macsweeney et al. 1990; Paisey et al. 1984; Puckette and Seymour 1967). Attempts have been made to relate the measurement to body weight (Gonticas et al. 1969), and the measurement is also shown to vary with race (Mittal et al. 1983). For practical purposes, values of heel pad thickness over 23 mm in men and 21.5 mm in women are suggestive of the diagnosis of acromegaly if local causes of skin thickening are excluded (Resnick 1995a). The use of ultrasound in the measurement of heel pad thickness has also been described (Gooding et al. 1985). However, radiological morphometry now has little role to play in the diagnosis and monitoring of acromegaly given the ready availability of accurate and sensitive biochemical assays for growth hormone.

3.8.2.2 Bone Changes

Acromegaly brings about many well-recognized radiological changes in the skeleton as a result of the effect of growth hormone in stimulating bone proliferation. The feet are commonly affected by the disease. The changes seen include enlargement of the tufts and bases of the terminal phalanges, overgrowth of the metatarsal heads often

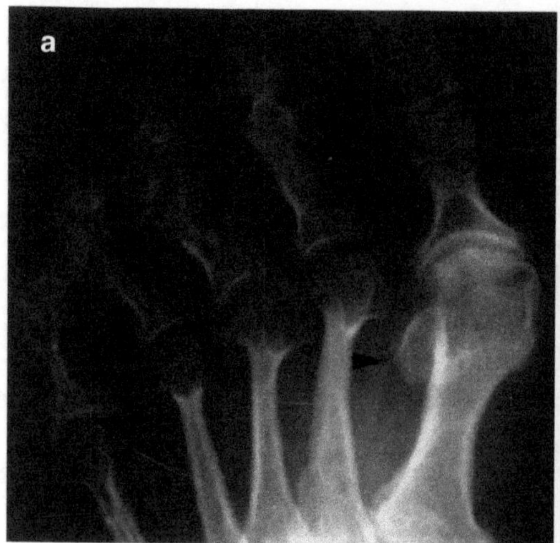

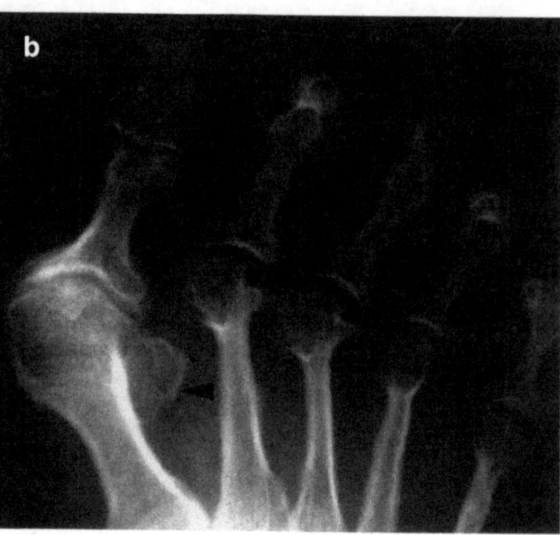

Fig. 13 (**a**, **b**) Dorsoplantar views of left (**a**) and right (**b**) feet. The typical features of acromegaly are shown. There is widening of the metatarsophalangeal joint spaces, with overgrowth of the metatarsal heads and hypertrophic beaking. There is also enlargement of the sesamoid bones (*arrowheads*) and proliferation of the terminal phalangeal tufts and bases

with hypertrophic beaking, and increase in the joint space, seen particularly at the metatarsal phalangeal joints (Fig. 13). In addition, there is enlargement of the sesamoid bones, and bone proliferation is seen at enthesis sites of tendinous and ligamentous attachments (Fig. 12). Ultrasound has been successfully used to monitor joint and soft tissue changes, including tendon thickness, in acromegaly (Colao et al. 1998, 1999). Despite the general picture of bone proliferation in acromegaly, the tubular bones in the foot may show thinning or penciling. This may be seen particularly in the shafts of the distal metatarsals and the phalanges. Doppman and colleagues have proposed that this is the result of remodeling along the plantar aspect of the metatarsals as a response to the thickened soft tissues overlying the bones during weight-bearing (Doppman et al. 1988).

3.9 Paget's Disease

Paget's disease is a common disease of unknown etiology. It is characterized by a combination of bone resorption and formation, resulting in disordered bone remodeling. The condition has a predilection for the axial skeleton and long bones of the leg (Guyer et al. 1981; Resnick and Niwayama 1995a) but can be seen in the small bones of the foot. It may affect one bone in isolation or show widespread bone involvement.

The radiological features reflect the pathophysiology of the disease, with distinct phases of the disease demonstrated radiologically. During the early osteolytic (hot) phase of the disease, the affected bone undergoes a process where resorption predominates, and bone lysis is seen radiologically. The mixed phase of Paget's disease involves processes of both resorption and proliferation occurring together. During this stage, remodeling of the bone occurs, and the radiological picture is characterized by coarsening of the bone trabeculae and cortical thickening. In its sclerotic (cool) phase, there is a diffuse increase in bone density with further cortical thickening and widening of the bone.

A number of complications of Paget's disease exist. The most serious one is the development of sarcoma within the pagetic bone. Fortunately, this is rare, with the most common sarcoma to develop being osteosarcoma. More commonly, pathological fractures are seen, particularly in the long bones where they often appear as stress fractures.

Involvement of Paget's disease in the foot is relatively unusual, although when seen, it seems to have a predilection for the os calcis (Fig. 14) (Korber et al. 1993; Resnick and Niwayama 1995a; Rubin et al. 1983). However, it may also be seen in the short bones of the foot (Fig. 15). The tibia is more commonly affected, and where it involves the distal tibia, the patient may present with chronic ankle pain (Neylon 1995).

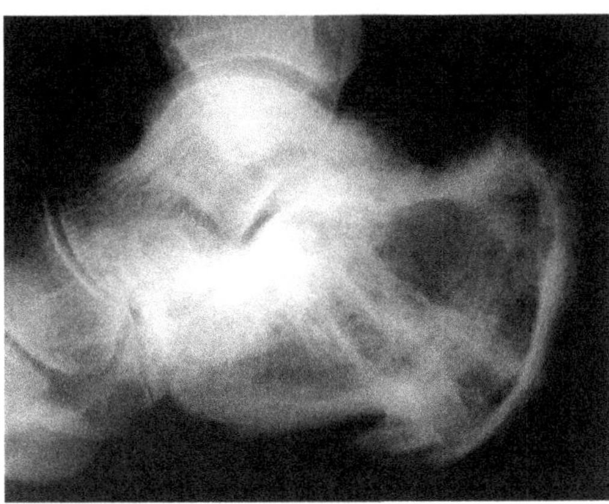

Fig. 14 Lateral radiograph of the calcaneus. There is coarsening of the trabecular pattern with bony expansion and cortical thickening. The appearance is that of Paget's disease

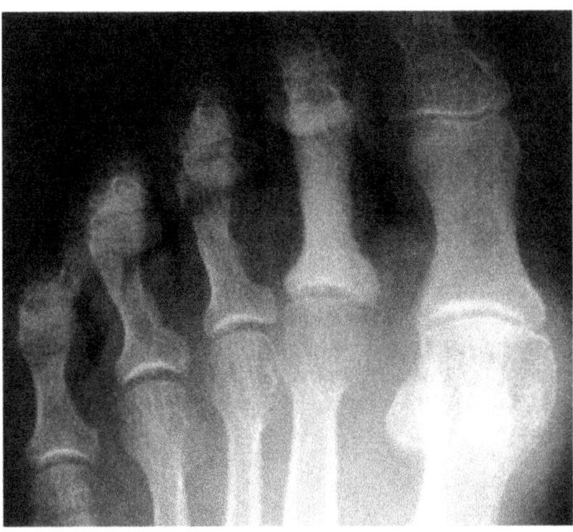

Fig. 15 Dorsoplantar radiograph of left foot. Paget's disease of the second proximal phalanx seen as sclerosis and mild expansion

3.9.1 Radiological Findings of Metabolic Bone Diseases

- Endosteal scalloping.
- Cortical thinning.
- Verticalization of trabeculae.
- A T score of less than −2.5 on DEXA.
- Recurrent metatarsal fractures (Harper 1989)—these can be seen in conditions like **hypophosphatasia**.
- Pseudofractures—in osteomalacia.
- Subligamentous and subtendinous changes are nonspecific and can be frequently noted in the inferior calcaneus (Patel et al. 2015)—in hyperparathyroidism or renal osteodystrophy.
- **Brown tumors** can rarely occur in bones of the foot—in both **primary and secondary hyperparathyroidism**. These appear as cyst-like lucencies. They are composed of highly vascular fibrous tissue that undergoes hemorrhage, giving rise to a brownish color and hence the name.
- Soft tissue and vascular calcifications are seen more frequently in secondary hyperparathyroidism from chronic renal disease.

3.9.2 Pseudotumors of the Foot and Ankle

These are more common than malignant neoplasms. These can be seen in metabolic conditions and include (Van Hul et al. 2011):

- **Gout**—The hallux is the most commonly involved site followed by the metatarsophalangeal and interphalangeal joints and the Achilles tendons (Gerster 2007). Tophus represents an amorphous or crystalline mass of urate with a surrounding layer of inflammatory tissue. They are isointense to muscle on T1WI and heterogeneously high signal intensity on T2WI (Fig. 16). They usually show heterogeneous enhancement on postcontrast images.
- **Pseudo-gout**—Caused by calcium pyrophosphate dihydrate (CPPD), can have a similar imaging appearance.
- **Tumoral calcinosis**—This can be primary or secondary. Unlike the primary form which

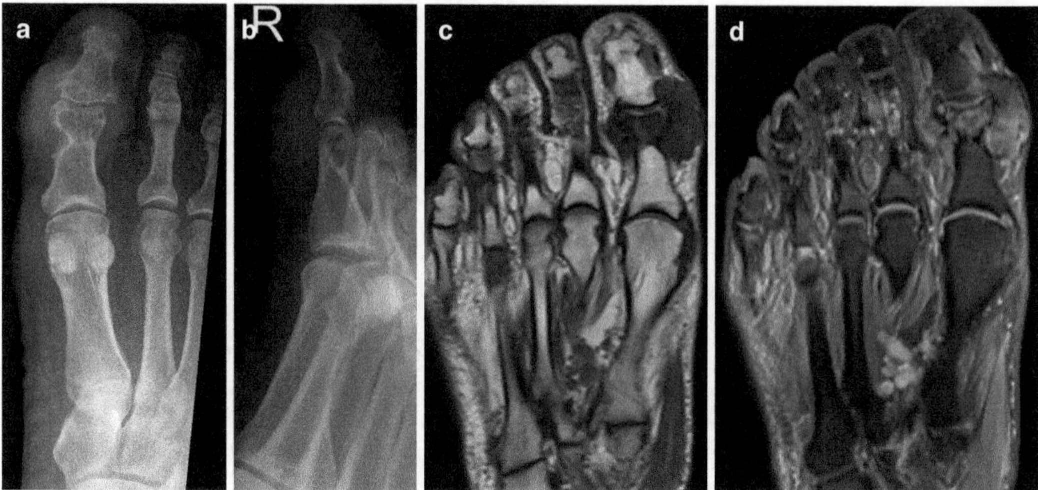

Fig. 16 Radiograph of the great toe (**a, b**) demonstrating characteristic erosions in the medial aspect of the distal proximal phalanx and base of the distal phalanx with associated soft tissue swelling. Axial T1 and proton density fat-saturated images of the foot demonstrating (**c, d**) a tophus around the first interphalangeal joint

presents early, the secondary form presents late as a result of chronic renal failure. Lobulated, calcified deposits in the periarticular locations are seen on imaging (Van Hul et al. 2011).

- **Amyloidosis**—Amyloid deposits can be seen as soft tissue masses within the joint capsule or in the skin. These are hypointense of T1WI and hypo- to isointense on T2WI (Van Hul et al. 2011).
- **Hemochromatosis**—Chondrocalcinosis may occur (Gerster 2007).
- **Hyperlipidemia**—Xanthomatous deposits may be seen in the Achilles tendon.

3.9.3 Diabetic Foot

Vasculopathy, neuropathy, infection, and immunosuppression lead to diabetic foot (Krishnamurthy et al. 1977). The main role of imaging is the following:

- Differentiation of soft tissue infection from osteomyelitis.
- Differentiation of osteomyelitis (Fig. 17) from neuroarthropathy (Figs. 18 and 19).

  Dynamic contrast-enhanced MR imaging can help to detect differences between the vascularization patterns of neuropathic arthropathy and osteomyelitis.

  WBC-labeled radionuclide imaging is helpful. A few days after the onset of symptoms of acute osteomyelitis, a triple-phase bone scan shows increased activity in the first two phases (angiographic and blood pool phases) and focal increased uptake in the late phase (Lipsky 1997) (Table 2).
- To detect abscess formation early.

The topic “diabetic foot” is discussed in more detail in another separate chapter.

3.9.4 Edema Versus Cellulitis

- Contrast enhancement is present in cellulitis and not in diabetes-related edema and neuropathic disease.

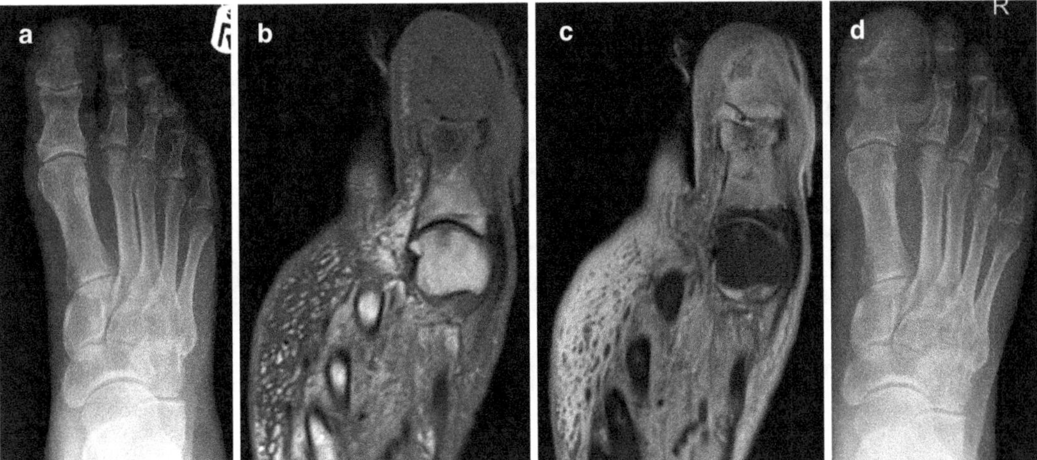

Fig. 17 Osteomyelitis of great toe in a diabetic patient—(**a**) Initial AP radiograph of the foot demonstrating subtle lucency and osteolysis in the tuft of the terminal phalanx of great toe. Axial T1 (**b**) and proton density fat-saturated (**c**) MRI images of the great toe demonstrating osteomyelitis changes (edema and loss of marrow fat signal) in the terminal and proximal phalanx of with extensive soft tissue inflammatory changes. Follow-up radiograph done after 3 months (**d**) demonstrates significant destruction of the terminal phalanx and proximal phalanx of great tor with significant soft tissue swelling

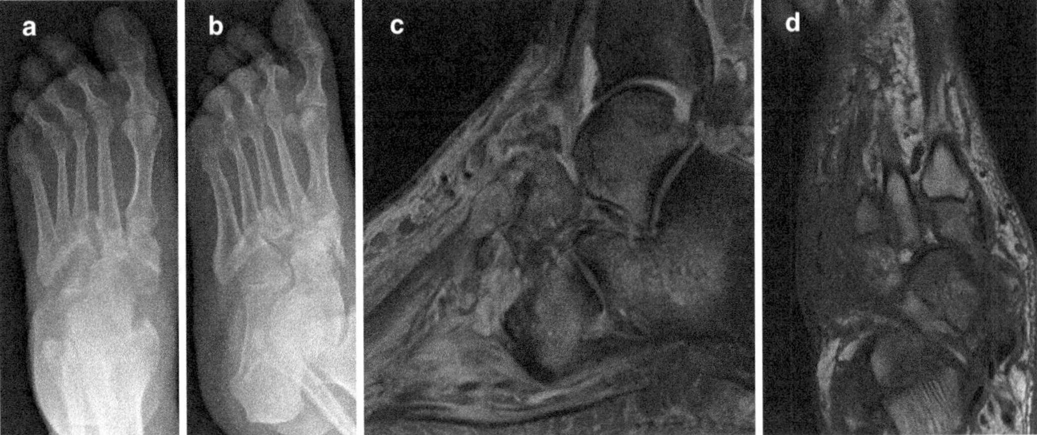

Fig. 18 Charcot foot: Anteroposterior (**a**) and oblique (**b**) radiograph of the foot demonstrating extensive joint space reduction, destruction of the tarsal bones with subluxation of the tarsometatarsal articulation suggesting a Charcot arthropathy. Sagittal PDFS (**c**) MRI image demonstrating significant edema in the tarsal bones and proximal metatarsals with destruction. Axial T1 (**d**) MRI image demonstrating preserved marrow fat in the tarsal bones, ruling out infection

3.9.5 Advances in Imaging

- CT perfusion
- MR perfusion without contrast
- Dynamic contrast-enhanced perfusion and arterial spin labeling perfusion
- Phosphorous imaging
- MR neurography and diffusion-tensor imaging
- Bone marrow planar scintigraphy
- SPECT and SPECT/CT
- Radiolabeled antibiotics

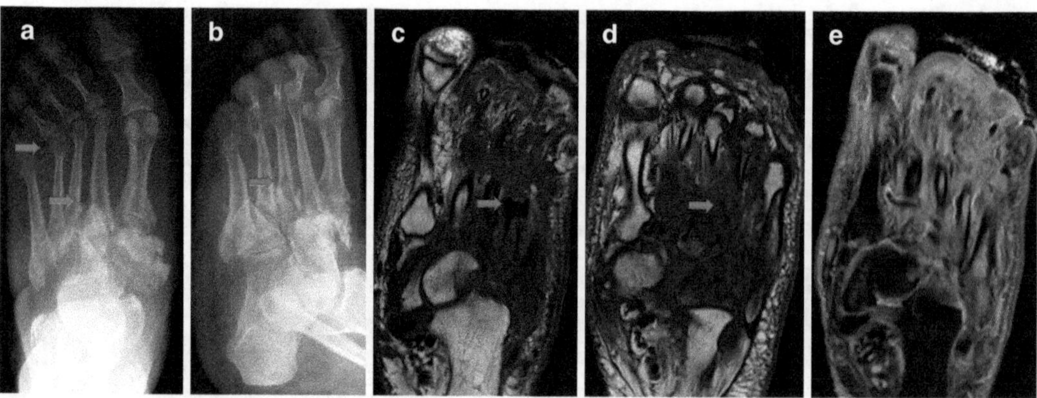

Fig. 19 Charcot foot with infection: AP (**a**) and oblique (**b**) radiograph of the foot demonstrating extensive changes of Charcot arthropathy in the midfoot. Note the presence of air lucencies in the adjacent soft tissues suggesting infection (blue arrows). Axial T1 (**c, d**) MRI images show changes of Charcot arthropathy with infection, note the loss of normal marrow signal in the tarsal bones and base of the third to fifth metatarsal. Air foci are seen in the surrounding soft tissue. Axial PDFS (**e**) MRI image of the foot demonstrating extensive marrow edema in the third to fifth metatarsals with surrounding soft tissue edema

Table 2 Difference between osteomyelitis and neuroarthropathy

Osteomyelitis	Neuroarthropathy
Sites adjacent to skin ulcers	Periarticular
Distal to the tarsometatarsal joint, in the calcaneus and malleolus	Tarsometatarsal and metatarsophalangeal joints
Sinus tract may be present	Absent

Acknowledgments We would like to acknowledge the authors of the first edition of this chapter.

References

Aggarwal ND, Singh GD, Aggarwal R et al (1986) A survey of osteoporosis using the calcaneum as an index. Int Orthop 10:147–153

Atkins RM, Duthie RB (1987) Algodystrophy (reflex sympathetic dystrophy or Sudeck's atrophy). In: Weatherall DJ, Ledingham JGG, Warrell DA (eds) Oxford textbook of medicine. Oxford University Press, pp 16.89–16.91

Bhargava SK, Gupta R, Lohchab VS et al (1983) Unusual radiological changes in metacarpals, metatarsals and phalanges in rickets. J Indian Med Assoc 81: 175–179

Canalis E (1993) Regulation of bone remodeling. In: Favus MJ (ed) Primer on the metabolic bone diseases and disorders of mineral metabolism. Raven, New York, pp 33–37

Cepollaro C, Gonnelli S, Pondrelli C et al (1998) Usefulness of ultrasound in Sudeck's atrophy of the foot. Cakif Tissue Int 62:538–541

Chalmers GW, Brown WR, Stienstra JJ (1998) Tumoral calcinosis-like lesion of the foot. A case report. J Am Podiatr Med Assoc 88:87–91

Chevrot A, Pallardy G, Ledoux-Lebard G (1978) Skeletal manifestations of hyperthyroidism (author's translation). J Radiol Electrol Med Nucl 59:167–173

Chew FS (1991) Radiologic manifestations in the musculoskeletal system of miscellaneous endocrine disorders. Radiol Clin N Am 29:135–147

Cockshott WP, Occleshaw CJ, Webber C et al (1984) Can a calcaneal morphologic index determine the degree of osteoporosis? Skelet Radiol 12:119–122

Colao A, Marzullo P, Vallone G et al (1998) Reversibility of joint thickening in acromegalic patients: an ultrasonography study. J Clin Endocrinol Metab 83:2121–2125

Colao A, Marzullo P, Vallone G et al (1999) Ultrasonographic evidence of joint thickening reversibility in acromegalic patients treated with lanreotide for 12 months. Clin Endocrinol 51:611–618

Crouzet J, Mimoune H, Beraneck L et al (1995) Hypophosphatemic osteomalacia with plantar neurilemoma. A review of the literature (100 cases). Rev Rhum Engl Ed 62:463–466

Darbois H, Boyer B, Dubayle P et al (1999) MRI symptomology in reflex sympathetic dystrophy of the foot. J Radiol 80:849–854

De Palma L, Serra F, Coletti V et al (1993) Foot alterations in the hemodialyzed patient. J Foot Ankle Surg 32:526–529

Doppman JL, Sharon M, Gorden P (1988) Metatarsal penciling in acromegaly: a proposed mechanism based on CT findings. J Comput Assist Tomogr 12:708–709

Edwards MC Jr, Spinner S (1994) Renal osteodystrophy with pedal involvement. J Am Podiatr Med Assoc 84:26–29
Fishco WD, Stiles RG (1999) Atypical heel pain. Hyperparathyroidism-induced stress fracture of the calcaneus. J Am Podiatr Med Assoc 89:413–418
Garver P, Resnick D, Niwayama G et al (1981) Epiphyseal sclerosis in renal osteodystrophy simulating osteonecrosis. AJR Am J Roentgenol 136:1239–1241
Genant HK (1997) Interpretation of bone densitometry. Rev Rhum Engl Ed 64(6 Suppl):20S–25S
Genant HK, Heck LL, Lanzi LH et al (1973) Primary hyperparathyroidism. A comprehensive study of clinical, biochemical and radiographic manifestations. Radiology 109:513–524
Genant HK, Kozin F, Bekerman C et al (1975) The reflex sympathetic dystrophy syndrome. A comprehensive analysis using fine-detail radiography, photon absorptiometry, and bone and joint scintigraphy. Radiology 117:21–32
Gerster JC (2007) Involvement of the foot in metabolic diseases. Praxis 96(34):1251–1256
Gonticas SK, Ikkos DG, Stergiou LH (1969) Evaluation of the diagnostic value of heel-pad thickness in acromegaly. Radiology 92:304–307
Gooding GA, Stress RM, Graf PM et al (1985) Heel pad thickness: determination by high-resolution ultrasonography. J Ultrasound Med 4:173–174
Guyer PB, Chamberlain AT, Ackery DM et al (1981) The anatomic distribution of osteitis deformans. Clin Orthop 156:141–144
Hamilton EB (1972) Hyperparathyroidism with chondrocalcinosis and periarticular calcification. Proc R Soc Med 65:1013
Han ZH, Palnitkar S, Rao DS et al (1996) Effect of ethnicity and age or menopause on the structure and geometry of iliac bone. J Bone Miner Res 11:1967–1975
Harper MC (1989) Metabolic bone disease presenting as multiple recurrent metatarsal fractures: a case report. Foot Ankle 9(4):207–209
Hayes CW, Conway WF (1991) Hyperparathyroidism. Radiol Clin N Am 29:85–96
Hodgskinson R, Njeh CF, Currey JD et al (1997) The ability of ultrasound velocity to predict the stiffness of cancellous bone in vitro. Bone 21:183–190
Jadav RB, Ray JG, Patsu AS, Kumar N, Paul J, Pradhan S (2014) Student poster abstracts. J Oral Maxillofac Pathol 18(Suppl 2):S36–S111
Jergas M, Schmid G (1999) The role of quantitative ultrasound versus other techniques in osteoporosis assessment. In: Njeh CF, Hans D, Fuerst T, Gluer C, Genant HK (eds) Quantitative ultrasound: assessment of osteoporosis and bone status. Dunitz, London, pp 245–281
Kalender WA, Felsenberg D, Louis O et al (1989) Reference values for trabecular and cortical vertebral bone density in single and dual-energy quantitative computed tomography. Eur J Radiol 9:75–80
Koch E, Hofer HO, Sialer G et al (1991) Failure of MR imaging to detect reflex sympathetic dystrophy of the extremities. AJR Am J Roentgenol 156:113–115
Korber J, McCarthy S, Marsden W (1993) Case report 782. Predominantly osteolytic Paget's disease of the calcaneus. Skelet Radiol 22:222–225
Kottamasu SR, Rao DS, Meema HE, Genant HK (1983) Radiology of metabolic bone disease: workshop report. Henry Ford Hosp Med J 31(4):239–243
Kozin F, Genant HK, Bekerman C et al (1976a) The reflex sympathetic dystrophy syndrome. II. Roentgenographic and scintigraphic evidence of bilaterality and of periarticular accentuation. Am J Med 60:332–338
Kozin F, McCarty DJ, Sims J et al (1976b) The reflex sympathetic dystrophy syndrome. I. Clinical and histologic studies: evidence for bilaterality, response to corticosteroids and articular involvement. Am J Med 60:321–331
Krishnamurthy GT, Brickman AS, Tubis M, Blahd WH (1977) Skeletal imaging in metabolic bone disease. Medical radionuclide imaging
Levine MA (1993) Parathyroid hormone resistance syndromes. In: Favus MJ (ed) Primer on the metabolic bone diseases and disorders of mineral metabolism. Raven, New York, pp 194–200
Lipsky BA (1997) Osteomyelitis of the foot in diabetic patients. Clin Infect Dis 25(6):1318–1326
MacSweeney JE, Baxter MA, Joplin GF (1990) Heel pad thickness is an insensitive index of biochemical remission in acromegaly. Clin Radiol 42:348–350
Mazess R, Chesnut CH III, Mcclung M et al (1992) Enhanced precision with dual-energy X-ray absorptiometry. Calcif Tissue Int 51:14–17
Meneghello A, Bertoli M (1983) Tendon disease and adjacent bone erosion in dialysis patients. Br J Radiol 56:915–920
Mittal RK, Ahuja IS, Ahuja GK (1983) Heel pad thickness in normal Nigerians and patients with acromegaly. East Afr Med J 60:156–159
Neylon TA (1995) Paget's disease of bone presenting as chronic ankle pain. J Am Podiatr Med Assoc 85:556–559
Paisey R, Jeans WD, Hartog M (1984) Is soft tissue radiology useful in acromegaly? Br J Radiol 57: 561–564
Panwar J, Mathew AJ, Jindal N, Danda D (2017) Utility of plain radiographs in metabolic bone disease–a case-based pictorial review from a tertiary centre. Pol J Radiol 82:333
Parfitt AM (1988) Bone remodeling: relationship to the amount and structure of bone, and the pathogenesis and prevention of fractures. In: Riggs BL, Melton LJ III (eds) Osteoporosis: etiology, diagnosis and management. Raven, New York, pp 45–93
Patel AA, Ramanathan R, Kuban J, Willis MH (2015) Imaging findings and evaluation of metabolic bone disease. Adv Radiol 2015:812794
Pitt MJ (1981) Rachitic and osteomalacic syndromes. Radiol Clin N Am 19:581–599
Pitt MJ (1991) Rickets and osteomalacia are still around. Radiol Clin N Am 29:97–118

Puckette SE Jr, Seymour EQ (1967) Fallibility of the heel-pad thickness in the diagnosis of acromegaly. Radiology 88:982–983

Resnick D (1995a) Pituitary disorders. In: Resnick D (ed) Diagnosis of bone and joint disorders. Saunders, Philadelphia, pp 1971–1994

Resnick D (1995b) Thyroid disorders. In: Resnick D (ed) Diagnosis of bone and joint disorders. Saunders, Philadelphia, pp 1995–2011

Resnick D, Niwayama G (1995a) Paget's disease. In: Resnick D (ed) Diagnosis of bone and joint disorders. Saunders, Philadelphia, pp 1923–1968

Resnick D, Niwayama G (1995b) Parathyroid disorders and renal osteodystrophy. In: Resnick D (ed) Diagnosis of bone and joint disorders. Saunders, Philadelphia, pp 2012–2075

Resnick D, Deftos LJ, Parthemore JG (1981) Renal osteodystrophy: magnification radiography of target sites of absorption. AJR Am J Roentgenol 136:711–714

Rubin RP, Adler JJ, Adler DP (1983) Paget's disease of the calcaneus. J Am Podiatry Assoc 73:263–267

Sherwood LM (1993) Hypoparathyroidism. In: Favus MJ (ed) Primer on the metabolic bone diseases and disorders of mineral metabolism. Raven, New York, pp 191–193

Van Hul E, Vanhoenacker F, Van Dyck P, De Schepper A, Parizel PM (2011) Pseudotumoural soft tissue lesions of the foot and ankle: a pictorial review. Insights Imaging 2(4):439–452

Veldman PH, Reynen HM, Arntz IE et al (1993) Signs and symptoms of reflex sympathetic dystrophy: prospective study of 829 patients. Lancet 342:1012–1016

WHO (1994) Assessment of fracture risk and its application to screening for postmenopausal osteoporosis. WHO Tech Rep Ser 843:1–129

Osteonecrosis and Osteochondrosis

Milko C. de Jonge and Maarten J. Steyvers

Contents

M. C. de Jonge (✉)
Department of Radiology, St. Antonius Hospital, Utrecht, The Netherlands
e-mail: milkodejonge@gmail.com

M. J. Steyvers
Department of Radiology, University Hospitals Leuven, Leuven, Belgium

1 Introduction

Osteonecrosis (ON) means bone death. The term describes the condition in which bone, due to whatever reason, is deprived of blood and thus oxygen, which leads to ischemia, leading to relatively fast cell death (2–3 h) (McCarthy 2006). This cell death is followed by a complex process of bone resorption and bone formation. Ultimately, it leads, often, to bone degradation and structural collapse (Assouline-Dayan et al. 2002). Interestingly, it is not the necrosis itself that will lead to the collapse, but this is predominantly due to the repair process, particularly the resorptive component of this repair, that leads to the subchondral fractures that are often seen (Glimcher and Kenzora 1979a, b, c). There are many synonyms of osteonecrosis in which the etiology of this disease is often reflected within the name like avascular necrosis, ischemic necrosis, and bone infarction. Aseptic necrosis is also used to emphasize the fact that the condition almost never results from infectious disease (Pearce et al. 2005). Bone infarction is usually reserved to describe osteonecrosis in the metaphysis or diaphysis of a long bone, while osteonecrosis is usually used to describe ischemic death in the epiphysis or subarticular zone. Although osteonecrosis is quite commonly seen in various parts of the skeleton (e.g., hip and shoulder), its incidence and prevalence in the foot and ankle are less common. The percentage in which osteonecrosis involves the foot or

Med Radiol Diagn Imaging (2023)

https://doi.org/10.1007/174_2023_405,
Published Online: 12 April 2023

ankle is roughly estimated to be around 3–4% (Cooper et al. 2010; Delanois et al. 1998; Issa et al. 2014). However, there is no definitive data that can be extracted from the literature, but if all the different types of osteonecrosis (including the osteochondrosis, see below) are considered, the percentage is most likely higher than the estimated figures.

Osteochondrosis is not completely synonymous with osteonecrosis. There are certainly similar pathophysiologic mechanisms that occur with cell death and repair, but very often, it will not lead to structural collapse and/or degradation of the involved bone (Gillespie 2010; Siffert 1981; Doyle and Monahan 2010; Ytrehus et al. 2007). Firstly, the term is usually reserved to describe injuries to the epiphysis, physis, and apophysis in the growing skeleton (Gillespie 2010). Secondly, the process is often reversible and self-limiting in which in later life no sequelae of the process can be seen. Apophyseal injuries can be considered a subset of osteochondrosis and are subsequently called apophysitis, which is a misnomer because inflammation is not the underlying etiology of the condition (Gillespie 2010). The cause of osteochondrosis and apophyseal injuries is multifactorial and most likely more complicated than in adults. It is even sometimes considered as a normal variation of normal ossification although the clinical symptoms in these patients are obviously not explained by this. In osteonecrosis, incidence and prevalence are unclear although foot and ankle problems in general are quite common in the pediatric population, especially in young athletes and the physically active.

2 Etiology and Risk Factors for Osteonecrosis

The ultimate decisive etiology of bone death is lack of oxygen due to vascular insufficiency. For some attributed risk factors, the pathogenesis is well defined, and for others, it is less clear why they predispose or can predispose for osteonecrosis. Roughly, we can classify three major pathways in which a bone becomes ischemic:

1. Trauma, in which the vessels to the specific bone are interrupted (e.g., in talar fractures)
2. Diseases or conditions that lead to occlusion of vessels (e.g., in sickle cell disease)
3. Conditions in which there is increase in intraosseous extravascular pressure where arterial inflow and/or venous outflow can be both obstructed (e.g., in corticosteroid use)

There is a unified concept of pathogenesis of osteonecrosis that emphasizes the role of vascular pathology and ischemia leading to cell death. Any of the specific circumstances mentioned above will lead ultimately to a decreased blood flow, leading to ischemia, osteocyte necrosis, repair, loss of structural integrity, and ultimately collapse (Ytrehus et al. 2007; Shah et al. 2015; Moon 2019).

Trying to identify the cause of the ischemia is obviously important for treatment reasons. However, in a significant number of cases, it is not clear what causes the osteonecrosis. The list of diseases and different etiologies that are associated with osteonecrosis is long, and it is not always clear whether some of these are the causative factors or if they are merely coincidental findings with at best a weak correlation (Ytrehus et al. 2007; Shah et al. 2015; Moon 2019) (Table 1). It is difficult to say which conditions

Table 1 Conditions leading to or associated with osteonecrosis

Trauma
Burns
Fractures
Dislocations
Vascular trauma
Kiënbock's disease
Nontraumatic conditions
Hematologic
Sickle cell anemia
Thalassemia
Disseminated intravascular coagulation
Polycythemia
Hemophilia

Table 1 (continued)

Metabolic/endocrinologic
Hypercholesterolemia
Gout
Hyperparathyroidism
Hyperlipidemia
Pregnancy
Cushing's disease
Chronic renal failure
Gaucher disease
Diabetes (in association with obesity)
Fabry disease
Gastrointestinal
Pancreatitis
Inflammatory bowel disease
Neoplastic
Marrow infiltrative disorders
Infectious
Osteomyelitis
Human immunodeficiency virus
Meningococcemia
Vascular/rheumatologic/connective tissue disorders
Systemic lupus erythematosus
Polymyositis
Polymyalgia rheumatica
Raynaud disease
Rheumatoid arthritis
Ankylosing spondylitis
Sjögren syndrome
Giant cell arthritis
Thrombophlebitis
Lipid emboli
Ehlers-Danlos syndrome
Orthopedic problems
Slipped capital femoral epiphysis
Congenital hip dislocation
Hereditary dysostosis
Legg-Calve-Perthes disease
Extrinsic dietary or environmental factors
Dysbaric conditions (caisson disease)
Alcohol consumption
Cigarette smoking
Iatrogenic
Corticosteroids
Radiation exposure
Hemodialysis
Organ transplantation
Laser surgery
Idiopathic

From: Assouline-Dayan Y, Chang C, Greenspan A, Shoenfeld Y, Gershwin ME. Pathogenesis and Natural History of Osteonecrosis. Semin Arthritis Rheum 2002;32(2):96, with permission

are the most prevalent in osteonecrosis in the foot and ankle. Talar osteonecrosis is in the majority of cases trauma related and seen after talar fractures in which the specific vascular supply of the talus is interrupted (Buchan et al. 2012; Tuthill et al. 2014; Pearce et al. 2005). On the other hand, the cause of Freiberg infraction, which is one of the commonest osteonecrosis conditions seen in the foot, is unclear and most likely multifactorial (Wax and Leland 2019).

Although osteonecrosis can be seen throughout the entire foot and ankle, specific bones are much more at risk than others. This is most likely because of their specific (vulnerable) vascular supply and/or their involvement in weight-bearing. The talus, navicular, and second metatarsal head are the most well-known, but osteonecrosis has also been described in the other metatarsals, sesamoids, and incidentally other tarsals (e.g., the medial cuneiform) (Moon 2019; Buchan et al. 2012; Couturier and Gold 2019; Heinen and Harris 2019; Nunes et al. 2021; Bartosiak and McCormick 2019) (Fig. 1).

In osteochondrosis, etiology is also considered to be multifactorial. The most common osseous structures involved are the navicular, calcaneal apophysis, second metatarsal head, and apophysis of the base of the fifth metatarsal. Rapid growth, anatomical characteristics, repetitive microtrauma, dietary factors, hereditary predisposition, hormonal imbalances, and vascular abnormalities have all been implied as etiologic factors that can contribute (Gillespie 2010; Siffert 1981; Doyle and Monahan 2010).

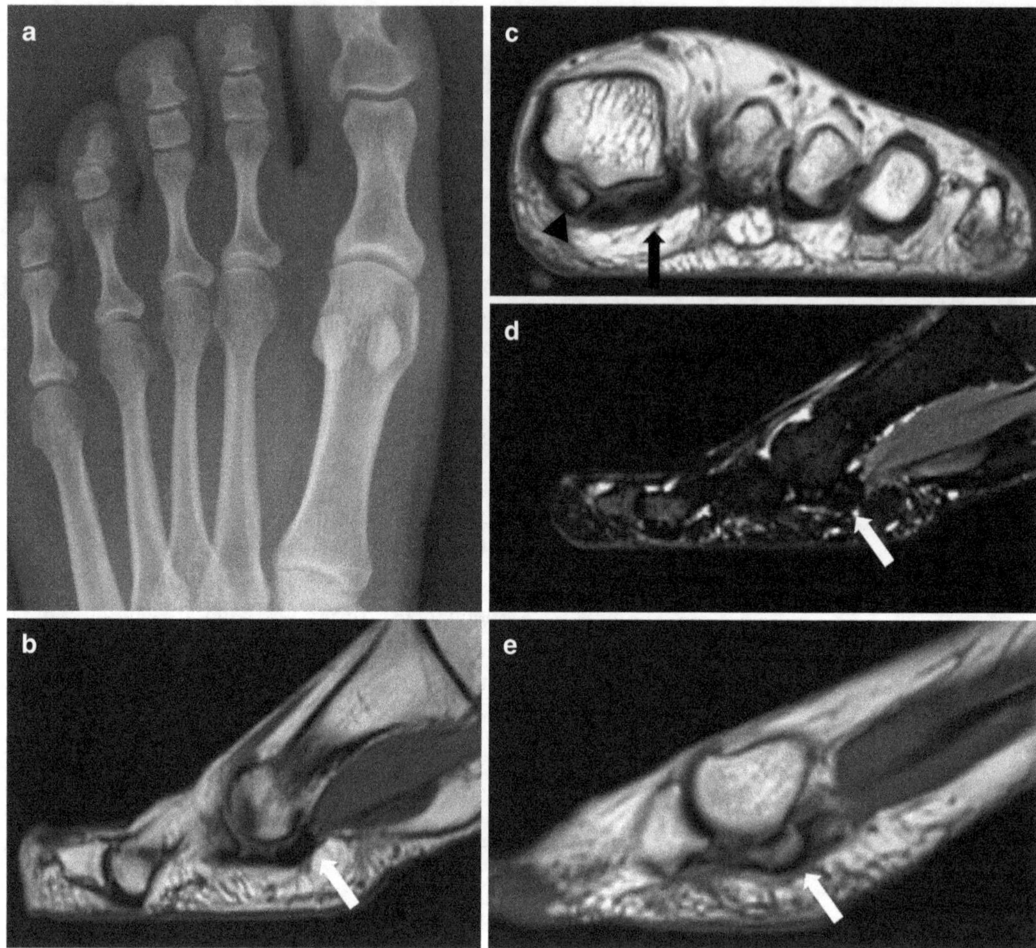

Fig. 1 Avascular necrosis of the lateral sesamoid of the hallux. A 34-year-old female with chronic plantar foot pain at the level of the hallux. AP radiograph (**a**), sagittal T1-weighted (**b**), coronal PD-weighted (**c**), sagittal STIR (**d**), and sagittal T1-weighted (**e**) MR images. The radiograph is unremarkable. The sagittal T1 and coronal PD images demonstrate the hypointense lateral sesamoid (arrows in **b**, **c**) compared to the normal medial sesamoid (arrowhead in **c** and arrow in **e**). There is no significant bone marrow edema in the sesamoid on the STIR (arrow in **d**)

3 Imaging of Osteonecrosis

Radiography is always the first imaging modality that should be used to evaluate patients with suspected osseous or articular pathology. Usually, images are acquired in two orthogonal planes although additional different views are often helpful. Normal ankle radiographs are comprised of at least an AP and lateral view. Whether this AP is a true AP or mortise view (AP view with 10°–15° endorotation) is not relevant for the evaluation of signs of osteonecrosis but is more important in trauma situations to evaluate the congruency of the ankle joint. Other additional views are of less importance for the diagnosis of osteonecrosis. Standard foot radiography protocols depend upon the institution but ideally should consist of three views: AP, ¾ AP, and lateral. The two most important features to evaluate are the bone structure/mineralization and the structural integrity of the different bones. Both can be difficult because there is considerable overlap between the osseous structures of the foot and ankle. A thorough clinical history or clinical information is mandatory to create awareness with the reporting radiologist. Unfortunately, this is very often missing, leading to either underreading or underreporting of subtle abnormalities. Early osteonecrosis is most often radiographically occult (Buchan et al. 2012; Pearce et al. 2005; Couturier and Gold 2019). Signs of osteonecrosis will become visible once a significant repair and remodeling process is initiated. Initially, this will lead to osteopenia of the involved bone compared to the surrounding bones. When new bone is laid over necrotic trabecular bone, areas of sclerosis will become evident, sometimes linear, creating the typical appearance of osteonecrosis (Buchan et al. 2012; Pearce et al. 2005; Couturier and Gold 2019). In case of collapse, the structural integrity of the bone changes, sometimes very subtle, beginning in the subchondral areas. Typical features of osteonecrosis in individual bones will be discussed in the appropriate sections dealing with the individual conditions.

Bone infarcts in the metaphysis or diaphysis of long bones can be seen as focal areas of sclerotic bone or popcorn-like sclerosis, not to be confused with chondroid tumors. Differentiation between these two is easier on MRI than on plain films. If, however, abnormalities are seen in more than one bone, the diagnosis of bone infarcts is readily made because multifocal chondroid lesions are extremely rare (Lafforgue and Trijau 2016).

Some of the osteochondroses (like Kohler disease) are relatively easily diagnosed on plain radiography, whereas others can be notoriously difficult and are usually diagnosed on MRI (like Sever's disease) (Gillespie 2010).

Computed tomography (CT) is not considered to be a primary imaging technique except in patients with metallic hardware in the foot and ankle, which would be unsuitable for MRI. Characteristics seen on CT will resemble those seen on radiography. Structural collapse and amount of collapse are better seen on CT than radiographs, so for secondary survey, once the diagnosis is made or suspected on plain films, CT can be used for this reason (Buchan et al. 2012; Couturier and Gold 2019) (Fig. 2).

In cases of suspicion of osteonecrosis with normal radiographs, MRI will be the next imaging modality (Gillespie 2010; Buchan et al. 2012; Pearce et al. 2005; Couturier and Gold 2019). The hallmark of all stages of osteonecrosis will be bone marrow edema (BME). BME must be detected on fat-saturated images as diffuse or patchy areas of high signal intensity. Basically, any fat saturation technique can be used, but short tau inversion recovery (STIR) is one of the most sensitive techniques. Another advantage of STIR is its relative insensitivity for magnetic field inhomogeneities as seen, e.g., in patients with metallic hardware in place. In early stages, BME could be the only finding and the corresponding T1-weighted (T1-W) images will be normal. Only in later stages or with a large amount of BME will the T1-W signal intensity change, initially with the formation of patchy areas of low signal intensity and later with a more profound hypointense appearance of the involved bone. Apart from the distal tibia, the characteristic "double-line sign," which is often seen in cases of shoulder and hip osteonecrosis, is not common in the foot and ankle (Couturier and Gold 2019) (Fig. 3). The double-line sign is a pathognomonic finding in AVN/osteonecrosis and is seen as a high signal intensity serpentine line bordered by a hypointense line. It represents a border between viable and nonviable bone tissue. Gadolinium administration is most of the times not necessary for the diagnosis but can be helpful if the clinical suspicion comprises more than osteonecrosis like infection or osteomyeli-

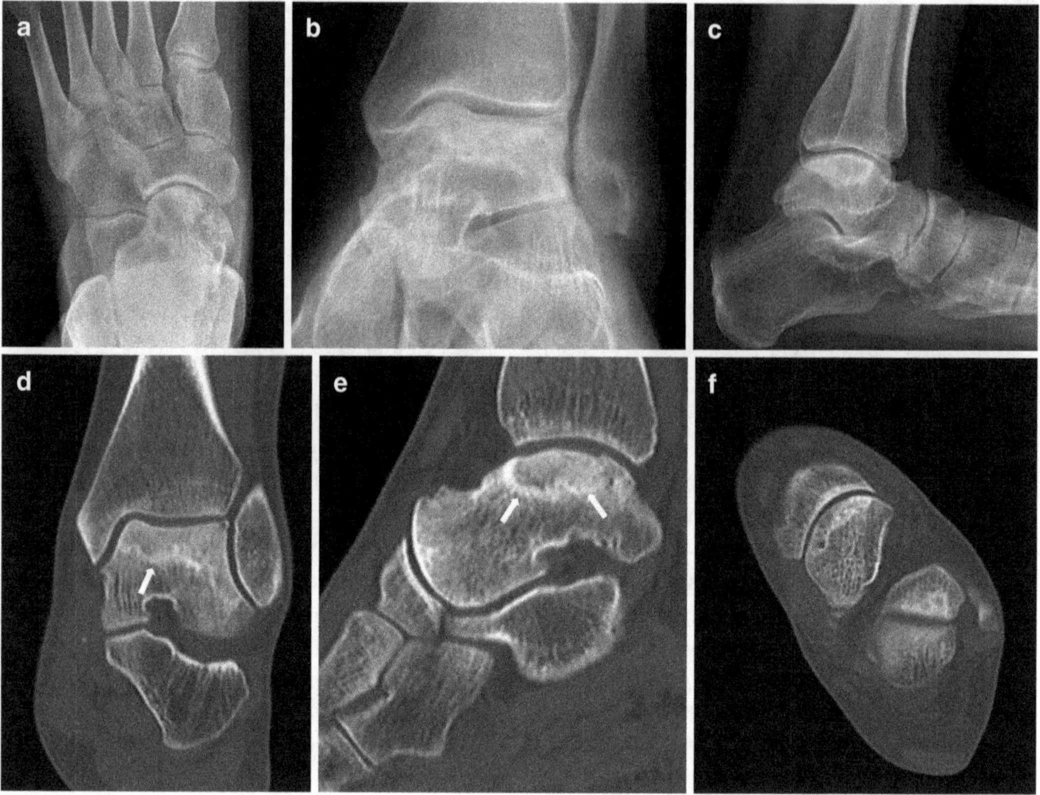

Fig. 2 Avascular necrosis of the talus. A 26-year-old female with chronic ankle pain after treatment for acute myeloid leukemia. AP radiograph of the foot (**a**), AP and lateral radiographs of the ankle (**b**, **c**), coronal multiplanar reconstruction (MPR) CT (**d**), sagittal MPR CT (**e**), and axial CT images (**f**) of the ankle. The radiographs demonstrate severe inhomogeneous bone structure of the talar dome with partial collapse and similar abnormalities in the anterior talus at the level of the talonavicular joint. CT was made for preoperative reasons, demonstrating the increased sclerosis of the talar dome with partial collapse of the articular surface and similar abnormalities in the anterior talus compatible with the radiographs. Compared to the radiographs, the CT very well visualizes the sharp sclerotic border between necrotic and viable bone tissue (arrows in **d** and **e**)

tis. The problem with BME as such is that it is very sensitive for osteonecrosis but there is a relative lack of specificity. There are many conditions that can cause BME in the foot and ankle like infection, trauma, overuse, malignancies, or bone marrow reconversion (yellow to red).

Nuclear medicine studies are not routinely recommended in case of suspicion of osteonecrosis. The sensitivity of scintigraphy is lower than that of MRI and the specificity is even lower (Buchan et al. 2012). The role of SPECT is unclear. It appears in some publications that the sensitivity and specificity are higher in osteonecrosis of the hip but its role in the foot and ankle is unclear (Agrawal et al. 2017). The role of positron emission tomography (PET)/CT or PET/MRI is likewise unclear to establish osteonecrosis in the foot and ankle.

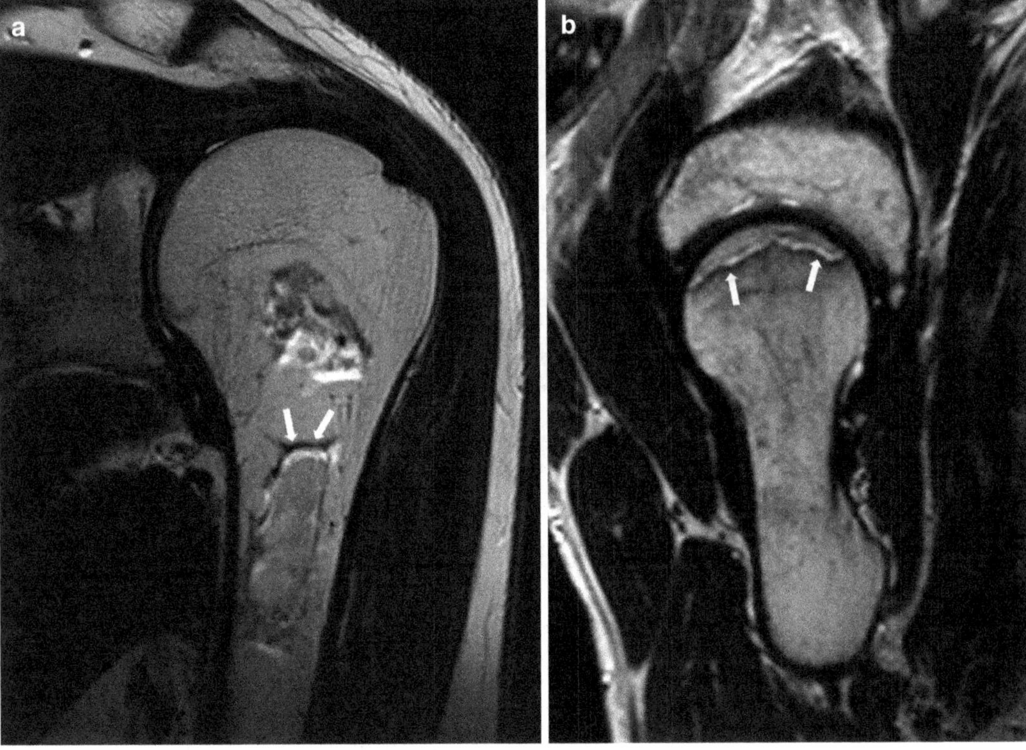

Fig. 3 Classic "double-line sign." Coronal T2-weighted MR image of the shoulder (**a**) and sagittal T2-weighted MR image of the hip (**b**) in two different patients demonstrating a bone infarct in the shoulder and avascular necrosis of the femoral head. Sharp outlined parallel low and high signal intensity lines are seen (white arrows) representing the classical "double-line sign"

4 Distal Tibia and Talus Osteonecrosis

Osteonecrosis of the distal tibia or tibia plafond is quite uncommon (Buchan et al. 2012; Heinen and Harris 2019). It is most often seen in the lateral tibial plafond, which is most likely due to the amount of vascularization which appears to be less on the lateral side compared to the medial side. Trauma seems to be the most common cause, especially the pronation external rotation injuries (Menck et al. 1992). Due to the lack of available literature, it is difficult to establish if the distal tibia is as prone as, e.g., the hip for developing osteonecrosis due to other causes although clinically we see much more osteonecrosis of the hip than of the tibia in daily clinical practice. So, logic dictates that the vulnerability of the two must be quite different, especially given the fact that both are very commonly injured in trauma. Nontraumatic osteonecrosis of the distal tibia has been described in case reports however (McLeod et al. 2017). Clinically, symptoms are a-specific and can be often contributed to the post-traumatic situation with healing fractures or due to soft tissue damage. Radiographs are also usually a-specific with changes that are normally seen in post-traumatic patients, which do not primarily point to osteonecrosis. Since osteonecrosis is often within the marrow cavity, the typical signs of osteonecrosis (in later stages) can be absent. Increased sclerosis can point to ON, but it is more

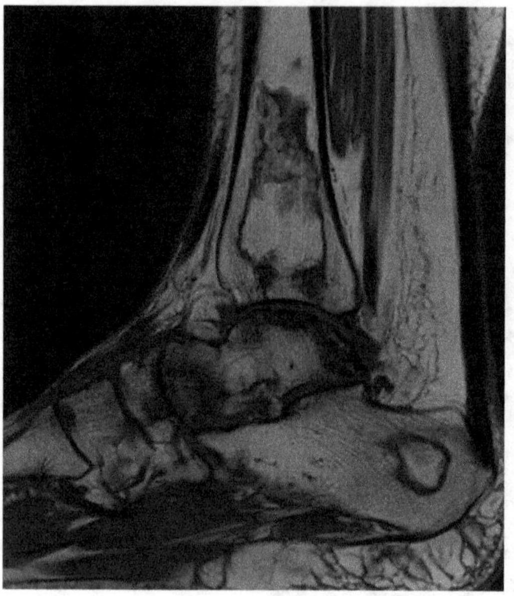

Fig. 4 Multiple bone infarcts and osteonecrosis. A 35-year-old female with chronic ankle pain and corticosteroid use. Sagittal T1-weighted MR image. Typical serpiginous configurations are seen in the distal tibia, talus, calcaneus, and navicular, representing multiple infarcts and osteonecrosis. There is discrete collapse of the talar dome

likely that this is seen due to the healing of fractures. MRI is the imaging modality of choice and will show the typical serpiginous configuration in later stages indicating ON (Figs. 4 and 5) (Buchan et al. 2012; Heinen and Harris 2019). Early stages will demonstrate areas of low signal intensity on T1-weighted images with high signal of T2-weighted fat-saturated images. Defects in the tibia plafond can be seen, but these could also be due to osteochondral defects which are very common in post-traumatic patients although they are more common in the talus.

Osteonecrosis of the talus is more common than in the distal tibia, but nevertheless it is still not very frequently seen. One reason for this is that the etiology is most often traumatic and talus fractures are rare compared to all the other ankle joint fractures, which are very commonly seen. The relative vulnerability for osteonecrosis of the talus stems from the intricate vascularization. The largest part of the talus is covered with cartilage because of its three articulations (with the tibia, calcaneus, and navicular bone). There is therefore only a relatively

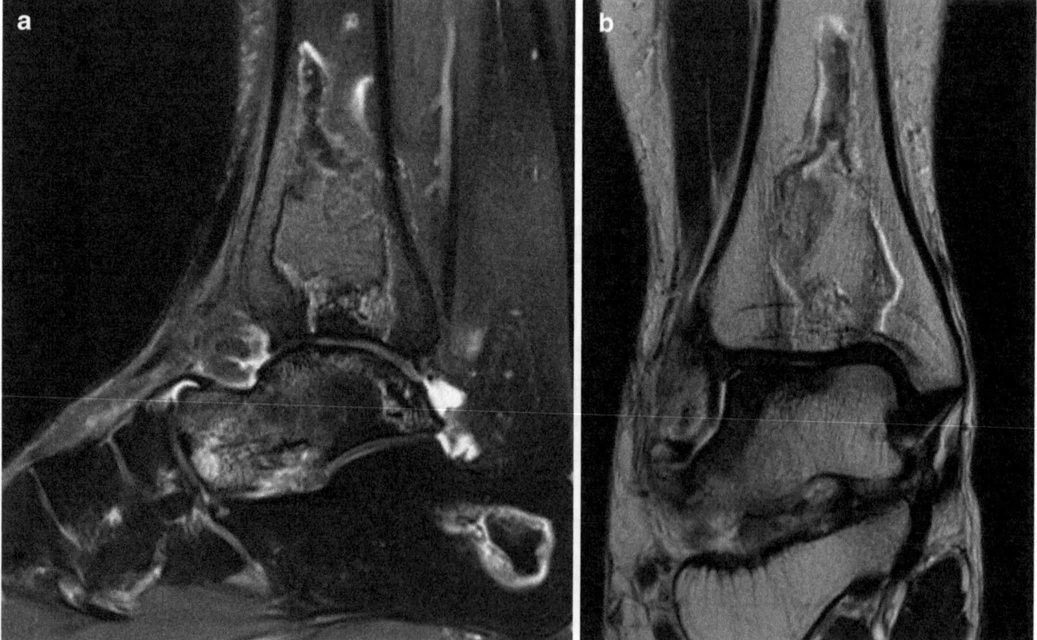

Fig. 5 Same patient as in Fig. 4. Sagittal STIR (**a**) and coronal PD-weighted (**b**) MR images. Multiple bone infarcts and osteonecrosis in the distal tibia, talus, calcaneus, and navicular

small amount of bone which is accessible for penetrating vessels, and therefore vulnerability to vascular disruption is high (Moon 2019; Pearce et al. 2005). Although idiopathic talar osteonecrosis is described as well as medication induced, the largest contributing factor to the development of osteonecrosis is trauma (Mankin 1992; Zizic et al. 1985) (Fig. 6). There is however a difference in region depending upon the etiology. In traumatic osteonecrosis, the anterolateral region is more prone to ON, whereas in other situations, the ON appears to be more located in the posterolateral region (Moon 2019). In post-traumatic situations, with talar neck fractures, the risk of ON is determined by the type of fracture (Moon 2019; Pearce et al. 2005). Typically, the Hawkins classification, later revised by Canale and Kelly,

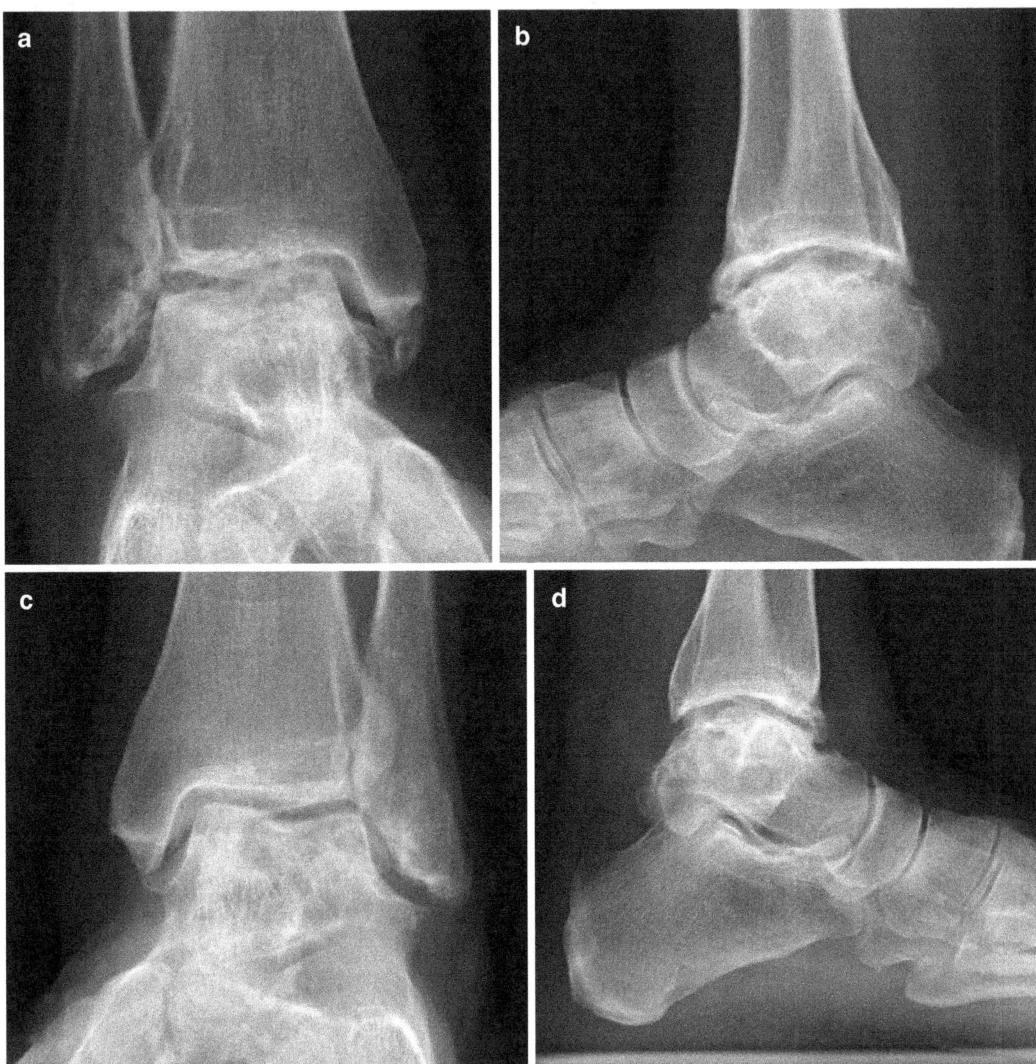

Fig. 6 Bilateral talar osteonecrosis. A 45-year-old female on corticosteroids with chronic ankle pain. Previous AVN of the hip. AP and lateral radiographs of the right (**a** and **b**) and left ankle (**c** and **d**). Both ankles demonstrate extensive abnormalities in both talus with ill-defined sclerosis, lucencies, and collapse of the talar dome

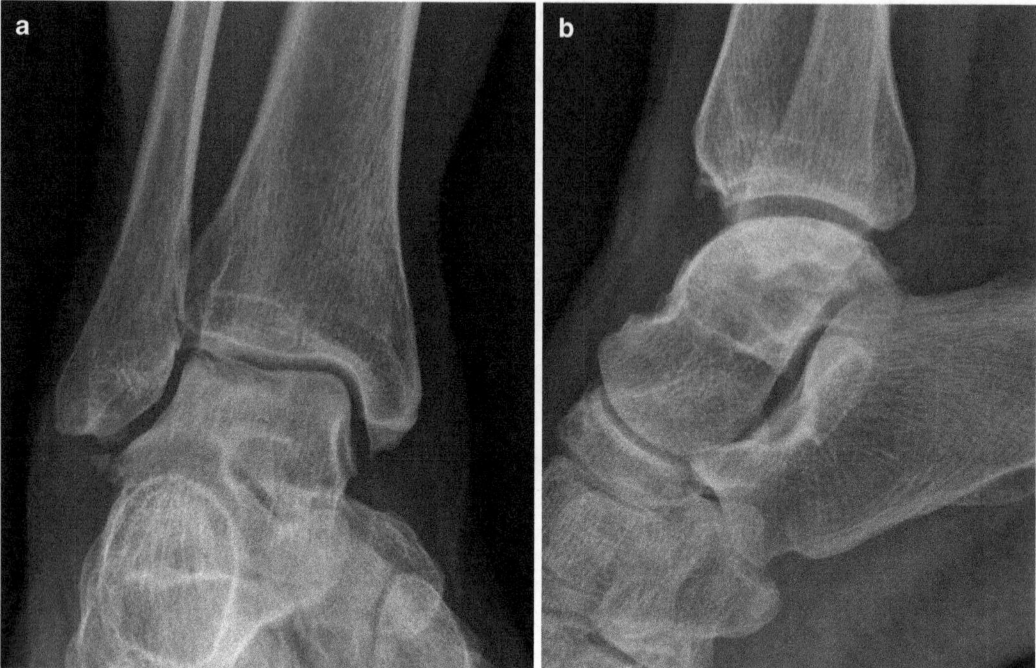

Fig. 7 Same patient as in Fig. 4. AP (**a**) and lateral (**b**) radiographs of the ankle. There is a focal abnormal appearance of the lateral talar dome, which was interpreted as an osteochondral defect (there was no information about corticosteroid use). The subsequent MRI (see Figs. 4 and 5) demonstrated extensive osteonecrosis and bone infarcts

is used to describe talar neck fractures (Hawkins 1970; Canale and Kelly Jr. 1978). Four types are described:

1. Nondisplaced talar neck fracture
2. Displaced fracture with subluxation or dislocation of subtalar joint
3. Displaced fracture with dislocation/subluxation of the subtalar joint and tibiotalar joint
4. Displaced neck fracture with dislocation/subluxation of the subtalar joint, tibiotalar joint, and talonavicular joint

Whereas the risk of developing ON is only around 10–15% in case of a type 1 fracture, in type 4 fracture, the risk is 100% (Pearce et al. 2005; Couturier and Gold 2019).

Radiographically, ON in the talus can be seen as increased sclerosis of the talar dome with, in later stages, collapse of the subarticular surface and collapse of the dome (Fig. 7). Radiographs are however not very sensitive, and in case of high suspicion, especially in post-traumatic patients who sustained a type 3 or 4 Hawkins talar fracture, MRI is indicated to demonstrate or rule out osteonecrosis (Buchan et al. 2012; Pearce et al. 2005). Differentiating focal AVN from osteochondral pathology can be difficult sometimes (Fig. 7). Whereas in AVN a double-line sign is described (like in hip and shoulder), osteochondral pathology can have a different appearance with hyperintense signal in between two hypointense lines, described as the so-called rim sign (Buchan et al. 2012; Couturier and Gold 2019). A rim sign indicates instability of an osteochondral fragment, whereas a double-line sign configuration does not (Couturier and Gold 2019) (Fig. 8).

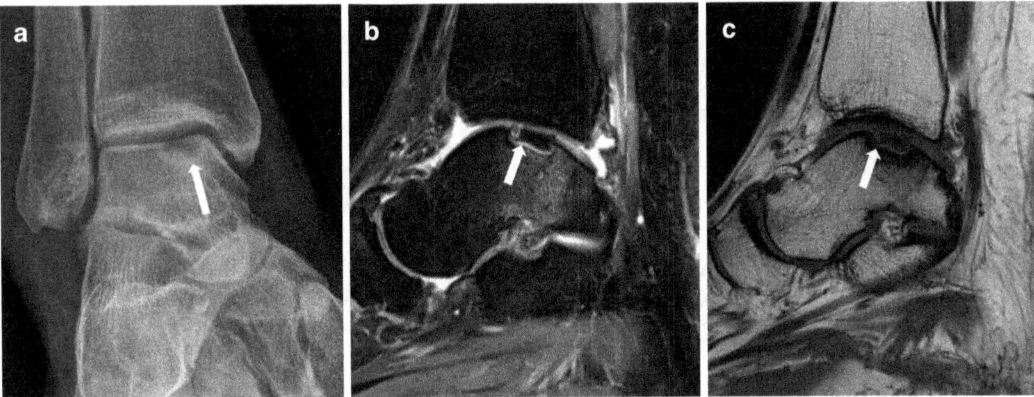

Fig. 8 Rim sign in osteochondral defect. A 26-year-old female with chronic ankle pain. No prior medical history. AP radiograph of the right ankle (**a**), sagittal STIR (**b**), and T1-weighted MR images (**c**) of the right ankle. A focal lucency is seen in the medial talar dome on the radiograph (arrow) surrounded by sclerosis. The MRI demonstrates a focal osseous lesion surrounded by a hyperintense line on STIR and T1, the so-called rim sign, which is virtually pathognomonic for an osteochondral defect and not osteonecrosis

5 Osteonecrosis of the Navicular Bone in Adults (Mueller-Weiss Syndrome)

Mueller-Weiss syndrome (MWS) refers to spontaneous osteonecrosis of the tarsal navicular in adults and is an uncommon cause of chronic medial midfoot pain (Haller et al. 1988; Reade et al. 1998; Samim et al. 2018; Ahmed et al. 2019). The eponym originates from Mueller's description of an adult with chronic deformation of the navicular in 1927 and radiologist Weiss's postulation that this condition was the result of an ischemic process in 1929 (Haller et al. 1988; Reade et al. 1998). It is a separate entity from Kohler disease (osteochondrosis of the navicular in the immature skeleton). Unlike Kohler disease, most patients with MWS are symptomatic at the time of radiographic diagnosis. MWS typically manifests with chronic dorsomedial midfoot pain, exacerbated during weight-bearing activity. Most commonly, it occurs bilaterally with a female predominance (Samim et al. 2018; Ahmed et al. 2019). Its true prevalence is unknown and likely underestimated, being misattributed to peri-navicular osteoarthritis. It is characterized by collapse of the lateral portion of the navicular, midfoot deformity, and finally secondary osteoarthritis. The dorsal and lateral aspects of the navicular are supplied by branches from the dorsalis pedis artery, whereas the plantar aspect is nourished by the medial plantar artery. Blood supply is organized in a circumferential centripetal fashion, leaving the central force-bearing part of the navicular with a tenuous blood supply, even becoming more compromised with increasing age (Samim et al. 2018; Ahmed et al. 2019). In MWS, chronic loading forces preferentially cause compression of the lateral half of the navicular. Any biomechanical predisposition, such as subtalar varus, leading to net lateral compression of the navicular may be a contributing factor. Delayed or suboptimal ossification of the navicular may be a second precondition. Compromised vascularization (e.g., smoking, diabetes) is another contributing factor. Regardless of the exact cause, the pathogenesis of MWS is probably multifactorial and related to chronic mechanical strain on a suboptimal ossified navicular, being predisposed to central ischemia owing to its arterial anatomy. Weight-bearing frontal and lateral radiographs and CT typically initially show a "comma-shaped" navicular with increased lateral density (Haller et al. 1988; Samim et al. 2018) (Figs. 9 and 10). Usually, over years, this

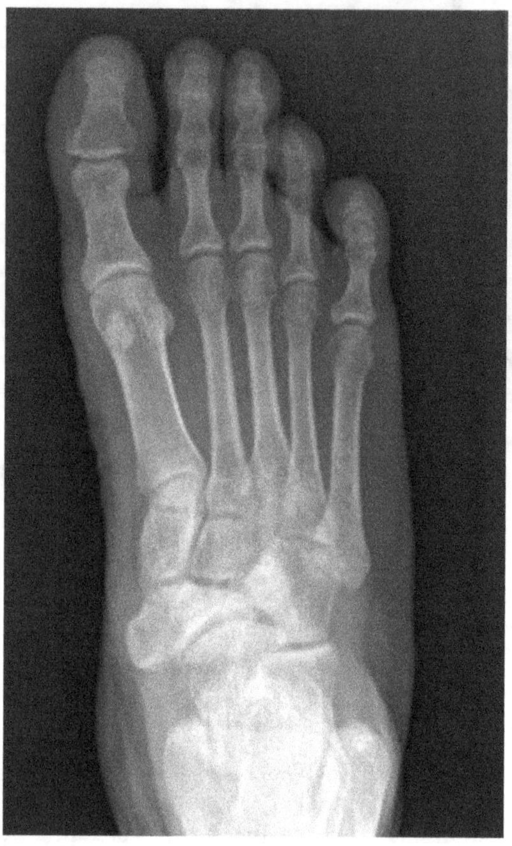

Fig. 9 Mueller-Weiss syndrome. Abnormal morphology of the navicular with comma-shaped appearance of the lateral portion indicative of osteonecrosis. (Image courtesy of Dr. R. Botchu)

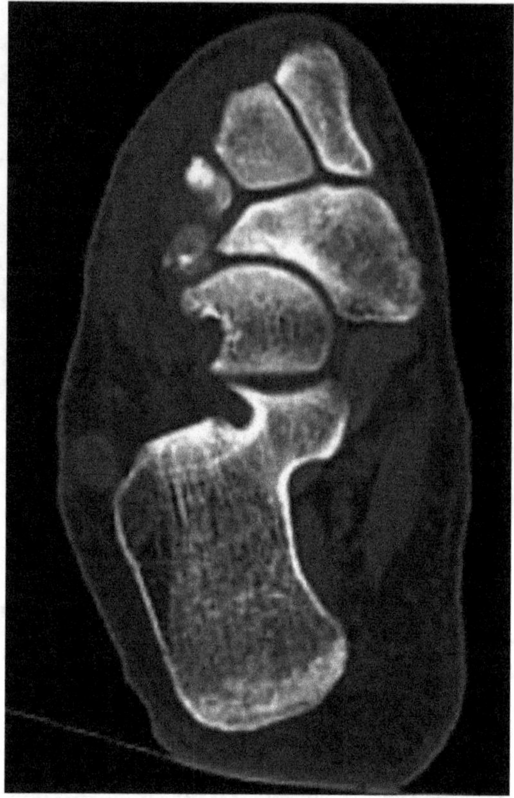

Fig. 10 Mueller-Weiss syndrome. Same patient as in Fig. 9. Axial CT image demonstrating a comma-shaped navicular with increased sclerosis of the lateral portion indicative of Mueller-Weiss syndrome. (Image courtesy of Dr. R. Botchu)

gradually progresses with increased lateral degenerative changes, flattening and fragmentation of the dorsolateral aspect, dorsal/medial protrusion of the medial navicular part, hindfoot varus, and forefoot deformity. If left untreated, peri-navicular osteoarthritis will develop with subsequent permanent disability. MRI can detect bone marrow edema (typically in the dorsolateral aspect of the navicular) already in the initial early stages, (more subtle) osteoarthritic changes, and T1 hypointensity consistent with sclerosis/necrosis (Haller et al. 1988; Samim et al. 2018). The differential diagnosis of a sclerotic navicular includes stress-adaptive sclerosis without other features of MWS, healing/callus formation following a (insufficiency) fracture, and/or osteomyelitis. Secondary osteonecrosis of the navicular can also occur in association with rheumatoid arthritis, renal failure, and SLE (Ahmed et al. 2019).

6 Osteonecrosis of the Metatarsals, E.g., Freiberg Disease and Infraction

Freiberg "disease" was initially described as osteochondrosis of the metatarsal heads, predominantly occurring in females aged 11–14 years (Freiberg 1914). However, the entity is not limited to adolescents, and the term Freiberg "infraction" (i.e., the combined infarction and fracture) refers to osteonecrosis of the metatarsal heads both in adolescents and adults (Wax and Leland 2019). The most common location is the dorsal aspect of the second metatarsal head (two-thirds of cases), followed by the third metatarsal (approximately the remaining one-third of cases), and seldomly the fourth or other metatarsals (Wax and Leland 2019; Aiyer and Hennrikus 2014). The second metatarsal is usually the longest and is subjected to the greatest repetitive ground forces during walking/running. Predisposing factors include a short first metatarsal and wearing high-heeled shoes with a narrow toe box. Hence, Freiberg infraction most commonly occurs in women in the third to seventh decades of life. Sometimes, it may be associated with underlying systemic disease such as diabetes and SLE (Wax and Leland 2019). Increased stress on the metatarsal head results in osteochondral shearing at the interface between mineralized and non-mineralized cartilage. This initially leads to small vascular compromise with subchondral fractures, progressing to subarticular osteonecrosis, collapse, and finally secondary osteoarthritis (Wax and Leland 2019). Clinical manifestations are dull aching forefoot pain increased by weight-bearing, soft tissue swelling around the metatarsal head, and decreased range of motion (Aiyer and Hennrikus 2014).

Radiographs are the first imaging modality, and changes in the second metatarsal head are quite commonly seen, also in non-symptomatic individuals, but the imaging appearance is quite typical especially in the later stages in which there is usually some degree of collapse of the articular surface of the head of the metatarsal with increased sclerosis and/or subarticular "loose" fragments (Couturier and Gold 2019; Wax and Leland 2019) (Fig. 11). MRI is the best imaging tool especially in the early stages with clinical symptoms, with subchondral bone marrow edema and serpentine linear signal abnormality as the earliest imaging findings (Lee and Saifuddin 2019). Subsequently, subtle metatarsal head flattening becomes apparent (Fig. 12). In later stages, abnormal density (typically mottled sclerosis and lucency and/or linear subchondral fissure lines with surrounding sclerosis) in the metatarsal head can be observed, and it is at this time, like mentioned above, that they are picked up on radiographs (Fig. 13). Concavity of the metatarsal head articular surface indicates advanced disease. Fragmentation and collapse of the central portion of the head may follow, and an unstable osteochondral fragment (usually located dorsally) is a late finding (Shane et al. 2013). It is worth mentioning that metatarsal head flattening can be a normal variant (in this case without subarticular imaging abnormalities), seen in about 10% of asymptomatic individuals (Jensen and De Carvalho 1987).

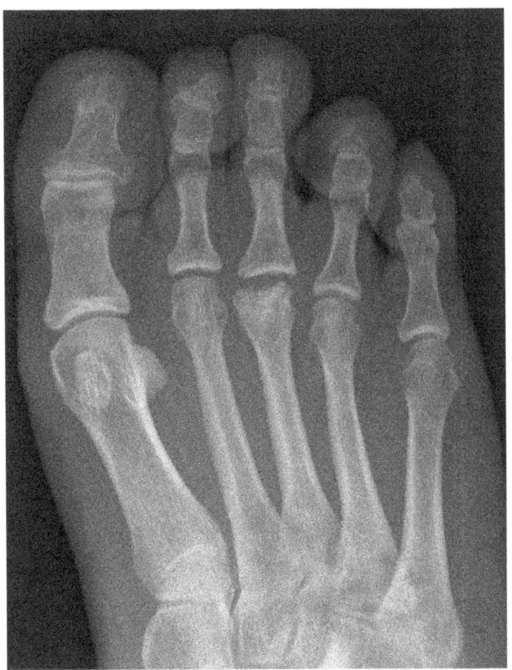

Fig. 11 Freiberg disease. A 35-year-old female with chronic metatarsalgia. AP radiograph of the right foot. An abnormal head is seen of the third metatarsal with irregular sclerosis and collapse of the articular surface compatible with long-standing osteonecrosis

Differential diagnoses include fracture of the metatarsal head or neck, rheumatoid arthritis, and soft tissue lesions (plantar plate injury, collateral ligament injury, Morton's neuroma, and

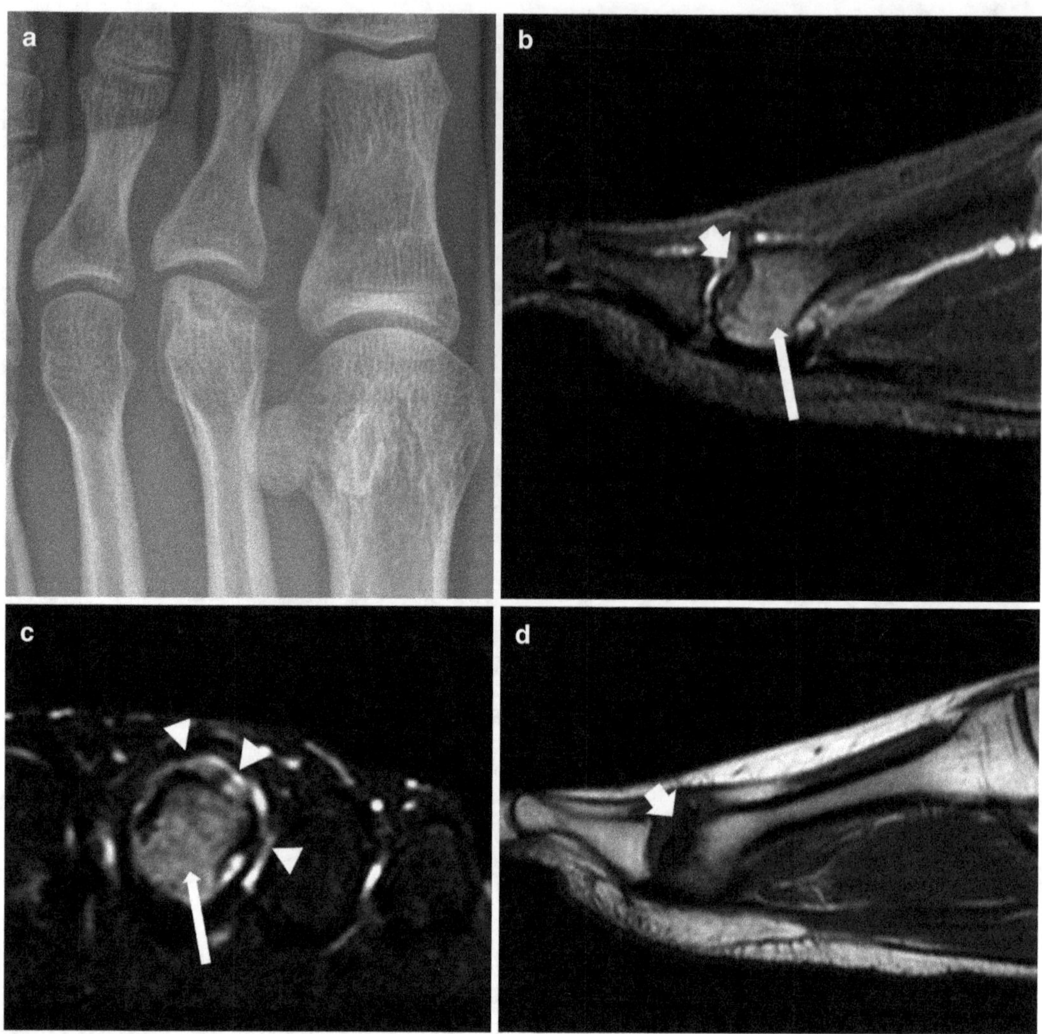

Fig. 12 Freiberg disease. A 19-year-old female with forefoot pain. ¾ radiograph (**a**), MRI images with sagittal STIR (**b**), coronal T2 fat-sat (**c**), and sagittal T1 (**d**). The radiograph clearly shows increased sclerosis, lucency, and partial collapse of the head of the second metatarsal. MRI demonstrates some synovitis (arrowheads in **c**), bone marrow edema (long arrows in **b** and **c**), and partial collapse of the central and dorsal portions of the articular surface of second metatarsal (short arrows in **b** and **d**)

intermetatarsal bursitis). A fracture of the metatarsal head or neck is typically located proximal to the area of Freiberg disease/infraction. Rheumatoid arthritis most commonly involves the fourth and fifth MTP joints in early disease and can be differentiated by the presence of marginal erosions and periarticular osteopenia. Plantar plate rupture may mimic Freiberg infraction, with prominent subchondral edema and dorsal MTP joint subluxation. Obviously, discontinuity of the plantar plate on MR clearly distinguishes both.

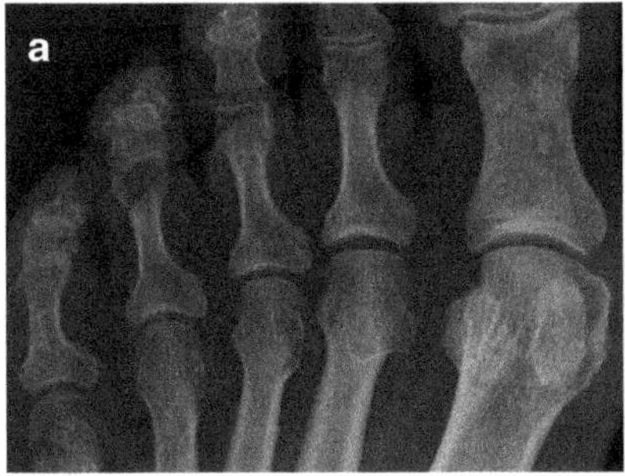

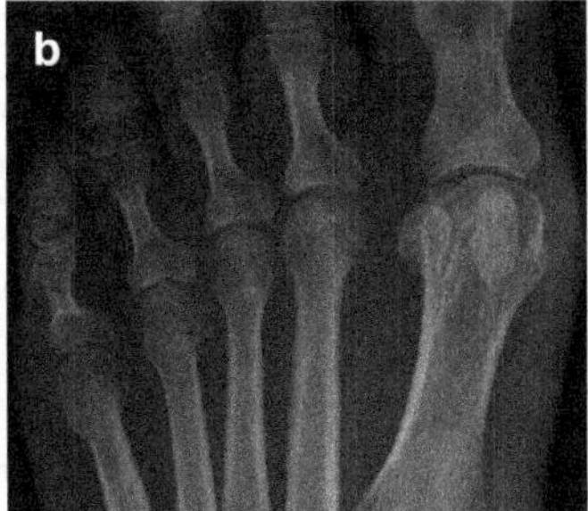

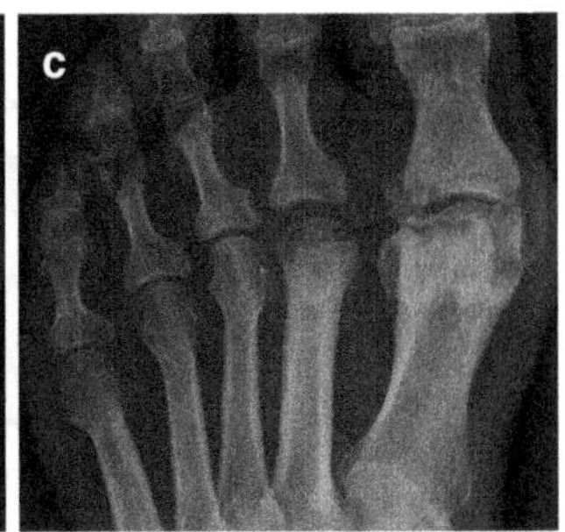

Fig. 13 Natural progression of Freiberg disease. A 50-year-old female with chronic forefoot pain. AP radiographs of the foot from 2017 (**a**), 2019 (**b**), and 2020 (**c**). Initial radiograph in 2017 normal, whereas in 2019, increased sclerosis and lucency of the head of the second metatarsal progressing to partial collapse in 2020. Discrete abnormal appearance of the head of the first metatarsal in 2019 with increasing abnormalities in 2020 with partial collapse indicative of a rare location of Freiberg

7 Osteochondrosis

7.1 Kohler Disease

Kohler disease refers to avascular necrosis of the navicular bone in the child. It was first described in 1908 by Alban Köhler, who reported on three children with medial midfoot pain and radiological abnormalities of the navicular (Köhler 1908). Its incidence is not well known, considering that not all patients with radiographic abnormalities are symptomatic. It is most often seen in children 2–10 years old (Borges et al. 1995), and boys are 2–6 times more likely affected than girls (Chan and Young 2019). Typically, the condition is unilateral, but in 15–20% of cases, it presents bilaterally (Chan and Young 2019). Although the etiology is not fully understood, it is likely multifactorial and it is thought to be caused by disruption of the vascular supply due to compression of the navicular bone prior to ossification. It is therefore often considered to be congenital. The navicular is the last tarsal bone to ossify, and it displays significant variability in the timing and pattern of ossification. In girls, it ossifies between 18 and 24 months, and between 30 and 36 months in boys. Additionally, one-third of the navicular bones ossify from multiple centers, and these patients typically show a delayed navicular ossification (Chan and Young 2019; Ferguson Jr and Gingrich 1957). As the child begins weight-bearing, the navicular becomes compressed between the already ossified talus and cuneiform bones. Increased pressure on the largely cartilaginous navicular could induce microtrauma to the delicate arterial supply, leading to ischemia and necrosis (Chan and Young 2019). The condition can be clinically silent and seen on foot and ankle radiographs of asymptomatic children. If symptomatic, patients typically present with dorsomedial foot pain, swelling, and/or limping in which they walk on the lateral side of the foot. In most circumstances, no specific event such as a (minor) trauma is recalled. The clinical diagnosis is supported by plain radiographs that show flattening, sclerosis (patchy or uniform), and fragmentation of the navicular, with soft tissue swelling (Aiyer and Hennrikus 2014; Chan and Young 2019) (Fig. 14). It is important to keep in mind that these findings may also reflect a normal variant in asymptomatic patients. There are limited indications for advanced imaging, but MRI shows bone marrow edema with/without central necrosis and surrounding inflammatory reaction (West and Jaramillo 2019). The differential diagnosis for Kohler disease includes osteomyelitis, arthritis, tarsal coalition, symptomatic accessory navicular bone, and posterior tibial tendinopathy. Unlike avascular necrosis of the navicular in adults, Kohler disease is almost always self-resolving.

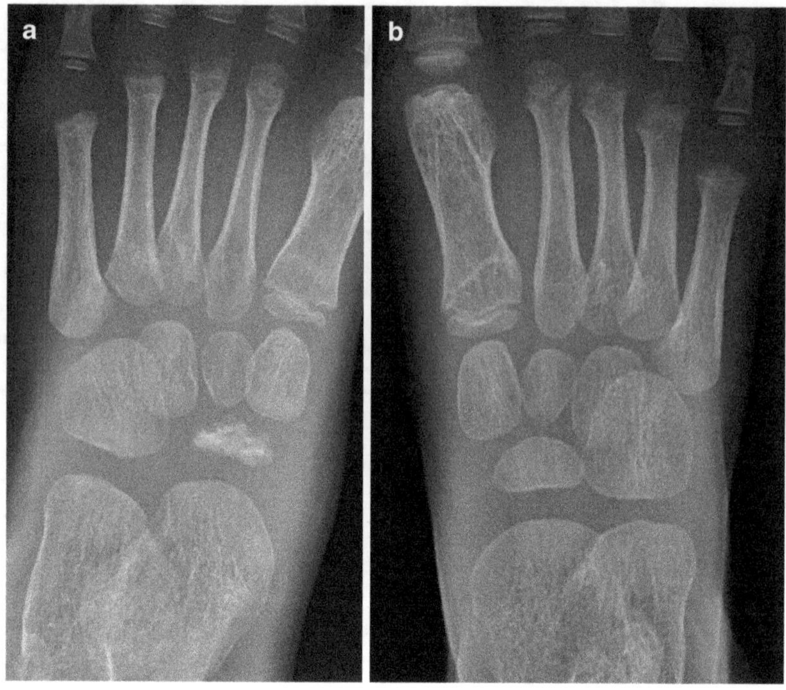

Fig. 14 Kohler's disease. A 5-year-old boy with left midfoot pain. AP radiographs of the left (**a**) and right foot (**b**). A small, fragmented, sclerotic navicular bone is seen in the left foot

Treatment is conservative. There are no indications for surgery, and symptoms are expected to show improvement in around 3 months (Chan and Young 2019).

7.2 Sever's Disease

Sever's disease is also described as an apophysitis of the skeletally immature posterior calcaneus. The posterior apophysis appears around age 7 and is fused around the age of 15 (Volpon and De Carvalho 2002). Typically, it is associated with athletic activity at a relatively early age. Its etiology is unclear; overuse with repetitive traction on the unfused calcaneal apophysis, stress fractures due to compression on the metaphysis (rather than traction), obesity, deformity of the foot, and even inflammation of the calcaneal apophysis have all been implicated. Although in general it is thought that it is more common in more active children, a recent study showed a higher incidence in less active patients. In this study by Martinelli et al., there was also a positive correlation with younger age but not with other previously assumed role-playing factors (Martinelli et al. 2019). The condition presents with a painful posterior calcaneus exacerbated by exercise at the age of 8–14 years. Radiographs are usually the first imaging modality. The condition can manifest radiographically as a fragmented, sclerotic apophysis of the calcaneal posterior process (West and Jaramillo 2019; Volpon and De Carvalho 2002) (Fig. 15). However, the latter are not reliable signs as they may also be present in asymptomatic children (West and Jaramillo 2019; Kose 2010). In one study, 50% of asymptomatic controls had a fragmented posterior calcaneal apophysis (Perhamre et al. 2013). Also, in many patients who are clinically suspected of Sever's disease, radiographs are usually normal (Scharfbillig et al. 2008). If radiographs are requested, it is therefore better to make comparative radiographs of the contralateral side (lateral view of the calcaneus suffices) to detect abnormalities and/or subtle differences. Overall, radiographs are rarely useful for the diagnosis of Sever's and are predominantly made to rule out other abnormalities. CT is not indicated in this young population; there is no advan-

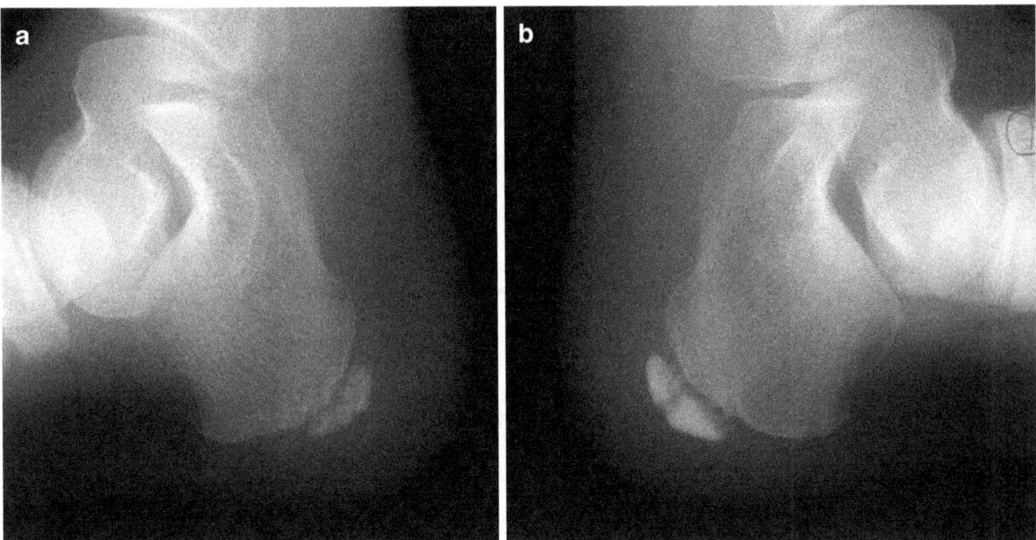

Fig. 15 Sever's disease. Lateral radiographs of both feet. There is an abnormal appearance of the calcaneal apophysis (**b**) with increased sclerosis, which is even more pronounced when compared to the other healthy side (**a**). (Image courtesy of Dr. R. Botchu)

tage over plain films. If imaging is sought, then MRI is the preferred imaging tool (West and Jaramillo 2019; Volpon and De Carvalho 2002). It shows bone marrow edema in and around the posterior apophysis together with associated abnormalities in the adjacent soft tissues (retrocalcaneal bursitis and Achilles paratenonitis) (Ogden et al. 2004) (Fig. 16). Additionally, MRI can aid to narrow the differential diagnosis, i.e., to exclude stress fractures, chronic Achilles tendinopathy, plantar fasciitis, juvenile idiopathic arthritis, tarsal tunnel syndrome, and Haglund syndrome. Based on the MRI findings, it was suggested by Ogden et al. that Sever's disease is an unrecognized stress fracture of the metaphysis due to compression, as MRI often shows this adjacent to the apophysis in patients with clinical Sever's disease (Ogden et al. 2004). Treatment is conservative, and the condition is self-limiting.

7.3 Iselin's Disease

Iselin's disease is a rarely reported and therefore most likely underdiagnosed apophysitis of the base of the fifth metatarsal (Iselin 1912). It is a traction apophysitis by the inserting peroneus brevis tendon. It is therefore considered to be an overuse injury and is most often seen in children who are engaged in sporting activities. The apophysis of the base of the fifth metatarsal appears around the age of 12–13 years, but it can be seen in younger children as well (at earlier ages in girls than in boys). Fusion is usually finished around 17–18 years of age (Gillespie 2010; Forrester et al. 2017). The condition is most likely to occur in a period with rapid growth. The typical clinical presentation is lateral foot pain on weight-bearing and swelling at the base of the fifth metatarsal. Especially in case of trauma, it can be very difficult to distinguish the condition from traumatic avulsions of the apophysis. The condition can be however also acute on chronic, and thorough patient history is important. Confirmation of clinical suspicion is made by obtaining radiographs. The apophysis is seen as an elongated fragment parallel to the long axis of the base of the fifth metatarsal (Gillespie 2010). It can be very challenging sometimes to call the position of the apophysis abnormal. Sometimes,

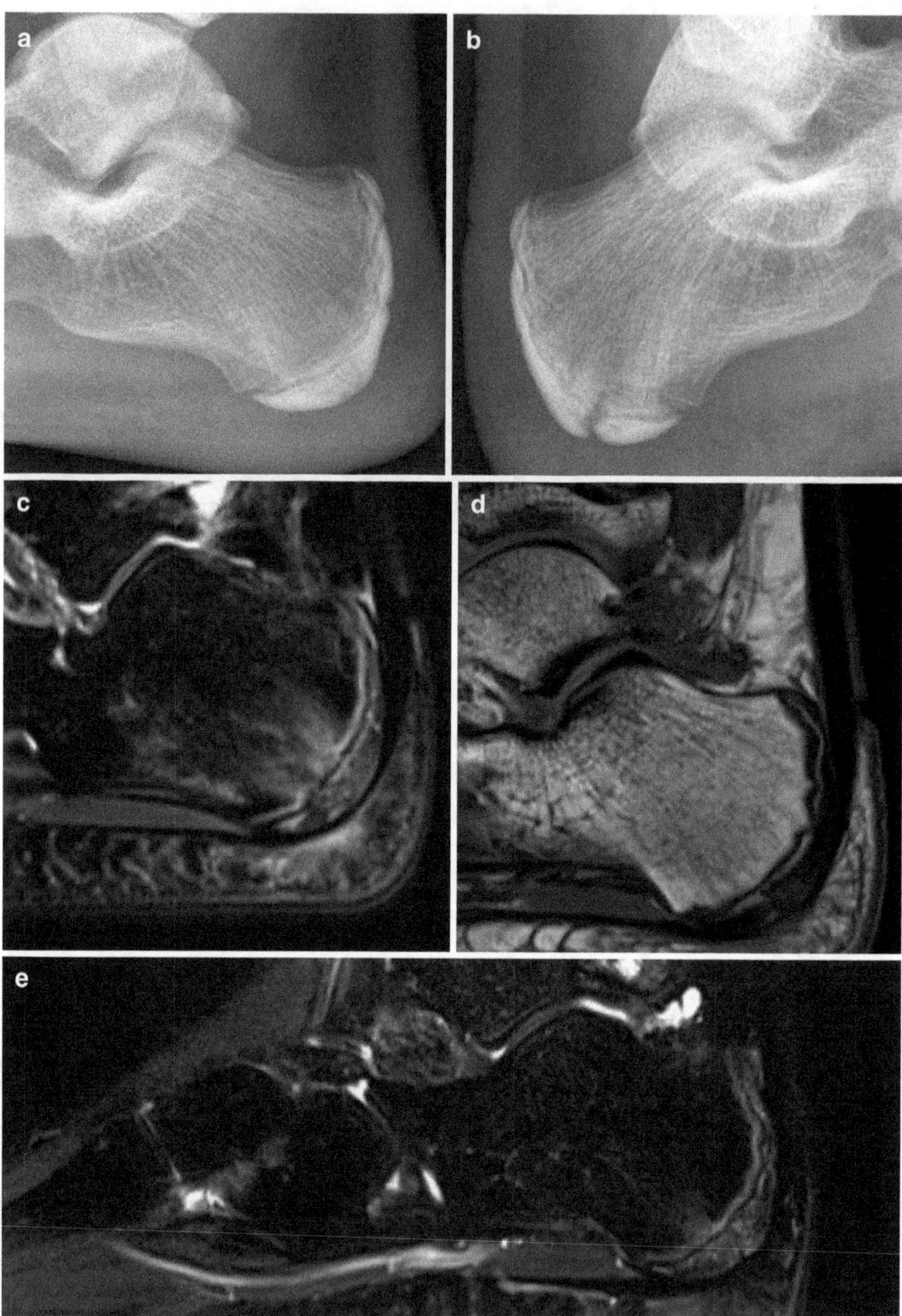

Fig. 16 Sever's disease. A 13-year-old girl with right-sided heel pain. Lateral radiographs of the right (**a**) and left calcaneus (**b**), sagittal STIR (**c**), and T1-weighted MR images (**d**) and sagittal STIR after 8-week treatment (**e**). The apophysis of the right calcaneus is unremarkable, also compared to the contralateral side. The MRI demonstrates bone marrow edema in the metaphysis of the calcaneus adjacent to the apophysis and edema in the subcutaneous fat on the plantar posterior side (**c**). No apparent abnormalities were seen on the T1. Conservative treatment was applied with 4-week plaster of paris after which the MRI was repeated. The reactive BME and subcutaneous fat edema are almost completely gone. There were no more clinical complaints at that time

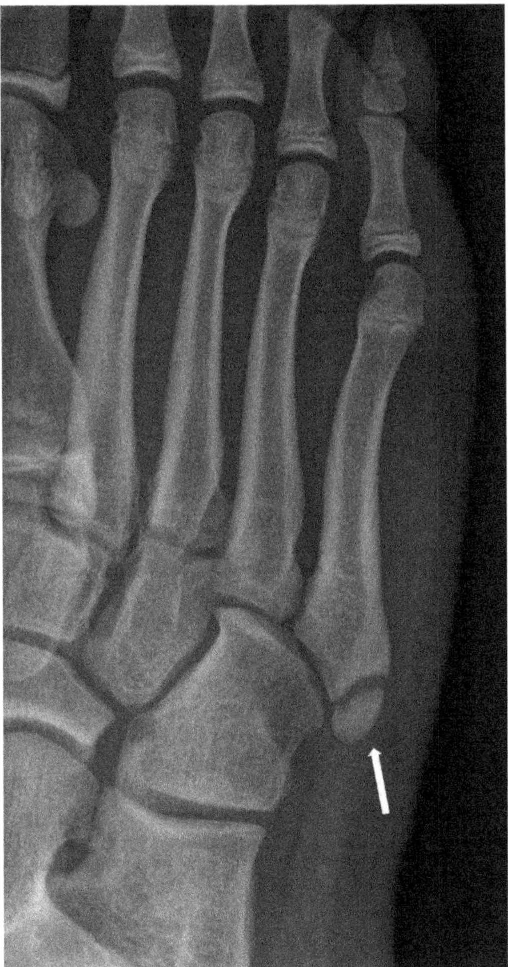

Fig. 17 Iselin's disease. A 14-year-old boy with chronic pain at level base fifth metatarsal. No history of trauma. ¾ radiograph of the right foot. There is thickening/hypertrophy of the apophysis of the base of the fifth metatarsal (arrow) with minimal cortical irregularities and minimal sclerosis

it seems to be quite far away from the rest of the bone. Comparative views in those cases of the contralateral side can be helpful. Other causes of lateral foot pain can be ruled out with plain films, especially fractures of the base of the fifth metatarsal. The described imaging findings on radiographs are an enlarged apophysis with fragmentation of the ossification, widening of the apophysis, and cystic changes around the apophysis (Gillespie 2010; Forrester et al. 2017) (Fig. 17).

References

Agrawal K, Tripathy SK, Sen RK, Santhosh S, Bhattacharya A (2017) Nuclear medicine imaging in osteonecrosis of the hip: old and current concepts. World J Orthop 8:747–753

Ahmed AA, Kandil MI, Tabl EA, Elgazzar A (2019) Müller-Weiss disease: a topical review. Foot Ankle Int 40:1447–1457

Aiyer A, Hennrikus W (2014) Foot pain in the child and adolescent. Pediatr Clin North Am 61:1185–1205

Assouline-Dayan Y, Chang C, Greenspan A, Shoenfeld Y, Gershwin ME (2002) Pathogenesis and natural history of osteonecrosis. Semin Arthritis Rheum 32:94–124

Bartosiak K, McCormick JJ (2019) Avascular necrosis of the sesamoids. Foot Ankle Clin 24:57–67

Borges JL, Guille JT, Bowen JR (1995) Köhler's bone disease of the tarsal navicular. J Pediatr Orthop 15(5):596– 598.

Buchan CA, Com B, Pearce DH, Lau J, White LM (2012) Imaging of postoperative avascular necrosis of the ankle and foot. Semin Musculoskelet Radiol 16:192–204

Canale ST, Kelly FB Jr (1978) Fracture of the neck of the talus. J Bone Joint Surg Am 60:143–156

Chan JY, Young JL (2019) Köhler disease. Avascular necrosis in the child. Foot Ankle Clin 24:83–88

Cooper C, Steinbuch M, Stevenson R, Miday R, Watts NB (2010) The epidemiology of osteonecrosis: findings from the GPRD and THIN databases in the UK. Osteoporos Int 21:569–577

Couturier S, Gold G (2019) Imaging features of avascular necrosis of the foot and ankle. Foot Ankle Clin 24(1):17–33

Delanois RE, Mont MA, Yoon TR, Mizell M, Hungerford DS (1998) Atraumatic osteonecrosis of the talus. J Bone Joint Surg Am 80-A(4):529–536

Doyle SM, Monahan A (2010) Osteochondroses: a clinical review for the pediatrician. Curr Opin Pediatr 22:41–46

Ferguson AB Jr, Gingrich RM (1957) The normal and abnormal calcaneal apophysis and tarsal navicular. Clin Orthop 10:87–95

Forrester RA, Eyre-Brook AI, Mannan K (2017) Iselin's disease: a systematic review. J Foot Ankle Surg 56:1065–1069

Freiberg AH (1914) Infraction of the second metatarsal bone: a typical injury. Surg Gynecol Obstet 19:191–193

Gillespie H (2010) Osteochondroses and apophyseal injuries of the foot in the young athlete. Curr Sports Med Rep 9:265–268

Glimcher MJ, Kenzora JE (1979a) The biology of osteonecrosis of the human femoral head and its clinical implications: I. Tissue biology. Clin Orthop Relat Res 138:284–309

Glimcher MJ, Kenzora JE (1979b) The biology of osteonecrosis of the human femoral head and its clinical implications: II. The pathological changes in the femoral head as an organ and in the hip joint. Clin Orthop Relat Res 138:283–312

Glimcher MJ, Kenzora JE (1979c) The biology of osteonecrosis of the human femoral head and its clinical implications: III. Discussion of the etiology and genesis of the pathological sequelae; comments on treatment. Clin Orthop Relat Res 138:273–312

Haller J, Sartoris DJ, Resnick D, Pathria MN, Berthoty D, Howard B, Nordtsrom D (1988) Spontaneous osteonecrosis of the tarsal navicular in adults: imaging findings. AJR Am J Roentgenol 151:355–358

Hawkins LG (1970) Fractures of the neck of the talus. J Bone Joint Surg Am 52:991–1002

Heinen AK, Harris TG (2019) Avascular necrosis of the tibial plafond following rotational ankle fractures. Foot Ankle Clin 24:113–119

Iselin H (1912) Wachstumsbescherden zur Zeit der knochem Entwicklung der Tuberositas metatarsi quinti. Deutsche Zeitschrift Chir 117:529–535

Issa K, Naziri Q, Kapadia BH, Lamm BM, Jones LC, Mont MA (2014) Clinical characteristics of early-stage osteonecrosis of the ankle and treatment outcomes. J Bone Joint Surg Am 96:e73

Jensen EL, De Carvalho A (1987) A normal variant simulating Freiberg's disease. Acta Radiol 28:85–86

Köhler A (1908) Ueber eine häufige, bisher anscheinend unbekannte Erkrankung einzelner kindlicher Knochen. MWW 55:1923–1925

Kose O (2010) Do we really need radiographic assessment for the diagnosis of non-specific heel pain (calcaneal apophysitis) in children? Skeletal Radiol 4:359–361

Lafforgue P, Trijau S (2016) Bone infarcts: unsuspected gray areas? Joint Bone Spine 83:495–499

Lee S, Saifuddin A (2019) Magnetic resonance imaging of subchondral insufficiency fractures of the lower limb. Skeletal Radiol 48:1011–1021

Mankin HJ (1992) Nontraumatic osteonecrosis of bone (osteonecrosis). N Engl J Med 326:1473–1479

Martinelli N, Spreafico A, Tramacere I, Marcolli D, Valli F, Curci D (2019) Prevalence and associated factors of Sever's disease in an athletic population. J Am Podiatr Med Assoc 5:351–356

McCarthy I (2006) The physiology of bone blood flow: a review. J Bone Joint Surg Am 88:4–9

McLeod JM, Ng A, Kruse DL, Stone PA (2017) Nontraumatic osteonecrosis of the distal tibia: a case presentation and review of the literature. J Foot Ankle Surg 56:158–166

Menck J, Bertram C, Lierse W (1992) Sectorial angioarchitecture of the human tibia. Acta Anat 143(1):76–73

Moon D (2019) Epidemiology, cause, and anatomy of osteonecrosis of the foot and ankle. Foot Ankle Clin 24:1–16

Nunes GA, De Souza MLAT, Braga BM, Marcatti MM, Bertolini FM, Oliveira O Jr (2021) Osteonecrosis of the intermediate cuneiform: a case report. Rev Bras Ortop (Sao Paulo) 56(3):394–398

Ogden JA, Ganey TM, Hill JD, Jaakkola JL (2004) Sever's injury: a stress fracture of the immature calcaneal metaphysis. J Pediatr Orthop 24(5):488–492

Pearce DH, Mongiardi CN, Fornasier VL, Daniels TR (2005) Avascular necrosis of the talus: a pictorial essay. Radiographics 25:399–410

Perhamre S, Lazowska D, Papageorgiou S, Lundin F, Klässbo M, Norlin R (2013) Sever's injury: a clinical diagnosis. J Am Podiatr Med Assoc 5:361–368

Reade B, Atlas G, Distazio J, Kruljac S (1998) Mueller-Weiss syndrome: an uncommon cause of midfoot pain. J Foot Ankle Surg 37:535–539

Samim M, Moukaddam HA, Smitaman E (2018) Imaging of Mueller-Weiss syndrome: a review of clinical presentations and imaging spectrum. AJR Am J Roentgenol 207:W1–W11

Scharfbillig RW, Jones S, Scutter SD (2008) Sever's disease: what does the literature really tell us? J Am Podiatr Med Assoc 3:212–223

Shah KN, Racine J, Jones LC, Aaron RK (2015) Pathophysiology and risk factors for osteonecrosis. Curr Rev Musculoskelet Med 8:201–209

Shane A, Reeves C, Wobst G, Thurston P (2013) Second metatarsophalangeal joint pathology and Freiberg disease. Clin Podiatr Med Surg 30:313–325

Siffert RS (1981) Classification of the osteochondrosis. Clin Orthop Relat Res 158:10–18

Tuthill HL, Finkelstein ER, Sanchez AM, Clifford PD, Subhawong TK, Jose J (2014) Imaging of tarsal navicular disorders: a pictorial review. Foot Ankle Spec 7(3):211–225

Volpon JB, De Carvalho FG (2002) Calcaneal apophysitis: a quantitative radiographic evaluation of the secondary ossification center. Arch Orthop Trauma Surg 122(6):338–341

Wax A, Leland R (2019) Freiberg disease and avascular necrosis of the metatarsal heads. Foot Ankle Clin 24:69–82

West EY, Jaramillo D (2019) Imaging of osteochondrosis. Pediatr Radiol 49:1610–1616

Ytrehus B, Carlson CS, Ekman S (2007) Etiology and pathogenesis of osteochondrosis. Vet Pathol 44:429–448

Zizic TM, Marcoux C, Hungerford DS, Dansereau JV, Stevens MB (1985) Corticosteroid therapy associated with ischemic necrosis of bone in systemic lupus erythematosus. Am J Med 79:596–604

Acquired Deformities of Foot and Ankle

Yet Yen Yan and Ankit Anil Tandon

Contents

Y. Y. Yan (✉)
Department of Radiology, Changi General Hospital, Singapore, Republic of Singapore
e-mail: yanyetyen@gmail.com

A. A. Tandon
Department of Radiology, Tan Tock Seng Hospital, Singapore, Republic of Singapore
e-mail: ankit_tandon@ttsh.com.sg

Abstract

This chapter aims to focus on soft tissue and structural ankle and foot deformities and will be categorized into hindfoot, midfoot, and forefoot. Only conditions that present as a deformity clinically or radiographically will be included in this review. Normal variants of the ankle and foot have not been discussed. Additionally, although trauma and degenerative changes are among the most common etiologies, these will be addressed in other chapters of this book.

Abbreviations

AP	Anteroposterior
CT	Computed tomography
DIPJ	Distal interphalangeal joint
MRI	Magnetic resonance imaging
MTPJ	Metatarsophalangeal joint
PIPJ	Proximal interphalangeal joint
SPECT	Single photon-emission computed tomography
US	Ultrasound

1 Hindfoot

1.1 Achilles Tendinopathy

Achilles tendon injuries which comprise 20% of large tendon injuries are common in both athletes and nonathletes. These often result from a combi-

Med Radiol Diagn Imaging (2023)
https://doi.org/10.1007/174_2023_384,
Published Online: 06 April 2023

nation of factors that include overuse, altered biomechanics, and tendon degeneration. Patients with chronic tendinopathy usually present with pain and a focal lump. Achilles tendon injuries can be categorized into abnormalities within the vicinity of the tendon, within the mid-portion of the tendon, and a group of abnormalities that can occur at the tendon insertion.

1.1.1 Mid-Substance Achilles Tendinopathy

Tendinosis is a degenerative condition associated with aging. Varying degrees of hypoxic, mucoid, calcific, and/or fatty degeneration occur with aging or with overuse, with hypoxic and mucoid degeneration being the most common causes of degeneration in ruptured Achilles tendons (Kannus and Jozsa 1991). With increasing severity, the Achilles tendon shows a disorganized collagen structure and decreased elasticity, with progression to microtears, intrasubstance tears, surface partial tears, and eventually complete tears. Hypoxic degenerative changes are deemed related to hypovascularity and ischemia in the critical zone of the tendon (Kannus and Jozsa 1991). Mucoid degeneration results in myxoid accumulation between the degenerated tendon fibers. Patients with predominant hypoxic degeneration frequently present with episodes of pain in the mid tendinous portion, in contradistinction to the usually silent presentation of mucoid degeneration.

On conventional radiography, the abnormal Achilles tendon would usually be more than 8 mm thick in the anteroposterior dimension (Fig. 1a)

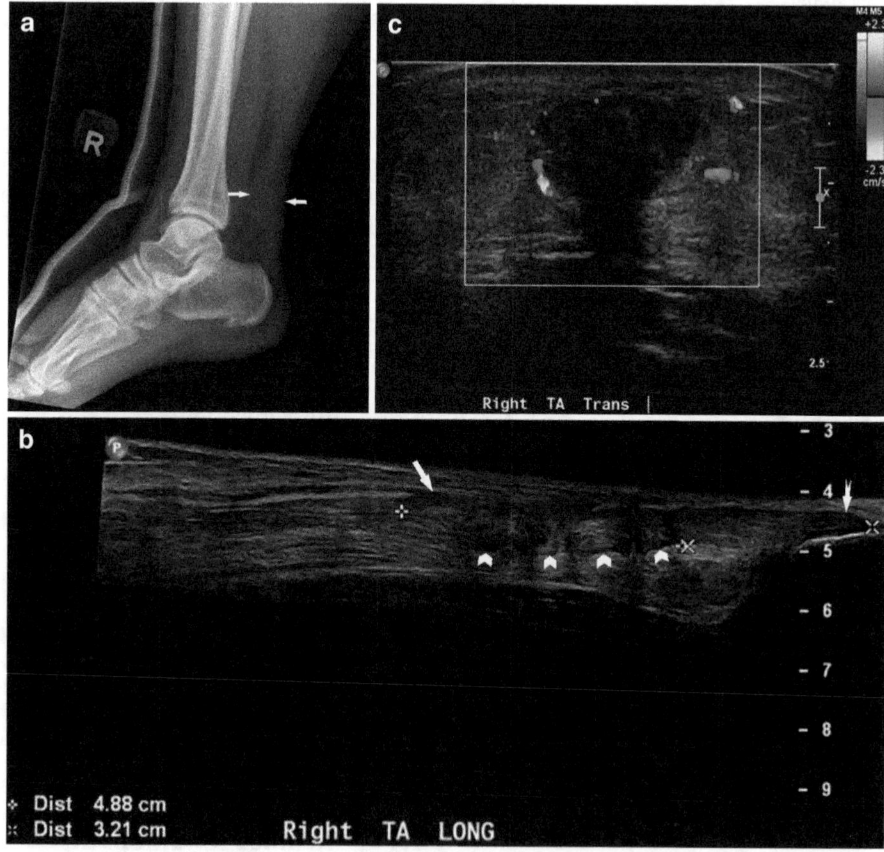

Fig. 1 A 61-year-old female with mid-substance Achilles tear and insertional Achilles tendinosis who presented with right ankle swelling. (**a**) Lateral right ankle radiograph shows midportion Achilles tendon thickening (arrows) suggestive of tendinosis and/or tear. (**b**) Longitudinal US of the right Achilles tendon demonstrates a high-grade partial to full thickness, full width tear of the midportion of the Achilles tendon starting 3.2 cm from its insertion and with the tendinous stump retracted 8.1 cm from its insertion (arrow). Heterogeneous echogenicities in the intervening gap spanning a length of a 4.9 cm is suggestive of a hematoma (chevron arrows). Heterogeneous appearance of the insertional Achilles tendon is suggestive of tendinosis (notched arrow). (**c**) Transverse US of the right Achilles tendon shows posterior acoustic shadowing of the retracted tendinous stump in keeping with a tear, with surrounding hypervascularity

and could show associated findings such as avulsion fracture, calcification, and heterotopic ossification (Yan et al. 2022). Intratendinous ossification is typically seen in patients with prior Achilles tendon rupture or chronic Achilles tendinopathy. On US, tendinosis can manifest as focal or diffuse thickening and hypoechogenicity, with tendon thickening ranging from 7 to 16 mm on transverse images (Fornage 1986). Partial tears can be difficult to differentiate from tendinosis as both appear hypoechoic (Fig. 1b, c). On MRI, hypoxic degeneration usually causes tendon thickening without internal signal alteration, while mucoid degeneration results in tendon enlargement with raised T2-weighted signal due to mucoid deposits and interstitial tears. Chronic Achilles tendinopathy, attenuation, and rupture (Fig. 2a, b) can be surgically treated with flexor hallucis longus tendon transfer procedure to improve tendon strength (Fig. 2c, d).

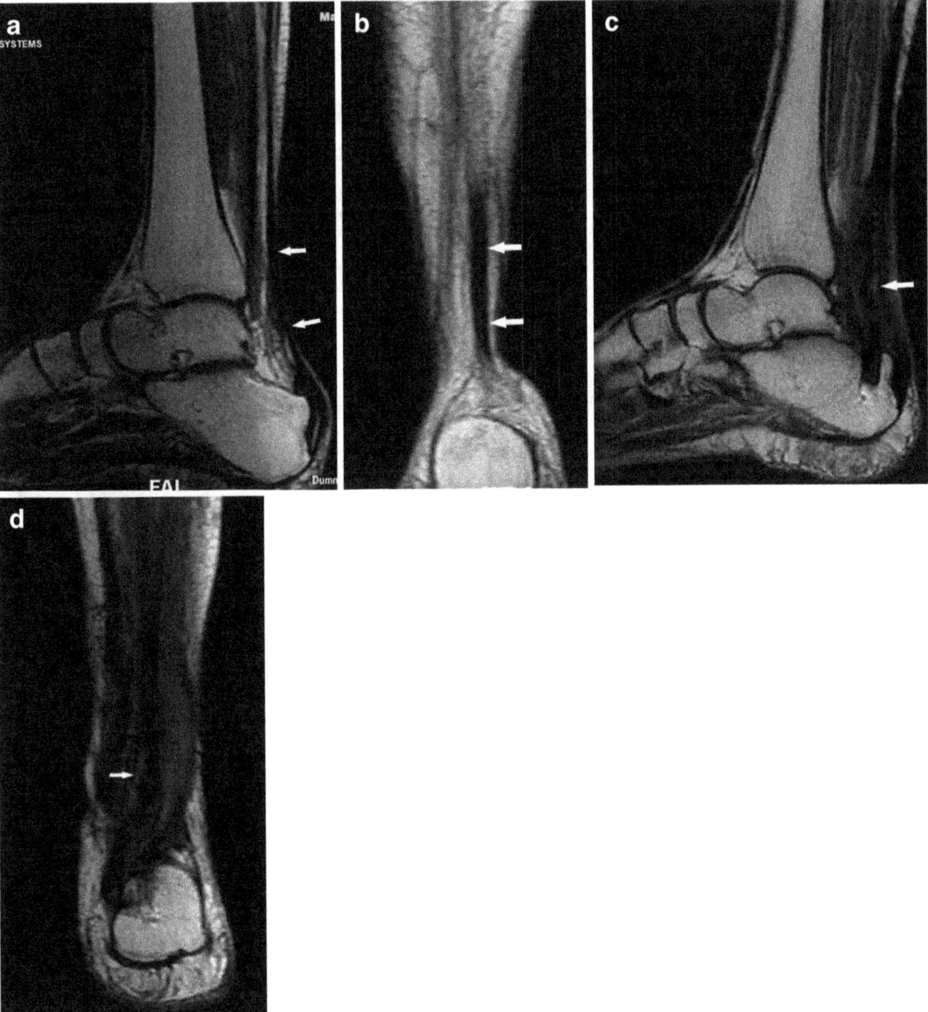

Fig. 2 A 45-year-old male with a right chronic mid-substance Achilles tendon partial tear who had undergone a flexor hallucis longus tendon transfer surgery. Pre-operative (**a**) sagittal and (**b**) coronal PD-W images demonstrate a chronically attenuated Achilles tendon (arrows) compatible with a chronic partial tear. (**c**) Sagittal and (**d**) coronal PD-W images of the same patient acquired 10 months after the surgery shows a markedly thickened flexor hallucis longus tendon graft demonstrating heterogeneously increased signal in keeping with tendinosis, with a more well defined linear intrasubstance raised signal delineating a superimposed partial tear (arrow). (Case courtesy: Adj Asst Prof Muhd Farhan Bin Mohd Fadil, Tan Tock Seng Hospital, Singapore)

1.1.2 Insertional Achilles Tendinopathy, Haglund Syndrome, and Bursitis

Insertional Achilles tendinopathy is frequently associated with adjacent soft tissue and bony abnormalities and is commonly due to overuse. Haglund's deformity is deemed as a predisposing factor of insertional Achilles tendinopathy. Insertional Achilles tendinopathy is also seen in patients with inflammatory arthropathy, corticosteroid use, diabetes, hypertension, obesity, gout, and those on fluroquinolone antibiotics. Patients typically present with stiffness and a palpable, painful bump at the Achilles tendon insertion (Burns et al. 2008). Haglund syndrome refers to posterosuperior calcaneal enlargement, retrocalcaneal bursitis, and insertional Achilles tendinopathy. The inflamed retrocalcaneal bursa is compressed between the Achilles tendon and calcaneus, and this incites a bony spurring reaction that precipitates Haglund deformity.

On conventional radiography, a positive parallel pitch line (PPL) on lateral radiographs is the main radiographic measure of Haglund syndrome (Fig. 3a). Additional radiographic measures include an increased Fowler-Philip angle

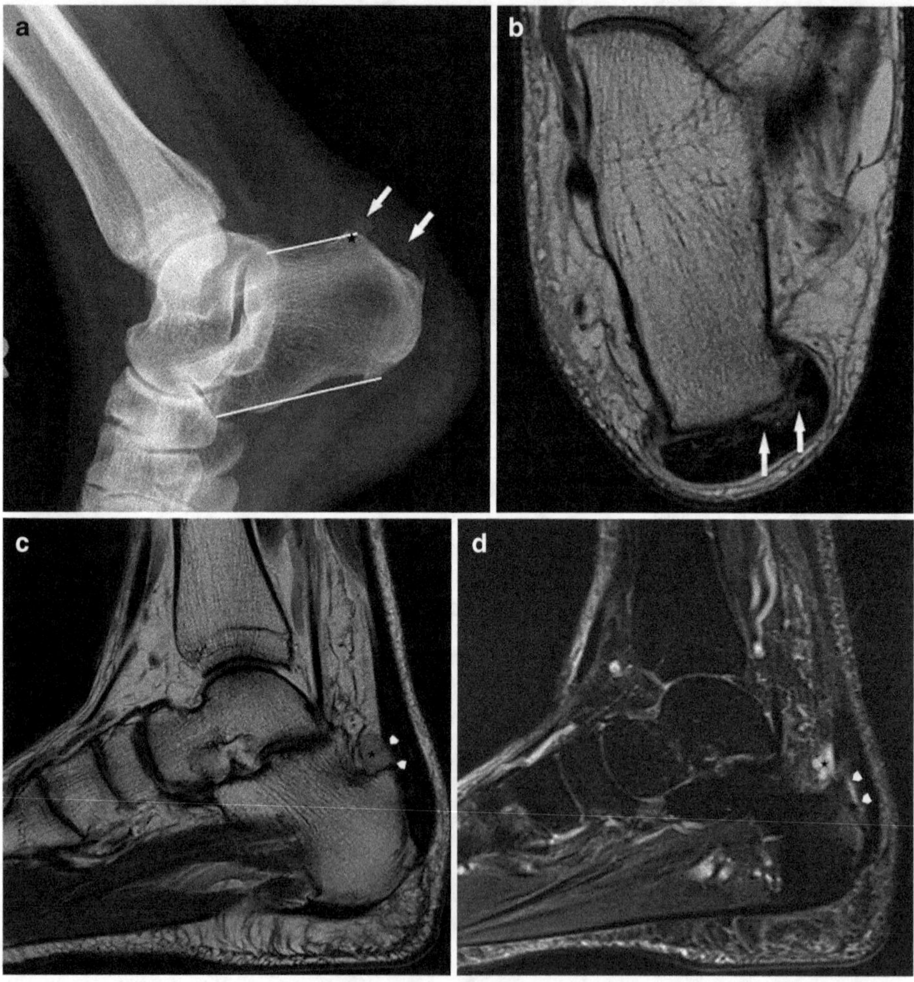

Fig. 3 A 57-year-old female with Haglund syndrome who presents with right heel pain. (**a**) Lateral right ankle radiograph shows a positive parallel pitch line in keeping with a Haglund deformity (star). Dystrophic ossification (arrow) is projected over the thickened distal Achilles tendon. (**b**) Axial PD-W, (**c**) sagittal PD-W, and (**d**) sagittal STIR reveal raised signal and thickening of the insertional Achilles tendon in keeping with moderate tendinosis. There is superimposed low grade partial tear of the deep fibers of the Achilles tendon just proximal to and at its insertion (pentagon arrows). The dystrophic ossification is better delineated on the radiograph. Retrocalcaneal bursal fluid is in keeping with bursitis (star). There is reactive marrow edema in the posterior calcaneal tuberosity

(normal range being 44°–69°) and Chauveaux-Liet angle (normal being ≤12°). The sensitivity and specificity of these radiographic assessments are low to moderate (sensitivity: PPL between 50% and 70%, Fowler-Philip as low as 0%, and Chauveaux-Liet as low as 56%; specificity ranging between 45% and 85%) (Desai et al. 2022), and should serve only as an adjunct to clinical evaluation (Tourné et al. 2018). On a lateral radiograph, retrocalcaneal bursitis can show a loss of the retrocalcaneal recess and effacement of Kager's fat. Achilles tendinopathy can appear as an indistinct interface between the Achilles tendon and Achilles fat pad (Pavlov et al. 1982). Achilles tendon enthesophytes or calcification/ossification within the distal Achilles tendon are common.

On US, retrocalcaneal bursitis can display a complex hypoechoic fluid with nodular echogenicities within, while insertional Achilles tendinopathy shows a fusiform heterogeneous thickening of the distal Achilles tendon (Sofka et al. 2006). CT can show the posterosuperior calcaneal enlargement of Haglund deformity and soft tissue abnormalities although it is rarely utilized. On MRI, retrocalcaneal bursitis can show enlarged bursal dimensions (>1 mm, 11 mm, and 7 mm in the anteroposterior, transverse, and craniocaudal directions, respectively) (Fig. 3c, d) (Bottger et al. 1998). On MRI, distal tendon thickening with ill-defined tendon signal heterogeneity can be seen. Partial tears demonstrate hyperintense defects on fluid sensitive sequences (Fig. 3b–d). Edema within enthesophytes correlates with more acute symptoms (Fig. 3d).

1.2 Calcaneal Spurs

Plantar and posterior calcaneal spurs comprise of non-pathological exostoses of the calcaneus and are the result of increased traction forces or an altered force transmission on the calcaneal entheses that are related to age and body weight (Menz et al. 2008). It is widely accepted that spur incidence increases with increasing age and body weight. Plantar calcaneal spur is more common than posterior spur, with a prevalence of 32% and 13%, respectively (Beytemür and Öncü 2018). There is increased spur incidences in females younger than 50 years than males (Toumi et al. 2014). The evidence for an increased incidence of calcaneal spurs in patients with osteoarthritis is weak (Menz et al. 2008). There is an association with insertional Achilles tendinopathy and plantar fasciitis. Most patients present with pain and tension in the heel region although 10% of spurs are asymptomatic (Başdelioğlu 2021). On conventional radiography, CT, and MRI, plantar calcaneal spur manifests as a bony spur on the lateral radiograph/sagittal image extending inferomedially from the calcaneus, while posterior calcaneal spur extends superiorly from the posterior calcaneal tuberosity.

1.3 Hindfoot Deformities

1.3.1 Hindfoot Varus

Hindfoot varus refers to adduction and rotation of the calcaneus under the talus, decreasing the normal talar plantar angulation and is frequently caused by muscle imbalances such as neurologic, traumatic, congenital, or idiopathic aetiologies. Hindfoot varus deformity may be associated with a cavovarus foot deformity (first ray plantarflexion, forefoot pronation, and hindfoot varus) (Fig. 4). Two thirds of adults with symptomatic cavovarus deformity have an underlying neurologic cause, predominantly Charcot-Marie-Tooth disease (Alexander and Johnson 1989). Patient can present with pain, hindfoot instability, and difficulty fitting into shoes. In the early stages, patients can have discomfort along the lateral foot border, metatarsalgia, and recurrent supination sprains. Subsequently, patients can have restricted ankle dorsiflexion and pain due to anterior ankle impingement or anteromedial ankle arthritis (Krause and Iselin 2012) (Figs. 4d and 5).

In conventional radiography weight-bearing AP projection, there is decreased almost parallel talocalcaneal angle (<15°), a line drawn through the talus will point laterally to the first metatarsal base, and the navicular bone will be subluxed medially with respect to the talar head. On the lateral projection, there is a decrease in the talocalcaneal angle (<25°) and a posterior position of the fibula. If there is an associated cavovarus deformity, additional radiographic features include an increased navicular height, a calcaneal pitch >30°, an increased Hibbs angle (>45°), an increased angle of Meary, a "flat-topped" talus and an open sinus tarsi area (lateral projection), as well as a medially concave talo–first metatarsal angle and fractures of the fifth metatarsal (AP projection) (Krause and Iselin 2012). Degenerative changes such as anterior tibial and talar osteophytes, decreased anteromedial ankle joint space, and osteochondral lesions should also be assessed.

CT can evaluate occult degenerative joint disease and tarsal coalitions and assists with preoperative planning. In long-standing hindfoot varus, MRI can assess cartilage degeneration, hindfoot arthritis, and the integrity of tendons. US can establish if tendons are torn.

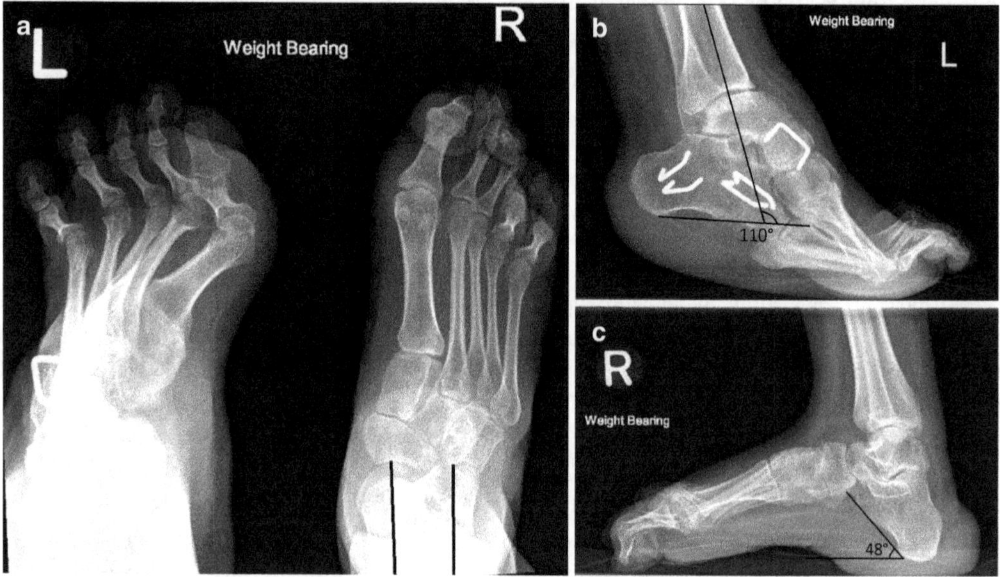

Fig. 4 A 29-year-old female with spina bifida, lumbosacral lipomeningomyelocele, and sacral tethered cord presented with bilateral cavovarus foot deformities and claw toes. Patient is status post left Dwyer's osteotomy and subsequent plantar fascia release, split tibialis anterior tendon transfer, Achilles tendon lengthening, wedge tarsectomy and posterior and medial capsular release, with internal fixation across the posterior calcaneus as well as the talonavicular and calcaneocuboid joints. (**a**) Bilateral AP weight-bearing feet radiographs show near parallel alignment of the talus and calcaneus indicative of hindfoot varus (better seen over the right). There is a left metatarsus adductus. Lateral weight-bearing (**b**) left and (**c**) right foot radiograph delineates a left calcaneotibial angle >90° in keeping with hindfoot equinus and right calcaneal pitch >30° compatible with pes cavus. In addition, there are diffuse hyperflexion deformities of the PIPJs and DIPJs of bilateral toes consistent with bilateral claw toes. (**d**) Blood pool phase of bone scan shows tracer uptake at the medial tibiotalar joint may be related to degenerative changes. Mild tracer activity in the left fifth metatarsal shaft may be due to stress changes. (**e**) CT shows accelerated severe degenerative changes of the tibiotalar joint in the form of marginal osteophytes, and subchondral cystic-like changes and sclerosis. Partial ankylosis of the subtalar, calcaneonavicular and calcaneocuboid joints. No residual equinus deformity post Achilles tendon lengthening

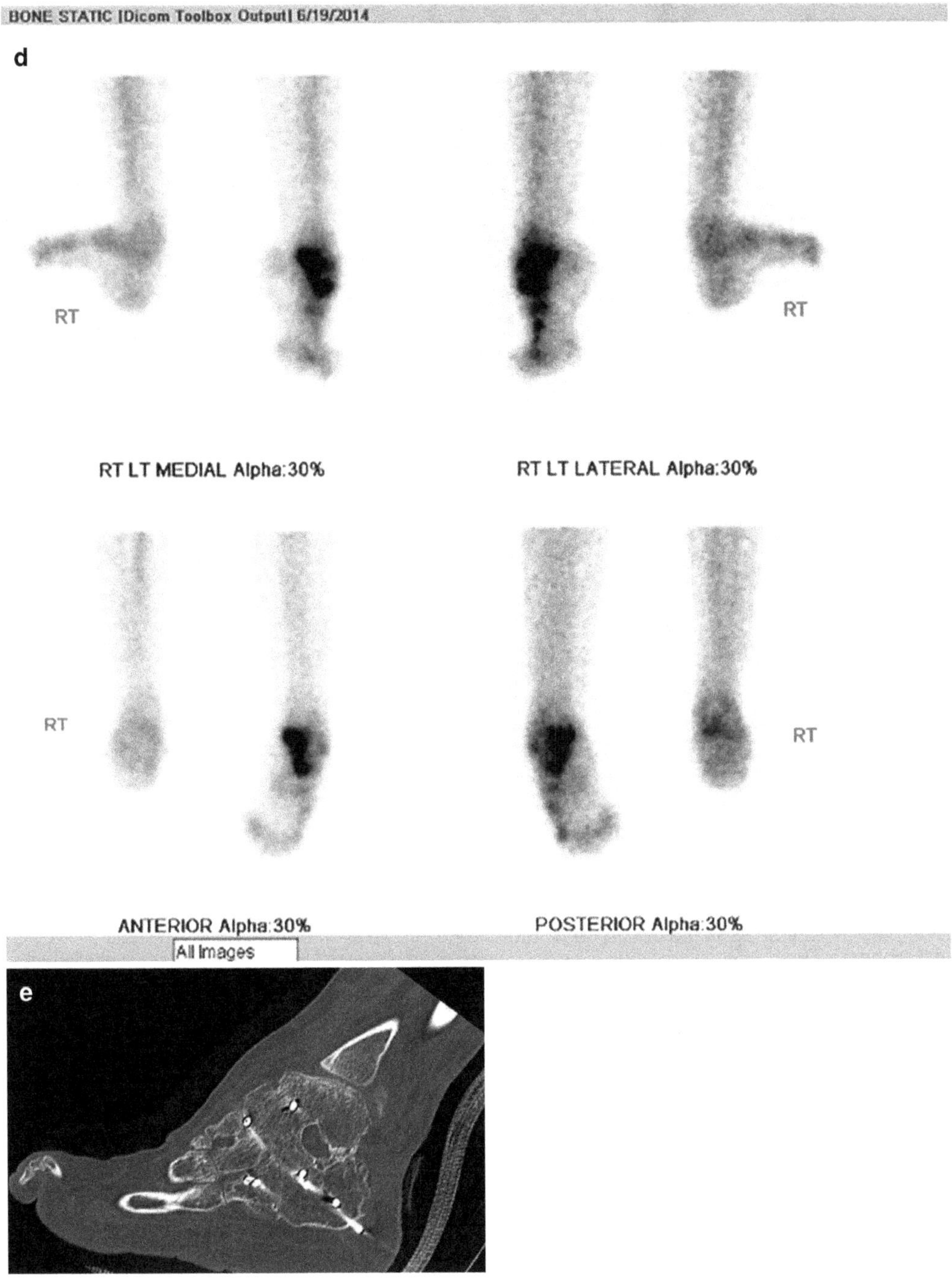

BONE STATIC [Dicom Toolbox Output] 6/19/2014

d

RT

RT

RT LT MEDIAL Alpha:30%

RT LT LATERAL Alpha:30%

RT

RT

ANTERIOR Alpha:30%

POSTERIOR Alpha:30%

All Images

e

Fig. 4 (continued)

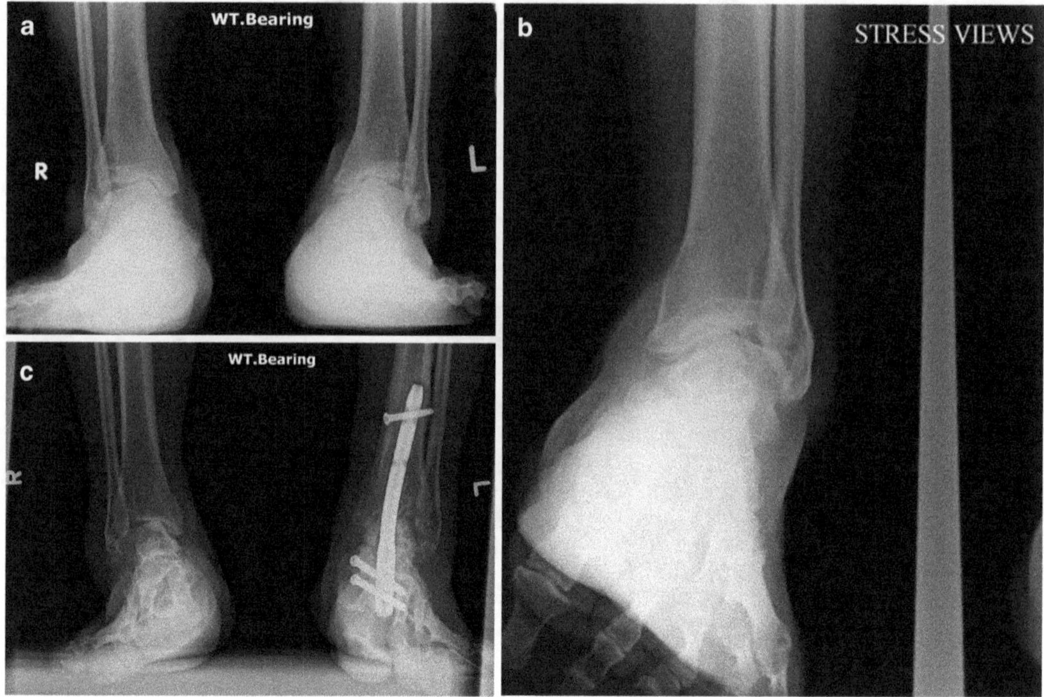

Fig. 5 A 43-year-old female with bilateral hindfoot varus who was subsequently treated with left ankle and subtalar joint fusion using screws and bone graft. (**a**) AP weight-bearing radiograph of both ankles reveals bilateral hindfoot varus with Takakura Stage IIIA osteoarthritis. (**b**) Stress AP view of the left ankle joint reveals further obliteration of the medial joint space. (**c**) AP weight-bearing radiograph of both ankles shows left ankle and subtalar joint fusion using screws and bone graft

1.3.2 Hindfoot Valgus

Hindfoot valgus is defined as the deviation of the mid-calcaneal axis away from the midline of the body. Hindfoot valgus can be categorized into congenital causes such as tarsal coalition or acquired causes such as posterior tibialis tendon dysfunction and inflammatory or osteoarthritis. Predisposing factors for hindfoot valgus include pes planus (Figs. 6 and 9), obesity, hypertension, diabetes, and participation in high-impact sports (Vulcano et al. 2013). Patients can present with hindfoot pain on weight-bearing, swelling, and tenderness in the region anterior and inferior to the lateral malleolus.

On conventional radiography, weight-bearing hindfoot alignment and long axial view radiographs show a tibiocalcaneal angle >10°, and foot weight-bearing radiographs show a talocalcaneal angle >40° and >45° in the AP and lateral radiographs, respectively. CT can assess occult degenerative tibiotalar and subtalar joint disease and tarsal coalitions. MRI can evaluate chondral wear, the tibiotalar and subtalar joints, as well as the surrounding supporting soft tissue structures of the hindfoot. An increased tibiocalcaneal angle >11° and a horizontal orientation of the calcaneofibular ligament on the sagittal plane can suggest hindfoot valgus (Lee et al. 2020).

1.3.3 Hindfoot Equinus

An equinus position refers to the superior elevation of the posterior part of the foot, with a plantar flexed lower anterior end (Fig. 4b). The ankle is unable to dorsiflex sufficiently to permit the heel to contact the supporting surface. Ankle equinus can be isolated, compensatory, or in combination with other lower limb deformities. Acquired equinus causes include poliomyelitis, trauma, burns, limb lengthening, limb disuse, while congenital equinus causes include cerebral palsy, Charcot-Marie-Tooth, clubfoot, muscular dystrophy, pes planus, and idiopathic toe walking. Equinus deformity is secondary to a bony abnormality with or without soft tissue involvement, whereas an equinus contracture is caused by only soft tissues (Gourdine-Shaw et al. 2010). Patients can complain of a myriad of symptoms such as lower back pain, knee pain, and ankle and foot pain owing to the body's compensatory positional response to equinus. On conventional radiogra-

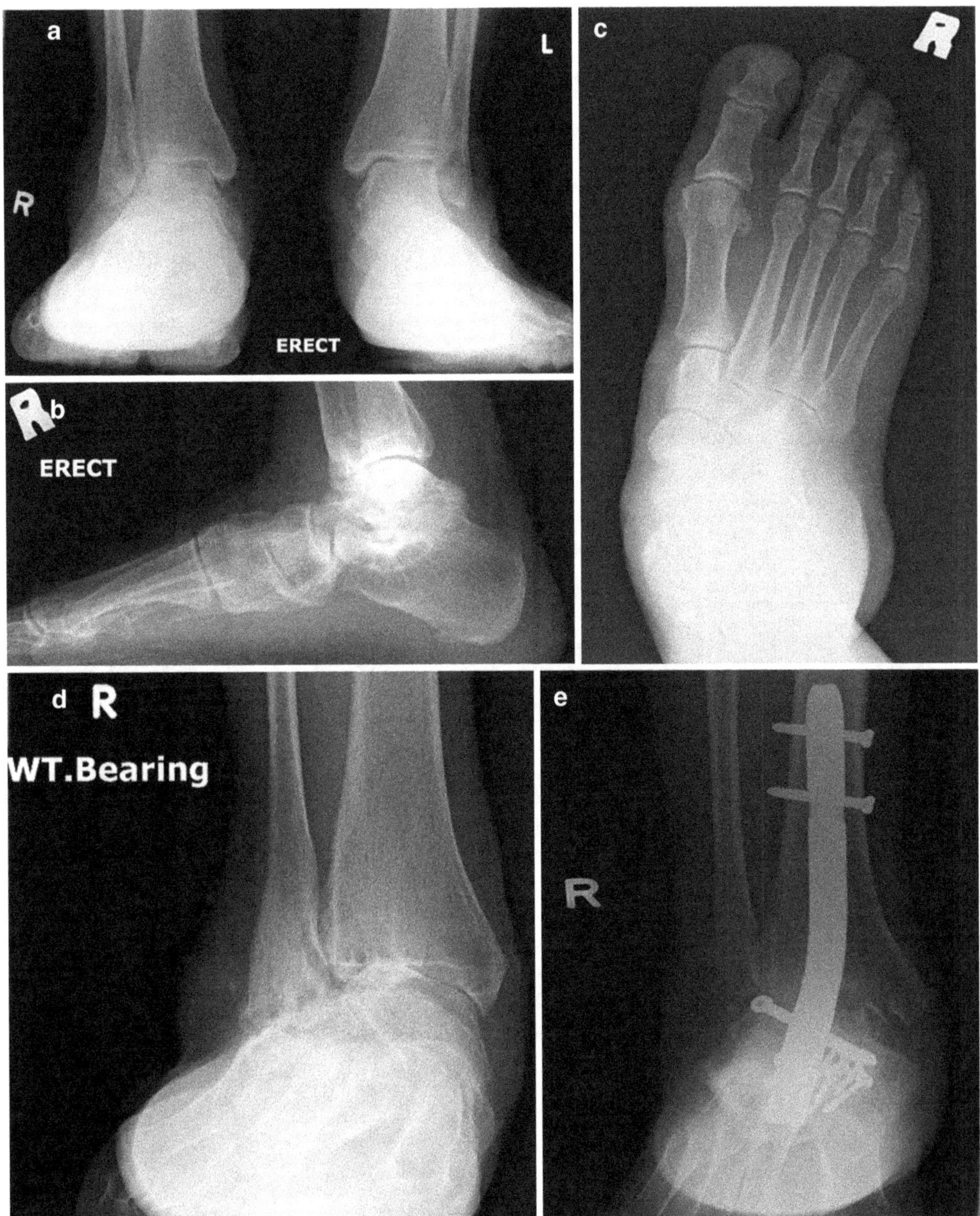

Fig. 6 A 63-year-old male with right hind foot valgus, pes planus, and ankle osteoarthritis. (**a**) AP weight-bearing radiograph of both ankles reveals right sided hind-foot valgus with ankle osteoarthritis. (**b**) Lateral and (**c**) AP weight-bearing radiographs of the right foot also show pes planus and collapse of medial longitudinal foot arch. (**d**) Follow-up weight-bearing radiograph of right ankle reveals significant progression of hindfoot valgus and ankle osteoarthritis. (**e**, **f**) Patient was treated with right pantalar fusion, distal fibular osteotomy, and medial cuneiform cotton osteotomy (latter was performed to correct pes planus and restore the foot arch). (Case courtesy: Adj Asst Prof Muhd Farhan Bin Mohd Fadil, Tan Tock Seng Hospital, Singapore)

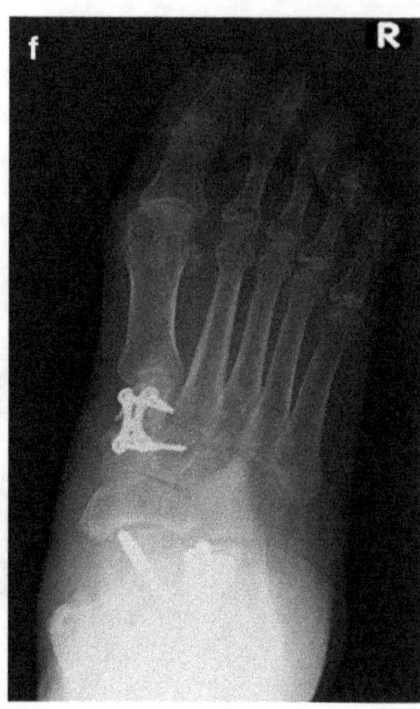

Fig. 6 (continued)

phy, the lateral weight-bearing radiograph shows a hyper plantarflexed calcaneus, a calcaneal-tibial angle >90° (Fig. 4b), and a decreased talocalcaneal angle (<25°) (Yablon et al. 2010).

2 Midfoot

2.1 Pes Planus

Pes planus has been termed as flatfoot, planovalgus foot, adult acquired flatfoot deformity and lately, progressive collapsing flatfoot deformity. Pes planus can be classified into developmental or acquired causes. Developmental flatfoot is normal in toddlers and is usually related to immaturity; however, it can be associated with tarsal coalition (Fig. 7), neuromuscular disease, and laxity syndromes (Fig. 8). Acquired flatfoot causes include

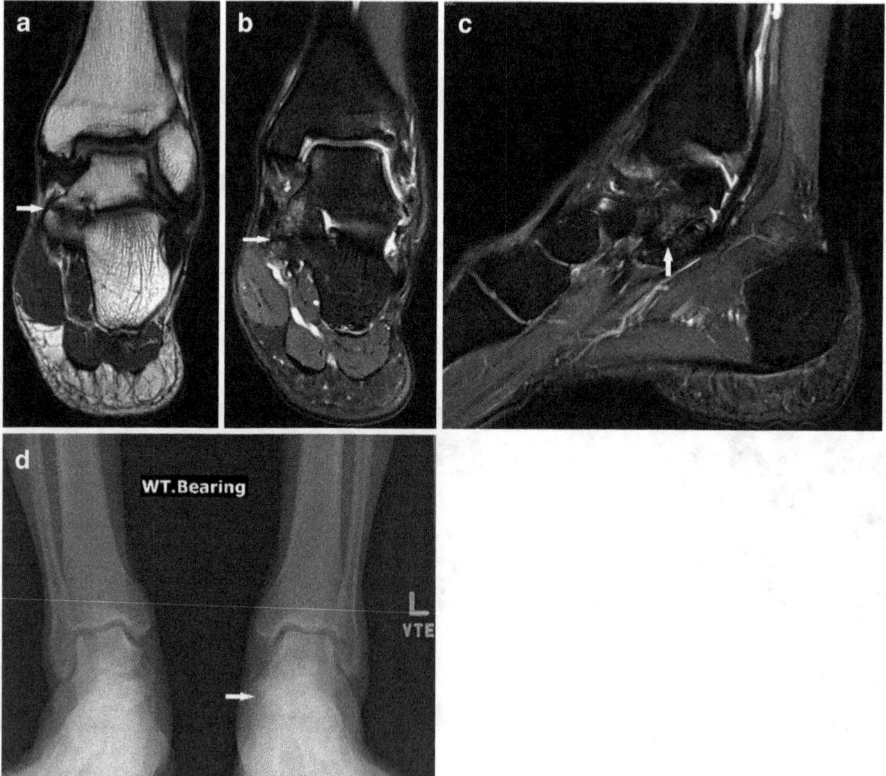

Fig. 7 A 23-year-old male with a rigid left flat foot secondary to tarsal coalition who presented with recurrent ankle sprains. (**a–c**) Coronal PD-W, coronal PD-W fat suppressed and sagittal PD-W fat suppressed images demonstrate a fibrocartilaginous talocalcaneal coalition involving the middle subtalar joint (arrow). There is non-osseous union with irregularity of the articular surface and narrowing of the intervening space with presence of marrow oedema in the talus and sustentaculum tali. There are degenerate chondral changes in the ankle joint. (**d**) AP weight-bearing radiograph of left ankle demonstrates abnormal articular orientation between medial talus and sustentaculum tali (arrow) at the medial aspect of subtalar joint

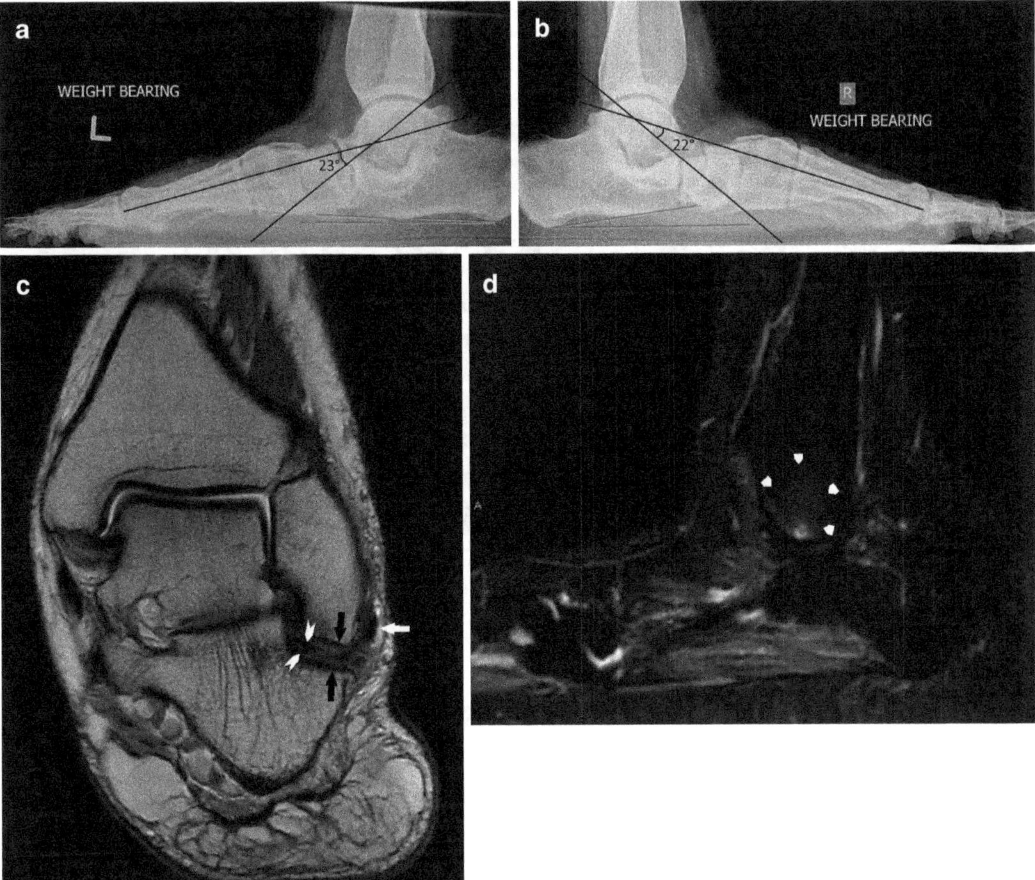

Fig. 8 A 21-year-old male patient of Marfan's syndrome presented with bilateral pes planus along with signs of hindfoot valgus and lateral hindfoot impingement. (**a**) Left and (**b**) right foot lateral weight-bearing radiographs show bilateral midfoot sag (increased Meary's angles convex downwards and decreased calcaneal pitch) compatible with pes planus. There are moderate degenerative changes in talonavicular joints bilaterally. (**c**) Coronal PD-W and (**d**) sagittal STIR MRI images demonstrate hindfoot valgus with obliteration of the calcaneofibular ligament (chevron arrows) in keeping with a complete tear. There are also flat neo-facets at the fibular tip and lateral calcaneus (black arrows) with subcortical fibular tip marrow edema (pentagon arrows) and cystic like changes consistent with lateral hindfoot impingement. Posterior tibialis tendon and spring ligament complex are intact (not shown). Peroneus longus and brevis tendons are dislocated laterally (white arrow) and show raised signal suggestive of tendinosis

posterior tibialis tendon degeneration (PTTD), trauma, neuropathic arthropathy, neuromuscular disease, and inflammatory arthritis, of which PTTD is the most common. Many patients are asymptomatic and approximately 1% can be symptomatic with a predilection toward females and a peak age of 55 years (Deland 2008). Symptomatic patients present with a medial based pain along the arch or under/on the inside of the ankle. With disease progression, patients may have lateral ankle pain in the calcaneofibular region, as well as increased pain with activity, unsteady gait, and abnormal shoe wear (Jackson III et al. 2022).

In a PTTD aetiology, there are four stages. In stage I, radiographs are usually normal and MRI can show raised signal and thickening of the posterior tibialis tendon in keeping with tendinosis or posterior tibialis tendon sheath fluid in keeping with tenosynovitis (Fig. 9). In stage II, radiographs show increased talonavicular uncoverage and talar-first metatarsal angle (AP weight-bearing), due to forefoot abduction, and decreased calcaneal pitch and increased Meary's angle (lateral weight-bearing radiograph) (Fig. 8a, b). In the presence of hindfoot valgus, the talocalcaneal angle is >40° and >45° in the AP and lateral

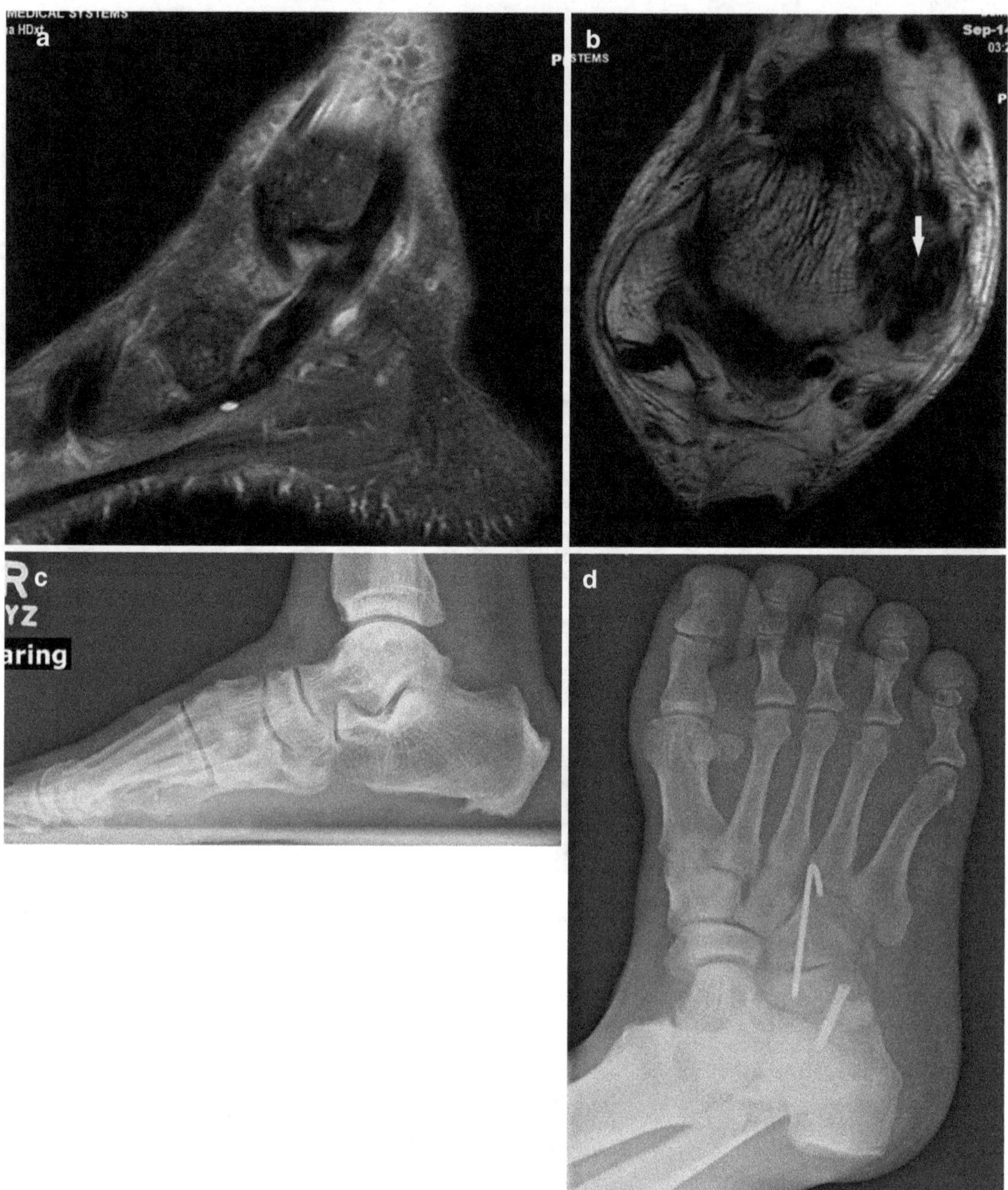

Fig. 9 A 54-year-old female with right pes planus secondary to Type 1 posterior tibialis tendon dysfunction (PTTD) who presented with pain along the medial aspect of foot and ankle on running. (**a**) Sagittal PD-W fat suppressed image demonstrates abnormal thickening and high signal within the posterior tibialis tendon in its inframalleolar course. (**b**) Axial PD-W images show interstitial splitting within the fibers of posterior tibialis tendon along with a small tear anteriorly (arrow). Images also demonstrate increase in diameter of the posterior tibialis tendon. Findings are in keeping with Type I PTTD. (**c**) Lateral weight-bearing radiograph of the right foot demonstrates pes planus. (**d**) Patient was treated with endoscopic gastrocnemius resection, Mosca osteotomy of calcaneum with iliac bone graft, and debridement of posterior tibialis tendon

radiographs, respectively. In stage IIA, there is <30% talonavicular uncoverage, whereas in stage IIB, talonavicular uncoverage is >30%. On MRI, apart from depicting posterior tibialis tendinosis, tears of the posterior tibialis tendon and spring ligament can be seen (Flores et al. 2019). Features of sinus tarsi syndrome may also be observed in stage IIB. In stage III, in addition to the imaging findings in stage II, there can be degenerative changes at the talonavicular, calcaneocuboid, and subtalar joints (Jackson III et al. 2022). In stage IV, radiographs can show lateral talar tilt with tibiotalar valgus and progressive asymmetric tibiotalar arthritis, and medial clear space widening. MRI can depict deltoid ligament tear and features of bony and soft tissue features of lateral hindfoot impingement (Fig. 8c, d) such as extra-articular subcortical bone marrow oedema, cystic changes, and sclerosis at specific locations at the talus, calcaneus or fibula, soft tissue edema at the most posterior aspect of the sinus tarsi and at the adjacent subfibular region, calcaneofibular ligament tear, peroneal tendon subluxation or dislocation as well as peroneal tenosynovitis, tendinosis, and tears.

2.2 Neuropathic Arthropathy

Neuropathic arthropathy is characterized by bony fragmentation, destruction, fractures as well as joint subluxation and instability. Consequently, bony deformities form, and in the foot, the most common deformity is the rocker bottom deformity on the plantar aspect of the midfoot. Neuropathic arthropathy can be due to alcoholism, syphilis, syringomyelia, peripheral nerve injuries, congenital insensitivity to pain, and leprosy but occurs most commonly in diabetic patients in the foot and ankle, of which the tarsometatarsal joints are most frequently involved (Fig. 10) (Yablon et al. 2010). Patients commonly

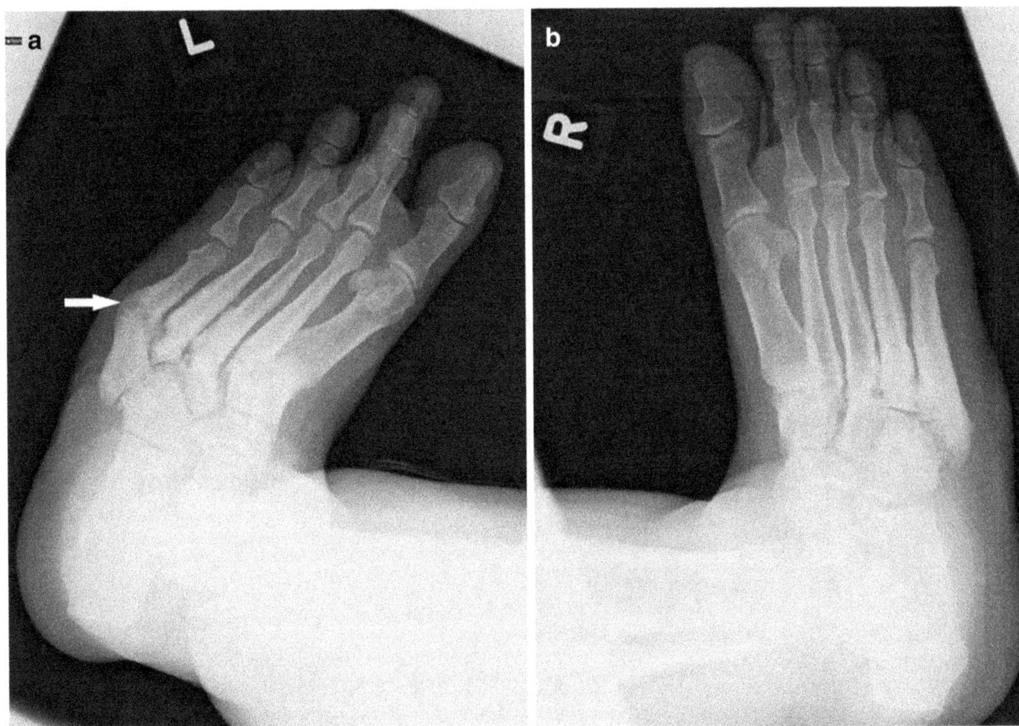

Fig. 10 A 58-year-old male driver with Eichenholtz stage 2 neuropathic arthropathy. He was also assessed for his ability to drive and was found to have poorly controlled diabetes mellitus, poor proprioception. Oblique radiographs of (**a**) left and (**b**) right foot demonstrate patchy areas of sclerosis and fusion in the midfoot and proximal metatarsals. There is also a healing fracture of fifth metatarsal shaft with callus formation (arrow)

present with erythema, warmth, and swelling of the lower extremity. Although this clinical presentation can mimic and can be difficult to differentiate from that of cellulitis or septic arthritis, fever and raised white blood cell count are not usually seen in neuropathic arthropathy. The Eichenholtz classification system has been utilized to detail the evolution of clinical and radiographic changes (Eichenholtz 1966). Whereas radiologically, disease patterns can be composed of hypertrophic, atrophic, and mixed types. The hypertrophic pattern can mimic osteoarthritis and is characterized by joint destruction, bony fragmentation and debris, sclerosis, and large osteophytes. The atrophic type can mimic septic arthritis and is shown by joint disorganization and bone resorption. Patients commonly present with a combination of both hypertrophic and atrophic types (Fig. 11a). Patients with advanced neuropathic joints and those with rocker bottom foot deformity often present with superimposed infection and osteomyelitis due to ulcerations, and MRI plays an important role in the assessment of superimposed infection (Fig. 11b, c).

On conventional radiography, weight-bearing radiographs, midfoot and hindfoot collapse, pes planus, and/or rocker bottom deformity should be assessed for. Midfoot collapse is evaluated by assessing the Meary's angle (<0° in the presence of pes planus) and AP talar-first metatarsal angle

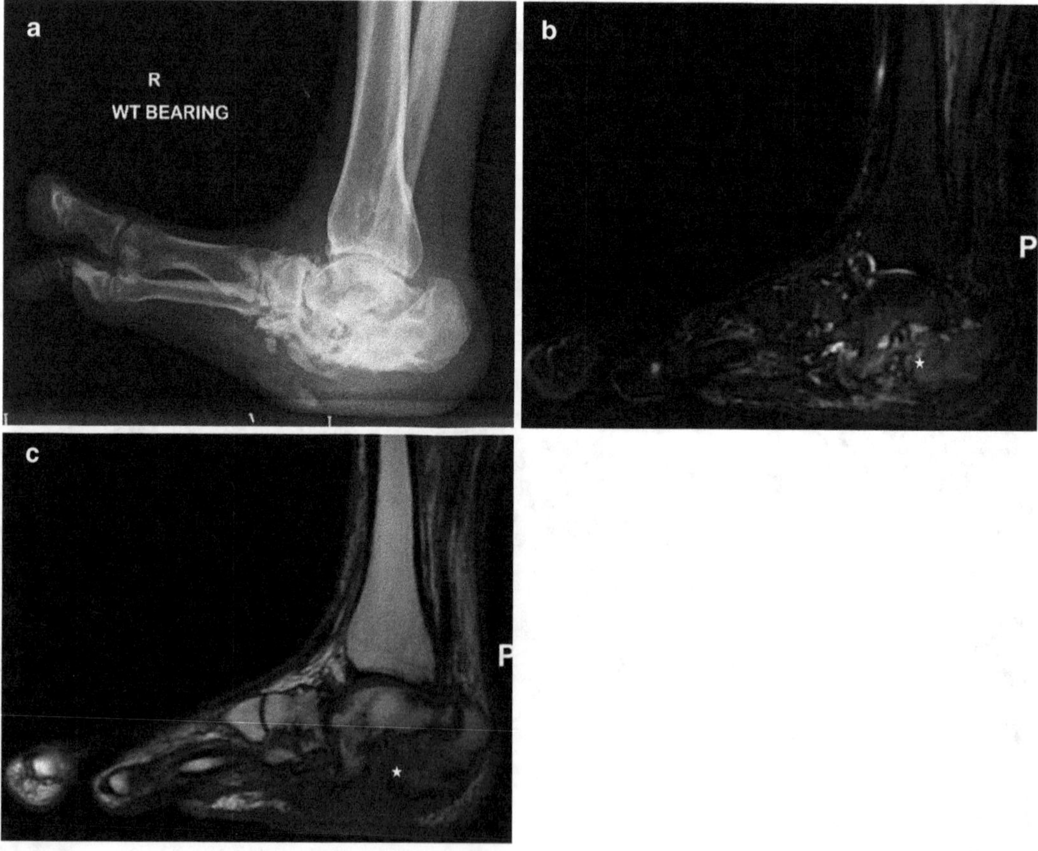

Fig. 11 A 56-year-old male diabetic with known Charcot's joints with rocker bottom foot deformity who presented with soft tissue swelling and ulcer at the plantar aspect of right mid foot. (**a**) Lateral weight-bearing radiograph of the right foot highlights the rocker bottom foot deformity and demonstrates disorganization of mid foot and subtalar joints. Patient had previous amputations to treat osteomyelitis. (**b**) Sagittal STIR and (**c**) T1-W images demonstrate destruction of anterior calcaneum and cuboid bones with altered marrow signal intensity, appearing hyperintense on STIR and hypointense on T1-W images, in the remnant cuboid, calcaneum (star) as well as inferior talus in keeping with osteomyelitis. Soft tissue changes are also noted in the region of bony destruction and plantar ulceration

and on the lateral radiograph the calcaneal-fifth metatarsal angle (>170° in the presence of pes planus). The presence of a hindfoot equinus deformity contributing to midfoot collapse can be evaluated on a lateral radiograph with an increased calcaneal-tibial angle (>90°) (Yablon et al. 2010). Presence of hindfoot varus or valgus can be assessed on the AP or lateral radiograph. On AP radiograph, the talocalcaneal angle is decreased in hindfoot varus (<15°) and increased in hindfoot valgus (>40°). On lateral radiograph, the lateral talocalcaneal angle is decreased in hindfoot varus (<25°) and increased in hindfoot valgus (>45°).

2.3 Pes Cavus

Pes cavus foot is defined as an increase in height of the medial longitudinal arch of the foot that does not flatten on weight-bearing. The cavovarus foot deformity is frequently used interchangeably with the pes cavus deformity as well as "claw foot" and "hollow foot" (Fig. 4). Clawing of the toes is frequently associated with a pes cavus deformity (Fig. 4b, c). The cavus foot is most commonly due to a neurological cause, Charcot-Marie-Tooth Disease being the commonest, with calcaneocavus feet predominantly caused by poliomyelitis, cerebral palsy, and myelomeningocele. Traumatic causes are rare. Pes cavus can be categorized into posterior, anterior, and combined (anterior and posterior) causes. Posterior deformity (hindfoot cavus or calcaneocavus), secondary to weakness of the gastrocnemius-soleus complex, is associated with vertical orientation of the calcaneus (the calcaneal pitch angle being >30°) and frequently involves a degree of varus alignment (Fig. 4c). Anterior deformity involves plantar flexion of the mid/forefoot and often an adduction component. The flexion can lower the forefoot globally or predominantly the first and/or second metatarsals. There is varying clinically presentation, from being asymptomatic to severe disease, with difficulty in fitting shoes, and wearing away the lateral border of the shoes and painful callosities over the dorsum of toes (Maynou et al. 2017).

On conventional radiography, the lateral weight-bearing radiograph shows an increased Meary's angle (>5°), a decreased Djian-Annonier angle <120°, and a Hibb's angle of >45° (Rosenbaum et al. 2014). A calcaneal pitch angle >30° is consistent with calcaneocavus. The apex of the deformity is typically in the midfoot at the transverse tarsal articulation or at the naviculocuneiform joint. MRI or US is rarely used. CT or SPECT-CT evaluates the hindfoot for presence, site, and severity of the degenerative changes or the presence of an associated lesion.

3 Forefoot

3.1 Hallux Valgus

Hallux valgus is a fixed abduction of the first MTPJ in the form of first metatarsal medial deviation, hallux lateral deviation, and a prominent metatarsal head. Hallux valgus can be complicated by inflammation of the medial bursa, synovitis of the MTPJ, chondral wear over the central and plantar metatarsal head and sesamoids, and/or entrapment of the medial dorsal cutaneous nerve. Patients can present with aching pain in the metatarsal head that is relieved by removal of shoes, and the metatarsal can be painful during ambulation. Hallux valgus is a common condition affecting 23% of adults aged 18–65 years and 36% of adults aged >65 years in the United States, with a predilection for women (Nix et al. 2010).

On conventional radiography AP weight-bearing radiograph, a hallux valgus angle >15°, 20°, and 40°, as well as an intermetatarsal angle >9°, 11°, and 18° indicate mild, moderate (Fig. 12), and severe deformities, respectively (Piqué-Vidal and Vila 2009). A metatarsus adductus angle >15° is also a predisposing factor for the development of hallux valgus. Degenerative changes of the first MTPJ, such as joint space narrowing and subchondral cyst formation, particularly in the central and plantar aspects of the first metatarsal head can be seen. There can be bony hypertrophy and cystic changes of the median eminence (Fig. 12c). In

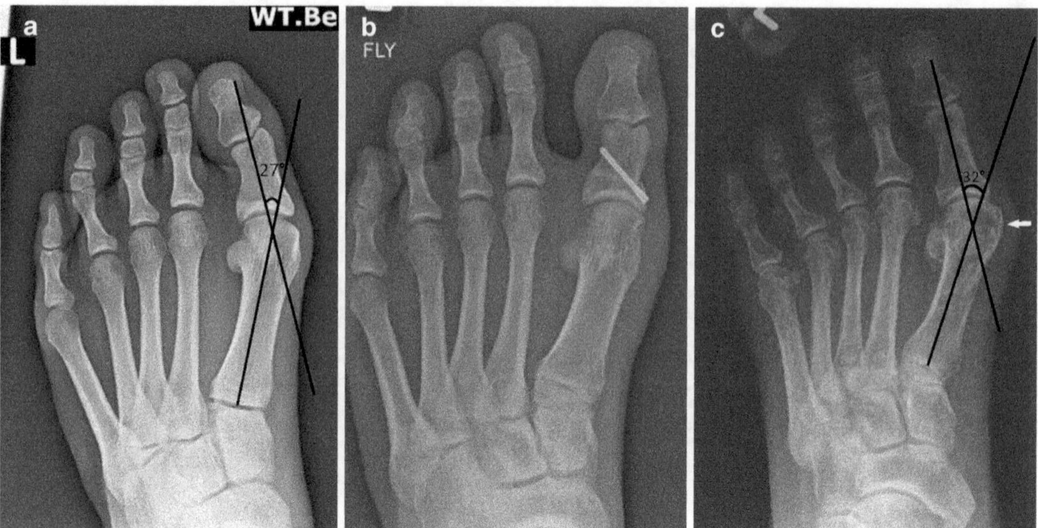

Fig. 12 Hallux valgus on AP weight-bearing radiographs. (**a**) A 19-year-old male with moderate left hallux valgus (hallux valgus angle 27°) presented with a bunion. (**b**) Patient was subsequently treated with Akin osteotomy with restoration of the normal alignment. (**c**) Another 79-year-old female with moderate left hallux valgus (hallux valgus angle 32°) presented with medial eminence hypertrophy (arrow)

post-operative radiographs, the extent of hallux sesamoid subluxation and persistent rounded appearance of the first metatarsal are risk factors.

MRI can evaluate alternative causes of pain such as degenerative changes of the MTPJ and injuries of the plantar plate, cartilage, and collateral ligaments as well as adventitial bursitis. CT and MRI can also assist in the assessment of hallux sesamoids subluxation.

3.2 Hallux Rigidus

Hallux rigidus is defined as degenerative arthritis of the first MTPJ and affects 2.5% of all patients over 50 years old (Ho and Baumhauer 2017). The cause of this condition is mostly idiopathic although trauma is one of the causes. There can be associated metatarsal head articular shape abnormality, metatarsus adductus, and hallux valgus interphalangeus (Coughlin and Shurnas 2003a). Patients present with pain and stiffness that aggravates with activities, especially with first MTPJ dorsiflexion, and/or numbness and paraesthesia. On conventional radiography AP weight-bearing view, decreased first MTPJ space and flattening and widening of the first metatarsal head with subchondral sclerosis may be seen. On the lateral weight-bearing view, there can be dorsal osteophytes over the base of the proximal phalanx and the metatarsal head, along with joint space narrowing. Hattrup and Johnson defined a classification system for hallux rigidus based on radiographs: grade 1—mild to moderate osteophyte formation but with good joint space preservation; grade 2—moderate osteophyte formation with joint space narrowing and subchondral sclerosis (Fig. 13); grade 3—marked osteophyte formation and loss of the visible joint space, with or

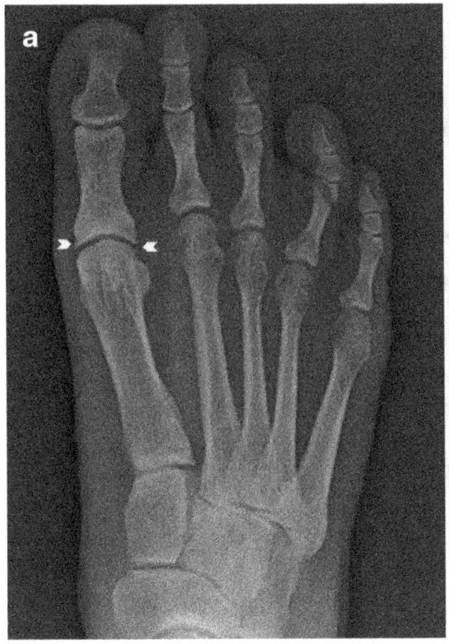

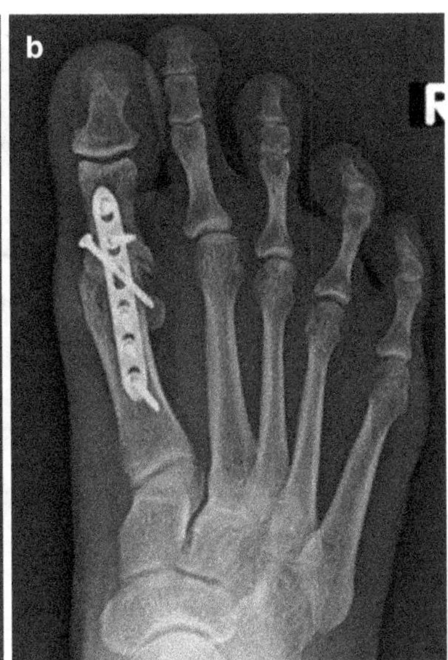

Fig. 13 A 51-year-old female with Hattrup and Johnson grade II hallux rigidus presented with worsening pain over the lateral aspect of the right first MTPJ. (**a**) Pre-operative right foot AP weight-bearing radiograph demonstrates moderate osteophyte formation (chevron arrows) with joint space narrowing of the first MTPJ. (**b**) Post-operative right AP weight-bearing radiograph shows a fused first MTPJ with implants in situ. (Case courtesy: Adj Asst Prof Muhd Farhan Bin Mohd Fadil, Tan Tock Seng Hospital, Singapore)

without subchondral cyst formation (Hattrup and Johnson 1988). An alternative grading system used is by Coughlin and Shurnass (2003b). CT and MRI are not routinely used in the evaluation.

3.3 Bunionette Deformity

Bunionette deformity is characterized by a bony prominence at the lateral aspect of the fifth metatarsal head. This condition tends to occur in women and is commonly bilateral. Predisposing factors include prominence of the metatarsal head, congenital plantarflexed or dorsiflexed metatarsals, increased fourth to fifth intermetatarsal angle, and lateral bowing of the metatarsal shaft. Congenital deformities such as splayfoot and brachymetatarsia and soft tissue abnormalities may be associated with bunionette deformities. Patients present with lateral forefoot pain, which is worsened by closed shoe wear (Fig. 14).

On conventional radiography, a fifth MTPJ angle $\geq 16°$, fourth to fifth intermetatarsal angle $\geq 9°$ fifth metatarsal lateral deviation angle $>8.1°$ and enlarged fifth metatarsal head width (normal fifth metatarsal head width averages 13 mm) can be seen in a symptomatic bunionette (Cooper 2010). Coughlin classification system is most commonly used. Type 1 refers to an enlarged fifth metatarsal head, type 2 refers to normal fourth to fifth intermetatarsal angle with increased lateral bowing of the fifth metatarsal shaft, and type 3 refers to an increased fourth to fifth intermetatarsal angle. Type 3 is the most common type in symptomatic bunionettes.

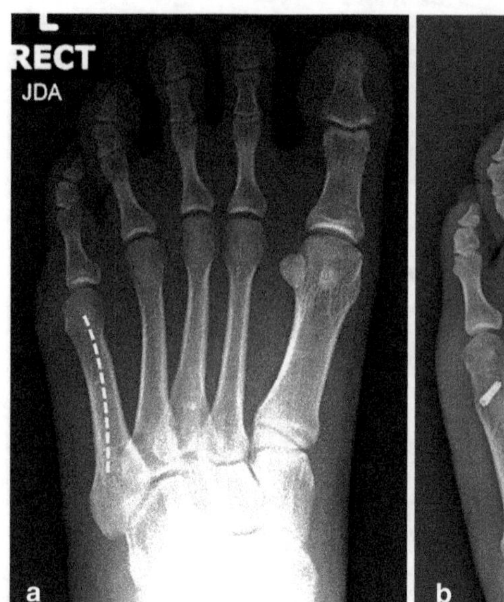

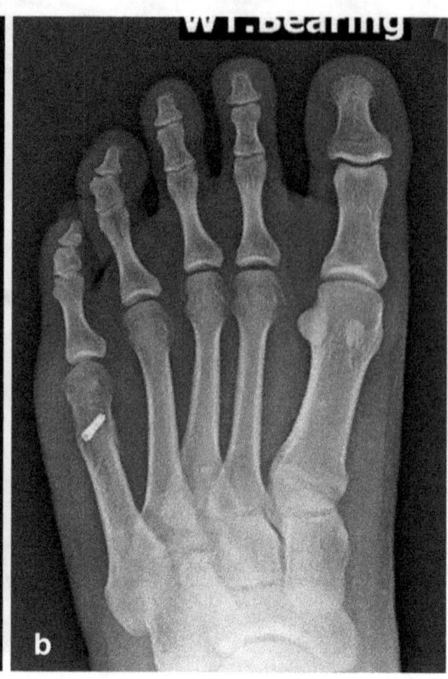

Fig. 14 A 34-year-old male with bunionette deformity presented with lateral forefoot pain and difficulty in wearing safety shoes at work. He was subsequently treated with Chevron osteotomy. (**a**) Pre-operative left foot AP weight-bearing radiograph shows lateral bowing of the fifth metatarsal with slight uncovering of the fifth MTPJ and mild soft tissue swelling lateral to it. (**b**) Post-operative left foot AP weight-bearing radiograph shows correction of deformity. (Case courtesy: Adj Asst Prof Muhd Farhan Bin Mohd Fadil, Tan Tock Seng Hospital, Singapore)

3.4 Other Toes Deformities

A hammer toe deformity is characterized by PIPJ hyperflexion with or without hyperextension at the MTPJ and/or the DIPJ (Fig. 15). Hammer toe deformity typically occurs in the fifth and sixth decades of life, is mostly due to excessively tight or high-heeled footwear, although it can be associated with a long second toe, hallux valgus, inflammatory arthritis, trauma, and muscle imbalance in neuromuscular disorders. Initially, a hammer toe is flexible. As the disease progresses, the deformity becomes fixed. Shoes can rub against the raised portion of the toe or toes, causing painful corns or calluses and even ulcerations leading to osteomyelitis.

Mallet toe is defined by an isolated flexion deformity of the DIPJ of the foot. Mallet toe is usually caused by an overly tight footwear. The mallet deformity is flexible initially and eventually becomes rigid. This may be associated with callous formation at the tip of the toe and pressure on and subsequent nail deformity of the nail. Mallet toe is usually caused by rupture of the distal aspect of the extensor tendon with an unopposed flexor tendon. It may also be associated with flexor digitorum longus tendon contracture, trauma, and a long digit.

The claw toe deformity is typified by MTPJ hyperextension with hyperflexion of the PIPJ and DIPJ of the foot (Fig. 4b, c). A claw toe is commonly associated with muscle imbalances in neuromuscular disorders, peripheral neuropathy in diabetes, trauma, synovitis/inflammatory arthritis, and usually involves all of the lesser toes. As the toes loses contact with the ground during

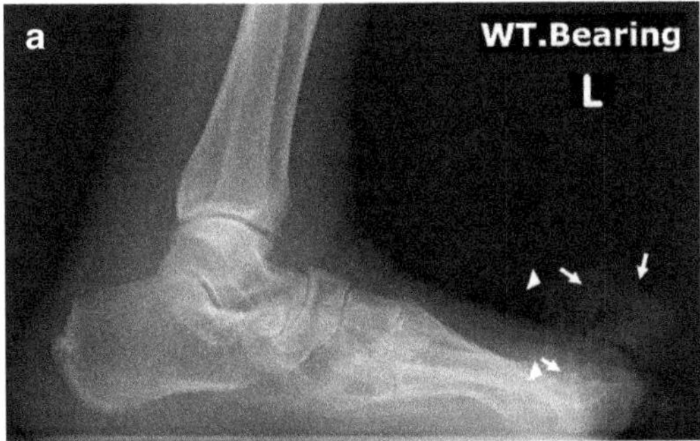

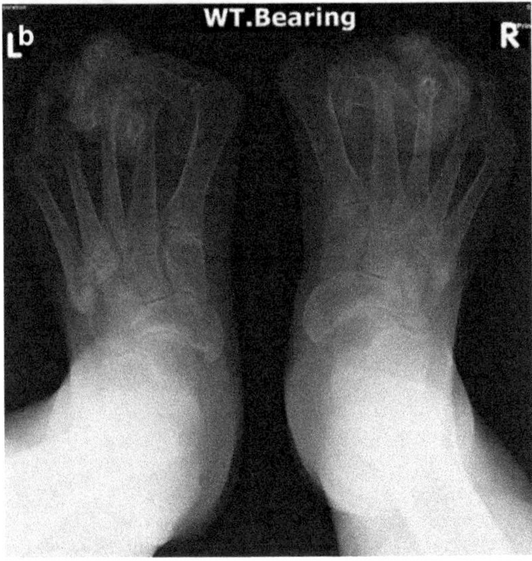

Fig. 15 A 67-year-old female with rheumatoid toes. (**a**) Left lateral weight-bearing foot radiograph shows hyperflexion at the PIPJ (triangular arrow) with hyperextension at the MTPJ (triangular arrow) of the third toe is compatible with hammertoe. Hyperflexion at the PIPJ and DIPJ (arrows) with hyperextension at the MTPJ (arrow) of the second toe is also in keeping with hammertoe. (**b**) AP weight-bearing radiographs demonstrate symmetrical Rheumatoid deformities of the toes in bilateral feet of the same patient

walking, increased force transmission to the metatarsal heads eventuates in metatarsalgia and soft tissue changes as well as increased risk of osteomyelitis (Malhotra et al. 2016).

Lesser toe deformities usually have a chronic, gradual onset and can present with significant morbidity including pain, callus formation, and ulcerations/infection. In the elderly, they can even lead to an unstable gait and increased risk of falls. On conventional radiography, MTPJ hyperextension and hyperflexion of the PIPJ and DIPJ can be seen when applicable in the various toe deformities. Bony erosion or periosteal reaction be seen if these deformities are complicated by osteomyelitis. MRI can evaluate for osteomyelitis, tendon tears, and plantar plate injuries.

3.5 Sesamoid Pathology

Sesamoids are osseous structures embedded within tendon and commonly include the hallux, lesser metatarsal and interphalangeal sesamoids (Guo et al. 2019). Although sesamoids are mostly asymptomatic, they can be fractured or undergo infection, inflammation, osteonecrosis, and degeneration. Of the hallux sesamoids, the medial hallux sesamoid is more commonly injured. Patients can present with acute or chronic pain. Differentiating between a bipartite/multipartite hallux sesamoid variant and a hallux sesamoid fracture can be challenging (Fig. 16).

On conventional radiography, acute fractures usually have more jagged and irregular margins and increased separation of the parts or comminution (Lee et al. 2019). The presence of callus formation on follow-up radiographs or absence of partition in previous radiograph is the most specific for a hallux sesamoid fracture. Additional axial projection through the hallux sesamoids can be useful. Technetium-99m bone scan or MRI can be useful for troubleshooting. Radioisotope uptake will be expected in a fracture within 24 h of a preceding trauma. MRI can demonstrate marrow edema arising from a recent fracture (Fig. 16c) and associated soft tissue injuries.

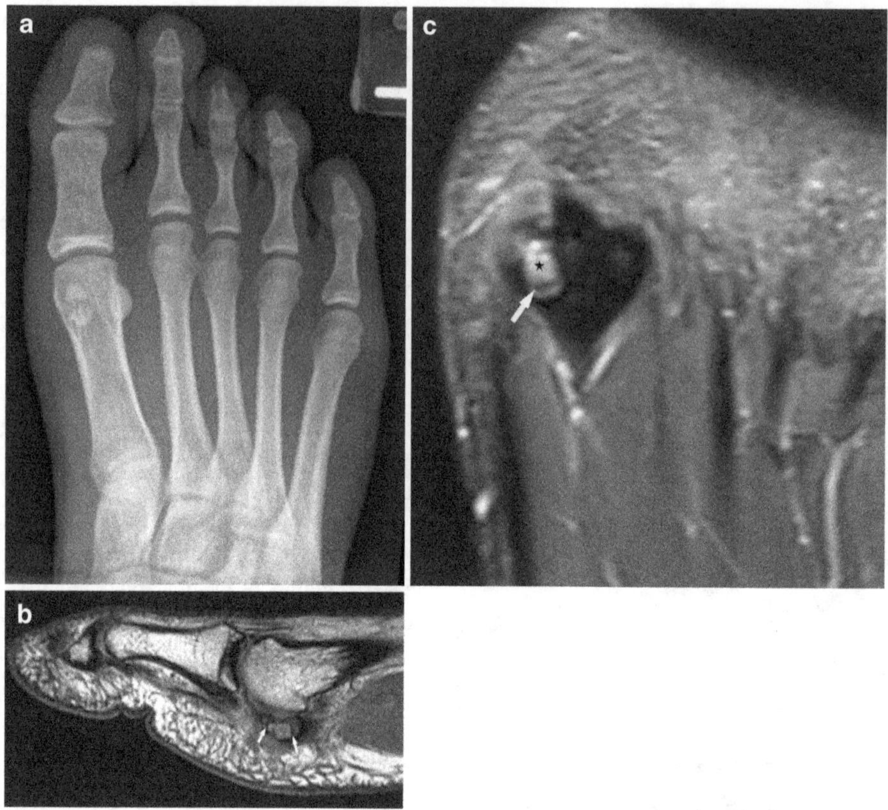

Fig. 16 A 19-year-old male presented with first metatarsal head region pain. (**a**) Left foot AP radiograph shows a bipartite medial hallux sesamoid without any discernible callus formation or fracture cleft. (**b**) Sagittal PD-W and (**c**) coronal STIR demonstrate fracture lines (arrows) in the proximal and distal counterparts of the bipartite medial hallux sesamoid with marked surrounding marrow oedema (star) suggestive of stress fractures

3.6 Osteochondrosis of the Metatarsal (Freiberg's Disease)

Freiberg disease, also termed as Freiberg infraction, is a painful osteochondrosis involving the metatarsal heads. The exact cause is unclear with major contributing factors including repetitive stress and improper shoe wear including high heels. Ischemic necrosis from repetitive trauma likely produces a disruption in the end-arterial blood supply to the metatarsal heads. This condition is bilateral in less than 10% of cases. Although Freiberg's disease usually affects the second metatarsal more than the third metatarsal, it can rarely involve the fourth or fifth metatarsals. There is a predilection for females (5:1 ratio relative to males) and adolescents (10–18 years) (Schade 2015). Patients present with pain on weight-bearing and swelling localized to the metatarsal head area of the forefoot.

On weight-bearing foot radiographs, early findings include a joint effusion with widening of the MTPJ space, and this progresses to subchondral sclerosis, cystic changes, and metatarsal head flattening (Fig. 17a, b). Oblique radiographs can assess subtle flattening at the dorsum of the metatarsal head. In advanced stages of the disease, findings include central joint depression, loose bodies, reactive thickening of the metatarsal shaft, and degenerative changes (Carter et al. 2022). A classification system by Smillie has been used for staging (Smillie 1967).

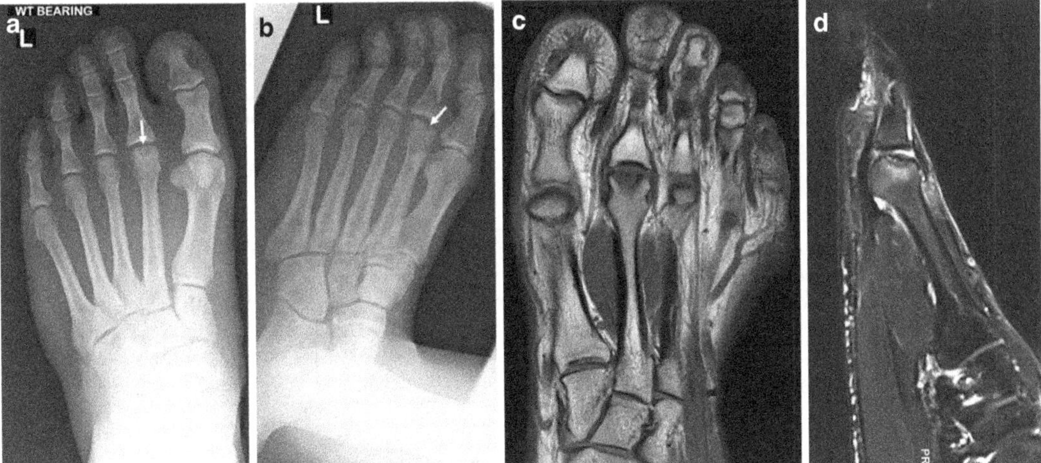

Fig. 17 A 33-year-old female patient with Freiberg disease of second metatarsal head. (**a**, **b**) AP and oblique radiographs of the left foot demonstrate cystic changes, sclerosis and flattening of the second metatarsal head (arrow). (**c**) Axial PD-W and (**d**) sagittal T2-W fat suppressed images through the second MTPJ of same patient demonstrate flattening of the central and dorsal aspect of second metatarsal head with bone marrow oedema and sclerosis along with early osteoarthritic changes

Stage 1: Subtle fracture cleft through the ischemic epiphysis.
Stage 2: Early collapse and central depression of the metatarsal head.
Stage 3: Increased central depression of the metatarsal head.
Stage 4: Loose body formation with displaced central fragment.
Stage 5: Flattened deformed metatarsal head with secondary arthritis, smaller loose bodies, and cortical thickening of metatarsal shaft.

MRI can help evaluate early stages of radiographically occult disease. In early stages, joint effusion and marrow edema can be seen. With disease advancement, there can be hypointense signal on T1-weighted images and mixed hypointense and hyperintense signals on T2-weighted images with metatarsal head flattening (Fig. 17c, d). Nuclear medicine bone scans can help assess for the early stages of the disease when the disease is radiographically occult. Early changes on bone scan include a photopenic area surrounded by increased radiotracer uptake. In later stages, these will be diffuse radiotracer avidity secondary to revascularization, bony repair, and progression to MTPJ arthritis.

4 Conclusion

Acquired deformities of the foot and ankle are commonly encountered in imaging. Familiarization with the various imaging features, diagnostic criteria, and commonly used classification systems of these soft tissue and bony structural abnormalities can aid the radiologist in clinching the diagnosis and serve a pivotal role in the management of these conditions.

References

Alexander IJ, Johnson KA (1989) Assessment and management of pes cavus in Charcot-Marie-tooth disease. Clin Orthop Relat Res 246:273–281

Başdelioğlu K (2021) Radiologic and demographic characteristics of patients with plantar calcaneal spur. J Foot Ankle Surg 60:51–54

Beytemür O, Öncü M (2018) The age dependent change in the incidence of calcaneal spur. Acta Orthop Traumatol Turc 52:367–371

Bottger BA, Schweitzer ME, El-Noueam KI et al (1998) MR imaging of the normal and abnormal retrocalcaneal bursae. AJR Am J Roentgenol 170:1239–1241

Burns P, Hyer CF, Neufeld S, Penner M (2008) Chronic Achilles tendon disorders. Foot Ankle Spec 1:300–304

Carter KR, Chambers AR, Dreyer MA (2022) Freiberg infraction. StatPearls Publishing

Cooper MT (2010) The bunionette deformity: overview and classification. Tech Foot Ankle 9:2–4

Coughlin MJ, Shurnas PS (2003a) Hallux rigidus: demographics, etiology, and radiographic assessment. Foot Ankle Int 24:731–743

Coughlin MJ, Shurnas PS (2003b) Hallux rigidus: grading and long-term results of operative treatment. J Bone Joint Surg Am 85:2072–2088

Deland JT (2008) Adult-acquired flatfoot deformity. J Am Acad Orthop Surg 16:399–406

Desai SS, Wong TT, Crockatt WK et al (2022) The 'Bauer bump:' ice hockey skates as a common cause of Haglund syndrome. Phys Sportsmed:1–6

Eichenholtz SN (1966) Charcot joints. Charles C. Thomas, Springfield, IL

Flores DV, Mejía Gómez C, Hernando F et al (2019) Adult acquired flatfoot deformity: anatomy, biomechanics, staging, and imaging findings. Radiographics 39:1437–1460

Fornage BD (1986) Achilles tendon: US examination. Radiology 159:759–764

Gourdine-Shaw MC, Lamm BM, Herzenberg JE, Bhave A (2010) Equinus deformity in the pediatric patient: causes, evaluation, and management. Clin Podiatr Med Surg 27:25–42

Guo S, Yan YY, Lee SSY, Tan TJ (2019) Accessory ossicles of the foot—an imaging conundrum. Emerg Radiol 26:465–478

Hattrup SJ, Johnson KA (1988) Subjective results of hallux rigidus following treatment with cheilectomy. Clin Orthop Relat Res 226:182–191

Ho B, Baumhauer J (2017) Hallux rigidus. EFORT Open Rev 2:13–20

Jackson JB III, Pacana MJ, Gonzalez TA (2022) Adult acquired flatfoot deformity. J Am Acad Orthop Surg 30:e6–e16

Kannus P, Jozsa L (1991) Histopathological changes preceding spontaneous rupture of a tendon. A controlled study of 891 patients. J Bone Joint Surg Am 73:1507–1525

Krause FG, Iselin LD (2012) Hindfoot varus and neurologic disorders. Foot Ankle Clin 17:39–56

Lee SYS, Tan TJ, Yan YY (2019) Fracture of a bipartite medial hallux sesamoid masquerading as a tripartite variant: a case report and review of the literature. J Foot Ankle Surg 58:980–983

Lee S, Oliveira I, Pressney I et al (2020) The horizontal calcaneofibular ligament: a sign of hindfoot valgus on ankle MRI. Skeletal Radiol 49:739–746

Malhotra K, Davda K, Singh D (2016) The pathology and management of lesser toe deformities. EFORT Open Rev 1:409–419

Maynou C, Szymanski C, Thiounn A (2017) The adult cavus foot. EFORT Open Rev 2:221–229

Menz HB, Zammit G, Landorf KB, Munteanu SE (2008) Plantar calcaneal spurs in older people: longitudinal traction or vertical compression? J Foot Ankle Res 1:7

Nix S, Smith M, Vicenzino B (2010) Prevalence of hallux valgus in the general population: a systematic review and meta-analysis. J Foot Ankle Res 3:1–9

Pavlov H, Heneghan MA, Hersh A et al (1982) The Haglund syndrome: initial and differential diagnosis. Radiology 144:83–88

Piqué-Vidal C, Vila J (2009) A geometric analysis of hallux valgus: correlation with clinical assessment of severity. J Foot Ankle Res 2:1–8

Rosenbaum AJ, Lisella J, Patel N, Phillips N (2014) The cavus foot. Med Clin North Am 98:301–312

Schade VL (2015) Surgical management of Freiberg's infraction: a systematic review. Foot Ankle Spec 8:498–519

Smillie IS (1967) Treatment of Freiberg's infraction. Proc R Soc Med 60:29–31

Sofka CM, Adler RS, Positano R, Pavlov H, Luchs JS (2006) Haglund's syndrome: diagnosis and treatment using sonography. HSS J 2:27–29

Toumi H, Davies R, Mazor M et al (2014) Changes in prevalence of calcaneal spurs in men & women: a random population from a trauma clinic. BMC Musculoskelet Disord 15:87

Tourné Y, Baray AL, Barthélémy R, Moroney P (2018) Contribution of a new radiologic calcaneal measurement to the treatment decision tree in Haglund syndrome. Orthop Traumatol Surg Res 104:1215–1219

Vulcano E, Deland JT, Ellis SJ (2013) Approach and treatment of the adult acquired flatfoot deformity. Curr Rev Musculoskelet Med 6:294–303

Yablon CM, Duggal N, Wu JS et al (2010) A review of Charcot neuroarthropathy of the midfoot and hindfoot: what every radiologist needs to know. Curr Probl Diagn Radiol 39:187–199

Yan YY, Dous YN, Ouellette HA et al (2022) Periarticular calcifications. Skeletal Radiol 51:451–475

Great Toe Metatarsalgia

Anish Patel

Contents

1 Introduction

Pain in the great toe in both the athletic and nonathletic populations can have a variety of different causes which cannot be reliably differentiated by means of history and clinical examination alone. Imaging plays a central role in the differential diagnosis of great toe pain (Fig. 1). Common causes of pain include fractures/stress fractures, degenerative and inflammatory arthritides, abnormalities of the sesamoid apparatus, plantar plate ruptures, and certain tumor and tumor-like pathologies. X-rays can be extremely useful in the initial investigation of great toe pain but often MRI will be required to make the diagnosis and determine the degree of pathological process which can have an impact on the management and the prognosis of such patients.

A. Patel (✉)
The Royal Orthopaedic Hospital, Birmingham, UK
e-mail: anish.patel4@nhs.net

Med Radiol Diagn Imaging (2023)
https://doi.org/10.1007/174_2023_385,
Published Online: 18 April 2023

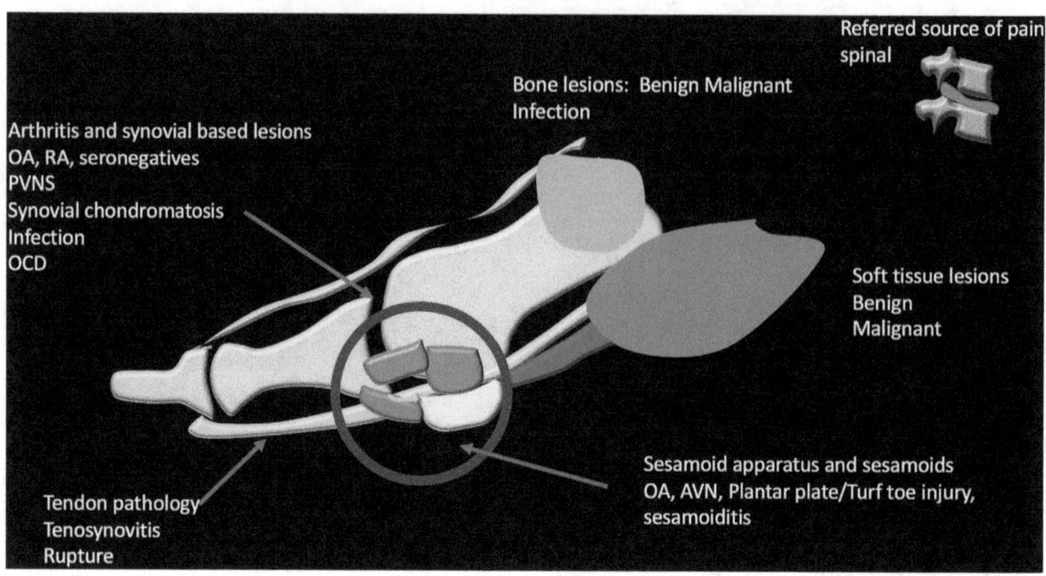

Fig. 1 Differential diagnosis of potential causes of great toe pain based on the anatomical structures of great toe

2 MRI Protocol

For optimal assessment of the great toe, we recommend a fluid sensitive fat suppressed sequence or an intermediate weighted sequence in at least two planes and T1-weighted sequences in at least one plane (usually the sagittal or coronal) or adapted to the site of pathology. A T1 fat suppresses postcontrast sequence is not routinely required but may help in certain circumstances such as to determine the extent of any inflammatory changes or if there is a solid or cystic mass lesion.

3 Sesamoid Pathology

The great toe has two sesamoids, the medial and the lateral also known as the tibial and fibular, respectively. The name is derived from the Arabic term semsem (sesame) which describes its shape. The bones are embedded in the medial and lateral heads of the flexor hallucis brevis tendons. An intersesamoid ligament attaches the two bones together, and they are attached to the metatarsal and the base of the proximal phalanx by the metatarso-sesamoid and the sesamoid phalangeal ligament, respectively. The plantar plate is part of the capsule which is deep to the sesamoid phalangeal ligament. The ligaments and tendons fuse to the capsule of the first metatarsophalangeal joint. The flexor hallucis longus tendon passes between the sesamoid bones and is in close proximity to the intersesamoid ligament (Figs. 2 and 3). The plantar surface of the sesamoids is lined with articular cartilage and articulates with the plantar aspect of the metatarsal. They stabilize the metatarsophalangeal joint (Ogata et al. 1986) during the toe off phase of gait and they also help distribute load forces especially the medial sesamoid and hence it is more susceptible to pathology (Helal 1981).

Bipartite sesamoid bones are seen in up to 30% of individuals and usually affect the medial sesamoid. Bipartite sesamoids are usually larger. The vascular supply varies, arising from the medial plantar artery and plantar arch in about

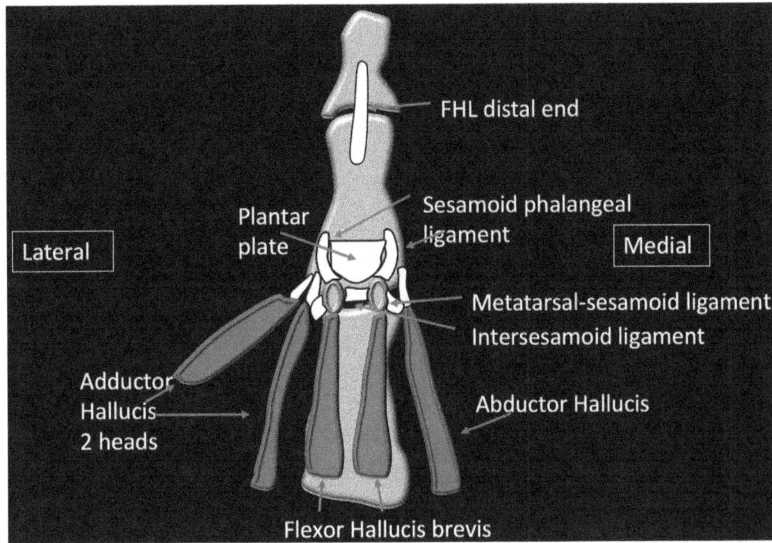

Fig. 2 Diagram showing the gross anatomy of the sesamoid apparatus as viewed from the plantar surface of the great toe

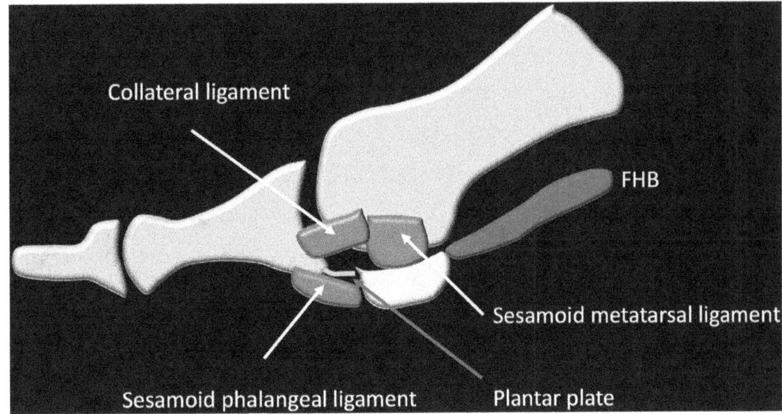

Fig. 3 Diagram showing the gross anatomy of the sesamoid apparatus in the sagittal view

half of all patients and from the planar arch alone and from the medial plantar artery alone is about a quarter of patients each. Poor healing can be observed following injury.

3.1 Sesamoid Fracture

Sesamoid fractures can be difficult to differentiate from bipartite sesamoid bones. Radiographic features which suggest a fracture include an irregular jagged outline to the sesamoid with no cortication with the ends of the fracture fitting together like pieces of a jigsaw. Unipartite sesamoid is also usually smaller than their bipartite counterparts which can also help (Fig. 4). If the diagnosis is in doubt on radiographs, a CT or MRI should be considered.

3.2 Turf Toe Injuries

Turf toe injuries were first described in the 1970s by Bowers in American football players. The use of flexible footwear on a surface which did not

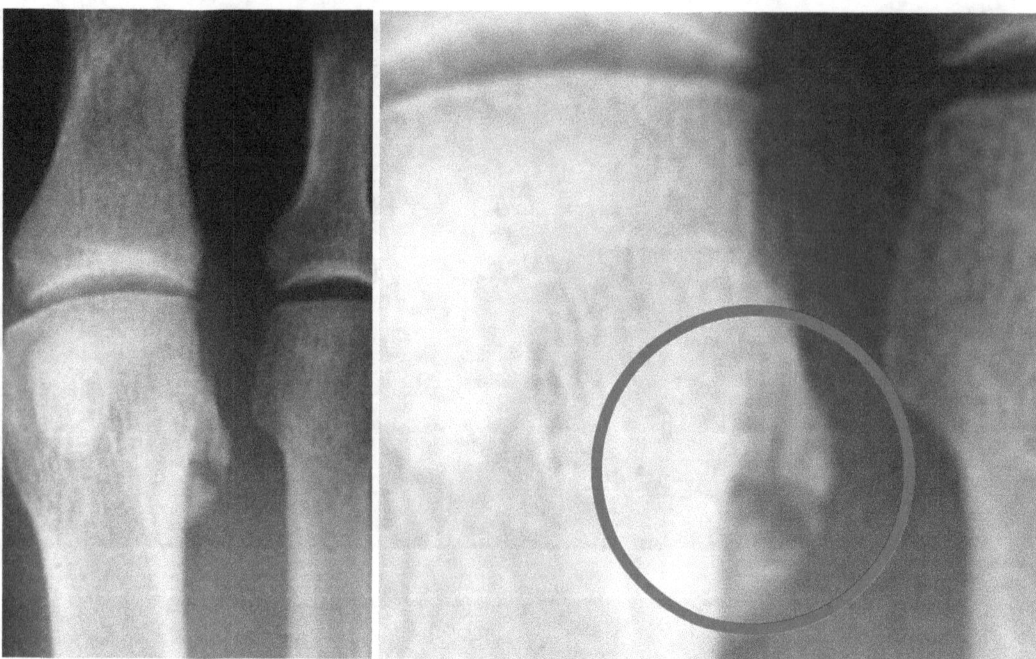

Fig. 4 Radiographs of the sesamoids with a magnified view (right) showing a transverse fracture of the medial sesamoid. Note the irregular, non-corticated margin and slight comminution

give way such as the artificial turf seen on American football pitches resulted in a forced toe hyperextension and subsequent injury of the capsuloligamentous structures of the plantar aspect of the great toe (Bowers and Martin 1976) (Fig. 5).

Turf toe is actually a spectrum of injuries which can be classified as:

Grade 1 Stretching of the capsuloligamentous structures. Mild injury.
Grade 2 Partial tears of the capsuloligamentous structures. Moderate injury.
Grade 3 Full thickness tears of the capsuloligamentous structures. Severe injury.

Radiographs can show proximal migration of the sesamoids in full thickness ligament injuries as they are retracted by the pull of the flexor hallucis brevis and fractures of the sesamoids. Radiographs of the contralateral side can help when the diagnosis is in doubt. MRI is the gold standard in imaging of suspected turf toe inju-

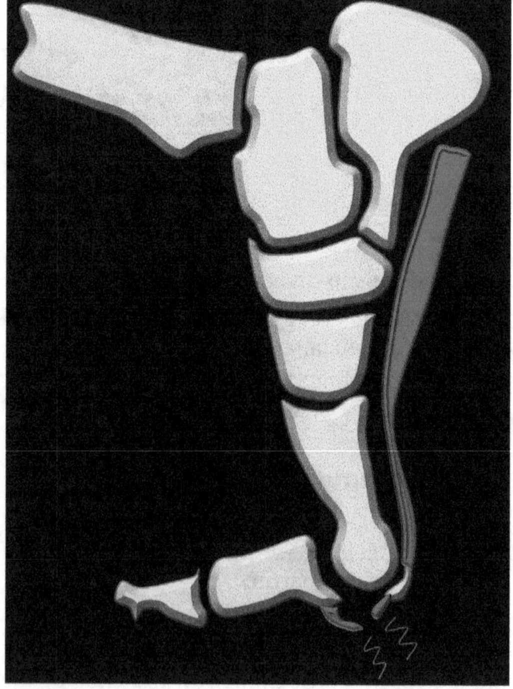

Fig. 5 Diagram showing the forced hyperextension mechanism of injury to the capsuloligamentous structures seen in turf toe injuries

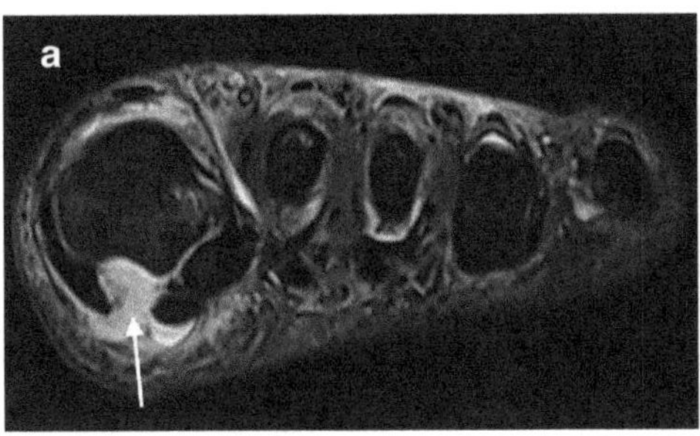

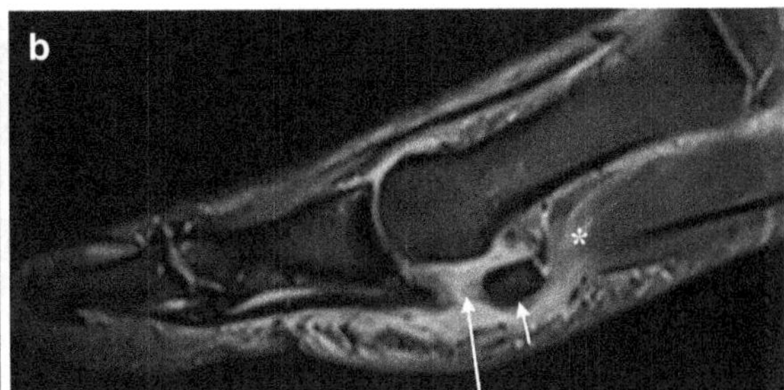

Fig. 6 (**a**) Short axis PDFS MRI of the MTP joint in a rugby player shows non visualization of the medial sesamoid at its expected location (arrow) with fluid and edema in the gap. (**b**) The coronal PDFS MRI in the same patient shows a full thickness rupture of the sesamoid phalangeal ligament from its sesamoid origin (long arrow) with proximal migration of the medial sesamoid (short arrow). There is also a strain of the flexor hallucis muscle belly with feathery edema (asterisk)

ries as it is best at showing the anatomy of the capsuloligamentous structures. It can show periligamentous edema, partial or full thickness tears. Tears most commonly involve the distal attachment of the plantar plate and the sesamoid phalangeal ligament. MRI can also show concomitant injuries such as fractures, tendon injures and can help decide the need for operative repair (Fig. 6).

3.3 Osteonecrosis of the Sesamoid

Osteonecrosis of the sesamoid typically involves the medial sesamoid and is more common in females between 18 and 29. The entity was initially described in 1924 (Ogata et al. 1986). Predisposing factors include cavus foot, tight Achilles tendon, high heeled shoes, a high medial arch, and chronic repetitive injury. Radiographs can show fragmentation and sclerosis of the sesamoid especially in the later stages of the disease. MRI in the early stage of the disease will show A decreased signal on T1-weighted and increased signal on T2-weighted sequences. In the later phase of disease, the sesamoid will show decreased signal on both T1- and T2-weighted sequences which reflects the necrosis and sclerosis (Waizy et al. 2008) (Fig. 7).

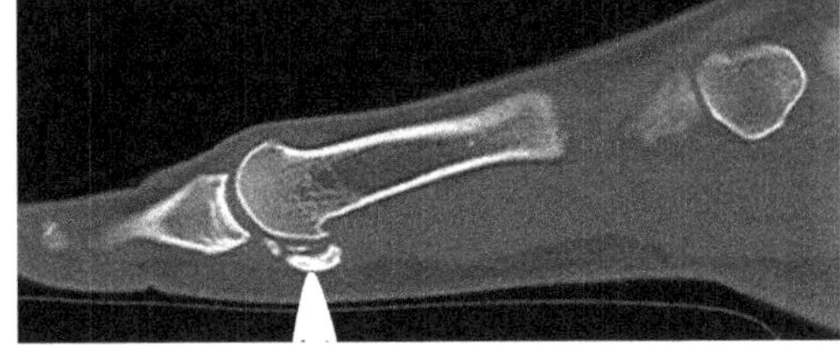

Fig. 7 Lateral radiograph showing fragmentation and sclerosis of the medial sesamoid (arrowhead) in keeping with later stage osteonecrosis

3.4 Sesamoiditis

Inflammation of the sesamoid apparatus can occur as a result of chronic overuse activities such as running and jumping but can also be seen in the context of arthritis and infection. Predisposing factors include cavus foot, tight Achilles tendon, high heeled shoes, and a high medial arch. The medial sesamoid is most frequently affected. A careful history and examination usually make the diagnosis. Radiographs can be normal but may show some soft tissue swelling, subluxation, or fractures of the sesamoid. MRI can be helpful as it will show bone marrow edema and periarticular inflammatory changes (Fig. 8). Differentiation from acute fractures can be difficult on MRI alone but a chronic history does point to a diagnosis of sesamoiditis hence a detailed history is important.

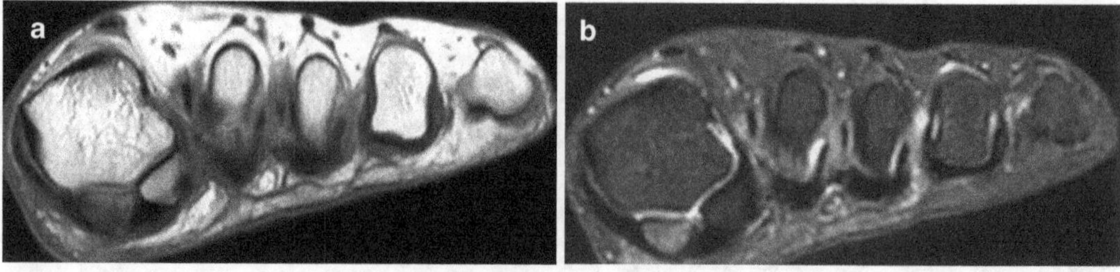

Fig. 8 (**a**) Short axis T1-weighted image. (**b**) Short axis PDFS weighted image shows edema in the medial sesamoid and peri-sesamoid inflammatory changes in a patient with a chronic history of medial sesamoid pain

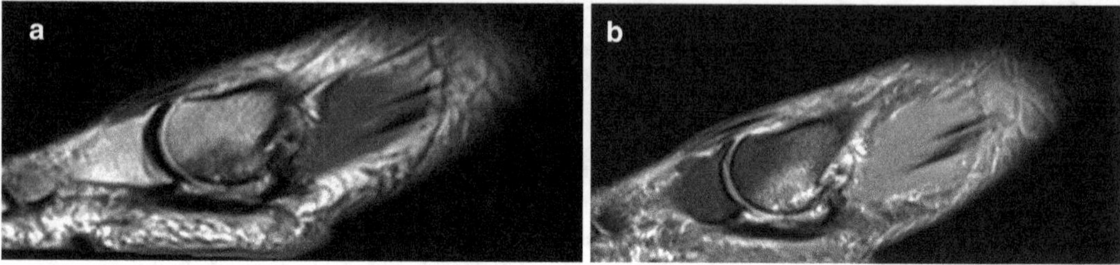

Fig. 9 (**a**) Sagittal T1-weighted and (**b**) Sagittal PDFS weighted image showing osteoarthritis of the medial sesamoid and the metatarsal head. There is loss of joint space with subchondral cyst formation and subchondral oedema

3.5 Osteoarthritis of the Sesamoids

Osteoarthritis of the sesamoid commonly occurs with concomitant osteoarthritis of the first metatarsophalangeal joint. Loss of the joint space, subchondral cysts, and marrow oedema and new bone formation are the typical radiographic findings (Fig. 9).

3.6 Inflammatory Arthritis of the Sesamoids

Rheumatoid arthritis involving the sesamoids is usually seen in longstanding rheumatoid arthritis affecting the first metatarsophalangeal joint. An inflammatory pannus results in articular cartilage destruction with erosion formation and joint space narrowing. Bone resorption and adjacent tenosynovitis are also features (Resnick et al. 1977).

The changes seen in other inflammatory arthritides, e.g., psoriasis, Reiter's syndrome, ankylosing spondylitis include whiskering or an irregular outline to the bone which reflects periosteal new bone formation (Resnick et al. 1977).

4 Stress Fractures and Stress Response

Stress fractures around the great toe can be seen in athletes and nonathletes alike. Repetitive submaximal loading usually results in host bone adaptation to the stress, however when the applied forces exceed the bones capability to repair, there is an imbalance between bone resorption and bone formation which can lead to an injury. Stress injuries are a spectrum ranging from marrow oedema alone (stress response) to an undisplaced incomplete fracture line to a clearly visible fracture. Stress injuries of the first metatarsal are seen less commonly than similar injuries to the second and third metatarsals (Kaiser et al. 2018).

The clinical history and examination will often raise the suspicion of a stress injury. Radiographs can often be normal in a stress response, when the injury is more severe there

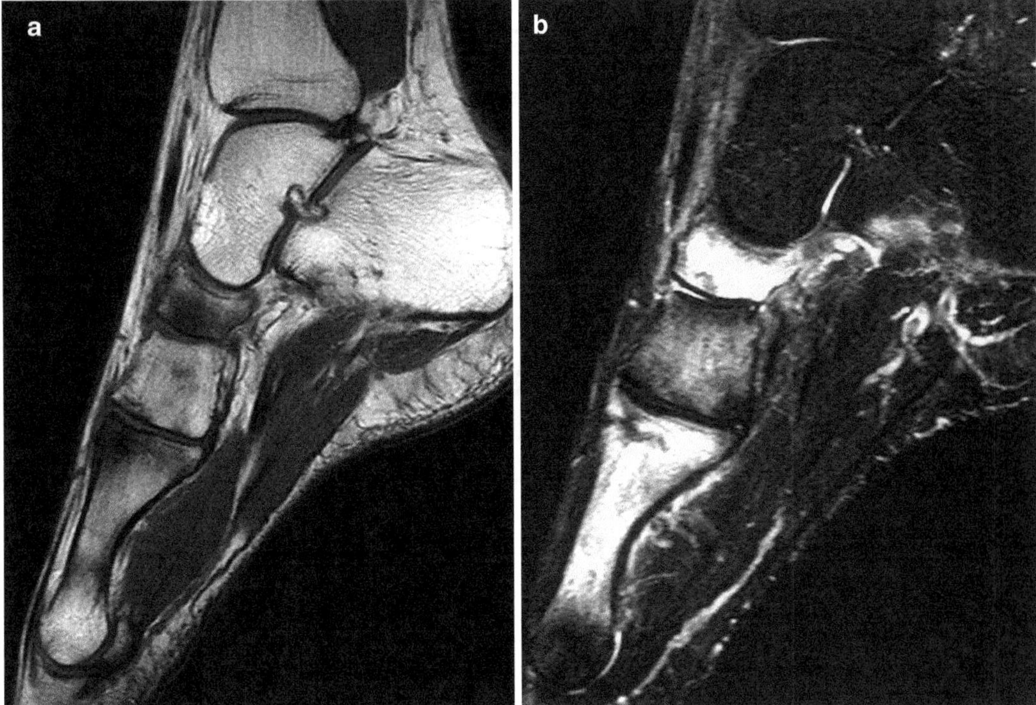

Fig. 10 (**a**) Sagittal T1-weighted and (**b**) Sagittal STIR images in a ballet dancer who complained of great toe pain. Multiple stress fractures (Grade 4b) in the first metatarsal base and the navicular

Table 1 Fredericson classification for the grading of stress injures

Grade of injury	MRI findings
0	No abnormality detected on MRI
1	Periosteal edema only
2	Periosteal edema and marrow edema on T2-weighted sequences
3	Periosteal edema and marrow edema on T1- and T2-weighted sequences
4a	As per 3 with intracortical signal change
4b	Visible fracture line

may be a smooth periosteal reaction, and eventually a visible fracture line and callous formation. MRI is the most sensitive modality to detect stress fractures/stress response (Fig. 10). It is not unreasonable to grade the injuries as per the Fredericson classification which was initially devised for stress injuries of the medial tibia (Fredericson et al. 1995) (Table 1). Stress injuries of the first metatarsal are seen less commonly than similar injuries to the second and third metatarsals (Kaiser et al. 2018).

5 Arthritis

5.1 Osteoarthritis

The great toe is the commonest site for foot osteoarthritis and is seen in up to 35–60% of adults over 65 years of age (Van Saase et al. 1989). It can be idiopathic or secondary to trauma, inflammatory conditions, infection, mechanical stress, sport and overuse injuries, obesity, and age among others. It results in the breakdown of the articular cartilage which in turn causes reduction of the joint space, subchondral cysts, subchondral sclerosis, and osteophytosis (Fig. 11).

Radiographs form the mainstay of diagnosis and can accurately assess the severity of the disease. One of the most frequently used scales to quantify the severity of osteoarthritis is the one proposed by Kellgren and Lawrence (1957) (Table 2). Hallux rigidus is a term given to a painful first metatarsal osteoarthritis and restriction of motion.

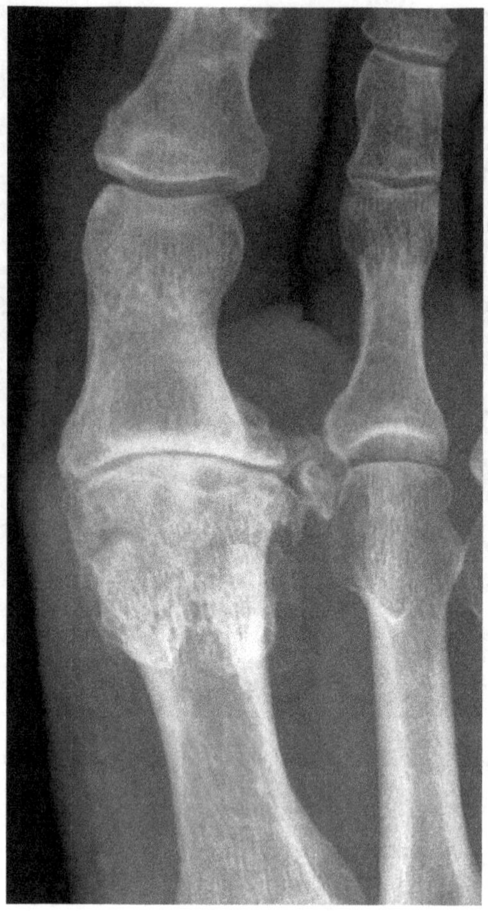

Fig. 11 AP radiographs showing classical osteoarthritis with loss of joint space, osteophyte formation, subchondral sclerosis, and cyst formation

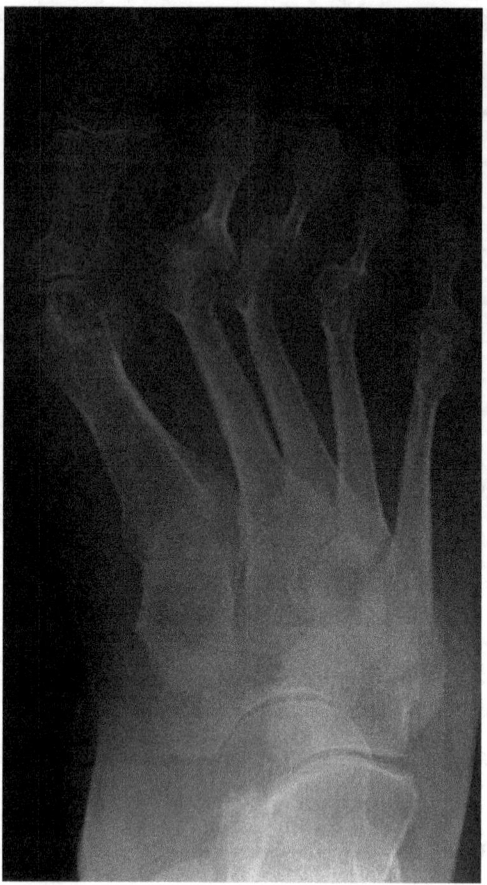

Fig. 12 AP radiographs of the foot showing MTP joint rheumatoid arthritis. There are periarticular erosions at the bare area of the first MTP joint with loss of joint space and periarticular osteopenia. There is also subluxation of the lesser MTP joints

Table 2 Kellgren and Lawrence's original system for the classification for the severity of osteoarthritis

Kellgren and Lawrence Scale	Radiographic changes
Grade 0	No changes of osteoarthritis
Grade 1	Doubtful joint space narrowing and possible osteophytic lipping
Grade 2	Definite osteophytes and possible joint space narrowing
Grade 3	Definite joint space narrowing, moderate osteophytes, subchondral sclerosis
Grade 4	Large osteophytes, marked narrowing of joint space, severe sclerosis, and definite deformity of bone ends

5.2 Rheumatoid Arthritis

Rheumatoid arthritis is a chronic progressive inflammatory condition with a predilection for joints. It has a prevalence of approximately 1%. An inflammatory pannus forms in joints and destroys the articular cartilage and bone. The foot is one of the commonest sites of disease along with the hands. There is a 3:1 female predilection, and the disease is commonest between the fourth and sixth decades of life.

Radiographs will classically show loss of joint space which is usually concentric, erosions which usually start at the bare area and periarticular osteopenia (Fig. 12). Ultrasound can be used to detect early disease prior to radiographic changes. In power doppler mode, ultrasound can assess the extent of inflammation/synovitis in involved joints and can be used to monitor the response to treatment. Ultrasound can also detect other associated conditions such as tenosynovitis, adventitial, and intermetatarsal bursitis.

5.3 Gout

Gout is a crystal arthropathy. It results in deposition of monosodium crystals in and around joints. It typically affects people over 40 years of age and has a male to female predilection of 20:1. Gout can affect any joint but is typically seen around the great toe MTP joint (75–90%) but is also common in the other joints of the feet and in the hands.

There are five stages of the disease.

1. Asymptomatic gout.
2. Acute gouty arthritis.
3. Intercritical gout (in between attacks).
4. Tophaceous gout.
5. Neuropathic gout.

Acute gout results in severe pain of the affected joint.

The radiographic features of gout do not manifest themselves in early disease. It can take many years for the radiographic to declare themselves, therefore, normal radiographs do not exclude gout.

The classical radiographic findings include joint swelling, well-defined periarticular marginal erosions which have a sclerotic border and over hanging edges, and a lack of periarticular osteopenia (Fig. 13a). The joint space is relatively preserved till the late stage of disease. Tophi are calcified masses that can be periarticular or in the bone when large the tophi can destroy large parts of the bone and joint (Fig. 13b).

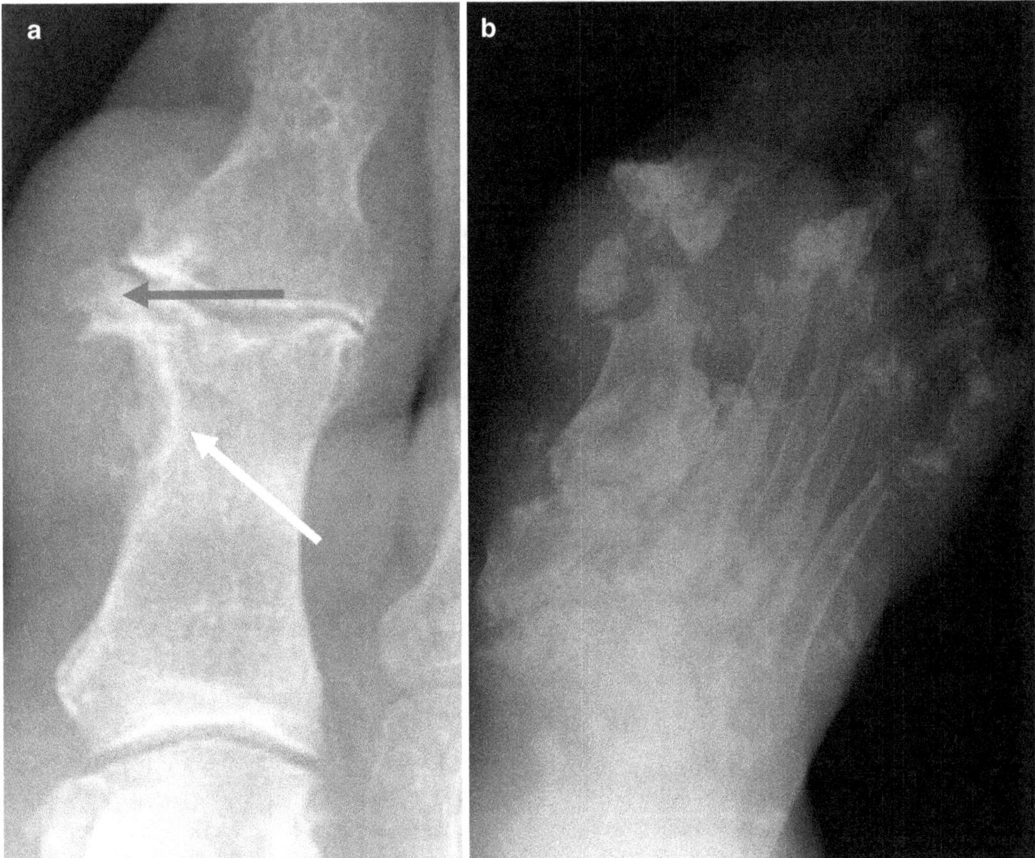

Fig. 13 (**a**) Radiographs showing gout of the IP joint of the great toe. There is a well-defined punched out marginal erosion with a sclerotic margin (white arrow) and an overhanging edge (red arrow).The joint space is relatively preserved. (**b**) Radiograph showing extensive tophus formation and bone destruction in advanced gout

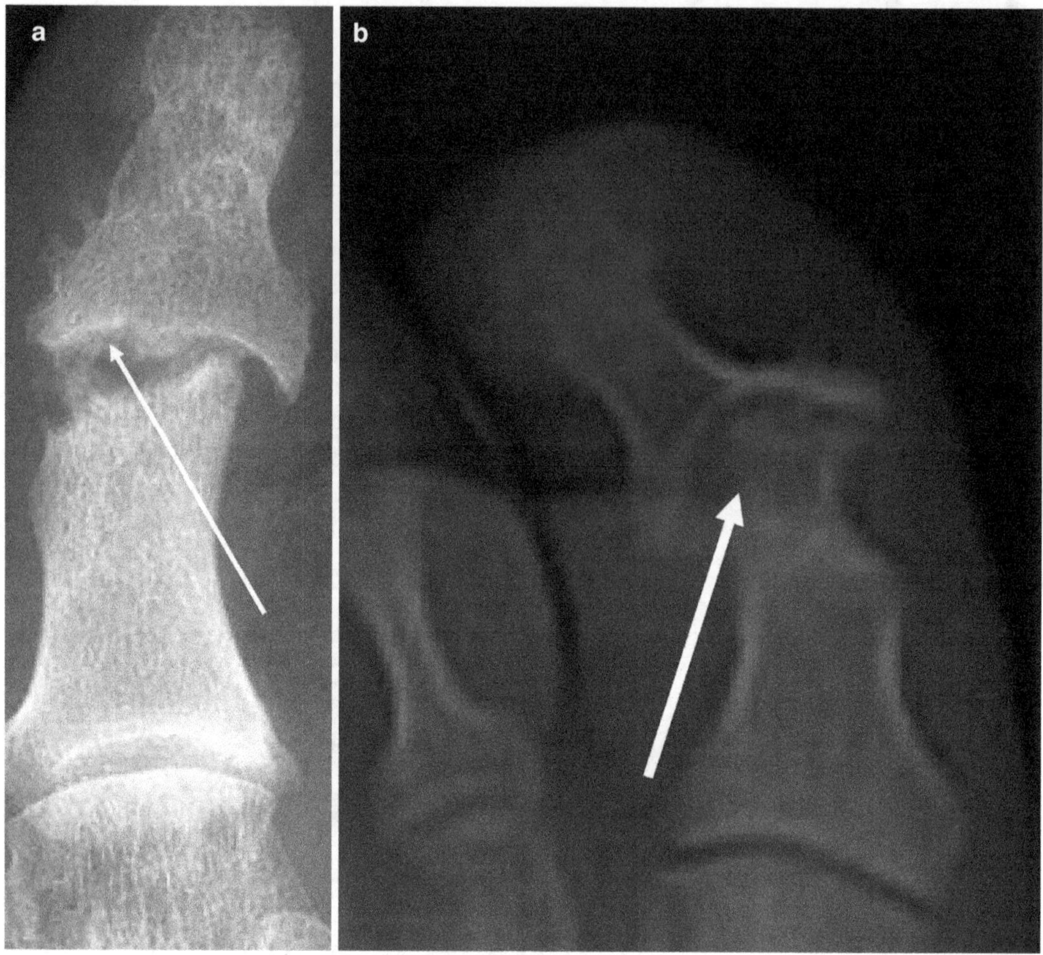

Fig. 14 (**a**) Radiographs showing the IP joint of the hallux showing erosion and marked joint destruction (white arrow). (**b**) Radiographs showing joint destruction and a "pencil in cup" deformity that is commonly seen in psoriatic arthritis (white arrow)

5.4 Psoriatic Arthritis

Psoriatic arthritis is an inflammatory arthritis associated with psoriasis. It is seen in about 20–30% of patients with psoriasis (Moll and Wright 1973). There are five subtypes:

Oligoarticular arthritis (five or fewer joints)
Poly-articular arthritis
Distal arthritis with involvement of the DIP's
Arthritis mutilans with severe joint destruction
Spondyloarthritis

The oligoarticular is the commonest subtype. Characteristic patterns on radiographs include erosions and joint destruction leading to a "pencil in cup" appearance. New bone formation and ankylosis can also be seen (Fig. 14).

6 Osteochondral Lesions

Osteochondral lesions commonly involve the knee, elbow, and talus. Lesions involving the great toe are uncommon and are mainly limited to case reports or small case series in the medical literature. An acute traumatic event, repetitive microtrauma, and local ischemia are implicated in the aetiology.

Radiographs can show an osteochondral defect in the bone with the presence of an osteochondral fragment which can either be non/mini-

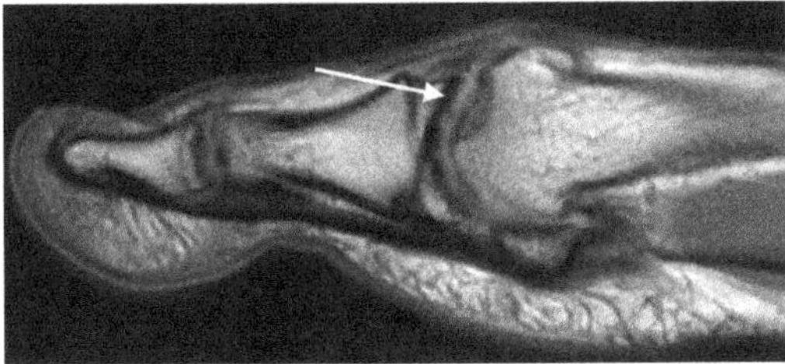

Fig. 15 T1-weighted MRI showing a deep metatarsal head osteochondral defect. The overlying cartilage looks irregular but not displaced (arrow)

mally displaced or displaced as a free osteochondral fragment in the joint.

Clanton and DeLee have classified lesions into four types.

Type I—depressed osteochondral fracture.
Type II—a fragment still attached.
Type III—a detached but nondisplaced fragment.
Type IV—a displaced, loose fragment (Clanton and DeLee 1982).

MRI can be used to determine the size of the defect and the stability of the fragment (Fig. 15). If there is fluid undermining the base of the osteochondral fragment, it increases the likelihood of an unstable fragment. Surgery is the preferred treatment method as non-operative management can predispose to hallux rigidus (Bartlett 1998).

7 Synovial Based Lesions

7.1 Primary Synovial Chondromatosis (PSC)

PSC is a benign lesion in which islands of metaplastic cartilage develop in the synovium of joints, tendon sheaths, and bursae (when it involves the tendon sheaths and bursae it is also known as extra-articular synovial chondromatosis or tenosynovial and bursal chondromatosis, respectively).

It is most common between the third and fifth decades. It most commonly affects the hip and knee. It is relatively uncommon around the great toe. Radiographs may show an intra-articular soft tissue mass. Calcification is present in 65–95% of cases and is chondroid in nature (Fig. 16). MRI demonstrates lobulated synovial masses which are high signal on fluid sensitive sequences due to its chondroid nature. Any calcification will be low signal on all sequences. Extra-articular synovial chondromatosis is also known as tenosynovial and bursal chondromatosis depending on if there is involvement of the tendon sheath or bursae. They are rare lesions but are most commonly seen in the hands and feet (Doral et al. 2007).

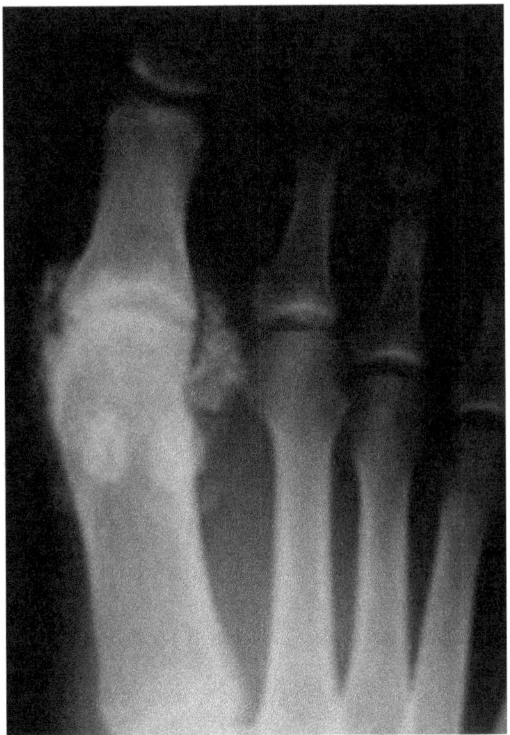

Fig. 16 AP radiograph of the foot showing chondroid calcification in the first MTP joint which is classical for primary synovial chondromatosis

7.2 Pigmented Villonodular Synovitis (PVNS)

PVNS is a benign fibrohistiocytic tumor characterized by villous proliferation of the synovium. There are two forms, the diffuse form and the focal form. It is usually seen in the third and fourth decades. Males and females are affected equally. It usually presents as a mono arthritis of a joint, there may be a large effusion

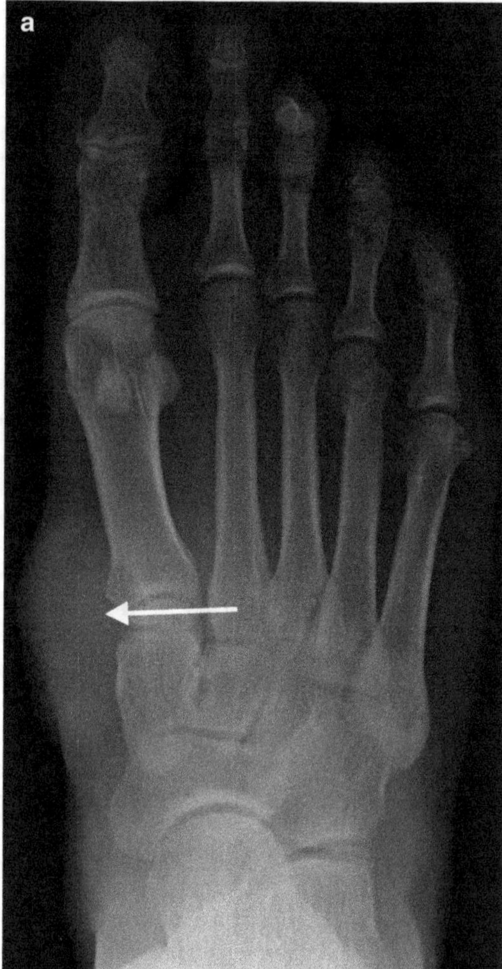

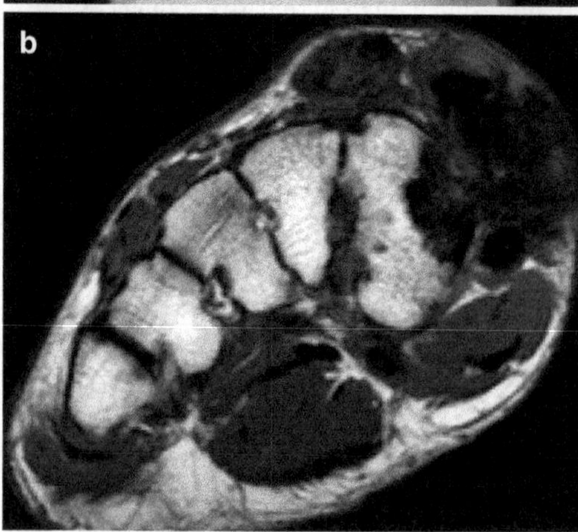

Fig. 17 (**a**) AP radiograph of the foot showing a soft tissue mass at the base of the great toe metatarsal without any calcification (white arrow). (**b**) Coronal T1-weighted MRI showing low signal lobulated masses around the first TMT joint in keeping with PVNS

or a hemarthrosis. Macroscopically it has the appearance of a red shaggy beard. Radiographs can show a soft tissue mass. Calcification is not a feature and can help differentiate it from other conditions such as synovial chondromatosis. MRI demonstrates a well-defined often lobulated soft tissue masses. Lesions are usually isointense/hypointense to skeletal muscle on T1-weighted sequences. On T2-weighted sequences, lesions can have a variable appearance but are usually hypointense to fat. Foci of low T2 signal represents areas of hemosiderin deposition which will produce the characteristic blooming artifact on gradient imaging (Fig. 17).

8 Benign Tumors

8.1 Osteoid Osteoma (OO)

OO is a benign bone forming tumor that occurs most frequently in children and young adults. There is a slight male preponderance. Clinical presentation is typically pain that worsens at night and is relieved by salicylates. Osteoid osteomas can be classified by their location as cortical, medullary (cancellous), subperiosteal, and rarely physeal. Typical sites are the shaft of the long bones, particularly the femur and tibia. They are seen in the foot in about 10% of cases and they are the commonest benign tumor of the foot. The most common appearance on radiographs is a cortical-based lucency which measures less than 2 cm. Central calcification occasionally may be visible within a radiolucent nidus. The nidus is surrounded by reactive sclerosis.

CT is the most useful modality for diagnosis. On CT, the nidus is well-defined, round or oval lesion with low attenuation. The nidus may or may not be mineralized. Reactive sclerosis ranges from mild cancellous sclerosis to extensive periosteal reaction and new bone formation (Fig. 18a). MRI will show the nidus, the associated surrounding sclerosis and cortical thickening. There is also usually fairly florid bone marrow, cortical and periosteal edema (Fig. 18b).

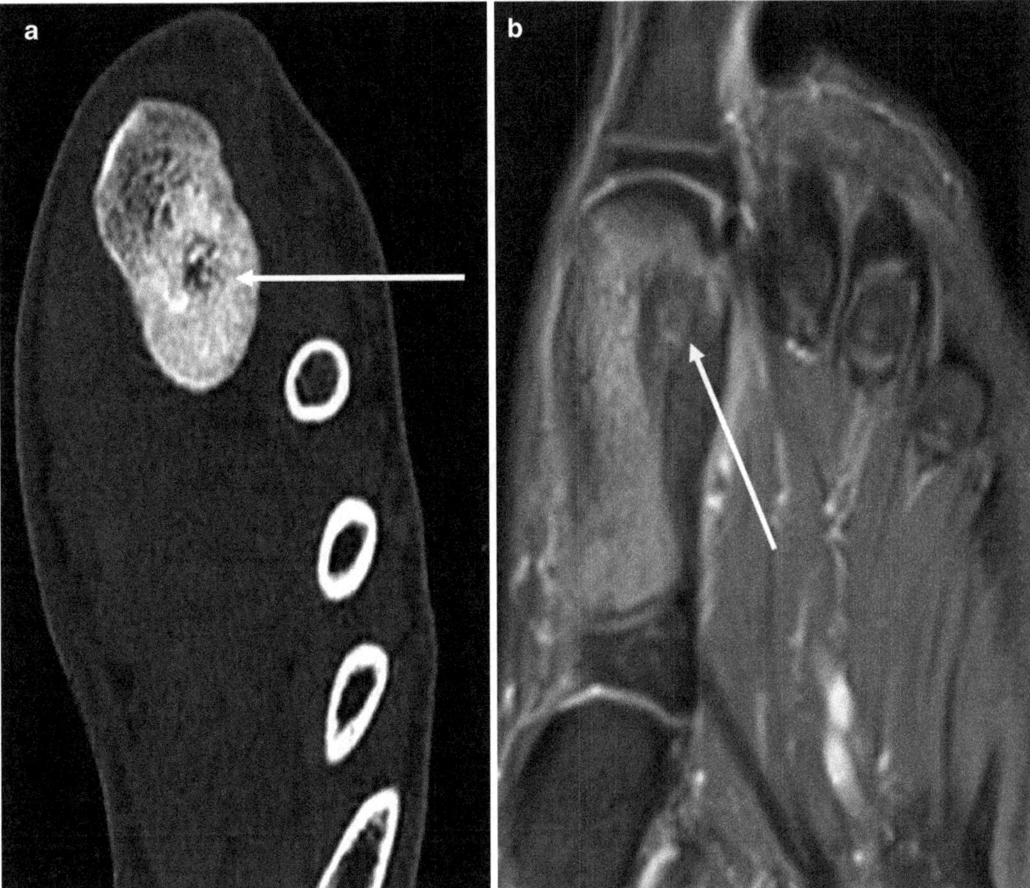

Fig. 18 (**a**) Reformatted CT images showing low attenuation OO in the cortex of the first metatarsal (white arrow) with extensive surrounding cortical sclerosis. (**b**) STIR MRI image showing nidus in the metatarsal and the surrounding bone marrow, cortical and periosteal edema

The differential diagnosis includes a stress fracture or cortical abscess.

8.2 Enchondroma

It is a benign tumor consisting of hyaline cartilage in medullary bone. It represents 12–24% of all benign bone tumors and 3–10% of all bone tumors (Flemming and Murphey 2000). Up to 50% are seen in the hands and feet and there may be multiple lesions. Radiographs show a lucent intramedullary lesion with or without chondroid matrix. When the chondroid matrix is present, the diagnosis is fairly clear without the need for further cross-sectional imaging. In the foot, lesions can expand the bone and cause endosteal scalloping. Unlike in the long bones, endosteal scalloping is not a feature of malignant transformation. In the foot, features concerning for malignant transformation include a rapid increase in size or the presence of cortical breakthrough and an associated extra-osseous mass. MRI will show a well-defined lobulated mass which is markedly hyperintense on T2-weighted sequences reflecting the high water content of the cartilage and there may be some low signal septae. When chondroid calcification is present, it will be low signal on all sequences (Fig. 19). Pain may be associated with complications such as a pathological fracture or malignant transformation.

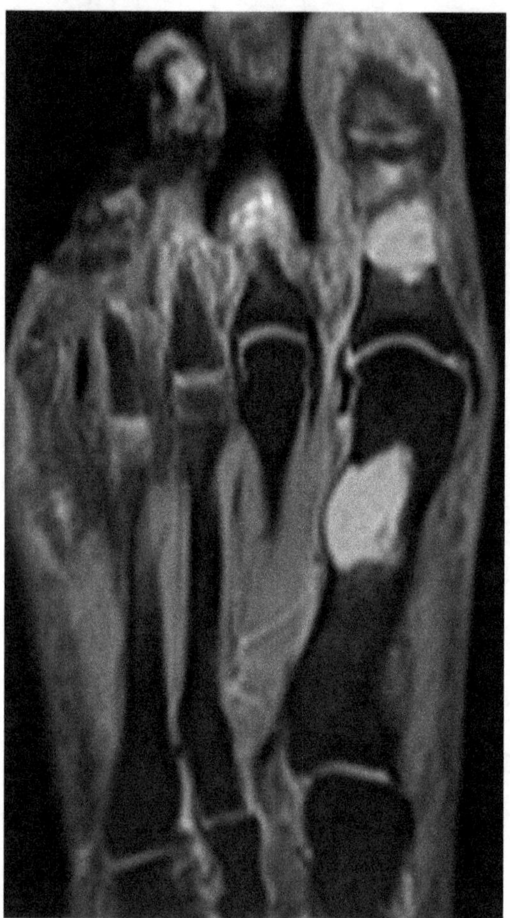

Fig. 19 STIR MRI showing multiple lobular masses in the great toe metatarsal and proximal phalanx in keeping with enchondromas

8.3 Osteochondroma

Osteochondromas are the most commonly identified primary bone tumor at all sites. They are a cartilage capped osseous excrescence and must demonstrate cortical and medullary continuity for a diagnosis to be made (Murphey et al. 2000).

They are most usually encountered in the first three decades of life, and there is no sex predilection. When symptomatic, presentation may be secondary to complications such as bone deformities, fractures, neurological or vascular complications. Most are metaphyseal in location and commonly occur around the knee, although they may appear from any bone. They are seen in the feet in about 10%. The radiographic appearance of solitary osteochondroma is frequently pathognomonic. Computed tomography may demonstrate the cortical and marrow continuity of the lesion with the parent bone. MR imaging also demonstrates this continuity clearly and is the best modality for assessing the effect of the osteochondroma on nearby structures. It is also the modality of choice for measuring the cartilage cap (Murphey et al. 2000) (Fig. 20). A cartilage cap thickness of greater than 2 cm is concerning for secondary chondrosarcoma, and a biopsy of the cartilage cap will be required. An overlying bursa can mimic the cartilage cap, however careful windowing on the MRI is usually sufficient to differentiate one for the other, when the diagnosis is still in doubt an ultrasound scan is a useful tool to differentiate the solid cartilage cap from a fluid filled bursa.

8.4 Giant Cell Tumor of Bone (GCTB)

GCTB is a tumor of bone composed of sheets of neoplastic ovoid mononuclear cells and large osteoclast-like giant cells. Ninety-five percent are benign and 5% can be malignant. It generally occurs in skeletally mature individuals with its peak incidence in the third decade. Most lesions are metaphyseal and extend to the subchondral bone. There is no matrix mineralization. GCTB is usually seen in in the long bones. Less than 5% occur in the feet.

Radiographs show a geographic eccentric lytic lesion which extends to the subchondral

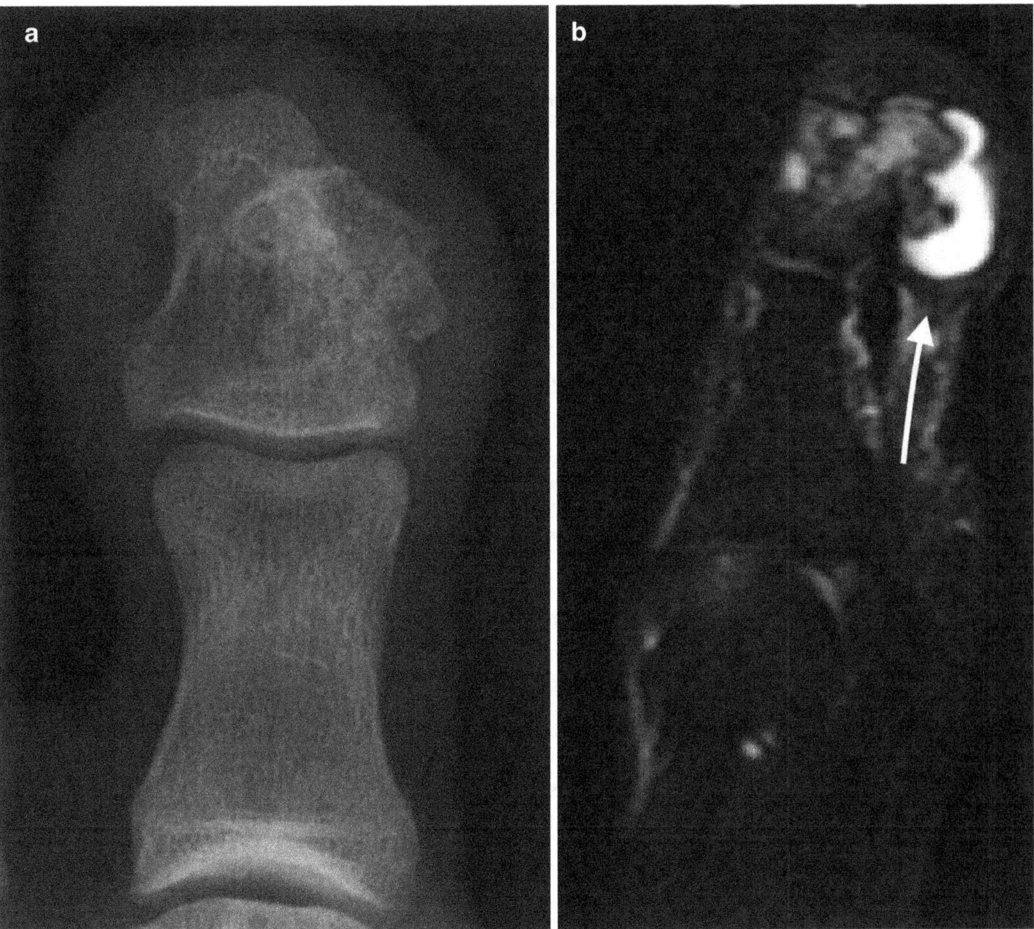

Fig. 20 (**a**) AP radiograph showing osteochondroma from the distal phalanx. It can be difficult to differentiate it from a subungual exostosis on this view. (**b**) Sagittal STIR MRI shows corticomedullary continuity and a cartilage cap

bone with expansion and thinning or possible destruction of the cortex. There is usually a non-sclerotic border. Matrix mineralization is not a feature (Fig. 21). MRI will define the extent of the tumor and is useful for surgical planning. Lesions are usually low to intermediate signal intensity on both T1- and T2-weighted sequences (Fig. 21). A soft tissue mass can be present. Secondary aneurysmal bone cyst formation with fluid-fluid levels are seen in approximately 15% of cases.

8.5 Giant Cell Tumor of Tendon Sheath (GCTTS)

GCTTS is also known as extra-articular PVNS. It is a benign synovial proliferation within the tendon sheath. It is commonly seen in the hands and feet. Peak incidence is between 30 and 50 years of age, and there is a female preponderance of 2:1. It is usually painless but occasionally can cause pressure effects when it grows sufficiently large. Pain may also occur if it compresses local nerves.

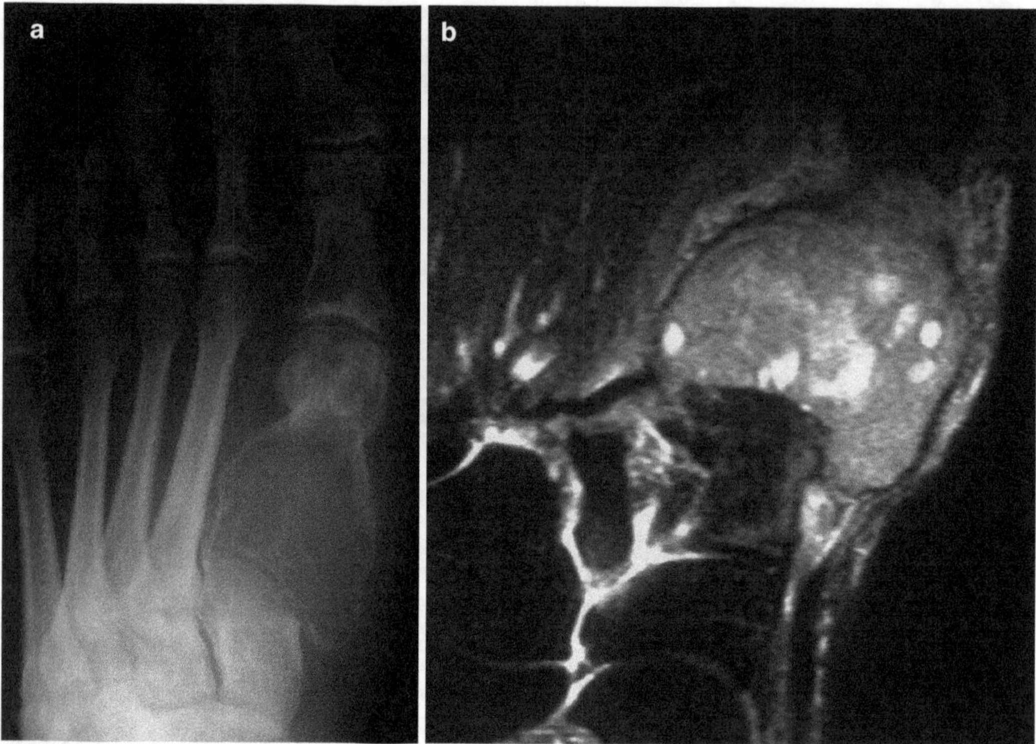

Fig. 21 (**a**) AP radiograph showing a lucent expansile lesion in the first metatarsal with extension to the subchondral bone. (**b**) STIR MRI showing an intermediate to low signal lesion with some cystic areas in keeping with a GCTB

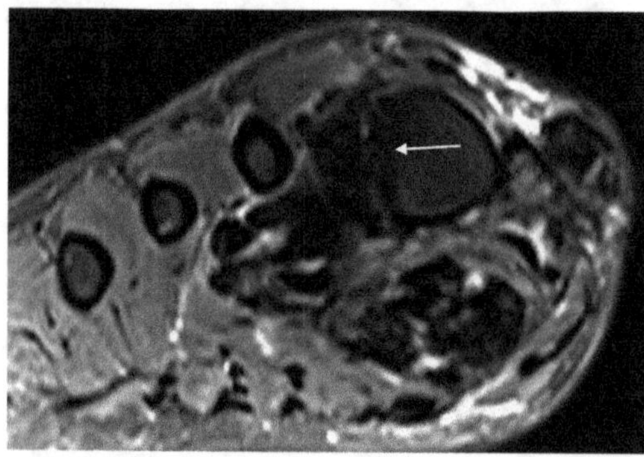

Fig. 22 Coronal STIR MRI shows lobulated soft tissue masses around the tendon sheath to the great toe which is causing bony pressure erosion (white arrow)

Radiographs may show a soft tissue mass. When the mass has been present for sometime and presses on bones, erosions may be seen. Calcification is rare. MRI will show a mass closely related to a tendon. It will be hypointense to skeletal muscle on T1-weighed sequences and hypointense to intermediate signal on the fluid sensitive sequences (Fig. 22). Hemosiderin in the lesion may lead to blooming artifact on gradient echo sequences.

9 Malignant Tumors

9.1 Osteosarcoma

Osteosarcoma is a malignant bone forming tumor. There are eight subtypes: conventional, telangiectatic, small cell, low-grade central, secondary, parosteal, periosteal, and high-grade surface (Lefkowitz and Hwang 2010). It is one of the commonest primary bone tumors. There is a bimodal age distribution with a peak in the second decade and a second peak in older adults. Up to 30% occur in those age >40 years. There is a slight male preponderance. There is an increased incidence in those with Li-Fraumeni, Rothmund-Thompson syndrome, and hereditary retinoblastoma.

In conventional osteosarcoma, 90% involve the metaphysis and 10% involve the diaphysis. Lesions can extend into the epiphysis, and the growth plate is not an effective barrier top tumor growth. Tumors involve the long bones usually. They are relatively infrequent in the foot overall but are the third commonest primary sarcoma in the foot.

The radiographic appearances can vary from purely lytic to purely sclerotic but most will show a mixed appearance with permeative margins, cortical destruction, soft tissue extension, and periosteal new bone formation. The latter may appear lamellated or spiculated and, if interrupted, will have Codman angles.

Parosteal osteosarcoma is a low-grade malignancy and is the commonest of the surface osteosarcomas, accounting for approximately 5% of all osteosarcomas. Radiographically, it appears as a dense lobulated mass attached to the outer cortex with a thin cleft between part of the mass and the cortex as it wraps around the bone due to periphery of the tumor being less mineralized. Intramedullary extension is best visualized on CT or MR imaging.

Periosteal osteosarcoma is an intermediate grade surface osteosarcoma. It accounts for approximately 2% of all osteosarcomas. It has a peak incidence in the second and third decades. Radiographs can demonstrate a cortically based lesion with a perpendicular (hair on end) periosteal reaction, Chondroid calcification can be seen (Fig. 23). There may be a visible soft tissue mass and saucerization of the outer cortex of the involved bone. MRI can demonstrate high T2 areas within the tumor which reflects the chondroblastic nature of the tumor.

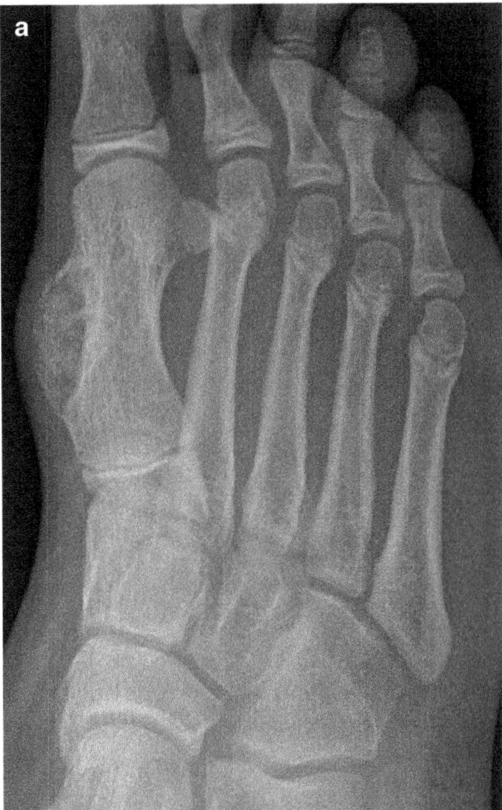

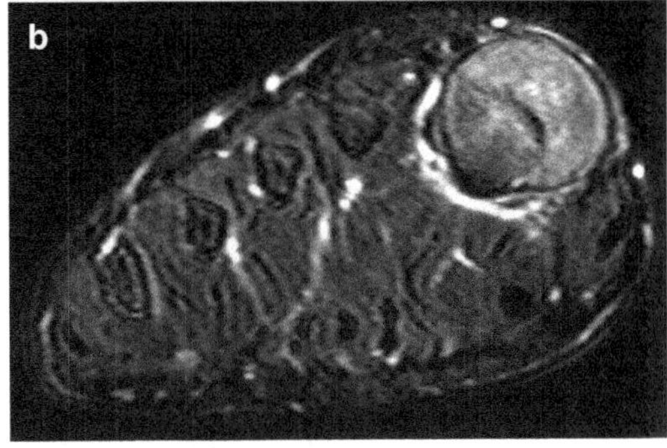

Fig. 23 (**a**) AP radiograph showing a bone forming surface lesion involving the medial aspect of the first metatarsal. (**b**) Coronal STIR MRI shows bone forming surface lesion. Biopsy confirmed periosteal osteosarcoma. Osteosarcomas are rare at this site

9.2 Ewing Sarcoma

Ewing sarcoma is a small round cell tumor which is characterized histologically by small round cells with round nuclei and inconspicuous nucleoli. The undifferentiated nature of the cells means that they can be difficult to diagnose without immunohistochemical techniques. Strong CD99 expression is seen in 95% of cases.

There is a slight male preponderance (Qureshi et al. 2007). The classic site in long bones is the diaphysis, but this is the site in only one-third of cases. Approximately 60% arise in the meta-diaphysis. As with most primary tumors of bone it is unusual in the foot but is the commonest primary bone sarcoma of the foot. Radiographs may show a lytic lesion with no matrix mineralization. The aggressive onion skin periosteal reaction seen in the long bones may not seen in the small bones of the foot due to their small size and therefore early presentation. MRI is the preferred modality for the local staging of the disease and to determine the presence and size of the soft tissue component (Fig. 24).

9.3 Chondrosarcoma

Chondrosarcoma is a malignant tumor of hyaline cartilage. They can be primary—which occurs in normal bone and secondary which occurs in a pre-existing cartilage lesion, e.g., enchondroma or osteochondroma. It is uncommon in the feet. The conversion of a foot enchondroma into a chondrosarcoma is >1%. In the context of enchondromatosis, e.g., Ollier's and Maffucci's syndrome, it is approximately 25% and in hereditary multiple exostosis is approximately 3% (Vázquez-García et al. 2011). Radiographs will show a lytic lesion with or without chondroid calcification (Fig. 25). As the foot bones are small in size, the presence of endosteal scalloping is not a sign of malignancy. Usually malignant lesions will demonstrate

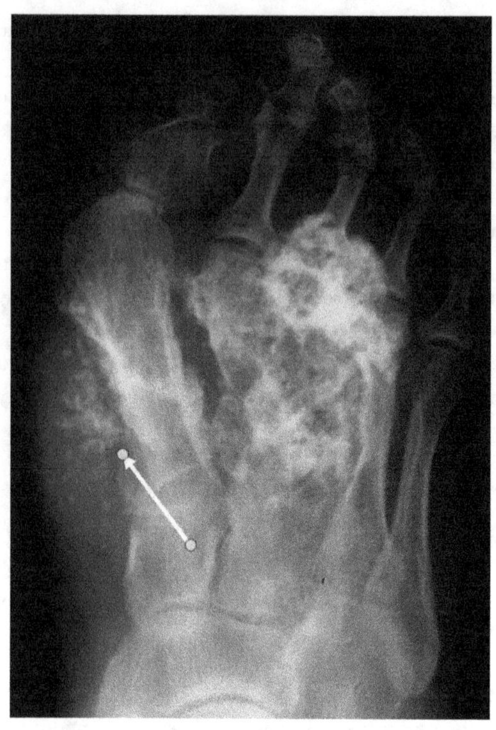

Fig. 25 AP radiograph of the foot showing a destructive lesion in the great toe metatarsal with a soft tissue component and chondroid calcification (white arrow) in keeping with a chondrosarcoma. Further lesions noted in the other metatarsals in this patient with known Ollier's disease

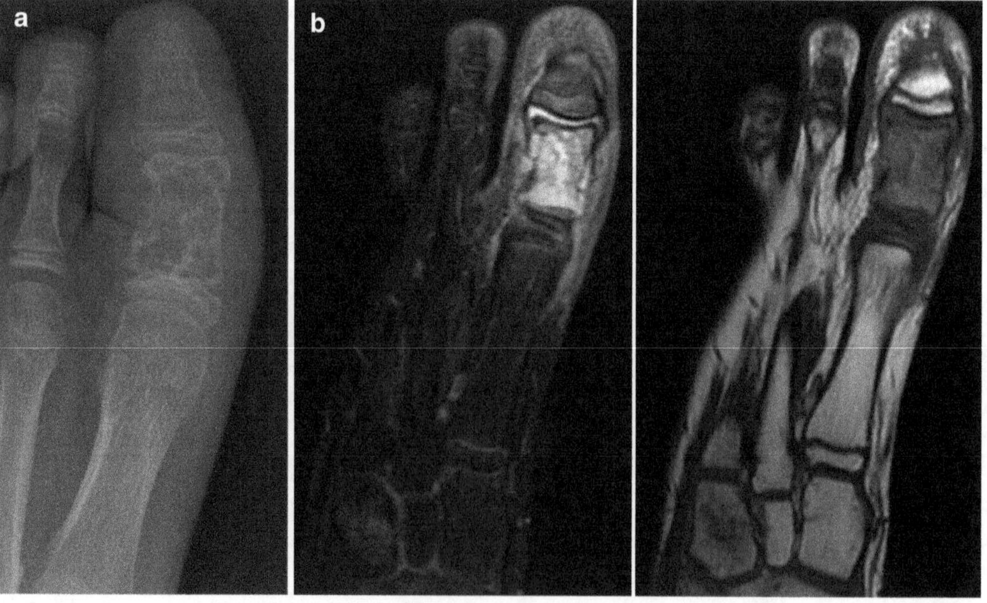

Fig. 24 (**a**) AP radiograph showing a lesion in the proximal phalanx which is permeative and lytic. There is destruction of the cortex and no matrix mineralization. (**b**) T1-weighted and STIR coronal images show a destructive lesion involving the whole bone with surrounding periostitis but no soft tissue mass. Biopsy confirmed Ewing's sarcoma. Infection would also be in the differential diagnosis

destruction of the cortex and extra-osseous extension. MRI will show a high T2-weighted signal which has a lobulated outline with destruction of the cortex and an extra-osseous soft tissue mass. Any chondroid calcification will below signal on all MRI sequences. In an osteochondroma, a cartilage cap over 2 cm is a sign of chondrosarcomatous transformation (Murphey et al. 2000).

9.4 Acral Metastasis

Metastatic lesions of the foot are uncommon. They usually present with foot pain and swelling and are usually have a very poor prognosis. The vast majority are from primary lung tumors followed by gastrointestinal and genitourinary tumors. The hindfoot was the commonest site of location (Greco et al. 2020).

Radiographs will show an aggressive lytic lesion in the bone with or without destruction of the cortex and an extra-osseous soft tissue mass. MRI will show marrow infiltration with loss of signal on T1-weighted sequence and will be hyperintense on fluid sensitive sequences. A soft tissue mass may be present (Fig. 26).

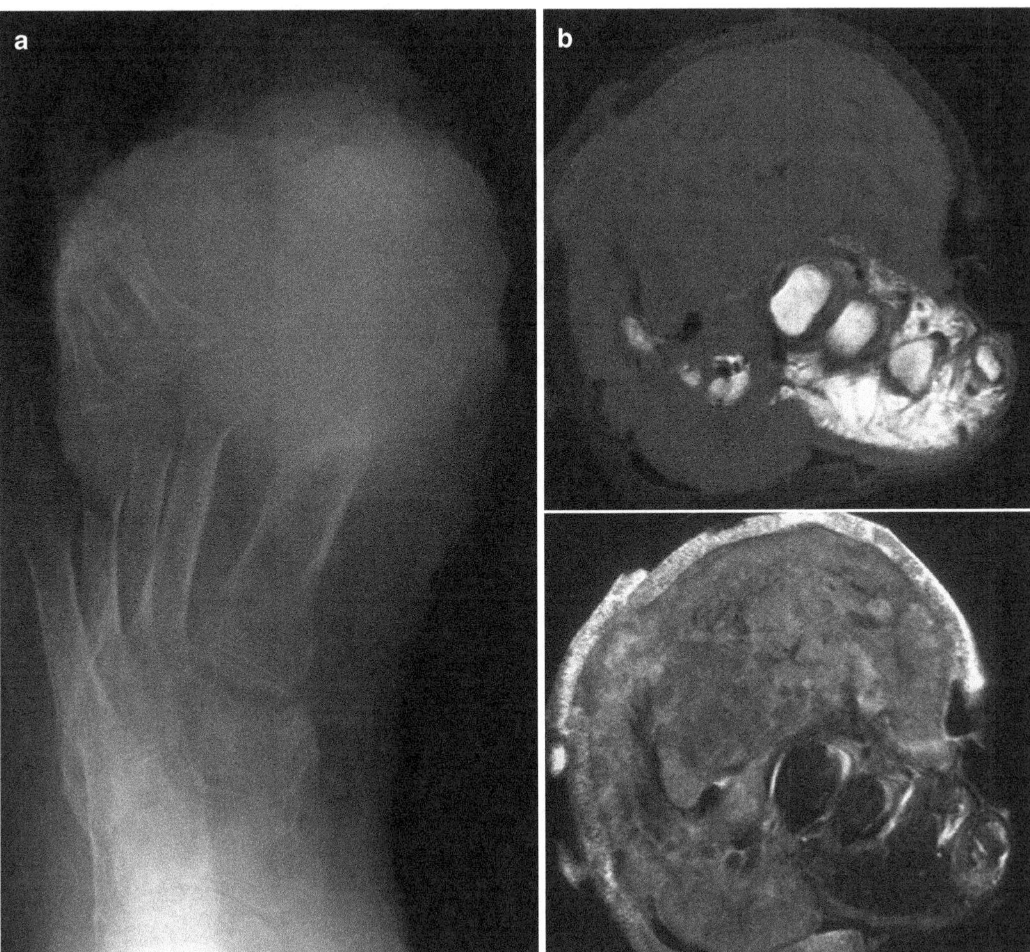

Fig. 26 (**a**) AP radiograph of the foot showing gross done destruction involving the great toe with massive soft tissue swelling. (**b**) T1-weighted and STIR coronal sequences showing gross bone destruction and a massive soft tissue mass in a patient with known lung cancer

10 Miscellaneous Lesions

10.1 Paget's Disease

Paget's disease is a relatively common disorder in which there is an imbalance in osteoclast mediated bone absorption and osteoclast mediated bone deposition. It is a metabolic condition of unknown aetiology. It can affect multiple bones and is much more common in patients over 85 years of age. The disease has three phases.

The osteolytic phase results in excessive bone resorption. In the mixed osteoclastic and osteoblastic phase, there is excessive resorption and compensatory bone formation. In the osteosclerotic phase, bone turnover is at normal levels and there is cortical thickening and thickened trabeculae. Most occur in the skull, pelvis, and long bones. It is rarely seen in the feet. It can be asymptomatic and discovered incidentally but can also resulted in deep seated pain often worse at night. Pathological fractures can occur, and malignant transformation is seen in about 0.3% of cases (Mangham et al. 2009). The osteoclastic–osteoblastic phase is when it is usually diagnosed. Radiographs will show cortical thickening, bone expansion, coarsening of the trabeculae, and loss of corticomedullary differentiation (Cortis et al. 2011) (Fig. 27).

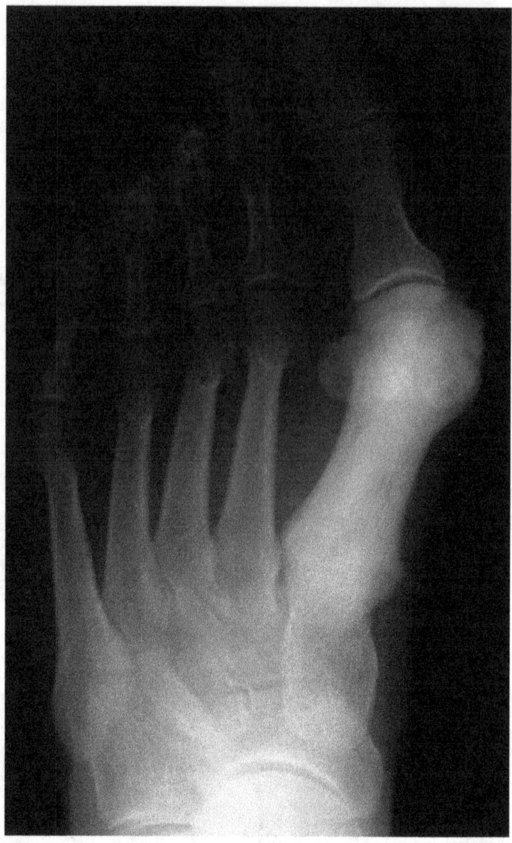

Fig. 27 AP radiograph of the foot showing expansion of the bone, loss of corticomedullary differentiation, and coarse trabeculae. Paget's is rare diagnosis in the foot

10.2 Tendon Abnormalities

Abnormalities of the tendons, namely the FHL tendon, e.g., tendinopathy, tendon tears, and tenosynovitis (Fig. 28) can present with pain especially after exercise. It is commonly seen in ballet dancers. MRI is the best modality to evaluate the tendons. Tears of the distal FHL tendon can also be seen in the context of a turf toe injury. Ruptures of the tendon can be classified by location. Tears can be classified into three zones.

Zone 1 is distal to the sesamoids. Zone 2 is rupture between the sesamoids and the knot of Henry. Zone 3 is proximal to the knot of Henry (Coughlin et al. 2007). In zone 3 tears, there is a risk of proximal retraction as there is no fibrous slip connection to the flexor digitorum longus.

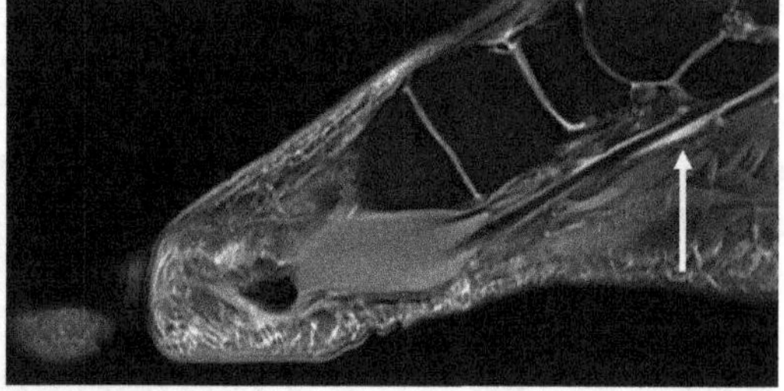

Fig. 28 PDFS sagittal showing tenosynovitis of FHL (arrow)

References

Bartlett DH (1998) Arthroscopic management of osteochondritis dissecans of the first metatarsal head. Arthroscopy 4:51–54

Bowers KD, Martin RB (1976) Turf-toe: a shoe-surface related football injury. Med Sci Sports 8:81–83

Clanton TO, DeLee JC (1982) Osteochondritis dissecans. History, pathophysiology and current treatment concepts. Clin Orthop Relat Res 167:50–64

Cortis K, Micallef K, Mizzi A (2011) Imaging Paget's disease of bone—from head to toe. Clin Radiol 66(7):662–672. https://doi.org/10.1016/j.crad.2010.12.016. Epub 2011 Apr 27. PMID: 21524738

Coughlin MJ, Mann RA, Saltzman CL (2007) Surgery of the foot and ankle. Mosby-Elsevier, Philadelphia, pp 1177–1178

Doral MN, Uzumcugil A, Bozkurt M, Atay OA, Cil A, Leblebicioglu G, Tetik O (2007) Arthroscopic treatment of synovial chondromatosis of the ankle. J Foot Ankle Surg 46:192–195

Flemming DJ, Murphey MD (2000) Enchondroma and chondrosarcoma. Semin Musculoskelet Radiol 4(1):59–71

Fredericson M, Bergman AG, Hoffman KL, Dillingham MS (1995) Tibial stress reaction in runners: correlation of clinical symptoms and scintigraphy with a new magnetic resonance imaging grading system. Am J Sports Med 23:472–481

Greco T, Cianni L, De Mauro D, Dughiero G, Bocchi MB, Cazzato G, Ragonesi G, Liuzza F, Maccauro G, Perisano C (2020) Foot metastasis: current knowledge. Orthop Rev (Pavia) 12(Suppl 1):8671

Helal B (1981) The great toe sesamoid bones: the lusor or lost souls of Ushaia. Clin Orthop 157:82–87

Kaiser P, Guss D, DiGiovanni C (2018) Stress fractures of the foot and ankle in athletes. Foot Ankle Orthop 3:247301141879007. https://doi.org/10.1177/2473011418790078

Kellgren J, Lawrence J (1957) Radiological assessment of osteo-arthrosis. Ann Rheum Dis 16(4):494–450

Lefkowitz RA, Hwang S (2010) Imaging characteristics of primary osteosarcoma: nonconventional subtypes. Radiographics 10065:1653–1673

Mangham DC, Davie MW, Grimer RJ (2009) Sarcoma arising in Paget's disease of bone: declining incidence and increasing age at presentation. Bone 44:431e6

Moll JM, Wright V (1973) Psoriatic arthritis. Semin Arthritis Rheum 3(1):55–78. https://doi.org/10.1016/0049-0172(73)90035-8

Murphey MD et al (2000) Imaging of osteochondroma: variants and complications with radiologic-pathologic correlation. Radiographics 20(5):1407–1434

Ogata K, Sugioka Y, Urano Y, Chikama H (1986) Idiopathic osteonecrosis of the first metatarsal sesamoid. Skelet Radiol 15(2):141–145. https://doi.org/10.1007/BF00350208. PMID: 3961520

Qureshi A, Qureshi GA, Hassan M (2007) A case of Ewing's sarcoma involving cervical spine. Am Eur J Sci Res 2(01):57–59

Resnick D, Niwayama G, Feingold ML (1977) The sesamoid bones of the hands and feet: participators in arthritis. Radiology 123(1):57–62

Van Saase JL, Van Romunde LK, Cats A, Vandenbroucke JP, Valkenburg HA (1989) Epidemiology of osteoarthritis: Zoetermeer survey. Comparison of radiological osteoarthritis in a Dutch population with that in 10 other populations. Ann Rheum Dis 48:271–280

Vázquez-García B, Valverde M, San-Julián M (2011) Enfermedad de Ollier: tumores benignos con riesgo de malignización. Revisión de 17 casos [Ollier disease: benign tumours with risk of malignant transformation. A review of 17 cases]. An Pediatr (Barc) 74(3):168–173. Spanish. Epub 2011 Jan 14. PMID: 21237730. https://doi.org/10.1016/j.anpedi.2010.10.012

Waizy H, Jäger M, Abbara-Czardybon M et al (2008) Surgical treatment of AVN of the fibular (lateral) sesamoid. Foot Ankle Int 29:231–236

Imaging of the Forefoot

Douglas Hoffman, Ryan C. Kruse,
Ramanan Rajakulasingam, and Rajesh Botchu

Contents

The original version of this chapter was revised. A few corrections were made to the chapter, including changes to the chapter title and order of authors. A correction to this chapter can be found at https://doi.org/10.1007/174_2023_446

D. Hoffman
Department of Orthopedics and Radiology, Essentia Health, Duluth, MN, USA

R. C. Kruse
Sports Medicine Department, University of Iowa, Iowa City, IA, USA

R. Rajakulasingam (✉)
Department of Radiology, Royal National Orthopedic Hospital, London, UK
e-mail: ramanan.rajakulasingam1@nhs.net

R. Botchu
Department of Radiology, Royal Orthopedic Hospital, Birmingham, UK

Med Radiol Diagn Imaging (2023), corrected publication 2023
https://doi.org/10.1007/174_2023_402,
Published Online: 03 May 2023

1 Introduction

Pain that arises from the second to fourth rays and interspaces is termed lesser metatarsalgia (LM). While the pain is commonly located at the plantar aspect of metatarsophalangeal joints (MTP), it can also be experienced more diffusely in the forefoot, including dorsally in some individuals. In this chapter, we review the forefoot anatomy and outline a systematic approach to the sonographic and MRI evaluation of LM. Both common and less common causes of LM will be discussed.

2 Epidemiology

Lesser metatarsalgia is relatively common and can affect individuals throughout the spectrum of ages. The prevalence of forefoot pain increases with age, with a prevalence of up to 36% in individuals over the age of 50 years old (Gates et al. 2019). Women tend to be more affected than men. In the younger population, LM is less common but is often associated with runners or activities requiring repetitive foot impact. It has been reported that the incidence of foot injuries in runners ranges from 5.7% to 39.3% (van Gent et al. 2007). The causes of LM are myriad, with reports of up to 23 distinct diagnoses (Scranton Jr. 1980). In a non-published review of the senior author's database of over 700 diagnostic ultrasound (US) examinations for LM, the 3 most common diagnoses were an interdigital neuroma, plantar plate abnormalities, and plantar fat pad abnormalities. However, it is important to note that the etiology of LM may arise from a single abnormality or multiple, concomitant injuries.

3 Imaging

While magnetic resonance imaging (MRI) has historically been the advanced imaging modality of choice for forefoot pain, there are notable characteristics of ultrasound (US) that offer advantages over MRI. First, the spatial resolution of US for superficial soft-tissue structures is superior to that of MRI. US can provides submillimetric resolution compared to a standard MRI, which typically provides a spatial resolution of 2–3 mm (Martinoli 2010). In the forefoot, pain generating pathologic structures may be very small and thus more readily identified with US. Another advantage of US compared to MRI is that imaging is not limited to specific anatomic planes. The optimal anatomic plane to image pertinent structures in the forefoot may be different for the first ray or interspace compared to the lesser rays or interspaces. US can easily adjust to the optimal planes of imaging to best evaluate the potential pain generators in LM. Finally, real-time feedback from the patient with the practitioner can provide important information regarding whether an abnormal appearing structure is symptomatic and thus is important feedback to help decipher pain-generating pathology from asymptomatic findings.

When MRI is needed, a dedicated high resolution surface coil, e.g., wrist or flex coil should be adopted. This is needed so a small field of view (8–10 cm) with a thin slice thickness (1.5–2 mm) can be acquired with appropriate signal to noise ratio. The toes should be resting in extension and brought to a neutral midline position. Side padding/forms of immobilization should be used to prevent motion. Sagittal plane images are usually planned of the second metatarsal, whereas short-axis sequences are planned of the perpendicular axis of the second toe. A typical lesser metatarsalgia protocol should involve axial and coronal T1 and fat-saturated (FS), sagittal PD and PD FS sequences. PD images better delineate the capsuloligamentous complex and cartilaginous surfaces when compared to T1 WI, hence their use in this protocol. Any further fat suppressed imaging, e.g., STIR is acquired in the best plane that can depict the observed pathology (Nouh et al. 2015). Intravenous (IV) contrast is rarely ever needed.

4 Normal Sonoanatomy

A detailed understanding of the normal sonographic appearance of forefoot structures is important in identifying pathology. A thorough sonographic evaluation of the forefoot requires imaging pertinent structures in both longitudinal and transverse views as well as imaging from both the dorsal and plantar approach. In addition, utilizing a protocol-based approach assures that all pertinent structures are systematically imaged. Table 1 outlines our protocol for the US evaluation of LM.

Table 1 Protocol for the sonographic evaluation of lesser metatarsalgia

Dorsal structures	Plantar structures
Metatarsophalangeal joints	Metatarsophalangeal joints
Metatarsal bones	Plantar plate
Metatarsal interspaces	Flexor tendons
	Plantar fat pad
	Metatarsal interspaces

The evaluation of LM typically begins with the MTP joints via a dorsal approach. A high-frequency transducer with a relatively short footprint is ideal due to the superficial location of the structures to be evaluated. Additionally, generous coupling gel can facilitate skin contact when various deformities are present. Light transducer pressure is necessary when using Doppler imaging as these small vessels can easily be compressed. The bony acoustic contours of the metatarsal head and proximal phalanx, as well as the dorsal synovial recess and capsule are readily imaged with US (Fig. 1a). In the normal state, a small amount of anechoic fluid within the joint can be present. Superficial to the capsule, the extensor digitorum longus (EDL) and brevis (EDB) tendons traverse over the MTP joint next to each other with the EDB lateral to the EDL (Fig. 1b). The EDL and EDB tendons insert onto the dorsal cortex of the distal phalanx and proximal phalanx, respectively. Proximal to the MTP joints, the dorsal cortex of the metatarsal diaphy-

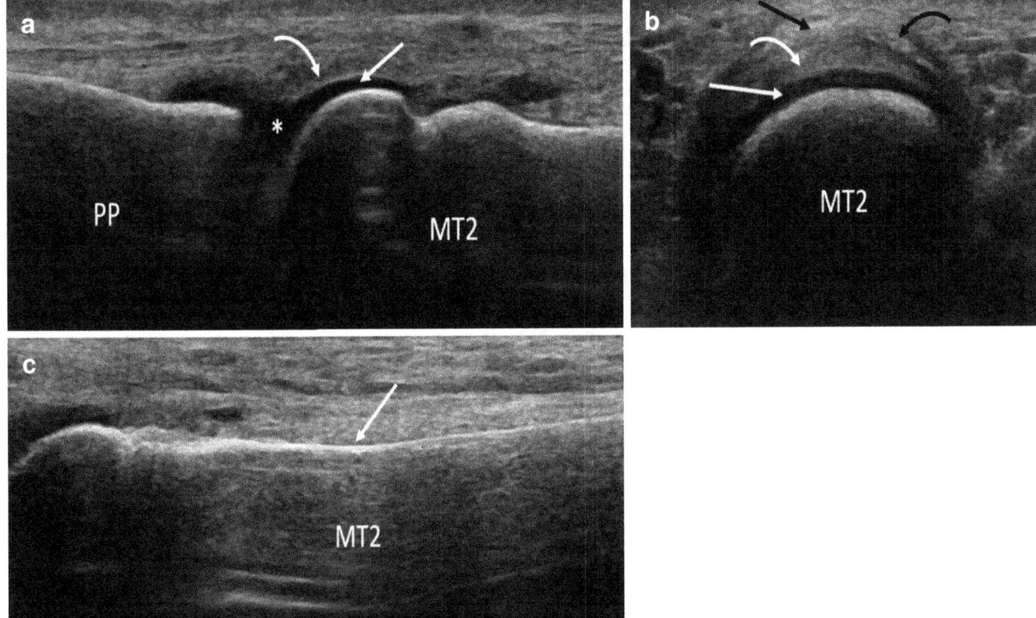

Fig. 1 Normal second metatarsophalangeal (MTP) joint and metatarsal diaphysis. (**a**) Normal longitudinal image of the MTP joint from the dorsal approach. Dorsal synovial recess (asterisk), joint capsule (curved arrow), and articular cartilage of the second metatarsal head (straight arrow). (**b**) Normal transverse image of the second MTP joint at the level of the metatarsal head showing the articular cartilage (straight white arrow), capsule (curved white arrow), extensor digitorum longus tendon (straight black arrow), and extensor digitorum brevis tendon (curved black arrow). (**c**) Normal longitudinal image of the second metatarsal diaphysis. The periosteum is visualized as a very thin hypoechoic line adjacent to the echogenic bony cortex (arrow). *MT2* second metatarsal bone, *PP* proximal phalanx

sis appears as a smooth hyperechoic line with posterior acoustic shadowing and reverberation artifacts. The periosteum appears as a very thin hypoechoic line that overlies the bony cortex (Fig. 1c).

Structures within the metatarsal interspaces consist of the intermetatarsal bursa (IB), superficial transmetatarsal ligament (STML), deep transmetatarsal ligament (DTML), and the interdigital neurovascular bundle (Fig. 2). The IB is located dorsal to the DTML while the interdigital neurovascular bundle is plantar to the DTML. The metatarsal interspaces are more completely evaluated with US from the dorsal approach since the IB, interdigital nerve (IN), and DTML can all be visualized. However, the IN should also be evaluated from the plantar approach as discussed below. From the dorsal longitudinal approach, applying a dorsally directed pressure with the thumb from the plantar aspect of the interspace will improve visualization of the IN since it widens the interspace as well as moves the IN from a plantar to a more dorsal position distal to the DTML (Fig. 3). The IN appears as a hypoechoic structure that is plantar to the DTML. The DTML is viewed as a small ovoid hyperechoic structure that becomes more conspicuous during plantar thumb pressure since it is the only structure within the interspace that remains stationary. The IB normally appears as small irregular hypoechoic structure dorsal to the DTML.

From a plantar approach, the bony contours of the metatarsal head and proximal phalanx are again visualized (Fig. 4). The articular cartilage appears as a thin, anechoic line overlying the metatarsal head. Spanning the plantar aspect of the MTP joint is the plantar plate. In the longitudinal view, the plantar plate appears as a well-defined, homogenous, slightly hyperechoic, curvilinear structure that attaches onto the plantar base of the proximal phalanx (Fig. 4a). At its distal attachment, a small hyperechoic triangle within the plantar plate is often present due to a high concentration of connective septa which serve to reinforce its attachment onto the proximal phalanx (Gregg et al. 2006). Dynamic imaging with flexion and extension of the MTP joint can often increase conspicuity of plantar plate tears. In the transverse plane, the plantar plate has a homogenous curvilinear appearance draping over the metatarsal head and should be imaged from the MTP joint to its attachment onto the proximal phalanx (Fig. 4b). Superficial to the plantar plate, the flexor digitorum longus (FDL) and flexor digitorum brevis (FDB) tendons are visualized both in the longitudinal and transverse planes.

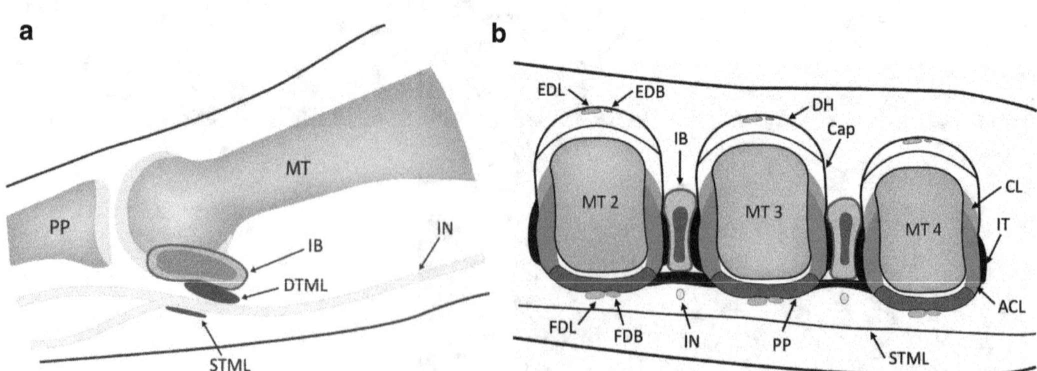

Fig. 2 Anatomy of the metatarsal interspaces. (**a**) Longitudinal illustration of the metatarsal interspace showing the metatarsal (MT) and proximal phalanx (PP) bones, intermetatarsal bursa (IB), deep transmetatarsal ligament (DTML) and superficial transmetatarsal ligament (STML), and interdigital nerve (IN). (**b**) Transverse view of the metatarsal interspaces which also includes the extensor digitorum longus (EDL) and extensor digitorum brevis (EDB) tendons, flexor digitorum longus (FDL) and flexor digitorum brevis (FDB) tendons, and interosseous tendons (IT), collateral (CL) and accessory collateral (ACL) ligaments, joint capsule (Cap), dorsal hood (DH), and plantar plates (PP)

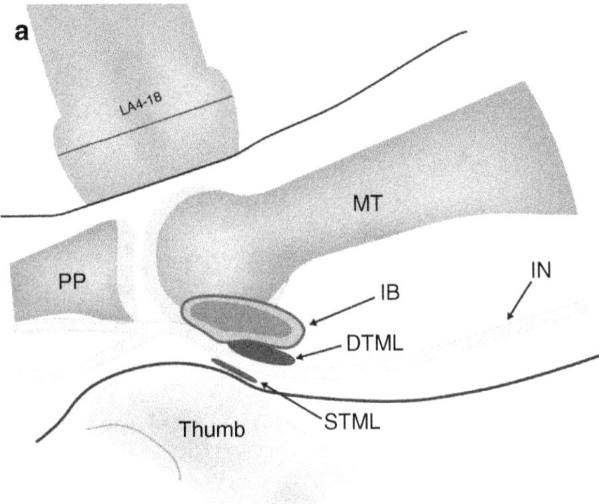

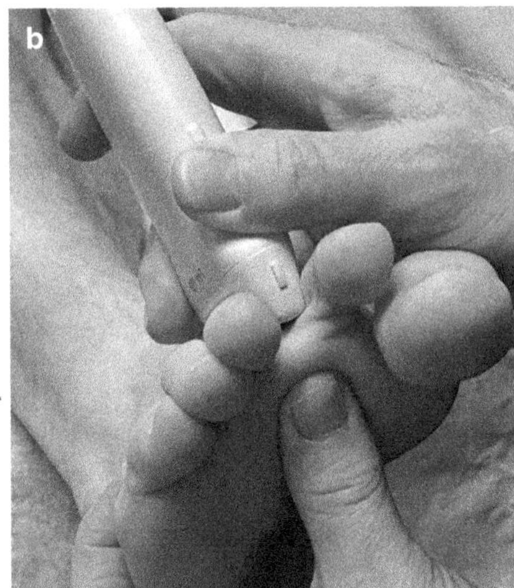

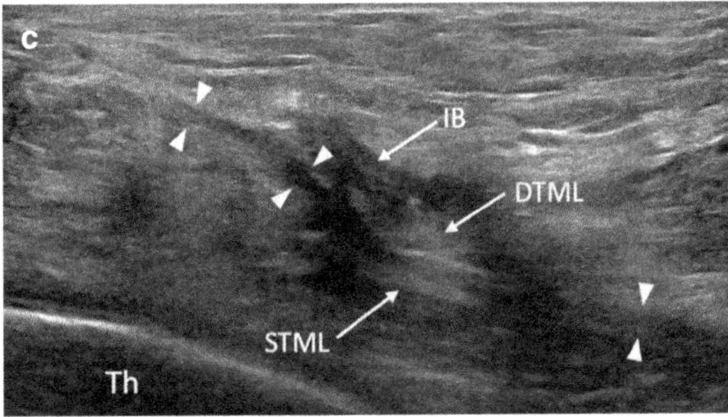

Fig. 3 Longitudinal view of the metatarsal interspace with thumb pressure from the plantar aspect. (**a**) Longitudinal illustration of the interspace showing that thumb pressure displaces the interdigital nerve (IN) more dorsally allowing better visualization with ultrasound. Note how the IN bends around the deep transmetatarsal ligament (DTML) and abuts the intermetatarsal bursa (IB) located just dorsally to the nerve. *PP* proximal phalanx, *MT* metatarsal bone, *STML* superficial transmetatarsal ligament. (**b**) Picture illustrating technique of applying thumb pressure to the plantar aspect of the interspace. (**c**) Corresponding normal sonogram of the interspace with thumb pressure. The IN appears hypoechoic and located between the arrowheads. *Th* thumb

The metatarsal interspace should also be view from the plantar approach. In the normal state, the IN is difficult to visualize from the plantar approach. In contrast, interdigital neuromas are more easily identified both in the longitudinal and transverse planes from the plantar approach. Finally, the plantar fat pad is normally viewed as a slightly hyperechoic homogenous tissue that is mildly compressible (Fig. 5). Both the epidermis and dermis are also easily visualized with US. In the plantar foot region, the epidermis often has a bilaminar hyperechoic appearance while the dermis typically appears more heterogenous due to the nonuniform distribution of collagen fibers (Mlosek and Malinowska 2013).

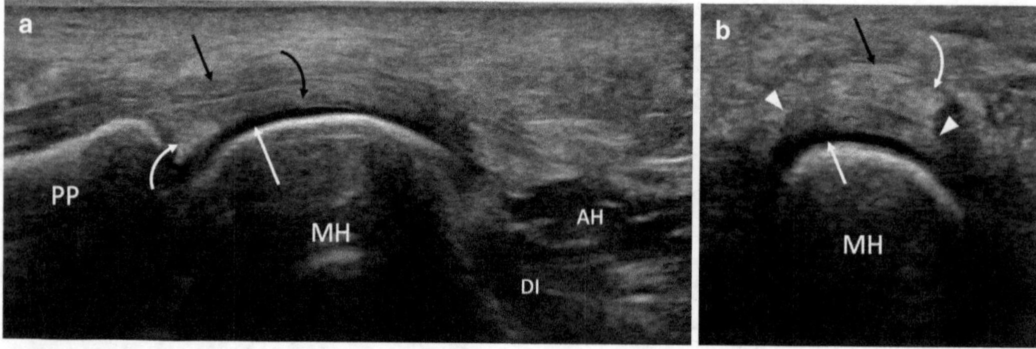

Fig. 4 Normal anatomy of the plantar MTP joint and plantar plate. (**a**) Longitudinal view showing the bony acoustic contours of the metatarsal head (MT) and proximal phalanx (PP), the plantar plate (curved black arrow), and flexor digitorum longus tendon (straight black arrow). Note the anechoic hyaline cartilage of the MT head (straight white arrow) and hyperechoic triangle within the plantar plate (curved white arrow) which is due to a high concentration of connective septa which reinforce its attachment onto the PP. (**b**) Transverse view of the plantar aspect of the MTP joint at the level of the MT head showing the flexor digitorum longus (straight black arrow) and flexor digitorum brevis (curved white arrow) tendons and plantar plate (arrowheads). Straight white arrow = hyaline cartilage of MT head

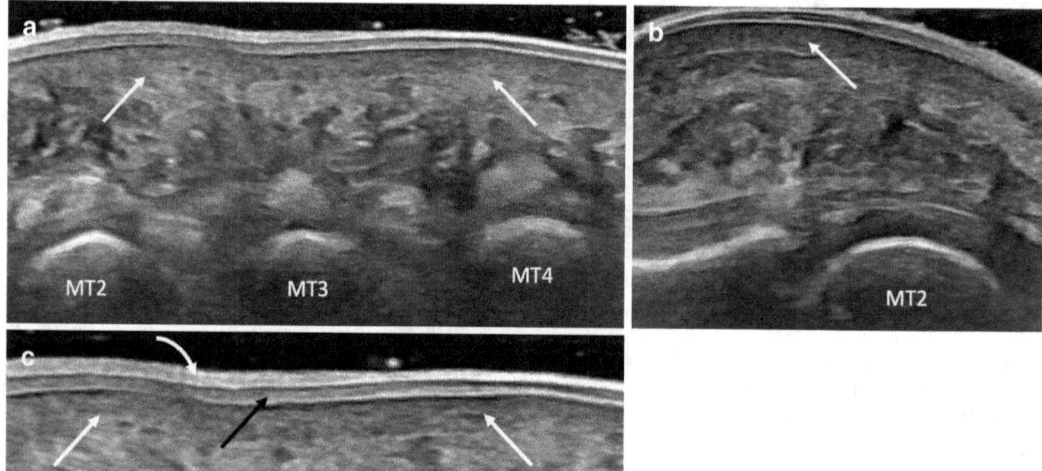

Fig. 5 Normal plantar fat pad. Transverse (**a**) and longitudinal (**b**) sonograms of the plantar fat pad beneath the lesser MTP joints. Note the fairly uniform hyperechoic adipose echotexture beneath the dermis (white arrows) due to the relative high density of echogenic fibrous septae. (**c**) Zoomed in image of the epidermis, dermis, and superficial subcutaneous tissue. Note that the epidermis in the plantar foot region is hyperechoic and has a bilaminar appearance in areas of increased skin thickness (curved arrow). The dermis appears as a relatively hyperechoic band (black arrow) in between the epidermis and subcutaneous tissue (white arrow)

5 Normal MRI Anatomy

The lesser MTP joints grossly follows the anatomy of the first MTPJ with a few exceptions. Firstly, the vertical axis of the lesser metatarsal heads are larger than the transverse axis. The distal condyles of the metatarsoglenoid head have two epicondyles on either side of the head which act as insertional sites for the MTP collateral ligaments (proper) and metatarsoglenoid

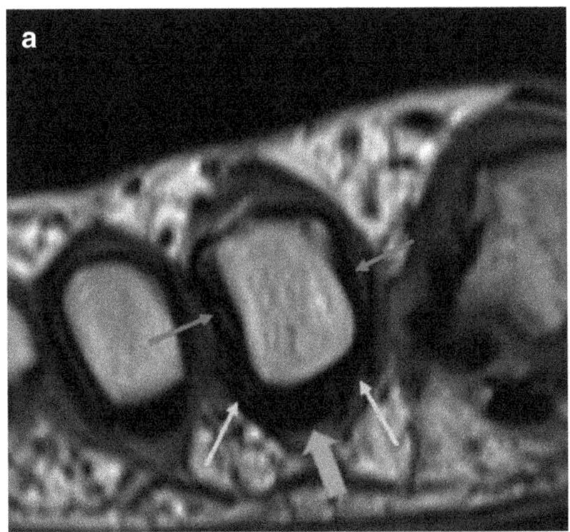

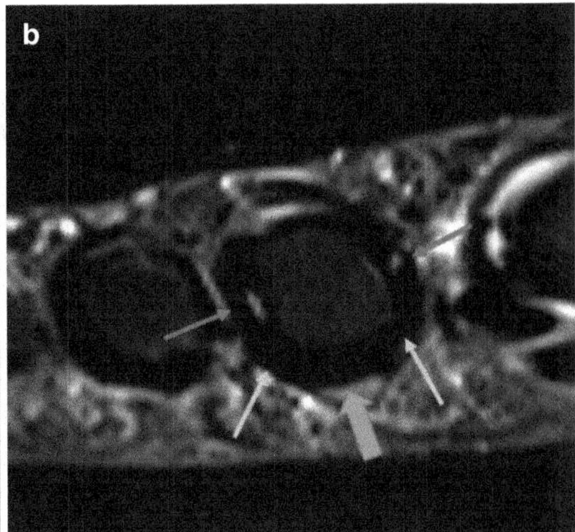

Fig. 6 Normal MRI anatomy of the plantar plate and MTPJ. T1 axial (**a**) and T2 stir (**b**) shows the accessory ligaments (red arrows) inserting into the margins of the plantar plate (orange arrow). The plantar plate hugs the plantar aspect of the metatarsal head. The underlying flexor tendon (blue arrow) is located within the fibrous pulley at the plantar margin of the plantar plate

(accessory) ligaments (Fig. 6). The proper collateral ligaments insert onto the medial and lateral phalangeal tubercles while the accessory ligaments insert onto the medial and lateral borders of the plantar plate. The plantar plate is the main stabilizer of the lesser MTPJs which acts a sling for the metatarsal head. It is a fibrocartilaginous structure that originates proximal to the articular surface and inserts onto the base of the proximal phalanx (Figs. 7 and 8). It is roughly 2–5 mm thick with a maximum length of roughly 23 mm.

The plantar plate is made up of type 1 collagen, and so shows low signal on all pulse sequences with a typical cradle appearance on short-axis sequences. A normal synovial recess with typical fluid signal undercutting the midline insertion of the plantar plate is considered a normal finding and should not be diagnosed as a tear (Linklater and Bird 2016). This measures roughly 2.5 mm and is commonly associated with attenuation of the midline distal portion of the plantar plate (Linklater and Bird 2016).

The undersurface of the plantar plate has a fibrous tunnel where the FDL and FDB tendons traverse (Figs. 7 and 8). FDL inserts onto the plantar aspect of the distal phalanges while FDB inserts onto the middle phalanges of the same toes. Dorsal and plantar interossei and lumbrical tendons insert on the tibial aspect of the bases of the proximal phalanges. The EDL and EDB tendons are visualized on the dorsal aspect of the lesser MTPJs and enclosed by the extensor hood which act as a fibro-aponeurotic sling.

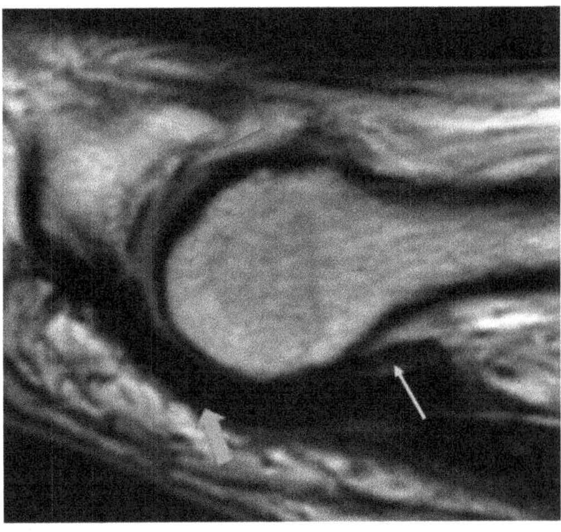

Fig. 7 Paracentral PD sagittal MRI shows normal anatomy of the plantar plate (blue arrow). The second MPTJ dorsal capsule is noted (red arrow). The flexor halluces brevis tendon (orange arrow) inserts on the proximal phalanx in confluence with the plantar plate

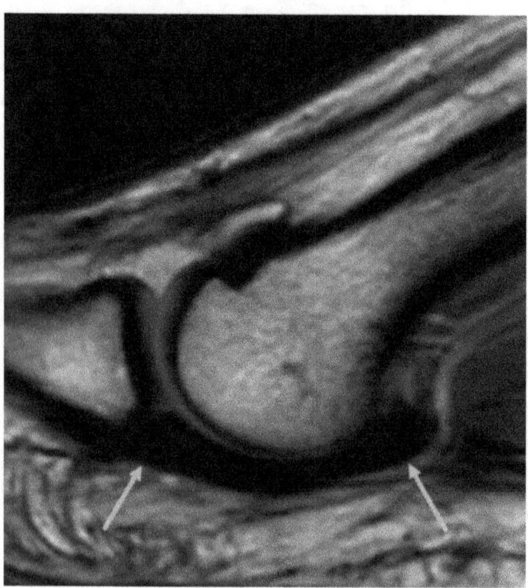

Fig. 8 Paracentral PD sagittal MRI shows an intact plantar plate (orange arrows). This exhibits uniformly low signal on all sequences, inserting onto the proximal phalanx plantar base

6 Common Pathology

6.1 Osteoarthritis

Osteoarthritis (OA) is a noninflammatory arthropathy, characterized by loss of articular cartilage and joint space narrowing. In the lesser MTP joints, capsular thickening often accompanies OA and can be an important clue to early joint degeneration on US. From the dorsal approach, both longitudinal and transverse views are important to fully evaluate for lesser MTP joint degenerative changes. Longitudinal US images will demonstrate bony irregularities and loss of the normal contours of the metatarsal head (Fig. 9). A small effusion and mild thickening of the dorsal synovial recess and capsule are also common. Hyperemia of the dorsal synovial recess is typically absent or mild. Capsular thickening is better assessed with transverse images and in some cases the enlarged capsule can encroach upon the interspace and mimic a symptomatic interdigital neuroma (Fig. 10). In the early stages of OA, early degenerative changes can often be better appreciated with US as compared to plain radiographs (Fig. 9).

On MRI, OA manifests as joint space narrowing, peripheral osteophytosis, subchondral cysts (low T1W SI and high STIR/T2W SI), and subchondral sclerosis (low SI on all pulse sequences) (Fig. 11) (Gregg et al. 2008). Over time the articulating portion of the metatarsal head loses is wavy contour and becomes more square shaped.

6.2 Avascular Necrosis

Avascular necrosis affecting the metatarsal head is typically called Freiberg's infarction. This is due to overloading of the subchondral bone plate with marrow edema leading eventually to ischemia and finally collapse (Ganguly et al. 2018). Avascular necrosis can be primary or post-traumatic. Common sonographic findings include bony fragmentation and irregularity of the metatarsal head and, less commonly, the proximal phalanx. Additionally, there may be a small effusion and hyperemia of the dorsal synovial recess indicating an associated synovitis (Fig. 9).

Edema like signal changes are usually early findings on MRI (Fig. 12). Subchondral collapse tends to happen later on with a T2 hyperintense stripe, paralleling the subchondral plate. The more symptomatic cases usually show a joint effusion, and the overlying cartilage maybe breeched with thinning, fissuring, or even loss. Subsequently, flattening of the metatarsal head and sclerosis occurs with secondary end stage osteoarthritis occurring with pronounced cystic change (Ganguly et al. 2018).

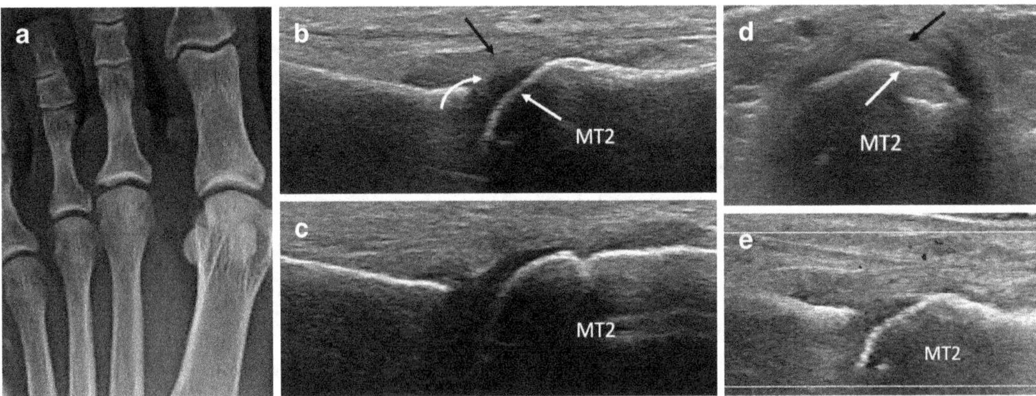

Fig. 9 Osteoarthrosis of the second MTP joint. A 43-year-old female with painful second MTP joint. Standing AP radiograph in (**a**) shows degenerative changes of the second MTP joint. Longitudinal sonogram (**b**), contralateral comparison (**c**), and transverse sonogram (**d**) show mild capsular thickening (black arrows) and loss of the normal contour of the metatarsal head (white arrows). There are also subtle irregularities of the articular cartilage of the metatarsal head (curved arrow). Longitudinal sonogram with Doppler (**e**) typically shows absent to minimal vascularity of the dorsal synovial recess

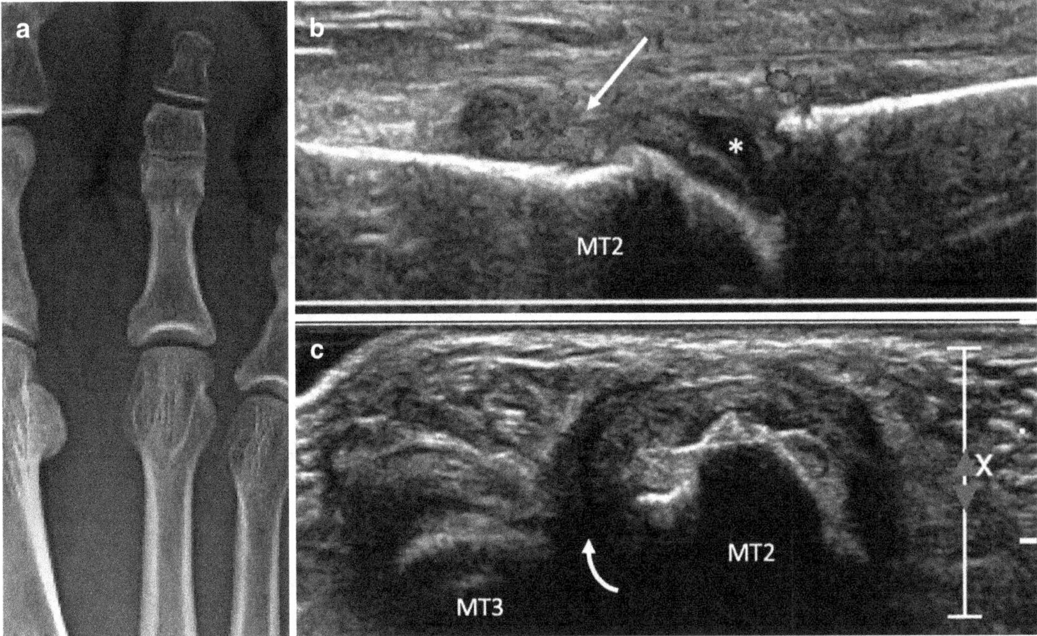

Fig. 10 Avascular necrosis of the second metatarsal head (Freiberg's infarction). A 14-year-old female with progression second MTP joint pain for 1 year. (**a**) Oblique radiograph showing increased sclerosis and flattening of the second metatarsal head. (**b**) Longitudinal sonogram shows irregularity and flattening of the second metatarsal head as well as synovial hypertrophy (asterisk). (**c**) Longitudinal sonogram with Doppler reveals increased vascularity of the dorsal synovial recess consistent with synovitis

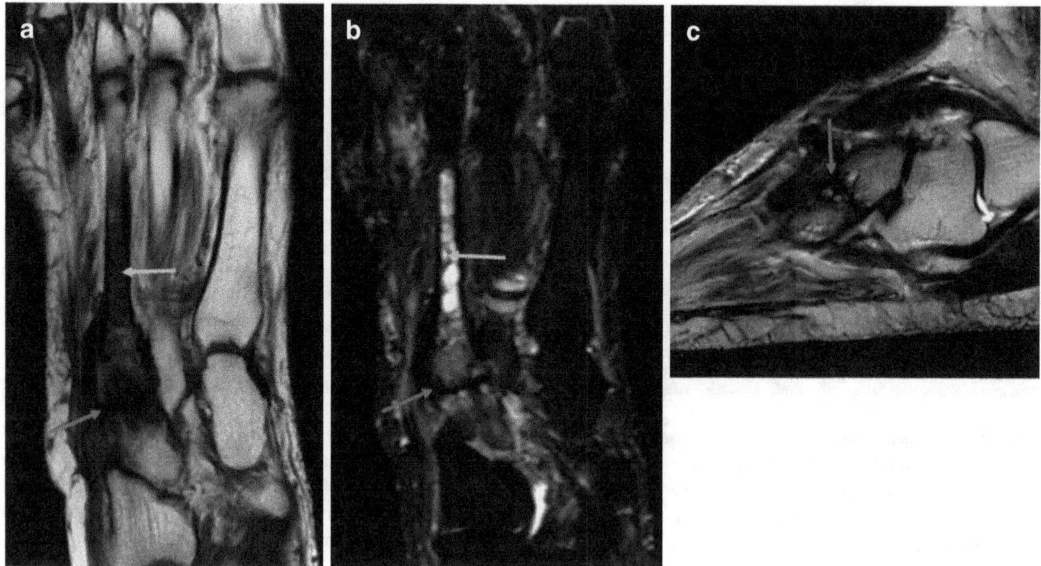

Fig. 11 Axial T1 (**a**), axial STIR (**b**), and sagittal T2 (**c**) show prominent degenerative marrow edema and subchondral cystic change at the third TMTJ consistent with pronounced osteoarthritis. There is further intra-osseous ganglion cystic change within the third metatarsal shaft itself (orange arrow)

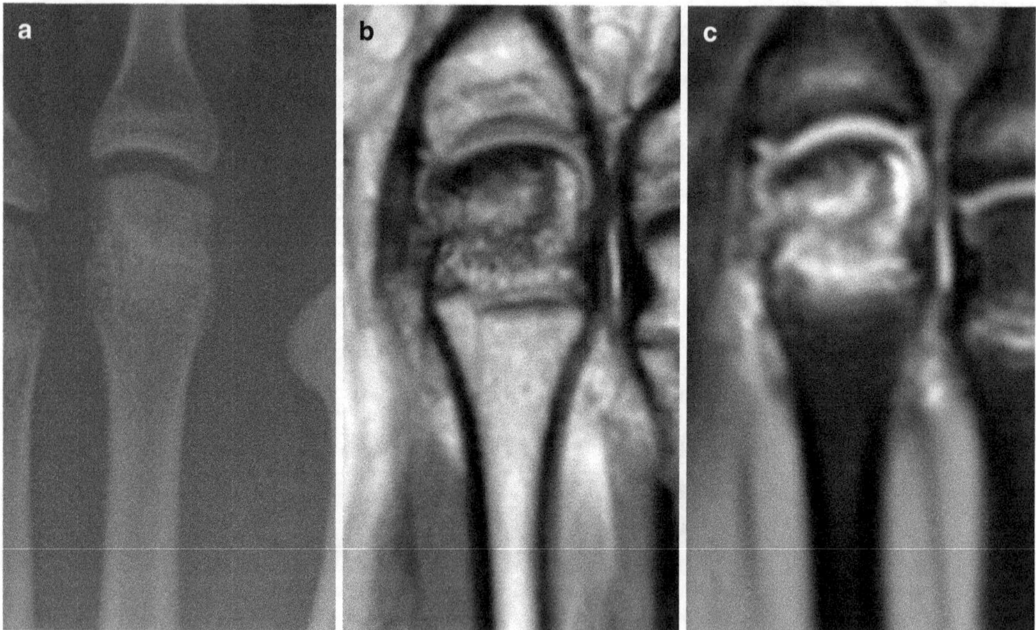

Fig. 12 AP radiograph (**a**) shows flattening and squaring of the second metatarsal head with ill-defined sclerosis in keeping with Freiberg's infarction. This is confirmed on MRI-PD axial (**b**) and PD SPAIR axial (**c**) confirms patchy marrow edema and subchondral cystic change without marrow infiltration. A small reactive joint effusion is present

7 Inflammatory Arthropathy

7.1 Rheumatoid Arthritis

Rheumatoid arthritis (RA) commonly involves the lesser MTP joints. In the early stages, US imaging reveals synovitis which appears as hypoechoic thickening with varying degrees of vascularity of the dorsal synovial recess (Fig. 13). In the more advanced stages, erosive changes and deformities are present (Fig. 14).

On MRI, the main imaging findings to suggest an underlying inflammatory arthropathy are proliferative synovitis such as pannus formation and secondary synovitis being a joint effusion. Pannus formation is typically seen in RA and displays low to intermediate signal on PD and T1-weighted sequences (König et al. 1990). SI may vary on T2W sequences and if bright, could be a sign of hypervascular pannus. Over time, chronic pannus develops hemosiderin and fibrous foci which shows up as low SI on all pulse

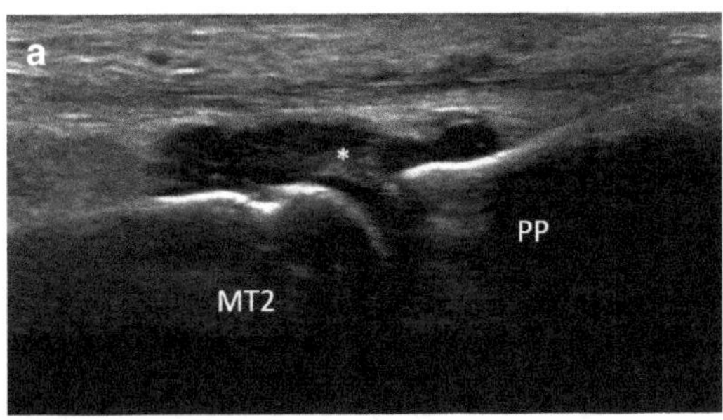

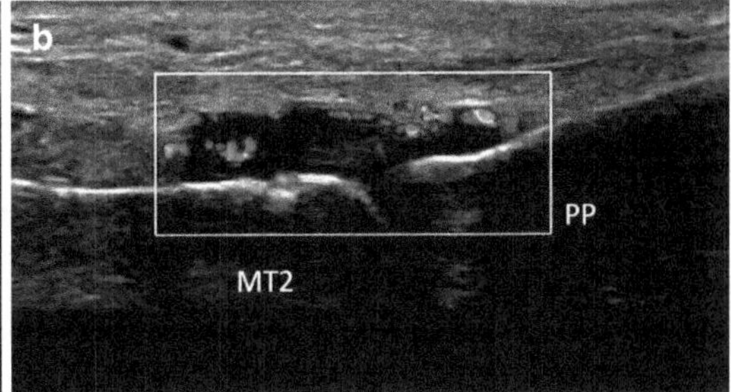

Fig. 13 Early rheumatoid arthritis (RA) with MTP joint synovitis. A 32-year-old female with early RA with primarily forefoot involvement. Longitudinal sonogram (**a**) with Doppler (**b**) shows hypoechoic enlargement of the dorsal synovial recess (asterisk) with moderate vascularity consistent with active synovitis. *MT2* second metatarsal, *PP* proximal phalanx

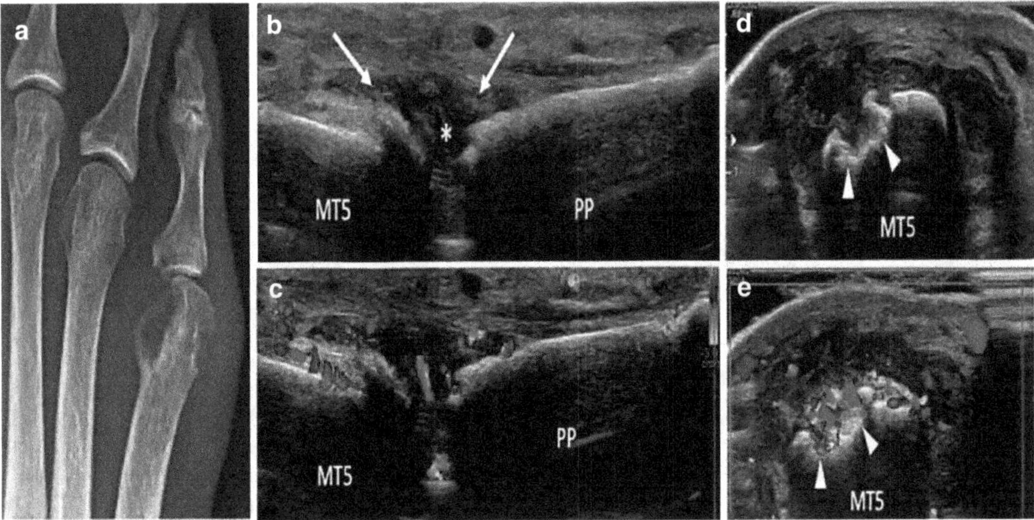

Fig. 14 Rheumatoid arthritis (RA) with active synovitis and erosive changes. A 56-year-old female with seropositive RA and painful fifth MTP joint. (**a**) AP radiograph of the lateral forefoot reveals extensive erosive changes of the fifth MTP joint. Longitudinal sonogram (**b**) with Doppler (**c**) shows synovial hypertrophy (asterisk) and capsular thickening (arrows) with vascularity. Erosive changes are also present at the articular surfaces of the proximal phalanx (PP) and metatarsal head (MT5). Transverse sonogram at the level of the fifth metatarsal head (**d**) with Doppler (**e**) also reveals synovial and capsular thickening as well as extensive erosive changes with vascularity (arrowheads). These findings are consistent with active synovitis and erosions

sequences (König et al. 1990). Bone erosions appear on MRI as sharply marginated areas of trabecular bone loss with small cortical defects. Although they are better seen following contrast administration, the combination of standard T1W sequences along with fine cut CT slices should be able to accurately delineate erosions.

7.2 Dactylitis

Dactylitis is another potential cause of forefoot pain and is defined as uniform swelling of a digit due to varying degrees of inflammation involving the subcutaneous tissue, tendon sheath (tenosynovitis), enthesis (enthesitis), and joints (synovitis). While there are multiple etiologies of dactylitis, psoriatic arthritis is the most common cause occurring in 16–49% of patients (Kaeley et al. 2018). Dactylitis may be the initial symptoms of psoriatic arthritis, and recurrent dactylitis may be the only manifestation of the disease for years (Ritchlin et al. 2009). The toes are more commonly affected than the fingers and the lesser toes more common than the great toe (Brockbank et al. 2005). Potential findings on US include the following: soft tissue edema and/or thickening with vascularity, peri-tendinitis or tenosynovitis of the extensor and flexor tendons, enthesitis of the flexor and extensor tendons, and synovitis of one or multiple joints (Fig. 15).

Tuberculous arthritis is another cause of dactylitis and usually has the classical Phemister triad of juxta articular osteoporosis, bone erosions, and progressive narrowing of the joint space (Berrady et al. 2014). This should be easily visualized on MRI (Fig. 16).

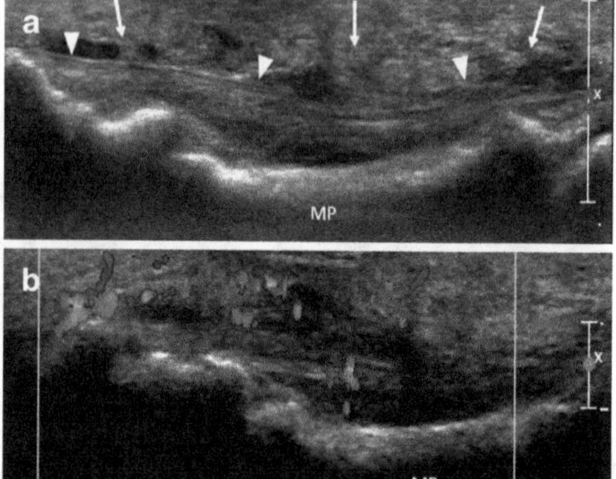

Fig. 15 Dactylitis in a patient with psoriatic arthritis. Longitudinal sonogram (**a**) shows soft tissue thickening, edema, and vascularity (arrows), and tenosynovitis of the flexor tendons (arrowheads). Doppler imaging (**b**) reveals vascularity of both the soft tissue and flexor tendon suggesting an active inflammatory process

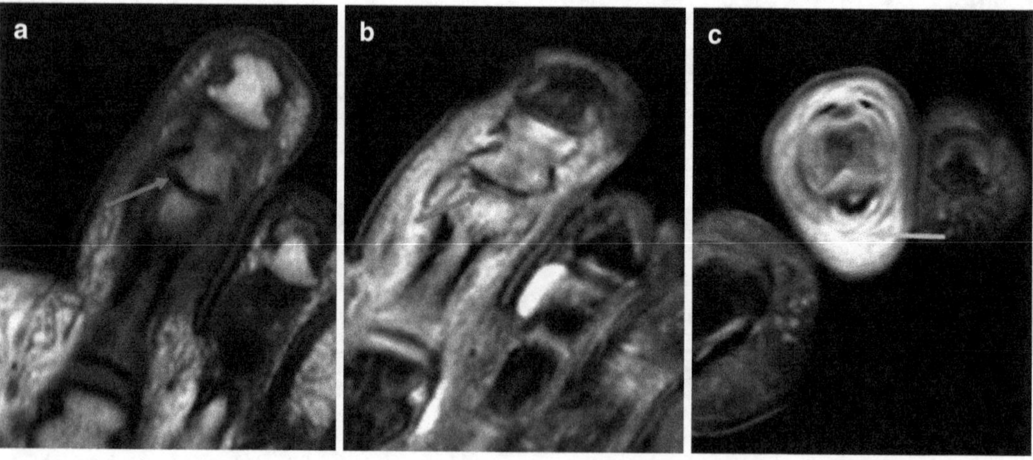

Fig. 16 Dactylitis in a patient with focal tuberculous arthritis. PD SPAIR coronal (**a**), PD SPAIR FS coronal (**b**), and PD SPAIR FS axial (**c**) show prominent marrow edema in the second toe PIPJ (red arrows) with gross soft tissue edema and swelling (orange arrow). Note how the PIPJ joint margin itself is relatively well preserved in comparison to the extent of surrounding changes, more typical of infection rather than malignancy

7.3 Gout

Gout is often associated with first MTP joint involvement. However, the lesser MTP joints may also be involved, with the spectrum of pathology ranging from asymptomatic urate deposition, acute or chronic synovitis, to tophaceous gout. Urate deposition within the MTP joint appears as multiple echogenic dots either scattered or in clusters and is often associated with synovial hypertrophy and varying degrees of vascularity (Fig. 17). Urate may also accumulate within the superficial portion of the articular cartilage of the metatarsal head resulting in a double white line appearance or "double contour sign." When identified, a "double contour sign" is highly suggestive of urate deposition disease, although not pathognomonic as it may also been seen with pseudogout (Löffler et al. 2014). A double contour sign should be distinguished from a cartilage interface artifact which occurs when fluid is adjacent to hyaline cartilage. The echogenic line above the articular cartilage characteristic of the cartilage interface artifact is dependent on the transducer's angle of incidence whereas a double contour sign is unaffected by the transducer position. Tophaceous gout also can affect the lesser MTP joints. Gouty tophi most often appear as heterogenous, hyperechoic masses, often circumscribed by a hypoechoic rim or halo, and varying degrees of internal and peripheral vascularity (de Ávila Fernandes et al. 2011) (Fig. 18).

On MRI, tophi occur as intermediate signal lesions on T1 WI but have variable signal on T2 WI (hypointense to hyperintense) that is thought to be related to the amount of calcification in the lesion (Ganguly et al. 2018). Enhancement is a nonspecific finding and usually homogenous (Ganguly et al. 2018).

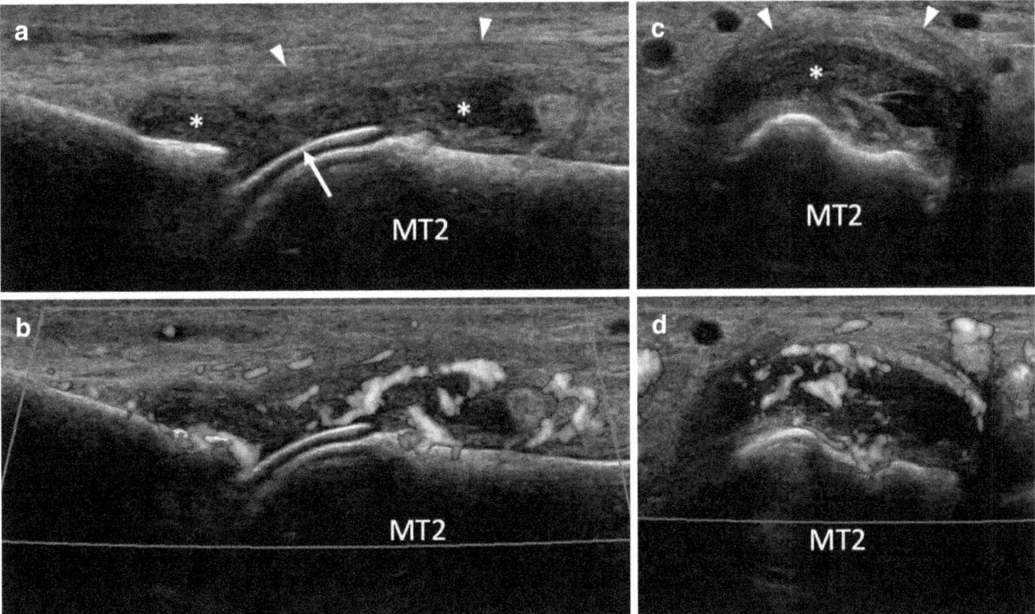

Fig. 17 Acute gout involving the second MTP joint. A 34-year-old male with previous history of painful second toe and now an acute onset of second MTP joint swelling and pain. Longitudinal sonogram (**a**) with Doppler (**b**) and transverse sonogram (**c**) with Doppler (**d**) show synovial hypertrophy with hyperechoic aggregates (asterisks) consistent with urate deposition, capsular thickening (arrowheads), and urate deposition on the superficial border of the hyaline cartilage of the metatarsal head (arrow) resulting in a "double contour sign." The presence of diffuse vascularity signals an active inflammatory process

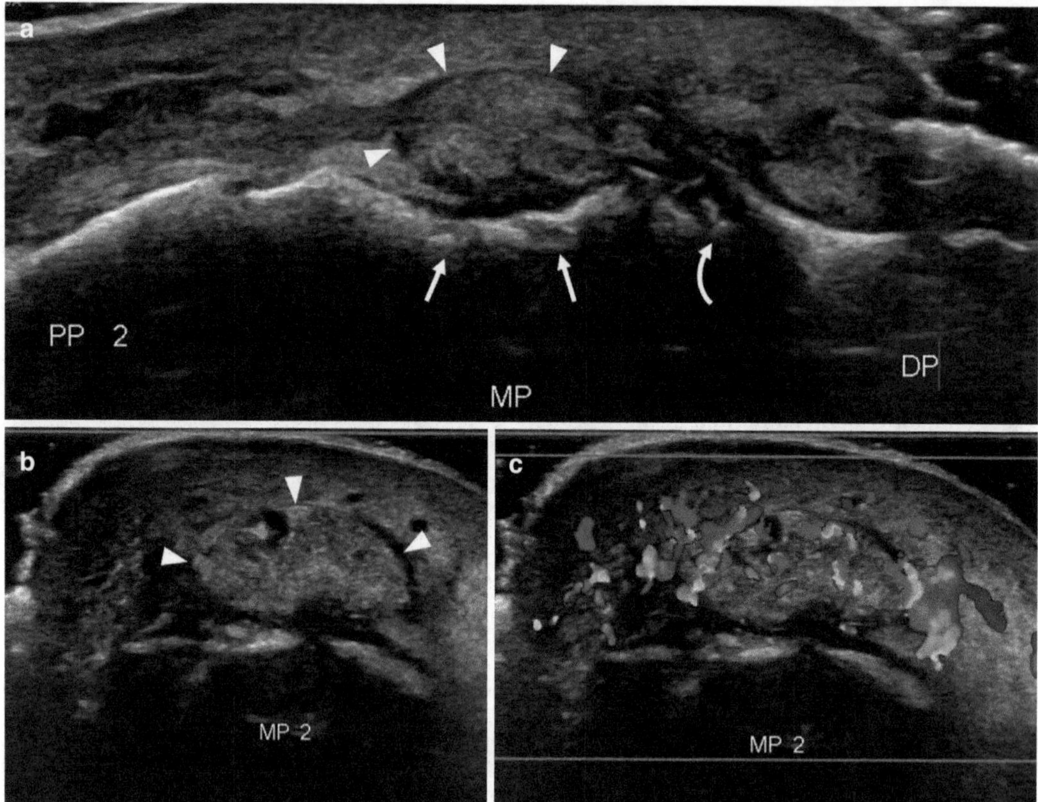

Fig. 18 Tophaceous gout of the second toe. A 75-year-old male with a painful swollen second toe. Longitudinal sonogram (**a**) of the second toe shows a tophus (arrowheads) dorsal to the middle phalanx (MP) with early bony destruction of the dorsal cortex of the MP (arrows) and destruction of the distal interphalangeal joint (curved arrow). Transverse image (**b**) of the tophus with Doppler (**c**) again shows bony destruction of the dorsal cortex of the MP and diffuse hypervascularity. *PP 2* second proximal phalanx, *DP* distal phalanx

8 Metatarsal Stress Fractures

Metatarsal stress fractures most commonly involve the second and third metatarsals (Gehrmann and Renard 2006). US has an important role in the diagnosis of an early stress fracture since it can often detect signs of bone stress injury before radiographs (Banal et al. 2006). US of metatarsal stress fractures is primarily performed from a dorsal approach. Early sonographic findings include periosteal thickening and hyperemia and hypoechoic soft tissue edema within the adjacent subcutaneous tissue (Hoffman et al. 2015) (Fig. 19). As a stress fracture progresses, a distinct cortical break is typically seen. US can also visualize callous formation as healing progresses.

On MRI, stress fractures are seen as low T1W SI linear lines which represent the fracture lines (Anderson and Greenspan 1996). This is typically surrounded by avid bone marrow edema, sometimes with periostitis, periosteal soft tissue edema and a neighboring joint effusion (Fig. 20). An adjacent periosteal bone reaction can occur, usually as a low signal stripe paralleling the cortical bone. Stress fractures are usually graded using the Fredericson grading system for tibial stress syndrome described on MRI (Fredericson et al. 1995). A grade 1 fracture shows periosteal edema, grade 2 shows high intrinsic marrow signal, grade 3 shows low T1W SI along with grade 2 features, and grade 4 shows intracortical signal change with/without a cortical fracture line.

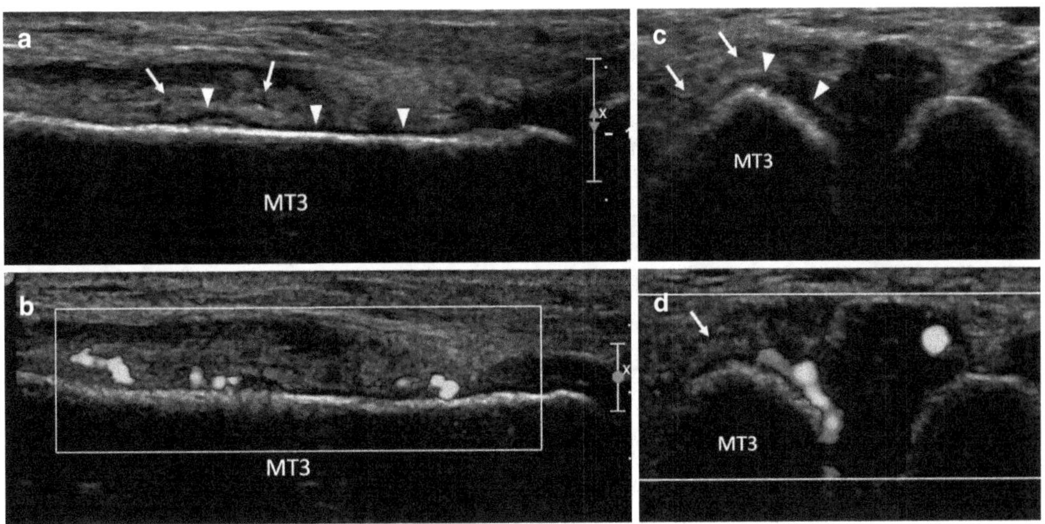

Fig. 19 Third metatarsal stress fracture. A 50-year-old female runner with swelling and pain over the third metatarsal bone. Both longitudinal and transverse images (**a** and **c**) with Doppler (**b** and **d**) show periosteal thickening (arrowheads) and hypervascularity and soft tissue edema within the dorsal subcutaneous tissue (arrows)

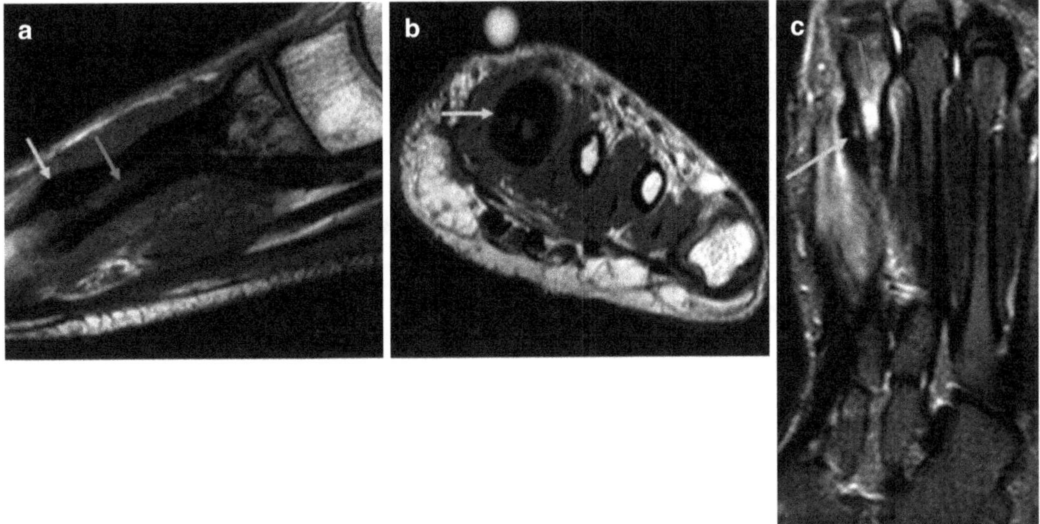

Fig. 20 Second metatarsal stress fracture. Sagittal T1 (**a**), coronal T2 (**b**), and axial STIR (**c**) MRI show prominent marrow edema within the second metatarsal shaft (red arrows). There is some cystic change associated with this with rather marked cortical thickening and new bone formation which is almost circumferential (orange arrow). The findings are typical for a stress fracture with persisting marrow edema

9 Metatarsal Interspaces

9.1 Interdigital Nerve Neuroma

An interdigital neuroma is a focal fusiform enlargement of the common digital plantar nerve located just distal to the deep transmetatarsal ligament but before the bifurcation into the proper digital nerves. Most commonly, interdigital neuromas occur within the third metatarsal interspace followed by the second interspace (Kay and Bennett 2003). Histologically, interdigital neuromas consist of varying degrees of nerve degeneration, epineural and perineural fibrosis, epineural and endovascular hyalinization, vessel obstruction, and bursal scarring (Giakoumis et al. 2013). Despite the terminology of neuroma, the mass refers to swelling of the common digital nerve with perineural fibrosis but a true neoplasm is not present.

The sonographic evaluation of an interdigital neuroma should ideally be performed from both the dorsal and plantar approach. The dorsal approach is advantageous in that there is potentially less image quality degradation compared to visualization through a thickened plantar skin or callus, if present. It also allows better visualization of the intermetatarsal bursa and therefore is the best view to differentiate an interdigital neuroma from an intermetatarsal bursopathy. However, this approach can be challenging if the interspace is narrow, particularly the second interspace. For the dorsal approach, the transducer is placed in a longitudinal orientation within respect to the metatarsal interspace. As discussed previously, dorsal displacement of the contents within the interspace with dorsally directed thumb pressure will improve visualization of the IN. From the dorsal approach, an interdigital neuroma is a spindle-shaped hypoechoic mass located directly beneath an irregular and hypoechoic intermetatarsal bursa just distal to the DTML (Fig. 21). Distinguishing an interdigital neuroma from the bursa may be difficult, and the term "neuroma-bursal complex" may be a more accurate reflection of the underlying pathology (Cohen et al. 2016). From the plantar approach, interdigital neuromas appear as a well-demarcated hypoechoic mass between the metatarsal heads. In the transverse view, manual compression of the metatarsal heads will displace the neuroma plantarly (Fig. 21b, e). Often, this

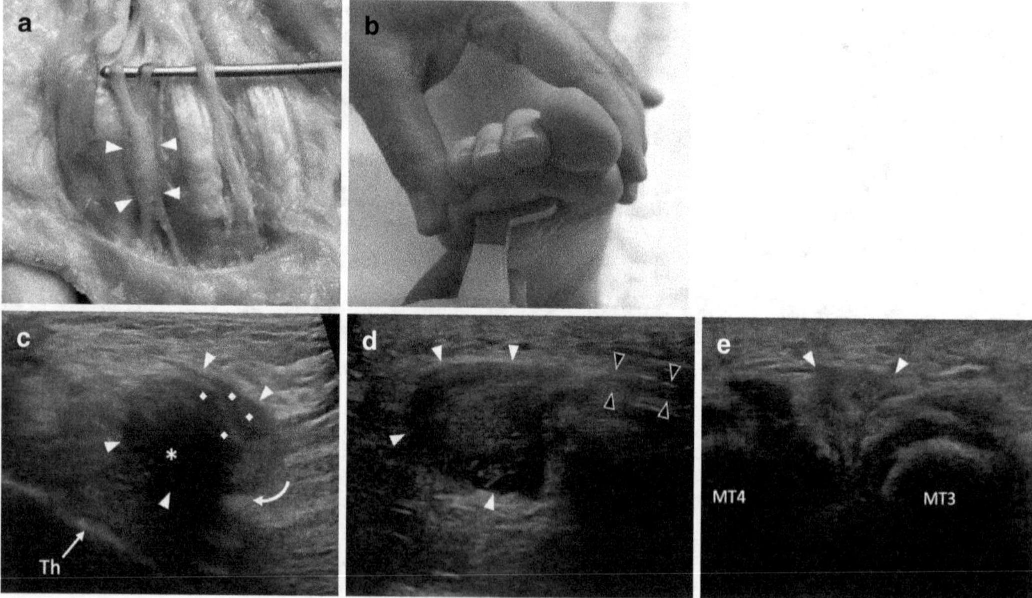

Fig. 21 Third metatarsal interspace interdigital neuroma. A 48-year-old female with pain arising from the third metatarsal interspace. The picture in (**a**) shows a cadaveric dissection of the plantar aspect of the third metatarsal interspace revealing a third interdigital neuroma (arrowheads). Longitudinal image (**c**) shows the interdigital neuroma (asterisk) and bursal tissue (diamonds) forming a "neuroma-bursal complex" (arrowheads). Note how dorsally directed thumb pressure (Th and arrow) displaces the neuroma-bursal complex more dorsally and therefore more conspicuous with ultrasound imaging. The deep transverse metatarsal ligament corresponds to the curved arrow. Distal is to the left of the image. The interdigital neuroma is also visualized from the plantar approach in both the longitudinal (**d**) and transverse (**e**) planes. In (**d**), the neuroma (white arrowheads) is in continuity with the common digital nerve (black arrowheads). By compressing the metatarsal heads in the transverse plane (**b**) the neuroma viewed in the transverse plane (**e**) is displaced plantarly (arrowheads) increasing its visualization. Distal is to the left in images (**c**) and (**d**)

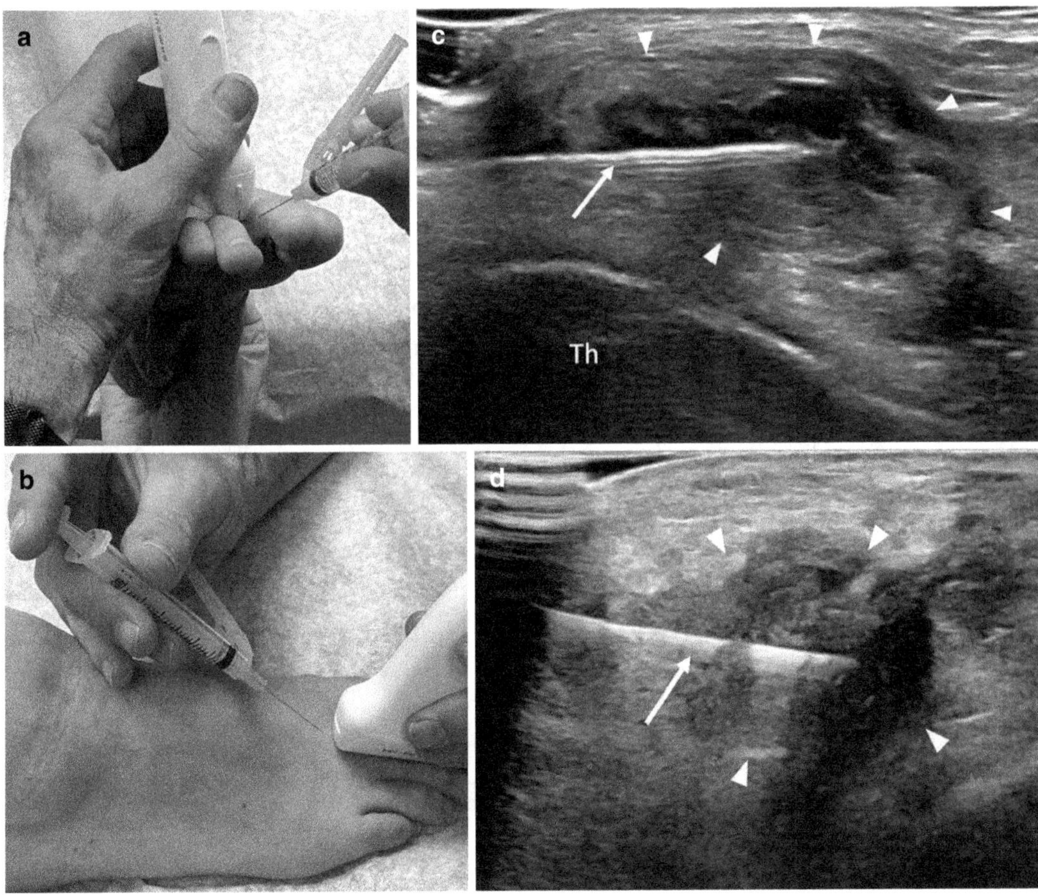

Fig. 22 Injection techniques for an interdigital neuroma. (**a**) An injection through the webspace in a distal to proximal longitudinal in-plane approach. With this approach, having an assistant apply thumb pressure to the interspace will increase the visualization of the interdigital neuroma. Corresponding sonogram (**c**) shows the needle (arrow) in the "neuroma-bursal complex" (arrowheads). Note the cortex of the thumb (Th) that is applying dorsally directed pressure to the interspace. Distal is to the right. (**b**) Dorsal approach to an interdigital neuroma injection and corresponding sonogram (**d**). This approach can easily be accomplished with a single provider

displacement is associated with a click corresponding to the Mulder's sign. In the longitudinal view, visualizing the common digital nerve in continuity of the neuroma will improve diagnostic confidence (Quinn et al. 2000) (Fig. 21d). The presence of an interdigital neuroma may also be an asymptomatic finding and correlating the neuroma with sonopalpatory pain will help direct treatment options (Symeonidis et al. 2012).

An ultrasound-guided injection into an interdigital neuroma can be performed either from a dorsal or plantar approach. The dorsal approach is typically performed in-plane either distal to proximal directly through the interspace or proximal to distal (Fig. 22). Alternatively, a plantar approach is typically done in-plane, longitudinal to the IN, distal to proximal.

On MRI, an interdigital neuroma is seen as a small mass usually isodense/slightly hyperintense to skeletal muscle on T1W sequences with intermediate T2W SI (Fig. 23) (Zanetti et al. 1997; Ashman et al. 2001). The latter is usually due to fibrous tissue. Sometimes an associated bursal complex is seen where there is bright T2 fluid surrounding the neuroma. It should be noted that intermetatarsal fluid is a common finding in the asymptomatic population but collections greater than 3 mm in transverse dimensions are

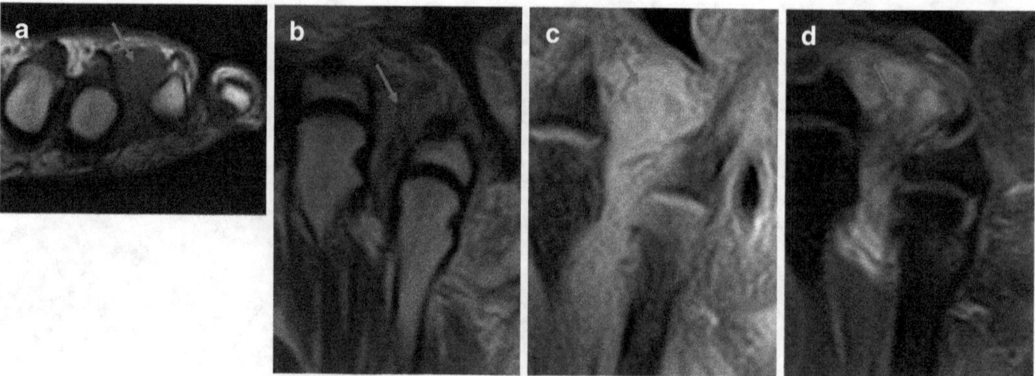

Fig. 23 Interdigital neuroma within the third-fourth metatarsal web space. Coronal T1 (**a**), axial T2 (**b**), axial T1 FS (**c**), and axial T1 FS postcontrast (**d**) MRI show a dumb bell shaped low T1 and intermediate T2 signal lesion in between the third and fourth metatarsal heads. It exhibits heterogenous FS signal and avid heterogenous contrast throughout

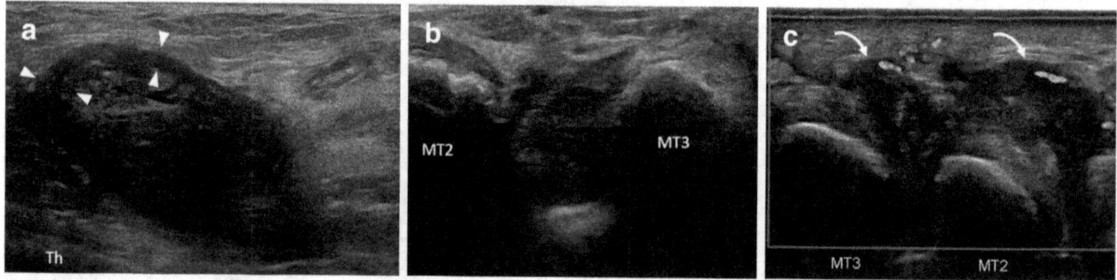

Fig. 24 Intermetatarsal bursopathy in a person with seropositive RA. Longitudinal (**a**) and transverse (**b**) images from a dorsal approach show thickening of the synovial-lined wall of the bursa (arrowheads) which is fill with thick hypoechoic fluid. In (**a**), to the left is distal. Image (**c**) is a transverse sonogram with Doppler from the plantar approach showing an intermetatarsal bursa in both the first and second interspaces and the pannus from the bursa that has eroded through the deep transverse intermetatarsal ligament and into the plantar fat pad (curved arrows). *MT2* second metatarsal head, *MT3* third metatarsal head. *Th* thumb

more likely to be associated with an interdigital neuroma (Zanetti et al. 1997; Ashman et al. 2001). IV contrast is typically not helpful as the varying maturation stages and degree of fibrosis give varying degrees of enhancement. However, it can improve the conspicuity of the neuroma if there is prominent surrounding fibrosis on standard imaging sequences (Zanetti et al. 1997; Ashman et al. 2001).

9.2 Intermetatarsal Bursopathy

An isolated intermetatarsal bura can be caused by both inflammatory and noninflammatory etiologies. Rheumatoid arthritis is the most common cause of an inflammatory bursopathy and may involve multiple interspaces (van Dijk et al. 2022). Best viewed from a dorsal approach due to its location dorsal to the DTML, an inflammatory bursopathy appears as a well-circumscribed, predominantly hypoechoic mass, which typically consumes most of the interspace (Fig. 24). In some cases, Doppler flow may be seen in the bursal walls. Compared to a noninflammatory bursopathy, an inflammatory bursopathy tends to have more of a rounded appearance and is minimally compressible.

Noninflammatory bursopathy can be mechanical, often from direct or repetitive trauma to the region, or postsurgical as a sequelae of a prior neuroma excision. In contrast to inflammatory bursopathy, noninflammatory bursopathy appears as a more irregularly shaped mass often associated with compressible anechoic fluid (Fig. 25).

On MRI, intermetatarsal fluid is noted to be a very common finding and is usually asymptomatic and physiological. If over 3 mm in thickness however, it can be a sign of a neighboring interdigital neuroma or if across a few metatarsals, maybe a feature of an underlying inflammatory arthropathy (Ganguly et al. 2018). It should be noted that the fluid-like signal should always remain dorsal to the intermetatarsal ligament along the plantar surface without extending into it. Postcontrast sequences display peripheral enhancement (Fig. 26), whereas neuromas centrally enhance (Ganguly et al. 2018).

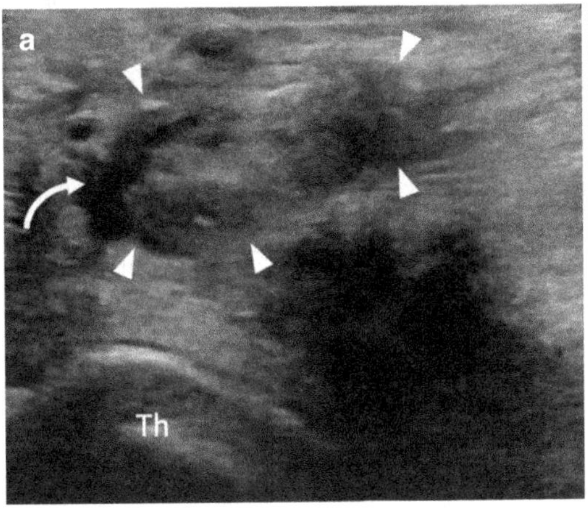

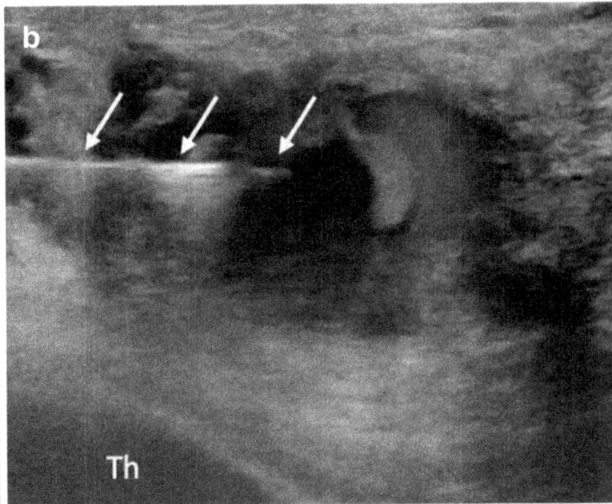

Fig. 25 Intermetatarsal bursopathy after surgical excision of an interdigital neuroma. (**a**) Longitudinal sonogram from the dorsal approach shows an irregular-shaped thickened bursa (arrowheads) with a small amount of compressible fluid (curved arrow). An US-guided corticosteroid injection (**b**) resulted in pain resolution (arrows indicate needle). In both images to the left is distal. *Th* thumb

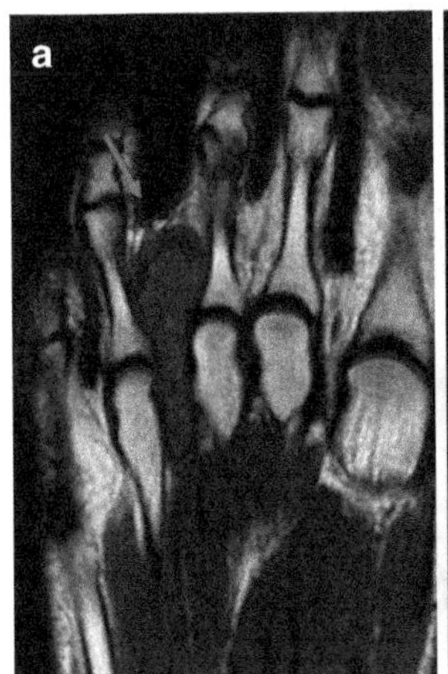

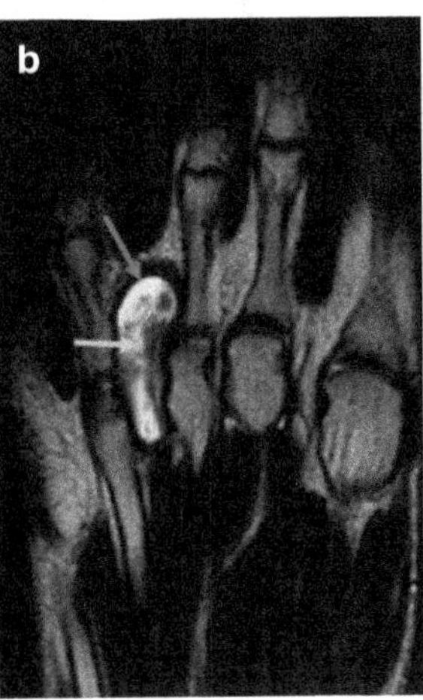

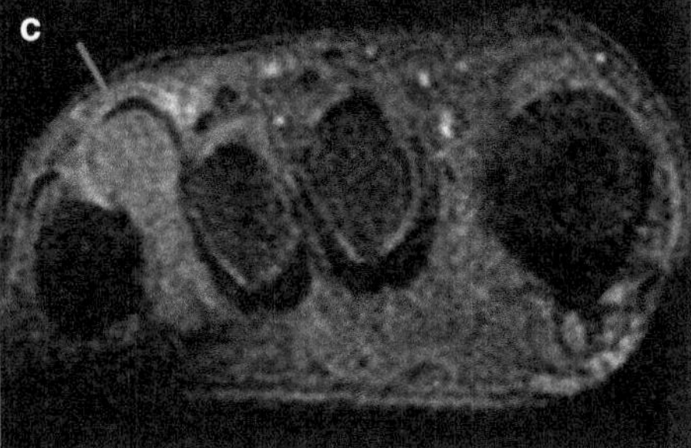

Fig. 26 Third-fourth intermetatarsal webspace bursopathy. Coronal T1 (**a**), Coronal T2 (**b**) and Coronal T1 FS postcontrast (**c**) MRI show a well-encapsulated fluid signal lesion in the third-fourth metatarsal web space. Intrinsic debris is noted (orange arrow) with no real appreciable enhancement post gadolinium

9.3 Plantar Fat Pad Miscellaneous Lesions

Abnormalities of the plantar fat pad are common and can either be a primary pain generator or occur in conjunction with other forefoot abnormalities such as plantar plate tears. Plantar fat pad thickening is the most common abnormality and is typically reactive due to biomechanical overload within the forefoot, such as is seen with hammertoe deformities. Histologically, this thickening is due to fibrotic changes with the fat pad (Studler et al. 2008). On US, the fat pad demonstrates hypoechoic thickening, occasionally with subtle hypervascularity (Fig. 27). An adventitial bursa may also develop within the plantar fat pad, often termed a submetatarsal bursopathy. Sonographically, a submetatarsal bursa appears as a well-demarcated area of increased hypoechogenicity, often with a small amount of fluid (Fig. 29). Compression will deform the bursa but volume is maintained. Repetitive trauma to a submetatarsal bursa may result in increased vascularity, suggesting inflammatory changes, and/or hemorrhage (Fig. 28d, e). A submetatarsal bursa is a common finding beneath the first and fifth MTP joints and is often asymptomatic. A submetatarsal bursa beneath the other lesser MTP joints is commonly symptomatic.

Although adventitial bursa are common in asymptomatic patients, they are typically smaller than those in symptomatic individuals. Bursitis typically occurs in the areas of maximal pressure, usually the heal and first and fifth metatarsal heads. It is the authors experience however that this is also present under the second metatarsal head which is a high weight-bearing area in patients with subsidence of the longitudinal foot arch and those with along second ray. MRI (Fig. 29) normally shows a fluid collection which

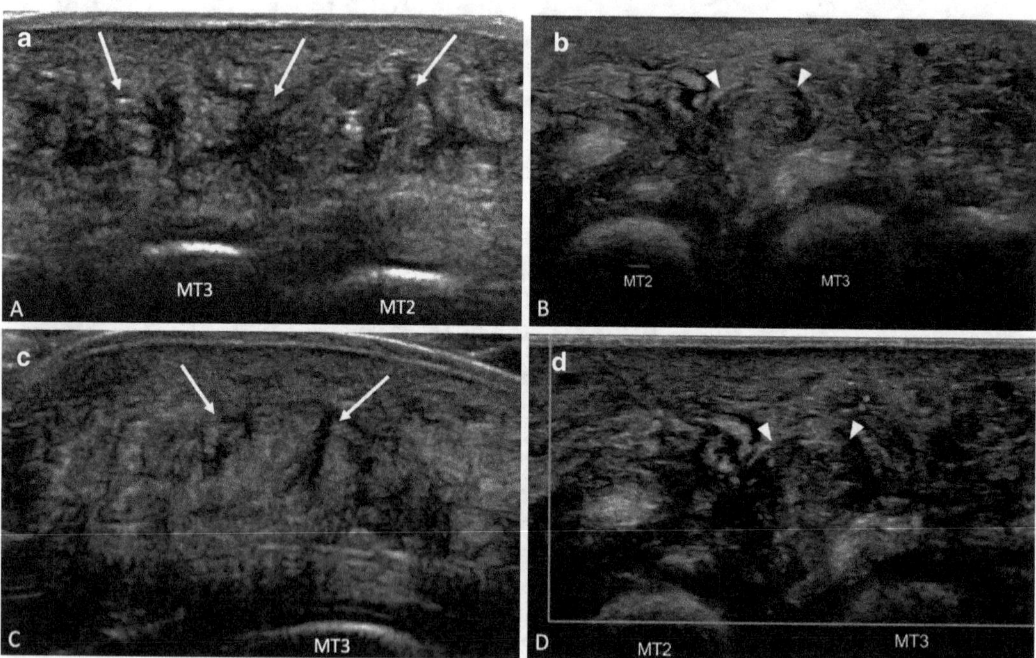

Fig. 27 Plantar fat pad fibrosis. Transverse (**a**) and longitudinal (**c**) sonograms of the plantar fat pad beneath the second and third MTP joints show diffuse thickening with interspersed hypoechoic tissue correlating with fat pad fibrosis (arrows). Sonograms (**b**) and with Doppler (**d**) also show hypoechoic thickening of the plantar fat pad beneath the second and third MTP joints associated with an interdigital neuroma (arrowheads) within the second metatarsal web space. Fat pad abnormalities often coexist with other forefoot pathology. *MT2* second metatarsal head, *MT3* third metatarsal head

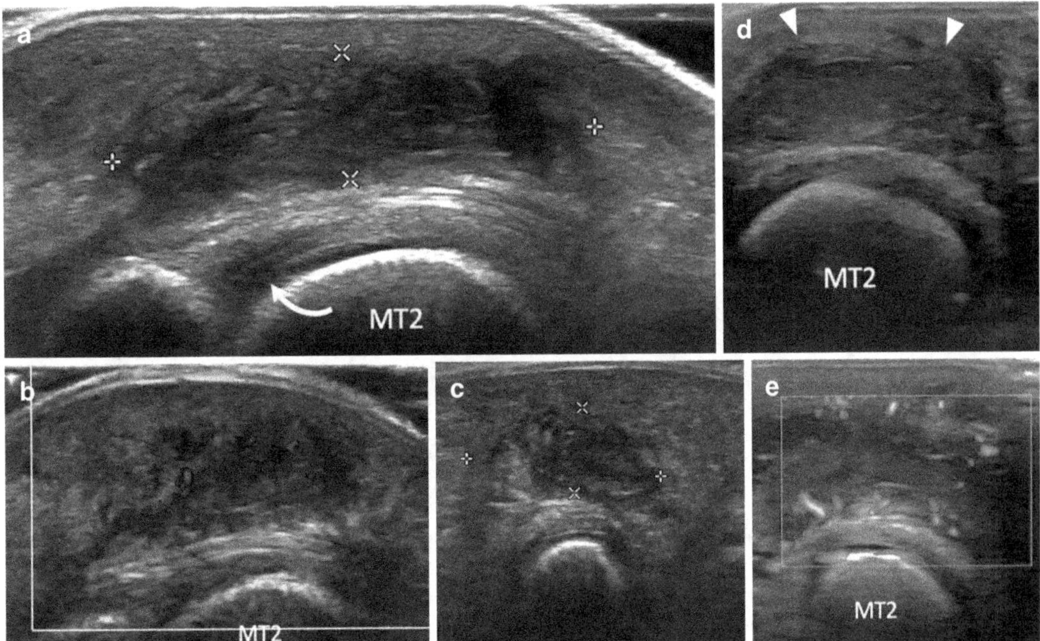

Fig. 28 Plantar fat pad adventitial (submetatarsal) bursopathy. Longitudinal sonogram (**a**) with Doppler (**b**) and transverse image (**c**) showing a fairly well-demarcated area of increased hypoechogenicity (between calipers) and mild vascularity beneath the second MTP joint. Note the early attritional appearing partial-thickness tear of the plantar plate (curved arrow in **a**). Sonograms (**d**) and (**e**) are longitudinal images with Doppler beneath the third MTP joint on a 52-year-old male with repetitive trauma to the forefoot from an exercise routine. Image (**d**) shows a well-demarcated hypoechoic bursa beneath the third MTP joint (arrowheads) with peripheral vascularity (**e**). An aspiration of the bursa revealed 2 cc of bloody fluid supporting the diagnosis of a hemorrhagic bursopathy

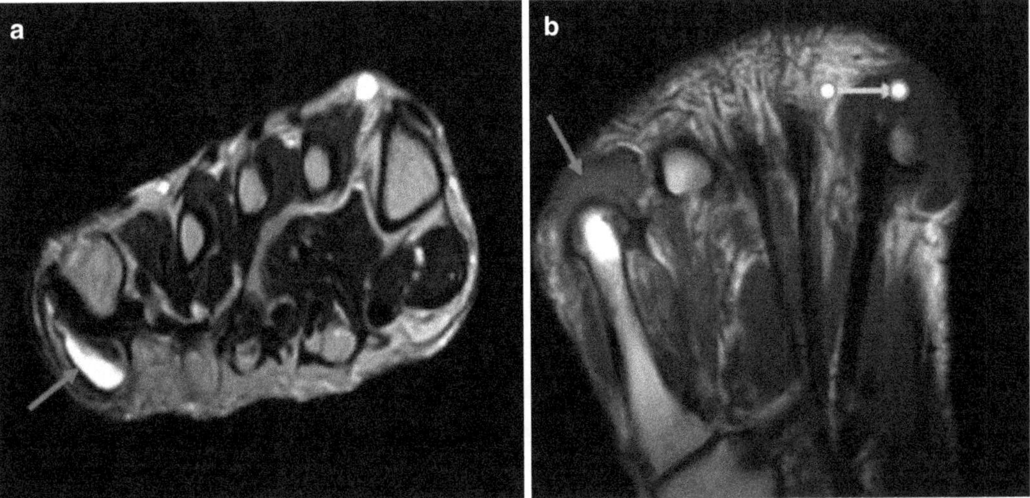

Fig. 29 Fifth metatarsal adventitial bursa. Coronal T2 (**a**) and axial T1 (**b**) show a fluid signal lesion deep to the fifth metatarsal head with some intrinsic synovitis. It closely related to and arising from the adventitial bursa. A similar but more prominent lesion is seen in the first metatarsal head

may exhibit rather heterogenous T2W SI due to the coexistence of fibrosis and inflammatory tissue, the latter especially so if in the plantar fat pad (Fig. 30).

Calluses and plantar warts are frequent causes of plantar forefoot pain and readily imaged with US. Sonographically, calluses primarily involve thickening of the epidermis, although there may be associated thickening of the underlying dermis and fat pad in more advanced cases (Fig. 31). Plantar warts most commonly appear as a fusiform shaped, hypoechoic mass that arises from the epidermis and ingrowth into the dermis and occasionally into the superficial subcutaneous

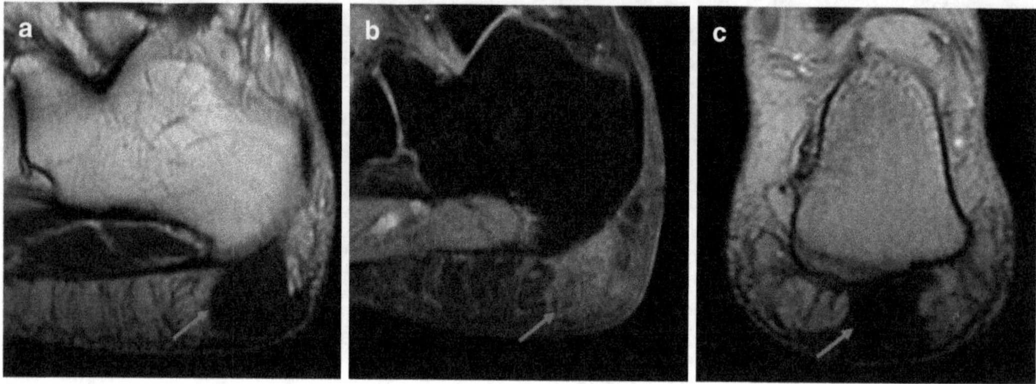

Fig. 30 Plantar adventitial bursa. Sagittal T1 (**a**), Sagittal T1 FS (**b**), and Coronal T2 (**c**) MRI show a low signal lesion centered over the plantar fat pad. There is mild increased signal on the T1 FS sequences which extends to the skin surface. The location and overall appearances are consistent with a bursa with some intrinsic fibrous reactive signal change

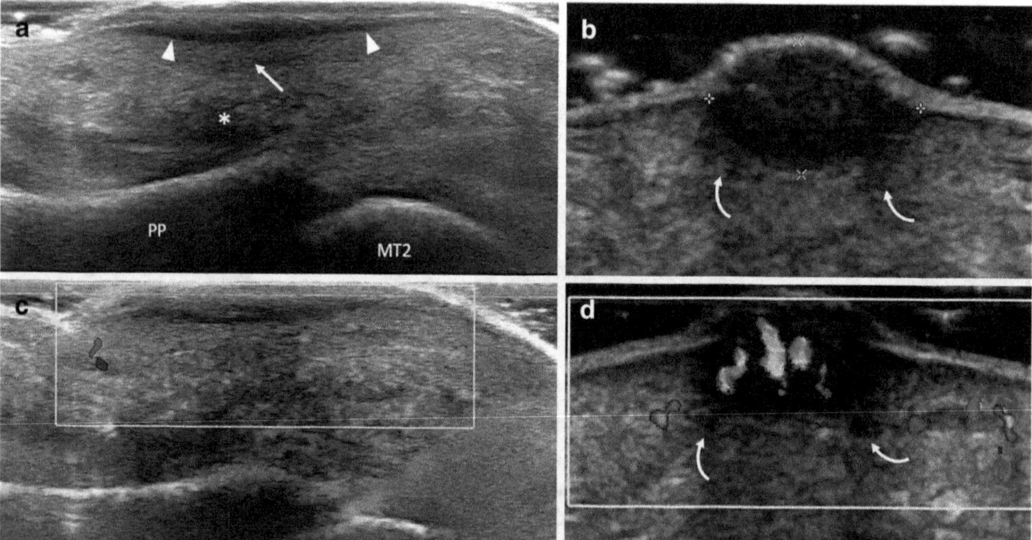

Fig. 31 Plantar fat pad callus and plantar wart. Longitudinal sonogram (**a**) with Doppler (**c**) shows a plantar callus beneath the second MTP joint. The callus appears as a hypoechoic thickening of the epidermal and dermal layers of the skin (arrowheads). Note the faint shadowing (arrow) and hypoechoic thickening of the underlying plantar fat pad (asterisks). Also note that the callus does not have internal vascularity (**c**). Image (**b**) is a longitudinal sonogram of a plantar wart showing a hypoechoic mass (between calipers) that extends beyond the epidermal layer and into the dermis. Doppler imaging (**d**) reveals arterial blood flow within the mass characteristic of a plantar wart. The deep border of a plantar wart is often irregular (curved arrows in both **b** and **d**) due to the viral-induced proliferation and ingrowth into the dermal tissue

tissue. Hypervascularity within the plantar wart is a common feature (Wortsman 2012) (Fig. 32). Plantar warts are not usually an indication for MRI but if done shows up as a deep, subcutaneous localized area of inflammatory soft tissue.

Foreign bodies (FB) within the plantar fat pad can be readily identified with US. Their appearance is based on the underlying FB material. Glass and metallic objects are brightly echogenic often with acoustic shadowing (Fig. 33). Wood splinters are also hyperechoic as compared to the surrounding fat pad but less bright than glass or metal. Acoustic shadowing is less common. Frequently, there is edema and

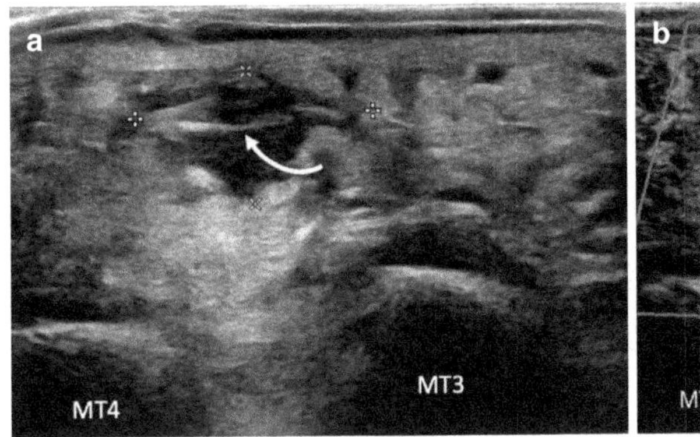

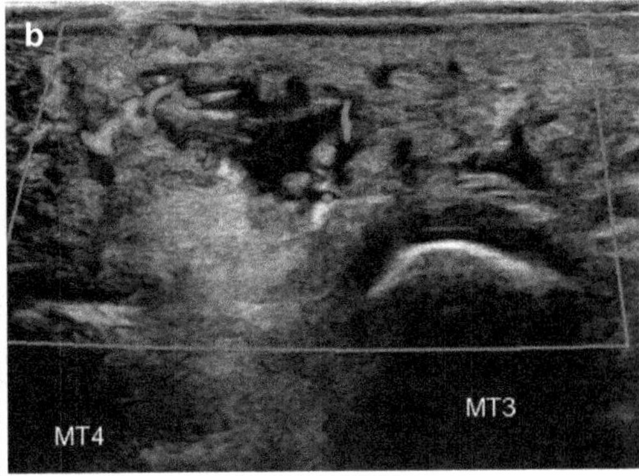

Fig. 32 Glass foreign body (FB) within the plantar fat pad beneath the third metatarsal interspace. A 38-year-old female with a painful plantar fat pad 1 week after stepping on some broken glass. Transverse sonogram (**a**) reveals an echogenic irregularly shaped FB (curved arrow) with surrounding fluid (between calipers). Doppler imaging (**b**) shows peripheral vascularity suggesting an inflammatory reaction. Surgical excision confirmed the presence of a small disc-shaped glass chard surrounded by purulent fluid consistent with a small abscess

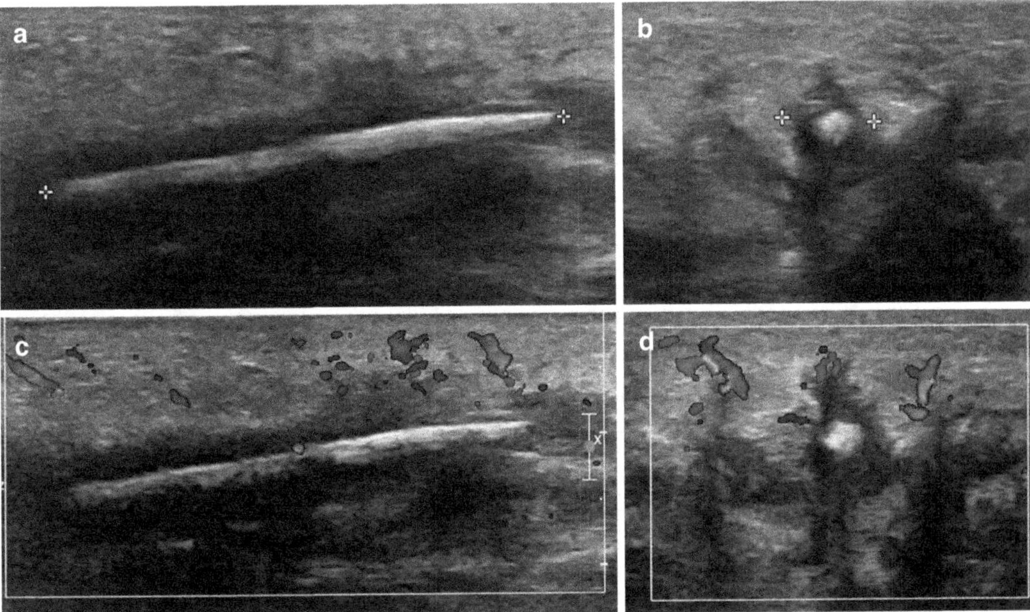

Fig. 33 Wood foreign body (FB) within the plantar fat pad beneath the second metatarsal interspace. A 29-year-old female stepped on toothpick that was hidden in a carpet. Longitudinal sonogram (**a**) with Doppler (**c**) and transverse image (**b**) with Doppler (**d**) show a FB lodged within the plantar fat pad (between calipers) with surrounding edema and vascularity. Ultrasound was utilized to guide a mini-hemostat to the FB for removal

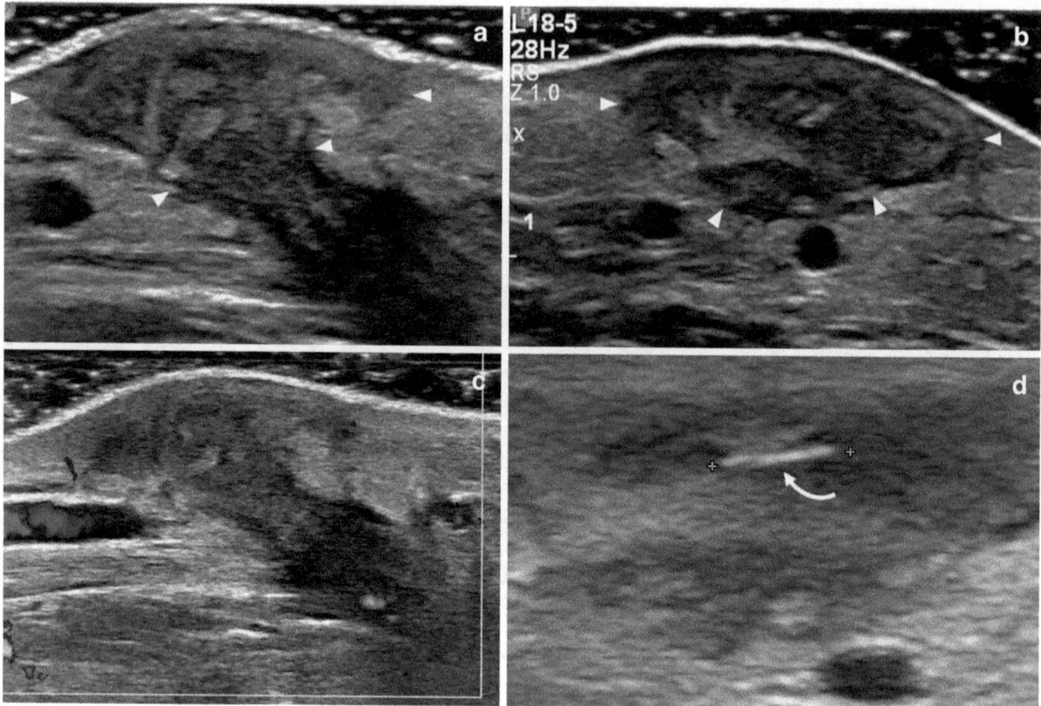

Fig. 34 Dorsal foot abscess with foreign body material. A 7-year-old male with painful dorsal foot mass over the third metatarsal interspace and no history of injury. Longitudinal (**a**) and transverse (**b**) sonograms show a well-demarcated mixed echogenic mass that extends from the dermis to the deep subcutaneous tissue (arrowheads). Longitudinal sonogram with Doppler (**c**) does not show vascularity. A longitudinal sonogram (**d**) revealed foreign body material (curved arrow). Surgical exploration confirmed the presence of an abscess and small fragments of rubber

vascularity of the subcutaneous tissue or fat pad surrounding the FB. On MRI, the appearances of foreign body reactions are variable. They are typically low on T1 WI while surrounding granulation tissue is often high signal on T2 WI. Adjacent perifascial soft tissues normally show heterogeneously high signal on fluid sensitive sequences and low signal on T1 WI with rather significant contrast enhancement (Ganguly et al. 2018; Peterson et al. 2002).

Abscess formation around the FB can also occur and be identified with US (Fig. 34). On MRI, abscesses usually show a well- or ill-defined fluid collection, which is often associated with reactive osseous edema. In cases where the FB is very small, changes in the fat pad may be a clue to the location of the FB.

10 Plantar Plate Degeneration and Tear

Plantar plate abnormalities of the lesser MTP joints generally arise from chronic attritional stresses and less commonly from an acute traumatic injury (Smith and Coughlin 2009). The plantar plate of the second MTP joint is the most often affected followed by the third MTP joint (Nery et al. 2014). Lesser plantar plate abnormalities may involve multiple joints and correlation with sonopalpation is important for determining clinical relevance. The sonographic evaluation of the plantar plates should include both longitudinal and transverse images. Early changes of an attritional plantar plate tear include an increase in hypoechogenicity and anechoic clefts at its

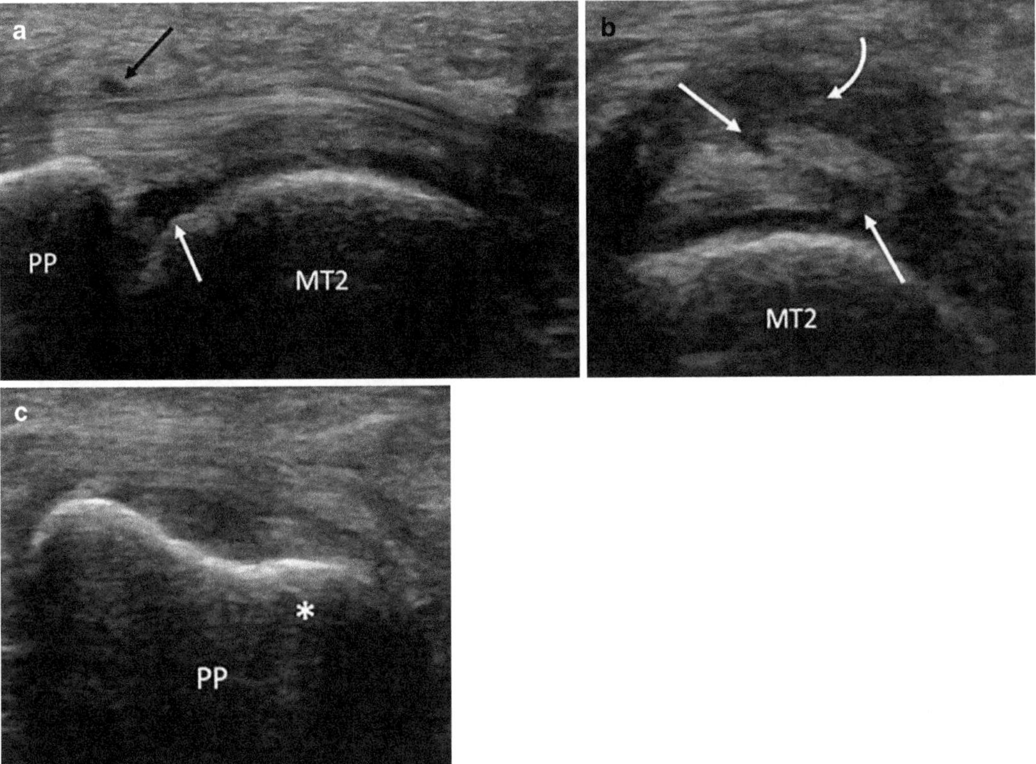

Fig. 35 Full-thickness plantar plate tear of the second MTP joint. Longitudinal (**a**) and transverse (**b**) sonograms of an obliquely oriented full-thickness tear of the plantar plate (white arrows) at its attachment onto the proximal phalanx (PP). Note that the full-thickness nature of the tear is best revealed on the transverse image (**b**). Also note that in the longitudinal image (**a**) there is a very small amount of fluid at the plantar surface of the flexor tendon suggesting a full-thickness tear (black arrow). (**c**) Is a transverse sonogram of the condyles of the PP which, in this case, shows that the bony cortex where the plantar plate attaches onto the lateral condyle is minimally altered (asterisk). Also note that the overlying flexor tendons are hypoechoic due to anisotropy (curved arrow). *MT2* second metatarsal head

enthesis representing partial-thickness tearing (Fig. 35). These early changes typically start at the insertion onto the lateral condyle of the proximal phalanx. As the tear progresses, fluid is often visualized adjacent to the plantar cortex of the proximal phalanx indicating a full-thickness tear (Fig. 37). It is important to image the plantar plate in orthogonal views to reveal the full extent of the tear. In addition, carefully following the plantar plate to its insertion onto the condyles of the proximal phalanx may reveal bony irregularities and hypertrophic changes of the condyles which is often an important pain generator (Fig. 36). This most often occurs at the lateral condyle of the second MTP joint. In the more advanced stages of plantar plate tears, MTP joint instability may ensue. Normally, the proximal phalanx and metatarsal head should be in the same sagittal plane. Dorsal displacement of the proximal phalanx relative to the metatarsal head is indicative of joint instability, and this can be dynamically assessed by applying a dorsally directed pressure to the proximal phalanx.

Acute tears of the plantar plates of the lesser MTP joints are uncommon but will often result in joint instability (Fig. 37). Radiographs are important to rule out associated fractures. The most sensitive sign of a plantar plate tear on MRI is high-signal intensity on fluid sensitive sequences (Yamada et al. 2017). The tear can be

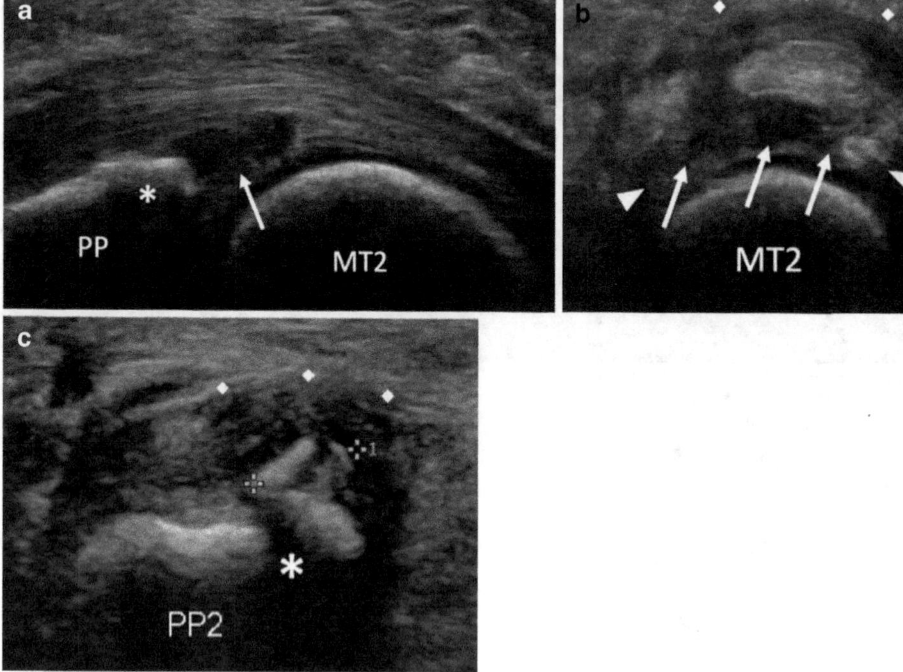

Fig. 36 Full-thickness plantar plate tear with advanced bony changes of the lateral condyle of the proximal phalanx (PP). Longitudinal (**a**) and transverse (**b**) sonograms show an extensive attritional appearing full-thickness plantar plate tear (arrows). In (**a**) there are mild cortical irregularities at the insertion of the plantar plate tear onto the lateral condyle of the PP (asterisk). The transverse sonogram in (**c**) of the condyles of the PP reveals extensive bony irregularity and a large bony projection of the lateral condyle (asterisk and between the calipers) with adjacent fat pad thickening (diamonds). These bony changes corresponded to the maximal location of tenderness with sonopalpation. Also note that the transverse image of the condyles of the PP (**c**) is the best plane to evaluate for these bony changes which are often underestimated on the longitudinal view (asterisk in **a**). Finally, despite the full-thickness tear, the plantar cortex of both the PP and MT in the longitudinal image (**a**) are in the same sagittal plane indicating the absence of dorsal instability of the PP in respect to the MT

either partial or complete with varying amounts of fluid interposed. Other indirect signs have also been described in literature including the pseudoneuroma sign (Umans et al. 2014, 2016). Here, there is a pericapsular ill-defined soft tissue thickening and inflammatory change which is eccentric to the intermetatarsal space. This can mimic a neuroma but are asymmetric in relation to the vertical axis of the intermetatarsal space (Umans et al. 2016). In addition, the signal changes are more ill-defined and nodular rather than mass like as seen in neuromas. Overt thickening and/or thinning of the interosseous tendon–collateral ligament complex is also a known indirect sign of plantar plate tears (Yamada et al. 2017).

Although not necessarily specific for MRI, Coughlin et al. (2011) proposed a classification system for grading plantar tears:

- Grade 0—Plantar plate degeneration without a discrete tear.
- Grade 1—Transverse tear adjacent to the proximal phalanx insertion, but involving <50% the insertion width (Fig. 38).
- Grade 2—As above but involving >50% of the insertion width.
- Grade 3—Extensive tear with vertical and/or longitudinal components.
- Grade 4—Extensive tear with both vertical and longitudinal components and a buttonhole deformity.

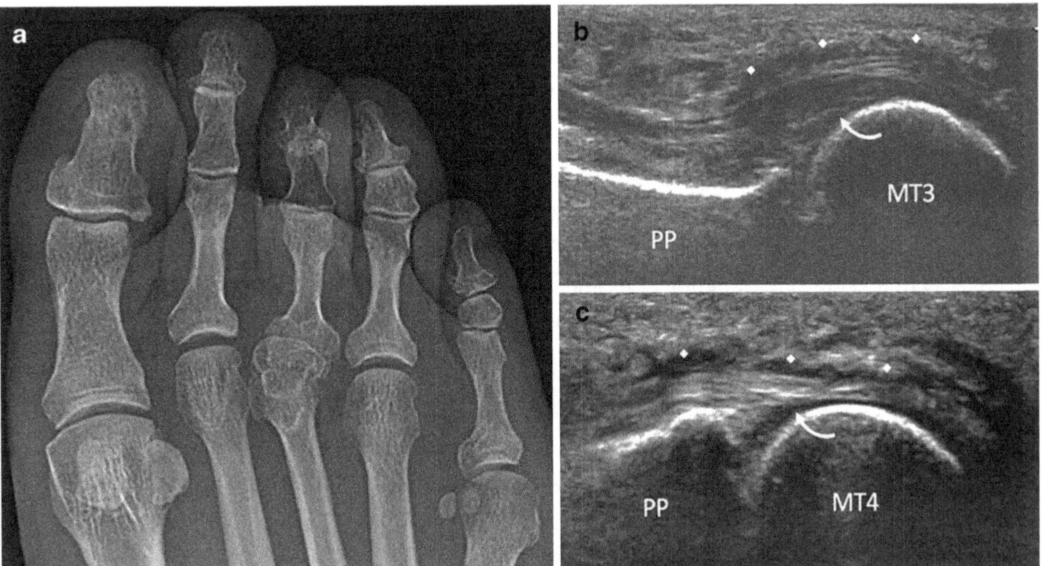

Fig. 37 Acute traumatic rupture of the plantar plates of the third and fourth MTP joints resulting in dorsal dislocation of the third MTP joint. AP radiograph (**a**) of the right foot showing dorsal dislocation of the third MTP joint. Longitudinal sonograms of the plantar plate of the third MTP joint (**b**) and fourth MTP joint (**c**) show complete rupture of the plantar plate with associated edema within the plantar fat pad (diamonds). The curved arrows in (**b**) and (**c**) show an absent plantar plate with the flexor tendons located adjacent to the metatarsal head. *MT3* third metatarsal head, *MT4* fourth metatarsal head

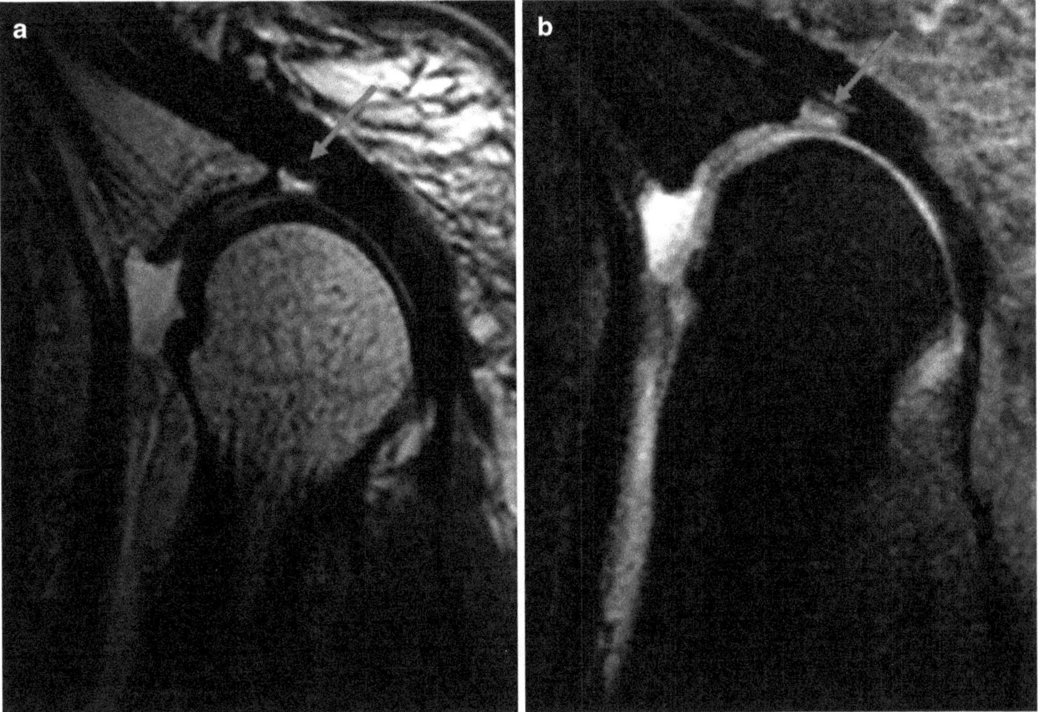

Fig. 38 Degenerate plantar plate tear. PD sagittal (**a**) and T1 sagittal FS (**b**) MRI shows a chronic attritional tear (red arrow) of the distal phalangeal attachment of the left fourth toe plantar plate. No soft tissue or marrow edema is seen

11 Mass Lesions

Forefoot masses encompass a broad spectrum of pathology. The most common mass in this region is a ganglion cyst which typically originates from the MTP joint and less commonly from a tendon (Longo et al. 2016). Occasionally, a ganglion cyst may originate from a midfoot joint and dissect its way to the forefoot. Ganglion cysts appear as encapsulated, hypoechoic or anechoic, non-compressible masses, often multilobulated or septated. There is no internal vascularity, although peripheral vascularity may be present. Increased through transmission is characteristic although not specific. The most common location for ganglion cysts in the forefoot includes the interspaces and on the plantar surface of the plantar plates (Fig. 39). On MRI, ganglion cysts appear as sharply delineated cysts which follow water-equivalent signal on all pulse sequences (Fig. 39). They can be uni/multilocular, have septations but will typically show peripheral rim enhancement on postcontrast sequences (Ganguly et al. 2018).

Nerve sheath tumors and tenosynovial giant cell tumors can occur in the forefoot (Zhang et al. 2013). Nerve sheath tumors appear as a well-defined, solid, hypoechoic mass that is in continuity with a peripheral nerve (Fig. 40). Hyperemia is common as is increased through transmission (Reynolds Jr et al. 2004). On MRI, typical benign peripheral nerve sheath tumors show a central area of low T2 and peripheral high T2 signal, known as the "target sign." Within the low central area of T2 signal, individual nerve bundles can sometimes be seen, termed the "fascicle," sign (Kakkar et al. 2015). However, these signs are not always seen in smaller lesions and indeed the lesion can exhibit more cystic signal internal reflective of the abundant myxoid content (Fig. 40).

Tenosynovial giant cell tumors in the forefoot most commonly appear as a homogenous hypoechoic mass adjacent to a tendon with abundant flow on Doppler imaging. The substance of the mass may appear as solid or cystic (Zhang et al. 2013). On MRI, they usually depict iso-hypointense signal to skeletal muscle on T1W

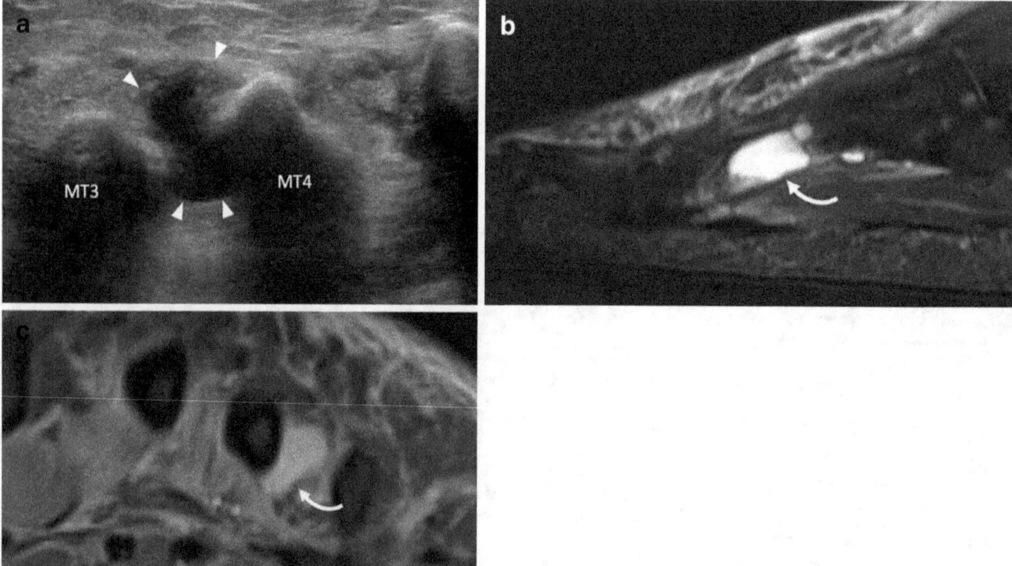

Fig. 39 Ganglion cyst within the third metatarsal interspace. A 39-year-old female referred for a presumed diagnosis of a third metatarsal interspace interdigital neuroma. Transverse sonogram (**a**) of the third interspace from a plantar approach reveals a ganglion cyst (arrowheads). Correlative MR images (**b**) and (**c**) confirm a ganglion cyst within the third MT interspace (curved arrow). *MT3* third metatarsal head, *MT4* fourth metatarsal head

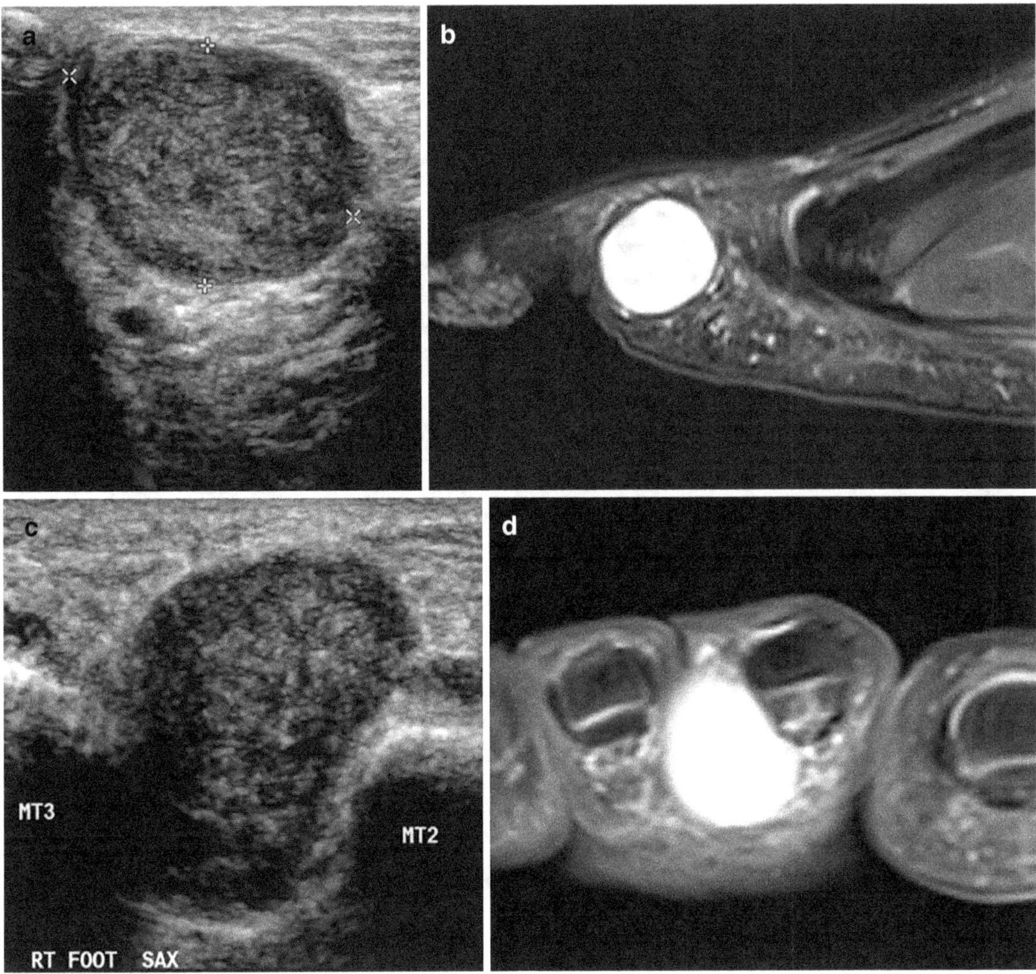

Fig. 40 Nerve sheath tumor within the second metatarsal interspace. A 43-year-old male with enlarging painful second MT interspace mass. Excisional biopsy revealed a schwannoma. Longitudinal sonogram (**a**) and transverse sonogram from a plantar approach (**c**) show a solid well-demarcated homogenous hypoechoic mass that fills the interspace (between calipers). Corresponding MR images (**b**) and (**d**) with intravenous gadolinium reveals a large enhancing mass within the interspace. Note that in the transverse US image (**c**) and corresponding coronal MR image (**d**) the schwannoma has a more plantar location within the interspace since it arises from the interdigital nerve which is located deep to the deep transverse metatarsal ligament

and heterogeneously hypointense on T2W sequences due to the paramagnetic effect of hemosiderin (Wang et al. 2017) (Fig. 41). Prominent heterogenous contrast enhancement has been described following gadolinium administration.

Plantar fibromatosis, also known as ledderhose disease is most commonly seen in patients with diabetes and epilepsy. On ultrasound, a plantar fibroma is typically seen as a small, well-circumscribed hypoechoic lesion. It usually arises from the medial and central band of the plantar fascia with some intrinsic color doppler flow (Fig. 42) (Nduka et al. 2021). On MRI, they are mainly of low signal intensity on T1- and T2 WI with variable postcontrast appearances (Fig. 43). Aggressive fibromatosis surrounds and entraps skeletal muscle with a high recurrence rate. The variable histologic composition results in variable MRI signal (Robbin et al. 2001).

Malignant tumors in this region are uncommon, with synovial sarcoma being the most com-

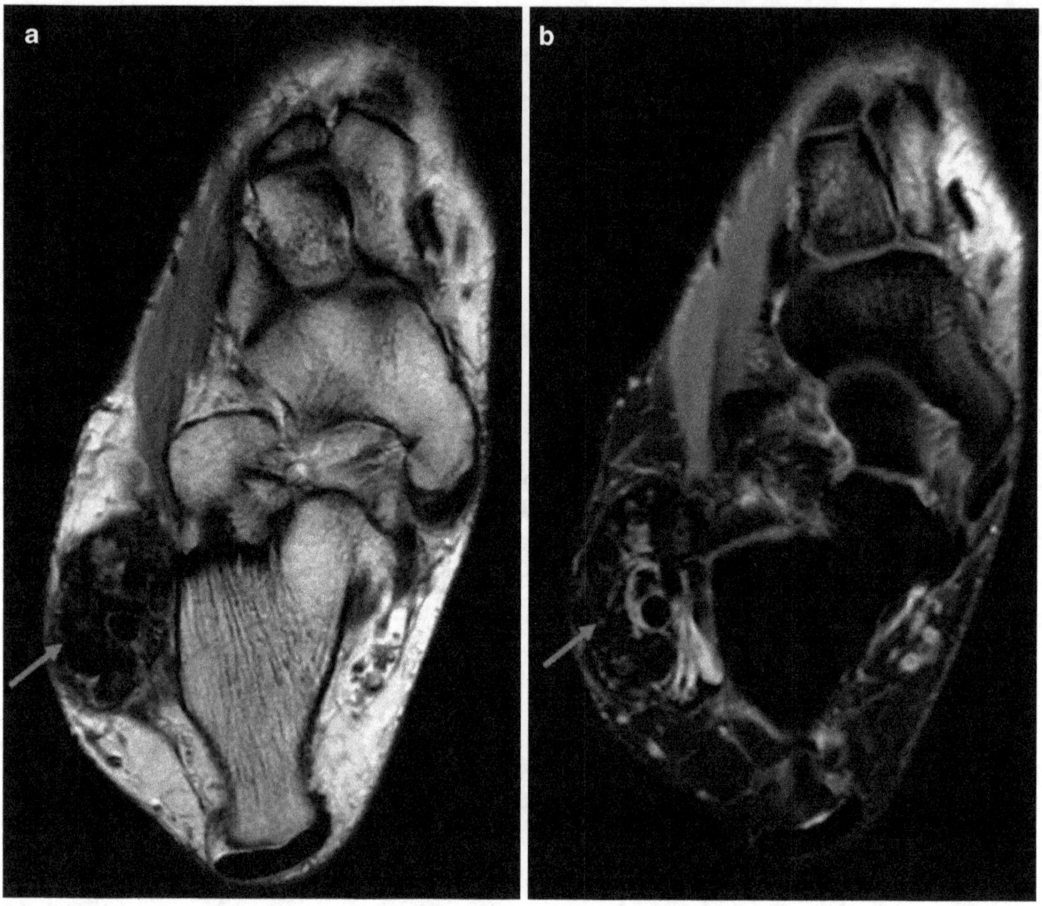

Fig. 41 Tenosynovial giant cell tumor. PD axial (**a**) and PD FS axial (**b**) show a diffuse low signal mass adjacent to the calcaneocuboid joint. It shows mildly heterogenous low signal throughout and is centered over the peroneal tendon sheath consistent with TCGCT

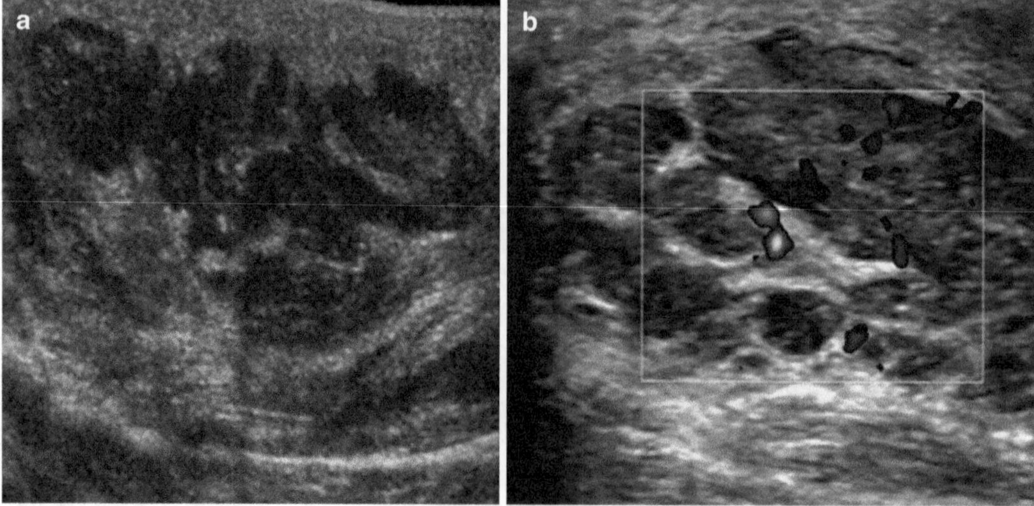

Fig. 42 Plantar fibromatosis. Ultrasound spot image (**a**) shows a diffuse hypoechoic echotexture mass centered over the plantar fascia. It has a lobular morphology with mild intrinsic neo vascularity on power doppler (**b**)

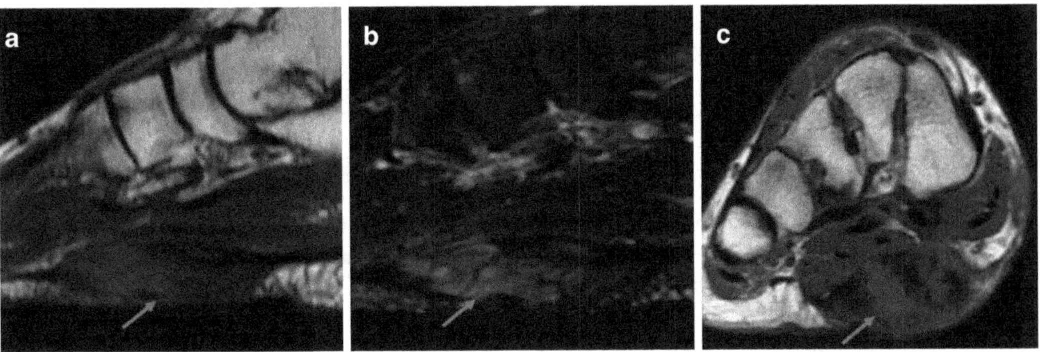

Fig. 43 Plantar fibromatosis. Sagittal T1 (**a**), sagittal STIR (**b**), and coronal T1 (**c**) show a low signal lesion centered over the central band of the plantar fascia. Show fibrous signal striations with mild heterogenous signal traverse through the lesion typical for fibromatosis

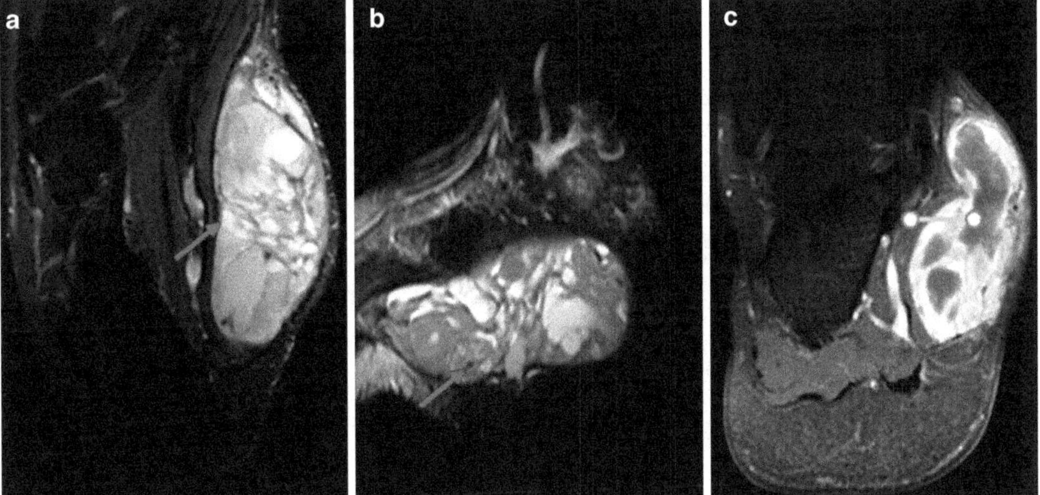

Fig. 44 Synovial sarcoma. PD SPAIR axial (**a**), sagittal PD SPAR (**b**), and coronal T1 FS post gad (**c**) show a heterogenous signal lesion within the medial foot soft tissues. It shows mixed signal throughout (red arrows) with hemorrhage, solid soft tissue, and cystic foci throughout. Postcontrast sequences reveals prominent central necrosis with peripheral rim enhancement (orange arrow), typical of synovial sarcoma

mon in a large case series (Kransdorf 1995). The sonographic appearance of malignant tumors may mimic other benign tumors, and tissue biopsy is often required for definitive diagnosis. Sonographic features that suggest malignancy include mixed, complex echogenicity, irregular borders, invasion of surrounding structures, and abundant vascularity (Wu and Hochman 2009). On MRI, synovial sarcoma is usually seen in the juxta-articular location with infiltrating margins. A triple signal pattern has been described, with areas of solid, cystic and hemorrhagic signal (Fig. 44) (Waldt et al. 2003). The more solid portion of the lesion tends to show avid enhancement and should be targeted during biopsy.

12 Conclusion

Disorders of the lesser metatarsals are common, with imaging playing a key role in determining the etiologies of LM. A systematic approach should be taken when performing US evaluation of this region, and a thorough understanding of the sonoanatomy is imperative in order to make an accurate diagnosis. In many cases, however, cross-sectional imaging in the form of MRI will be needed for further characterization. Radiologists should be aware of the US and MRI appearances of the most common entities causing lesser metatarsalgia, with many conditions mimicking each other, especially an interdigital neuroma. It is reassuring however that most are in fact benign and easily characterized with appropriate clinical history and various pathognomonic imaging features.

References

Anderson MW, Greenspan A (1996) Stress fractures. Radiology 199:1–12

Ashman CJ, Klecker R, Yu J (2001) Forefoot pain involving the metatarsal region: differential diagnosis with MR imaging. Radiographics 21:1425–1440

Banal F, Etchepare F, Rouhier B, Rosenberg C, Foltz V, Rozenberg S et al (2006) Ultrasound ability in early diagnosis of stress fracture of metatarsal bone. Ann Rheum Dis 65(7):977–978

Berrady MA, Hmouri I, Benabdesslam A, Berrada MS, El Yaacoubi M (2014) Tuberculosis arthritis of the metatarsal phalangeal: a rare location. Pan Afr Med J 17:323. https://doi.org/10.11604/pamj.2014.17.323.4220. PMID: 25328618; PMCID: PMC4198287

Brockbank JE, Stein M, Schentag CT, Gladman DD (2005) Dactylitis in psoriatic arthritis: a marker for disease severity? Ann Rheum Dis 64(2):188–190. https://doi.org/10.1136/ard.2003.018184

Cohen SL, Miller TT, Ellis SJ, Roberts MM, DiCarlo EF (2016) Sonography of Morton neuromas: what are we really looking at? J Ultrasound Med 35(10):2191–2195. https://doi.org/10.7863/ultra.15.11022. Epub 2016 Aug 25. PMID: 27562973

Coughlin MJ, Baumfeld DS, Nery C (2011) Second MTP joint instability: grading of the deformity and description of surgical repair of capsular insufficiency. Phys Sportsmed 39:132–141

de Ávila Fernandes E, Kubota ES, Sandim GB, Mitraud SA, Ferrari AJ, Fernandes AR (2011) Ultrasound features of tophi in chronic tophaceous gout. Skeletal Radiol 40(3):309–315. https://doi.org/10.1007/s00256-010-1008-z

Fredericson M, Bergman AG, Hoffman KL, Dillingham MS (1995) Tibial stress reaction in runners: correlation of clinical symptoms and scintigraphy with a new magnetic resonance imaging grading system. Am J Sports Med 23:472–481

Ganguly A, Warner J, Aniq H (2018) Central metatarsalgia and walking on pebbles: beyond Morton neuroma. AJR Am J Roentgenol 210(4):821–833. https://doi.org/10.2214/AJR.17.18460. Epub 2018 Feb 22. PMID: 29470159

Gates LS, Arden NK, Hannan MT, Roddy E, Gill TK, Hill CL, Dufour AB, Rathod-Mistry T, Thomas MJ, Menz HB, Bowen CJ, Golightly YM (2019) Prevalence of foot pain across an international consortium of population-based cohorts. Arthritis Care Res (Hoboken) 71(5):661–670. https://doi.org/10.1002/acr.23829. PMID: 30592547; PMCID: PMC6483849

Gehrmann RM, Renard RL (2006) Current concepts review: stress fractures of the foot. Foot Ankle Int 27(9):750–757. https://doi.org/10.1177/107110070602700919

Giakoumis M, Ryan JD, Jani J (2013) Histologic evaluation of intermetatarsal Morton's neuroma. J Am Podiatr Med Assoc 103(3):218–222. https://doi.org/10.7547/1030218. PMID: 23697728

Gregg J, Silberstein M, Schneider T, Marks P (2006) Sonographic and MRI evaluation of the plantar plate: a prospective study. Eur Radiol 16(12):2661–2669. https://doi.org/10.1007/s00330-006-0345-8. Epub 2006 Jul 4. PMID: 16819605

Gregg JM, Schneider T, Marks P (2008) MR imaging and ultrasound of metatarsalgia—the lesser metatarsals. Radiol Clin North Am 46(6):1061–78, vi–vii. https://doi.org/10.1016/j.rcl.2008.09.004. PMID: 19038613

Hoffman DF, Adams E, Bianchi S (2015) Ultrasonography of fractures in sports medicine. Br J Sports Med 49(3):152–160. https://doi.org/10.1136/bjsports-2014-094217

Kaeley GS, Eder L, Aydin SZ, Gutierrez M, Bakewell C (2018) Dactylitis: a hallmark of psoriatic arthritis. Semin Arthritis Rheum 48(2):263–273. https://doi.org/10.1016/j.semarthrit.2018.02.002

Kakkar C, Shetty CM, Koteshwara P, Bajpai S (2015) Telltale signs of peripheral neurogenic tumors on magnetic resonance imaging. Indian J Radiol Imaging 25(4):453–458. https://doi.org/10.4103/0971-3026.169447. PMID: 26752825; PMCID: PMC4693395

Kay D, Bennett GL (2003) Morton's neuroma. Foot Ankle Clin 8(1):49–59. https://doi.org/10.1016/s1083-7515(03)00004-4

König H, Sieper J, Wolf KJ (1990) Rheumatoid arthritis: evaluation of hypervascular and fibrous pannus with dynamic MR imaging enhanced with Gd-DTPA. Radiology 176(2):473–477. https://doi.org/10.1148/radiology.176.2.2367663. PMID: 2367663

Kransdorf MJ (1995) Malignant soft-tissue tumors in a large referral population: distribution of diagnoses by age, sex, and location. AJR Am J Roentgenol 164(1):129–134. https://doi.org/10.2214/ajr.164.1.7998525. PMID: 7998525

Linklater JM, Bird SJ (2016) Imaging of lesser metatarsophalangeal joint plantar plate degeneration, tear, and repair. Semin Musculoskelet Radiol 20(2):192–204.

https://doi.org/10.1055/s-0036-1581115. Epub 2016 Jun 23. PMID: 27336453

Löffler C, Sattler H, Peters L, Löffler U, Uppenkamp M, Bergner R (2014) Distinguishing gouty arthritis from calcium pyrophosphate disease and other arthritides. J Rheumatol 42. https://doi.org/10.3899/jrheum.140634

Longo V, Jacobson JA, Dong Q, Kim SM (2016) Tumors and tumor-like abnormalities of the midfoot and forefoot. Semin Musculoskelet Radiol 20(2):154–166. https://doi.org/10.1055/s-0036-1581118. Epub 2016 Jun 23. PMID: 27336450

Martinoli C (2010) Imaging of the peripheral nerves. Semin Musculoskelet Radiol 14(5):461–462. https://doi.org/10.1055/s-0030-1268395

Mlosek RK, Malinowska S (2013) Ultrasound image of the skin, apparatus and imaging basics. J Ultrason 13(53):212–221. https://doi.org/10.15557/JoU.2013.0021. Epub 2013 Jun 30. PMID: 26675386; PMCID: PMC4613587

Nduka JC, Lam K, Chandrasekar CR (2021) Diagnosing plantar fibromas - beware of sarcomas. Foot (Edinb) 49:101736. https://doi.org/10.1016/j.foot.2020.101736. Epub 2020 Sep 8. PMID: 33268229

Nery C, Coughlin MJ, Baumfeld D, Raduan FC, Mann TS, Catena F (2014) Prospective evaluation of protocol for surgical treatment of lesser MTP joint plantar plate tears. Foot Ankle Int 35(9):876–885. https://doi.org/10.1177/1071100714539659. Epub 2014 Jun 23. PMID: 24958766

Nouh MR, El-Gawad EAA, Abdulsalam SM (2015) MRI utility in patients with non-traumatic metatarsalgia: a tertiary musculoskeletal center observational study. Egypt J Radiol Nucl Med 46(4):1057–1064. https://doi.org/10.1016/j.ejrnm.2015.08.004

Peterson JJ, Bancroft LW, Kransdorf MJ (2002) Wooden foreign bodies: imaging appearance. AJR Am J Roentgenol 178:557–562

Quinn TJ, Jacobson JA, Craig JG, van Holsbeeck MT (2000) Sonography of Morton's neuromas. AJR Am J Roentgenol 174(6):1723–1728. https://doi.org/10.2214/ajr.174.6.1741723. PMID: 10845513

Reynolds DL Jr, Jacobson JA, Inampudi P, Jamadar DA, Ebrahim FS, Hayes CW (2004) Sonographic characteristics of peripheral nerve sheath tumors. AJR Am J Roentgenol 182(3):741–744. https://doi.org/10.2214/ajr.182.3.1820741. PMID: 14975979

Ritchlin CT, Kavanaugh A, Gladman DD, Mease PJ, Helliwell P, Boehncke WH, de Vlam K, Fiorentino D, Fitzgerald O, Gottlieb AB, McHugh NJ, Nash P, Qureshi AA, Soriano ER, Taylor WJ, Group for Research and Assessment of Psoriasis and Psoriatic Arthritis (GRAPPA) (2009) Treatment recommendations for psoriatic arthritis. Ann Rheum Dis 68(9):1387–1394. https://doi.org/10.1136/ard.2008.094946. Epub 2008 Oct 24. PMID: 18952643; PMCID: PMC2719080

Robbin MR, Murphey MD, Temple T et al (2001) Imaging of musculoskeletal fibromatosis. Radiographics 21:585–600

Scranton PE Jr (1980) Metatarsalgia: diagnosis and treatment. J Bone Joint Surg Am 62(5):723–732. PMID: 7391095

Smith BW, Coughlin MJ (2009) Disorders of the lesser toes. Sports Med Arthrosc Rev 17(3):167–174. https://doi.org/10.1097/JSA.0b013e3181a5cd26

Studler U, Mengiardi B, Bode B, Schöttle PB, Pfirrmann CW, Hodler J, Zanetti M (2008) Fibrosis and adventitious bursae in plantar fat pad of forefoot: MR imaging findings in asymptomatic volunteers and MR imaging-histologic comparison. Radiology 246(3):863–870. https://doi.org/10.1148/radiol.2463070196. Epub 2008 Jan 14. PMID: 18195378

Symeonidis PD, Iselin LD, Simmons N, Fowler S, Dracopoulos G, Stavrou P (2012) Prevalence of interdigital nerve enlargements in an asymptomatic population. Foot Ankle Int 33(7):543–547. https://doi.org/10.3113/FAI.2012.0543. PMID: 22835390

Umans H, Srinivasan R, Elsinger E, Wilde GE (2014) MRI of lesser metatarsophalangeal joint plantar plate tears and associated adjacent interspace lesions. Skeletal Radiol 43:1361–1368

Umans RL, Umans BD, Umans H, Elsinger E (2016) Predictive MRI correlates of lesser metatarsophalangeal joint plantar plate tear. Skeletal Radiol 45:969–975

van Dijk BT, Dakkak YJ, Matthijssen XME, Niemantsverdriet E, Reijnierse M, van der Helm-van Mil AHM (2022) Intermetatarsal bursitis, a novel feature of juxtaarticular inflammation in early rheumatoid arthritis related to clinical signs: results of a longitudinal magnetic resonance imaging study. Arthritis Care Res (Hoboken) 74(10):1713–1722. https://doi.org/10.1002/acr.24640. Epub 2022 Jul 16. PMID: 33973415

van Gent RN, Siem D, van Middelkoop M, van Os AG, Bierma-Zeinstra SM, Koes BW (2007) Incidence and determinants of lower extremity running injuries in long distance runners: a systematic review. Br J Sports Med 41(8):469–80; discussion 480. https://doi.org/10.1136/bjsm.2006.033548. Epub 2007 May 1. PMID: 17473005; PMCID: PMC2465455

Waldt S, Rechl H, Rummeny E, Woertler K (2003) Imaging of benign and malignant soft tissue masses of the foot. Eur Radiol 13:1125–1136

Wang C, Song RR, Kuang PD, Wang LH, Zhang MM (2017) Giant cell tumor of the tendon sheath: magnetic resonance imaging findings in 38 patients. Oncol Lett 13(6):4459–4462. https://doi.org/10.3892/ol.2017.6011. Epub 2017 Apr 7. PMID: 28599446; PMCID: PMC5452996

Wortsman X (2012) Common applications of dermatologic sonography. J Ultrasound Med 31(1):97–111. https://doi.org/10.7863/jum.2012.31.1.97. PMID: 22215775

Wu JS, Hochman MG (2009) Soft-tissue tumors and tumorlike lesions: a systematic imaging approach. Radiology 253(2):297–316. https://doi.org/10.1148/radiol.2532081199. PMID: 19864525

Yamada AF, Crema MD, Nery C, Baumfeld D, Mann TS, Skaf AY, Fernandes ADRC (2017) Second and third metatarsophalangeal plantar plate tears: diagnostic performance of direct and indirect MRI features using surgical findings as the reference standard. AJR Am J Roentgenol 209(2):W100–W108. https://doi.org/10.2214/AJR.16.17276. Epub 2017 Jun 1. PMID: 28570126

Zanetti M, Strehle JK, Zollinger H, Hodler J (1997) Morton neuroma and fluid in the intermetatarsal bursae on MR images of 70 asymptomatic volunteers. Radiology 203:516–520

Zhang Y, Huang J, Ma X, Wang X, Zhang C, Chen L (2013) Giant cell tumor of the tendon sheath in the foot and ankle: case series and review of the literature. J Foot Ankle Surg 52(1):24–27. https://doi.org/10.1053/j.jfas.2012.09.008. Epub 2012 Oct 22. PMID: 23085383

Tumors and Tumorlike Lesions

J. D. Fitzpatrick, Christine Azzopardi, D. A. Ritchie, A. M. Davies, and D. Vanel

Contents

1 Introduction

Musculoskeletal tumors and tumorlike lesions present a significant diagnostic challenge both clinically and radiologically. This is exacerbated in the foot and ankle where the proximity of multiple anatomical structures and tissues and the paucity of intervening fat or subcutaneous tissue create more uncertainty. The significant increase in availability and quality of advanced cross-sectional imaging over the years, particularly MRI, means that imaging is relied upon even more than before. However, imaging should not be considered in isolation as it is only one part of the diagnostic pathway. An understanding of the clinical context is vital if the reporter is to give a helpful, accurate, and specific differential diagnosis. With this in mind, this chapter begins by introducing the important non-imaging background/context including summaries of the relevant aspects of anatomy, epidemiology, clinical presentation, and management. Having established this important context, a more in-depth discussion of the imaging of these lesions is presented including specific imaging modalities, importance of a systematic approach to image interpretation, staging, biopsy, and follow-up. Finally, an illustrated review of lesions is presented, which is organized by the tissue of origin according to the latest WHO classification of soft tissue and bone tumors (5th edition, 2020).

2 Non-imaging Background

2.1 Relevant Anatomy

The anatomy of the foot and ankle is complex, with multiple tendons, muscles, and neurovascular bundles, which are closely opposed to and overlap each other. Both the foot and ankle are

J. D. Fitzpatrick · C. Azzopardi (✉) · A. M. Davies
The Royal Orthopaedic Hospital, Birmingham, UK
e-mail: chrsitine.azzopardi1@nhs.net

D. A. Ritchie
Royal Liverpool University Hospitals, Liverpool, UK

D. Vanel
Institut Gustave Roussy, Villejuif, France

Med Radiol Diagn Imaging (2023)

https://doi.org/10.1007/174_2023_394,
Published Online: 09 June 2023

divided into compartments by fascial planes, which may limit the spread of neoplasm or infection, although fascial defects caused by traversing tendons can compromise this (Singer et al. 2016; Ledermann et al. 2002). A clear understanding is helpful when reporting imaging studies, and particularly important when performing image-guided biopsies to avoid cross-compartmental contamination.

The foot is divided into dorsal and plantar compartments. The plantar compartment is further subdivided into medial, central, and lateral compartments, by two intermuscular septa which arise from the plantar aponeurosis. The dorsal compartment contains all the dorsal muscles and tendons. The plantar medial compartment contains the muscles and tendons of the great toe. The plantar lateral compartment contains the muscles and tendons of the fifth toe. The plantar central compartment contains the remaining plantar muscles, namely flexor digitorum brevis, flexor digitorum longus tendons, quadratus plantae, adductor hallucis, and lumbricals (Singer et al. 2016; Ledermann et al. 2002).

The ankle is divided into four main compartments: anterior, posterior, medial, and lateral. The anterior compartment is delineated anteriorly by the superior extensor retinaculum and contains tibialis anterior, extensor hallucis longus, extensor digitorum longus, and dorsalis pedis. The posterior compartment contains the Achilles and plantaris tendon. The medial compartments are delineated by the flexor retinaculum and contain posterior tibial tendon, flexor digitorum longus tendon, flexor hallucis longus tendon, and posterior tibial artery, nerve, and vein. The lateral compartment is delineated by the superior peroneal retinaculum and contains the peroneus longus and brevis tendons (Singer et al. 2016).

2.2 Epidemiology

Neoplasia of the foot and ankle is proportionally more common than would be expected from the proportionate mass of this region compared to the rest of the body (Ozdemir et al. 1997; Ruggieri et al. 2014; Chou et al. 2009; Toepfer et al. 2018). However, as musculoskeletal tumors are rare throughout the body, the incidence of true neoplastic tumors is small (Toepfer et al. 2018). Finding the true incidence/prevalence of tumors and tumorlike lesions of the foot and ankle is complicated by a variety of confounding factors and biases in the epidemiological studies (Toepfer et al. 2018; Hochman and Wu 2017). This includes variation in the nature of the institution studied, where musculoskeletal tumor referral centers would be expected to have a very different caseload than general hospitals. Inclusion/exclusion criteria are also significantly different between studies, with variation as to whether tumorlike lesions (pseudotumors) or metastases are included having an obvious effect on the proportion of malignant tumors being reported. The requirement in several studies for histopathological diagnosis for inclusion favors overreporting of malignant masses, as benign "don't touch" lesions would not be included (Toepfer et al. 2018). Many of the studies also have small numbers of cases, decreasing statistical significance.

Accordingly, the reported proportion of malignant tumors (bone and soft tissue) in the foot and ankle varies widely from as low as 9% (Kim et al. 2014) to as high as 42% (Sarkar et al. 1996). Soft tissue tumors have a higher rate of malignancy than bone tumors (Toepfer et al. 2018). The incidence of individual tumor diagnoses is also variable between studies. Nonetheless, these studies do provide useful information of the relative frequency of certain diagnoses.

The most common benign bone tumors are osteoid osteoma, osteochondroma, enchondroma, simple bone cyst (SBC), aneurysmal bone cyst (ABC), and giant cell tumor of bone (GCTB) (Ruggieri et al. 2014; Murahashi et al. 2021; Mascard et al. 2017; Azevedo et al. 2013).

The most common malignant bone tumors are chondrosarcoma, osteosarcoma, Ewing's sarcoma, and bone metastases (Ruggieri et al. 2014; Murahashi et al. 2021; Mascard et al. 2017; Azevedo et al. 2013).

The most common tumorlike soft tissue lesions are ganglion cysts and Morton's neuromas (Tay et al. 2021). The most common benign soft tissue tumors are lipoma, fibromatosis, vascular malformations/hemangioma, schwannoma, and giant cell tumor of tendon sheath (GCTTS)/pigmented villonodular synovitis (PVNS) (Ruggieri et al. 2014; Murahashi et al. 2021; Mascard et al. 2017; Azevedo et al. 2013).

The most common malignant soft tissue tumors are synovial sarcoma, pleomorphic undifferentiated sarcoma (PUS; previously known as malignant fibrous histiocytoma), and myxofibrosarcoma (Ruggieri et al. 2014; Murahashi et al. 2021; Mascard et al. 2017; Azevedo et al. 2013; Tay et al. 2021).

Some very rare tumors (including epithelioid sarcoma) demonstrate a predilection for the foot and may appear falsely reassuring on imaging (Toepfer et al. 2017, 2018; Nishimura et al. 2010; Saad et al. 2021).

While a broad understanding of these relative frequencies is useful, its application to any particular lesion in any particular individual is limited by the fact that the likelihood of a particular diagnosis is heavily influenced by patient-specific factors, including age and past medical history (see Sect. 3.2).

2.3 Clinical Presentation

Masses in the foot and ankle are a common cause of presentation. The small volume of subcutaneous tissue in the foot and ankle means that the masses are often palpable and this, along with the wearing of shoes causing discomfort, often enables early detection. Nonetheless, due to the prevalence of nonmalignant masses in the foot and a lack of awareness of the relatively rarer malignant masses, the latter can be underappreciated or misdiagnosed (Murahashi et al. 2021; Young et al. 2013).

The UK guidelines advise that any soft tissue mass that is (1) increasing in size, (2) greater than 5 cm, or (3) painful should be treated as malignant until proven otherwise and therefore should be urgently assessed with ultrasound or directly referred to a local sarcoma service (Dangoor et al. 2016).

2.4 Management

Due to rarity, heterogeneity, and difficulty in differentiating benign from malignant musculoskeletal tumors, if there is suspicion or uncertainty for malignancy, then they should be referred to a specialist center (Bouchard et al. 2017). In the United Kingdom, these are centralized as bone and/or soft tissue sarcoma centers. Multidisciplinary teams (MDTs) comprising radiologists, surgeons, oncologists, pathologists, specialist nurses, and MDT coordinators are vital to the thorough and efficient assessment of these lesions with subsequent decisions on further imaging, biopsy, diagnosis, and treatment (Dangoor et al. 2016; Cavalcante et al. 2021).

The management strategy varies widely depending on local aggressiveness and malignant potential, in conjunction with the patient's age, fitness, and clinical presentation. Some benign lesions are discovered incidentally but have highly characteristic or pathognomic imaging appearances and can therefore be regarded as "leave me alone"/"do not touch" lesions that do not require any further follow-up (Hegde et al. 2022; Helms 2019). Others may require further imaging or biopsy to exclude a more concerning pathology.

Benign tumors which are not locally aggressive nor symptomatic can often be discharged. Benign tumors with a rare future risk of malignant change may be followed up clinically or with imaging. Benign tumors which are symptomatic or locally aggressive may be managed surgically or with systemic therapy. For example, giant cell tumors may be managed with curettage and cement or with denosumab therapy (Singer et al. 2016). Osteoid osteomas and similar symptomatic bone lesions may be amenable to image-guided ablation, including radiofrequency (RFA) or cryoablation (Khan et al. 2015) (Fig. 1).

Malignant tumors with curative intent are normally treated surgically with or without radiotherapy or chemotherapy (Singer et al. 2016). Sarcomas should be resected with wide margins when possible. Options include function-preserving/limb salvage surgery, but the complex

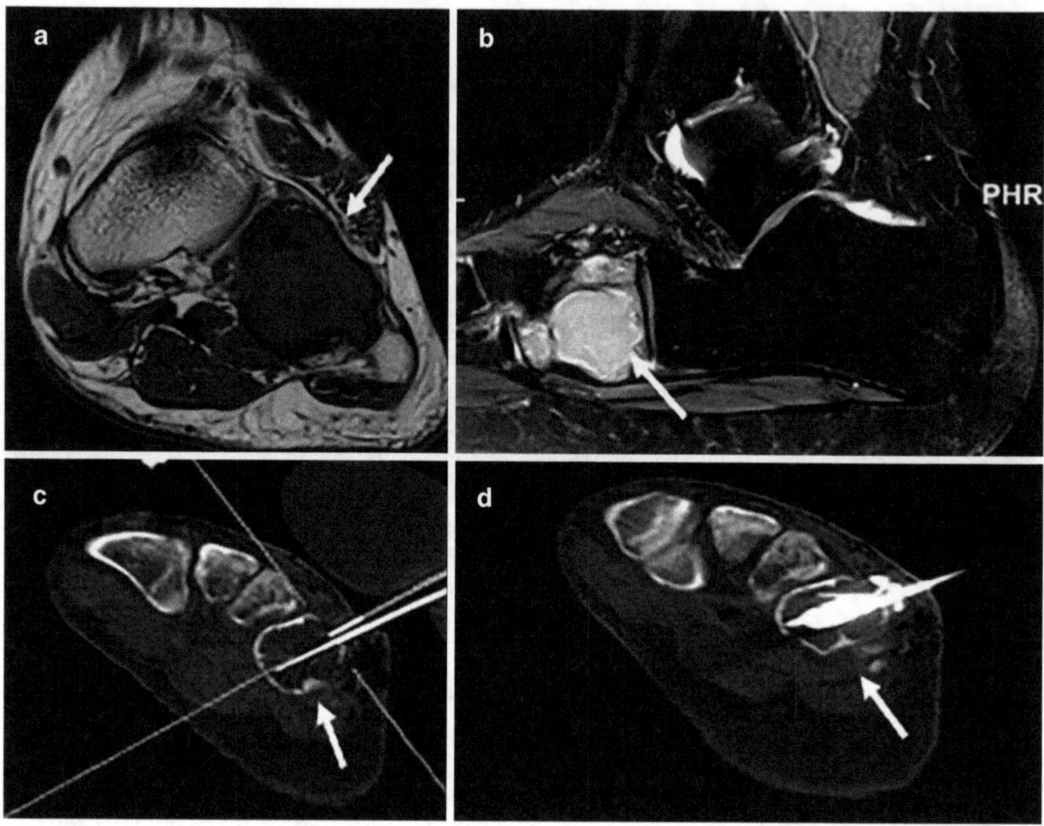

Fig. 1 High T2-weighted (**b**) and low T1 signal-weighted (**a**) lesion on MRI in keeping with a benign fibro-osseous lesion in the cuboid (**c**). This was biopsied and followed by cryoablation (**d**)

anatomy and close arrangement of important neurovascular structures in the foot and ankle mean that this is often not possible and a more radical resection may be required (Singer et al. 2016). Amputation is often performed as reconstruction is made more challenging by the small volume and surface area of soft tissue. Also, function is easier to preserve in the foot and ankle than some other regions with the use of a prosthesis (Murahashi et al. 2021). A planned positive margin may be left if the above options are not appropriate, after discussion with the patient regarding the potential negative implications for disease prognosis (Khan et al. 2015). If the malignant nature of a foot or ankle mass is not appreciated, then it may undergo an inadequate (unplanned, "whoops") excision, often in a non-specialist institution (Khan et al. 2015). The consequences of this can be marked, as if the surgical margins are insufficient, then more aggressive surgery and adjuvant radiotherapy or chemotherapy may be required, and a worse prognosis can result (Toepfer et al. 2018; Murahashi et al. 2021; Bouchard et al. 2017; Thacker et al. 2008; Davis et al. 1997; Latt et al. 2010).

Treatment with adjuvant radiotherapy is standard for all intermediate- and high-grade sarcomas and shows similar results to radical resection, with the added benefit of functional preservation (Yang et al. 1998).

Neoadjuvant chemotherapy is now routinely used in almost all bone sarcomas with the exception of chondrosarcoma (Khan et al. 2015). Chemotherapy is not standard for soft tissue sarcomas (Khan et al. 2015).

3 Imaging

3.1 Imaging Modalities

Radiography should be the initial imaging investigation for suspected bone tumors. It is useful as an adjunct for soft tissue tumors as it can demonstrate tissue calcification and reactive bone changes (Hochman and Wu 2017). For bone tumors, the radiograph remains a predictor of the histological nature of a tumor, although detection depends to a degree on the radiographic technique and the size, location, and aggressiveness of the lesion. It is usually possible to characterize the aggressiveness of a bone tumor from the radiograph, but when analyzing the radiographic features in the foot, some modifications must be borne in mind. Lesions in the foot do not have to achieve a large size to become symptomatic. The small size of many bones means that involvement of an entire bone is not uncommon. Early bone destruction and periosteal reaction are more easily detected in the small, thin tubular bones of the forefoot than in the larger bones of the midfoot and hindfoot. Soft tissue lesions will only be seen if they display mass effect, bone or joint involvement, or mineralization (e.g., synovial sarcomas, or phleboliths in hemangiomas).

Ultrasound (US) is an important imaging technique in the assessment of soft tissue masses in the foot and ankle and is the imaging method of choice for small superficial lesions. The limited depth of the soft tissues allows the use of high-frequency probes providing high-resolution imaging. US is readily available, differentiates cystic from solid lesions, and assists biopsy, while color flow Doppler techniques allow the assessment of vascular lesions (Hochman and Wu 2017). US-guided biopsies are commonly performed for soft tissue tumors (Kaminsky et al. 1997).

Computed tomography (CT) with fast high-resolution thin-slice techniques and multiplanar image reformatting is sensitive in detecting matrix mineralization and demonstrating fine cortical detail. CT lacks the soft tissue contrast of MRI and uses ionizing radiation, but it is useful for situations where high special resolution is key, such as identifying the lucent nidus in osteoid osteoma. CT is accurate in defining the attenuation of lesions and is therefore helpful in detecting lesion mineralization or fat (Hochman and Wu 2017). Dual-energy CT can demonstrate monosodium urate in gouty tophi (Fritz et al. 2016; Desai et al. 2011). CT-guided biopsy is key to the diagnosis of many bone tumors.

MR imaging has an established role in imaging tumors and tumorlike conditions, particularly in local staging. MR imaging is also the most sensitive imaging technique for lesion detection. MRI is undoubtedly superior to CT at defining the intra-osseous, soft tissue, and extracompartmental spread of tumors as well as their relationship to important neurovascular and articular structures (Bloem et al. 1988). Care should be taken in the interpretation as the sensitivity of MR imaging is such that many incidental findings are discovered, which have no clinical relevance. Appropriate coil selection and slice thickness are required for lesion coverage and high-quality images. Protocols vary with anatomical site and lesion extent (Hochman and Wu 2017). Where an aggressive bone sarcoma of the distal tibia or fibula is suspected, a large field-of-view T1-weighted sequence of the whole bone in the longitudinal plane is required to exclude skip metastases. Compartmental anatomy is often best defined in the transverse plane. T1-weighted, fat-suppressed T2-weighted, or STIR sequences all demonstrate the margin between an osseous tumor and normal marrow, although peri-tumoral edema may obscure the tumor margin. Fat-suppressed T2-weighted or STIR sequences are required to demonstrate the soft tissue extent. Supplementary MRI sequences are used in certain circumstances, for example metal artifact reduction techniques when metallic prosthesis is in situ (Talbot and Weinberg 2016; Ariyanayagam et al. 2015). T2* gradient-echo sequences can demonstrate blooming artifact in PVNS. Intravenous gadolinium contrast may be used to differentiate cystic and solid lesions (Hochman and Wu 2017). As many structures in the foot do not lie in orthogonal planes, oblique planes may be required for optimal evaluation. On MR imaging, as most lesions display nonspecific intermediate signal intensity (similar to muscle) on T1 weighting and high signal intensity on T2 weighting, tissue characterization based on signal intensities alone is not usually possible. In addition, the signal intensity and homogeneity will also vary with the type of tumor matrix as well as with the presence of hemorrhage and necrosis. However, some lesions may have characteristic findings. Cystic lesions such as ganglia and simple bone cysts display homogeneous low signal intensity on T1 weighting and very high signal intensity on T2 weighting and show either no or rim enhancement. Lipomas usually have a characteristic homogeneous pattern with a signal intensity equal to that of fat on all pulse sequences. Hemangiomas also contain fatty tissue but typically also have serpentine vascular structures. Some lesions produce a low/intermediate signal intensity on both T1 weighting and T2 weighting, including pigmented villonodular synovitis due to hemosiderin (Bravo et al. 1996) and fibromatosis due to high collagen content (Morrison et al. 1994). The detection of fluid-fluid levels (sedimentation effect) in an expansile bone lesion in an adolescent is highly suggestive of an aneurysmal bone cyst, although fluid-fluid levels may also be seen in other lesions including giant-cell tumor and chondroblastoma.

Nuclear medicine. Isotope bone scan usually with ^{99m}Tc-methylene diphosphonate is highly sensitive but relatively nonspecific and with limited anatomical resolution. In malignant bone tumors, the main role of scintigraphy lies in the detection of metastatic disease. Scintigraphy is of limited value in the assessment of benign bone tumors but may play a significant role in the detection of osteoid osteomas. *PET-CT* is not yet routine for sarcoma workup (Dangoor et al. 2016).

3.2 Image Interpretation

A definitive diagnosis of bone and soft tissue masses may be made by imaging alone in certain cases, for example with certain pathognomonic features (e.g., lucent nidus in osteoid osteoma). However, often the diagnosis cannot be stated with certainty and in order to provide a clinically useful report, and to positively influence the diagnostic and therapeutic pathway, it is important to give a considered differential diagnosis that is as narrow as possible. In order to do this efficiently and consistently, one must have a systematic approach to image interpretation (Helms 2019; Radiology Assistant 2022; UW Radiology 2022).

3.2.1 Bone Lesion Interpretation

3.2.1.1 Clinical

Before assessing any imaging studies, it is important to have relevant clinical information. The age of the patient is important, with some diagnoses virtually unheard of in certain age groups. It is worth noting that the age range for some foot tumors may differ from the same tumor at more proximal sites. It is also important to be aware of any preexisting lesion or hereditary condition such as multiple enchondromatosis (Ollier's disease).

3.2.1.2 Location in Skeleton

Some bone tumors have a predilection for a particular bone. Chondroblastoma, giant cell tumor, and osteoid osteoma/osteoblastoma commonly arise in the anterior talus (Boo et al. 2020), and simple bone cysts and intra-osseous lipomas in the calcaneus (Azzopardi et al. 2021).

3.2.1.3 Location Within the Bone Itself

The location of a tumor within a bone can also be described in longitudinal (epiphysis vs. metaphysis vs. diaphysis) and transverse (centric vs. eccentric vs. juxtacortical) planes. However, the small length and cross section of most bones in the foot can make the differentiation of these characteristics challenging or impossible. Nevertheless, the calcaneus has identifiable sites that correspond to the physeal zones. The calcaneal apophysis and the subarticular portions of the upper and anterior calcaneus correspond to the epiphysis equivalent zone, the bone adjacent to the metaphyseal zone, and the central calcaneus to the diaphyseal zone. Chondroblastoma frequently occurs in the apophysis posteriorly and adjacent to the posterior calcaneal facet, both epiphyseal equivalent sites. Giant cell tumors are also found at the sites of old apophyses and occur most commonly in the anterior and posterior margins of the calcaneus. Osteoid osteoma appears most often in the subtalar region, and simple bone cysts and lipomas usually in the anterior third of the calcaneus. Of the malignant bony lesions, metastases and Ewing's sarcoma tend to occur centrally in the body and at the tuberosity of the calcaneus, but osteosarcoma has no predilection for site.

Radiographic appearance remains one of the key ways of narrowing the imaging diagnosis and provides a wealth of information that more "advanced" imaging modalities like MRI are unable to differentiate. CT is able to give similar findings, but with a higher dose of ionizing radiation. *Lytic or sclerotic* helps narrow the differential diagnosis significantly. *Zone of transition* (wide or narrow; ill-defined or well-defined) is a marker of local aggressiveness (wide is aggressive, narrow is benign) and is often a marker of malignancy, although locally aggressive nonmalignant pathologies like giant cell tumor of bone or osteomyelitis will also have a wide zone of transition. *Periosteal reaction* is another marker of local aggressiveness and can range across solid, lamellated, spiculated, and Codman's in order of increasing aggressivity. *Cortical destruction* is often caused by malignant and locally aggressive pathology, but can also be caused by more benign pathology, although this is normally limited to endosteal scalloping (e.g., fibrous dysplasia) rather than full-thickness erosion. *Matrix* can be used to identify the histopathological type and can be described as chondroid (popcorn/rings and arcs), osteoid (cloud-like/ill-defined amorphous), or fibrous (ground glass). *Multiplicity* is a key feature to note as this can affect the likelihood of certain diagnoses (e.g., metastases) or the requirement for biopsy/treatment (Helms 2019; Radiology Assistant 2022; UW Radiology 2022; Costelloe and Madewell 2013).

3.2.2 Soft Tissue Lesion Interpretation

Location can help identify particular diagnoses. Of the soft tissue masses, Morton's neuroma is by far the most common mass in the forefoot and typically arises in the third or second intermetatarsal web spaces. Plantar fibromatosis is the most common lesion in the plantar region and, by definition, arises in the plantar fascia. Ganglion cysts and lipomas are the most common lesions in the midfoot and hindfoot. Soft tissue sarcomas are less common in the forefoot. When a mass is in contact with a tendon, a giant cell tumor of the tendon sheath should be considered (Longo et al. 2016). Any mass deep to the deep fascia should be investigated by the appropriate sarcoma unit (Khan et al. 2015).

Size of tumor has been shown to be a statistically significant marker of malignancy for soft tissue masses. The UK referral guidelines use 50 mm as a cutoff (Dangoor et al. 2016), but there is evidence that a cutoff value of 40 mm is more appropriate in the foot and ankle, which may reflect the earlier detection of masses due to the thinner layer of soft tissue in this region (Murahashi et al. 2021; Tay et al. 2021). Increasing size is also justification for further investigation (Khan et al. 2015).

Specific imaging features depend upon the imaging modality but include cystic vs. solid and degree of vascularity. Most soft tissue lesions are isointense to muscle on T1W images and relatively hyperintense on T2W images. The differential can be narrowed when masses demonstrate either T1W hyperintensity (fat, proteinaceous fluid, methemoglobin, melanin, gadolinium) or T2W hypointensity (calcification, fibrous tissue, hemosiderin). Inhomogeneity, necrosis, hemorrhage, irregular margins, surrounding soft tissue edema, and invasion of surrounding structures are suspicious for malignancy. However, it is important to understand that soft tissue sarcomas can have a nonaggressive, well-defined appearance on MRI (Hochman and Wu 2017).

Increasing age and male sex are also significant predictors of soft tissue malignancy (Tay et al. 2021).

3.3 Biopsy

Biopsy is a key stage in the diagnostic pathway for many lesions and frequently results in an alteration in the patient's management (Singer et al. 2016; Toomayan et al. 2005). Minimally invasive procedures are preferable (Khan et al. 2015), and therefore image-guided percutaneous biopsy is often the technique of choice. The technique is quick and safe and has a low risk of complications and tumor seeding. Percutaneous biopsy has an accuracy rate of over 90% in most series (Stoker et al. 1991). Incisional/excisional biopsy may be necessary on rare occasions, for example for some small superficial lesions (Dangoor et al. 2016). Discussion between the radiologist and orthopedic surgeon, as part of a multidisciplinary/interdisciplinary team, is important in choosing the appropriate biopsy site and route (Khan et al. 2015; Rammelt et al. 2020). If the mass is superficial, then often the shortest route is the best, but care should be taken to ensure that the biopsy tract remains within a single compartment and to avoid neurovascular structures via an approach that can be resected at the definitive surgical procedure (Singer et al. 2016). Any open incision for biopsy should be in line with the definitive incision for further surgery, and meticulous homeostasis should be achieved to avoid local spread of tumor (Khan et al. 2015). Samples are then sent for histopathological diagnosis according to the 2020 WHO classification and grading (Dangoor et al. 2016; WHO Classification of Tumours Editorial Board 2020).

3.4 Staging

The objective of staging is to define the tumor in terms of histological grade and anatomical extent. For local staging, wide field-of-view MRI should be performed (see Sect. 3.1). Confirmed soft tissue or bone sarcoma should be staged with a CT chest to exclude pulmonary metastases. Rarely, a plain chest radiograph may be acceptable depending on the grade of the lesion and the demographics of the patient. CT abdomen/pelvis are not routine in most cases but may be considered in certain cases including lower limb tumors or certain histological subtypes (Dangoor et al. 2016). Isotope bone scan is used in some centers for the exclusion of bone metastases. PET-CT is not yet routine (Dangoor et al. 2016). In the foot and ankle, although lesions confined to a single ray or one of the three compartments of the plantar side of the midfoot are intracompartmental, many lesions of the hindfoot and midfoot are extracompartmental due to the lack of anatomical boundaries (Anderson et al. 1999). Imaging is therefore crucial in detecting extracompartmental spread and deciding surgical management. A malignancy distal to the metatarsophalangeal joint may require ray resection, whereas lesions of the hindfoot may require below-knee amputation.

There are numerous musculoskeletal staging systems. The original was the Enneking/MSTS (Musculoskeletal Tumor Society) staging system, which is still in use and is often favored by oncological orthopedic surgeons. It covers both bone and soft tissue tumors and is based upon anatomical, radiological, and pathological features (Enneking et al. 1980; Murphey and Kransdorf 2021). Extracompartmental involvement or metastases upstage the lesion.

The most frequently used system currently is the American Joint Committee on Cancer (AJCC) staging system (8th edition, updated 2017). It is applicable to both bone and soft tissue sarcomas and incorporates the pathological grade of the tumor. Non-primary lesions and primary lymphoma or multiple myeloma are not included (Murphey and Kransdorf 2021).

3.5 Follow-Up

There are several guidelines for the follow-up of sarcomas (Roberts et al. 2016; von Mehren et al. 2018; Noebauer-Huhmann et al. 2015; ESMO/European Sarcoma Network Working Group 2014a, b), but there is a lack of controlled studies

(Tavare et al. 2018). ESSR guidelines are for clinical and radiological follow-up with foot and ankle radiographs and chest radiographs at 3-month intervals for 3 years, 6-month intervals for the next 2 years, and then annually until 10 years posttreatment (Noebauer-Huhmann et al. 2015). Local radiographs, local MRI, and chest radiographs/CT are recommended. Recurrence and metastases can occur after 10 years, and there is no universally accepted stopping point (Tavare et al. 2018). The lungs are the most frequent site of metastases in sarcoma and are therefore a key part of follow-up imaging (Roberts et al. 2016). CT chest and bone scintigraphy are indicated for suspected lung and bone metastases.

Knowledge of the preoperative appearance is important, as recurrent masses will typically have similar imaging characteristics (Garner et al. 2009). For this reason, comparison should always be made with preoperative and initial postoperative imaging. However, radiation-induced sarcomas can have different histological compositions and therefore imaging appearances compared to the original tumor (Lewis et al. 1997). There can be confusion between recurrent masses and nonmalignant findings including seroma, hematoma, lymphocele, scarring, and radiation-induced pseudotumor (Tavare et al. 2018). Ultrasound can be used to problem solve. Postcontrast MRI and PET-CT may also help increase diagnostic confidence (Tavare et al. 2018). T1-weighted fat-suppressed and gradient-echo MRI sequences may help differentiate hemorrhage from local tumor recurrence.

3.6 Illustrated Review

Diagnoses are listed according to the latest (2020) WHO Classification of bone and soft tissue musculoskeletal tumors. Changes and reclassifications from previous editions represent the emerging importance of genetics to histopathological diagnosis and management (WHO Classification of Tumours Editorial Board 2020; Murphey and Kransdorf 2021).

3.6.1 Bone Tumors and Tumorlike Lesions

3.6.1.1 Chondrogenic Tumors

Chondroblastoma is a rare, benign but locally aggressive lesion (Kennedy et al. 2016). In the foot, there is a male predominance of over 80%, and presentation tends to be later (mean 26 years) than in other parts of the skeleton (mean 17 years) (Fink et al. 1997; Huvos and Marcove 1973). The lesion favors an epiphyseal/apophyseal location, which accounts for the high incidence in the posterior subchondral regions of the talus and calcaneus and calcaneal apophysis (Kennedy et al. 2016; Fink et al. 1997; Reda 2018). It typically presents with pain (Singer et al. 2016). Radiographically, lesions are typically lytic, with well-defined, often sclerotic margins. Chondroid matrix mineralization is only present in around half of the lesions in the hand and foot. Endosteal scalloping or expansion are present in the majority (Cavalcante et al. 2021; Murai et al. 2018; Davila et al. 2004). Subchondral fractures are frequent but often radiographically occult. On MRI, there is typically perilesional edema with intralesional low/intermediate T1 signal (Murai et al. 2018; Davila et al. 2004). On T2-weighted MR images, variable amounts of intermediate/low signal intensity tissue are commonly found and attributed to hemosiderin, calcifications, and hypercellularity of the chondroblasts (Jee et al. 1999). Fluid-fluid levels and secondary ABC may be present (Reda 2018). Most will demonstrate moderate uptake on bone scan (Murai et al. 2018; Weatherall et al. 1994). It is generally considered a benign diagnosis but, like giant cell tumors of bone, it has been reported to rarely metastasize to the lung. Clear cell chondrosarcoma can have a similar imaging appearance and should be considered if there are any aggressive features (Singer et al. 2016). Treatment is normally surgical with curettage and bone grafting (Dhatt et al. 2012). Recurrence rates of 10–30% have been reported (Reda 2018) (Fig. 2).

Enchondroma (chondroma) is a benign cartilaginous neoplasm of the medullary cavity that is much less common in the foot and ankle than the

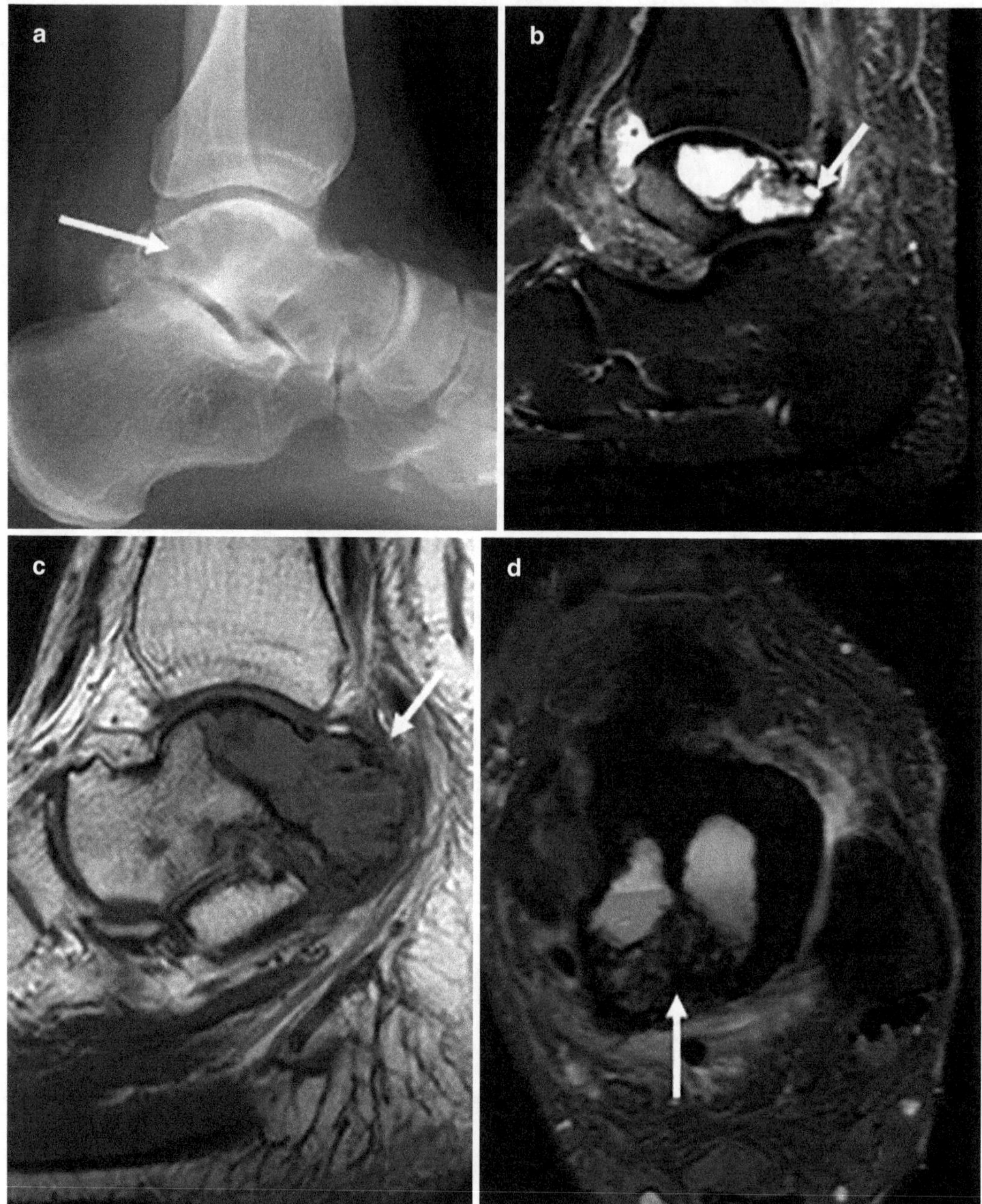

Fig. 2 A lucency seen in talus on the X-ray (**a**). This demonstrates high signal on STIR (**b**) and intermediate signal on T1 (**c**) with fluid-fluid levels suggestive of secondary ABC (**d**). There is marked perilesional oedema. Findings are in keeping with chondroblastoma

digits of the hand. However, it remains one of the most common benign bone tumors of the foot (Unni 1986; Campanacci 2013) and most commonly affects the tubular bones (Cavalcante et al. 2021; Khan et al. 2015). Involvement of the phalanges is more common than of the metatarsals or distal tibia and fibula, and rare in the hindfoot. Lesions usually present with a painless swelling or pathological fracture in the second and third decades (Reda 2018). Radiographs typically display a well-defined, expansile lesion in the metaphyseal region that, unlike in the rest of the body (except the hands), may be entirely lytic without the classical punctate, stippled, or ring-and-arc calcifications. In larger lesions, endosteal scalloping can be seen. *Periosteal chondroma* is uncommon and usually displays a rim of reactive bone (Ricca et al. 2000). Cartilage tumors often have characteristic MR appearances. On T1 weighting, unmineralized components display homogeneous low to intermediate signal intensity, but on T1 weighting, thin low signal intensity septa are noted between the lobulated high T2 signal intensity cartilage. Following intravenous contrast, there is typically septal and peripheral enhancement. Mineralized components show low signal intensity on all sequences. The risk of sarcomatous transformation in a solitary foot lesion is very rare but may be as high as 5% for large lesions in a long bone such as the distal tibia. The risk of malignant transformation in multiple enchondromatosis (Ollier's disease) or Maffucci's syndrome (enchondromatosis and soft tissue hemangiomas) is significantly higher at >20%. Large or symptomatic lesions may need surgical treatment with curettage with or without bone grafting (Khan et al. 2015; Kennedy et al. 2016; Reda 2018).

Osteochondroma (exostosis) is probably a developmental growth plate aberration rather than a true bone tumor but is classified with the benign chondrogenic tumors. It is one of the most common benign bone tumors of the foot and ankle. However, the majority of osteochondromas of the ankle and foot are located in the distal tibia and fibula, and the metatarsals are most commonly involved in the foot. Most present with a slow-growing, hard lump or symptoms from pressure effects on adjacent structures. Malignant degeneration of the cartilage cap is 1% in solitary lesions, but 5–25% in hereditary multiple exostosis (HME) (Lee et al. 1987). Radiographically, the lesions may be sessile or pedunculated and grow away from the physis. The cartilage cap may show variable stippled or ring-shaped calcifications. Continued growth after maturity or pain should raise the possibility of sarcomatous degeneration. MR imaging is useful in excluding bursitis and allows accurate assessment of the cartilage cap. After skeletal maturity, a cartilage cap thickness of more than 1.5 cm, or a growing cap, is suspicious for malignant transformation (Murphey et al. 2000) (Fig. 3).

Subungual exostosis is a benign diagnosis that is generally accepted to be separate from true osteochondromas in that it lacks marrow continuity and cartilage cap (Singer et al. 2016). It is a fibrocartilaginous proliferation deep to the nail bed which undergoes endochondral ossification to form trabeculated bone (Kennedy et al. 2016). They most frequently involve great toe, often with a history of prior trauma, although the pathogenesis is not clear. Radiographically, they appear as a well-defined bony outgrowth extending away from the distal phalanx. They are normally excised if painful, including the nail bed if this is involved (Kennedy et al. 2016) (Fig. 4).

Chondromyxoid fibroma (CMF) is a rare benign cartilage tumor. It typically occurs in the second or third decades with discomfort and local swelling. The tibia is the most commonly involved bone, and in the foot, the lesion most commonly occurs in the metatarsals and phalanges (Reda 2018; Mirra 1989). Radiographs typically show a lytic, slow-growing, well-defined, expansile, eccentric lesion often with sclerotic margins (Reda 2018; O'Connor et al. 1996). Matrix calcification is uncommon. In the small tubular bones of the foot, lesions often extend from the metaphysis into the diaphysis or epiphysis. Occasionally, chondromyxoid fibroma can appear more aggressive with cortical breach (Reda 2018). On MR imaging, lesions display low signal intensity on T1 weighting and hyperintense signal intensity on T2 weighting due to chondroid and myxoid matrices (Reda 2018). The margin of the lesion usually displays a low signal intensity on all sequences, reflecting new periosteal bone. Treatment is with curettage and bone grafting, with reported recurrence rates of 15–30%, or with resection and reconstruction for larger lesions (Reda 2018) (Fig. 5).

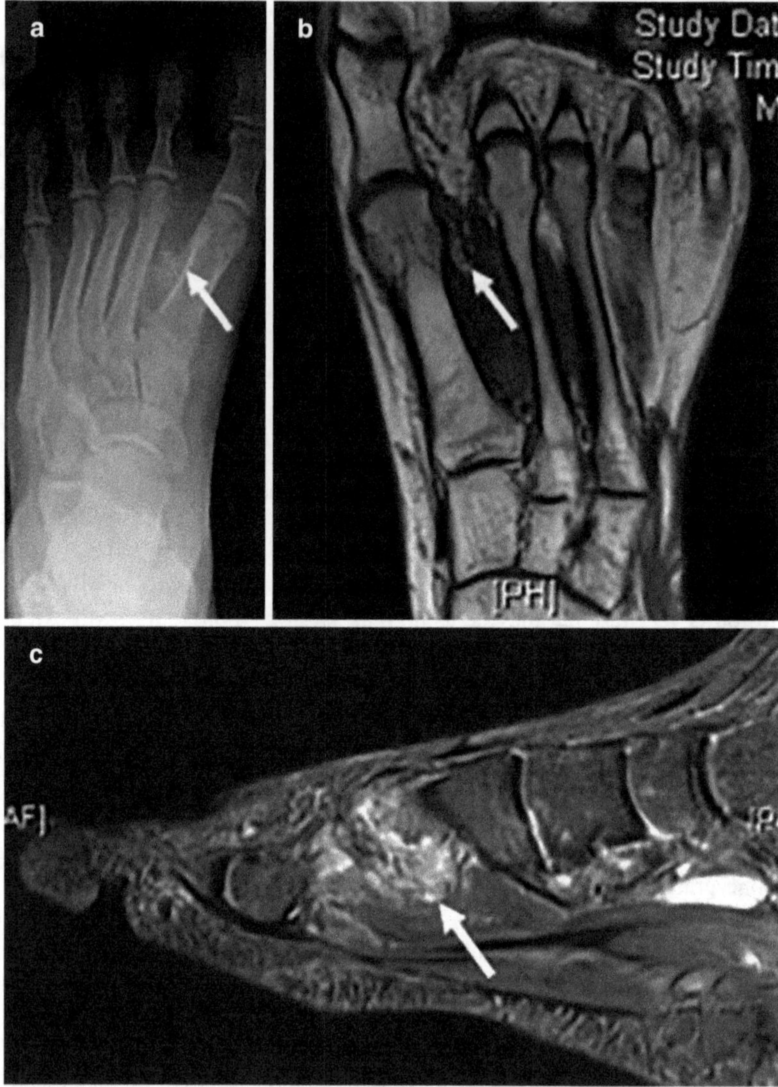

Fig. 3 A bony exostosis is seen to arise from the first metatarsal on the DP radiograph (**a**). This appears in continuity with the medulla and demonstrates a cartilage cap which is bright on T2 (**c**) and low on T1 (**b**) and is in keeping with a small osteochondroma

Chondrosarcoma is one of the most common bony malignancies of the foot and ankle. They may be primary or arise from an enchondroma or osteochondroma (Murai et al. 2018; Kilgore and Parrish 2005). The majority involve the distal tibia and fibula, and in the foot, lesions are most commonly found in the calcaneus, talus, and metatarsals (Cavalcante et al. 2021; Bovée et al. 1999). Chondrosarcoma of the ankle and hindfoot are more likely to metastasize than phalangeal chondrosarcoma, which only rarely metastasizes and behaves as a locally aggressive lesion (Bovée et al. 1999). The majority of lesions are centrally located with a geographic pattern of bone destruction, although a more aggressive permeative pattern may also be found. In a large study of 75 lesions of the foot, endosteal erosion, cortical destruction, and expansion were present in over 90%, ill-defined margins and a soft tissue mass in 80%, and mineralization in 74% (Ogose et al. 1997). In the feet and hands, lesions are smaller than elsewhere in the skeleton, ranging between 2 and 5 cm (maximal size). On MR imaging, the signal characteristics are similar to enchondroma, although chondrosarcoma should be suspected where there is cortical destruction, periosteal reaction, and soft tissue infiltration (Hottya et al. 1999). Differentiating low-grade

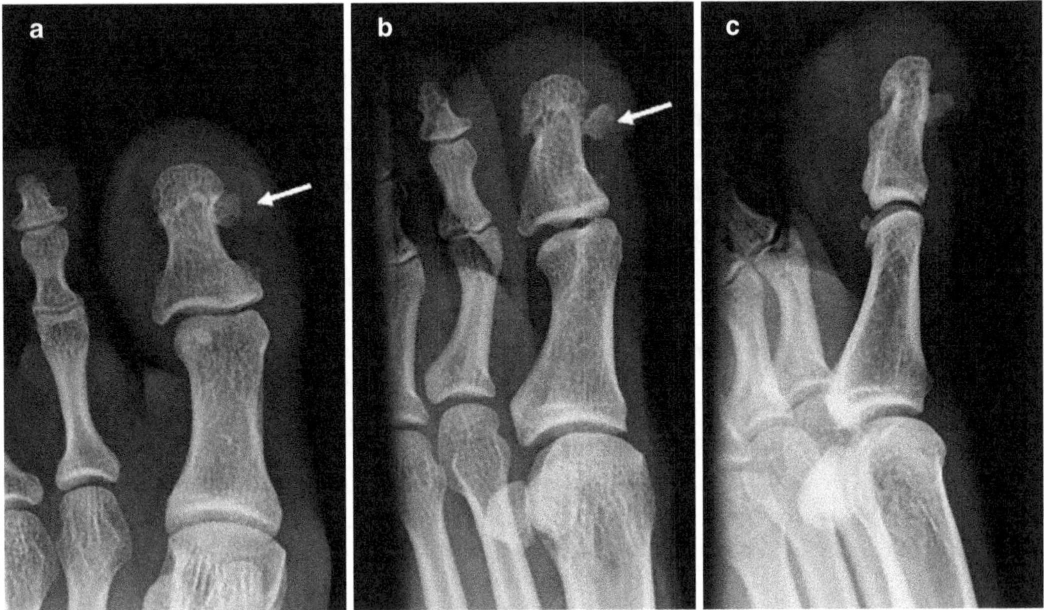

Fig. 4 A small bony exostosis is seen to arise from the distal phalanx of the big toe (white arrow images **a**, **b**). Image **c** is a lateral X-ray which shows the exostosis is subungual in nature

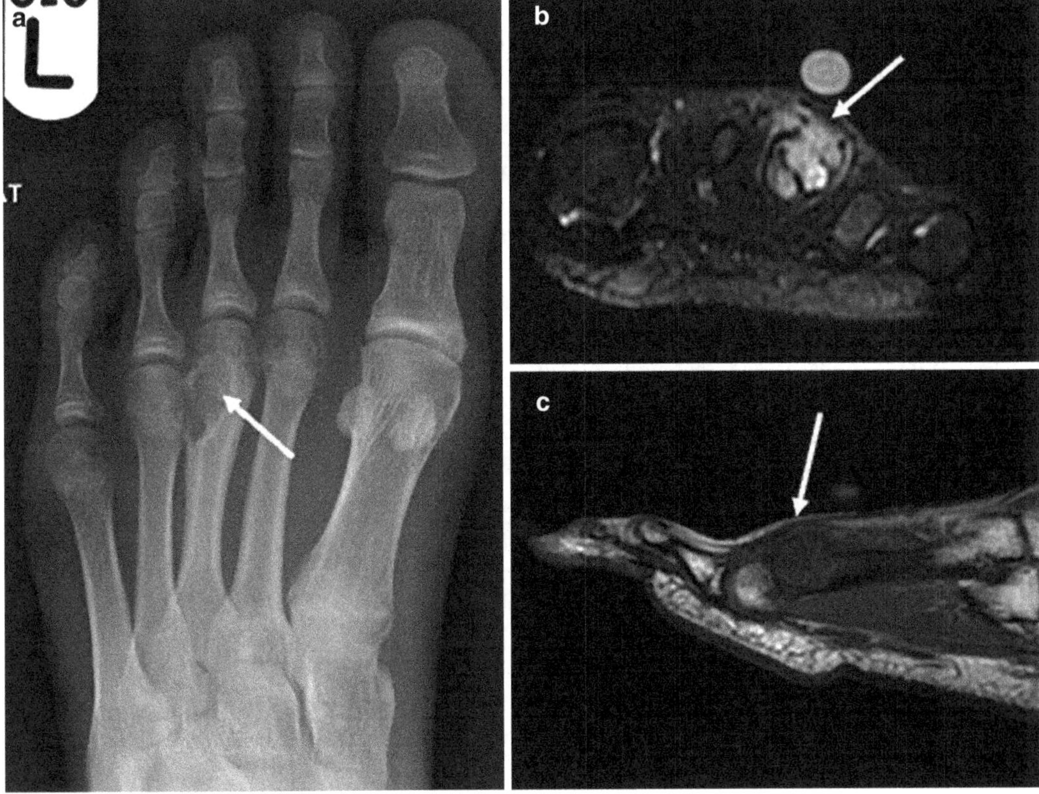

Fig. 5 Lytic eccentric and expansile lesion in the third metatarsal on X-ray (**a**) which is intermediate to bright signal on T2 weighted imaging (**b**) and intermediate signal on T1 (**c**). This was in keeping with a Chondromyxoid fibroma of the third metatarsal on biopsy

chondrosarcomas and enchondromas can be challenging. Bone uptake in chondrosarcomas is greater than that in the anterior superior iliac spine (ASIS) in 82% of cases, whereas in enchondromas, it is usually less than that in the ASIS (Murai et al. 2018; Soldatos et al. 2011). Peripheral lesions are much less common than central lesions and usually arise from preexisting osteochondroma rather than the periosteum. The variants periosteal and clear cell chondrosarcoma of the foot and ankle have been reported but are extremely rare (Fig. 6).

3.6.1.2 Osteogenic Tumors

Osteoid osteoma is one of the most common benign tumors of the foot and ankle, with the majority found in the talus, calcaneus, and distal tibia (Ruggieri et al. 2014; Reda 2018; Unni 1986; Mirra 1989; Huvos 1987). They are more common in men, with the majority of patients being in the second or third decade (Greenspan et al. 2007). Patients usually complain of a dull constant bone pain that is worse at night and relieved by salicylates/NSAIDs (Khan et al. 2015; Reda 2018; Monroe and Manoli 1999). Lesions of the phalanges may present with swelling rather than pain (Barca et al. 1998). Most talar lesions are subperiosteal and located at the superior aspect of the talar neck. In cortical lesions, radiography usually reveals a lucent or mineralized nidus with surrounding sclerosis that is less than 1.5 cm in size. However, in intramedullary and subperiosteal lesions, surrounding sclerosis may be absent and the nidus occult (Kennedy et al. 2016). CT is superior to MRI to identify the precise location of the nidus, is more cost effective, and helps plan arthroscopic or percutaneous resection or CT-guided thermal ablation. MRI shows extensive bone marrow edema on fluid-sensitive sequences (Reda 2018). On contrast-enhanced, fat-suppressed, T1-weighted MR images, the noncalcified nidi show homogeneous enhancement, whereas the calcified lesions show a ring enhancement sign. Bone scintigraphy may reveal the "double-density sign" where the central nidus shows greater uptake than the inflammatory response in the surrounding bone (Murai et al. 2018; Youssef et al. 1996; Temple et al. 1998). While they would normally resolve spontaneously within 10 years, the majority are treated to relieve pain. Curettage and resection are options for treatment, but minimally invasive ablation (radiofrequency, cryoablation) is the treatment of choice (Cavalcante et al. 2021; Khan et al. 2015; Kennedy et al. 2016). Minimally invasive techniques are associated with shorter recovery time and hospital stay (Reda 2018) (Fig. 7).

Osteoblastoma is an uncommon bone tumor but has a predilection for the foot and ankle. Third decade of life is most common, with a 2:1 male predominance. Some 40% affect the talus, and half of these are in a subperiosteal location on the dorsal aspect of the talar neck (Reda 2018; Unni 1986; Temple et al. 1998). A similar preference is found with osteoid osteoma, and indeed they may be indistinguishable histologically, although osteoblastoma is more aggressive and locally destructive (Cavalcante et al. 2021). Although osteoid osteomas tend to be less than 1 cm in size and osteoblastomas tend to be larger than 2 cm, an arbitrary value of 1.5 cm can be used as a dividing line for lesions that are indistinguishable by other criteria (Cavalcante et al. 2021; McLeod et al. 1976). Radiologically, subperiosteal lesions are often associated with a soft tissue mass and matrix mineralization (Cavalcante et al. 2021; Kennedy et al. 2016; Temple et al. 1998). Intramedullary lesions tend to have a geographic pattern of bone destruction, with variable margins and little if any mineralization. Perilesional osteopenia is common (Reda 2018). Occasionally, lesions can be locally aggressive with infiltration of adjacent structures. The term "aggressive osteoblastoma" is controversial; most show a tendency to recur but not to metastasize (Miyayama et al. 1993). Rarely, true osteosarcomatous transformation with metastases has been recorded (Kennedy et al. 2016; Reda 2018; Temple et al. 1998). Curettage and minimally invasive ablation have been successful in treatment, but larger lesions may require excision and reconstruction (Kennedy et al. 2016; Reda 2018).

Osteosarcoma is one of the most common bony malignancies of the foot and ankle. It has a bimodal age distribution peaking in ado-

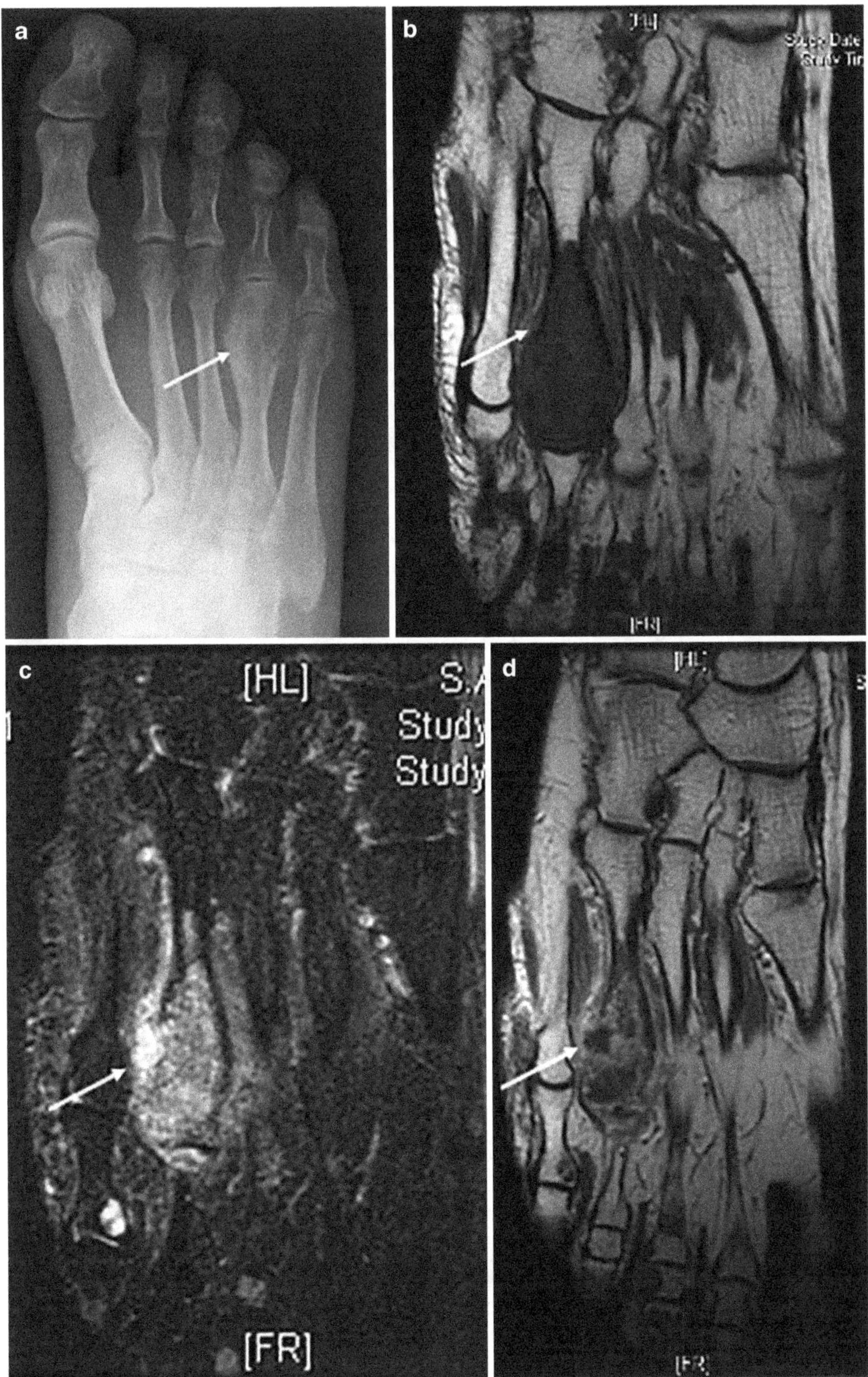

Fig. 6 Lytic, mildly expansile lesion in the fourth metatarsal is seen on X-ray (**a**). This returns low signal on T1 (**b**) and heterogenous signal on both STIR and T2 imaging (**c, d**). Findings are in keeping with low grade chondrosarcoma on a background of Ollier's disease

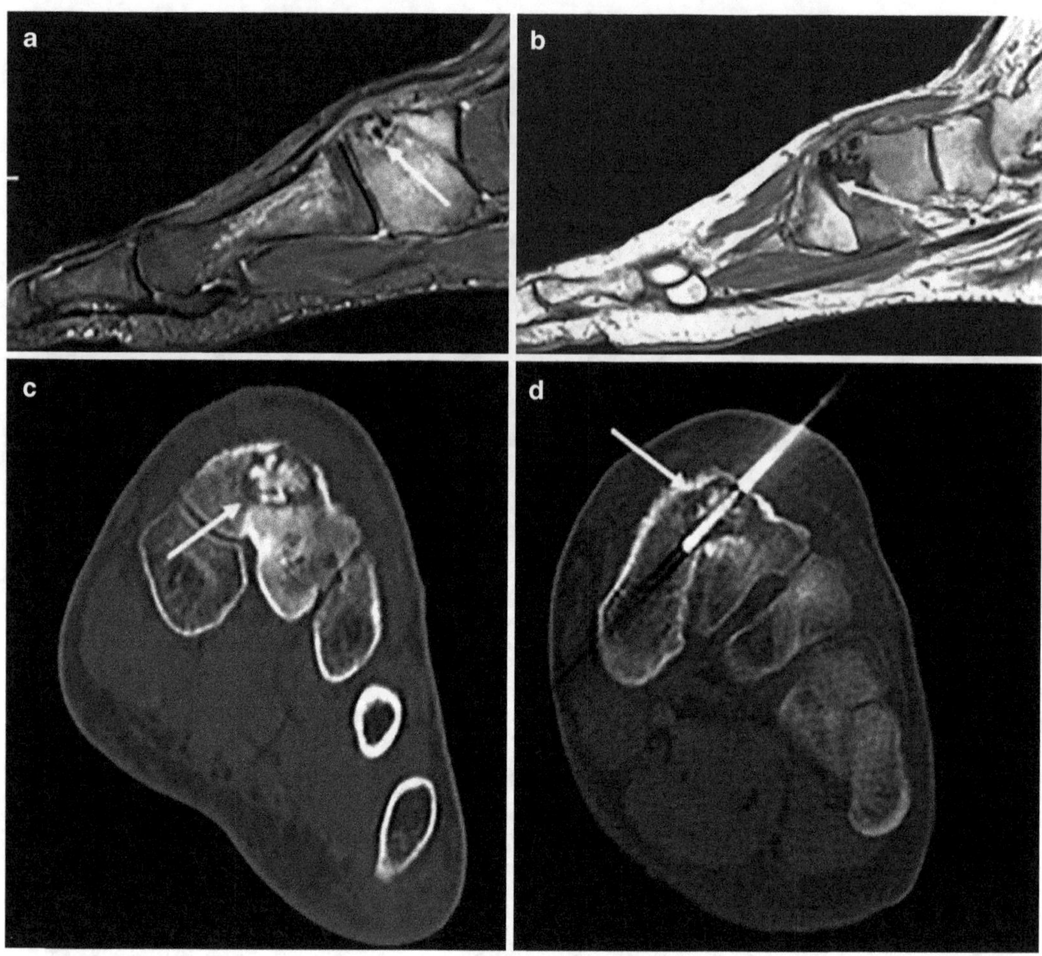

Fig. 7 Classic nidus of an osteoid osteoma with marked perilesional oedema seen on STIR (**a**) and T1 (**b**) sagittal images. The nidus is more clearly defined on the coronal CT image (**c**) and appears to be involving the cortex of the medial cuneiform with cortical thickening. This was biopsied and ablated under CT guidance (**d**)

lescence and elderly adults (Singer et al. 2016; Rammelt et al. 2020). Most lesions in the foot and ankle are intra-osseous, osteoblastic, and high grade. Metastatic disease is common and results in a poor prognosis of 65% mortality at 2.5 years (Choong et al. 1999). Approximately 66% are located in the distal tibia, and of the remainder, 75% are located in the tarsus and 75% in the calcaneus. Patients present with pain and often swelling, but the diagnosis is often delayed. In the foot, it tends to present later than osteosarcoma at other sites, with a mean age of 35 years. Radiographically, there is an aggressive moth-eaten or permeative pattern of bone destruction and usually soft tissue extension. Occasionally, slow-growing lesions may be expansile with well-defined margins (Lee et al. 2000). Amorphous or cloud-like mineralization is common, and a lamellated or spiculated periosteal reaction is often present. On MR imaging, lesions typically display low to intermediate signal intensity on T1 weighting and inhomogeneous high signal intensity on T2 weighting. Mineralized foci often display low signal on all sequences (Murai et al. 2018) (Fig. 8). They may spread within a bone, resulting in a skip lesion, and can metastasize with lung being the most common location (Singer et al. 2016). *Parosteal osteosarcoma* of the foot and ankle is very rare (Johnson et al. 1999).

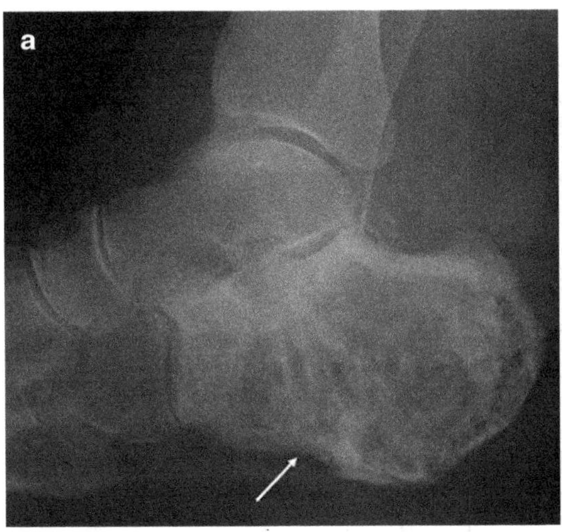

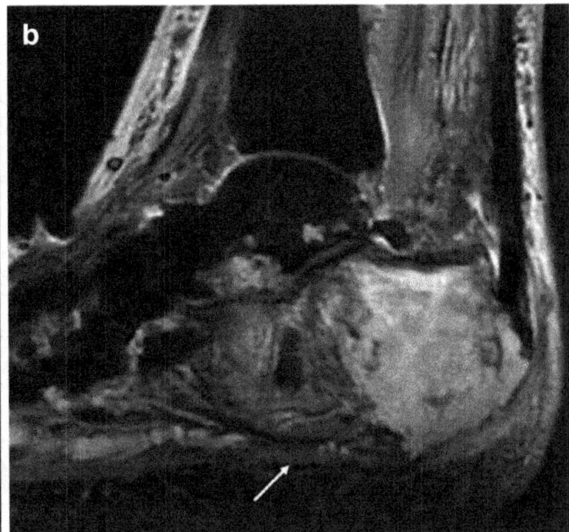

Fig. 8 The lateral calcaneal X-ray demonstrates a lytic lesion with coarsened trabeculae (**a**). There is however an area of irregularity and sclerosis which was more clearly demonstrated on MRI. The sagittal STIR image (**b**) confirms osteosarcoma changes on a background of Paget's disease

3.6.1.3 Fibrogenic Tumors

Desmoplastic fibroma is a very rare (Böhm et al. 1996), locally aggressive, primary bone tumor that can be considered the intra-osseous counterpart of fibromatosis (see soft tissue section). Most cases present in the second and third decades, with an equal sex incidence. Lesions usually present with pain or swelling or occasionally with pathological fracture. Radiographically, a geographic pattern of bone destruction, narrow zone of transition, and internal pseudotrabeculation are the most consistent features (Taconis et al. 1994). Cortical breakthrough and soft tissue infiltration are present in up to 48% of lesions, but periosteal reaction is uncommon. The MR features are mainly nonspecific, but foci of low to intermediate signal intensity on T2 weighting are often present and reflect the fibrous, relatively acellular components of the tumor (Vanhoenacker et al. 2000).

Fibrosarcoma is a malignant bone lesion which most commonly occurs in the ankle and hindfoot, and involvement of the forefoot is very rare. Radiographically, it has a variable growth rate ranging from a geographic pattern of bone destruction to a more aggressive moth-eaten or permeative pattern with extensive bone destruction and soft tissue infiltration (Link et al. 1998). The lack of mineralization helps distinguish them from osteochondroma or chondrosarcoma, although occasionally some mineralization may be present. Lesions usually display nonspecific intermediate signal intensity on T1 weighting and inhomogeneous high signal intensity on T2 weighting, although if the collagen content is high, then a predominantly lower signal intensity on T2 weighting may be noted. Foci of hemorrhage and necrosis may be present. Undifferentiated pleomorphic sarcoma (UPS—discussed in Sect. 3.6.2) can also rarely involve bone, in which case its imaging features are very similar to that of fibrosarcoma (Antonescu et al. 2000).

3.6.1.4 Vascular Tumors

Hemangiomas of the bones of the foot and ankle are rare. Most are asymptomatic, but some may present with pain and swelling (Cavalcante et al. 2021; Hoffmann and Israel 1990). Radiographs usually show a well-defined, often expansile, lytic lesion with a coarse latticelike trabecular pattern, without a sclerotic rim. They may contain detectable fat on CT and MR imaging. Unlike soft tissue hemangioma, phleboliths are not typical (Cavalcante et al. 2021; Peterson et al. 1992).

Angiosarcoma is a rare, malignant, vascular tumor, which is similar to and difficult to differentiate from *hemangioendothelioma* and *hemangiopericytoma* which are usually of intermediate aggressiveness and may be benign, whereas angiosarcoma is an aggressive malignant tumor with a poor prognosis (Bakotic et al. 1999). They are associated with previous radiotherapy and chronic lymphedema (Stewart-Treves syndrome). They can present as growing red or bruise-like masses. In bony lesions, intermediate or low-grade lesions may present with lytic areas and a honeycombing appearance, whereas aggressive lesions demonstrate a permeative pattern of bone destruction and soft tissue infiltration. In hemangioendothelioma, multicentricity is common (Cavalcante et al. 2021), and the small bones of the foot may be extensively involved (Boutin et al. 1996). Prominent serpentine structures on cross-sectional imaging are suggestive. Ultrasound may reveal an inhomogeneous lesion containing cystic foci, and Doppler studies may reveal arteriovenous shunting. MR imaging may show prominent vessels of variable signal intensity (depending on the blood flow) and fluid-fluid levels, but unlike hemangiomas, there is no fatty overgrowth. They can contain hemorrhage and areas of necrosis (Singer et al. 2016).

3.6.1.5 Osteoclastic Giant Cell-Rich Tumors

Nonossifying fibroma (NOF) and *fibrous cortical defect* (FCD) are histologically identical self-limiting benign fibrous tumors that are common in the distal tibia and fibula (Unni 1986). They develop due to failure of normal ossification of fibrous tissue within the bone. The incidence is likely underestimated as they tend to be asymptomatic but are present somewhere in the skeleton in up to 40% of children (Reda 2018; Betsy et al. 2004). Although FCDs and smaller NOFs are often incidental findings, larger NOFs may present with a pathological fracture. Radiography typically reveals an eccentric, ovoid, lytic lesion with a well-defined, sclerotic margin and often a multiloculated "bubbly" appearance in larger lesions (Reda 2018). Cross-sectional imaging is not usually required, but CT may show thinning of the cortex and MR imaging may display low signal intensity on T2 weighting due to an abundance of collagen. Lesions often enhance with intravenous contrast. The natural history is to resolve spontaneously. Distal tibial lesions and lesions involving more than 50% cortical diameter are at higher risk of fracture in which case curettage and bone grafting can be considered (Kennedy et al. 2016; Reda 2018; Arata et al. 1981).

Aneurysmal bone cysts (ABCs) are benign lesions that can be locally aggressive. They occur predominantly in the metaphyseal region of long bones. Their origin is unknown but may be related to intra-osseous vascular malformation (Reda 2018). The majority of lesions are primary and occur in the first and second decades (Cavalcante et al. 2021). Later presentation should suggest that the ABC is secondary to an underlying lesion, which may be benign or malignant, including giant cell tumor or chondroblastoma. Lesions are more commonly found in the distal tibia and fibula than in the foot. In the foot, it is more common in the calcaneus and metatarsals (Khan et al. 2015; Reda 2018). In the initial phase, radiography shows a markedly expansile, metaphyseal, eccentric, lytic lesion contained by a thin layer of periosteal new bone. In the healing phase, there is maturation of the periosteal bone and consolidation of the lesion. MR imaging shows a lobulated, expansile, heterogeneous, and multiseptate lesion with fluid-fluid levels containing foci of variable signal depending on the age of the blood products (Figs. 9 and 10). In the active phase, the thin rim of intact periosteal tissue gives a low signal on all sequences. MR imaging is more sensitive than CT at detecting intralesional fluid-fluid levels. In primary lesions, intravenous contrast confirms rim and septal enhancement, whereas in secondary lesions, the enhancement pattern depends on the extent and nature of the underlying lesion. Telangiectatic osteosarcoma also demonstrates fluid-fluid levels, and aggressive imaging features such as a solid soft tissue component or cortical destruction should prompt further investigation (Singer et al. 2016; Cavalcante et al. 2021; Reda 2018). Due to locally aggressive behavior, it can be treated with curettage with or without bone grafting (Khan et al. 2015). Local recurrence rates are in the range of 20–30%. Wide resection of bone has lower recurrence rates but higher morbidity (Reda 2018).

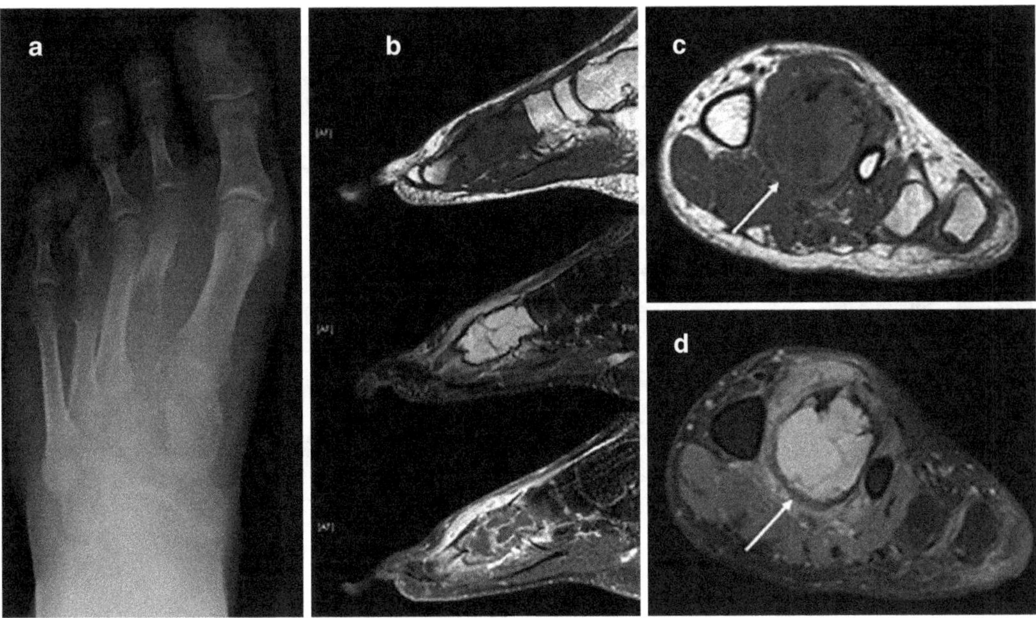

Fig. 9 A 30-year-old female presents with a painful foot. The DP X-ray (**a**) shows a lytic appearance to the second metatarsal. On Sag MR images (**b**) the second metatarsal appears expanded with high T2 signal and low T1 signal with some enhancement on post contrast imaging. Coronal T1 (**c**) and STIR (**d**) shows low T1 signal (**c**) and high T2 signal (**d**). This was in keeping with an aneurysmal bone cyst (ABC) of the proximal second metatarsal. At this age, a giant cell tumour and giant cell reparative granuloma would be included in the differential diagnosis

Giant cell tumor of bone (GCTB) is a benign but locally aggressive tumor. They typically occur in the third and fourth decades of life (Reda 2018; Murai et al. 2018; Frassica et al. 1993). Lesions usually present with pain and swelling and often a pathological fracture. In the foot and ankle, the majority occur in the distal tibia, talus, or calcaneus (Reda 2018). Calcaneal lesions are often found posteriorly at the site of the apophysis, although they may also occur in the subarticular portion of the anterior calcaneus. GCTBs of the small bones of the foot tend to occur in younger patients, present more aggressively with more bone destruction, are more likely to recur locally after resection, and show a more aggressive behavior than giant cell tumors of large bones (Reda 2018; Biscaglia et al. 2000). On radiographs, they typically are lytic, expansile, and eccentric, extending from the subchondral bone to the metaphysis (Reda 2018; Murai et al. 2018; Chakarun et al. 2013). The majority of lesions have an ill-defined geographic pattern of bone destruction, although they can have a more aggressive moth-eaten pattern with cortical destruction and soft tissue infiltration. As cystic components and hemorrhage are common, MR images typically show an inhomogeneous appearance, with foci of variable signal intensity (low to intermediate T1 and intermediate to high T2 signal) and often fluid-fluid levels. Fluid-fluid levels can be seen with a secondary ABC (Reda 2018; Selek et al. 2007). On bone scan, it often demonstrates increased uptake peripherally with central photopenia due to necrosis or osteolysis (Murai et al. 2018; Hudson et al. 1984). They are generally benign but locally aggressive tumors that can locally recur but have been reported to rarely metastasize to the lungs (Singer et al. 2016). The very rare multicentric giant cell tumor has a tendency to involve the feet but does not seem to carry an increased risk of pulmonary metastases (Cummins et al. 1996). They are normally treated with curettage and bone grafting. Generally, recurrence rate is around 20%, but this decreases to around 5% with the use of adju-

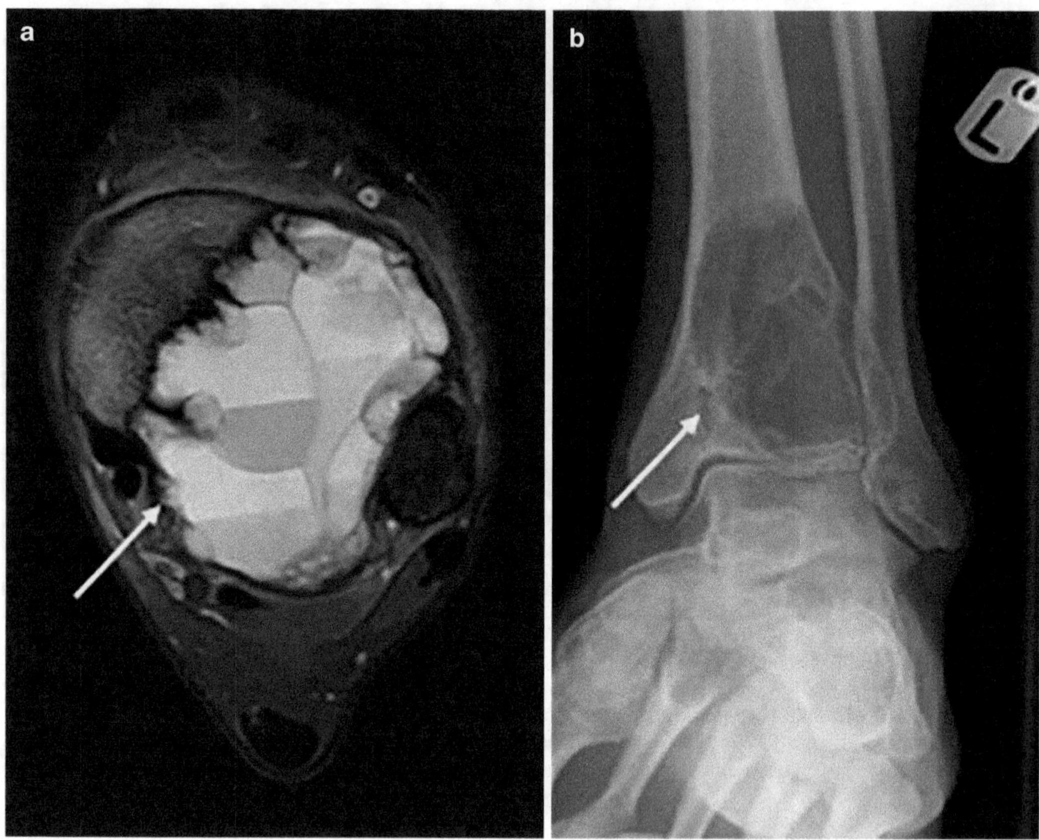

Fig. 10 Lytic expansile lesion in the distal tibia on X-ray (**b**). Typical features with fluid-fluid levels on MRI axial STIR image (**a**), in keeping with an aneurysmal bone cyst (ABC) distal tibia

vant treatments such as denosumab. However, when looking at the foot and ankle specifically, recurrence rates are higher (Reda 2018) (Fig. 11).

3.6.1.6 Other Mesenchymal Tumors

Fibrous dysplasia is a benign medullary fibro-osseous lesion, in which bone-forming tissue is unable to develop into mature lamellar bone (Cavalcante et al. 2021). In its monostotic form, only 3% of lesions occur in the foot and ankle mostly in adolescents and young adults (Schajowicz 2012). In the less common polyostotic form, however, the majority of patients show involvement of the foot. Polyostotic disease tends to present in the first decade with pain or pathological fracture or with endocrine problems (McCune-Albright syndrome). Monostotic disease more commonly presents in the second decade as an incidental finding or after innocuous trauma. Both forms of the disease have an equal sex distribution, although there is a predilection for girls in Albright's syndrome. Radiographs show a well-defined, expansile, medullary lesion often with a sclerotic margin. The matrix is classically ground glass but is variable, ranging from lucent to sclerotic (Kennedy et al. 2016). MR imaging shows a hypointense or isointense signal intensity compared with muscle on T1 weighting and a variable signal intensity on T2 weighting depending on the cellularity and fibrous and mineralized components (Cavalcante et al. 2021; Isefuku et al. 1999). Treatment with curettage and bone grafting may be required if there is a risk of fracture (Reda 2018) (Fig. 12).

Unicameral bone cyst (UBC; also known as simple bone cyst, SBC) is uncommon in the foot and ankle but does have a predilection for the calcaneus, classically at the ankle of Gissane

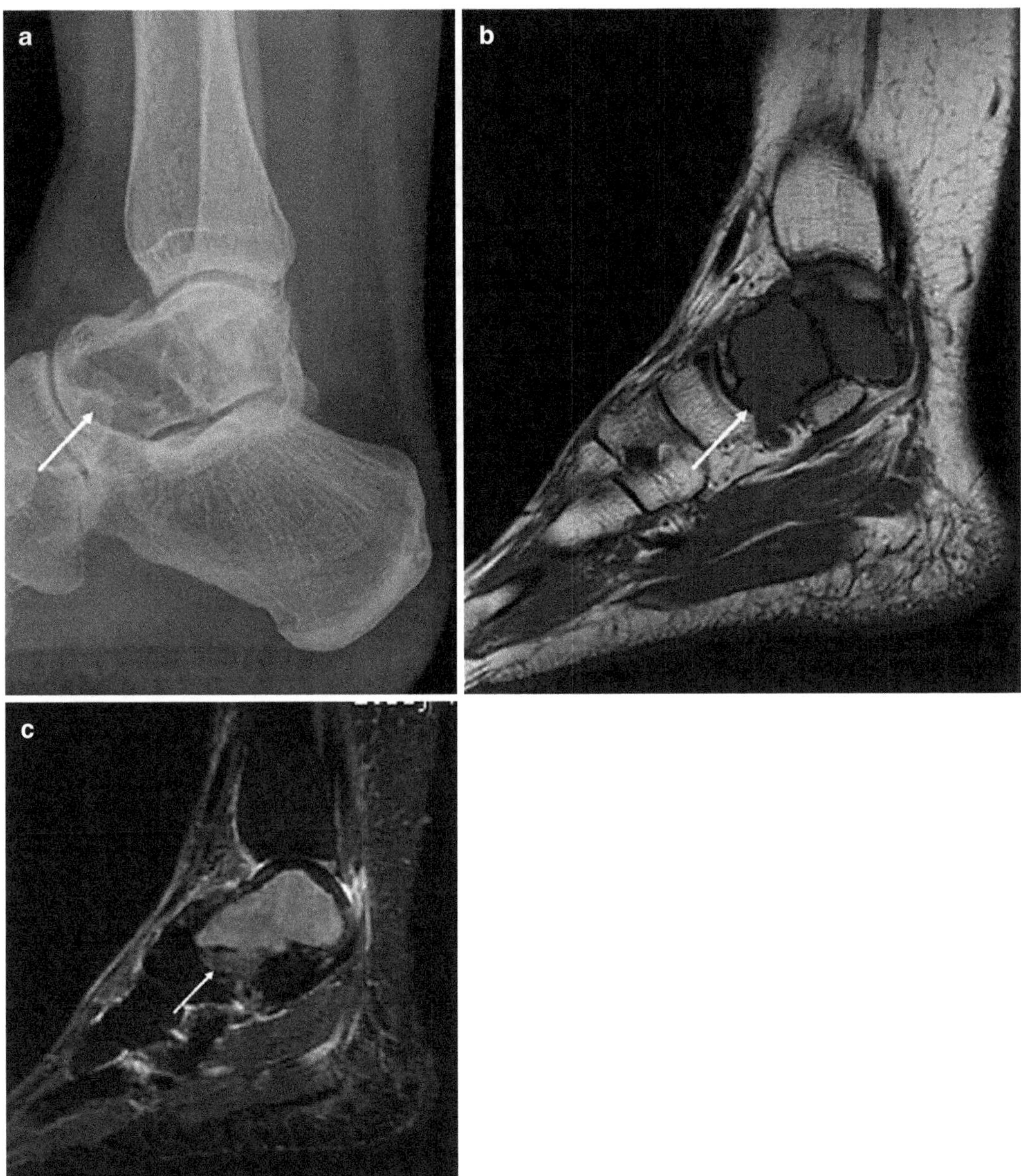

Fig. 11 Lytic lesion in talus (**a**). This returns low signal on T1 (**b**) and heterogenous low signal on STIR (**c**). Biopsy demonstrates GCT (giant cell tumor of bone) of the talus

(Cavalcante et al. 2021; Reda 2018). It is most common in the second decade of life, with a 2–3:1 male predominance (WHO Classification of Tumours Editorial Board 2020; Kaelin 1995). Some lesions present incidentally, whereas others present with chronic pain probably due to microfractures. Radiographs reveal a well-defined lytic lesion often with a sclerotic rim. The "fallen fragment sign" whereby there is a pathological fracture through the lesions with a bone fragment within the cyst is pathognomonic but not always present (Singer et al. 2016; Cavalcante et al. 2021). Pseudocysts can appear similar but are less well-defined, and internal trabeculations are often present (Stukenborg-Colsman et al. 1999). On CT and MR imaging, lesions often display fluid characteristics, although the density and signal intensity may be greater than water

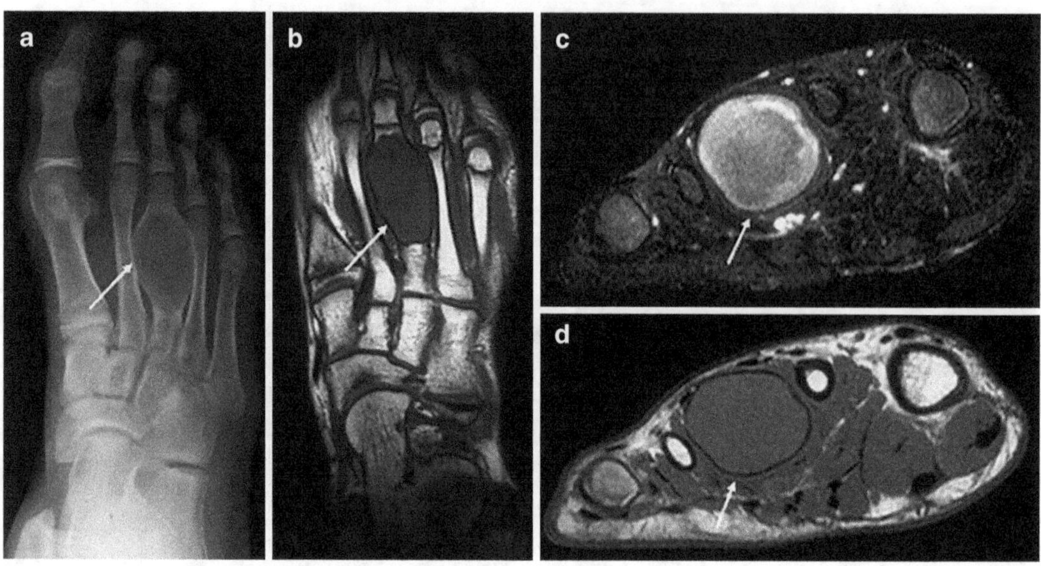

Fig. 12 Lytic lesion with ground-glass matrix in the third metatarsal on X-ray (**a**) typical of fibrous dysplasia. Nonspecific features on MRI with low T1 signal (**b**, **d**) and heterogenous T2 signal on PD FS imaging (**c**). The X-ray features are diagnostic of fibrous dysplasia

due to their high protein content. UBCs that are small with low risk of pathological fracture may be observed or discharged. Larger cysts with risk of significant pathological fracture may undergo curettage and bone grafting (Khan et al. 2015; Kennedy et al. 2016; Reda 2018) (Fig. 13).

Intra-osseous lipoma is a rare benign tumor composed of mature adipose cells. However, 13–24% of intra-osseous lipomas occur in the foot and ankle, with a predisposition for the calcaneus (Reda 2018; Mirra 1989; Milgram 1988; Weinfeld et al. 2002). Lesions appear most frequently in the fourth decade, show no sexual predilection, and are often incidental findings. In the calcaneus, the lesion usually occurs anteriorly and is characterized by a well-defined, radiolucent lesion with a thin sclerotic rim (Cavalcante et al. 2021; Kennedy et al. 2016). There may be a central stippled or course calcific density representing an area of fat necrosis histologically. Intralesional trabeculation may be seen (Singer et al. 2016; Kennedy et al. 2016). On MRI, the signal intensity is similar to subcutaneous fat on all sequences, although calcific foci will give a low signal on all sequences, and areas of necrosis and cyst formation will give a low signal intensity on T1 weighting and high signal intensity on T2 weighting. They may spontaneously resolve with observation. If there is risk of fracture, then curettage with bone grafting can be considered (Kennedy et al. 2016; Reda 2018) (Fig. 14).

Primary liposarcoma of bone is very rare and controversial but has been recorded in the calcaneus (Murari et al. 1989).

Metastases to the foot and ankle are rare due to less red marrow in this location, with a reported incidence of less than 1% of all metastatic disease (Singer et al. 2016; Khan et al. 2015; Reda 2018). However, it is likely that the true incidence is higher as many probably go unrecognized in disseminated disease. 50% of metastases are secondary to colorectal, renal, or lung primaries, while another 25% are due to uterine, bladder, or breast cancer (Singer et al. 2016). Occasionally, a foot or ankle metastasis may present without a known primary. In the foot, the tarsal bones are more commonly involved than the forefoot, and the majority of these occur in the calcaneus and talus (Murai et al. 2018; Maheshwari et al. 2008). Involvement of several foot bones is common and may result in massive bone loss. Radiographically, most metastases are purely osteolytic in 80%, but prostatic metastases are usually sclerotic, and breast, bladder, and gastrointestinal primaries may be lytic, sclerotic, or mixed (Murai et al. 2018; Libson et al. 1987).

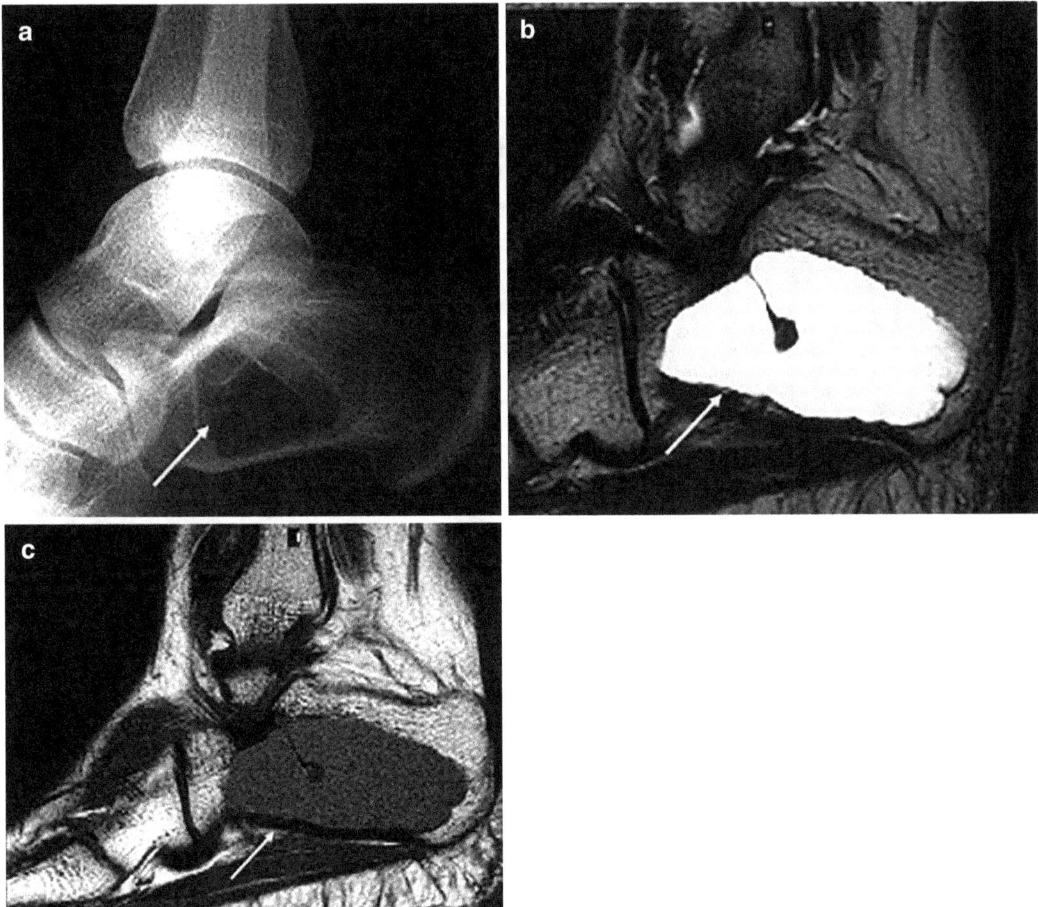

Fig. 13 Lytic lesion in the anterior calcaneus on X-ray (**a**). The MRI is diagnostic as it returns high T2 signal (**b**) and low T1 signal (**c**) typical of a simple bone cyst anterior calcaneus. This is an incidental finding of little clinical significance. This is also a typical site for an intra-osseous lipoma, but the MRI shows that it contains fluid and not fat

Although the lesions may be expansile, cortical destruction is normally present. The MR imaging features are variable but normally demonstrate low T1 signal, high T2 signal, avid contrast enhancement, and soft tissue extension (Singer et al. 2016). Metastases from thyroid and renal cell carcinoma are highly vascular and therefore may demonstrate flow voids on MRI (Murai et al. 2018) (Fig. 15).

Adamantinoma is a rare, low-grade, malignant tumor of unknown origin that has a preference for the tibia. In a large review of 200 patients, there was involvement of the distal tibia in 58 cases and the distal fibula in 9 cases. Only 2 cases were recorded in the foot, one in a metatarsal, and the other in a cuneiform (Moon and Mori 1986).

3.6.1.7 Hemopoietic Tumors

Primary lymphoma of bone (PLB) is defined as osseous involvement without systemic disease for 6 months. Secondary lymphoma represents systemic disease with spread to the bone. Primary disease has a better prognosis (Murai et al. 2018; Kirsch et al. 2006). Primary lymphoma has a wide age range but usually peaks in the fifth decade and is more common in males (2:1). Lesions are more common in the distal tibia than the foot. Of the foot bones, the calcaneus is most commonly involved (Skorman and Martin 1999). Radiographically, lesions typically show an aggressive moth-eaten or permeative pattern of destruction and are predominantly lytic, although up to a third may have a mixture of lysis and scle-

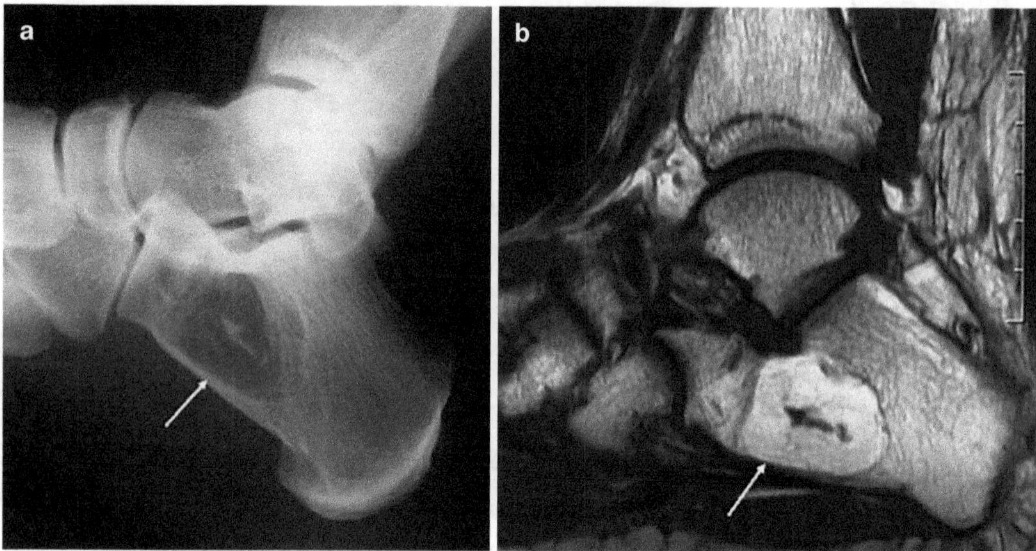

Fig. 14 Mixed lucent sclerotic lesion on radiograph (**a**). The lesion has signal features similar to subcutaneous fat on T2 sagittal MR image (**b**). This is typical of an intra-osseous lipoma in the anterior calcaneum

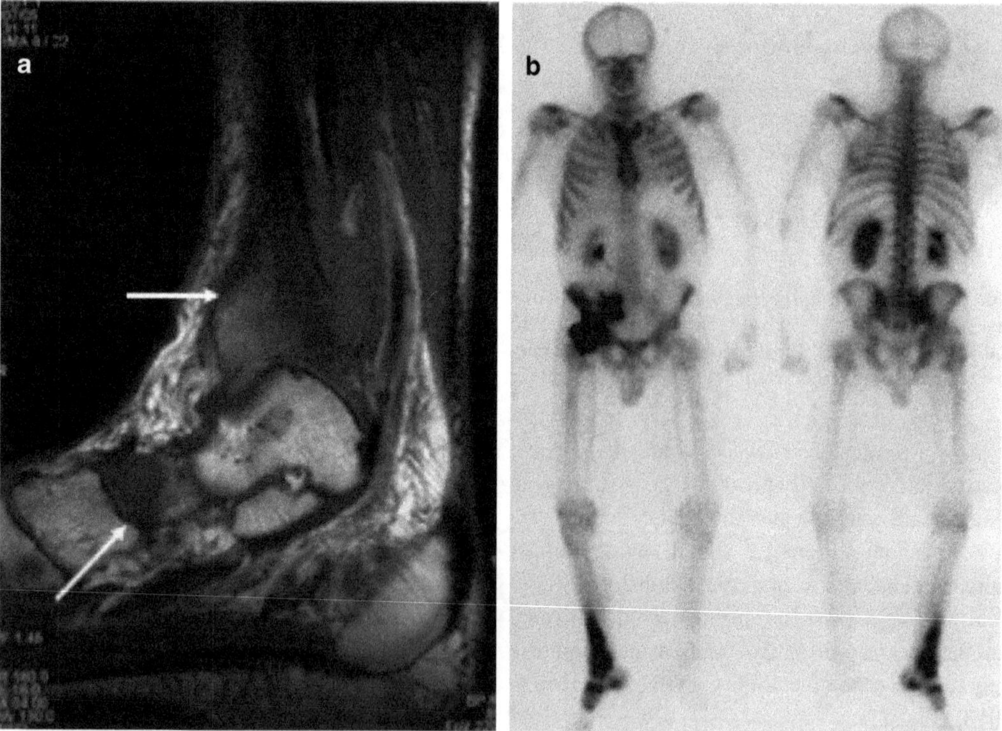

Fig. 15 Metastatic transitional carcinoma tibia. The MRI confirms an extensive lesion in the tibia with low signal change on the sagittal T1 image (**a**). There are further lesions in the talus, calcaneus, and navicular. Multiple lesions at this age are always suggestive of metastatic disease as was proven in this case. The bone scan (**b**) shows considerable activity over the right hip and right hemipelvis in keeping with further metastatic disease

rosis. Periosteal reaction and soft tissue extension are common. Sequestra may also be present. On MR imaging, most lesions are isointense or hypointense to skeletal muscle on T1 weighting and inhomogeneous and predominantly hyperintense on T1 weighting (White et al. 1998). Relative paucity of cortical destruction relative to the degree of marrow replacement and soft tissue extension is characteristic (Murai et al. 2018).

Multiple myeloma in the foot and ankle is rare, accounting for less than 2% of all myelomas and less than 1% of all malignant bone tumors of the foot and ankle (Unni 1986; Campanacci 2013; Mirra 1989). Myeloma of the foot and ankle usually indicates widespread involvement with marrow reconversion. Radiographically, lesions are osteolytic with a geographic pattern of bone destruction and variable margins.

Langerhans cell histiocytosis is very rare in the foot and ankle (Reisi et al. 2021). In its localized form, it is known as *eosinophilic granuloma.* Patients present between the ages of 5 and 15 years with a slight male predominance. In the early phase, lesions often have an aggressive pattern of bone destruction, with ill-defined margins and lamellated periosteal reaction simulating Ewing's sarcoma, whereas in the later healing phase, they have well-defined sclerotic margins simulating a benign bone tumor. The MR imaging appearances are nonspecific.

3.6.1.8 Undifferentiated Small Round Cell Sarcomas

Ewing's sarcoma is a highly aggressive round cell tumor. Lesions are most commonly found in the distal tibia and fibula and to a lesser extent the calcaneus and metatarsals (Ruggieri et al. 2014; Adkins et al. 1997). Lesions usually present with a painful swelling in the second decade. There is a slight male predominance (1.7:1) and a shorter duration of symptoms for forefoot lesions than hindfoot lesions. Survival is much better in patients who present with localized disease and forefoot lesions. For the 50% who have metastases at presentation, the prognosis is very poor (Adkins et al. 1997). Radiographically, lesions typically show an aggressive moth-eaten or permeative pattern of bone destruction (Cavalcante et al. 2021), usually with a soft tissue mass (Fig. 9), although atypical features are more commonly found in the tarsal bones (Baraga et al. 2001). In particular, tarsal lesions less commonly demonstrate permeative bone destruction, periosteal reaction, or soft tissue mass (Mascard et al. 2017; Schatz et al. 2010). Purely osteosclerotic lesions are more common in the calcaneus. On MR imaging, lesions are usually hypointense or isointense with muscle on T1 weighting and hyperintense and inhomogeneous on T1 weighting. The lack of mineralized matrix helps differentiate it from osteosarcoma (Fig. 16).

3.6.1.9 Tumorlike/Nonneoplastic Lesions

Bizarre parosteal osteochondromatous proliferation (BPOP, also known as Nora lesions) is an uncommon, parosteal, tumorlike lesion that is typically found on the surfaces of the proximal phalanges and metatarsal and metacarpal bones. It is most common in the third and fourth decades, has an equal sex incidence, and usually presents with a painless swelling (Cavalcante et al. 2021; Harty et al. 2000). Initially, the lesion is an immature mass of mineralization within the parosteal soft tissues with no clear osseous attachment, but as it matures, radiographs show attachment to bone with a pedunculated or sessile base but without medullary continuity (Nora et al. 1983). CT can help to demonstrate this when radiographs are equivocal (Meneses et al. 1993). Rapid growth and pain can occur and can mimic a more aggressive lesion. Despite this, aggressive imaging features should not be seen. In the differential diagnosis, it is parosteal osteosarcoma and florid reactive periostitis. Histologically, they are composed of bizarrely organized bone, hyaline cartilage, and fibroblasts without atypia or high mitotic index (Singer et al. 2016; Cavalcante et al. 2021) (Fig. 17).

Mature bone infarcts have a typical appearance, with densely mineralized foci within the medullary cavity. However, in the early stages, radiographs may show nonspecific mottled bone rarefaction, sometimes with mild reactive sclerosis mimicking infection or malignancy. MR imaging is helpful as it demonstrates a central focus of high or intermediate signal surrounded

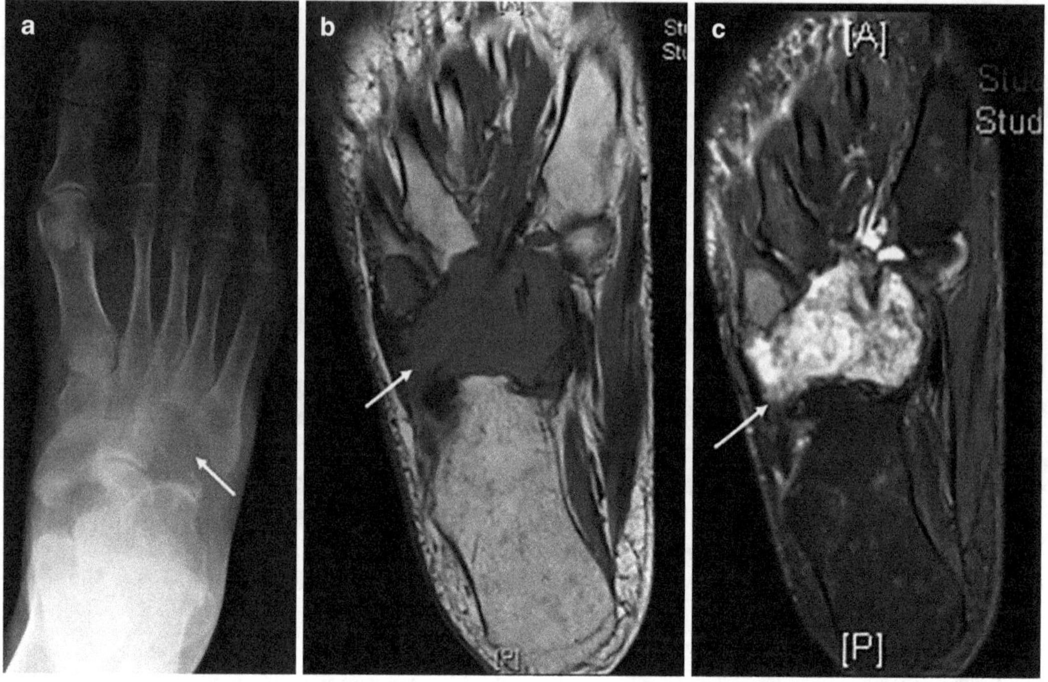

Fig. 16 Local recurrence of the soft tissue Ewing's sarcoma destroying the cuboid bone. The differential diagnosis would also have to include a radiation-induced sarcoma. This appears as a destructive lesion of the cuboid on X-ray (**a**) and is low signal to intermediate signal on T1 (**b**) and heterogenous but predominantly high signal on T2 (**c**) weighted imaging

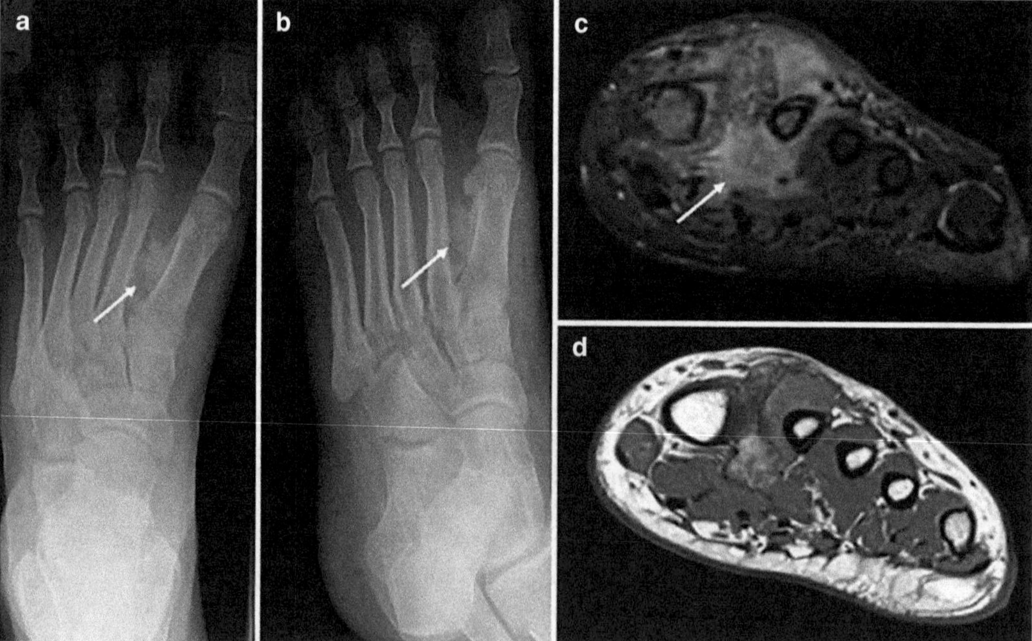

Fig. 17 Florid reactive periostitis first metatarsal best appreciated on the radiographs (**a**, **b**) white arrows. This is part of the spectrum of reactive surface lesions of bone including BPOP (bizarre parosteal osteochondromatous proliferation). T1 coronal (d) and post contrast images (**c**) are non specific and the radiograph is more diagnostic

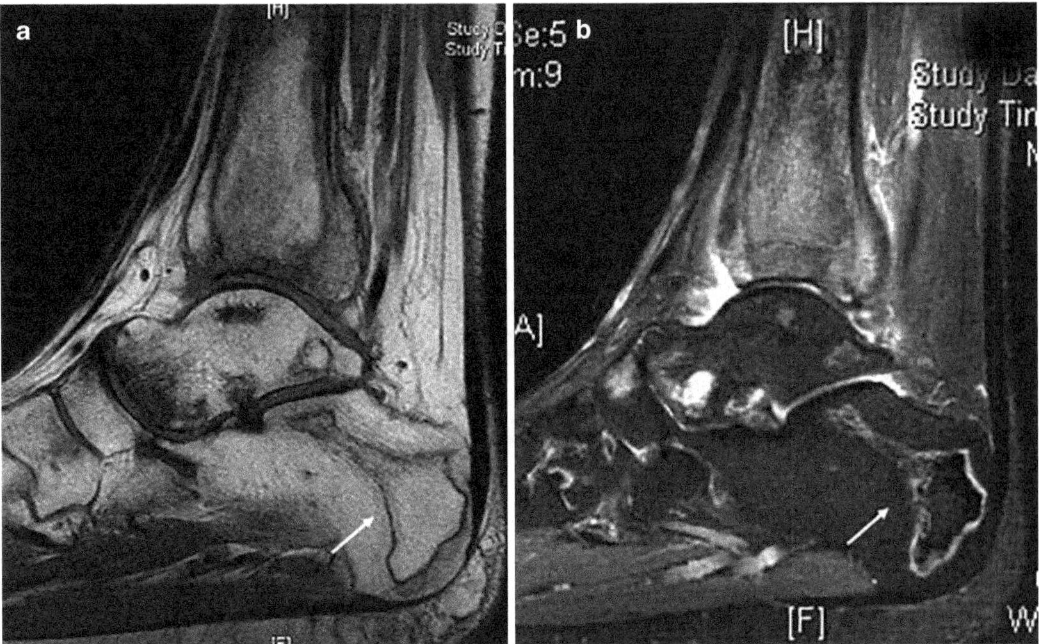

Fig. 18 Sagittal PD (**a**) and STIR (**b**) MR images demonstrate a low signal serpiginous line in the calcaneum in keeping with a bone infarct

by a thin, serpentine, low-signal border (Abrahimzadeh et al. 1998) (Fig. 18).

Giant cell reparative granuloma is a rare, benign, reactive, intra-osseous lesion with a predilection for the hands and feet (Murphey et al. 2001). In the foot, most lesions occur in the metatarsals, and the majority present in the third decade (Ratner and Dorfman 1990). Radiographically, the lesion is typically a solitary, lytic, expanded metaphyseal lesion occasionally extending into subarticular bone and more frequently extending into the diaphysis. Extension into soft tissues is unusual unless it is located in a distal phalanx or when a pathological fracture occurs. A common differential diagnosis, giant cell tumor of bone (GCTB), tends to occur in slightly older patients, and soft tissue infiltration is more common (Murphey et al. 2001).

Intra-osseous ganglia are juxta-articular cystic lesions that are much less common than their soft tissue counterparts. In a large study reviewing 213 cases in the literature, 18% were found in the medial malleolus, 3% in the lateral malleolus, and 8% in the foot (Murff and Ashry 1994). Most patients present in mid-adult life with intermittent pain. Radiographs show a well-defined, nonexpansile, radiolucent, juxta-articular lesion with a well-defined sclerotic margin.

There are several other lesions that may mimic bone tumors, including gout, infection, Paget's disease, and stress fractures, which are discussed in other chapters.

3.6.2 Soft Tissue Tumors and Tumorlike Lesions

3.6.2.1 Adipocytic Tumors

Lipomas are common benign lesions. The majority present in middle-aged patients as a superficial soft tissue mass around the ankle or heel (Kirby et al. 1989). Lipomatous variants, heterogeneous lipomas, and lipoblastoma are much less common but have been recorded in the foot and ankle. Radiographically, lipomas may appear as a soft tissue mass of low (fatty) density and rarely bone erosion (Braunschweig et al. 1992). Simple lipomas are easily diagnosed on CT and MR imaging as they are homogeneous, do not enhance, and have similar density and signal characteristics to subcutaneous fat (Hochman and Wu 2017). Simple lipomas containing various connective tissue elements, spindle cell and pleomorphic variants of lipoma, may contain foci of enhancing and nonenhancing non-lipomatous tissue that may be indistinguishable from atypical lipoma (well-differentiated liposarcoma). Angiolipoma is indistinguishable from intramuscular angioma, and both may contain serpentine structures, heterotopic bone, and phleboliths. Perineural fibrolipoma rarely occurs in the foot and may be associated with macrodactylia fibrolipomatosis (Donley et al. 1996).

Liposarcoma usually presents as a painless mass in the fifth and sixth decades and is rare in children. Myxoid and well-differentiated liposarcomas (atypical lipomas) are the most common subtypes and carry a better prognosis than the more aggressive round cell, pleomorphic, and dedifferentiated subtypes (Werd et al. 1995). Nonetheless, well-differentiated liposarcomas do have the potential to dedifferentiate and metastasize. On cross-sectional imaging, nodular components, large size, septations thicker than 2 mm, and subfascial location suggest that further investigation is required. On MR imaging, well-differentiated lesions always contain demonstrable fat, whereas the remaining subtypes may not (Singer et al. 2016). Well-differentiated liposarcomas tend to have thick enhancing septa or nodules, whereas lipomas have thin septa that display only slight if any enhancement (Hochman and Wu 2017).

3.6.2.2 Fibroblastic/Myofibroblastic Tumors

Musculoskeletal fibromatoses are a spectrum of benign fibroblastic/myofibroblastic neoplasms which can be locally aggressive. The fibromatoses are classified as superficial or deep (Guillou and Folpe 2010). They classically demonstrate infiltrative growth, a tendency for local recurrence, and do not metastasize. *Deep fibromatosis* has a more locally aggressive nature and higher recurrence rate (Singer et al. 2016; Lee et al. 2006). *Superficial fibromatosis* is known as *plantar fibromatosis* in the foot (Ledderhose disease) and is one of the most common benign soft tissue tumors of the foot and ankle. There is a predilection for males and advancing age (Hochman and Wu 2017; Guillou and Folpe 2010). Lesions can be multiple and bilateral and can be associated with fibromatosis in the hands (Dupuytren contracture) and penis (Peyronie disease) (Bouchard et al. 2017). Patients usually present with one or more firm, fixed, subcutaneous nodules measuring around 2 cm in size on the plantar side of the foot. They occur along the medial or central band of the plantar fascia. When affecting the medial band, it may impinge upon a digital branch of the nerve to the great toe (Zgonis et al. 2005). Small lesions may remain asymptomatic, but larger, deeper, infiltrating lesions often require wide resection. Ultrasound shows a well-defined, inhomogeneous, hypoechoic mass superficial to the medial slip of the plantar aponeurosis. On MR imaging, lesions are well-defined superficially against the subcutaneous fat, but the infiltrative deep margin often blends imperceptibly with the deep aponeurosis (Morrison et al. 1994). However, the tissues deep to the aponeurosis are invaded in only 15% of patients. The signal characteristics vary with the phase of the disease (Woertler 2005). On T2 weighting, most lesions in the involutional or residual phase display only a slightly hyperintense signal intensity compared with skeletal muscle due to the high collagen content, whereas in the cellular proliferative phase, a higher signal intensity on T2 weighting is typical. Uniform low signal on all sequences is in keeping with established fibrous tissue without associated cellularity. Enhancement is variable and more marked in the proliferative phase. Flexor tendon sheaths can be involved leading to motion deficits (Singer et al. 2016). Treatment for superficial fibromatosis is normally conservative with NSAIDs, corticosteroid injection, or physiotherapy. Surgery with resection and fasciectomy is reserved for lesions which are refractory to conservative treatment (Veith et al. 2013).

Fibroma of the tendon sheath is an uncommon, benign, fibroblastic proliferation of the tendon sheaths. It usually presents as a slow-growing mass and is more common in men in the third to fifth decades. Radiographs may demonstrate a soft tissue mass and occasionally bony involvement. On MR imaging, lesions tend to display mainly intermediate signal intensity on both T1 weighting and T2 weighting.

Nodular fasciitis (pseudosarcomatous fibromatosis/fasciitis) is a benign soft tissue lesion that is rare in the foot and ankle, accounting for only 1% of benign soft tissue lesions of the foot and ankle (Kransdorf 1995). On MR imaging, lesions are usually well-defined but can be irregular. Myxoid and cellular lesions display high signal intensity on T2 weighting, whereas lesions with a predominantly fibrous histology display low to intermediate signal intensity on all sequences. Lesions typically enhance.

Calcifying aponeurotic fibroma (juvenile aponeurotic fibroma) is a rare, locally aggressive but self-limiting fibroblastic lesion that is found in the palms and soles of children and adolescents (Yee et al. 1991). The majority of cases involve the deep spaces of the sole. The cellular histology, aggressive growth pattern, and tendency to recur may lead to a misdiagnosis of fibrosarcoma. The imaging appearances are similar to fibromatosis (Chalatsis et al. 2022).

Dermatofibrosarcoma protuberans (DFSP) is a rare, slow-growing, low/intermediate-grade malignancy that originates in the dermal layer of the skin with low metastatic potential but with local aggressivity and potential for local recurrence (Singer et al. 2016). They are most common in the third to fifth decades (Cione et al. 1999). They are normally painless but may ulcerate. Large lesions may infiltrate deeper structures and will require imaging. Cutaneous components and lobular architecture with low to intermediate T1 signal and high T2 signal with intense internal enhancement are typical (Singer et al. 2016).

Fibrosarcoma is a malignant fibroblastic tumor that most commonly presents in the fifth and sixth decades. The long-term prognosis is guarded, with a 5-year survival rate of less than 40%. The infantile form usually occurs in the first 5 years of life and carries a better prognosis (Laffan et al. 2009; Cecchetto et al. 2001). Radiography may show a soft tissue mass and occasionally bony involvement. On MR imaging, the signal characteristics are nonspecific, with intermediate signal intensity on T1 weighting and inhomogeneous, intermediate signal intensity on T2 weighting. Post-gadolinium, they often have marked rim enhancement and may have an appearance of a spoked wheel (Bouchard et al. 2017).

3.6.2.3 So-Called Fibrohistiocytic Tumors

Pigmented villonodular synovitis (PVNS) is a benign but locally aggressive tumor of the synovium of joints or tendon sheaths. It may be diffuse and intra-articular, but in the foot and ankle, the localized extra-articular form is more common and is often termed *giant cell tumor of the tendon sheath* (GCTTS) (Kransdorf 1995). The uncommon diffuse extra-articular variant of GCTTS is a rare, locally aggressive neoplasm in the foot and ankle with significant recurrent and occasionally malignant potential (Somerhausen and Fletcher 2000). Patients usually present in early/middle adulthood with a painless slow-growing nodular soft tissue mass related to a tendon sheath or joint capsule or mechanical joint pain. Radiographs typically show an unmineralized soft tissue density opacity, normal bone density, and often corticated erosions. On ultrasound, lesions are typically solid, homogeneously hypoechoic with high Doppler blood flow internally (Murai et al. 2018). On MR imaging, hemosiderin-laden synovial tissue exerts a paramagnetic effect that shortens T1 and T2 relaxation times, resulting in low/intermediate signal intensity on both T1-weighted and T2-weighted sequences (Papp et al. 2007). Its low T2 signal intensity sets it apart from most other soft tissue tumors, although gouty tophi and amyloid can have similar T2 appearance (Murai et al. 2018). On gradient-echo (GE) sequences, the effect is exaggerated due to increased magnetic susceptibility. This results in areas of very low signal intensity and "blooming" artifact on T2-weighted GE sequences (Murphey et al. 2008). There may be erosion of adjacent bones. Typically, lesions show marked enhancement following intravenous contrast administration (Singer et al. 2016; Bravo et al. 1996; Kennedy et al. 2016). The disease can be progressive and so the treatment is normally surgical synovectomy, with a recurrence rate as high as 30% (Reda 2018; Stevenson et al. 2013). Radiotherapy can be used as an adjuvant treatment, but evidence of its effectiveness is not clear (Reda 2018; Mollon et al. 2015). In advanced or recurrent cases, reconstructive surgery may be considered (Khan et al. 2015) (Fig. 19).

Deep benign fibrous histiocytoma is a common benign soft tissue tumor (Kransdorf 1995). It usually presents in young to middle-aged adults as a protuberant nodular mass in the skin and is multiple in up to one-third. Imaging will usually be performed in the uncommon deep variety as they may mimic a more aggressive process. On MR imaging, lesions display intermediate signal intensity on T1 weighting and an inhomogeneous variable signal intensity on T1 weighting.

3.6.2.4 Vascular Tumors

Hemangioma/vascular malformation are relatively common benign soft tissue tumors of the foot and ankle. They may be true neoplasms or nonneoplastic vascular malformations (Singer et al. 2016). Malformations may be subdivided according to the speed of flow into capillary, lymphatic, venous, and arteriovenous malformations and arteriovenous fistulas. Symptomatic lesions tend to present in the first four decades with a swelling that may vary in size. Imaging is not usually required for superficial lesions but may be required for deep lesions. Radiographs may show a soft tissue mass that occasionally involves bone. Phleboliths are almost pathognomonic, but not always present (Singer et al. 2016). Hyperemia can cause bone demineralization (Murai et al. 2018). Angiography is helpful in confirming the type and extent of the lesion and the suitability for embolization (Mitty 1993). On ultrasound, appearances are variable, but lesions are usually inhomogeneous with a mixed echopattern due to vascular and nonvascular elements (Derchi et al. 1989). *Arteriovenous* malformations typically demonstrate high flow on Doppler, whereas slow-flowing *venous* lesions may give little or no Doppler signal. On T1-weighted MR images, lesions are predominantly low/intermediate signal intensity. On T2 weighting, lesions display very high signal intensity from the vascular components separated by low signal intensity fibrous elements. Intralesional fat manifests as high T1 signal and low signal on fat-suppressed sequences. Enhancement of the non-lipomatous

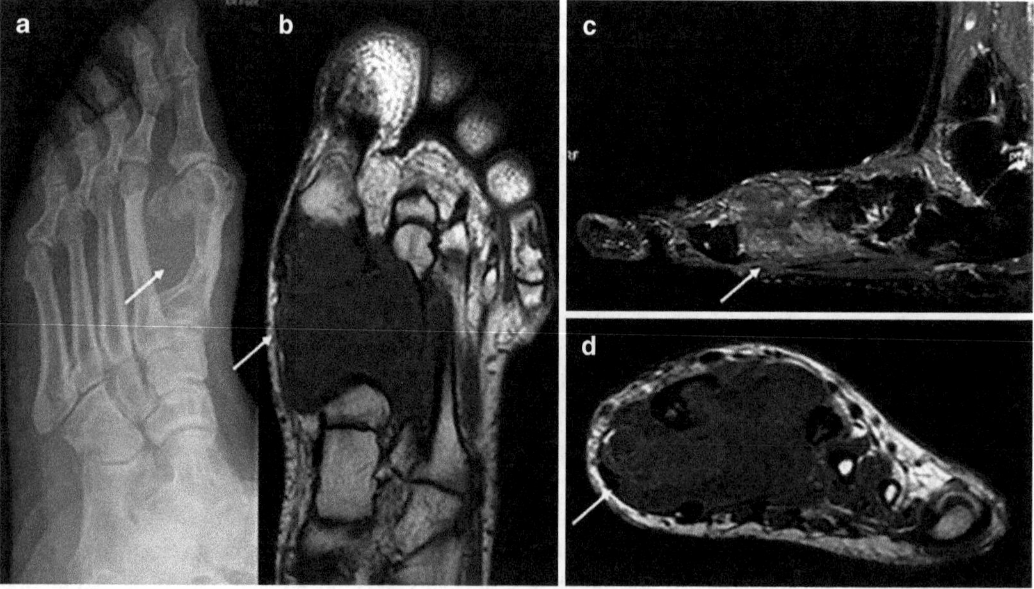

Fig. 19 The MRI images (**b**, **c**, **d**) show a soft tissue mass arising over the dorsum and medial aspect of the midfoot. There is erosion of the adjacent bone as seen on the radiograph (**a**). Much of the mass is low signal intensity on the T2W images

components is variable (Moukaddam et al. 2009). The vessels have a characteristic serpentine or circular appearance depending on the imaging plane and path of the vessel. The fast-flowing blood of an arteriovenous malformation results in flow voids on all sequences. Hemangioma often contains slow-flowing blood or pooling within dilated venous channels that give high signal intensity foci on T1 weighting and phleboliths that give low signal intensity on all sequences (Fig. 20). Soft tissue hemangiomas may be associated with syndromes including Klippel-Trenaunay-Weber, Maffuci, and Osler-Weber-Rendu (hereditary hemorrhagic telangiectasia) (Singer et al. 2016).

Kaposi's sarcoma has a strong predilection for the foot (Berlin 1995). Although classified as a vascular sarcoma, it is almost always located within the cutaneous tissues and is usually regarded as a skin tumor. AIDS-related Kaposi's sarcoma usually occurs in young adults and carries a poor prognosis, whereas the chronic (classic) form of Kaposi's sarcoma (often associated with lymphoreticular neoplasms) presents in later life and has a better prognosis. Imaging is only required for deep lesions, and the appearances are similar to the intermediate and malignant vasoformative tumors.

3.6.2.5 Pericytic (Perivascular) Tumors

Glomus tumors (glomangioma) are uncommon benign tumors of the foot that arise from neuromyoarterial glomus bodies and are usually located in the deepest layer of the dermis of the nail bed. Patients are usually women between the ages of 20 and 40 years and present with pain and cold sensitivity (Khan et al. 2015). Examination may reveal a characteristic small, red-blue, superficial nodule. US may show a small hypoechoic mass, but subungual lesions may be overlooked (Fornage 1988). X-ray may show scalloping of the terminal phalanx but is often unremarkable (Khan et al. 2015; Kennedy et al. 2016). On MR imaging, lesions are usually around 4 mm in size, encapsulated, and homogeneous and display high signal intensity on T2 weighting and marked enhancement (Drapé et al. 1996). The signal intensity on T1 weighting is variable depending on the histological variations of the lesion.

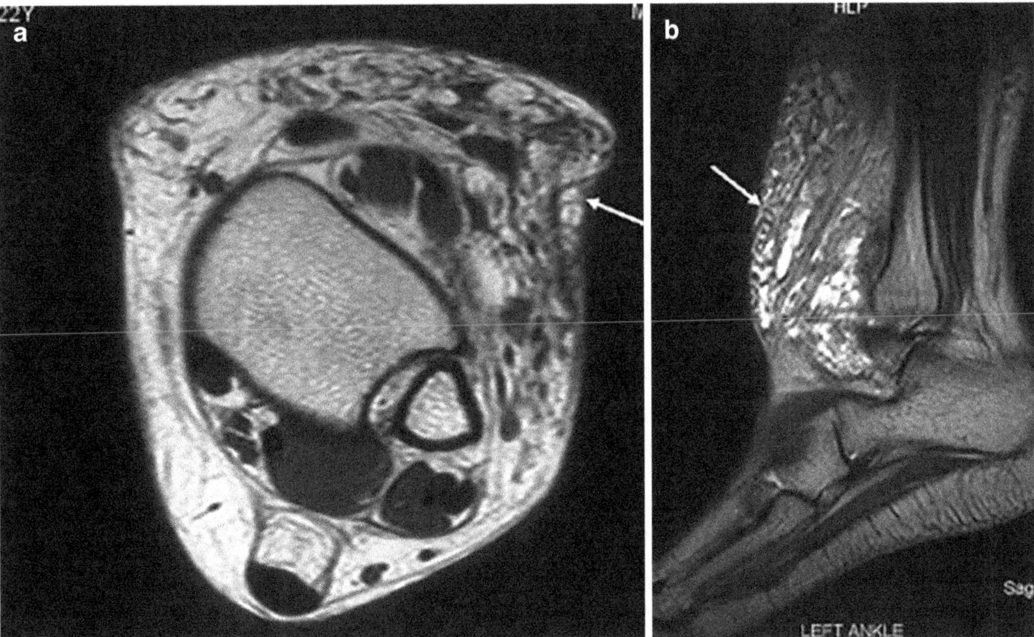

Fig. 20 Axial T1 (**a**) and sagittal STIR (**b**) demonstrate an ill-defined mass in the anterior aspect of the lower shin containing fat and serpiginous vessels typical of hemangioma/AVM

3.6.2.6 Smooth Muscle Tumors

Leiomyoma is an uncommon, benign, smooth muscle tumor (Kransdorf 1995). Deep lesions are much less common than superficial lesions but may mimic a sarcoma and therefore are more likely to be imaged. Deep leiomyomas are more likely to display fibrosis and mineralization. The mineralization varies from small flecks to large clumps of calcification and is readily shown on radiographs or CT. On MR imaging, lesions are typically homogeneous and isointense to skeletal muscle on T1W and heterogeneously hyperintense on T2W (Szolomayer et al. 2017).

Leiomyosarcomas are very rare neoplasms arising from smooth muscle cells. Patients most commonly present with a painless, slow-growing mass in the fifth–sixth decades. Rarely, leiomyosarcoma may arise in the wall of a vessel (Bégin et al. 1994). Radiography may show a soft tissue mass and bony involvement, but calcifications are rare. CT may show foci of decreased attenuation due to necrosis and cystic change. MR imaging typically shows a nonspecific, inhomogeneous, enhancing mass with necrosis, although more superficial lesions tend to be small, well-defined, and homogeneous.

3.6.2.7 Skeletal Muscle Tumors

Rhabdomyosarcoma is the most common childhood sarcoma in the pediatric foot and ankle (Rammelt et al. 2020; La et al. 2011). The alveolar subtype is more common than the embryonic subtype in extremity lesions and tends to occur in an older age group (10–25 years) than the embryonic subtype (0–15 years). Radiography may show a nonspecific soft tissue mass and sometimes with bony involvement (Suzuki et al. 1997). MR imaging shows an ill-defined, inhomogeneous, nonspecific mass, isointense on T1 weighting and hyperintense on T2 weighting. Prominent vascularity, intralesional hemorrhage, and necrosis are typical of the alveolar subtype and explain its inhomogeneous enhancement. On the other hand, embryonic lesions are less necrotic and display a more homogeneous enhancement pattern.

3.6.2.8 Chondro-Osseous Tumors

Synovial osteochondromatosis is a rare, benign soft tissue tumor around the foot and ankle. From a histopathological standpoint, it is listed under the chondrogenic bone tumor section of the 2020 WHO classification, but it is discussed here within the soft tissue tumor section due to its imaging appearance and its extra-osseous location. Synovial metaplasia produces multiple, round, intrasynovial, cartilaginous nodules that may ossify. It is more common in men and presents in middle age with joint swelling if intra-articular and a soft tissue mass if extra-articular. The disease is progressive, and secondary osteoarthritis in joints is common. Radiographs may show a soft tissue mass with variable mineralization, and well-defined bony erosions and scalloping are occasionally seen. Loose bodies are usually smooth and round or oval shaped and are often of similar size, although a dominant nodule may be present. On MR imaging, non-mineralized lesions give an intermediate signal intensity on T1 weighting and a very high signal intensity on T2 weighting (Kramer et al. 1993). Differentiation from synovial fluid can be achieved by using intravenous Gd-DTPA as the nodules enhance if they are attached to and derive a vascular supply from the synovium. However, the majority of cases contain foci of low signal intensity on both T1 weighting and T2 weighting due to calcification of cartilaginous nodules. Ossified nodules containing fatty marrow are less common. Chondrosarcomatous degeneration is very rare but has been reported in the ankle (Ontell and Greenspan 1994).

Extraskeletal chondromas are uncommon, benign, extra-osseous, and extrasynovial lesions composed mainly of mature hyaline cartilage (Bancroft et al. 2008). They have a propensity for the extremities and are most commonly found in men in the fourth to sixth decades (Kransdorf 1995; Chung and Enzinger 1978). They tend to occur near tendon sheaths and joint capsules. Radiographs often show a soft tissue mass containing chondroid mineralization (Hondar Wu et al. 2006). The uncalcified cartilaginous components of the lesions display intermediate signal intensity on T1 weighting and very high signal intensity on T2 weighting, whereas the mineralized components display low signal intensity on all sequences (Hochman and Wu 2017).

Extraskeletal chondrosarcomas are much less common than the skeletal equivalent and are normally of higher grade, but with similar imaging appearances. On MR imaging, lesions tend to appear ill-defined and inhomogeneous. Myxoid components typically display foci of very high signal intensity on T2 weighting, whereas the mineralized components of mesenchymal lesions display signal voids on all sequences (Murphey et al. 2003).

Extraskeletal osteosarcoma is a rare, aggressive, malignant mesenchymal osteoid-forming neoplasm (Kransdorf 1995). Plain radiographs show dense cloud-like mineralization in 50%. MR imaging shows an ill-defined, inhomogeneous lesion with predominantly intermediate signal intensity on T1 weighting and high signal intensity on T2 weighting. Mineralized foci result in low signal intensity on all sequences (Mc Auley et al. 2012).

3.6.2.9 Peripheral Nerve Sheath Tumors

Benign nerve sheath tumors most commonly affect young adults in the third and fourth decades with no gender predilection (Singer et al. 2016). *Schwannomas* are well-encapsulated tumors that arise from the Schwann cells of the nerve sheath and contain cellular and myxoid elements. As they grow, schwannomas displace the nerve fibers eccentrically and thus can be surgically removed without sacrificing the nerve. *Neurofibromas* are nonencapsulated lesions that separate the nerve fibers and cause fusiform enlargement of the nerve. Resection of a neurofibroma therefore typically requires sacrifice of the nerve (Singer et al. 2016). Benign nerve sheath tumors usually present with a soft tissue mass that may cause pain or neurological symptoms (Beggs 1997). The posterior tibial nerve/tarsal tunnel is the most common location in the foot and ankle (Kwon et al. 2009). Plexiform neurofibromas are pathognomonic of neurofibromatosis type 1. Between 3% and 13% of patients with neurofibromatosis will develop a malignant peripheral nerve sheath tumor, whereas malignant transformation of a solitary neurofibroma is rare and of schwannoma is extremely rare (Michelson and Sinclair 1994). Plain radiography may show a soft tissue mass, and mineralization is uncommon. On ultrasound, neurofibroma is elongated along the nerve axis, whereas schwannoma is eccentric often with cysts. On CT, both schwannoma and neurofibroma are usually hypodense to muscle. On MR imaging, both lesions are homogeneous and isointense or slightly hyperintense to muscle on T1 weighting and strongly enhance with intravenous Gd-DTPA. On T2 weighting, both lesions are mainly hyperintense but show inhomogeneity with foci of variable signal intensity. A fibrous pseudo-capsule, cystic change, necrosis, and hemorrhage are all more common in schwannoma than neurofibroma. Classic MRI findings suggestive of PNSTs are the "target," "string," and "split fat" signs (Fig. 21). The target sign describes the low T2 signal intensity fibrous central component against the high T2 signal peripheral myxoid component and is more commonly seen in neurofibroma than schwannoma but can be seen in both as well as malignant PNSTs (Singer et al. 2016).

Malignant peripheral nerve sheath tumors (MPNSTs) are associated with neurofibromatosis type 1 in around 70% (Kransdorf 1995). It is clear that most, if not all, MPNSTs in NF1 patients arise from preexisting neurofibromas. MPNST presents earlier in NF1 patients (mean 29 years) than in non-NF1 patients (mean 34 years) with a soft tissue mass that may cause neurological symptoms in the affected nerve. Sudden enlargement of a preexisting neurofibroma is an ominous finding suggestive of malignant transformation. Imaging features are nonspecific, and differentiation from benign nerve sheath tumors may be difficult. Ultrasound and CT show irregular, inhomogeneous masses with necrotic and cystic foci and occasionally calcification. On MR imaging, lesions are often irregular and larger than 5 cm, although in the foot and ankle, lesions tend to present earlier. Lesions are typically inhomogeneous, particularly on T2 weighting due in part to hemorrhage, necrosis, cystic change, and mineralization.

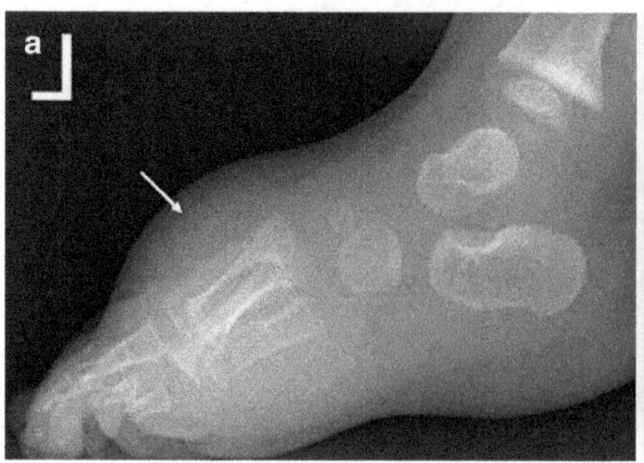

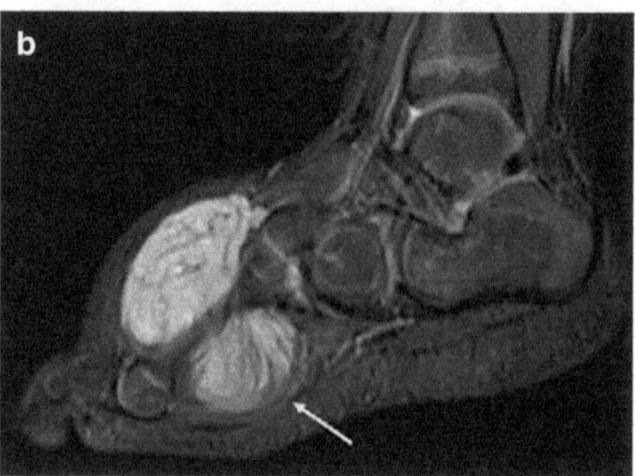

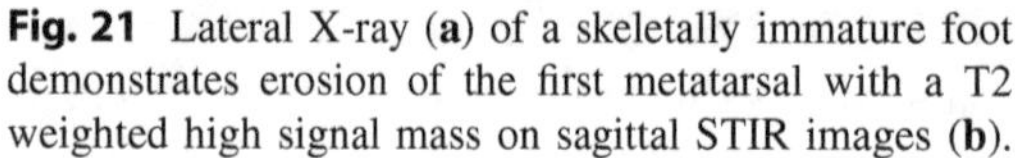

Fig. 21 Lateral X-ray (**a**) of a skeletally immature foot demonstrates erosion of the first metatarsal with a T2 weighted high signal mass on sagittal STIR images (**b**). This is in keeping with a nerve sheath tumour causing erosion of the adjacent metatarsal

Intra-osseous MPNSTs can occur and appear similar to other aggressive intra-osseous tumors (Singer et al. 2016).

3.6.2.10 Tumors of Uncertain Differentiation

Myxomas are benign tumors that can be subcutaneous or intramuscular in location. Intramuscular lipomas can occur sporadically or secondary to a syndrome (e.g., Mazabraud syndrome). Ultrasound typically shows a well-defined hypoechoic lesion, although occasionally some internal echoes may be present. On MR imaging, lesions are well-defined, homogeneous, and hypointense on T1 weighting and markedly hyperintense on T2 weighting. A rim of peritumoral fat may help to differentiate from more aggressive myxomatous tumors. Enhancement is variable, but intense solid enhancement would not be expected (Singer et al. 2016).

Synovial sarcoma is one of the most common soft tissue malignancy in the foot and ankle (Khan et al. 2015; Rammelt et al. 2020). Despite the name, it appears not to arise from synovium, hence the classification in the "tumors of uncertain differentiation" (Singer et al. 2016; Hochman and Wu 2017). It commonly presents with a mass arising from the tendons, tendon sheaths, or bursal structures and is rarely intra-articular, but articular spread from juxta-articular sites is common in the foot and ankle. Locoregional lymph node involvement is relatively common (Khan et al. 2015). Small lesions may be homogeneous, well-defined, and slow growing and mistakenly considered as benign (Kennedy et al. 2016; Blacksin et al. 1997). If they are mistaken for cysts or ganglia, then attempted aspiration or excision can contaminate the surgical bed and negatively affect prognosis (Singer et al. 2016). Favorable factors include age <25 years, size <5 cm, prominent mineralization, and no histological evidence of poor differentiation, and the estimated 5-year survival rate is 60% (Bergh et al. 1999). Radiographs may show a well-defined, round or lobulated, soft tissue mass. Calcifications may be present and vary from fine stippling to dense opacities. Small calcifications may be missed on MR imaging. On MR imaging, lesions are typically characterized by a fairly well-defined, lobulated, heterogeneous, juxta-articular mass. This can lead to them being misdiagnosed as ganglion cysts (Bouchard et al. 2017). On T1 weighting, lesions usually display low/intermediate signal intensity, although small foci of high signal intensity intratumoral hemorrhage are common. On T2 weighting, a heterogeneous pattern of variable signal intensity is typically found in most lesions (Hochman and Wu 2017; Kennedy et al. 2016). Due to their periarticular position, they can be contiguous with bone and cause pressure erosion or frank infiltration. Classical MRI signs include the "triple sign" and "bowl of grapes sign." The triple sign describes the presence of low, intermediate, and high signal intensity on long TR pulse sequences due to fibrous tissue, calcium, hemorrhage, and necrosis, but is not pathognomonic (Singer et al. 2016; Murphey et al. 2006; Jones et al. 1993). The bowl of grapes sign describes loculations and septations in the mass (Singer et al. 2016; Jones et al. 1993).

Undifferentiated pleomorphic sarcoma (UPS, previously known as malignant fibrous histiocytoma) is one of the most common soft tissue malignancies in the foot and ankle (Hughes et al. 2019). Lesions are more common in men in the fifth–seventh decades, although the rare angiomatoid type is more common in young adults (Chow et al. 1998). Clinically, the lesion presents as a nonspecific, enlarging, painless mass. Radiography may reveal a soft tissue mass and may detect mineralization. On MR imaging, lesions are typically inhomogeneous, with poorly defined margins and variable signal intensity depending on the different components. Myxoid change and necrosis give low signal intensity on T1 weighting and high signal intensity on T2 weighting. Fibrous tissue and mineralization tend to give low or intermediate signal intensity on all sequences. Recent hemorrhage may give high signal intensity on all sequences, whereas fluid-fluid levels are often found with older hemorrhage. Inhomogeneous enhancement is typical.

Clear cell sarcoma is rare, but the foot and ankle are relatively common sites of occurrence, accounting for as much as 8% of all foot and ankle soft tissue sarcomas (Kransdorf 1995). It most commonly appears in the second to fourth decades, is more common in women, and usually presents with a mass arising from a tendon, ligament, or aponeurosis. Clear cell sarcoma usually metastasizes to lungs, bone, and lymph nodes and has a poor prognosis. Radiographs usually show a nonspecific, unmineralized soft tissue mass. Osseous involvement is infrequent (De Beuckeleer et al. 2000). On MR imaging, the majority of lesions are well-defined and homogeneous and thus may give a false impression of a benign lesion. On T1 weighting, most lesions are slightly hyperintense compared with muscle, reflecting a high melanin content in the lesion. Similarly, the low/intermediate signal intensity on T2 weighting in some cases may be due to the "melanin" effect, but most cases display high signal intensity on T2 weighting. This probably reflects either low melanin content, high extracellular water content, or other factors including the type of stromal tissue (Mavrogenis et al. 2013).

Epithelioid sarcoma is an uncommon soft tissue sarcoma. It presents in young adults, more commonly men, with a hard, slow-growing, soft tissue mass. Metastatic spread most commonly involves the lymphatic system and to a lesser extent the lungs. Plain radiographs may show a soft tissue mass containing speckled calcifications or ossification (Lo et al. 1977). On MR imaging, the majority show nonspecific intermediate signal intensity on T1 weighting and high signal intensity on T2 weighting, but some also display evidence of hemorrhage. Superficial lesions tend to be homogeneous with clear margins, but the deeper lesions can appear heterogeneous and infiltrative (Saad et al. 2021).

3.6.2.11 Tumorlike/Nonneoplastic Lesions

Morton's neuroma is a very common nonneoplastic lesion of the forefoot due to perineural fibrosis of a plantar digital nerve at the plantar aspect of the transverse intermetatarsal ligament, secondary to chronic compression and irritation (Hochman and Wu 2017). Lesions usually present with a burning sensation and most commonly involve the second or third intermetatarsal web spaces. There is a marked propensity in women, and they are associated with high-heeled and narrow-toed footwear (Singer et al. 2016). However, it is also common in asymptomatic patients (Zanetti et al. 1997). Ultrasound typically shows an ovoid, hypoechoic, noncompressible mass between the metatarsal heads, but lesions smaller than 5 mm may be missed (Kaminsky et al. 1997). On MR imaging, the lesions are best visualized on coronal sequences (relative to the body) (Hochman and Wu 2017). They typically display low signal intensity on T1 weighting and low to intermediate signal on T2 weighting and may enhance with intravenous gadolinium contrast administration (Fig. 22). Associated fluid within the intermetatarsal bursae is common, but collections with a transverse diameter of 3 mm or less can be considered physiological (Longo et al. 2016). The neuroma component tends to be more plantar relative to the

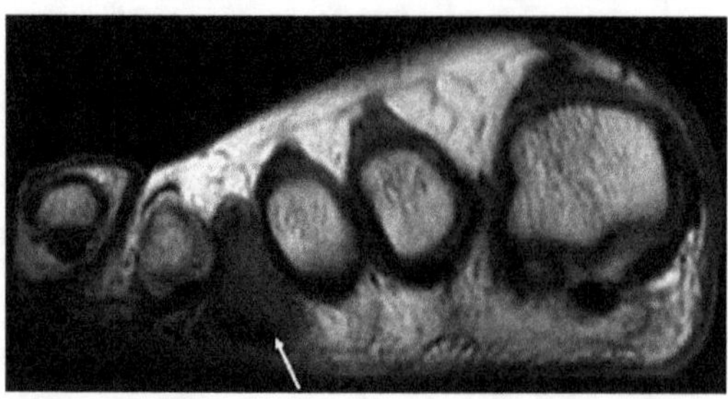

Fig. 22 A low signal intensity soft tissue mass is seen to arise adjacent to the base of the fourth metatarsal with extension into the intermetatarsal space in keeping with a Morton's neuroma

intermetatarsal bursae (Singer et al. 2016). Surgical excision is associated with a high rate of recurrence (Kennedy et al. 2016). A more favorable clinical outcome can be expected after surgical intermetatarsal neurectomy when a Morton's neuroma has a transverse measurement larger than 5 mm on MRI scans (Biasca et al. 1999).

Ganglion (cyst) is the most common soft tissue mass in the foot and ankle (Ortega et al. 2002). They usually arise from the surface of joint capsules or tendon sheaths but are not lined by synovium (Longo et al. 2016). Patients present with a painless mass but may spontaneously disappear or rupture (Khan et al. 2015). Ultrasound typically demonstrates a unilocular or multilocular, anechoic or hypoechoic, cystic lesion, often with a protrusion extending toward a joint, with which they can sometimes be seen to communicate. Communicating this can be helpful for surgeons considering resection. They are normally non-compressible (Longo et al. 2016). MR imaging usually demonstrates an encapsulated, septate, multilobulated lesion of low signal intensity on T1 weighting and very high signal intensity on T2 weighting. However, if the protein content is high, then the signal intensity on T1 weighting may be isointense with muscle. Peripheral rim or septal enhancement may occur (Petscavage-Thomas et al. 2014). On aspiration, a thick, gel-like fluid is obtained, although the viscosity of this can make aspiration difficult (Khan et al. 2015). Recurrence post-aspiration is common (Kiehn and Gutowski 2004) (Fig. 23).

Idiopathic tumoral calcinosis is a tumorlike lesion that is rare in the foot and ankle. Patients usually present in the first two decades with a slow-growing, juxta-articular, soft tissue mass that may ulcerate and drain chalklike material (Slomovitz et al. 1990). Similar appearances may be seen in various metabolic disorders including chronic renal failure. Radiographs demonstrate well-defined, juxta-articular, lobulated, calcific masses with linear radiolucencies and fibrous septations that may occasionally erode bone. CT may show a uniformly calcified mass or cystic lesion with calcific walls and fluid-fluid levels. On MR imaging, lesions show low signal intensity on all sequences but may have diffuse or focal areas of high signal intensity on T2 weighting if the lesions are inflammatory or contain fluid (Fig. 24).

Myositis ossificans is a benign, mineralizing, intramuscular mass that is usually post-traumatic but rarely occurs in the foot (De Maeseneer et al. 1997).

Granuloma annulare is a benign, inflammatory dermatosis that is most commonly found around the foot and ankle. The subcutaneous form is usually seen in children and presents with a rapidly growing nodule. Lesions tend to regress over time but may progress to a more generalized form and may recur following excision (Davids et al. 1993). Ultrasound shows an ill-defined mass hypoechoic to subcutaneous fat. MR imaging reveals an ill-defined mass that is hypointense on T1 weighting and hypointense or isointense on T2 weighting.

Epidermal inclusion (sebaceous) cysts are common, benign, superficial subcutaneous lesions. They may occur as a result of traumatic implantation of epidermal cells into dermal tissue, squamous metaplasia, hair follicle obstruction, or congenital factors (Kennedy et al. 2016; Fisher et al. 1998; Kim et al. 2011). They are normally slow growing and painless. On ultrasound, lesions are well-defined, iso- to mildly hyperechoic, with uniform internal echoes, and a hypoechoic halo, with increased transmission. A characteristic finding is scattered internal hypoechoic clefts (Kim et al. 2011). If ruptured,

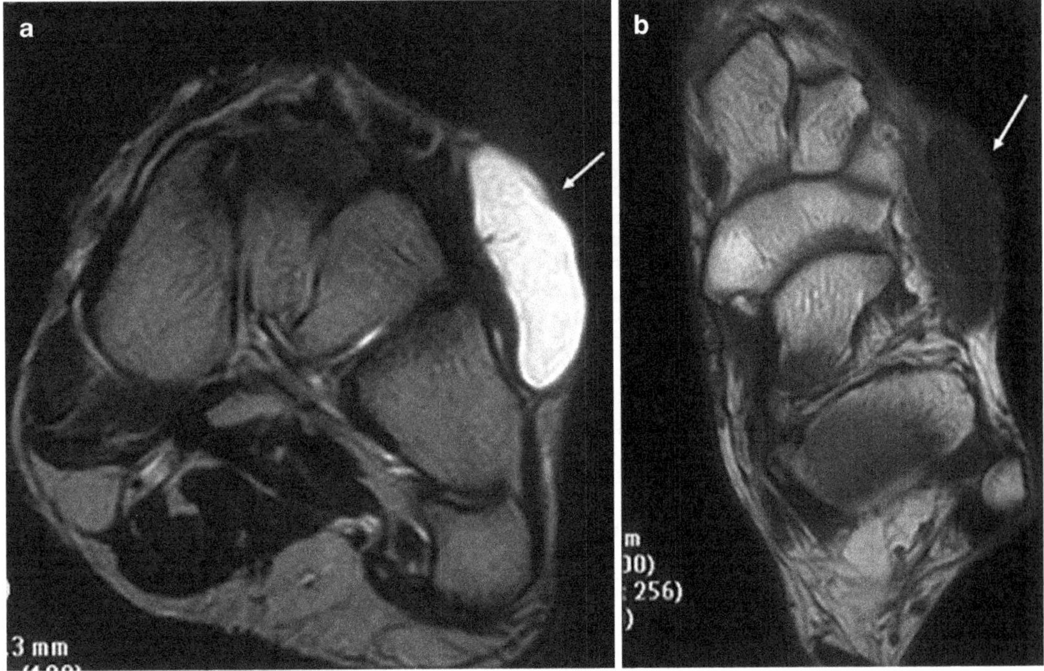

Fig. 23 Ganglion foot. The MRI shows a superficial lobulated soft tissue mass hyperintense on coronal T2 (**a**) and hypointense on axial T1 (**b**). Features suggest either a cystic or a myxoid lesion. It is difficult to know from these images if it is arising from an adjacent tendon sheath

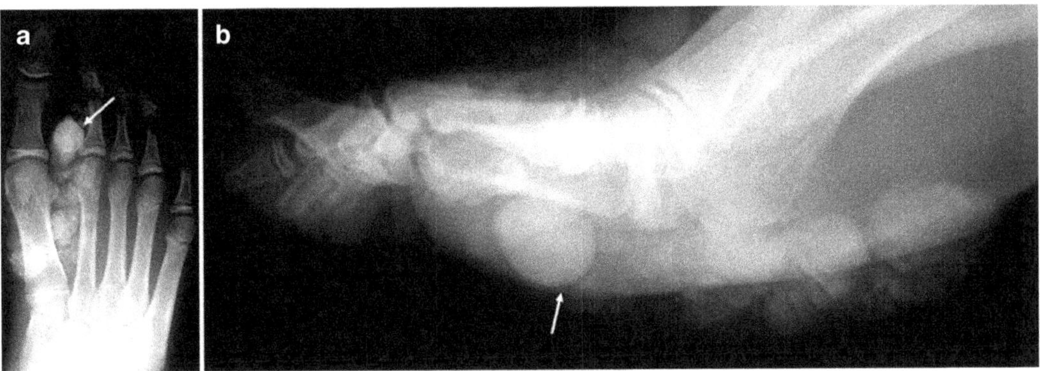

Fig. 24 Idiopathic tumoral calcinosis. Chalky/amorphous mineralization in the soft tissue seen on radiographs (**a**, **b**). A very similar appearance is found in association with chronic renal failure, which is also known as tumoral calcinosis or metastatic calcification

it may be ill-defined, without a halo, and with increased vascularity (Yuan et al. 2012). On MRI, lesions typically display low signal intensity on T1 weighting and high signal intensity on T2 weighting, although the hypointense keratin clusters may result in an inhomogeneous appearance (Longo et al. 2016). A differential diagnosis, particularly for a ruptured epidermal inclusion cyst, is a soft tissue reaction to a retained foreign body (Horton et al. 2001).

Subcutaneous *rheumatoid nodules* and *mycetoma* are discussed in the relevant chapters.

References

Abrahim-zadeh R, Klein RM, Leslie D, Norman A (1998) Characteristics of calcaneal bone infarction: an MR imaging investigation. Skeletal Radiol 27(6):321–324. https://doi.org/10.1007/s002560050389

Adkins CD, Kitaoka HB, Seidl RK, Pritchard DJ (1997) Ewing's sarcoma of the foot. Clin Orthop 343:173–182

Anderson MW, Temple HT, Dussault RG, Kaplan PA (1999) Compartmental anatomy: relevance to staging and biopsy of musculoskeletal tumors. Am J Roentgenol 173(6):1663–1671. https://doi.org/10.2214/ajr.173.6.10584817

Antonescu CR, Erlandson RA, Huvos AG (2000) Primary fibrosarcoma and malignant fibrous histiocytoma of bone—a comparative ultrastructural study: evidence of a spectrum of fibroblastic differentiation. Ultrastruct Pathol 24(2):83–91. https://doi.org/10.1080/01913120050118558

Arata MA, Peterson HA, Dahlin DC (1981) Pathological fractures through non-ossifying fibromas. Review of the Mayo Clinic experience. J Bone Joint Surg Am 63(6):980–988

Ariyanayagam T, Malcolm PN, Toms AP (2015) Advances in metal artifact reduction techniques for periprosthetic soft tissue imaging. Semin Musculoskelet Radiol 19(4):328–334. https://doi.org/10.1055/s-0035-1563734

Azevedo CP, Casanova JM, Guerra MG, Santos AL, Portela MI, Tavares PF (2013) Tumors of the foot and ankle: a single-institution experience. J Foot Ankle Surg 52(2):147–152. https://doi.org/10.1053/j.jfas.2012.12.004

Azzopardi C, Patel A, James S, Botchu R, Davies M (2021) A radiological diagnostic approach to tumours and tumour-like lesions of the calcaneus. Br J Radiol 94(1127):20210330. https://doi.org/10.1259/bjr.20210330

Bakotic BW, Robinson M, Williams M, Van Woy T, Nutter J, Borkowski P (1999) Aggressive epithelioid hemangioendothelioma of the lower extremity: a case report and review of the literature. J Foot Ankle Surg 38(5):352–358. https://doi.org/10.1016/s1067-2516(99)80007-6

Bancroft LW, Peterson JJ, Kransdorf MJ (2008) Imaging of soft tissue lesions of the foot and ankle. Radiol Clin North Am 46(6):1093–1103, vii. https://doi.org/10.1016/j.rcl.2008.08.007

Baraga JJ, Amrami KK, Swee RG, Wold L, Unni KK (2001) Radiographic features of Ewing's sarcoma of the bones of the hands and feet. Skeletal Radiol 30(3):121–126. https://doi.org/10.1007/s002560100349

Barca F, Acciaro AL, Recchioni MD (1998) Osteoid osteoma of the phalanx: enlargement of the toe—two case reports. Foot Ankle Int 19(6):388–393. https://doi.org/10.1177/107110079801900609

Beggs I (1997) Pictorial review: imaging of peripheral nerve tumours. Clin Radiol 52(1):8–17. https://doi.org/10.1016/s0009-9260(97)80299-1

Bégin LR, Guy P, Mitmaker B (1994) Intramural leiomyosarcoma of the dorsal pedal vein: a clinical mimicry of ganglion. Foot Ankle Int 15(1):48–51. https://doi.org/10.1177/107110079401500110

Bergh P, Meis-Kindblom JM, Gherlinzoni F et al (1999) Synovial sarcoma: identification of low and high risk groups. Cancer 85(12):2596–2607. https://doi.org/10.1002/(sici)1097-0142(19990615)85:12<2596::aid-cncr16>3.0.co;2-k

Berlin SJ (1995) Statistical analysis of 307,601 tumors and other lesions of the foot. J Am Podiatr Med Assoc 85(11):699–703. https://doi.org/10.7547/87507315-85-11-699

Betsy M, Kupersmith LM, Springfield DS (2004) Metaphyseal fibrous defects. J Am Acad Orthop Surg 12(2):89–95. https://doi.org/10.5435/00124635-200403000-00004

Biasca N, Zanetti M, Zollinger H (1999) Outcomes after partial neurectomy of Morton's neuroma related to preoperative case histories, clinical findings, and findings on magnetic resonance imaging scans. Foot Ankle Int 20(9):568–575. https://doi.org/10.1177/107110079902000906

Biscaglia R, Bacchini P, Bertoni F (2000) Giant cell tumor of the bones of the hand and foot. Cancer 88(9):2022–2032. https://doi.org/10.1002/(sici)1097-0142(20000501)88:9<2022::aid-cncr6>3.0.co;2-y

Blacksin MF, Siegel JR, Benevenia J, Aisner SC (1997) Synovial sarcoma: frequency of nonaggressive MR characteristics. J Comput Assist Tomogr 21(5):785–789. https://doi.org/10.1097/00004728-199709000-00025

Bloem JL, Taminiau AH, Eulderink F, Hermans J, Pauwels EK (1988) Radiologic staging of primary bone sarcoma: MR imaging, scintigraphy, angiography, and CT correlated with pathologic examination. Radiology 169(3):805–810. https://doi.org/10.1148/radiology.169.3.3055041

Böhm P, Kröber S, Greschniok A, Laniado M, Kaiserling E (1996) Desmoplastic fibroma of the bone. A report of two patients, review of the literature, and therapeutic implications. Cancer 78(5):1011–1023. https://doi.org/10.1002/(SICI)1097-0142(19960901)78:5<1011::AID-CNCR11>3.0.CO;2-5

Boo S, Saad A, Murphy J, Botchu R (2020) Tumours of the talus—a pictorial review. J Clin Orthop Trauma 11(3):410–416. https://doi.org/10.1016/j.jcot.2020.03.021

Bouchard M, Bartlett M, Donnan L (2017) Assessment of the pediatric foot mass. J Am Acad Orthop Surg 25(1):32–41. https://doi.org/10.5435/JAAOS-D-15-00397

Boutin RD, Spaeth HJ, Mangalik A, Sell JJ (1996) Epithelioid hemangioendothelioma of bone. Skeletal Radiol 25(4):391–395. https://doi.org/10.1007/s002560050102

Bovée JV, van der Heul RO, Taminiau AH, Hogendoorn PC (1999) Chondrosarcoma of the phalanx: a locally aggressive lesion with minimal metastatic potential: a report of 35 cases and a review of the literature. Cancer 86(9):1724–1732. https://doi.org/10.1002/(sici)1097-0142(19991101)86:9<1724::aid-cncr14>3.0.co;2-i

Braunschweig IJ, Stein IH, Dodwad MI, Rangwala AF, Lopano A (1992) Case report 751: spindle cell lipoma causing marked bone erosion. Skeletal Radiol 21(6):414–417. https://doi.org/10.1007/BF00241825

Bravo SM, Winalski CS, Weissman BN (1996) Pigmented villonodular synovitis. Radiol Clin North Am 34(2):311–326, x–xi

Campanacci M (2013) Bone and soft tissue tumors: clinical features, imaging, pathology and treatment. Springer Science & Business Media

Cavalcante MM, Silveira CRS, da Costa CR et al (2021) Tumors and pseudotumors of foot and ankle: bone lesions. Foot Edinb Scotl 49:101845. https://doi.org/10.1016/j.foot.2021.101845

Cecchetto G, Carli M, Alaggio R et al (2001) Fibrosarcoma in pediatric patients: results of the Italian Cooperative Group studies (1979-1995). J Surg Oncol 78(4):225–231. https://doi.org/10.1002/jso.1157

Chakarun CJ, Forrester DM, Gottsegen CJ, Patel DB, White EA, Matcuk GR (2013) Giant cell tumor of bone: review, mimics, and new developments in treatment. Radiographics 33(1):197–211. https://doi.org/10.1148/rg.331125089

Chalatsis GP, Mitrousias V, Siouras A et al (2022) Calcifying aponeurotic fibroma at the sole of the foot in a 5 year old girl. A case report with 5 years follow up. Foot Ankle Surg Tech Rep Cases 2(2):100180. https://doi.org/10.1016/j.fastrc.2022.100180

Choong PF, Qureshi AA, Sim FH, Unni KK (1999) Osteosarcoma of the foot: a review of 52 patients at the Mayo Clinic. Acta Orthop Scand 70(4):361–364. https://doi.org/10.3109/17453679908997825

Chou LB, Ho YY, Malawer MM (2009) Tumors of the foot and ankle: experience with 153 cases. Foot Ankle Int 30(9):836–841. https://doi.org/10.3113/FAI.2009.0836

Chow LT, Allen PW, Kumta SM, Griffith J, Li CK, Leung PC (1998) Angiomatoid malignant fibrous histiocytoma: report of an unusual case with highly aggressive clinical course. J Foot Ankle Surg 37(3):235–238. https://doi.org/10.1016/s1067-2516(98)80117-8

Chung EB, Enzinger FM (1978) Chondroma of soft parts. Cancer 41(4):1414–1424. https://doi.org/10.1002/1097-0142(197804)41:4<1414::aid-cncr2820410429>3.0.co;2-o

Cione JA, Lynn B, Boylan J (1999) Dermatofibrosarcoma protuberans. A rare case involving the pediatric foot. J Am Podiatr Med Assoc 89(8):419–423. https://doi.org/10.7547/87507315-89-8-419

Costelloe CM, Madewell JE (2013) Radiography in the initial diagnosis of primary bone tumors. Am J Roentgenol 200(1):3–7. https://doi.org/10.2214/AJR.12.8488

Cummins CA, Scarborough MT, Enneking WF (1996) Multicentric giant cell tumor of bone. Clin Orthop 322:245–252

Dangoor A, Seddon B, Gerrand C, Grimer R, Whelan J, Judson I (2016) UK guidelines for the management of soft tissue sarcomas. Clin Sarcoma Res 6(1):20. https://doi.org/10.1186/s13569-016-0060-4

Davids JR, Kolman BH, Billman GF, Krous HF (1993) Subcutaneous granuloma annulare: recognition and treatment. J Pediatr Orthop 13(5):582–586

Davila JA, Amrami KK, Sundaram M, Adkins MC, Unni KK (2004) Chondroblastoma of the hands and feet. Skeletal Radiol 33(10):582–587. https://doi.org/10.1007/s00256-004-0762-1

Davis AM, Kandel RA, Wunder JS et al (1997) The impact of residual disease on local recurrence in patients treated by initial unplanned resection for soft tissue sarcoma of the extremity. J Surg Oncol 66(2):81–87. https://doi.org/10.1002/(sici)1096-9098(199710)66:2<81::aid-jso2>3.0.co;2-h

De Beuckeleer LH, De Schepper AM, Vandevenne JE et al (2000) MR imaging of clear cell sarcoma (malignant melanoma of the soft parts): a multicenter correlative MRI-pathology study of 21 cases and literature review. Skeletal Radiol 29(4):187–195. https://doi.org/10.1007/s002560050592

De Maeseneer M, Jaovisidha S, Lenchik L et al (1997) Myositis ossificans of the foot. J Foot Ankle Surg 36(4):290–293; discussion 331. https://doi.org/10.1016/s1067-2516(97)80075-0

Derchi LE, Balconi G, De Flaviis L, Oliva A, Rosso F (1989) Sonographic appearances of hemangiomas of skeletal muscle. J Ultrasound Med 8(5):263–267. https://doi.org/10.7863/jum.1989.8.5.263

Desai MA, Peterson JJ, Garner HW, Kransdorf MJ (2011) Clinical utility of dual-energy CT for evaluation of tophaceous gout. Radiographics 31(5):1365–1375.; discussion 1376-1377. https://doi.org/10.1148/rg.315115510

Dhatt SS, Bhagwat KR, Kumar V, Dhillon MS (2012) Chondroblastoma in a metatarsal treated with autogenous fibular graft: a case report. J Foot Ankle Surg 51(3):356–361. https://doi.org/10.1053/j.jfas.2012.01.004

Donley BG, Neel M, Mitias HM (1996) Neural fibrolipoma of the foot: a case report. Foot Ankle Int 17(11):712–713. https://doi.org/10.1177/107110079601701113

Drapé JL, Idy-Peretti I, Goettmann S, Guérin-Surville H, Bittoun J (1996) Standard and high resolution magnetic resonance imaging of glomus tumors of toes and fingertips. J Am Acad Dermatol 35(4):550–555. https://doi.org/10.1016/s0190-9622(96)90678-7

Enneking WF, Spanier SS, Goodman MA (1980) A system for the surgical staging of musculoskeletal sarcoma. Clin Orthop 153:106–120

ESMO/European Sarcoma Network Working Group (2014a) Bone sarcomas: ESMO Clinical Practice Guidelines for diagnosis, treatment and follow-up. Ann Oncol 25 Suppl 3:iii113–iii123. https://doi.org/10.1093/annonc/mdu256

ESMO/European Sarcoma Network Working Group (2014b) Soft tissue and visceral sarcomas: ESMO

Clinical Practice Guidelines for diagnosis, treatment and follow-up. Ann Oncol 25 Suppl 3:iii102–iii112. https://doi.org/10.1093/annonc/mdu254

Fink BR, Temple HT, Chiricosta FM, Mizel MS, Murphey MD (1997) Chondroblastoma of the foot. Foot Ankle Int 18(4):236–242. https://doi.org/10.1177/107110079701800410

Fisher AR, Mason PH, Wagenhals KS (1998) Ruptured plantar epidermal inclusion cyst. AJR Am J Roentgenol 171(6):1709–1710. https://doi.org/10.2214/ajr.171.6.9843324

Fornage BD (1988) Glomus tumors in the fingers: diagnosis with US. Radiology 167(1):183–185. https://doi.org/10.1148/radiology.167.1.2831563

Frassica FJ, Sanjay BK, Unni KK, McLeod RA, Sim FH (1993) Benign giant cell tumor. Orthopedics 16(10):1179–1183. https://doi.org/10.3928/0147-7447-19931001-15

Fritz J, Henes JC, Fuld MK, Fishman EK, Horger MS (2016) Dual-energy computed tomography of the knee, ankle, and foot: noninvasive diagnosis of gout and quantification of monosodium urate in tendons and ligaments. Semin Musculoskelet Radiol 20(1):130–136. https://doi.org/10.1055/s-0036-1579709

Garner HW, Kransdorf MJ, Bancroft LW, Peterson JJ, Berquist TH, Murphey MD (2009) Benign and malignant soft-tissue tumors: posttreatment MR imaging. Radiographics 29(1):119–134. https://doi.org/10.1148/rg.291085131

Greenspan A, Jundt G, Remagen W (2007) Differential diagnosis in orthopaedic oncology. Lippincott Williams & Wilkins

Guillou L, Folpe AL (2010) Chapter 3—Fibroblastic and fibrohistiocytic tumors. In: Folpe AL, Inwards CY (eds) Bone and soft tissue pathology. W.B. Saunders, pp 43–96. https://doi.org/10.1016/B978-0-443-06688-7.00004-3

Harty JA, Kelly P, Niall D, O'Keane JC, Stephens MM (2000) Bizarre parosteal osteochondromatous proliferation (Nora's lesion) of the sesamoid: a case report. Foot Ankle Int 21(5):408–412. https://doi.org/10.1177/107110070002100509

Hegde G, Azzopardi C, Patel A, Davies AM, James SL, Botchu R (2022) "Do-not-touch" lesions of bone revisited. Clin Radiol 77(3):179–187. https://doi.org/10.1016/j.crad.2021.11.012

Helms CA (2019) Fundamentals of skeletal radiology. Accessed 21 Feb 2022. https://www.uk.elsevierhealth.com/fundamentals-of-skeletal-radiology-9780323611657.html

Hochman MG, Wu JS (2017) MR imaging of common soft tissue masses in the foot and ankle. Magn Reson Imaging Clin N Am 25(1):159–181. https://doi.org/10.1016/j.mric.2016.08.013

Hoffmann DF, Israel J (1990) Intraosseous frontal hemangioma. Head Neck 12(2):160–163. https://doi.org/10.1002/hed.2880120212

Hondar Wu HT, Chen W, Lee O, Chang CY (2006) Imaging and pathological correlation of soft-tissue chondroma: a serial five-case study and literature review. Clin Imaging 30(1):32–36. https://doi.org/10.1016/j.clinimag.2005.01.027

Horton LK, Jacobson JA, Powell A, Fessell DP, Hayes CW (2001) Sonography and radiography of soft-tissue foreign bodies. AJR Am J Roentgenol 176(5):1155–1159. https://doi.org/10.2214/ajr.176.5.1761155

Hottya GA, Steinbach LS, Johnston JO, van Kuijk C, Genant HK (1999) Chondrosarcoma of the foot: imaging, surgical and pathological correlation of three new cases. Skeletal Radiol 28(3):153–158. https://doi.org/10.1007/s002560050492

Hudson TM, Schiebler M, Springfield DS, Enneking WF, Hawkins IF, Spanier SS (1984) Radiology of giant cell tumors of bone: computed tomography, arthro-tomography, and scintigraphy. Skeletal Radiol 11(2):85–95. https://doi.org/10.1007/BF00348795

Hughes P, Miranda R, Doyle AJ (2019) MRI imaging of soft tissue tumours of the foot and ankle. Insights Imaging 10(1):60. https://doi.org/10.1186/s13244-019-0749-z

Huvos AG (1987) Bone tumors: diagnosis, treatment and prognosis, 2nd edn. W.B. Saunders. Accessed 14 Feb 2022. https://www.osti.gov/biblio/6324679

Huvos AG, Marcove RC (1973) Chondroblastoma of bone. A critical review. Clin Orthop 95:300–312. https://doi.org/10.1097/00003086-197309000-00039

Isefuku S, Hatori M, Ehara S, Hosaka M, Ito K, Kokubun S (1999) Fibrous dysplasia arising from the calcaneus. Tohoku J Exp Med 189(3):227–232. https://doi.org/10.1620/tjem.189.227

Jee WH, Park YK, McCauley TR et al (1999) Chondroblastoma: MR characteristics with pathologic correlation. J Comput Assist Tomogr 23(5):721–726. https://doi.org/10.1097/00004728-199909000-00016

Johnson K, Davies AM, Mangham DC, Grimer RJ (1999) Parosteal osteosarcoma of a metatarsal with intramedullary invasion. Skeletal Radiol 28(2):111–115. https://doi.org/10.1007/s002560050485

Jones BC, Sundaram M, Kransdorf MJ (1993) Synovial sarcoma: MR imaging findings in 34 patients. AJR Am J Roentgenol 161(4):827–830. https://doi.org/10.2214/ajr.161.4.8396848

Kaelin A (1995) Kyste essentiel des os. Cah Enseign SOFCOT 52:167–179

Kaminsky S, Griffin L, Milsap J, Page D (1997) Is ultrasonography a reliable way to confirm the diagnosis of Morton's neuroma? Orthopedics 20(1):37–39. https://doi.org/10.3928/0147-7447-19970101-07

Kennedy JG, Ross KA, Smyth NA, Hogan MV, Murawski CD (2016) Primary tumors of the foot and ankle. Foot Ankle Spec 9(1):58–68. https://doi.org/10.1177/1938640015620634

Khan Z, Hussain S, Carter SR (2015) Tumours of the foot and ankle. Foot Edinb Scotl 25(3):164–172. https://doi.org/10.1016/j.foot.2015.06.001

Kiehn MW, Gutowski KA (2004) A recurrent foot ganglion managed with extensor digitorum brevis muscle flap coverage. J Foot Ankle Surg 43(6):423–425. https://doi.org/10.1053/j.jfas.2004.09.009

Kilgore WB, Parrish WM (2005) Calcaneal tumors and tumor-like conditions. Foot Ankle Clin 10(3):541–565, vii. https://doi.org/10.1016/j.fcl.2005.05.002

Kim HK, Kim SM, Lee SH, Racadio JM, Shin MJ (2011) Subcutaneous epidermal inclusion cysts: ultrasound (US) and MR imaging findings. Skeletal Radiol 40(11):1415–1419. https://doi.org/10.1007/s00256-010-1072-4

Kim KJ, Lee SK, Chi YJ et al (2014) Treatment of tumours and tumour-like lesions in the foot and ankle—a single institution analysis. BSBT 2014. https://doi.org/10.14257/IJBSBT.2014.6.1.18

Kirby J, Shereff MJ, Lewis MM (1989) Soft-tissue tumors and tumor-like lesions of the foot. An analysis of eighty-three cases. J Bone Joint Surg Am 71-A(4):621

Kirsch J, Ilaslan H, Bauer TW, Sundaram M (2006) The incidence of imaging findings, and the distribution of skeletal lymphoma in a consecutive patient population seen over 5 years. Skeletal Radiol 35(8):590–594. https://doi.org/10.1007/s00256-006-0085-5

Kramer J, Recht M, Deely DM et al (1993) MR appearance of idiopathic synovial osteochondromatosis. J Comput Assist Tomogr 17(5):772–776. https://doi.org/10.1097/00004728-199309000-00020

Kransdorf MJ (1995) Benign soft-tissue tumors in a large referral population: distribution of specific diagnoses by age, sex, and location. AJR Am J Roentgenol 164(2):395–402. https://doi.org/10.2214/ajr.164.2.7839977

Kwon JH, Yoon JR, Kim TS, Kim HJ (2009) Peripheral nerve sheath tumor of the medial plantar nerve without tarsal tunnel syndrome: a case report. J Foot Ankle Surg 48(4):477–482. https://doi.org/10.1053/j.jfas.2009.03.005

La TH, Wolden SL, Su Z et al (2011) Local therapy for rhabdomyosarcoma of the hands and feet: is amputation necessary? A report from the Children's Oncology Group. Int J Radiat Oncol Biol Phys 80(1):206–212. https://doi.org/10.1016/j.ijrobp.2010.01.053

Laffan EE, Ngan BY, Navarro OM (2009) Pediatric soft-tissue tumors and pseudotumors: MR imaging features with pathologic correlation. Radiographics 29(4):e36. https://doi.org/10.1148/rg.e36

Latt LD, Turcotte RE, Isler MH, Wong C (2010) Case series. Soft-tissue sarcoma of the foot. Can J Surg J Can Chir 53(6):424–431

Ledermann HP, Morrison WB, Schweitzer ME (2002) Is soft-tissue inflammation in pedal infection contained by fascial planes? MR analysis of compartmental involvement in 115 feet. Am J Roentgenol 178(3):605–612. https://doi.org/10.2214/ajr.178.3.1780605

Lee JK, Yao L, Wirth CR (1987) MR imaging of solitary osteochondromas: report of eight cases. AJR Am J Roentgenol 149(3):557–560. https://doi.org/10.2214/ajr.149.3.557

Lee EY, Seeger LL, Nelson SD, Eckardt JJ (2000) Primary osteosarcoma of a metatarsal bone. Skeletal Radiol 29(8):474–476. https://doi.org/10.1007/s002560000237

Lee JC, Thomas JM, Phillips S, Fisher C, Moskovic E (2006) Aggressive fibromatosis: MRI features with pathologic correlation. AJR Am J Roentgenol 186(1):247–254. https://doi.org/10.2214/AJR.04.1674

Lewis JJ, Leung D, Heslin M, Woodruff JM, Brennan MF (1997) Association of local recurrence with subsequent survival in extremity soft tissue sarcoma. J Clin Oncol 15(2):646–652. https://doi.org/10.1200/JCO.1997.15.2.646

Libson E, Bloom RA, Husband JE, Stoker DJ (1987) Metastatic tumours of bones of the hand and foot. A comparative review and report of 43 additional cases. Skeletal Radiol 16(5):387–392. https://doi.org/10.1007/BF00350965

Link TM, Haeussler MD, Poppek S et al (1998) Malignant fibrous histiocytoma of bone: conventional X-ray and MR imaging features. Skeletal Radiol 27(10):552–558. https://doi.org/10.1007/s002560050436

Lo H, Kalisher L, Faix J (1977) Epithelioid sarcoma: radiologic and pathologic manifestations. Am J Roentgenol 128(6):1017–1020. https://doi.org/10.2214/ajr.128.6.1017

Longo V, Jacobson JA, Dong Q, Kim SM (2016) Tumors and tumor-like abnormalities of the midfoot and forefoot. Semin Musculoskelet Radiol 20(2):154–166. https://doi.org/10.1055/s-0036-1581118

Maheshwari AV, Chiappetta G, Kugler CD, Pitcher JD, Temple HT (2008) Metastatic skeletal disease of the foot: case reports and literature review. Foot Ankle Int 29(7):699–710. https://doi.org/10.3113/FAI.2008.0699

Mascard E, Gaspar N, Brugières L, Glorion C, Pannier S, Gomez-Brouchet A (2017) Malignant tumours of the foot and ankle. EFORT Open Rev 2(5):261–271. https://doi.org/10.1302/2058-5241.2.160078

Mavrogenis A, Bianchi G, Stavropoulos N, Papagelopoulos P, Ruggieri P (2013) Clinicopathological features, diagnosis and treatment of clear cell sarcoma/melanoma of soft parts. Hippokratia 17(4):298–302

Mc Auley G, Jagannathan J, O'Regan K et al (2012) Extraskeletal osteosarcoma: spectrum of imaging findings. Am J Roentgenol 198(1):W31–W37. https://doi.org/10.2214/AJR.11.6927

McLeod R, Dahlin D, Beabout J (1976) The spectrum of osteoblastoma. Am J Roentgenol 126(2):321–325. https://doi.org/10.2214/ajr.126.2.321

Meneses MF, Unni KK, Swee RG (1993) Bizarre parosteal osteochondromatous proliferation of bone (Nora's lesion). Am J Surg Pathol 17(7):691–697. https://doi.org/10.1097/00000478-199307000-00006

Michelson JD, Sinclair M (1994) Sarcomatous degeneration of neurofibromatosis presenting in the foot. Foot Ankle Int 15(7):400–403. https://doi.org/10.1177/107110079401500710

Milgram JW (1988) Intraosseous lipomas: radiologic and pathologic manifestations. Radiology 167(1):155–160. https://doi.org/10.1148/radiology.167.1.3347718

Mirra JM (1989) Bone tumors. Clin Radiol Pathol Correl. Accessed 14 Feb 2022. https://ci.nii.ac.jp/naid/10018825163/

Mitty HA (1993) Musculoskeletal neoplasms role of angiography in diagnosis and intervention. Semin Interv Radiol 10(04):277–283. https://doi.org/10.1055/s-2008-1074731

Miyayama H, Sakamoto K, Ide M et al (1993) Aggressive osteoblastoma of the calcaneus. Cancer 71(2):346–353. https://doi.org/10.1002/1097-0142(19930115)71:2<346::aid-cncr2820710213>3.0.co;2-j

Mollon B, Lee A, Busse JW et al (2015) The effect of surgical synovectomy and radiotherapy on the rate of recurrence of pigmented villonodular synovitis of the knee: an individual patient meta-analysis. Bone Jt J 97-B(4):550–557. https://doi.org/10.1302/0301-620X.97B4.34907

Monroe MT, Manoli A (1999) Osteoid osteoma of the lateral talar process presenting as a chronic sprained ankle. Foot Ankle Int 20(7):461–463. https://doi.org/10.1177/107110079902000712

Moon NF, Mori H (1986) Adamantinoma of the appendicular skeleton—updated. Clin Orthop 204: 215–237

Morrison WB, Schweitzer ME, Wapner KL, Lackman RD (1994) Plantar fibromatosis: a benign aggressive neoplasm with a characteristic appearance on MR images. Radiology 193(3):841–845. https://doi.org/10.1148/radiology.193.3.7972835

Moukaddam H, Pollak J, Haims AH (2009) MRI characteristics and classification of peripheral vascular malformations and tumors. Skeletal Radiol 38(6):535–547. https://doi.org/10.1007/s00256-008-0609-2

Murahashi Y, Iba K, Teramoto A et al (2021) Clinical features of bone and soft tissue tumors of the foot and ankle: results from a retrospective single-center case-series. J Orthop Sci 26(5):885–890. https://doi.org/10.1016/j.jos.2020.08.016

Murai NO, Teniola O, Wang WL, Amini B (2018) Bone and soft tissue tumors about the foot and ankle. Radiol Clin North Am 56(6):917–934. https://doi.org/10.1016/j.rcl.2018.06.010

Murari TM, Callaghan JJ, Berrey BH, Sweet DE (1989) Primary benign and malignant osseous neoplasms of the foot. Foot Ankle 10(2):68–80. https://doi.org/10.1177/107110078901000205

Murff R, Ashry HR (1994) Intraosseous ganglia of the foot. J Foot Ankle Surg 33(4):396–401

Murphey MD, Kransdorf MJ (2021) Staging and classification of primary musculoskeletal bone and soft-tissue tumors according to the 2020 WHO update, from the AJR special series on cancer staging. AJR Am J Roentgenol 217(5):1038–1052. https://doi.org/10.2214/AJR.21.25658

Murphey MD, Choi JJ, Kransdorf MJ, Flemming DJ, Gannon FH (2000) Imaging of osteochondroma: variants and complications with radiologic-pathologic correlation. Radiographics 20(5):1407–1434. https://doi.org/10.1148/radiographics.20.5.g00se171407

Murphey MD, Nomikos GC, Flemming DJ, Gannon FH, Temple HT, Kransdorf MJ (2001) Imaging of giant cell tumor and giant cell reparative granuloma of bone: radiologic-pathologic correlation. Radiographics 21(5):1283–1309. https://doi.org/10.1148/radiographics.21.5.g01se251283

Murphey MD, Walker EA, Wilson AJ, Kransdorf MJ, Temple HT, Gannon FH (2003) From the archives of the AFIP. Radiographics 23(5):1245–1278. https://doi.org/10.1148/rg.235035134

Murphey MD, Gibson MS, Jennings BT, Crespo-Rodríguez AM, Fanburg-Smith J, Gajewski DA (2006) From the archives of the AFIP: imaging of synovial sarcoma with radiologic-pathologic correlation. Radiographics 26(5):1543–1565. https://doi.org/10.1148/rg.265065084

Murphey MD, Rhee JH, Lewis RB, Fanburg-Smith JC, Flemming DJ, Walker EA (2008) Pigmented villonodular synovitis: radiologic-pathologic correlation. Radiographics 28(5):1493–1518. https://doi.org/10.1148/rg.285085134

Nishimura Y, Yamaguchi Y, Tomita Y et al (2010) Epithelioid sarcoma on the foot masquerading as an intractable wound for > 18 years. Clin Exp Dermatol 35(3):263–268. https://doi.org/10.1111/j.1365-2230.2009.03363.x

Noebauer-Huhmann IM, Weber MA, Lalam RK et al (2015) Soft tissue tumors in adults: ESSR-approved guidelines for diagnostic imaging. Semin Musculoskelet Radiol 19(5):475–482. https://doi.org/10.1055/s-0035-1569251

Nora FE, Dahlin DC, Beabout JW (1983) Bizarre parosteal osteochondromatous proliferations of the hands and feet. Am J Surg Pathol 7(3):245–250. https://doi.org/10.1097/00000478-198304000-00003

O'Connor PJ, Gibbon WW, Hardy G, Butt WP (1996) Chondromyxoid fibroma of the foot. Skeletal Radiol 25(2):143–148. https://doi.org/10.1007/s002560050051

Ogose A, Unni KK, Swee RG, May GK, Rowland CM, Sim FH (1997) Chondrosarcoma of small bones of the hands and feet. Cancer 80(1):50–59

Ontell F, Greenspan A (1994) Chondrosarcoma complicating synovial chondromatosis: findings with magnetic resonance imaging. Can Assoc Radiol J 45(4):318–323

Ortega R, Fessell DP, Jacobson JA, Lin J, van Holsbeeck MT, Hayes CW (2002) Sonography of ankle ganglia with pathologic correlation in 10 pediatric and adult patients. Am J Roentgenol 178(6):1445–1449. https://doi.org/10.2214/ajr.178.6.1781445

Ozdemir HM, Yildiz Y, Yilmaz C, Saglik Y (1997) Tumors of the foot and ankle: analysis of 196 cases. J Foot Ankle Surg 36(6):403–408. https://doi.org/10.1016/s1067-2516(97)80089-0

Papp DF, Khanna AJ, McCarthy EF, Carrino JA, Farber AJ, Frassica FJ (2007) Magnetic resonance imaging of soft-tissue tumors: determinate and indeterminate lesions. J Bone Joint Surg Am 89(Suppl 3):103–115. https://doi.org/10.2106/JBJS.G.00711

Peterson DL, Murk SE, Story JL (1992) Multifocal cavernous hemangioma of the skull: report of a case and review of the literature. Neurosurgery 30(5):778–781; discussion 782

Petscavage-Thomas JM, Walker EA, Logie CI, Clarke LE, Duryea DM, Murphey MD (2014) Soft-tissue myxomatous lesions: review of salient imaging features with pathologic comparison. Radiographics 34(4):964–980. https://doi.org/10.1148/rg.344130110

Radiology Assistant. The radiology assistant: bone tumors. Accessed 21 Feb 2022. https://radiologyassistant.nl/musculoskeletal/bone-tumors

Rammelt S, Fritzsche H, Hofbauer C, Schaser KD (2020) Malignant tumours of the foot and ankle. Foot Ankle Surg 26(4):363–370. https://doi.org/10.1016/j.fas.2019.05.005

Ratner V, Dorfman HD (1990) Giant-cell reparative granuloma of the hand and foot bones. Clin Orthop 260:251–258

Reda B (2018) Cystic bone tumors of the foot and ankle. J Surg Oncol 117(8):1786–1798. https://doi.org/10.1002/jso.25088

Reisi N, Raeissi P, Harati Khalilabad T, Moafi A (2021) Unusual sites of bone involvement in Langerhans cell histiocytosis: a systematic review of the literature. Orphanet J Rare Dis 16(1):1. https://doi.org/10.1186/s13023-020-01625-z

Ricca RL, Kuklo TR, Shawen SB, Vick DJ, Schaefer RA (2000) Periosteal chondroma of the cuboid presenting in a 7-year-old-boy. Foot Ankle Int 21(2):145–149. https://doi.org/10.1177/107110070002100209

Roberts CC, Kransdorf MJ, Beaman FD et al (2016) ACR appropriateness criteria follow-up of malignant or aggressive musculoskeletal tumors. J Am Coll Radiol 13(4):389–400. https://doi.org/10.1016/j.jacr.2015.12.019

Ruggieri P, Angelini A, Jorge FD, Maraldi M, Giannini S (2014) Review of foot tumors seen in a university tumor institute. J Foot Ankle Surg 53(3):282–285. https://doi.org/10.1053/j.jfas.2014.01.015

Saad A, Kho J, Almeer G, Azzopardi C, Botchu R (2021) Lesions of the heel fat pad. Br J Radiol 94(1118):20200648. https://doi.org/10.1259/bjr.20200648

Sarkar MR, Schulte M, Bauer G, Hartwig E, Von Baer A (1996) Primary bone and soft tissue tumours of the foot. Oncological and functional considerations. Foot Ankle Surg 2(4):261–270. https://doi.org/10.1016/S1268-7731(96)80010-5

Schajowicz F (2012) Tumors and tumorlike lesions of bone and joints. Springer Science & Business Media

Schatz J, Soper J, McCormack S, Healy M, Deady L, Brown W (2010) Imaging of tumors in the ankle and foot. Top Magn Reson Imaging 21(1):37–50. https://doi.org/10.1097/RMR.0b013e31820ef556

Selek H, Ozer H, Turanli S, Erdem O (2007) Giant cell tumor of the talar neck. J Am Podiatr Med Assoc 97(3):225–228. https://doi.org/10.7547/0970225

Singer AD, Datir A, Tresley J et al (2016) Benign and malignant tumors of the foot and ankle. Skeletal Radiol 45(3):287–305. https://doi.org/10.1007/s00256-015-2278-2

Skorman SE, Martin R (1999) Primary lymphoma of the calcaneus with recurrence in the distal tibia: a case report. J Foot Ankle Surg 38(4):278–282. https://doi.org/10.1016/s1067-2516(99)80070-2

Slomovitz M, Nixon B, Mott RC (1990) Tumoral calcinosis of the foot: case report and literature review. J Foot Surg 29(3):278–283

Soldatos T, McCarthy EF, Attar S, Carrino JA, Fayad LM (2011) Imaging features of chondrosarcoma. J Comput Assist Tomogr 35(4):504–511. https://doi.org/10.1097/RCT.0b013e31822048ff

Somerhausen NS, Fletcher CD (2000) Diffuse-type giant cell tumor: clinicopathologic and immunohistochemical analysis of 50 cases with extraarticular disease. Am J Surg Pathol 24(4):479–492. https://doi.org/10.1097/00000478-200004000-00002

Stevenson JD, Jaiswal A, Gregory JJ, Mangham DC, Cribb G, Cool P (2013) Diffuse pigmented villonodular synovitis (diffuse-type giant cell tumour) of the foot and ankle. Bone Jt J 95-B(3):384–390. https://doi.org/10.1302/0301-620X.95B3.30192

Stoker D, Cobb J, Pringle J (1991) Needle biopsy of musculoskeletal lesions. A review of 208 procedures. J Bone Joint Surg Br 73-B(3):498–500. https://doi.org/10.1302/0301-620X.73B3.1670457

Stukenborg-Colsman C, Wülker N, Wirth CJ (1999) Cystic bone lesions of the calcaneus and the talus: report of five cases. Foot Ankle Surg 5(1):33–38. https://doi.org/10.1046/j.1460-9584.1999.51120.x

Suzuki Y, Ehara S, Shiraishi H, Nishida J, Murooka G, Tamakawa Y (1997) Embryonal rhabdomyosarcoma of foot with expansive growth between metatarsals. Skeletal Radiol 26(2):128–130. https://doi.org/10.1007/s002560050206

Szolomayer LK, Talusan PG, Chan WF, Lindskog DM (2017) Leiomyoma of the foot and ankle: a case series. Foot Ankle Spec 10(3):270–273. https://doi.org/10.1177/1938640016670243

Taconis WK, Schütte HE, van der Heul RO (1994) Desmoplastic fibroma of bone: a report of 18 cases. Skeletal Radiol 23(4):283–288. https://doi.org/10.1007/BF02412362

Talbot BS, Weinberg EP (2016) MR imaging with metal-suppression sequences for evaluation of total joint arthroplasty. Radiographics 36(1):209–225. https://doi.org/10.1148/rg.2016150075

Tavare AN, Robinson P, Altoos R et al (2018) Postoperative imaging of sarcomas. AJR Am J Roentgenol 211(3):506–518. https://doi.org/10.2214/AJR.18.19954

Tay AYW, Tay KS, Thever Y, Hao Y, Yeo NEM (2021) An epidemiological review of 623 foot and ankle soft tissue tumours and pseudo-tumours. Foot Ankle Surg 27(4):400–404. https://doi.org/10.1016/j.fas.2020.05.004

Temple HT, Mizel MS, Murphey MD, Sweet DE (1998) Osteoblastoma of the foot and ankle.

Foot Ankle Int 19(10):698–704. https://doi.org/10.1177/107110079801901009

Thacker MM, Potter BK, Pitcher JD, Temple HT (2008) Soft tissue sarcomas of the foot and ankle: impact of unplanned excision, limb salvage, and multimodality therapy. Foot Ankle Int 29(7):690–698. https://doi.org/10.3113/FAI.2008.0690

Toepfer A, Harrasser N, Dreyer F, Mogler C, Walther M, von Eisenhart-Rothe R (2017) Epithelioid sarcoma of the plantar fascia mimicking Morbus Ledderhose—a severe pitfall for clinical and histopathological misinterpretation. Foot Ankle Surg 23(4):e25–e30. https://doi.org/10.1016/j.fas.2017.03.013

Toepfer A, Harrasser N, Recker M et al (2018) Distribution patterns of foot and ankle tumors: a university tumor institute experience. BMC Cancer 18(1):735. https://doi.org/10.1186/s12885-018-4648-3

Toomayan GA, Robertson F, Major NM (2005) Lower extremity compartmental anatomy: clinical relevance to radiologists. Skeletal Radiol 34(6):307–313. https://doi.org/10.1007/s00256-005-0910-2

Unni K (1986) Dahlin's bone tumors. Osteochondroma, pp 11–23

UW Radiology. Online musculoskeletal radiology book. Accessed 21 Feb 2022. https://rad.washington.edu/about-us/academic-sections/musculoskeletal-radiology/teaching-materials/online-musculoskeletal-radiology-book/

Vanhoenacker FM, Hauben E, De Beuckeleer LH, Willemen D, Van Marck E, De Schepper AM (2000) Desmoplastic fibroma of bone: MRI features. Skeletal Radiol 29(3):171–175. https://doi.org/10.1007/s002560050589

Veith NT, Tschernig T, Histing T, Madry H (2013) Plantar fibromatosis—topical review. Foot Ankle Int 34(12):1742–1746. https://doi.org/10.1177/1071100713505535

von Mehren M, Randall RL, Benjamin RS et al (2018) Soft tissue sarcoma, version 2.2018, NCCN clinical practice guidelines in oncology. J Natl Compr Cancer Netw 16(5):536–563. https://doi.org/10.6004/jnccn.2018.0025

Weatherall PT, Maale GE, Mendelsohn DB, Sherry CS, Erdman WE, Pascoe HR (1994) Chondroblastoma: classic and confusing appearance at MR imaging. Radiology 190(2):467–474. https://doi.org/10.1148/radiology.190.2.8284401

Weinfeld GD, Yu GV, Good JJ (2002) Intraosseous lipoma of the calcaneus: a review and report of four cases. J Foot Ankle Surg 41(6):398–411. https://doi.org/10.1016/s1067-2516(02)80087-4

Werd MB, DeFronzo DJ, Landsman AS, Surprenant M, Sakoff M (1995) Myxoid liposarcoma of the ankle. J Foot Ankle Surg 34(5):465–474. https://doi.org/10.1016/S1067-2516(09)80022-7

White LM, Schweitzer ME, Khalili K, Howarth DJ, Wunder JS, Bell RS (1998) MR imaging of primary lymphoma of bone: variability of T2-weighted signal intensity. AJR Am J Roentgenol 170(5):1243–1247. https://doi.org/10.2214/ajr.170.5.9574594

WHO Classification of Tumours Editorial Board (2020) Soft tissue and bone tumours. Accessed 21 Feb 2022. https://publications.iarc.fr/Book-And-Report-Series/Who-Classification-Of-Tumours/Soft-Tissue-And-Bone-Tumours-2020

Woertler K (2005) Soft tissue masses in the foot and ankle: characteristics on MR Imaging. Semin Musculoskelet Radiol 9(3):227–242. https://doi.org/10.1055/s-2005-921942

Yang JC, Chang AE, Baker AR et al (1998) Randomized prospective study of the benefit of adjuvant radiation therapy in the treatment of soft tissue sarcomas of the extremity. J Clin Oncol 16(1):197–203. https://doi.org/10.1200/JCO.1998.16.1.197

Yee DY, Mott RC, Nixon BP (1991) Calcifying aponeurotic fibroma. J Foot Surg 30(3):279–283

Young PS, Bell SW, MacDuff EM, Mahendra A (2013) Primary osseous tumors of the hindfoot: why the delay in diagnosis and should we be concerned? Clin Orthop 471(3):871–877. https://doi.org/10.1007/s11999-012-2570-6

Youssef BA, Haddad MC, Zahrani A et al (1996) Osteoid osteoma and osteoblastoma: MRI appearances and the significance of ring enhancement. Eur Radiol 6(3):291–296. https://doi.org/10.1007/BF00180597

Yuan WH, Hsu HC, Lai YC, Chou YH, Li AFY (2012) Differences in sonographic features of ruptured and unruptured epidermal cysts. J Ultrasound Med 31(2):265–272. https://doi.org/10.7863/jum.2012.31.2.265

Zanetti M, Strehle JK, Zollinger H, Hodler J (1997) Morton neuroma and fluid in the intermetatarsal bursae on MR images of 70 asymptomatic volunteers. Radiology 203(2):516–520. https://doi.org/10.1148/radiology.203.2.9114115

Zgonis T, Jolly GP, Polyzois V, Kanuck DM, Stamatis ED (2005) Plantar fibromatosis. Clin Podiatr Med Surg 22(1):11–18. https://doi.org/10.1016/j.cpm.2004.08.002

Orthopedic Hardware

Han Hong Chong and Maneesh Bhatia

Contents

H. H. Chong
University Hospitals of Leicester NHS Trust, Leicester, UK

M. Bhatia (✉)
University Hospitals of Leicester NHS Trust, Spire Leicester and Nuffield Health Leicester, Leicester, UK
e-mail: maneeshbhatia@yahoo.com

1 Introduction

With the advancement in medical device, there has been a tremendous increase in the usage of hardware in treating different orthopedic pathologies. Most clinicians are capable of recognizing an "orthopedic hardware" on a plain radiograph; however, they are often put off by the entire range or classifications of the hardware.

This chapter covers the assessment of foot and ankle orthopedic hardware used for trauma, reconstruction, fusion, and arthroplasty.

2 Basic Assessment of Common Orthopedic Hardware

Broadly speaking, orthopedic hardware can be divided into:

- Internal fixation using Kirschner wires (K-wire), staples, plates, and screws
- External fixation or frame
- Replacement/arthroplasty
- Fusion/arthrodesis using screws or plates

To interpret orthopedic hardware, it is important to first understand the underlying pathology being treated. Adequate preoperative imaging is essential in guiding orthopedic surgeon diagnosing the underlying disorder and choosing the appropriate surgical approach (Berquist 1994).

Med Radiol Diagn Imaging (2023)

https://doi.org/10.1007/174_2023_391,
Published Online: 06 April 2023

2.1 Plain Radiography (X-Ray)

Plain radiograph, commonly known as X-ray, remains the commonest imaging request by a clinician. As a general rule, it is crucial to assess a limb with a minimum of two orthogonal views, commonly an anteroposterior (AP) view and a lateral view. For foot and ankle radiograph, the standing view provides the most adequate information.

Without the need for advanced imaging, plain radiograph often provides enough information to aid the clinician in clinical assessment and decision. In different pathologies, there are several important markers:

- Fracture fixation: callus formation, cortical thickening, implant position, lucency around hardware suggesting loosening, hardware fracture
- Arthroplasty: implant alignment and congruency, lucency around the implant
- Arthrodesis: nonunion, malunion, issues with hardware (positioning, failure, or breakdown)

Serial radiographic studies are useful in monitoring change in hardware position or progression of radiolucency.

2.2 Computed Tomography (CT)

The complexity of the foot and ankle may warrant a CT scan for the evaluation of orthopedic hardware in relation to surrounding bony integrity. Two main indications for CT scan are assessment of fracture healing and bone stock as part of revision planning. It is important to consider the risk of metal artifact, and metal suppression imaging may be required based on the clinical question.

2.3 Ultrasonography (USS)

USS is an inexpensive and easily available modality in comparison with CT or magnetic resonance imaging (MRI). It is useful for assessing soft tissue status (i.e., ligament injury, tendonitis), collection (hematoma, abscess), and vascular disorders (venous thromboembolism).

2.4 Magnetic Resonance Imaging (MRI)

MRI is sensitive in detecting and staging soft tissue pathology and evaluating complications such as nonunion, infection, and avascular necrosis. It is, again, important to consider the risk of metal artifact causing local image distortion. Metal suppression imaging may be required to reduce the distortion and aids clinical assessment.

2.5 Other Imaging Modalities

Radionuclide bone scans, arthrogram, tenography, and diagnostic/therapeutic injections are all alternative techniques to gain further information in diagnosis and treatment planning.

3 Trauma Hardware

Any serious injury to the bones, joints, and/or soft tissue induced by an external source is referred to as orthopedic trauma. These injuries can be the result of a sudden incident, such as a vehicle accident or a fall. Trauma can also be produced by repetitive overuse, for example, second metatarsal stress fractures in a runner.

3.1 Forefoot Trauma

The forefoot consists of all the phalanges and metatarsals. The flexibility of the forefoot joints allows forward propulsion in the terminal stance phase of gait. Any hardware implanted in the forefoot is aimed to achieve a pain-free, near-normal gait.

Metatarsal fractures are the most common fracture site of the foot, often resulting from direct traumatic force (crush injuries, motor vehicle accident) or indirect force (inversion or eversion injuries) (Iwamoto and Takeda 2003; Rammelt et al. 2004). Fractures of the fifth metatarsal base may result from the pull of peroneus brevis along with the long plantar ligament and the plantar aponeurosis (Theodorou et al. 2003).

There are many techniques described in forefoot trauma surgical correction, ranging across the use of K-wires, cerclage wire, interfragmentary screw, plating, external fixation, or intramedullary fixation (Fig. 1). As a rule of thumb, percutaneous K-wire is used to maintain alignment if fracture can be reduced adequately using closed technique. Open reduction and internal fixation is indicated in fractures that are irreducible, closed, and displaced and with joint involvement and complex pattern (Mandracchia et al. 2006). Interfragmentary screw provides anatomical fixation and static compression to promote primary bone healing, commonly used in two-fragment fracture. Plate fixation is used in conjunction with either interfragmentary screw in shaft fracture to increase stiffness or multi-fragmentary fracture as a bridging construct. Intramedullary fixation using screw or rod has increasing popularity recently in the metatarsal shaft or neck fracture. The hardware acts as an internal splint to allow secondary bone healing.

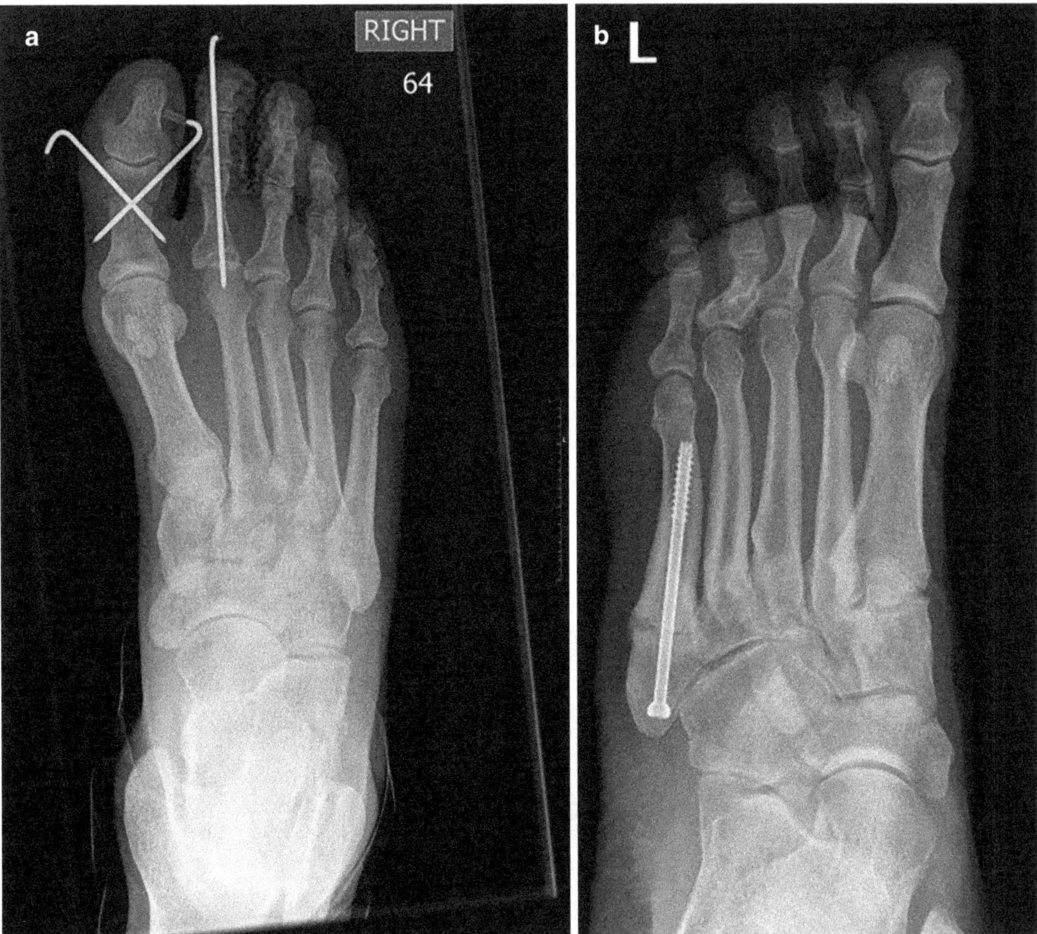

Fig. 1 Different types of orthopedic hardware in forefoot fractures. (**a**) K-wire fixation of first and second toe proximal phalanx fracture; (**b**) oblique view of left foot demonstrating interfragmentary screw fixation of fifth metatarsal base fracture

Complications of forefoot fixation include malunion, nonunion, hardware fracture, or loosening of hardware. Comparison of most recent imaging with postoperative imaging is crucial in aiding the clinician to identify any changes or progression.

3.2 Midfoot Trauma

The midfoot consists of navicular, cuboid, and three cuneiforms. It forms the arch of the foot with multiple ligamental attachments between the bones. The complex construct of midfoot provides a stable weight-bearing foot, rigid base during push-off, and flexibility when walking on uneven ground.

Tarsal fractures are relatively uncommon and mostly result from high-energy trauma such as motor vehicle accident. Mismanaged tarsal fracture, however, can lead to significant morbidity in the long term.

Tarsometatarsal (TMT) fracture dislocation is known as a Lisfranc injury, where the articulation between the medial cuneiform and the base of the second metatarsal has been disrupted. The typical radiological finding is widening between the bases of the first and second metatarsals. CT scan is often required to assess the extent of the injury and surgical planning (Moracia-Ochagavía and Rodríguez-Merchán 2019). Displaced or unstable Lisfranc injury warrants surgical treatment to achieve anatomical reduction. In a significant swollen foot, temporary stabilization with K-wire or an external fixator may be required to allow soft tissue settling along with reducing the risk of infection and compartment syndrome (Fig. 2a, b). Several definite fixation techniques have been described: transarticular screws, dorsal bridge plate, and primary arthrodesis of the first, second, and third TMT joints (Fig. 2c); none was shown to be majorly superior to another (Moracia-Ochagavía and Rodríguez-Merchán 2019; Alcelik et al. 2020; Boksh et al. 2020). While assessing postoperative imaging, pay attention to the hardware position, foot alignment, and signs of TMT joint arthritis.

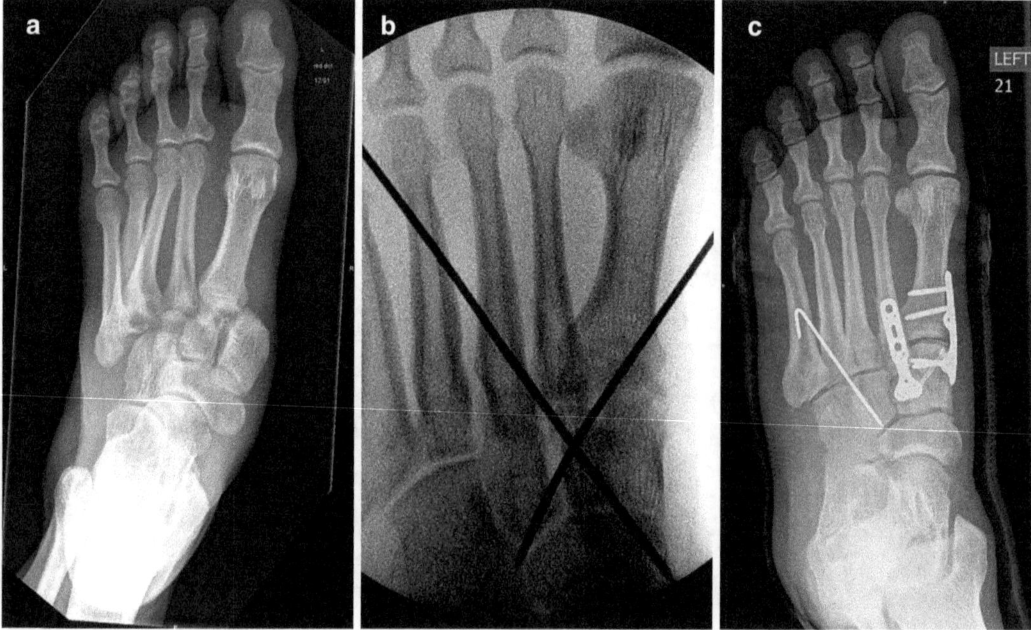

Fig. 2 Homolateral Lisfranc fracture-dislocation of the left foot in a young patient. (**a**) AP view of left foot at initial presentation; (**b**) intraoperative fluoroscopy showing temporary reduction and stabilization using K-wire; (**c**) definite fixation using plating of medial column and K-wire fixation of lateral column

Other tarsal bone fractures (navicular, cuneiform, cuboidal) can be subtle and easily missed in initial diagnosis. Depending on the severity and associated injuries, surgical fixation of the navicular includes the use of screw, plates, or external fixator (Patel 2018) (Fig. 3).

3.3 Hindfoot Trauma

The hindfoot consists of talus and calcaneus, making up the subtalar joint, talonavicular joint, and calcaneocuboid joint. It functions to distribute weight to the foot while weight-bearing and to permit complex foot movements in coordination with the ankle joint, especially inversion/eversion and axial rotation. The integrity of the joints will guide the choice of hardware in hindfoot surgery.

Calcaneal fracture is the commonest fracture of the tarsal bones, with 75% intra-articular involvement. The applied surgical anatomy of the calcaneus is complex due to the multifaceted nature and its articulations with the talus and cuboid. CT scan is required to allow three-dimensional assessment of the fracture for surgical planning. Choice of orthopedic hardware is pins, screws, or low-profile plate depending on the severity of fracture (Razik et al. 2018; Allegra et al. 2020) (Fig. 4). While assessing the postoperative imaging, it is essential to assess the hardware position in relation to surrounding joints and sinus tarsi, calcaneal alignment, and signs of infection.

Talus fracture, on the other hand, is rare but devastating with a high risk of nonunion due to the vascular supply complexity. CT scan is best to determine the degree of displacement, comminution, and joint congruity. External fixation may be required to stabilize a reduced talus fracture and/or dislocation if definite surgery needs to be delayed (i.e., soft tissue injury, hemodynamically unstable). Anatomical reduction and internal fixation remain the standard of treatment with screws or modern low-profile plates (Schwartz et al. 2020) (Fig. 5). The important radiological findings to look out for are hardware position, mal/nonunion, avascular necrosis, and post-traumatic arthritis.

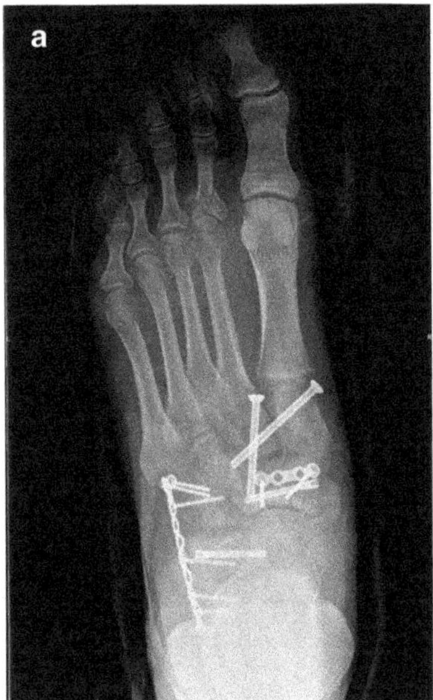

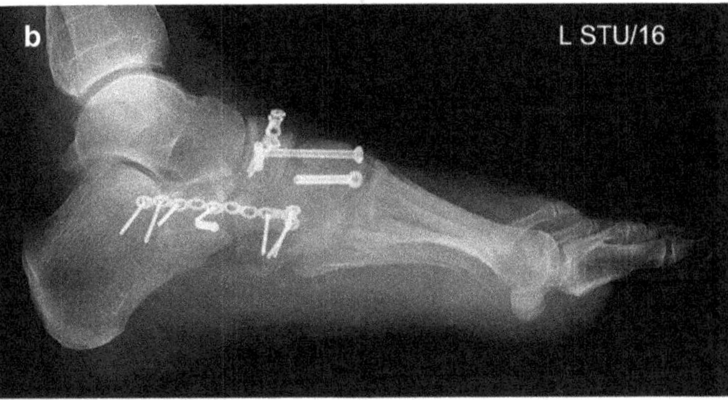

Fig. 3 Open reduction and internal fixation of cuneiform, navicular, and calcaneal process fracture using screw and plate construct. (**a**) AP view; (**b**) lateral view

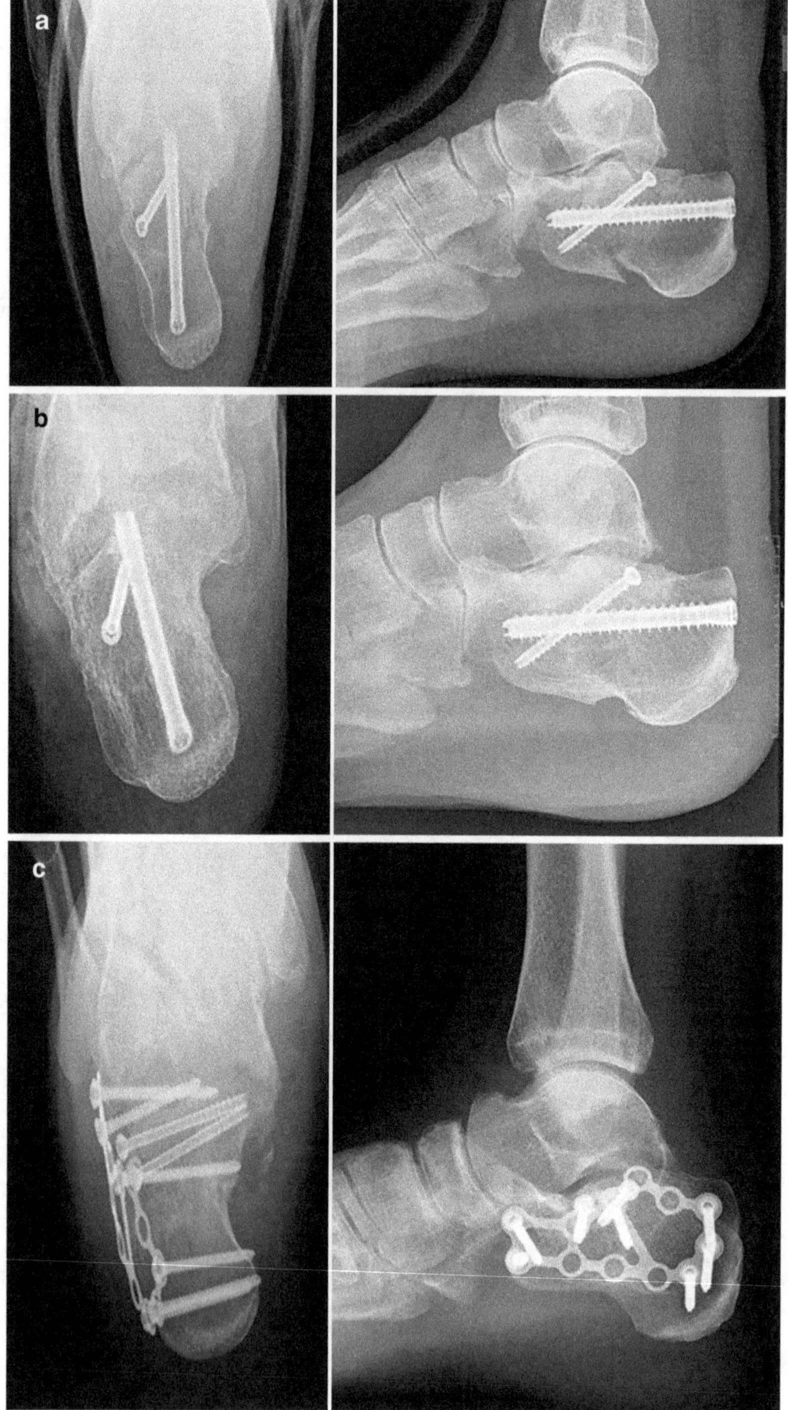

Fig. 4 Calcaneal fracture fixation using different orthopedic hardware. (**a**) Fracture fixation using two interfragmentary screws; images taken at 6 weeks postoperatively; (**b**) union of calcaneal fracture at 9-month follow-up; (**c**) fracture fixation using low-profile calcaneal plating

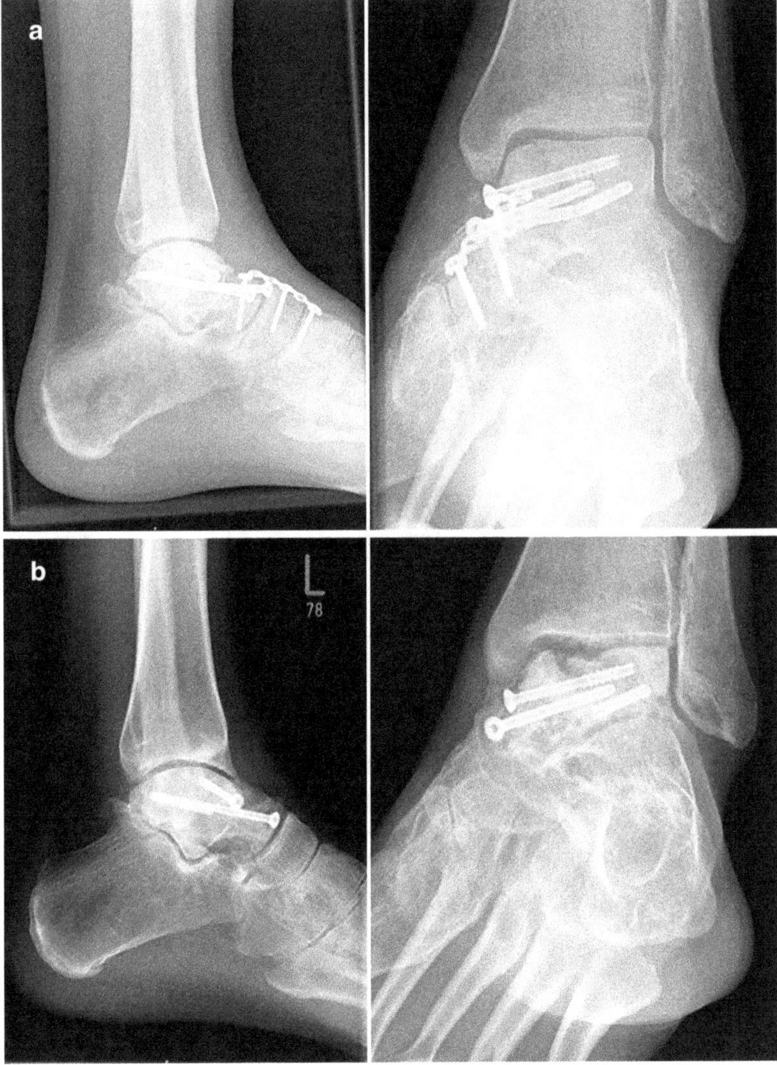

Fig. 5 Talar neck fracture fixation and potential complications. (**a**) Plain radiograph 6 weeks after surgery showing talus neck screw fixation with talar-navicular-cuneiform plating for augmentation. One of the talus fixation screws has cracked, as seen; (**b**) 4 years postoperatively after hardware removal revealed a broken screw, collapsed medial talar dome, and development of post-traumatic arthritis

3.4 Ankle Trauma

Ankle joint, or tibiotalar joint, is a hinge joint that consists of the tibia, fibular, and talus. It forms the kinetic linkage between the lower limb and the ground, allowing for a stable weight-bearing gait. The type of orthopedic hardware in the ankle joint goes by the principle of fixation, reconstruction, replacement, or fusion.

Most ankle fractures occur with the foot in eversion or inversion position, followed by either rotational deforming force or translational deforming force (Okanobo et al. 2012); axial force may also occur in a certain setting. Fracture fragment can be subcategorized into lateral malleolus, medial malleolus, posterior malleolus, and tibia plafond (pilon fracture).

Temporary external fixator is often deployed to allow soft tissue monitoring or complex wound prior to definite fixation. Circular frame is reserved for complex fracture with associated extensive soft tissue injuries. Lateral malleolus is traditionally fixed with screws and plates; recently, fibular nailing has returned into fashion with a lower complication rate and equivalent outcome (Asloum et al. 2014). Medial malleolus is commonly fixed with partially threaded cancellous screws for compression; in vertical shear

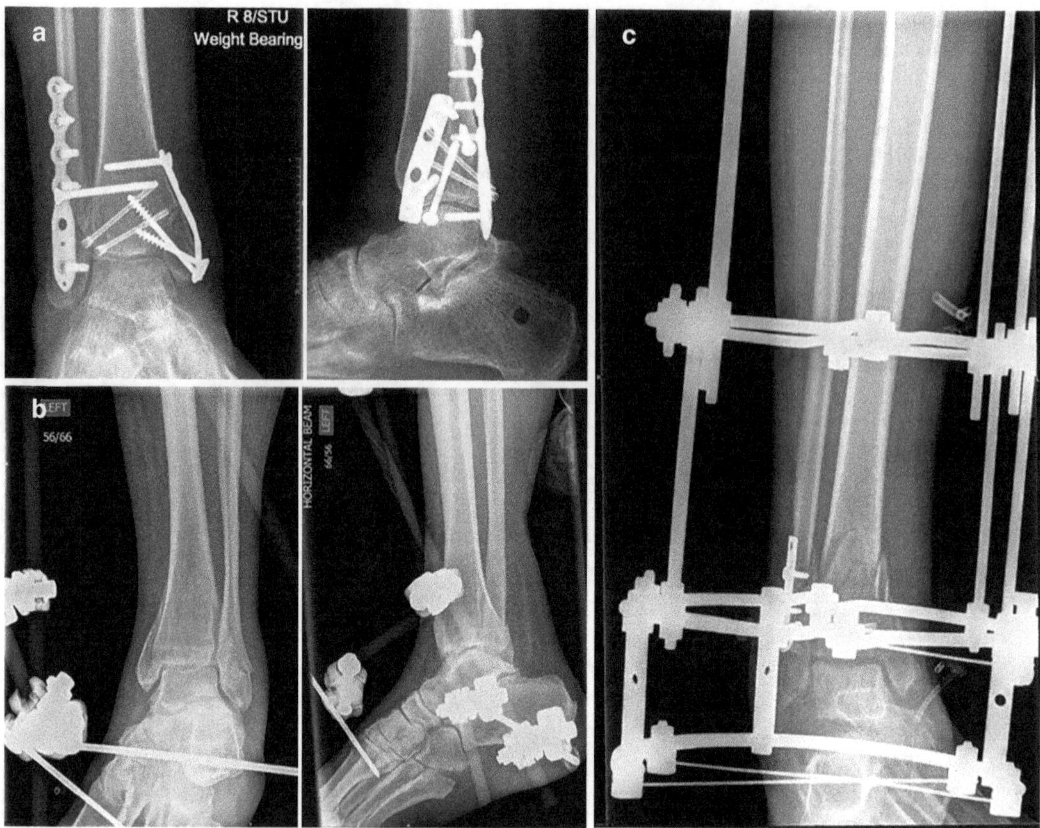

Fig. 6 Different types of orthopedic hardware in ankle fractures. (**a**) Posterior fixation of fibula and posterior malleolus using screws and plate construct, medial malleolus plating, and syndesmosis screw fixation; (**b**) temporary external fixator of ankle fracture; (**c**) circular frame construct for comminuted, non-reconstructable ankle pilon fracture

type, buttress plate will be the choice of hardware.

In the past, posterior malleolus was fixed through a percutaneous screw in either AP or PA direction. This led to high-risk malreduced fragment due to the difficulty to assess under fluoroscopy. Recent literature supports posterior approach to visualize the fragment directly and fixed with plates (O'Connor et al. 2015). Finally, there is a trend of fixing syndesmosis (distal tibiofibular joint) from syndesmotic screw (cortical screw) to TightRope suture button fixation (Wright et al. 2019). Figure 6 shows the different orthopedic hardware used in ankle fractures.

Complications following ankle fracture are common. Involvement of articular surface or malreduced fracture will lead to a higher risk of arthritis development. Mal/nonunion may occur with poor reduction or implant failure—most often medial malleolus (Gourineni et al. 1999). Other signs to look for are hardware fracture (common in syndesmotic screw but often asymptomatic), progression of deformity, and infection.

4 Elective Hardware

Elective foot surgeries are those that are planned because they are not an emergency. They can be done for cosmetic purposes or to alleviate pain and discomfort for medical reasons. Bunionectomy, hammertoes, arthritis of the foot and ankle, and a range of different procedures are examples of elective foot surgery.

4.1 Hallux Valgus (Bunion)

Weight-bearing AP and lateral plain radiograph of the foot are useful for the assessment of the deformity using these radiological measurements: hallux valgus angle (HVA, normal <15°), intermetatarsal angle (IMA, normal <9°), distal metatarsal articular angle (DMAA, normal <10°), and sesamoid position (Robinson and Limbers 2005).

Surgical planning of hallux valgus greatly depends on the severity of the deformity, joint congruency, and underlying hypermobility of the first tarsometatarsal joint. Surgical treatment involves soft tissue release, bunion resection, first metatarsal osteotomy, proximal phalanx osteotomy, or arthrodesis in severe deformity (MTP joint or first TMT joint) (Fig. 7). Screws, plates, and staples are the most commonly used hardware.

While assessing the postoperative imaging, the clinician should pay attention to several key points: union of osteotomy, hardware position, loss of reduction/recurrence, hallux varus, and avascular necrosis of metatarsal head (Lehman 2003; Edwards 2005; Rothwell and Pickard 2013). Serial imaging is often required to evaluate progression and complications. CT scan may be used to assess bone stock as part of revision surgery planning, while MRI is useful to assess early signs of avascular necrosis.

4.2 Hallux Rigidus (First Metatarsophalangeal Arthritis)

First metatarsophalangeal joint (MTPJ) arthrodesis remains the reference standard treatment for

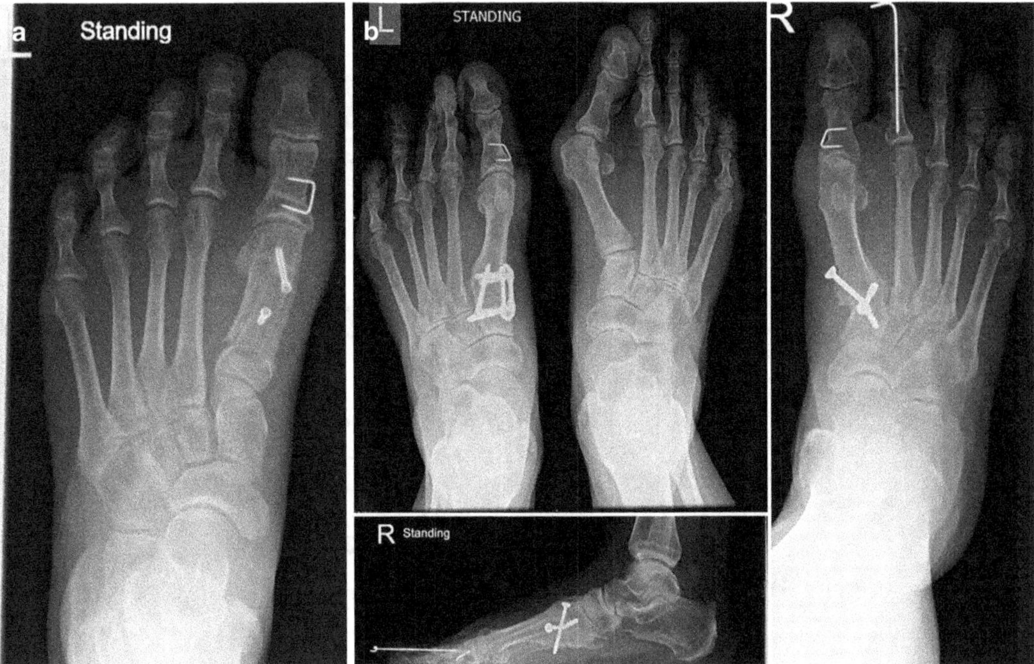

Fig. 7 Different types of orthopedic hardware for hallux valgus and potential findings. (**a**) Two interfragmentary cannulated screws for metatarsal scarf osteotomy, and 90° staples for proximal phalanx Akin osteotomy; (**b**) Top left: previous Lapidus treatment fusing first tarsometatarsal joints for hyperlaxity hallux valgus and Akin osteotomy on the left foot, with severe hallux valgus on the right foot; right and bottom left: plain radiograph of the right foot demonstrating two screws was used in the Lapidus operation, one of which failed after 6 weeks of weight-bearing. Also note the Akin osteotomy for the first proximal phalanx and the K-wire for the fusion of the second proximal interphalangeal joint

end-stage hallux rigidus (Anderson et al. 2018). Common orthopedic hardware used includes screw (cortical or cannulated), dorsal plates, and, less frequently, K-wires or clips (Fig. 8a) (Kannan et al. 2021). In postoperative imaging, the clinician should pay attention to the fusion of the intended joint, hardware failure (fracture or backing out), or radiolucency around hardware suggesting loosening.

MTPJ arthroplasty was first introduced back in the 1950s, evolving from simple silicone designs to complex metallic and ceramic implants (Stibolt et al. 2019). The aim of arthroplasty is the same as of any joint replacement principles: reduce pain, maintain joint kinematics, longevity, and ability to revise if it fails. Despite the advancement of medical device, survival rate of MTPJ arthroplasty remains inferior in comparison to hip and knee replacement (Majeed 2019; França et al. 2021). Two known MTPJ arthroplasties are hemiarthroplasty or total arthroplasty (Fig. 8b). Key points in postoperative imaging assessment are joint congruency, hardware position, and radiolucency around the hardware (for example, Cartiva implant).

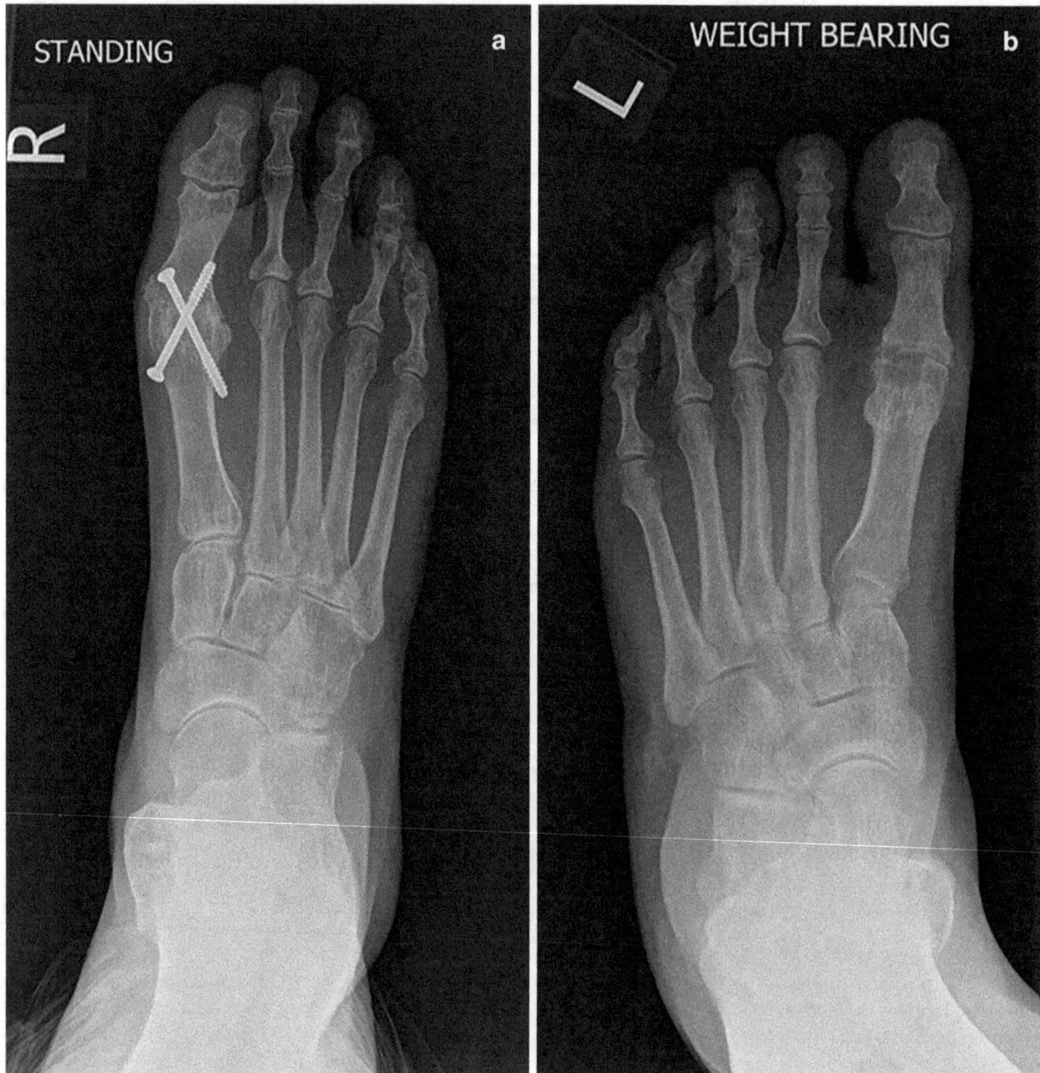

Fig. 8 Different types of orthopedic hardware in treating hallux rigidus. (**a**) Crossed interfragmentary screws; (**b**) Cartiva hemiarthroplasty of MTPJ

4.3 Lesser Toe Deformities

Lesser toe deformities are usually diagnosed clinically. Commonly known pathologies are curly toe (overlapping toes) in children, hammertoe, claw toe, mallet toe, and bunionette deformity of the fifth metatarsal. Treatment may be conservative if asymptomatic. In symptomatic, fixed contracture deformity, resection arthroplasty and corrective fixation may be required with K-wire or modern intramedullary implant (Fig. 9). Postoperative imaging assessments are loss of reduction, mal/nonunion, joint subluxation, or metalwork failure. Bunionette deformity of fifth metatarsal is similar to hallux valgus of the great toe, including twist-off screws for Weil's osteotomy.

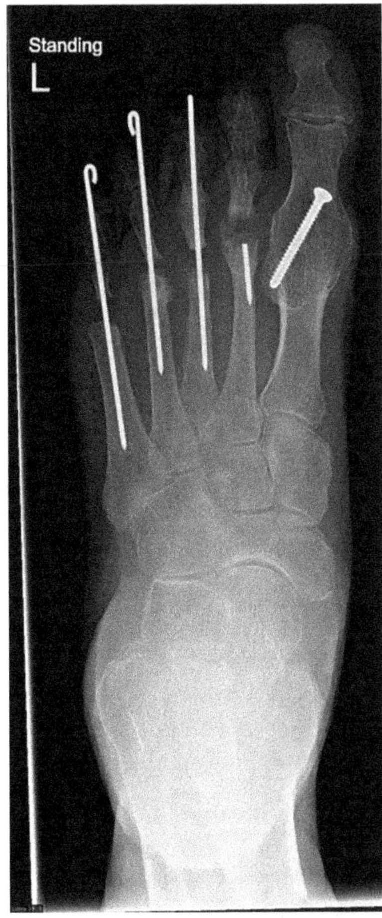

Fig. 9 Forefoot reconstruction surgery for fixed flexion-dislocation deformity of lesser toes. Resection arthroplasty (Stainsby procedure) was performed on the lesser toes with temporary fixation using K-wire. Note the first metatarsophalangeal joint fusion with screw fixation, and broken K-wire in the second toe metatarsal from previous Stainsby procedure

4.4 Midfoot Arthrodesis

Midfoot arthrodesis remains the standard of surgical intervention in patients with painful midfoot joints or deformity when all conservative treatments have failed. Common indications include osteoarthritis, deformity (flatfoot, cavus foot), and Charcot arthropathy. The number of constructs described for midfoot arthrodesis includes (but not limited to) screws, pins, K-wires, staples, plates, and external fixation. The choice of construct will depend on patient factors, anatomical factors, and fixation factors. Three basic principles to midfoot arthrodesis are fusion, correction, or interposition (Horisberger and Valderrabano 2014) (Fig. 10). Postoperative imaging assessments are infection, mal/nonunion, hardware failure, loss of alignment, and adjacent joint arthritis.

4.5 Hindfoot Arthrodesis

Hindfoot arthrodesis, also known as triple arthrodesis, is the surgical fusion of the talocalcaneal, talonavicular, and calcaneocuboid joint. The basic pathologies for hindfoot arthrodesis include Charcot arthropathy, arthritis (osteoarthritis, rheumatoid arthritis, post-traumatic), end-stage adult flatfoot, and neuromuscular disorder. Common hardware used to achieve hindfoot arthrodesis are screws, plates, or staples and, rarely, external fixator (Fig. 11). Complications are similar to any arthrodesis surgery: infections, mal/nonunion, adjacent joint arthritis, and hardware failure.

4.6 Ankle Arthroplasty

End-stage ankle arthritis can be debilitating to a patient's ability to carry out daily activities and

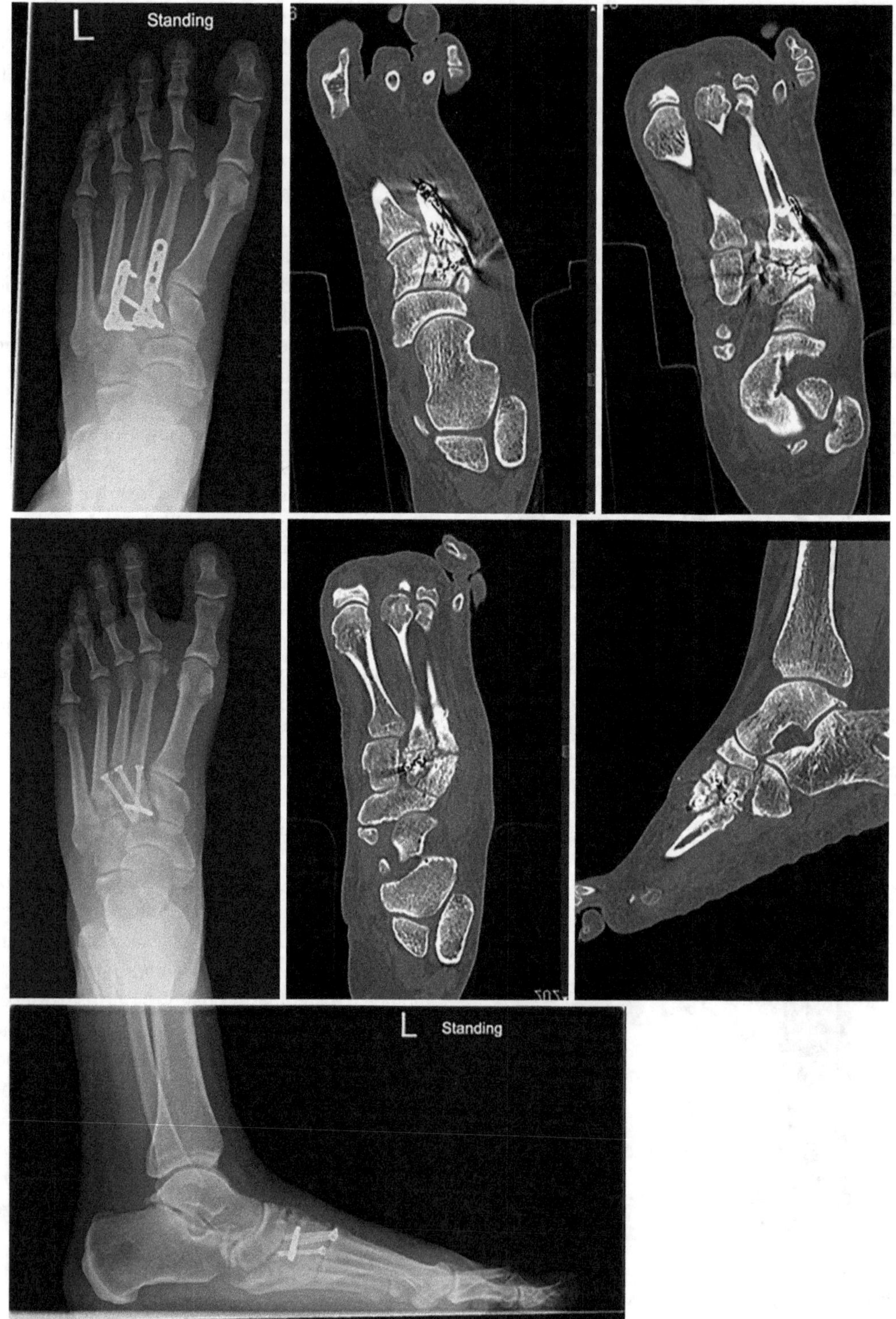

Fig. 10 Case example of midfoot arthrodesis with nonunion in a rheumatoid patient. Top three images show plain radiograph of the initial second and third TMTJ arthrodesis using plating system and 9-month postoperative CT scan showing no bony formation across the joints. The patient then underwent revision surgery using compression screws as shown in the bottom AP and lateral plain radiograph, limited by broken hardware from initial surgery. Subsequent CT scan 12 months post-revision surgery shows persistent nonunion across second and third TMTJ

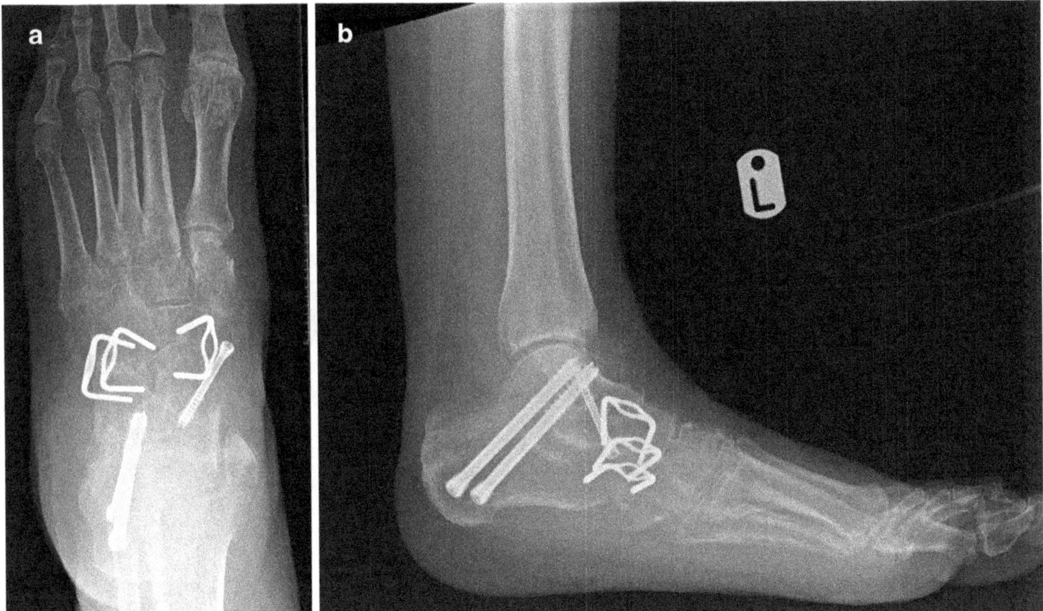

Fig. 11 Triple arthrodesis (fusion of subtalar, calcaneocuboid, and talonavicular joints) in hindfoot arthritis using screws and orthopedic staples. (**a**) AP view; (**b**) lateral view

quality of life. Although ankle arthrodesis has been the mainstream treatment of end-stage ankle arthritis, total ankle replacement (TAR) has shown equivalent clinical outcome in recent literature. This is due to the introduction of third-generation three-component mobile-bearing implants (Zaidi et al. 2013).

Indications for TAR are elderly patients with end-stage arthritis, low physical demands, adequate bone stock, satisfactory soft tissue coverage and blood supply, and ideally normal alignment. Absolute contraindications are active or chronic infection, insensate foot, severe multiplanar deformity, osteonecrosis of talus, and poor soft tissue coverage (Hayes et al. 2016).

There are at least seven known designs to date, which differ in bearing (fixed vs. mobile), constraint (semi- vs. non-constraint), and material (titanium, cobalt-chromium). While assessing the postoperative imaging, a few key points a clinician need to pay attention to are the following (Mulcahy and Chew 2015) (Fig. 12):

- Ideally, AP and lateral weight-bearing radiograph in neutral position
- Tibiotalar component alignment in coronal plane
- Tibiotalar component alignment in sagittal plane
- Bearing height
- Radiolucency around component suggesting loosening
- Fracture

4.7 Ankle Arthrodesis

Indications for ankle arthrodesis are end-stage ankle arthritis or failed arthroplasty. Contraindications are active infection, osteonecrosis of the talus, peripheral neuropathy, and active smoking (high risk of nonunion). It may be performed arthroscopically or as an open approach. Multiple hardware has been described, ranging across screws, plate, intramedullary nail, and

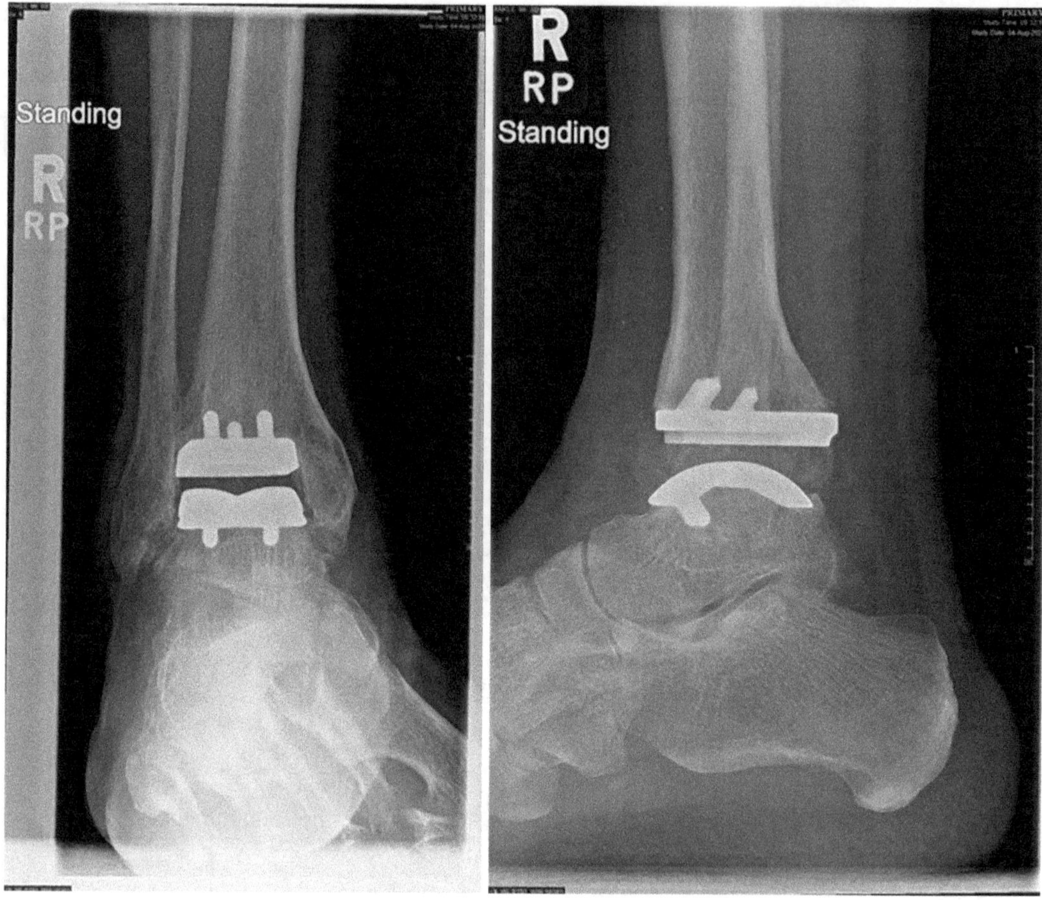

Fig. 12 AP and lateral view of a right ankle arthroplasty

external fixator (Fig. 13) (Marsh et al. 2020). Bone graft may be required if osteopenia is present.

The complications of ankle arthrodesis vary with the type of procedure, patient compliance, and underlying comorbidities. Radiological signs to look out for in postoperative imaging include mal/nonunion, infections, alignment, loosening of hardware, and fracture. Serial radiographs, CT scan, and MRI may help in monitoring progression.

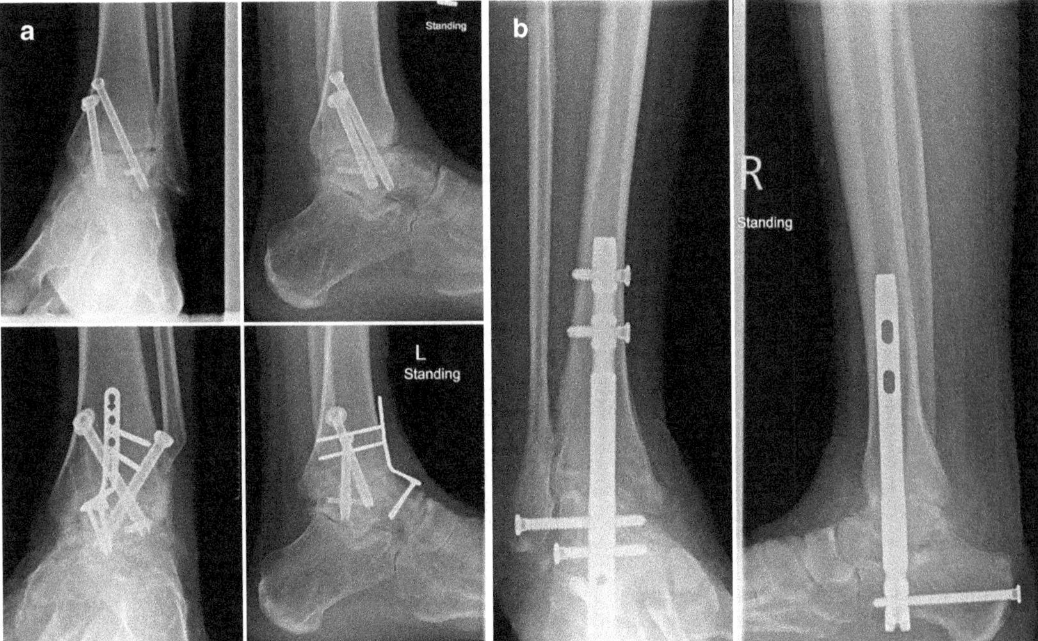

Fig. 13 Different types of orthopedic hardware for ankle arthrodesis. (**a**) Compression screw ankle arthrodesis was seen on the top two plain radiographs in a patient who had previously suffered a talus fracture (broken screw in situ) and developed post-traumatic arthritis. At 1 year, the patient had nonunion of the intended arthrodesis joint and a visible joint line. As shown in the bottom two plain radiographs, he underwent revision surgery with crossed compression screws and anterior plating. (**b**) Alternative method of ankle arthrodesis using hindfoot nailing system

References

Alcelik I, Fenton C, Hannant G et al (2020) A systematic review and meta-analysis of the treatment of acute Lisfranc injuries: open reduction and internal fixation versus primary arthrodesis. Foot Ankle Surg 26:299–307. https://doi.org/10.1016/j.fas.2019.04.003

Allegra PR, Rivera S, Desai SS et al (2020) Intra-articular calcaneus fractures: current concepts review. Foot Ankle Orthop 5:247301142092733. https://doi.org/10.1177/2473011420927334

Anderson MR, Ho BS, Baumhauer JF (2018) Current concepts review: hallux rigidus. Foot Ankle Orthop 3:247301141876446. https://doi.org/10.1177/2473011418764461

Asloum Y, Bedin B, Roger T et al (2014) Internal fixation of the fibula in ankle fractures. A prospective, randomized and comparative study: plating versus nailing. Orthop Traumatol Surg Res 100. https://doi.org/10.1016/j.otsr.2014.03.005

Berquist TH (1994) Imaging Atlas of Orthopedic Appliances and Prostheses. Lippincott Williams & Wilkins

Boksh K, Sharma A, Grindlay D et al (2020) Dorsal bridge plating versus. Transarticular screw fixation for Lisfranc injuries: a systematic review and meta-analysis. J Clin Orthop Trauma 11:508–513

Edwards WHB (2005) Avascular necrosis of the first metatarsal head. Foot Ankle Clin 10:117–127

França G, Nunes J, Pinho P et al (2021) Is arthrodesis still the best treatment option for first metatarsophalangeal joint arthritis?—a systematic review of arthrodesis and arthroplasty outcomes. Ann Joint 6:5. https://doi.org/10.21037/aoj-20-88

Gourineni PVRKV, Knuth AE, Nuber GF (1999) Radiographic evaluation of the position of implants in the medial malleolus in relation to the ankle joint space: anteroposterior compared with mortise radiographs. J Bone Joint Surg Am 81:364–369. https://doi.org/10.2106/00004623-199903000-00008

Hayes BJ, Gonzalez T, Smith JT et al (2016) Ankle arthritis: you can't always replace it. J Am Acad Orthop Surg 24:e29–e38

Horisberger M, Valderrabano V (2014) Midfoot arthrodesis. In: European surgical orthopaedics and traumatology. Springer, Berlin, pp 3547–3565

Iwamoto J, Takeda T (2003) Stress fractures in athletes: review of 196 cases. J Orthop Sci 8:273–278

Kannan S, Bennett A, Chong HH et al (2021) A multicenter retrospective cohort study of first metatarsophalangeal joint arthrodesis. J Foot Ankle Surg 60:436–439. https://doi.org/10.1053/j.jfas.2020.05.015

Lehman DE (2003) Salvage of complications of hallux valgus surgery. Foot Ankle Clin 8:15–35

Majeed H (2019) Silastic replacement of the first metatarsophalangeal joint: historical evolution, modern concepts and a systematic review of the literature. EFORT Open Rev 4:77–84. https://doi.org/10.1302/2058-5241.4.180055

Mandracchia VJ, Mandi DM, Toney PA et al (2006) Fractures of the forefoot. Clin Podiatr Med Surg 23:283–301

Marsh A, Kooner S, Conlin C et al (2020) Arthroscopic ankle arthrodesis: a review of current concepts and technique. Tech Foot Ankle Surg 19:19–25

Moracia-Ochagavía I, Rodríguez-Merchán EC (2019) Lisfranc fracture-dislocations: current management. EFORT Open Rev 4:430–444. https://doi.org/10.1302/2058-5241.4.180076

Mulcahy H, Chew FS (2015) Current concepts in total ankle replacement for radiologists: features and imaging assessment. Am J Roentgenol 205:1038–1047

O'Connor TJ, Mueller B, Ly TV et al (2015) "A to P" screw versus posterolateral plate for posterior malleolus fixation in trimalleolar ankle fractures. J Orthop Trauma 29:e151–e156. https://doi.org/10.1097/BOT.0000000000000230

Okanobo H, Khurana B, Sheehan S et al (2012) Simplified diagnostic algorithm for Lauge-Hansen classification of ankle injuries. Radiographics 32:E71. https://doi.org/10.1148/rg.322115017

Patel NG (2018) Navicular fractures: aetiology and management. Orthop Trauma 32:423–427. https://doi.org/10.1016/j.mporth.2018.09.007

Rammelt S, Heineck J, Zwipp H (2004) Metatarsal fractures. Injury 35:77–86. https://doi.org/10.1016/j.injury.2004.07.016

Razik A, Harris M, Trompeter A (2018) Calcaneal fractures: where are we now? Strategies Trauma Limb Reconstr 13:1–11

Robinson AHN, Limbers JP (2005) Modern concepts in the treatment of hallux valgus. J Bone Joint Surg Br 87:1038–1045

Rothwell M, Pickard J (2013) The chevron osteotomy and avascular necrosis. Foot 23:34–38

Schwartz AM, Runge WO, Hsu AR, Bariteau JT (2020) Fractures of the talus: current concepts. Foot Ankle Orthop 5:247301141990076. https://doi.org/10.1177/2473011419900766

Stibolt RD, Patel HA, Lehtonen EJ et al (2019) Hemiarthroplasty versus total joint arthroplasty for hallux rigidus: a systematic review and meta-analysis. Foot Ankle Spec 12:181–193

Theodorou DJ, Theodorou SJ, Kakitsubata Y et al (2003) Fractures of proximal portion of fifth metatarsal bone: anatomic and imaging evidence of a pathogenesis of avulsion of the plantar aponeurosis and the short peroneal muscle tendon. Radiology 226:857–865. https://doi.org/10.1148/radiol.2263020284

Wright DJ, Bariteau JT, Hsu AR (2019) Advances in the surgical management of ankle fractures. Foot Ankle Orthop 4:247301141988850. https://doi.org/10.1177/2473011419888505

Zaidi R, Cro S, Gurusamy K et al (2013) The outcome of total ankle replacement: a systematic review and meta-analysis. Bone Joint J 95B:1500–1507

Correction to: Imaging of the Forefoot

Douglas Hoffman, Ryan C. Kruse,
Ramanan Rajakulasingam, and Rajesh Botchu

Correction to:
Chapter "Imaging of the Forefoot" in:
D. Hoffman et al., Med Radiol Diagn Imaging,
https://doi.org/10.1007/174_2023_402

This chapter was inadvertently published without incorporating a few author corrections. The below listed corrections have now been carried out in the chapter.

1. Chapter title was changed from "Ultrasound and MRI of Lesser Metatarsalgia" to "Imaging of the Forefoot."
2. Order of authors was changed from "Ryan Kruse, Ramanan Rajakulasingam, Douglas Hoffman, and Rajesh Botchu" to "Douglas Hoffman, Ryan C. Kruse, Ramanan Rajakulasingam, and Rajesh Botchu."
3. The word "oedema" was changed to "edema" throughout the chapter for consistency.
4. In the first line of the section "6.2 Avascular Necrosis," the abbreviation "AVN" was expanded to "Avascular necrosis."
5. The word "parosteal" was changed to "periosteal" in the sentence "This is typically surrounded by avid bone marrow edema…."
6. The term "Morton's neuroma" was changed to "interdigital neuroma" throughout the chapter for consistency.

The updated original version of this chapter can be found at https://doi.org/10.1007/174_2023_402

Med Radiol Diagn Imaging (2023)
https://doi.org/10.1007/174_2023_446,
Published Online: 24 August 2023

Printed in the USA
CPSIA information can be obtained
at www.ICGtesting.com
LVHW080801160724
785622LV00005BA/23